# Drugs are NOT the Devil's Tools

## How Discrimination and Greed Created a Dysfunctional Drug Policy and How It Can Be Fixed

David Bearman, M.D.

Foreword by Judge James Gray

Volume 1 of 2

ISBN 978-1-883423-32-2
Volume 1 of 2

First Edition
10 9 8 7 6 5 4 3 2 1

Book Design by Carmen Lodise

Cover Design by Cathy Feldman

Book Production by Blue Point Books

To order this book in quantity for your organization please contact:
Blue Point Books
bpbooks@west.net 800-858-1058

Published by Blue Point Books
P.O. Box 91347
Santa Barbara, CA 93190-1347
www.bluepointbooks.com

Printed in United States of America

# Foreword

## by Judge James P. Gray

Welcome to a realistic and intelligent yet down-to-earth discussion of one of the most critical issues in our country, which is the background, hype and perpetuation of the policy of Drug Prohibition. In fact, I believe that this is the biggest failed policy in our country's history, second only to slavery. That is a large claim, but as you pour through Dr. David Bearman's book, the odds are strong that you will agree with that assessment.

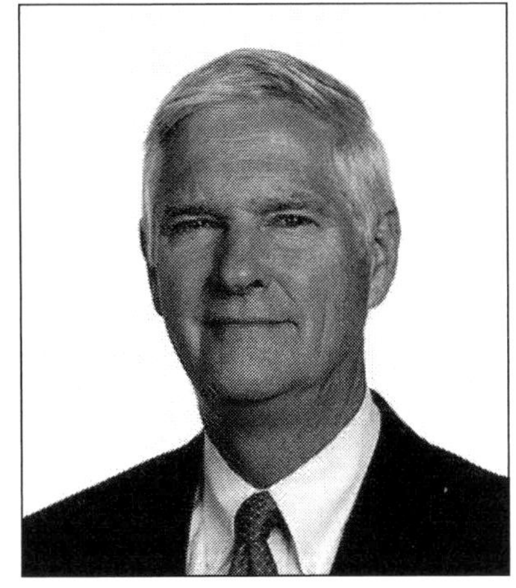

*James P. Gray is a retired judge of the Superior Court in Orange County, California. He is the author of* Why Our Drug Laws Have Failed: A Indictment of the War on Drugs *(Temple University Press,* 2nd edition, 2012*) and was the 2012 Libertarian candidate for U.S. vice president, along with Governor Gary Johnson as the candidate for president.*

Increasingly through my career in the criminal justice system as a Navy JAG attorney, federal prosecutor in Los Angeles and trial court judge for 25 years in Orange County, California, it became apparent to me that we couldn't employ a worse system if we tried. Today, drugs are more available both for us as adults and our children than ever before, and they are also stronger and less expensive. In fact, it is easier now for teenagers to purchase marijuana, ecstasy or any other illicit drug – if they want to – than it is alcohol. Why? Because the sellers of illicit drugs don't ask for i.d.! Don't just rely upon me for that conclusion, ask the next ten teenagers you find, and that is what they will tell you!

So on April 8, 1992, I did something quite unusual for a trial court judge: I held a press conference and told anyone who would listen that our policy of Drug Prohibition had failed, and that we had to put our heads together to find a better way. And I have continued actively speaking about this issue ever since.

As a result of my involvement in drug policy reform, I have met some of the best people I have ever known who were similarly involved. Some of them have been to prison, some are still drug addicted, and some, like me, have never used any form of illicit drugs. But, since many of them arrived at my same conclusions from vastly different experiences, it was genuinely reinforcing to me that we were on the right track.

One of the people at the top of this list is David Bearman, M.D. From my own observations and interactions with this gentle man, I have seen him to be an intelligent and caring medical professional, with an insightful understanding of addiction medicine. So when he asked me to write an introduction to his book, I hastened to agree.

And, as you will see, what an insightful book it is. Yes, fortunately, there are many fine books on the market that discuss the history and abject failures of Drug Prohibition, but with his theme of a timeline, Dr. Bearman insightfully provides more insights than most of them.

In the first place, he shows that there has never been a civilization in the history of mankind that has not been without some form of mind-altering and addictive substance, including mine, which is alcohol. So the idea of a "drug-free society" is a bureaucratic but entirely counterproductive pipedream. As Dr. Bearman points out, people in all walks of life are drawn to these substances for a variety of reasons, and most of them use those substances responsibly.

But when the government tries to control what adults put into their bodies, major problems develop. Of course, the drugs themselves can be a problem, but, as former New Mexico Governor Gary Johnson says, only about 10 percent of our drug problems are caused by the drugs themselves, while about 90 percent of the problems are caused by the drug money! So those are self-inflicted wounds.

Dr. Bearman hammers these points home time and again with concrete examples, showing first in his timeline how so many problems were caused by Alcohol Prohibition, and then how they were repeated by Drug Prohibition. But, all importantly, he also provides viable alternatives to this failed and hopeless policy, many of which are presently being employed successfully in other parts of the world. And that should genuinely bring you hope.

So congratulations to Dr. Bearman for publishing this pivotal book, and congratulations to you, as the reader, for choosing to share his insights. You are in for a lasting treat!

*Judge Gray can be contacted through his website: www.JudgeJimGray.com.*

# Preface

The origin of U.S. drug policy is a spider web woven of the intertwining motives of greed, discrimination, and religiosity. The connection between modern drug policy and historical events may not be crystal clear at first glance. The object of this book is to lay bare how these factors have played significant roles in influencing and providing a foundation for contemporary substance policy.

We'll also explore the joint propositions that psychoactive states may actually be good for you and that they have played a positive role in human development. We'll document how present drug policy, especially the so-called "War on Drugs", is needlessly expensive, illogical, and has an extremely negative impact on our freedoms. Finally, we'll put forth some sensible alternatives to our present policies, ones that are both more effective and humane.

## Marginalizing "Them" in "Us" vs. "Them"

The book identifies drug laws as just one more tool, and an effective one, in marginalizing discriminated-against groups. The tactic of demonizing drugs and those who are accused of using them has been used throughout history against numerous groups, including but not limited to pagans, witches, Aztecs, Incas, Native Americans, Irish, Germans, Chinese, Blacks, Sikhs, Mexicans, Puerto Ricans, Catholics, Jews and Italians. We will track this history of drugs as a tool of marginalization from the Middle Ages to the present.

## Fear of Change

Examination of the dynamics affecting drug laws through the ages reveals an admixture of elements, several centered on fear. Such fear is more pronounced in times of power shifts resulting from large economic changes that have generated instability in society. Finally, stir in the residue of differences in attitudes and experiences among ancient societies regarding the use of wine, beer, distilled spirits and other substances in both everyday use and celebratory functions. This combination of ingredients forms the basis for today's dysfunctional, costly, unconstitutional "wrong-headed" drug policy mess.

## It Is More about Greed than Health

Our drug regulations are not really about substance abuse, they are about how great wealth is generated and protected. We'll point out that famous names in America history have ties to drug distribution. The Bush family and Forbes family transported opiates to India in the 19th century. Elihu Yale earned his fortune working for the British East Indian Company. Joe Kennedy was a bootlegger. In the 1930s, Lammot du Pont of petrochemical giant DuPont, feared competition from hemp for many of DuPont's products – nylon, rayon, tetraethyl lead, cellophane, and sulfites used in paper making. He worked hard to make marijuana and hemp illegal in the Marijuana Controlled Substance Act of 1937. Even before this, William Randolph Hearst had used marijuana to vilify Hispanics. These were not necessarily bad people, and in many cases they were breaking no laws. For many it was "just business."

## What Role Do Altered States Play in Human Development?

What if altered states are as normal as apple pie? Who amongst us did not as a child spin around until dizzy, fall on the ground and watch the clouds above whiz around in a kaleidoscopic display. Some may have found that decreasing your oxygen supply by choking yourself or being choked, led to an altered state you found strangely pleasant. This is not for me, yet surveys show that fully 25% of the general population has experienced this phenomenon. Meditation, yoga, biofeedback and talking in tongues are all ways to achieve altered states of consciousness.

Throughout history, human kind has used a wide variety of mind-altering substances. This has to at least raise the question, Why? Integrative medicine specialist and author, Dr. Andrew Weil, points out that the indigenous peoples of the Amazon make an effort to have their children use psychoactive drugs so they can experience altered states of consciousness. This is not because they want their offspring to use drugs; it is to experience and understand altered states in the hope that they will be able to reproduce that experience naturally, without drugs.

## Are Altered States Actually Good For You?

The suggestion that alternative states of consciousness are necessary and/or normal for well-adjusted human existence has been put forth by among others, Thomas Sasz, Ph.D., Norman Taylor, Ph.D. and Dr. Andrew Weil, which raises the question of whether altered states are a survival mechanism to address our difficult existence.

Throughout history, elites and priesthoods have used psychoactive drugs. The people of the Middle Ages drank a lot of fermented beverages in large part because of the health risks of drinking water. The first American colonists were awash in alcohol, as were the founding fathers and mothers of this country. Native Americans ceremonially consumed several different psychoactive substances. American icon, John Chapman (aka Johnny Appleseed), was planting apples for hard cider. Citizens of the world have experienced and sought altered states from numerous psychoactive substances for millennia.

Ponder this proposition: Does our current legalistic approach to the age-old consumption of psychoactive drugs make human existence more difficult to endure? Is it historically and biologically a more natural state for humankind to be happier and better adjusted if they routinely and/or ceremonially use mind-altering drugs? If the issue of substance use were framed in that context, then having a substance dependency problem could just be a variant of normal that is caused both by genetic and cultural factors.

So, who has substance abuse problems? We will spell out how people with post-traumatic stress disorder (PTSD), people with genetically low levels of dopamine and/or an endocannabinoid deficiency, and people with an elevated dopamine transporter level are more likely to face this problem. People with low free-dopamine run an increased risk of attention deficit disorder (ADD), anxiety, panic attacks, anger management issues, migraine headaches, among other co-morbid conditions. Should we treat those humans suffering from conditions responsive to cannabis and cannabinoids by arresting them and throwing them in jail? We've done that for over 50 years and we'll document that this approach hasn't been of much benefit.

## Forces That Have Shaped Drug Policy; Logic is Out the Window

We'll explain why do we treat some drugs differently than others? Even more fundamentally, what is a drug? A "drug" could be aspirin, milk thistle, penicillin, ephedra, sugar, saline, water, spices, or even food. As a doctor I wonder why some problems with drug abuse are seen as medical problems, but others as legal ones. Looking for a scientific or pharmaceutical explanation for the reason some drugs are perceived in certain ways (e.g., good/bad, legal/illegal, medicine/social lubricant, accepted by society/not accepted) and not others was futile. It just didn't make sense. That's why it's necessary to dig into history to understand such distinctions.

## Current Drug Policy Has Not Served America Well

This book examines why U.S. policymakers have chosen a drug policy route that has repeatedly proven unsuccessful. This drug policy has compromised the Constitution, has shattered families, and has ignored the underlying causes of substance abuse. By turning a blind eye to the underlying causes of substance abuse, we make early intervention and prevention much more difficult. U.S. drug policy also has enriched our enemies, has marginalized the economic power of hemp, and has stood in the way of expanding our understanding of the human mind. U.S. drug policy is more expensive and less humane than possible alternative policy approaches. We document that not only are our policies failing, but they are counter-productive. We can do much better.

## The Search for Alternative Approaches Has Been Stymied

In twenty-first century America, a widespread, open, public discussion of an alternative substance control policy, one which downplays a criminal justice approach to substance abuse in favor of treatment and prevention, has not been tolerated.

Since at least the time of alcohol prohibition, the acceptance of drug use, as opposed to drug abuse, has been condemned by politicians of both major parties – Republican and Democrat. There has been some support from Greens and Libertarians, the occasional Libertarian-leaning Republican, and an occasional gay or minority Democrat for a medical and/or non-criminal justice approach to regulation of psychoactive social drugs.

At one point during the 2012 election, the Libertarian ticket of former two-term New Mexico Governor Gary Johnson and Orange County California Superior Court Judge Jim Gray were polling 8% of the vote, although their final tally was 1%. They held that government prohibition of drugs is an inappropriate use of government power, that it is a tool to limit our liberty. In their view, they are comparable to Thomas Jefferson who said, "If people let government decide which foods they eat and medicines they take, their bodies will soon be in as sorry a state as are the souls of those who live under tyranny".

## We Can Change

Historical context is important to framing the right questions to come up with better answers. In the big picture, that means understanding that "drugs" is an arbitrary category. We must come to grips with a reality stretching back beyond recorded history and treat "drugs" as part of social reality. American society and law have come to understand this with coffee, tea, nicotine, alcohol and excessive eating. We must recognize that not only do drugs often serve a positive social purpose, but that the percentage of abusers is ten percent or less. Further, that the motives for using drugs may well be positive or have significant positive elements. This framing can be useful in developing both prevention, intervention and treatment approaches.

As a society we need policies that can help decrease substance abuse and to make getting treatment for substance abuse as easy as it is to be arrested for possession.

## In Summary:

It is my hope that rehearsing how America arrived at this difficult place in public policy provides the basis for moving beyond it.

**David L. Bearman, M.D.**
October 2014

# Dedication

This book is dedicated to my wonderful wife and children. Lily Maestas Bearman, Samantha Bearman, and Benjamin Bearman. And to all those persons willing to look beyond cultural dogma to think for themselves. and to examine the evidence about America's so-called "War on Drugs."

.

# Table of Contents

# DRUGS ARE NOT THE DEVIL'S TOOLS

## How Discrimination and Greed Created a Dysfunctional Drug Policy and How It Can Be Fixed

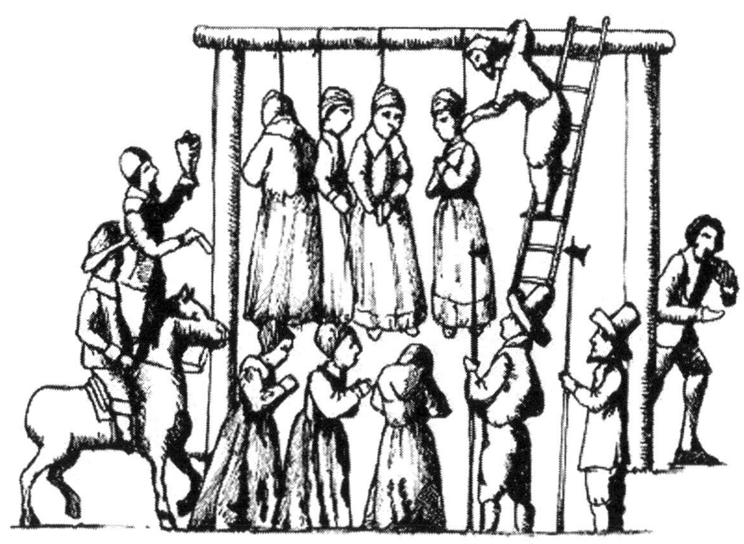

# CHAPTER I
# Introduction to a Witch Hunt

"Government is not reason, it is not eloquence; it is force, the fire of a troublesome servant and a fearful master. Never for a moment should it be left to irresponsible action."

**George Washington**
Revolutionary War Hero
and President of the United States, 1789-97

## Cost and Priorities

Every U.S. President from Richard Nixon to George W. Bush has declared a "War on Drugs." This has resulted in a massive allocation of manpower, materials, and money for what has turned out to be predominantly a war on minorities, the poor, and the Constitution. For nearly nine decades, towering amounts of public resources have been poured into "modern" America's ineffectual drug policy.

The U.S. Federal Bureau of Investigation (FBI), Central Intelligence Agency (CIA), Drug Enforcement Agency (DEA, and its predecessors), the U.S. military, state and local police, and countless prosecutors at all levels of government have devoted enormous energy, time, and the public's money in this fruitless effort. There is precious little to show for this immense expenditure of human and financial national treasure, other than the increasing numbers of crowded prisons that stand as monuments of failure.

Estimates of total cost vary widely. According to conservative estimates, federal, state, and local governments easily contribute

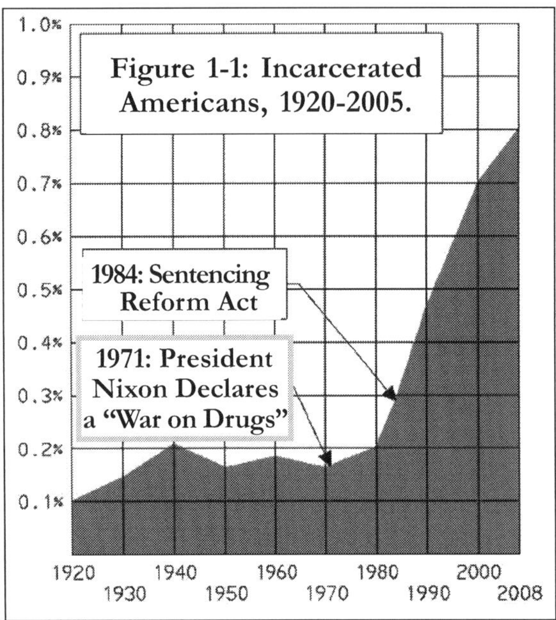


*The number of incarcerated Americans has sharply increased annually since U.S. President Richard M. Nixon declared a "War on Drugs." Estimates of the total cost of such incarcerations vary considerably, but easily exceed $50 billion per year.*

over $50 billion **annually** in resources toward prosecuting the "War on Drugs".[1,2] The related cost to U.S. taxpayers and the economy is much greater. Financial costs associated with the drug war include: drug testing, lost work time, family disruption, crime, lost tax revenue, and ignoring alternative policies that might generate tax revenues. These associated costs exceed another $100 billion (with a "b") dollars, that is, $100,000,000,000.00.[3,4,5] And that does not count the lost opportunity cost of putting the energy and money dedicated to fighting the so-called "War on Drugs" to more productive expenditures.

At any moment in 2007, the United States had 2.4 million people in prison. This is over four times the number in 1970, when the Controlled Substances Act was passed by the U.S. Congress and signed into law by President Richard M. Nixon. Our rate of incarceration is three-to-eight times that of any other developed nation. For Blacks and Hispanics, the incarceration rates are even worse, exceeding the rate of incarceration of Blacks in South Africa at the height of apartheid. Our current drug laws and their enforcement created this costly mess.

The comparative growth of the prison industrial complex versus education in California during the 1980s and '90s dramatically illustrates these misplaced spending priorities. Between 1985 and 2000, California increased its expenditures on prisons by more than 250%. In contrast, over the same span, expenditures on higher education in constant dollars actually decreased.[7] From 1984-1994, California prisons had a 209% increase compared to 15% in State University spending. In that time, California built 21 new prisons and one state university.[8] Our drug laws and the three strikes legislation with many 'criminals' getting 25-to-life for a non-violent third conviction are major

> **We must stop politicizing medical problems. We must stop building prisons instead of schools. We must begin to rebuild lives.**[6]
>
> **Joycelyn Elders, M.D.**
> U.S. Surgeon General, 1993-94

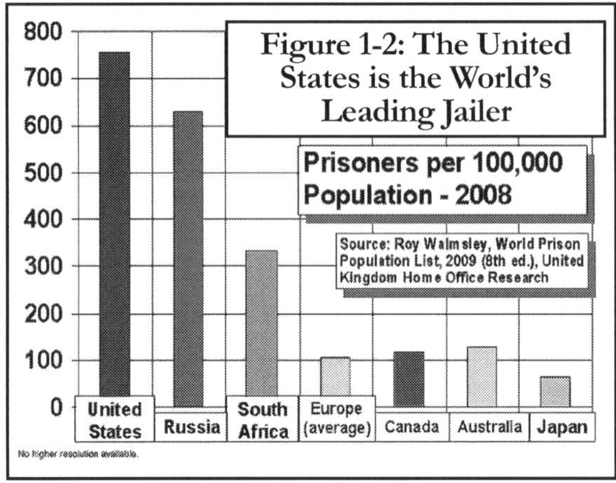


> **Jails and prisons are the complement of schools; so many less as you have of the latter, so many more you must have of the former.**[9]
>
> **Horace Mann**
> Noted 19th-century education reformer

contributors to the demand for more jail and prison cells.

Incarcerating substance policy violators with more serious criminals compounds our folly. By placing citizens convicted of illicit drug use in jail, we just increase the likelihood of them engaging in more serious crime in the future. Since many who have been incarcerated have mental health problems arising from growing up in dysfunctional families and suffering physical, verbal and/or sexual abuse, we are applying the wrong treatment to address their substance abuse.

**… the drug war, and the prohibitionist ideology which fuels it, is not about rational policy, and it's certainly not about science, compassion, health or human rights. Rather, it's become a sort of dogma – a secular fundamentalism – that sees itself as immune from critical examination, and that views people like us (i.e., drug policy reformers) as heretics.** [10]

**Ethan Nadelmann**
executive director, Drug Policy Alliance

By making substance use and abuse a criminal justice issue, we have created a criminal industrial complex, a giant industry of prison workers, contractors, and investors who are dependent on the illegality of drugs for financial gain. In California the most powerful group lobbying the state legislature is the prison guards union. For them, draconian drug laws are good for business.

## Is This Madness or What?

What has been done in our name? Our government has woven an ungainly web of drug laws devoid of much medical, legal, pharmacological, or Constitutional sense. American drug policies assault our intelligence, our freedom, our common sense and our families. Prohibition policies with onerous penalties did not exist in colonial times or during the first century and a quarter of the Republic. Where did these policies come from? How did we arrive at this "Alice-in-Wonderland" situation?

Contemporary U.S. drug policies destroy families, demonize "others," misallocate human and governmental resources, trample Constitutional guaranties, and ignore Americans' deeply held ethical and moral principals. The energy that powers this action must come from a powerful source. The force infusing this impressive energy into the anti-some-drug movement is fear and hostility toward "them" that are different — different language, geographic origin, culture, nationality, skin color and/or religion. Add to this amalgam greed and power and you have a potent motivational mixture for major policy mischief.

## Xenophobia

Prohibitionists claim their position is based on "truth" and morality. But their own arguments demonstrate that drug prohibition is based not on

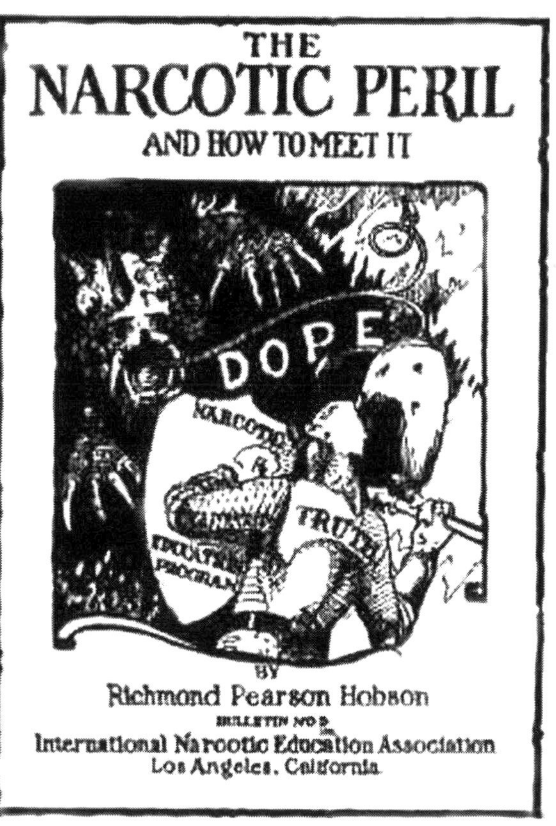


*Richard Hobson was an effective racist and Congressman from Alabama, 1907–1915. After leaving Congress, Hobson became very active in the cause of banning drugs and alcohol, earning the nickname "The Father of American Prohibition".*

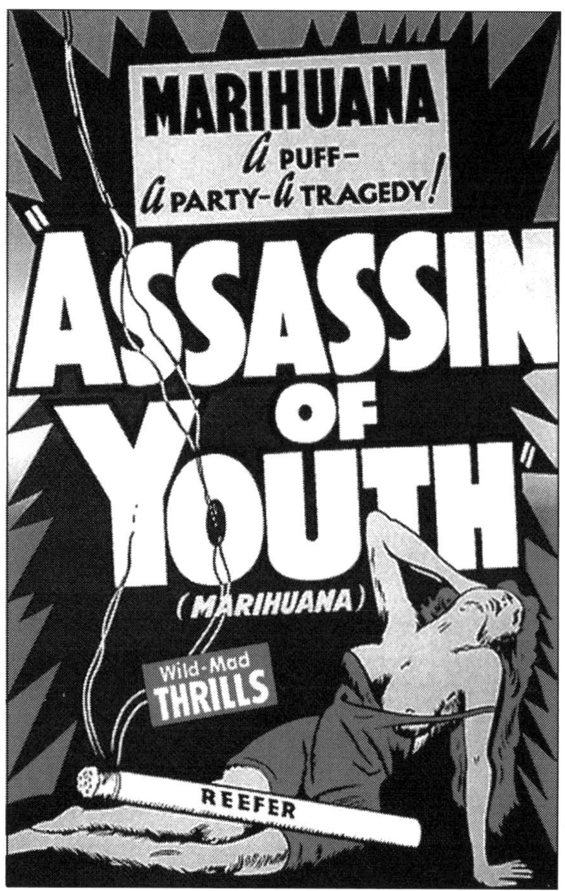


Assassin of Youth *(1937) is an exploitation film directed by Elmer Clifton about the supposed ill effects of cannabis. The film's title refers to an article of the same year by Harry J. Anslinger, the first commissioner of the U.S. Treasury Department's Federal Bureau of Narcotics, that appeared in* The American Magazine *and was reprinted in* Reader's Digest *in 1938. That article briefly mentions several stories from his "Gore file" of tragedies allegedly caused by marijuana.*

---

science, but is a symbolic, ideological, political act. Its bases are demons, discrimination, and commerce, plus a particular moral religious viewpoint. [11] The approach of Hamilton Wright, Richmond Pearson Hobson and Harry Anslinger, key figures within the drug prohibition movement, was the so-called "morality of social improvement."

"Morality of social improvement" is a more elegant way of saying, "if we could just stop these people ('them') from using drugs (or at least their drugs), then we'd have heaven on earth." The method for implementing this madness in our alleged free society: criminalization and punishment. Support for drug prohibition in the U.S. has largely been drummed up by negative, bigoted, stereotypical

**The myth of drugs as the assassin of youth is one of the cornerstones of drug prohibitionist rhetoric.**

Drugs as the despoiler of the young has been effective in generating fearful images of degradation of youth, most particularly innocent young women. Prohibited drugs are portrayed as threatening the Western way of life. [12]

**"It is, however, the criminalization of drugs, rather than their inherent dangers, that most prevents me from serving as "watcher" over my children's safety and mental health. Certainly, the hostile policies of America have kept me from discussing drug use in as honest and nuanced a way as I would like to have with my kids, for fear that their naïve interpretations and adolescent gossip might lead to serious stigmatization, despite our being a drug-free household."**

**"Criminalization further assures that if my kids ever do mess with drugs, I will be helpless to assure "quality control" and maximize their safety. They will be left to procure their substances from whatever unsavory sources, in whatever dosages, for use in whatever environments, because they will lack my cooperation and guidance – guidance that could lead me to prison and loss of custody. American law thus throws up a huge wall between me and my children and all but assures that the spiritual possibilities of their drug use, if it transpires, will be seriously compromised."** [13]

**Lawrence Bush**

"Drugs and Jewish Spirituality" in *Hallucinogens: A Reader* (2002)

depictions of the "other": Irish, German, Arab, Jew, Chinese, Sikh, Black or Hispanic alike, whomever, as drug abuser. [14]

"They" and everything about "them" has all been demonized here – their culture, food, odor, work habits and among other things, a particular drug, stereotypically associated with "them." All of this is done within the moral context of "us" protecting our youth, our women, our jobs, our "way of life."

We generate fear and loathing through our demonization. As a result of our fear, more and more of our freedom and rights are being usurped by the government. American Founding Father Benjamin Franklin was prophetic when he said, "Those who would give up essential liberty for safety deserve neither liberty nor safety." [15] The contrast between the '30s when U.S. President Franklin D. Roosevelt famously said "we have nothing to fear but fear itself" and the approach of the George W. Bush administration, "be afraid, be very afraid", is reflected in more restrictions on rights of Americans than existed during WWII.

The media emphasis on the negative gives us a skewed view of the dangers out there. In the July 2007 *Wisconsin State Journal*, columnist Bill Wineke pointed this phenomenon out in an article "It's Not News that Our Kids Do Good." He observed that when kids did good that was rarely news, but when they were bad it was news. "We regularly see reports from Lutherans, Baptists, Jews and any number of secular youth organizations reporting on good things their kids are doing. Not all of these kids are angels. Some of the same kids who go on mission trips may end up getting drunk at illegal parties later in the year. Some do things in the dark they hope their parents will never learn about. We don't have 'good kids' and 'bad kids.' We have only 'our kids.' And despite the challenges they face, by and large, they're kids we can feel proud of." [16]

America has criminalized what is at worst a medical problem and at best a medicine and a means to spiritual insight. All drugs, of course, are not criminalized – over the counter drugs, vitamins and most medicinal herbs are legal. We have some laws regarding age of use for alcohol and tobacco but breaking one of these laws is rarely a felony and carries little stigma. While the taxes on alcohol are low, those on tobacco are high enough to offer some deterrent to smoking. If you don't pay those more or less reasonable taxes then you are committing a felony.

America's "War on Drugs" rhetoric has lead people to accept collateral damage that would be impermissible in other civilian law enforcement or public health efforts. Drugs are portrayed as a plague but as Ethan Nadelmann pointed out, "Drug control is not like disease control for the simple reason that there is no popular demand for AIDS or cancer. On the other hand, mind-altering drugs of many stripes have been popular for eons." [17]

Our drug laws are but one of the levers of power that is used to marginalize those who we fear and/or are different from us. Our present policy, the fruits of this heritage, not only ignores the enormous social, financial, and constitutional cost of our current drug policy approach but it is scientifically illogical. From almost any vantage point and by any measuring stick, the U.S. drug policies, in force at least since 1914, have been an abysmal failure.

The so-called "War on Drugs" is more accurately a "War on People," specifically those people who use drugs the general populace doesn't approve of. For example, even though Blacks and Hispanics have a slightly lower rate of illicit drug use than Whites, both ethnic groups have a much higher likelihood of arrest, persecution and jail than Whites. [18] The drug war does great harm to the U.S. Constitution, the American family, harmony within the American community, respect for law and order, and the American sense of fair play.

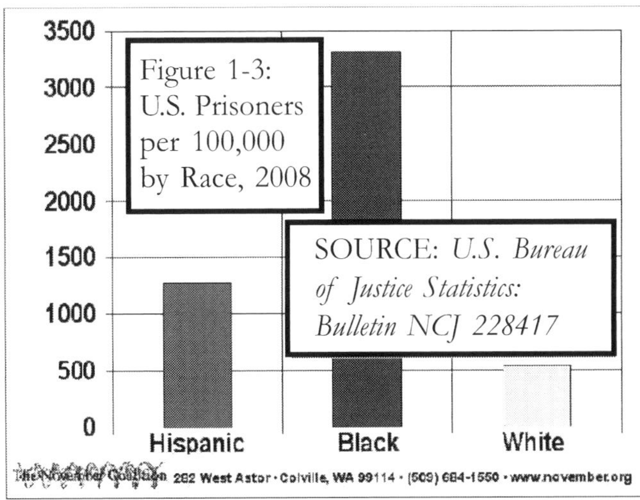

**Figure 1-4: Discriminated Against Groups**
**Where Drug Policy and/or Drugs Have Played a Role in That Discrimination**

| Discriminated Against Group | Key Time Periods | Drug(s) |
|---|---|---|
| • Native Americans | 1492 to present | Alcohol, peyote |
| • Blacks | 1500's to present | Cocaine, marijuana |
| • Irish | 1300's to 1960's | Alcohol |
| • Chinese | 1500's to 1960's | Opium |
| • Catholics | 1830's to 1933 | Alcohol |
| • Jews | 1880's to 1933 | Cocaine, Alcohol |
| • "Hindoos" | 1910 to 1914 | Hashish |
| • Mexicans | 1912 to present | Marijuana |
| • Germans | 1850 to 1950 | Alcohol (beer) |
| • Italians | 1918 to 1950 | Alcohol |
| • Jazz Musicians | 1916 to present | Heroin, marijuana, Benzedrine |
| • Puerto Ricans | 1930 to present | Marijuana |
| • Communists | 1921 to 1960 | All |
| • Beatniks | 1948 to 1963 | Heroin, marijuana, Benzedrine |
| • Hippies | 1963 to 1985 | LSD, marijuana, mushrooms |
| • Rock Musicians | 1964 to present | Heroin, LSD, marijuana, alcohol |
| • Liberals | 1980 to present | Marijuana, MDMA, cocaine |
| • Rap musicians | 1985 to present | Cocaine, heroin, alcohol |

## Drug Policy Change Would Be a Good Idea

Throwing people in jail is poor treatment for physical or mental health maladies. America needs a new paradigm. U.S. drug policy, like health care policy, generally just makes prevention an afterthought, damning it with faint praise. Prevention should be the top priority. Prevention should focus on family, love, effective parenting, community, understanding, early intervention, counseling, and then treatment; all based on science and common sense.

Instead of demonizing substance use, and having our drug policy heavily influenced by the fallout of slavery and its lingering modern manifestations of discrimination and racism, a comprehensive policy is needed that recognizes the difference between substance use and abuse. America needs a policy that understands and incorporates the pathophysiology and the psychological dynamics of substance abuse. We must not only apply this understanding in family and community oriented drug-abuse prevention and psychological treatment, but this medical family-values approach must be adequately funded.

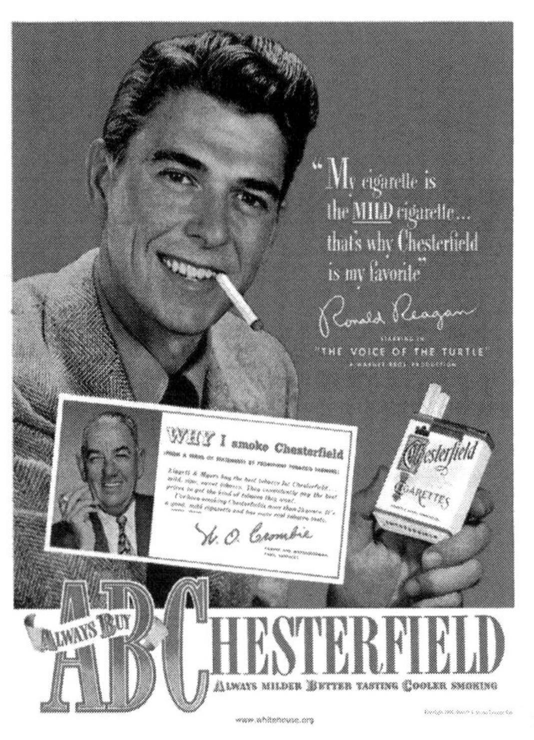

*The late President Ronald Reagan endorsed tobacco consumption in the 1940s. This advertisement stands as an ironic contrast to his wife Nancy's later simplistic slogan: "Just Say No" to drugs.*

**"We have passed laws which are worse than ineffective. Not only do drug prohibition laws have limited utility but they erode the very freedoms this country stands for. Is this because as a society we have chosen to emphasize superstition, demonization and propaganda over facts?**

**Drug policy touches a broad spectrum of issues: the Bill of Rights, religious freedom, mental health, proper expenditure of taxpayer dollars, States' rights, doctor-patient relationships, personal privacy, illegal search & seizure, forfeiture, parenting, discrimination and science vs. superstition, abuse of government authority, and capricious actions of state medical boards."** [19]

David L. Bearman, M.D.
"Medical Marijuana: Why This Issue is More Important to Health Care Than Just Cannabis"
Session Abstract for the Annual Meeting of the American Public Health Association.
November 8, 2005

These alternatives will be explored as the book moves through history.

Our current criminal justice drug-policy approach lumps almost all consumption of illicit drugs as abuse, making absolutely no distinction amongst use, misuse and abuse. There are some exceptions to that. The public does seem to wink at sharing some prescription drugs while giving lip service to concerns about under-age use of nicotine and ethyl alcohol. The public is pretty forgiving in situations involving alcohol and/or tobacco possession and use laws (as opposed to abuse involving other drugs). Confusing the mere use of a substance with abuse tends to complicate even framing the "problem" in a way that it can be effectively addressed. It has become a cliché that if the wrong question is asked, the wrong answer follows.

Our present approach toward those who use drugs in a personally destructive manner almost always only addresses the symptom, excessive inappropriate substance use, not the underlying causes of such behavior. And then, if cause is addressed at all, it's most likely to be addressed criminally, not medically. We must address the underlying social and psychological dynamics which contribute to substance abuse if we hope to make any progress in applying humane, effective substance abuse prevention, intervention and treatment techniques and strategies.

## Current U.S. Drug Policy Doesn't Work

The social and psychological cost of our present drug policy is too great. The strain on our mores and ethics, the shattering of families and the waste of human capital are excessive. American Drug Policy is worse than ineffective. There is an enormous amount of "collateral damage" to our current drug policy. Present U.S. drug control policy is causing dry rot in the timbers of the Constitution which supports our democratic republic. Implementation of our current policy has destroyed the lives of not only the convicted, but millions of innocent family members. *Shattered Lives: Portraits from America's Drug War* (1998) [20] is a book by Mikki Norris, Chris Conrad and Virginia Resner that paints a sad picture of the deleterious effects of drug policy, not drugs themselves, on people and their families.

The "drug war" is aided and abetted by the mainstream media's complicity. Not only are loaded words used (e.g. junkie, pusher, depraved, pot, weed, dope fiend), but mainstream media rarely puts so-called drug-related crime in context. That context is that almost all drug-related crime is caused by the illegality of the drugs themselves. U.S. politicians have proved particularly adept at confusing the collateral damage of the "drug war" with drugs themselves.

Yet, it is the drug prohibition policy itself which is responsible for the lion's share of what we have labeled the drug problem. Drug prohibition funds organized crime at home and terrorism abroad. Modern U.S. Drug Policy provides a barrier to adequate funding of treatment and to research into the fundamental causes of substance abuse. The problems and lack of success of our drug policy is then used to justify increasing drug war spending.[21]

## A Public Health Approach

The public health policies of the United States must be more compassionate, fair, and reasonable. Addressing a mental health issue with the rhetoric of demons, smacks of anachronistic medieval thinking. Unless we approach the issue of substance abuse treatment and prevention with a comprehensive, common sense, theoretically well-founded and well funded approach, we will continue to see large scale problems related to our substance abuse policy, on both the micro and macro level.

---

**The definition of insanity is doing the same thing over and over, and expecting different results.[22]**

Attributed to Benjamin Franklin and Albert Einstein, as well as to Rita Mae Brown and an old Chinese Proverb.

---

Just such a comprehensive approach to intervention and prevention for children at high risk for chemical dependency is laid out in a 1995 study entitled "Dual Diagnosis Intervention Planning Study", which I headed when I was the medical director of the Santa Barbara Regional Health Authority. This study was funded by a Robert Wood Johnson Foundation grant and published in the *Journal of Psychoactive Drugs* in 1997.[23]

The report lays out the importance of a comprehensive, holistic, family-focused intervention to stop the vicious cycle of chemical dependency occurring in families where one or both parents has a dual mental health and chemical dependency diagnosis. While the mix of services needed is not set in concrete, it is related to the mental health needs and need for structure of the victims of substance abuse.

Research by Dr. Ira Chasnoff has clearly demonstrated the value to the family and the child's development from this kind of comprehensive intervention.[24] The headline of a story on Chasnoff and his study says it succinctly: "Slow Development in Crack Babies May Be Caused By Condition of Urban Poverty, Says New Study".[25]

The list of likely helpful interventions is long and expansive. It includes mental and physical health services, Head Start, anger management counseling, career planning, job training, self-esteem building, parent effectiveness training, career counseling, spirituality and more.

This multi-pronged approach requires coordination of government and community support to effectively fund, organize and combine the potpourri of institutions and services needed to repair the damage inflicted from PTSD generating events (e.g., growing up in a dysfunctional family, child abuse, rape). Science recognizes a genetic predisposition to alcohol, but this can also be true for other abused substances.[26, 27, 28, 29, 30, 31, 32]

Meaningful intervention requires intergovernmental cooperation and public-private partnerships. The clogged arteries of bureaucratic cooperation are deleterious to the health of our communities. This multi-pronged approach is not a new concept. In the 1960s, the U.S. Housing and Urban Development's Office of Economic Opportunity and the Community Health Service of the U.S. Public Health Service endorsed community health centers. These centers had multiple services under one roof to encourage interagency cooperation and a comprehensive approach to health and mental health problems.

For several years, Santa Barbara County (Calif.) had a federally funded MISC program. This was a cooperative arrangement among County mental health, probation, criminal justice and community social service agencies to work together on difficult cases. Cooperative efforts that surmount bureaucratic barriers and resist the urge for agency "turf" protection and worries about government job security should be encouraged.

Implementing an effective multi-faceted approach to drug abuse treatment and prevention is costly. The only thing more expensive than taking this more comprehensive prevention, intervention and treatment tact is continuing our present approach. America cannot afford to continue the status quo. Instead of spending the funds currently being used in the present criminal justice approach, these should be applied to create a milieu to improve people, families, and the community. This would be a better, more effective expenditure of U.S. resources.

Unless we change our current failed substance abuse policy, we are doomed to spend ever increasing amounts of tax dollars on this area and still have generation after generation suffer from PTSD, ADHD, OCD, bipolar disorder, panic attacks, substance abuse and other related problems. And we are shredding the Constitution in the bargain. Sending people with these maladies to jail, as we frequently do today, further wastes human and financial resources in a futile effort which not only does little to address the problem but sows the seeds for these problems to continue on to the next generation.

U.S. substance policy should be life affirming, not fear mongering. The focus should be on increased nurturing, coming from parents and adult role models that have achieved a feeling of self-worth. There must be affirmations of personal worth to all people, particularly children coming from community and community institutions such as church, school and law enforcement.

America can do much better. But even with a new, more effective approach, the United States must be realistic about expectations. It must be recognized that while the rate of substance abuse can lowered and the vast majority of abusers can be effectively treated by improving family dynamics, promoting a supportive community, creating a loving environment, taking a comprehensive, multiple modalities approach and providing a variety of treatment opportunities, a goal of completely eliminating substance abuse is a fool's errand. Passing laws to try to achieve that goal marks the end of freedom and liberty.

**Figure 1-5: Services Required in a Comprehensive Approach to Treating Drug Abuse**

— Drug Treatment
— Career Counseling
— Parent effectiveness training
— Job skills training
— Anger management
— Techniques & strategies for successfully negotiating life with ADHD
— Mentoring
— Treatment of physical & mental health problems
— Treatment of any symptoms of Post Traumatic Stress Disorder
— Spirituality
— Life planning & decision-making skills

SOURCE: D. Bearman, K. Clayton et.al., "Breaking the Cycle of Dependency: Dual Diagnosis and AFDC Families". *Journal of Psychoactive Drugs,* October 1997.

## Policy of Folly

The present ineffective approach is not based on the relative harm of various drugs to the public's health. On the basis of deaths caused, tobacco is the most lethal drug. "Tobacco kills 650 per 100,000 users, alcohol 150, heroin 80, and cocaine 4."[33] It's known that every year, over 400,000 Americans die as the result of tobacco use. Alcohol abuse results in the deaths of another 110,640 Americans, including 16,653 alcohol-related traffic deaths. And alcohol is a contributing factor in more than half of all homicides and rapes, 62 percent of assaults, and 30 percent of suicides.[34] Illegal drug use causes at least another 3,562 deaths.[35] Moreover, there are an estimated 100,000 deaths/year related to prescription drug misuse. Why is the focus on those drugs which cause relatively less harm? This is examined in subsequent chapters.

## Reefer Madness

The movie *Reefer Madness* is a classic piece of drug-war propaganda. Hitting the "big screen" in 1935, it portrayed how a bunch of high school kids got hooked on the devil's weed, marijuana, and fell into a life of crime and deprivation. The film is now shown on college campuses as a fund-raiser for drug reform groups, or at nearby theaters as a midnight show. As the actors' eyes bug out, high school girls are "ruined." And as the piano player maniacally plays on, the 35-ish drug pushers prey on the high school kids as the movie theater rocks with laughter.

Marijuana was not the first demonized drug nor is it likely to be the last. The basis for our current approach to the abuse and recreational use of substances is found not in a modern, medical, scientific or logical approach; but in a culturally embedded, hysterical approach. This hysteria goes deep into our past where demons roam.

Conflicts amongst religions over the meaning and purpose of life have been a driving force in the creation of demons. The history of conflict and discrimination between and amongst religions started thousands of years ago. Divining the meaning of life is a matter of faith. The phrase "a leap of faith" means faith must be used to bridge

**Figure 1-6: Annual Causes of Death in the United States**

|  |  |
|---|---|
| Tobacco | 435,000 (1) |
| Poor Diet & Physical Inactivity | 365,000 (1) |
| Alcohol | 85,000 (1) |
| Microbial Agents | 75,000 (1) |
| Toxic Agents | 55,000 (1) |
| Motor Vehicle Crashes | 26,347 (1) |
| Adverse Reactions to Prescription Drugs | 32,000 (1) |
| Suicide | 30,622 (2) |
| Incidents Involving Firearms | 29,000 (1) |
| Homicide | 20,308 (2) |
| Sexual Behaviors | 20,000 (1) |
| All Illicit Drug Use, Direct & Indirect | 17,000 (2) |
| Non-Steroidal Anti-Inflammatory Drugs (such as Aspirin) | 7,600 (3) |
| Marijuana | 0 (4) |

SOURCE: www.drugwarfacts.org/causes/htm. Note: Drug War Facts footnotes these numbers as follows:

(1) Sources: Mokdad, Ali H., PhD, James S. Marks, MD, MPH, Donna F. Stroup, PhD, MSc, Julie L. Gerberding, MD, MPH, "Actual Causes of Death in the United States, 2000," Journal of the American Medical Association, March 10, 2004, Vol. 291, No. 10, pp. 1239, 1241.
(2) Source: Hoyert, Donna L., PhD, Heron, Melonie P., PhD, Murphy, Sherry L., BS, Kung, Hsiang-Ching, PhD; Division of Vital Statistics, "Deaths: Final Data for 2003," National Vital Statistics Reports, Vol. 54, No. 13 (Hyattsville, MD: National Center for Health Statistics, April 19, 2006), p. 5, Table C.
(3) Source: Robyn Tamblyn, PhD; Laeora Berkson, MD, MHPE, FRCPC; W. Dale Jauphinee, MD, FRCPC; David Gayton, MD, PhD, FRCPC; Roland Grad, MD, MSc; Allen Huang, MD, FRCPC; Lisa Isaac, PhD; Peter McLeod, MD, FRCPC; and Linda Snell, MD, MHPE, FRCPC, "Unnecessary Prescribing of NSAIDs and the Management of NSAID-Related Gastropathy in Medical Practice," Annals of Internal Medicine (Washington, DC: American College of Physicians, 1997), September 15, 1997, 127:429-438, from the web at http://www.acponline.org/journals/annals/15sep97/nsaid.htm, last accessed Feb. 14, 2001, citing Fries, JF, "Assessing and understanding patient risk," Scandinavian Journal of Rheumatology Supplement, 1992;92:21-4.
(4) Source: Drug Abuse Warning Network (DAWN), available on the web at http://www.samhsa.gov/; also see Janet E. Joy, Stanley J. Watson, Jr., and John A. Benson, Jr., "Marijuana and Medicine: Assessing the Science Base," Division of Neuroscience and Behavioral Research, Institute of Medicine (Washington, DC: National Academy Press, 1999), available on the web at http://www.nap.edu/html/marimed/; and US Department of Justice, Drug Enforcement Administration, "In the Matter of Marijuana Rescheduling Petition" (Docket #86-22), September 6, 1988, p. 57.

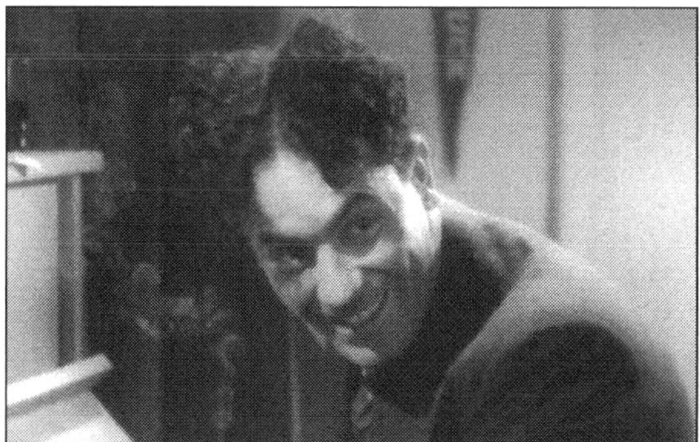

*Derisive laughter was not the intended response when the film was made.* Reefer Madness *was just another weapon in the long selective demonization of drugs; a demonization closely linked to commerce and discrimination. "Reefer Madness" is now another name for current U.S. drug policies.*

ADULTS ONLY!
The Sweet PILL that MAKES LIFE BITTER!
WOMEN CRY FOR IT - MEN DIE FOR IT!
"REEFER MADNESS"
SEE
DRUG-CRAZED ABANDON
YOUTHFUL MARIHUANA VICTIMS
WHAT ACTUALLY HAPPENS

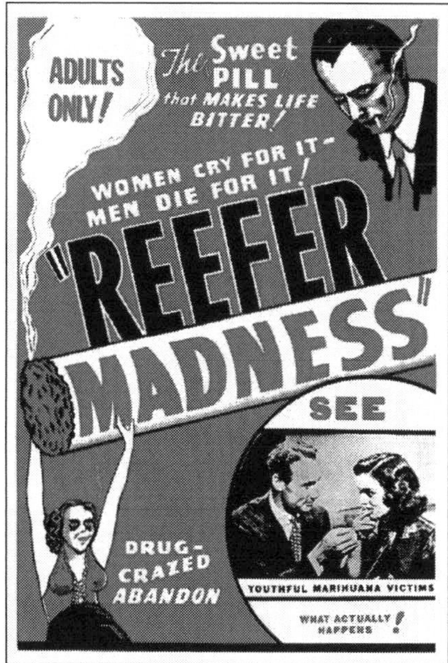

*This 1935 movie was produced as a propaganda piece against marijuana but has become a parody.*

the logic gap needed to answer the questions "Why are we here" and "what is the meaning of life." Unfortunately, throughout history religions big and small have used coercive tactics to generate faith. Faith is not supposed to work that way; that's why it's called "faith."

## The Cultural Attic

The foundation of our modern drug policies goes back to antiquity and the roots of our cultural heritage. In America, the so-called "melting pot", this heritage is not uniform and therein lays the rub. The clues as to how we got to today's illogical, costly, dysfunctional drug policy place are found by rummaging through our cultural attic. What we find is that our drug policy arises from an amalgam composed of remnants from European history prior to Columbus' "discovery" of America, combined with the subsequent 500-year history of demonization, discrimination and commerce in the Americas.

Columbus and the conquering Spanish conquistadors brought the spice trade, greed, witch hunting, and the Inquisition with them. They also brought Christianity as the state religion to the New World. Soon British, Dutch and French colonists brought yet more European cultural influences; influences which had been passed down through the ages by song, story and habit from one generation to the next.

Imported cultural factors, in combination with important post-1492 influences in the New World, produced America's cultural milieu. These historical influences created a pool of cultural primordial ooze out of which today's modern drug policy fiasco arises. These long ago cultural precursors still affect present day attitudes towards "them" and "their" drugs.

A FIFTH COLUMN SOWING DESTRUCTION IN THE YOUTH OF AMERICA ---
"DEVIL'S HARVEST"
A GOOD GIRL UNTIL SHE LIGHTS A "REEFER"
THE TRUTH ABOUT MARIJUANA
THE SMOKE OF HELL!

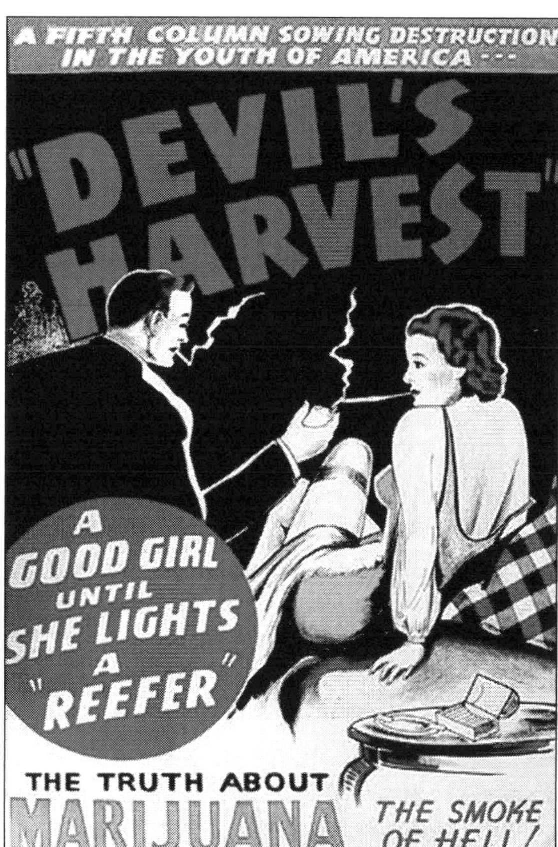

*The attempt to connect demons to anti-drug hysteria is clear from many of the posters produced in mid-20th-century America.*

Sadly, it's all too clear that cultural remnants of the past profoundly affect thought and action in today's world. The conflicts in the Balkans and the Middle East have graphically taught us the painful lesson that far too many people today carry grudges from hundreds of years ago that can, and do, dramatically influence the contemporary world. Religious conflicts, both European and American, the economic philosophy of Mercantilism, slavery, and the so-called triangular trade created historic remnants still affecting the United States.

From the post-Revolutionary War period into the 19th century, the United States saw the growth of both the Abolition and the Temperance movements, the rise of Manifest Destiny, and increasing Nativism. They are part of the American historical attic of concepts and events which have impacted our national thought. Events of the latter part of the 19th century also helped shape our "drug" policies. The Civil War, patent medicine, Reconstruction, the closing of the frontier, immigration, economic and professional forces, and the rise of the United States as an international power all influenced the ineffectual and self-defeating drug criminalization policy path that was taken.

## "Them" and "Us"

Myriad threads of our culturally influenced historical thoughts and concepts are woven into the tapestry of today's drug laws. This fabric includes fear of those from different clans, tribes, religions, classes, regions and cultural backgrounds. Throughout U.S. history, far too many Americans have seen their lives as "us" and "them." Demonizing some drugs is just one more tool to use for demonizing and marginalizing "them."

American drug policy is disproportionately derived from the dark side of the American psyche. The roots of our approach go back millennia. These roots grow in the fertile psychic soil of irrational fears. These fears arise from a combination of demonic iconic imagery, concern about ceremonial chemistry mixed with a fear of the "others".

Today's "them" and "us" are represented by the wedge issues, the red states and the blue states, the liberals and the fundamentalists. Seeing issues as a simple dichotomy eliminates all subtlety and shades of gray. Use of a divisive wedge issue approach removes controversial matters from intellectual inquiry. If you are not with me, you're against me, does not make for a thoughtful productive atmosphere.

Demonizing one's opponent is all too often an effective way of avoiding confronting real facts and issues. Unfortunately, it's also been a good way of avoiding accepting responsibility for a problem or an untoward outcome. Use of demonization and discrimination frequently confounds the situation with irrational, *ad hominem*, rigid rhetoric. This presents a real barrier to developing sophisticated, nuanced, cooperative approaches to problem solving.

The influence of discrimination is compounded by the impact of commerce. Who makes money at whose expense clearly affects policy. There are winners and losers with any policy and those with the financial power try to keep it. One strategy is to create public policy which supports the financial empires of the powers that be. Spices, tobacco, coca, tea, sugar, hemp, opium, alcohol – for centuries – have all been important commercial commodities. The role of money, jobs, and the economy have had a significant influence in shaping U.S. drug policy.

## The Founding Fathers Must be Shaking Their Heads

In devising today's substance abuse policies, we have strayed from many of the basic values of the country's founding fathers. Serious tinkering with the Constitution started with the income tax in 1913. The first federal drug prohibition law, the 1914 Harrison Narcotic Tax Act, as the name says, was a tax law, not technically a federal prohibition. Alcohol prohibition required a constitutional amendment. Current drug prohibition laws are not sanctioned by a constitutional amendment and are inconsistent with the Constitution drafted by our forefathers.

Prior to 1919, federal criminalization of substance abuse and use was practically unheard of in the United States because of Constitutional issues. States rights advocates defended the legal prerogatives of the state against federal incursion. Somehow the Supreme Court has found its way around the Ninth and Tenth amendments which preserve all rights to the several states not specifically granted by the Constitution to the federal government. The court has pretty much ignored the original 1925 commerce clause ruling regarding the state's right to regulate the practice of medicine. In 1925, in *Linder v. United States* (268 US 5), the U.S. Supreme Court ruled that Congress may not overreach into the practice of medicine in the states. In plain English, the rule of law is that Congress lacks the Constitutional authority to control the practice of medicine within a state. [36]

And our modern policies continue to eviscerate the Constitution. No doubt our policy of random student and employee urine testing – when one has done nothing wrong – is an anathama to the writers of the Bill of Rights. In his July 2006 "American Heritage" article "What would the Founding Fathers Do?", conservative writer Richard Brookhiser states flatly, "The Founders would not have fought a war on drugs." [37]

By overturning the Ninth Circuit Court of Appeals' *Raich v. Ashcroft* decision, the U.S. Supreme Court, in their 2005 *Gonzales v. Raich* decision, strained the Tenth Amendment and States rights. A plain reading of the Tenth Amendment and knowledge of its history suggests that the founding fathers would agree with the two written dissents in the case, one by Justice Clarence Thomas, and the other by Justice Sandra Day O'Connor, joined by Chief Justice William Rhenquist. They criticized the majority for usurping rights reserved for the States. [38] San Francisco Bay area attorney Bill Panzer pointed out at the time that after 200 years of jurisprudence, relying on the plain meaning of the Bill of Rights would get you laughed out of legal circles as a naif.

In overturning *Raich v. Ashcroft*, the U.S. Supreme Court ignored two pro-States' rights decisions from the 1990s which they themselves -- these very same nine justices, had made. These decisions had trimmed the sails of *Wickard v. Filburn*, the WWII - era decision that supported the federal government's power to limit the production of wheat even when the wheat was for local or family consumption.

By defining the effect on interstate commerce extremely broadly, *Wickard v. Filburn* allowed for an expansion of the power of the federal government beyond the reach contemplated by the Founding Fathers. In her dissent in *Gonzales v. Raich* (545 U.S. 1, 2005), Justice Sandra Day O'Connor made clear that the Ninth and Tenth amendments to the Constitution do not permit this over-reaching of federal power. [39]

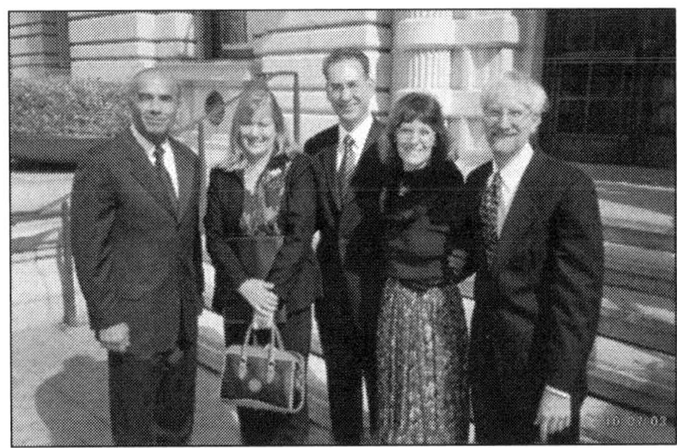

*Left to right: attorney David Michael, plaintiff Diane Monson, attorney Randy Barnett, lead plaintiff Angel Raich, and Robert Raich (Angel's ex-husband) on the steps of the Ninth Circuit Court of Appeals in San Francisco after oral arguments in 2003.*

The Fourth Amendment prohibits illegal search and seizure. Tell that to the high school students whose lockers are searched without cause or the chess team members who are required to take a urine test to participate in this or any extracurricular activity. We have a recent no knock Supreme Court decision which allows police to enter your house without knocking. If the government can invade your house without knocking and test your bodily fluids without probable cause, the Fourth Amendment affords little protection against abuse by the authorities.

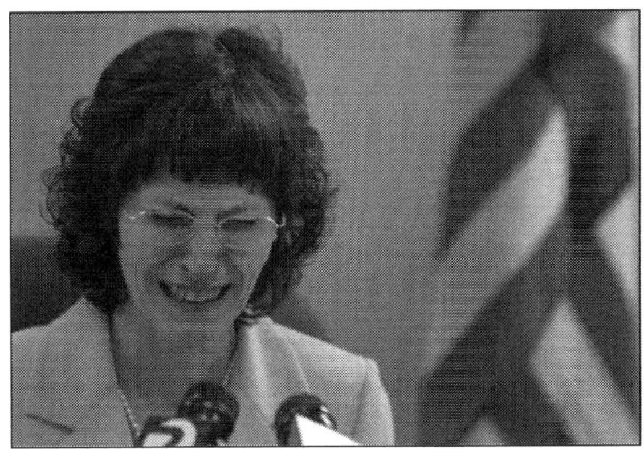

*Angel Raich's brain cancer is kept under control with cannabis. The U.S. Supreme Court said if she is ever arrested, she should try that as a defense. In the meantime, over the objections of its conservative members, the Court stretched the Commerce Clause and diminished States' rights in the 2005* Gonzales v. Raich *case.*

**"Arbitrary arrest and arbitrary searches conducted under the infamous writs of assistance and general warrants were among the bitterest grievances against George III recited in the American Declaration of Independence. When they established their independence Americans were determined that no government of their own creation should ever engage in these forms of despotism. Accordingly, they imposed heavy restraint upon police activity in the Fourth Amendment to the Constitution."** [40]

**Alan Barth**

in *The Rights of Free Men,* 1984

We seem to be basing more and more of our public policy on the mistaken belief that the United States was founded as a Christian nation. Actually, most of the founders were Deists, who believed in "povidence only through reason and experience." John Adams said, "The doctrine of the divinity of Jesus has made a convenient cover for absurdity." As president, Adams signed the Treaty of Tripoli, which states, "The United States of America is not in any sense founded on the Christian religion." [41]

Garry Wills notes, "Not only were our first six presidents Deists and not Christian, but the list of the founders who were Deists also includes Benjamin Rush, John Witherspoon, David Rittenhouse, Philip Freneau, Joel Barlow, Aaron Burr, James Wilson, Gouverneur Morris and more. . . . What our founders really believed will remain a scandal to the rank and file of professing American Christians." [42]

## Soak Thoroughly in 10,000 Years of History

There is a long prologue to America's Prohibitionist drug policy. This book places drug policies in that larger perspective. By understanding the role of drugs, demonization, discrimination and entheogens in the bigger historical picture, we get a much clearer idea of how we came to this pass in American drug policy. It allows an understanding of why we have devised a policy that does not sit on a rational base. In order to grasp how we got in this quagmire and how to get out of it, we need to go back 10,000 years.

The use of entheogens and mind-altering substances is almost universal. Only the Bushmen and the Eskimoes, had no intoxicants native to their culture. Like the Eskimoes who found plenty of substance problems once alcohol was introduced to their culture by Europeans, the Bushmen of Africa took to another intoxicant, tobacco. The Bushmen became so enamored with tobacco that they traded cattle, animal skins and other valuables for it. [43]

U.S. drug policy, such as it is, is a maze of counterproductive inconsistencies, which sprang from Western Europe's long heritage of those with the power using drugs, superstitions and myths as some of the tools to demonize, discriminate, dominate, scapegoat, marginalize and control people seen as different. Some have described this process as *othering*, generating fear and loathing towards the others.

## Measure Success or Failure of Drug Policy by Rational Analysis

America needs to assess drug policy success by the standards of basic human sanity: analytically, empirically scientifically, socially, financially, ethically, morally, and practically. Does it work? Is it cost-effective? What are the social consequences? And we must ask, "Are there other better ways to deal with this issue." We must examine our assumptions. It is well past time to reframe the question and

> **"I have examined all the known superstitions of the world, and I do not find in our particular superstition of Christianity one redeeming feature. They are all alike, founded on fables and mythology. The day will come when the mystical generation of Jesus, by a supreme being as his father in the womb of a virgin, will be classed with the fable of the generation of Minerva in the brain of Jupiter."** [44]
>
> **Thomas Jefferson**
> Principle author of the Declaraiton of Independence,
> Third President of the United States (1801-09).
> in an 1823 letter to John Adams

consider new paradigms for addressing substance use and abuse.

U.S. drug policy efforts are sabotaged by considering substance use to be synonymous with substance "abuse." Use is not abuse. By unnecessarily bringing this confusion into the discussion it is impossible to sort out normal behavior from that which might be considered pathological or at least behavior in need of some therapeutic intervention. Looking at substance use or abuse as a criminal matter or a matter of moral weakness has not been a particularly practical, useful, humane or cost effective approach to the situation.

We torture the English language to try to justify the unjustifiable. Not clearly understanding or defining what we mean by the so-called "drug problem" makes it all but impossible to come to a practical coherent, appropriate, effective solution. By applying the same old frame to defining the "problem"; potentially beneficial prevention, intervention and treatment approaches are more difficult to identify and implement.

If we do not understand the problem we are dealing with, it is difficult to be conscious of and/or develop other, more constructive policy and program options. The relationship of people to their drug consumption cannot be ignored. What is the consumer's motive for substance consumption? Is it a healthy motive? If not did it arise from being raised in a dysfunctional family or other Post-Traumatic Stress Disorder-generating situation? If there is a genuine drug related behavior problem, what kind of interventions might be helpful to curb this substance abuse? Is it really abuse?

How we cast or frame drug abuse and whether we distinguish "use" from "abuse" influences policy decisions. U.S. President Richard M. Nixon once declared that, "people drink alcohol to relax but people smoke marijuana to get high." [45] Was there some distinction there between relax and high, and if so, what is it? Nixon is not talking pharmacology; he is couching his choice of words in cultural bias.

## Current Drug Policy is Unsuccessful

America's present drug policy works poorly, if at all. Many say the present policy is counter-productive in controlling substance abuse and does unnecessary harm. There certainly is no harm in reviewing the current status of the so-called "War on Drugs" to see if a dramatic change of direction is needed. The contemporary U.S. approach pays only lip service to seriously considering the motivation for substance use and abuse. Hackneyed reasons like lack of willpower, drug use makes one a tool of the devil, a slave to drugs, or just being labeled a bad person, sometimes pass as an explanation for substance abuse. Worse yet, these reasons have been an excuse for punishment in lieu of pursuing a policy

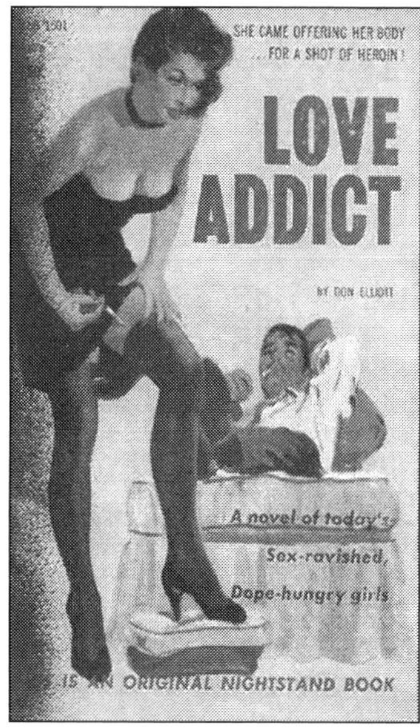


*Lurid tales of moral destruction were popular in pulp novels and an important part of anti-drug propaganda.*

emphasizing prevention, early intervention and treatment.

Prohibition has failed – again. Instead of treating the demand for illegal drugs as a market, and addicts as patients, policymakers the world over have boosted the profits of drug lords and fostered narco-states that would frighten Al Capone. Finally, a smarter drug-control regimen that values reality over rhetoric is rising to replace the "war" on drugs.[46]

## Is There a Choice?

Sadly, we are avoiding the real solution to America's large substance-abuse problem, a solution to which the vast majority of people can sign on. The real solution is to have loved children, raised in a healthy, supportive family environment, by happy, reasonably well adjusted parents, with positive self-images, in a community with adequate social services and ample opportunities in well-paying jobs.[47,48]

A quixotic dream to be true, but embracing this kind of policy would result in a different and much better set of public funding and policy choices. Basically, common sense tells us that people do better in life when they have a positive self-image, they know that someone cares about them, and there is hope and opportunity for a better future.

## Summary

Cultural forces steeped in history, not only tolerate, but power the demonization of the "others." These historical discriminatory forces, combined with commercial influences, made U.S. drug policy what it is today. The present drug policy of the United States relentlessly marginalizes and demonizes the "others" at the expense of all Americans' rights and pocketbooks. Worse yet, precious few societal resources and limited action is devoted toward implementing adequate, effective drug-abuse prevention, intervention and treatment.

A deeper understanding of the forces which have shaped our contemporary drug policy makes that failed policy more comprehensible. It also frees us to refocus our resources and priorities to policies which are both more effective and truer to the best of American values and tradition than existing U.S. drug policy.

If one tries to view current drug policy through the prism of science, it defies logic. Demons, discrimination and dollars is a far better framework for understanding the foundation of U.S. drug policy than searching for reasons in the public health arena. The recurrent theme undergirding U.S. drug policy is that "they" (the "others") are demonic, threaten the very foundations of our civilization, are corrupting our youth and engage in exploiting and despoiling innocent young women.

As society becomes more complex and unwieldy, the search for simple answers to complicated problems is an enticing fantasy. Unfortunately most of the simple answers have all been tried. In order to find solutions to complex problems, the first step is to take some responsibility, the second is to be willing to compromise and the third is to realize our foes on any issue are not demons. Are they?

**Sophisticated answers are needed; ones that reflect the best American values.**

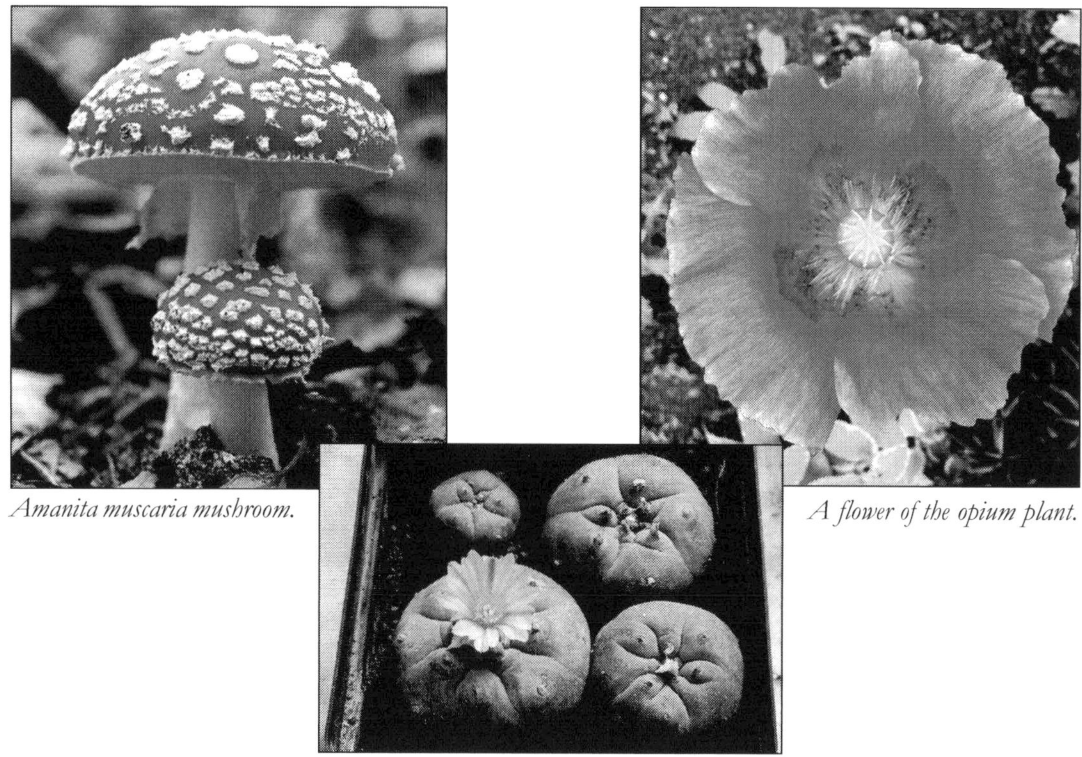

*Amanita muscaria mushroom.*

*A flower of the opium plant.*

*The peyote cactus in bloom.*

# CHAPTER II
# Ceremonial Drug Use: Religion, Shamans and Soma

## Paganism: The Foundation of Modern Religions

Spirituality and religion are very old. Psychotropic plants were crucial elements of the first religions, often collectively referred to as paganism. Religion is a good place to start exploring the origins of American drug policy. Sadly, spirituality and religion is another venue for "us" demonizing "them."

Humans have sought to explain existence from before written history. From the beginning of time, humans have struggled to answer the BIG questions: Why are we here? How did we get here? Where are we going? How did the world begin? Was the world always here? Was the world created from nothing? What does it all mean?

Each generation bases its answers, concepts, values, mores, customs and culture on what came before. When it comes to religion, entheogens are the most important plants in the world. Ancient religious concepts have profoundly influence modern religions. Some of these concepts were associated with or generated by spiritual flights fueled by entheogens.

Entheogens are plants that are used to create a spiritual experience and/or gain spiritual insight. Almost all pagan religions relied on psychotropic drugs for important aspects of their religious practices and beliefs. All subsequent religions arise from the historical residue of paganism. There is incorporation of some rituals and concepts of what came before into today's rituals and holidays.

## What! You Use That Drug in Your Holy Rituals?

For thousands of years, drugs, mind-altering substances, entheogens (whatever designation the reader is comfortable using to call psychotropic chemicals) have played a role in divining the meaning of existence, seeking the spiritual path and celebrating the important seasons and events of life. Use of entheogens is one way for a person to gain independent spirituality and a unique covenant with a power greater than oneself.

And for thousands of years the choice of one's ritualistic drug has been used as a lightning rod for attacking the credibility of another's spiritual beliefs. Today, the employment of most altered states of consciousness, particularly those that are drug-induced, to achieve a spiritual oneness with nature and/or a higher being or force is seen by many in Western culture as a challenge to the more hierarchical organized forms of religion.

This tradition of using entheogens to gain divine insight continues to this day for some humans both individually or in spiritual groups. The use of drugs such as peyote, kava-kava, cannabis, salvia, ayahuasca – the so-called vine of the soul – for achieving a spiritual oneness is still found worldwide. These and other entheogens are used to gain spiritual insight, albeit with controversy as to whether this is proper and acceptable.

## What is Beyond the Abyss?

As far as it is known, humans are the only animals that have the keen awareness of our own mortality. Humans have great curiosity about the meaning of life. Or as the announcer on the "Guy Noir, Private Eye" segment of the radio show *A Prairie Home Companion* says it: "Guy Noir, probing for the answers to life's persistent questions."

These are the big questions he posed: Where does life come from? Where are we going? How can I find happiness? What is the meaning of life? With no meaning, life can be very depressing.

Humans have developed belief systems, sometimes called religion sometimes not, to both explain how the Earth and its inhabitants got here and to give meaning to the life each person lives. Philosophy, thought, contemplation, and prayer — sometimes aided and abetted by drugs, sometimes not, have been used to try and unravel life's mysteries.

No one here on earth truly knows what comes next. This is why this type of religious belief requires faith. Indeed, the Zorastrians may be right that there is a heaven, the Islamic fundamentalists martyrs may have 72 virgins waiting for them, and the Baptists may have the best seats in heaven, but no one truly knows. People hope for an afterlife.

Most humans want an afterlife, but there clearly is doubt of its existence. Because of this doubt, some people hope against hope to live forever. The late novelist William Soroyan, author of many novels, plays and literary pieces, including the 1939 play, *The Time of Your Life*, expressed this thought shortly before his death in 1981: "I know that everyone has to die but I was hoping in my case an exception would be made."

Film auteur and former stand-up comedian, Woody Allen, says he makes movies simply to take his mind off the existential horror of being alive; that's "because it's much more pleasant to be obsessed over how the hero gets out of his predicament than it is over how I get out of mine." [1] Allen says, "Your perception of time changes as you get older, because you see how brief everything is. I don't want to depress you, but it's a meaningless little flicker." [2]

Allen expresses modern existential angst thusly: "I don't want to gain immortality through my work; I want to gain immortality by not dying."

Still, as comedian Bill Maher insightfully observed in *Religulous*, his 2008 documentary on the foibles of religion, pronouncements by religious figures of what, if anything, comes after life, are based on human thought and human perception. Maher notes that these prognosticators of what comes next are our fellow humans. They know no more of what comes next than other humans; than you or I. They may have more belief or more faith but they are not dead and have never been dead. Therefore, they are just speculating as to what comes next, based on their beliefs, hopes, dreams, and interpretation of history.

## Drugs: An Integral Part of the History of Religion, Magic and Medicine

From before the dawn of recorded history, spiritual and recreational drug use has been a part of every culture, save possibly two. The Eskimos near the Arctic Circle and Bushmen of the Kalahari Desert are the only pre-historic societies known not to have had psychotropic drugs as part of their indigenous culture. However, they are the exception. For example, a 60,000-year-old grave site excavated at Shandihar Iraq contained *Ephedra vulgaris*. Ephedra is an amphetamine-like drug that has a long medicinal history. [3] And the spiritual use of cannabis dates to prehistoric times. It played a significant role in the religions and cultures of Africa, the Middle East, India and China. [4]

### Middle East, India and China

According to the religious scholar, William A. Embolden:

> "Shamanistic traditions of great antiquity in Asia and Near East have as one of their most important elements the attempt to find God without a vale of tears; that cannabis played a role in this, at least in some areas, is born out in the philology surrounding the ritualistic use of the plant. Whereas Western religious traditions generally stress sin, repentance, and mortification of the flesh, certain older non-Western religious cults seem to have employed cannabis as a euphoriant, which allowed the participant a joyous path to the Ultimate; hence such appellations as 'heavenly guide'." [5]

Embolden's assessment regarding cannabis is echoed by the late Richard E. Schultes, the famous Harvard professor of psychoactive plants, when he wrote in an article entitled "Man and Marijuana":

> "...that early man experimented with all plant materials that he could chew and could not have avoided discovering the properties of cannabis (marijuana), for in his quest for seeds and oil, he certainly ate the sticky tops of the plant. Upon eating hemp the euphoric, ecstatic and hallucinatory aspects may have introduced man to an other-worldly plane from which emerged religious beliefs, perhaps even the concept of deity. The plant became accepted as a special gift of the gods, a sacred medium for communion with the spiritual world and as such it has remained in some cultures to the present." [6]

An archaeological find, reported in a 2008 issue of the *Journal of Experimental Botany*, confirms the long medicinal use of cannabis. Excavation of the Yaghai tombs in China revealed the 2700-year-old grave of a Caucasoid shaman. He was buried with the tools of his trade, which included a large cache of cannabis, extremely well preserved by climatic and burial conditions. Botanical examination, phytochemical investigation, and DNA analysis revealed that this material contained tetrahydrocannabinol, the psychoactive component of cannabis, its oxidative degradation product, cannabinol, other metabolites, and its synthetic enzyme, tetrahydrocannabinolic acid synthase. It is safe to conclude that the cannabis was employed 2700 years ago by this Chinese culture as a medicinal or psychoactive agent, or as an aid to divination. [7]

## Gods, Goddesses and Celebrating the Natural World

### Paganism

Paganism is the name for the many religions that pre-historic humans employed to explain the inexplicable. These ancient spiritual traditions were based on the intimate relationship people had with the natural world that dominated their lives. Paganism often relied on magic to explain that which logic couldn't explain: Who lives and who dies; why is the weather good sometimes and brutal others; what is the tribe's place among the stars; and, other such profound questions.

Each generation bases its answers to these questions on the concepts, values, mores and customs they inherit. With successive generations, some of these rituals and concepts are incorporated as so, while others are slightly revised and new material added or dropped off. Still, ancient religious concepts have profoundly influenced modern religions; modern religions arose from the historical residue of paganism. Some of these concepts were associated

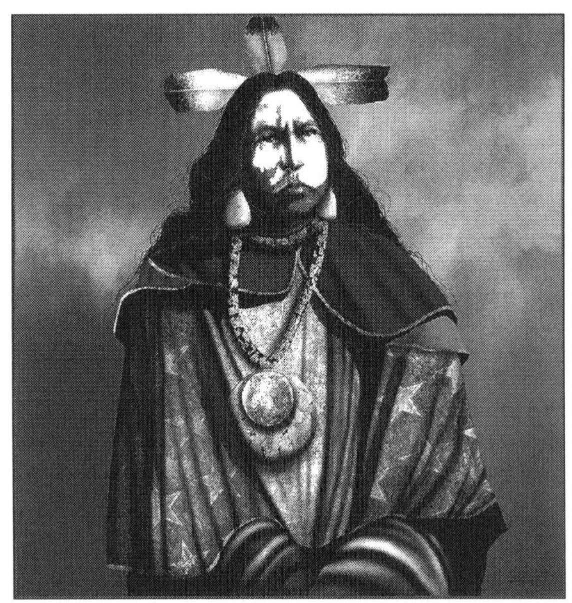

*Indigenous cultures from around the globe had some variation or other of the shaman, a link between our earthly realm and the ethereal world of spirits.*

with or generated by spiritual flights fueled by entheogens.

## Connected to Nature – the Sun, the Moon, the Earth, the Stars

Paganism regarded all nature as sacred and connected. These belief systems recognized that the right balance in the natural world is essential to survival. As a means of promoting survival, pagans worshipped a myriad of gods and goddesses to insure fertility (human and animal), good planting and an abundant harvest. "Ancient cave paintings and carvings reveal that from the beginning of recorded history and surely before, man has associated magic rituals with important life events -- death, birth, hunting .... To this day, magic is used to explain phenomena which are beyond the understanding of man."[8]

In ancient times, each tribe or community had its own sorcerer, wizard, or shaman. The shaman's role was to assist the tribe or the village to deal with disease, bad weather, war, death and birth. They did this through complex rituals associated with sacred objects. Their special knowledge was carefully transmitted from one generation to another through a secret initiation.[9]

Shamans have and had extensive practical knowledge about the local flora and fauna, including entheogens — psychoactive plants — so-called "magical" herbs. They used these special herbs for religious, medical, mystical, and magical purposes.[10,11] Shamanism unites the three principle strands of the role of drugs in society – religion, magic, and medicine.

There are indigenous healers in many contemporary cultures. In Russia, these healers are known as *felchers*, in Mexico and Central America, *curanderos*. Mushrooms and tincture of cannabis are part of the therapeutic armamentaria of the *curanderos*. The rain forest cultures still have shamans. One might characterize some modern day healers and religious leaders as contemporary shamans.

There are numerous scientists and organizations (for example, The Society of Economic Botany, the International Society of Ethnobiology, The American Anthropological Association and Shaman Pharmaceutical, Inc.) that recognize the tropical rain forest as a great source of new medicines and researchers still study tropical plants for sources of

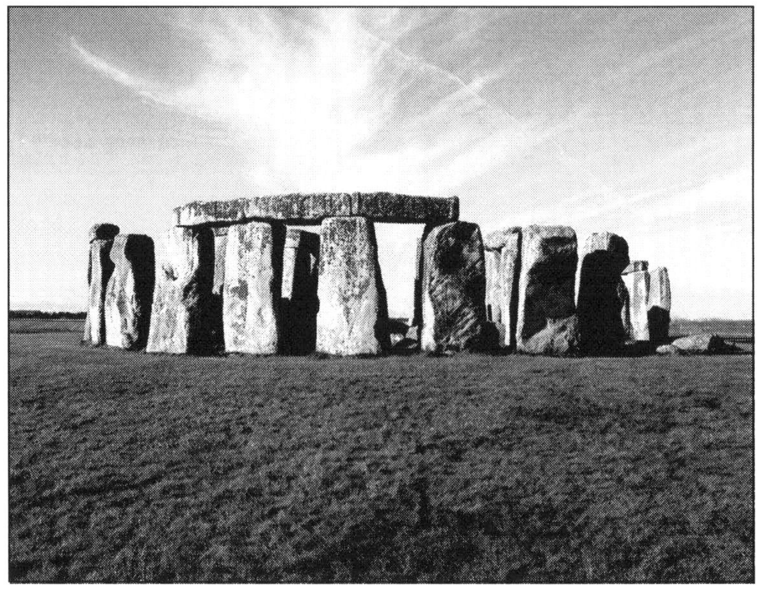

*Stonehenge is the name of this prehistoric monument in Wiltshire, England. It was probably established before 2000 B.C. and is thought to be a sacred place for healing and burial ceremonies and as a calculator of eclipses of the sun. It was built by peoples known as the Druids, who revered mistletoe among other plants.*

new pharmaceuticals. And why not? Over 100 pharmaceutical products currently being prescribed are derived from plants. Seventy-five percent of these pharmaceuticals were discovered by studying traditional medicines. [12]

## Goddess Worship

A central tenant of most ancient religions was the worship of The Goddess. In ancient times, such Goddess worship was almost universal. Numerous prehistoric, pear-shaped feminine form artifacts found in multiple cave sites throughout the world testify to the ubiquity of the ancient practice of goddess worship. Worship of goddesses is seen as representing the importance and sacredness of fertility: human, animal or plant. Fertility was essential to human survival. The most ancient goddess figures were a generalized representation of the force of nature as sacred, not of any specific goddess deity. [13]

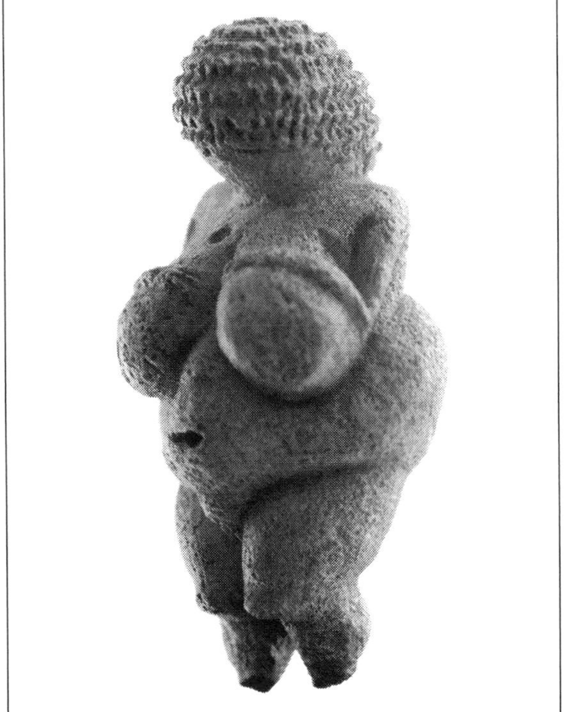

*Upper Paleolithic Earth Goddess, estimated to have been carved 24,000–22,000 BC.*

Over time, specific goddesses emerged around the world. By 1700 B.C., Isis was being worshipped in Egypt as the daughter of the moon. The Babylonian goddess Istar emerged circa 1500 B.C. The Greeks worshipped Diana as the goddess of the moon and Aphrodite as the goddess of sexual love. The great mother goddess was worshipped throughout Asia. She was known by many names: Astarte, Cybele, Anahita.

The gradual change from worshipping the pagan goddess (i.e. nature and the Earth), and the gods and goddesses of pantheism, to monotheism started about 10,000 years ago when human society evolved from hunter-gatherers to farmers. Efforts to change the gender of the god head went on for thousands of years as a male-oriented monotheism fought to marginalize the more female dominated pagan theology. This also meant marginalizing the pagans' shamans, gods, and their goddesses, and entheogens as spiritual and healing potions.

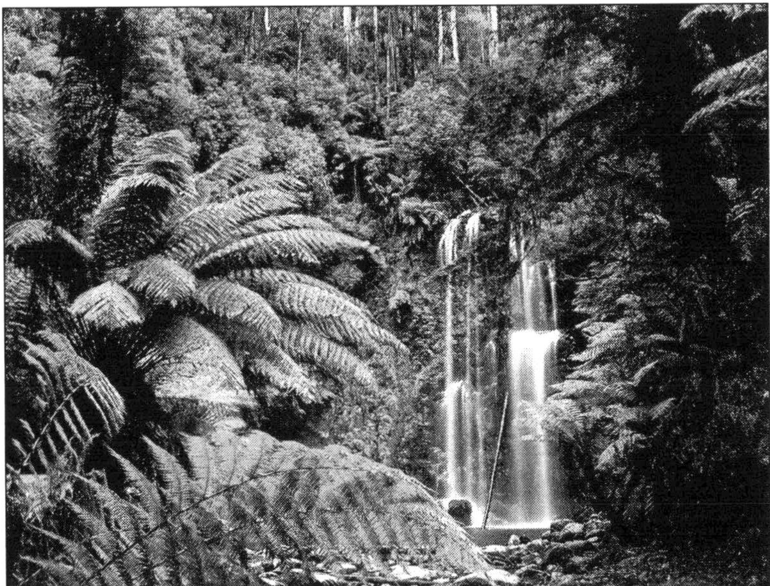

*Nature's chemical factory, the rain forest, is being destroyed at a disastrous rate.*

Paganism preceded and also coexisted with early Judaism and later with Christianity. Ancient Judaism contained such trappings of paganism as animal sacrifice. Since Christianity took its roots from Judaism, it follows that paganism is a foundation for Judeo-Christian thought and that many of today's accepted religious concepts developed and grew from these ancient drug-induced spiritual experiences.

It is no surprise that many of the trappings of today's mainstream religions incorporate ancient Jewish lore and teaching, plus

**Figure 2-1: Clinically Used Drugs from Tropical Rainforest Plants**

| Compound Name | Plant Source | Therapeutic Category |
|---|---|---|
| *Atropine/Hyoscyamine | Solanaceae, Australian cork tree) | Anticholinergic |
| *Camphor | Camphor tree | Rubefacient |
| *Chymopapain | Papaya | Proteolytic; Mucolytic |
| *Cocaine | Coca | Local anesthetic<br>Stimulant |
| * (a) L-Dopa | Velvet Bean | Antiparkinsonism |
| *Emetine | Rubiaceae, Iepcac | Amebicide; Emetic |
| Gossypol | | Cotton<br>Male contraceptive |
| *Physostigmine | Ordeal Bean | Anticholinesterase |
| Picrotoxin | Fish berry | Analeptic |
| *Pilocarpine | Ritaceae, Jaborandi | Parasympathomimetic |
| *Quinine | Yellow cinchona | Antimalarial; |
| *Scopolamine | Recurved thorinapple | Sedative |
| *Tubocurarine | Curare | Skeletal muscle paralyzer |
| *Vinblastine | Madagascan periwinkle | Antitumor agent |
| Yohimbine | Pausinystalia yohimba | Adrenergic blocker,<br>Aphrodisiac |

* currently used in the United States (a) now also synthesized commercially

Definitions:

Parasympathominetic – mimics actions of parasymptomatic (vegetative) nervous system
Anticholinesterase – keeps acetelcholine around longer
Rubefacient - irritant
Anticholinergic – interferes with effects of acetylcholine
Antipyretic – brings temperature down
Sedative – hypnotic – relaxation or sleep
Durietic - causes increased urination
Aletylcholine – a neurotransmitter

SOURCES: Farnsworth, N.R. Screening Plants for New Medicines. [14] In *Biodiversity*; Wilson, E.O., ed.; National Academy Press: Washington D.C., 1988 and Soejarto, D.D.; Farnsworth, N.R., *Perspectives in Biology and Medicine*, 1989, 32, 244-256. [15]

**Figure 2-2: Some Representative Plant-Derived Medicinal Compounds**

| Compound | Type | Source | Disease Treatmented/Use |
|---|---|---|---|
| Artemisinin | Terpenoid | Artemisia annua | Antimalarial |
| Camptothecin | Alkaloid | Camptotheca acuminate | Breast, colon cancer, etc. |
| Colchine | Alkaloid | Colchicum autumnale | Antitumor agent, gout |
| Digitalin | Glycoside | Digitalis purpurea | Cardiotonic |
| Docetaxel (Taxotere) | Terpenoid | Taxus sp. | Antitumor agent |
| Etoposide | Glycoside | Podophyllum peltatum | Antitumor agent |
| Irinotecan | Alkaloid | Camptotheca acuminate | Anticancer, antitumor |
| Paclitaxel (Taxol) | Terpenoid | Taxus sp. | Breast, colon cancer, etc. |
| Quinine | Alkaloid | Cinchona ledgeriana | Antimalarial, antipyretic |
| Reserpine | Alkaloid | Rauvolfia serpentine | Antihypertensive, tranquilizer |
| Theobromine | Alkaloid | Theobroma cacao | Diuretic |

SOURCE: www.hortpurdue,edu/newcrop/proceedings1990/v1-491.html

myths and rituals from pantheism, Greek and Roman mythology and naturalistic religions, which we have lumped together as paganism. (Note: "pagan" means country in Latin. The pagan worshippers of nature were country folk.)

Notwithstanding efforts at marginalizing ancient nature-based religions, pagan celebrations, rituals and beliefs comprise a large portion of the foundation of our contemporary spirituality, mores and ethics. Contemporary rituals, holidays and celebrations of life, death, union, spring, harvest, winter and summer solstice, and other important seasonal and life events have their roots in ancient religious thought.

## Go Ahead: They're Good For You

This notion that drugs can create a positive internal contemplative or spiritual environment is not limited to ancient times. Botanist Norman Taylor, Ph. D., author of *Narcotics Nature's Dangerous Gifts* (1963) and Dr. Andrew Weil, integrative medicine guru and author of *The Natural Mind* (1998), see a very important role in human existence for altered states of consciousness. Both see altered states as necessary for normal human living. Taylor postulates the use of mind-altering substances as a way to take a break from the weight of fate and the anxiety created by the unanswerable questions. In support of the normalcy of altered states, Weil points out that almost all children seek altered states by such common means as holding their breath, choking each other to near unconsciousness, and/or spinning around until they get dizzy.

Taylor says escape from reality is important because everyone knows each person and their loved ones are going to die. Humans need a break from the crush of existential angst. Weil takes a more upbeat view of the essential role of altered states. He believes that altered states are psychologically good for people. He cites the inhabitants of the Amazon who favor a natural high. They believe altered states are so important that in order to know this experience, teenagers should use drugs to experience these altered states. Having had the drug-induced altered reality experience(s), their elders hope that in the future their offspring will be able to achieve an altered state of mind without drugs.

In the 1960s and 1970s, Timothy Leary, Ph.D., once a Harvard faculty member, shook the foundations of the establishment by asking people to abandon the superficiality of accepted middle class goals. He urged people to be seekers, to drop out of the rat race and look into themselves. He promoted the use of LSD to gain these insights. His mantra was "Tune in, Turn on, Drop out." Noted theologian and comparative religious expert and author Huston Smith stated that Leary was promoting looking for the divine within each of us.

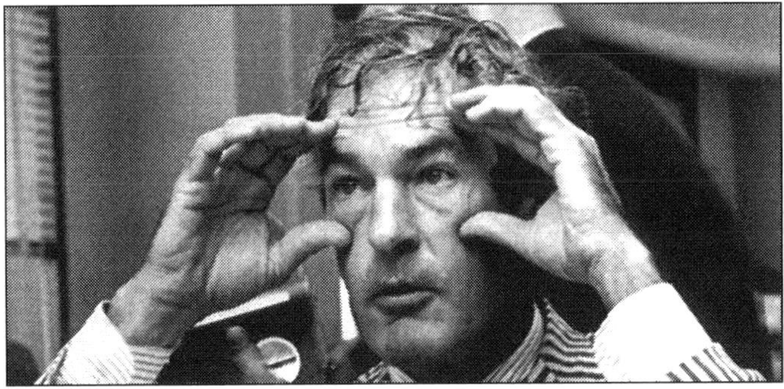

*Harvard professor and '60s guru, Dr. Timothy Leary, put it this way, "You have to go out of your mind to get into your head." Noted comparative religion authority Houston Smith described Leary's thesis about psychedelics as the drugs that bring out the gods within us, the divine spirit within us all that emanates beyond ourselves.* [16]

## Soma: From Ambrosia to Rhubarb

Originally thought of as the one true entheogen, Soma is probably best thought of as the name of a class of plants known to the ancients, which were used to acquire altered states of mind. In these altered states, people made contact with the local deity or deities and sought their advice.

It has become a real detective story to try and nail down what is the true Soma. Many plants and drugs can rightly claim the title Soma. Because different peoples had different sacred plants, there may not even be a one true Soma. To this day, there is no consensus on what the original Soma was. It is unlikely it will ever be known for certain. There are, however, many candidates:

### Ambrosia

The ambrosia of Greek and Roman mythology is similar to Soma. The gods and goddesses consumed ambrosia. According to this mythology, the eating and/or drinking of this nectar makes them gods and conferred immortality. Some texts believe the Greeks' ambrosia was honey. [17,18,19,20]

## Amanita muscaria

The red-with-white-flecks topped mushroom, *Amanita muscaria*, is perhaps the most credible of all the Soma candidates.

Over 50 years ago, R. Gordon Wasson, one of the first modern ethnobotanists, felt he had good evidence that the mushroom, *Amanita muscaria*, was the Soma. Before deciding on *A. muscaria*, Wasson considered and rejected several psychoactive plants as candidates for Soma.

Wasson came to his conclusion through researching ancient texts out of Asia. [21] The *Rig Veda* and the *Avesta* are the religious works of the Indian Hindus and Iranian Zoroastrians, respectively. In both religions, there is reference to a plant, which is believed to have hallucinogenic properties and was used in religious ceremonies. It is referred to as Soma in the *Rig Veda* and Haoma in the *Avesta*.

These religions derived from the Aryans, who were a warrior and grain-growing people whose homeland was somewhere in Central Asia. After leaving their homeland, they split into several groups approximately 4000 years ago. One group, the Indics, settled in the Valley of the Indus, which is now Afghanistan, and another settled in what is now Iran and became the Iranian Zoroastrians.

Both groups orally passed on their religious knowledge. Only hundreds of years later was it written down and preserved to the present. Both had a tribal religion with a hereditary priesthood, with a full complement of gods, including one called Soma. The *Rig Veda* specifically states that Soma can only be found growing in the mountains, which is where *Amanita muscaria* can only be found in the latitude of the Indus Valley. However, these mountains were not accessible to the Aryans, which only deepens the mystery.

Another clue is that Soma could be consumed in two forms: 1. Consumed directly, by either eating the raw mushroom or drinking its juices or 2. Taken in the urine of the person who has ingested the Soma. Here score a point for *Amanita muscaria*.

Dried *Amanita muscaria* can be freshened with water and macerated with a stone pestle that brings forth

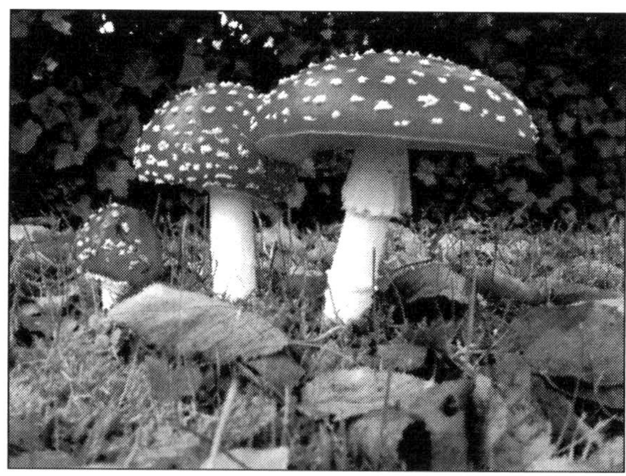

Amanita Muscaria. *The plant must be properly prepared in order for it to be effective as a hallucinogen. Some people have become ill and nauseous to the point of vomiting when consuming* Amanita muscaria. *Siberian shamons recommend cooking or drying before consumption.*

### Rg Veda or Rig Veda and Soma

The Rig Veda is several ancient Indian texts, composed roughly between 1700-1100 B.C. [22] The *Rg Veda* (aka *Rgveda Samhita*, *Rigveda* or *Rig Veda*), is the oldest and most important source of Indian (as in India) religion. This spiritual document is a collection of 1,028 hymns written in Sanskrit and contained in the Four Books of Wisdom. These hymns were seen as too sacred to be written down, so for centuries they were passed down by oral tradition.

The *Rgveda Samhita* is not dated. Scholars agree that the *Rig Veda* was written sometime between 1100 B.C. and 3000 B.C. The *Rgveda Samhita* discusses Soma at some length. An entire book is devoted to Soma, and six hymns and poetry about Soma are found in other books of the *Rig Veda* (*The Verse of Verses*).

The god, Soma, was very important to the Vedic people. "Soma was at the same time a god, a plant, and the juice of that plant." [23] Soma was believed to extend and improve life, produce happiness (*mada*) and even lead to immortality. Vedic priests were the primary consumers of Soma. Soma was praised for its energizing and intoxicating qualities. It was exalted for bringing heightened, often ecstatic, awareness.

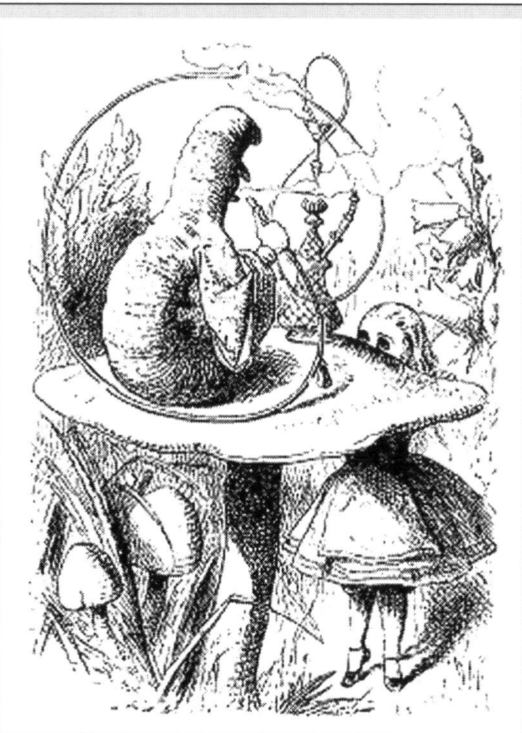

## Not Alice, Too

Fly agaric distorts one's perception of size. It's the mushroom Alice ate in Lewis Carroll's *Alice's Adventures in Wonderland.*[24] One of the hallucinations it causes is to make things look larger, so that's how Alice had the illusion that she got smaller and was able to slip under the door.

Patrick Harding of Sheffield University in England points out that Mordecai Cooke was a friend of the author of *Alice's Adventures in Wonderland,* Charles Dodgson (aka Lewis Carroll). Carroll was likely familiar with Cooke's 1862 book, *A Plain and Easy Account of British Fungi*, which contained mention of the recycling of urine containing fly agaric.

Harding wrote in *The Aerodynamics of Reindeer to the Thermodynamics of Turey,* "This inability to judge size – macropsia – is one of the effects of fly agaric... Very likely this is the basis of the episode in Alice where she eats the mushroom, where one side makes her grow very tall and the other very small."[25]

name, fly agaric, because people used to put it in a glass of milk to kill flies. The fly is supposed to drink the mushroom-adulterated milk, get high, fly around in a frenzy, then drop dead in mid-flight.

Intriguingly, the *A. muscaria* mushroom is thought by some historians to be the basis for many Christmas myths and traditions, a topic that is explored in the next chapter.

## Psilocybin Mushrooms

Terence McKenna is the author of *The Food of the Gods* (1992). His theory was that psilocybin mushrooms are the Soma. He disputes Wasson's evidence and said he was not convinced as to fly agaric's spiritual affects.[26]

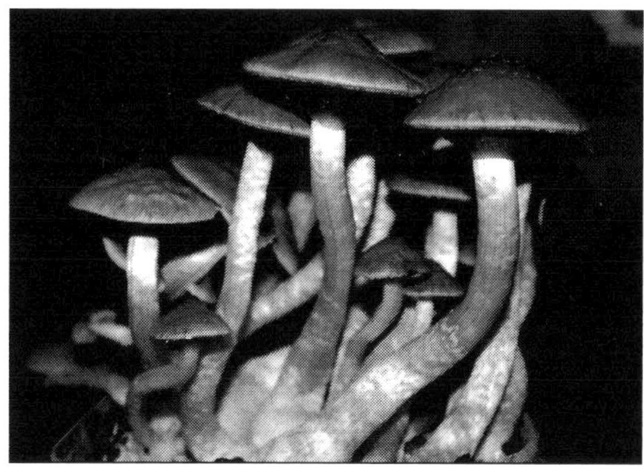

*Author Terence McKenna theorized that psilocybin mushrooms, known in the West as "magic mushrooms" or "shrooms", are the Soma. Over 40 species have been identified in the genus* Psilocybe *and they are found throughout the planet at almost any altitude.*

---

## Peganum Harmala or Rue

In 1989, David Flattery and Marint Schwartz put forth *Peganus harmala* (harmal or wild rue) as Soma. Richard Rudgley makes a strong case for wild *Peganum harmala* as the Soma of the Indo-Iranians. Rue contains several hallucinogenic compounds including harmine. It grows in the right geographic area, the Iranian plateau and Asia Steppes, for the Soma or haoma mentioned in the Zoroastrian sacred writings. The hallucinations caused by the harmaline, harmine and tetrahydroharmine all found in rue are consistent with the visions described in the *Avesta.* Rue looks like an all-purpose Middle Eastern plant. It not only is used to provide the red die used in Persian and Turkish rugs, but the hallucinations it causes are said to be the inspiration for the geometric designs in those rugs.[27]

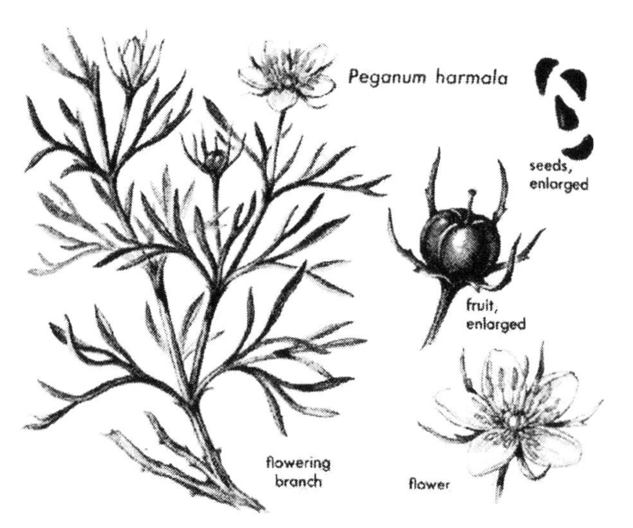


### A Spiritual Experience with Rue

A 3rd-century A.D. description of rue-induced hallucinations comes from a Zoroastrian spiritual quest. The spiritual quest required ingestion of soma. The quest was necessary because of the decline of Zoroastrianism caused by the invasion of Persia by Alexander the Great.

The most righteous man was selected to take this quest. He prepared by washing his hands, being perfumed, prayer and then he consumed three cups of a rue based liquid. His soul traveled to the other world. He sees heaven and hell and describes them in terms that sound very contemporary. He described heaven as the "all-glorious light of space, much perfumed with basil, all-bedecked, all admired and splendid, full of glory and every joy and every pleasure, with which no one was satiated" [28]

In the vision, Hell was not so good. He saw "the soul of a man who from head to toe remained stretched upon a rack; and a thousand demons trampled upon him, and ever smote him with great brutality and violence." [29] Seeing wavy and geometric figures is quite consistent with visions of the sun.

The story line and visions vary from culture to culture. Set, setting and previous experience and the drug itself all can influence the psychotropic visions that people experience. One can postulate that in a drug related spiritual vision the spiritual seekers are influenced in what they see by their cultural expectations.

a tawny yellow juice. That, however, could be many different plants.

*A. muscaria* was used by Koryak Shamans in Siberia until the 17th century when it was replaced by alcohol, which had been introduced to the Koryak people by the Russians. [30] The mushroom gets its

## Cannabis

Cannabis is a candidate for being the Soma and/or spiritual drug for Zoroastrians, Buddhists, and possibly early Christians and Jews. Zoraster (c.628-c.551 B.C.) was the first to mention cannabis in a sacred text, the *Zend-Avesta*. Cannabis was considered the principle religious sacrament for Zoroastrian priests. [31]

The role of cannabis is even better known in the Indian religious tradition. In the 5th century B.C., Siddhartha allegedly ate only hemp and its seeds for the six years prior to becoming the Buddha. [32]

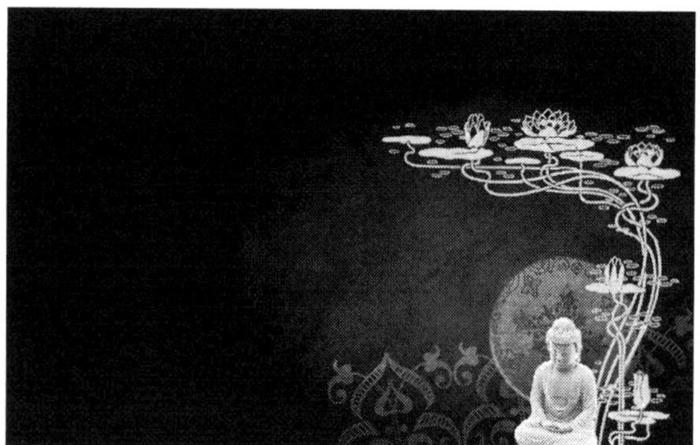

*It is said Siddhartha ate only hemp and its seeds for six years before he realized he was the Buddha.*

According to the *Vedas*, the four seminal books of the Hindu faith, the god Shiva brought cannabis down from the Himalayas for the pleasure of mankind. [33] More controversially, some scholars argue that Jesus may have used cannabis to heal and that some of the oils which Jews, including Jesus, were anointed with contained hemp seed oil as one of its constituents. [34]

## Peyote

Peyote is a spiritual plant with deep roots in religious practices in what is now northern Mexico and the present day U.S. Southwest. From at least 600 A.D., peyote was widely used by the Navajo and Huichol populations as a way of achieving spiritual insight. The Huichol Indians of the Nayarit and Jalisco states in Mexico view peyote as the very heart of their indigenous religion. To the Huichol, peyote symbolized life, health, accomplishment and good fortune. In their art, peyote is represented by a hexagon, the Peyote Mandala.[35]

Peyote and San Pedro *(Echinopsis pachanoi)*, a psychoactive cactus found in many South American countries, both contain mescaline as their principal visionary alkaloid. Mescaline was first isolated from the peyote cactus in Germany in 1896 and brought to popular attention in 1954 in Aldous Huxley's book, *The Doors of Perception.*

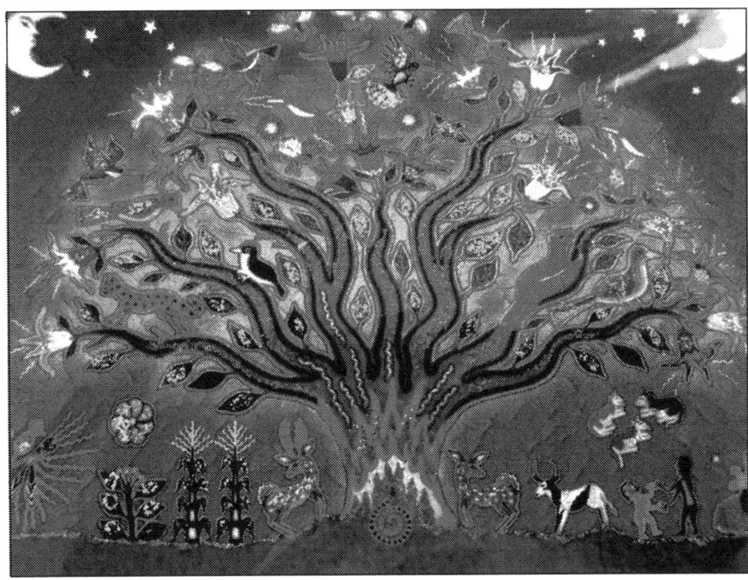

*The art of the Huichol Indians of Mexico includes many totems and symbols. For example, the deer is their totem for their spirit guide and spiritual leader. The salamander gets the Rain Mother to rain by prodding the clouds. The wolf represents the Huichol people and the hexagon represents peyote, while the serpent is thought to protect corn.* [36]

## Opium

Opium has been used in potions throughout history and been part of many religious rites. Part of its claim to being Soma is based on the finds in Turkmenistan. Ancient sacred shrines were discovered there. In these shrines, remnants of pottery that contain ephedra and opium have been found.

## Tobacco

Tobacco was used by Native American shamans, medicine men, and holy men to produce hallucinatory visions for spiritual journeys. These shamans believed that the tobacco-induced visions put them in intimate contact with the ethereal spirits.

Tobacco-induced visions also helped shamans heal diseases. To Native Americans, disease was caused by an intrusion of evil spirits or loss of the soul. Being in a tobacco-induced trance was thought to aid in either removing the evil spirit or finding the wandering soul. The indigenous people of the Americas claim that tobacco was a gift from their ancestors and their gods.

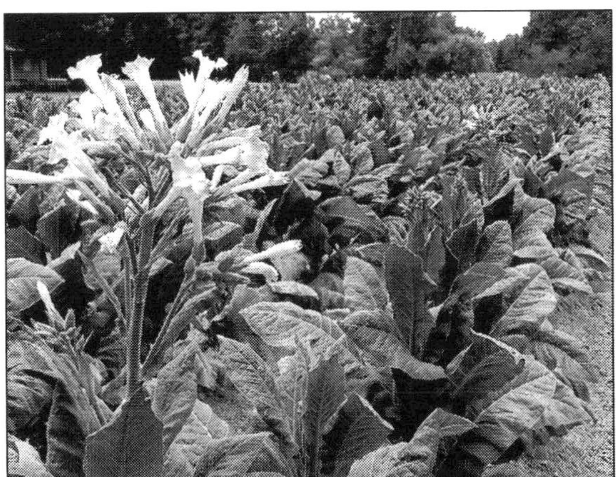

*A tobacco field in bloom.*

For a number of South American Indian shamans, *Nicotiana rustica* not *N. tabaccum* tobacco is their only ritual intoxicant. (For other tribes, tobacco is just the most prominent entheogeny in their ecstatic pharmacopoeias.) The nicotine content in *N. rustica* is many times higher than *N. tabacum*. This makes it able to trigger the desired ecstatic trance, so *N. rustica* is the shamanic intoxicant, while *N. tabacum* is the ancestor of modern tobacco blends.

## Ephedra

Ephedra, a stimulant, is a sympathominetic drug, which was included in Shen Neng's first pharmacopeia. Not only does it have medicinal value, but archeological research reveals that an Aryan Soma drink consisted of a mixture of opium, cannabis and ephedra.

## Ephedra and Cannabis

An early 21st-century Russian excavation in Turkmenistan's Kara Kum desert, unearthed archaeological finds dating from the second millennium B.C. These findings have led to the speculation that between 2000 and 1000 B.C., the haoma, the Iranian Soma, was a composite psychoactive drink composed of ephedra and cannabis (in one case, with ephedra and opium in another).

A big complex, which contained a large shrine used as a sacred fire temple, was found in Gonur South. The shrine had two parts: a public area used for public worship, and private areas used by the priesthood. The private rooms set aside for the priesthood contained three ceramic bowls. An analysis of their contents docu-mented traces of both cannabis and ephedra.

Ten ceramic pots and a number of pottery stands and strainers that have also been associated with making psychoactive beverages were found in another room. Anthropologists believe this shrine was likely dispensing the entheogenic drink to worshippers from all over Margiana in the first half of the second millennium B.C.

The discovery in the shrines of the remains of opium, cannabis and ephedra in ritual vessels show that Soma or haoma in its Iranian form may be considered as a composite psychoactive substance comprising cannabis and ephedra in one instance, and opium and ephedra in another. Work at Kara Kum and another shrine, Togouk, suggests that Soma may have never really existed, except in the minds of the priest, and that the plants used during the religious ceremonies have always been substitutes for this mythical Soma.

## Ayahuasca

Ayahuasca (or ayajuasca) is a vine found in Peru with psychoactive powers. It is also known as ayai, yage, caapi, hausca and natem. Among shamans and *curanderos*, it is considered to be a master plant whose use can connect one to spiritual realms and lead to healing and insight. Archaeological finds suggest it has been used in spiritual ceremonies for at least 4,000 years.[37] Like rue, ayahuasca also contains harmine and the usual hallucinatory patterns are similar to rue.

## Rhubarb?

What is the deal with rhubarb? It turns out that some authorities say, "well maybe an alcoholic drink was made from rhubarb" and was used as a substitute for Soma when the real Soma (if there indeed was a single Soma) was unavailable.

## Other Soma Candidates

Other suggested candidates for Soma include alcohol, mead, pomegranate, Chicory, and Blue lotus. However, these don't quite meet all the criteria for time, place and spiritual effect.

Humans have been very creative when it comes to seeking altered states. It seems likely that whatever the first Soma was, most if not all of these psychotropic plants were entheogens used in some spiritual ceremonies or efforts to attain spiritual insight.

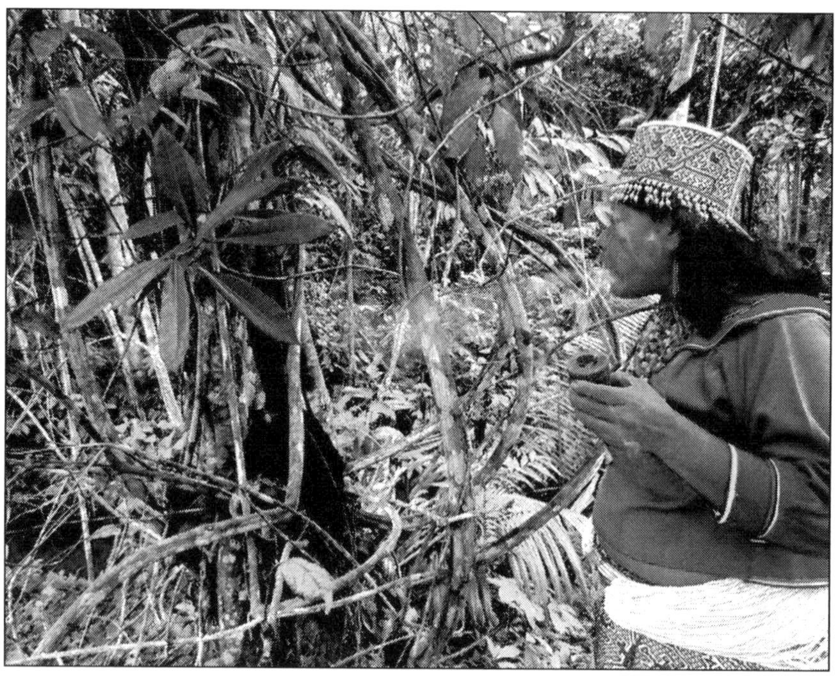

*Ayahuasca (or ayajuasca) is a vine found in Peru with psychoactive powers. It is also known as ayai, yage, caapi, hausca and natem. Among shamans and curanderos, it is considered to be a master plant whose spirits can connect one to spiritual realms and lead to healing and insight. Archaeological finds suggest it has been used in spiritual ceremonies for at least 4,000 years. Like rue, ayahuasca also contains harmine and the usual hallucinatory patterns are similar to rue.*

## The Search for Authentic Spirituality

A wide range of religions see divinity in nature, in all of creation. These include: Taoism, Zen Buddhism, paganism, Native American religions including the Native American Church, and some other forms of Christianity such as Creation Spirituality. Nature-based religions are a spiritual belief system that affirms life, the body, sex, nature and the universe. The spiritual force of these belief systems can be very powerful whether based in Christianity, Islam, Judaism or pantheism.

The belief that nature and the universe are divine is believed to have been first written up by the Greek philosopher Heraclitus of Ephesus.[38] For over 1500 years, well before the time of Constantine the Great, the 4th-century Roman emperor who embraced Christianity, efforts were made to marginalize these naturalistic belief systems.

American drug policy has profoundly influenced differences in finding, expressing and achieving spirituality and the route to moral, ethical insight, a oneness with God, and the relationship of humans to nature. These differences have led to the marginalization of people with belief systems unacceptable to those in power. In the West, achieving a spiritual state with drugs is often portrayed as insincere, cultist, hedonistic, or as a sham to get around repressive U.S. laws. These laws make the practice of the ritual use of many entheogens (e.g., kava kava, cannabis, LSD, peyote, ayajuasca, salvia divinorum, psilocybin mushrooms) forbidden, or at least very difficult to legally obtain and consume.

The wide variety of ethnogenic herbs and plants used to derive a spiritual experience represent a powerful competitor to more conventional religions for the spiritual hearts and minds of people. The worry of more conventional religions is that, if a person can discover the meaning of the cosmos and develop a spiritual connection with the Almighty by use of these plants, then all the structure and pomp of an organized religion is not needed. The use of "mind-altering" substances in a religious, spiritually related context is frequently deplored, often demonized. People who use entheogens have been, and are now, often portrayed as demons, vilified, and found in violation of the law.

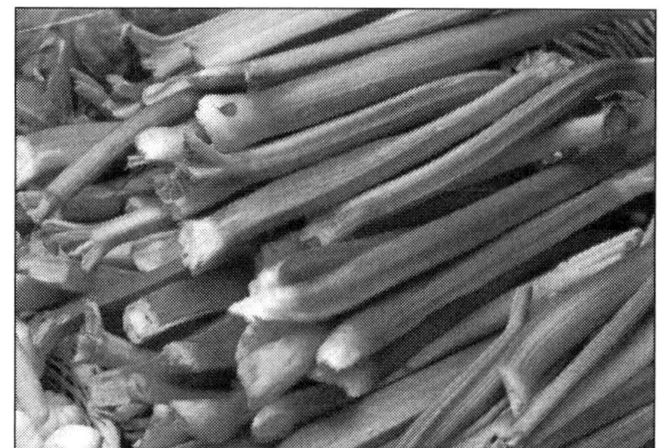

*Rhubarb is one of the more unlikely candidates for Soma. Can someone gain enlightenment from rhubarb, even rhubarb wine? This sounds a little bit like the myth in the 1970s that someone could get high from drying banana skins, scraping off the stuff on the inside of the peel and smoking it. It was called "Mellow Yellow" I don't know about rhubarb as Soma, but the banana story is urban myth.*

The use of substances to obtain spiritual insight is one of the bones of contention that most contemporary mainstream Christian, Judaic, and Islamic religions have with psychotropic substances. For their followers; the road to enlightenment is not littered with herbs, but obeisance to the orthodoxy of a hierarchical, male-dominated, frequently government-allied "faith".

In his 1970 book, *The Late Great Planet Earth*, Evangelical Christian author Hal Lindsey points out that Revelation 18:23 references sorcery. Lindsey said, "The word 'sorceries' comes from the Greek word 'pharmakeia,' which is the word from which we get our English word 'pharmacy.' Sorceries means a kind of occult worship or black magic associated with the use of drugs. This word is mentioned several times in the Book of Revelation." Lindsey went on to connect the psychedelic-ingesting youth of his time with demons, noting: "These drugs reduce a man's thinking and mentality to a point where he is easily demon-possessed."[39]

Chris Bennet, in his December 2007 *High Times* article on Christians and cannabis, quotes Jesus, "Nothing that enters a man from outside can make him 'unclean' by going into him. Rather, it is what comes out of a man that makes him 'unclean'" (Mark 7:18). Bennet suggests that this is what Frederic Madeleine had in mind in his 1988 book, *The Drug Controversy and the Rise of Antichrist*, where Madeleine depicts the enforcers of prohibition as the true practitioners of the "sorcery" referred to in The Book of Revelation. Like Lindsey, Madeleine noted that the word was derived from *pharmakeia*, "an occult

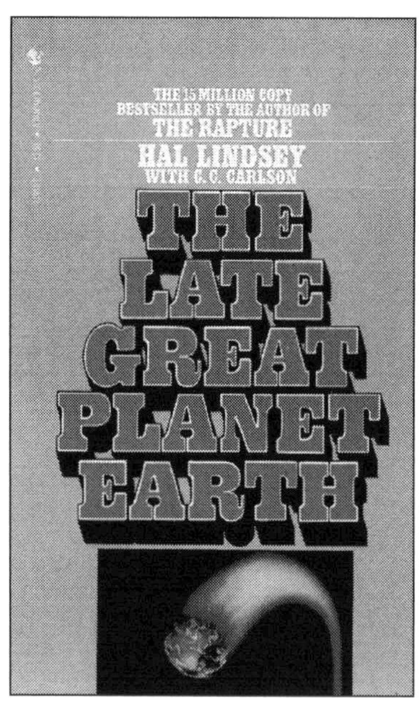


*In his 1970 book,* The Late, Great Planet Earth, *Hal Lindsey held that the modern word "pharmacies" was related to the Greek word for "sorceries", which is "a kind of occult worship or black magic associated with the use of drugs". The book sold nearly 30 million copies and further demonized the use of "illegal" drugs.*

science involving secret knowledge about drugs and herbs," but differed in his interpretation of what this meant. "Although some have suggested that the use of illegal drugs is sorcery," Madeleine continued, "I suggest instead that control of drugs is part of a system of sorcery, reinvented by the corrupt minds of men in high places.[40]

This sectarian dispute of how to attain spiritual insight does not take place unfettered in the market place of ideas. Laws, misinformation and disinformation have been used in a systematic, fairly successful attempt to marginalize and demonize psychotropics use as a spiritual tool. Yes, mainstream America has difficulty in accepting the use of psychotropics to assist in gaining spiritual insight and a oneness with nature, our fellow beings and the illusive life force. I s this "the force", the energy, the power to which George Lucas was alluding to in the *Star Wars* movie series, when his characters offer the salutation: "May the force be with you"?

## Religious Conflicts: Mine's Better Than Yours!

Few things are more emotional than our spirituality and our relationship to the life force, nature, the All Mighty, Jehovah, Christ, God, Buddha, what have you. There are many different roads to spiritual insight. Some take the main route; others the path less traveled. Whether our faith, our spiritual insight, our road is well-taken is simply a personal decision based more on faith than evidence.

Still, most religions have many general similarities. All too often, humans have focused on the differences among religions rather than celebrating the commonality of humanity and sharing a love and understanding for fellow inhabitants of the planet.

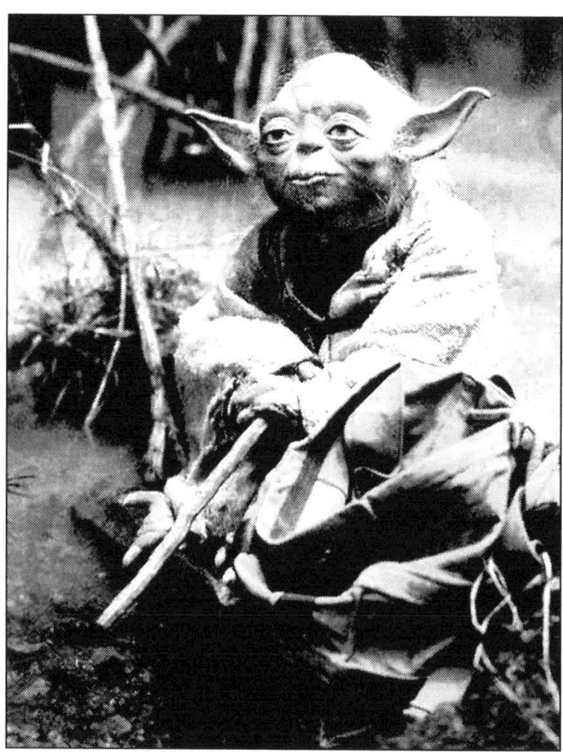

*Yoda was the most powerful Jedi Master in the* Star Wars *movies by filmmaker George Lucas. He taught Luke Skywalker, eventually the Grand Master of the New Jedi Order, in the ways of "the Force".*

Sadly, religion has usually been another venue for "us" demonizing "them." In this life, once a group has collectively found THE answer to a spiritual quest, the desire is to preserve its rightful place in society. Fear, rational or not, of losing this answer, of it being wrong, or having this answer taken away can generate a lot of, at the very least, hostility toward "them" that are different from us; those who, by their very difference represent a visible challenge to "our" faith and other aspects of "our" culture. What if "they" are right and "we" are wrong? "They" are trying to make our life devoid of meaning.

Religion has a long, sad history of applying illogic, torture and demonization in its followers' perception, treatment and persecution of non-believers, infidels, pagans, Jews, Christians and Muslims, or the like. In modern times, drug usage and drug policy have been an important strategy for marginalizing one religion or another or the orthodox wing of a religion attacking liberal practitioners of that faith.

## A Witch Hunting We Shall Go: Get the Scapegoats!

America's cultural attic includes the European witch hunts of the Renaissance era (1450-1650). There is a reason why today's drug laws and their propagation and enforcement is likened to a witch hunt. It is also not only the hysteria and lies but the "demonization" and discrimination against the minority position. It is the exercise of control by powerful governmental sources and the scapegoating of the "other."

There are modern concerns about the mystical, magical and medical use of drugs. Fear and hysteria have been used to construct and constrict the view of what can be socially acceptable ways of achieving spiritually. There is definitely prejudice against the use of drugs for communing with nature and exploring spirituality.

Today some formerly popular pejoratives have gone out of style. For example: radical, nigger, spic, rag head; only drug dealer remains politically correct. This has given rationalization for a whole host of unsavory actions and prohibitions previously shunned by Americans: the loss of protections provided by the Fourth and Fifth Amendments that have been obliterated to justify the constitutionality of urine screenings; the weakening of States' rights in *Gonzales vs. Raich* — the list goes on and on.

Witch hunts or ascribing bad outcomes to the supernatural power of witches is just an extreme form of scapegoating; of making someone else take the blame for some undesirable outcome. The scapegoat is the sacrificial victim. If we blame "them", then "we" can put off taking responsibility to actually do something constructive to solve the problem at hand. Girard describes the scapegoat as someone set apart from the dominant culture, set apart from the perceived mainstream of religion, ethnicity, sex, social class, or race. Making someone a scapegoat allows them to be seen as less than human. [41] The rhetoric around scapegoating is full of these degrading and repugnant invectives.

The motives for witch-hunting are many, complex and often conflicting. The roots go deep into antiquity, to a time when a vengeful male god concept began to ascend over the warm, loving female goddess embraced by most ancient cultures. Cruelty, hysteria, mob thinking, willingness to ignore science and human decency characterize both witch hunts and contemporary drug policy.

---

**"All religions provide at least some of their members with what members of the religion interpret as authentic experiences of non-empirical reality. This is done through the use of some means of reaching a trance state ... an 'altered state of consciousness.' The means of doing this include music, dance, meditation, pain and drugs."** [42]

**Serena Nanda and Richard L. Warms**

*Cultural Anthropology,* 2006 edition.

---

POGO:
WE HAVE MET THE ENEMY AND HE IS US
Walt Kelly

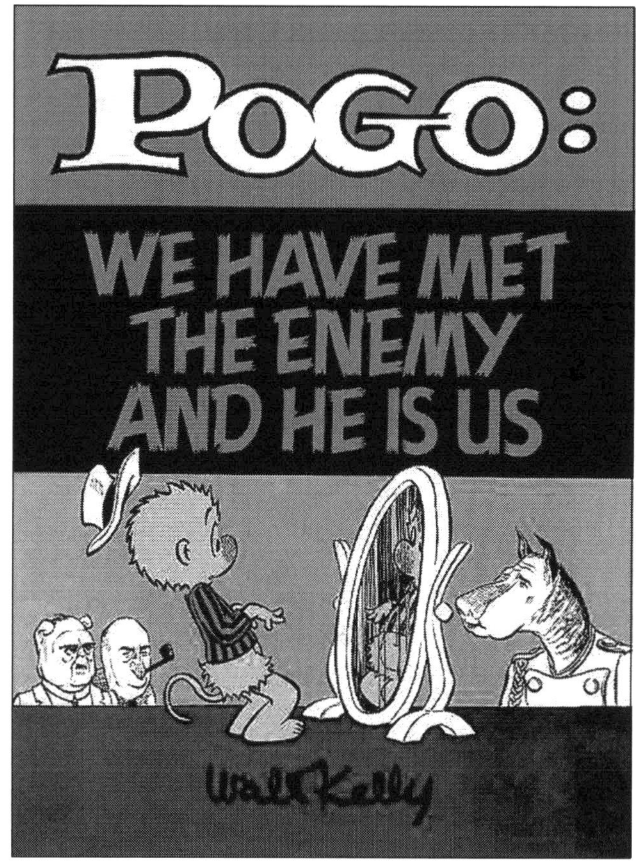

*Walt Kelley (1913-1973) was a political satirist whose popular cartoon strip, Pogo, ran in major newspapers for many years (1948-1975 and 1989 to 1990). This poster portrays U.S. President Richard Nixon's attorney general, John Mitchell, smoking a pipe, Federal Bureau of Investigation Director J. Edgar Hoover as a dog, and Spiro Agnew, Nixon's vice president (who was later forced to resign for corruption) as a hyena.*

## What Does This Mean Today?

What does all this ancient history have to do with modern day drug control policies? It documents how long the use of illogic and demonization of "them" has been with "us". It provides historical perspective and context to how onerous, impractical, and illogical policies have been directed by some humans toward others in order to push them to the margins of society.

History reveals a pattern of denying the essential humanity and dignity of any person or group we label as "them", the enemy, the different, the scapegoat. Prohibition and drug policy have been two of the levers in the tool kit of bigotry. Policies affecting control of entheogens have historically arisen more from hysteria than from science or reason. In response to real or imagined harm, the help offered has too frequently been in the form of punishment rather than treatment and/or prevention. In truth, too often humanity is its own worst enemy.

In some ways, contemporary drug-policy struggles reflect the religious struggles of the past. This conflict between punishment-versus-treatment policy, often comes down to taking the loving, nurturing approach of naturalistic religion as opposed to the punishing approach of an angry, aggressive male god. Drug enforcement officials appear to purposely and maliciously suggest that drug use and drug abuse are synonymous. There seems to be little interest in developing a real understanding of the root causes of substance abuse or assessing the cost-effectiveness of our present criminal approach. Such analysis is essential for adequate planning, implementing and funding scientifically based and tested, effective drug-abuse treatment and prevention programs.

We gloss over the damage done to the Constitution, our historical American values and the national psyche by oppressive federal drug policy. Make no mistake, the U.S. Constitution is under attack and the drug laws are the stalking horse for its destruction. The Bill of Rights is in tatters and serious attempts are being made to tear down the wall between church and state.

## Intellectual Honesty is the Best Policy. Right?

In a July 2006 article in *Playboy Magazine*, "Honesty is the Best Policy", Sam Harris, author of the book *The End of Faith: Religion, Terror and the Future of Reason* (2006), makes a plea for intellectual honesty. He describes the difference between scientific and religious thought. "The core of science is not controlled experiments or mathematical modeling; it is intellectual honesty. When considering the truth of a proposition, one is either engaged in a dispassionate weighing of evidence and logical arguments or one isn't. Religion is the one area of our lives in which people imagine some other standard of basic human sanity applies."

---

**"Religion is the one area of our discourse in which it is considered noble to pretend to be certain about things no human being could possibly be certain about."** [43]

**Sam Harris**

*Samharris.org*, April 20, 2013

---

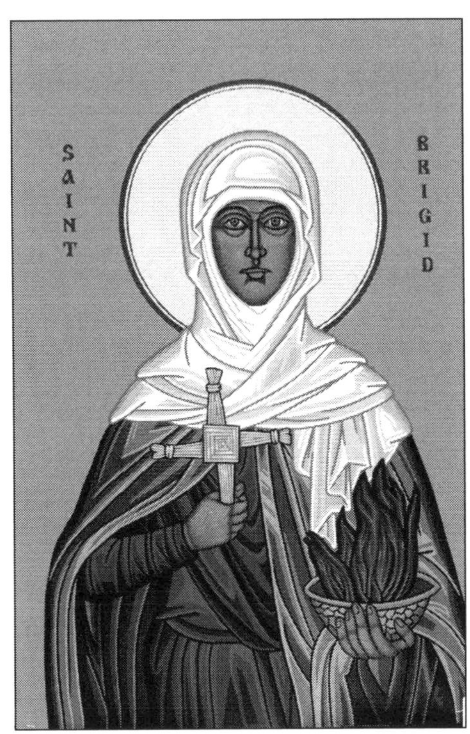


*The Catholic St. Brigit of Kildare (451–525) is thought to have been syncretised with the pagan goddess Brighid.* [1] *Here she is holding Brigid's Cross, which is still believed to protect a house from fire and evil.*

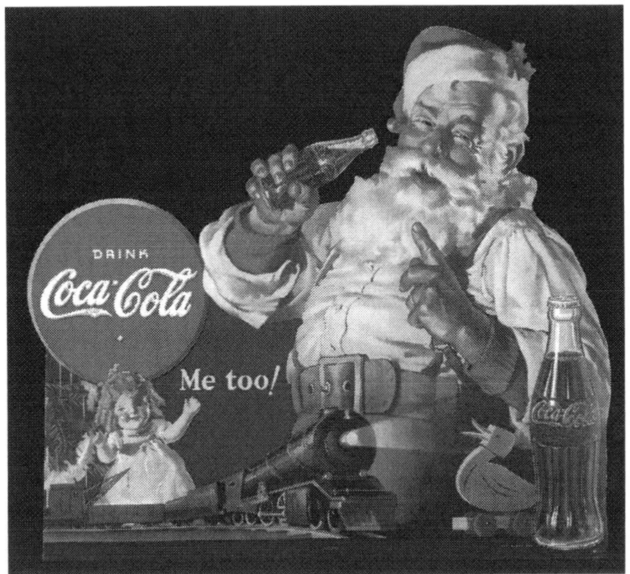


*Santa Claus, or St. Nicholas or Kris Kringle, is a mythical character from Europe's pre-Christian past. He is loosely based on a real man, a wealthy Turk named Nicholas, who gave away all his money and became Bishop of Myra. Santa Claus arises from a combination of myths and legends from many cultures. Coca-Cola Company advertising of the 1930s established Santa as that rotund, white-bearded character seen today. His red and white coloration may be an allusion to the entheogen,* Amanita muscaria.

# CHAPTER III
# Christianity, Entheogens & Holidays

## Christianity Emerges

In the 100 years between the middle of the 1st century BC to the middle of the 1st century AD, several religions of the east arrived in Rome. "They were called mystery religions because they were secretive, often shrouded in a body of rituals not to be revealed to the uninitiated. For the most part, they were brought to the Empire by traders, merchants, and slaves." [2]

Christianity was lumped in with the other mystery religions of its day. "To many in the first and second centuries AD, such Christian beliefs and rituals as monotheism, baptism, and the Eucharist (which sounded like cannibalism) were just as bizarre as those found in other cults. Contrary to much of the then prevailing wisdom and today's Christian church, Christianity gave all its members equal status and thus cut across all social and ethnic barriers." [3] These admirable values of equity changed in modern times to a more male-dominated, power-oriented institution.

In the years following the death of Jesus of Nazareth, different factions of his supporters worked to institutionalize their vision of his teachings. In the first century after his demise, there was not a sharp demarcation between Christianity and Judaism. There were Christian-Judeo sects and Judeo-Christian sects. And the disciples were not all on the same page; some wanted Jews to accept Christ as the Messiah, while others set about starting up their own church. And in the 4th century AD, the Emperor of Rome, Constantine the Great, shaped Christianity to enhance his power. It took several centuries to get to the sharper distinctions seen in the contemporary world.

In the 1st century after Christ and well into the Middle Ages, there was a concerted effort to expand the followers of Christianity. This went forth on many fronts; intellectual, spiritual and political. Early on, the Christians were seen by the Romans as "them." The Romans were concerned about their growing numbers and power. In that climate, the Romans could justify feeding the Christians to the lions as good public policy.

In fact though, the Romans were much more tolerant regarding the practice of religion than most ancient conquering emperors or the way the Romans are usually portrayed in Hollywood movies. True, the Romans did feed more than a few Christians to the lions. However, compared to most other dominant cultures in history, the Roman Empire exhibited broad religious tolerance in the three centuries after the birth of Christ.

First, the state religion of the Roman Empire was not very demanding. Participating in the Roman worship of the gods was not particularly onerous. It merely required the sprinkling of a little incense and then only on formal occasions. This act demonstrated allegiance to the emperor and the empire. It was more a patriotic than a religious act. The official religion was little more than a ceremonial pledge of allegiance, akin to singing the national anthem. [4,5,6] The Romans worshipped Olympian gods, and after Emperor Augustus (27 BC – AD 14), the emperor himself was considered divine. [7]

The Romans allowed the practice of most of the religions that existed within their expansive realm. Even during state celebrations, the Romans tolerated Persian Mithraism and the worship of the Egyptian gods Isis and Osiris, as long as their followers performed the formal sprinkling of incense at the altar of the Roman gods. The Jews refused to sacrifice to the Roman idols, but except for periods after Jewish insurrections, they were rarely persecuted. The Jews kept their beliefs to themselves and the authorities more often than not left them alone. The Romans tolerated any religion that would tolerate others and that respected Roman traditions. [8]

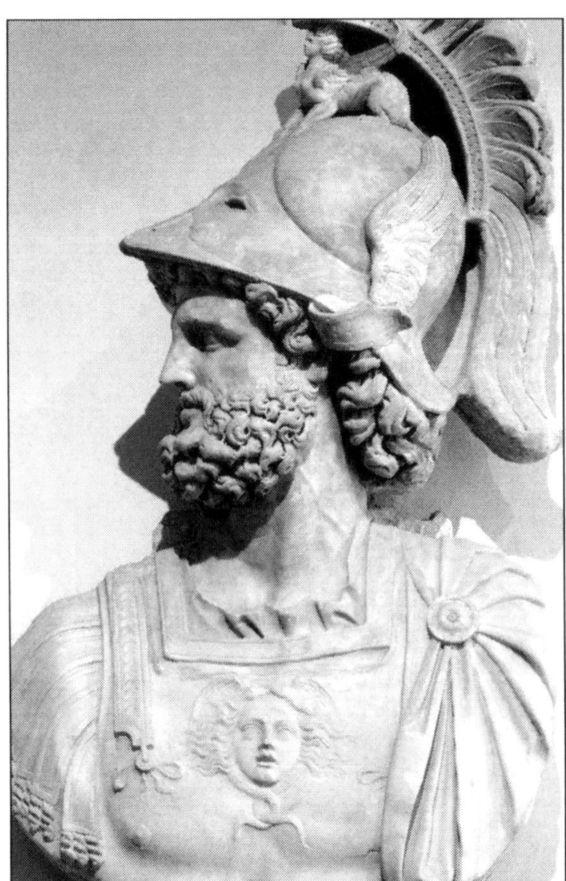

*Mars was the Roman god of war and agriculture. The month of March, which began and ended the season for military campaigning and farming, is named in his honor.*

## Christians and Roman Conflict

Christians earned the enmity of the Romans because they didn't follow the Roman's rules. They did not keep their beliefs to themselves and were disrespectful of the Romans' religious practices. The monotheistic Christians not only refused to burn the requisite incense, they insulted the Roman worshippers and their pantheon of gods and even defaced their idols. And why not? After all, the Christians saw all gods other than their own not as products of pagan imagination, but as actual demons. [9] And they flaunted this conviction.

Historian William Lecky describes the abrasive actions of early Christians toward the dominant

Roman culture in the book *A History of European Morals from Augustus to Charlemagne* (1869). [10]

> "Proselytizing with an untiring energy, pouring a fierce stream of invective and ridicule upon the gods on whose favor the multitude believe all national prosperity to depend, not infrequently insulting worshippers, and defacing the idols, they soon stung the pagan worshippers to madness, and convinced them that every calamity that fell upon the empire was the righteous vengeance of the gods. Nor was the skeptical politician more likely to regard with favor a religion whose development was plainly incompatible with the whole religious policy of the empire. The new church, as it was then organized, must have appeared to him essentially and fundamentally intolerant. To permit it to triumph was to permit the extinction of religious liberty in an empire which comprised all the leading nations of the world, and tolerated all their creeds." [11]

The Romans deemed the Christian's actions as a display of unpatriotic and irreverent behavior toward the Romans and their religion, notwithstanding there was no systematic or official persecution of the Christians in the Roman lands during the 1st and 2nd centuries AD. [12] The Christians, however, were quite unpopular amongst the Romans and candidates to be scapegoated and possibly punished for any calamity. But when Nero came to power, things dramatically changed for the worse. Nero was responsible for much of the cruel tortures and punishments associated with the Roman's persecution of the Christians.

> **"The poor have access to justice in the same way that the Christians had access to lions when they were dragged into a Roman arena."** [13]
>
> **Judge Earl Johnson**
>
> California Court of Appeals (c. 1985)

Nero was the prime suspect when Rome burned in 64 A.D; he remained so to the day he died and onward to the present time. To divert suspicion away from himself, Nero blamed the Christians.

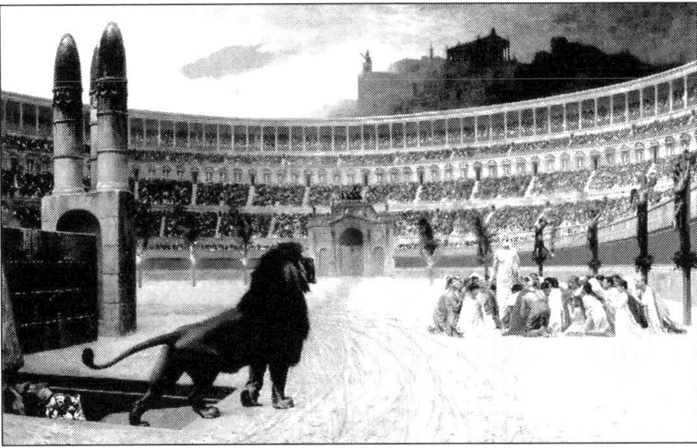

*In the 1st to the 3rd centuries, the Romans fed serious criminals and some Christians to large beasts in amphitheaters, including the Coliseum. The practice, however, was not nearly as popular as portrayed in some Hollywood movies and is little documented by contemporary historians.*

Through the acts of this insane man, the Christians were subjected to barbarous persecution. Nero's heinous acts were principally confined to the city of Rome. [14,15]

The fact that the most egregious atrocities occurred in Rome does not mean Christians elsewhere in the Empire had a picnic. It became common throughout the Empire to demonize the practice of the Christians. Roman authorities claimed the Christians indulged in secret orgies, that they worshipped a god with an ass's head and that early Christians killed babies for sacramental purposes. Similar changes have been used throughout history to demonize one religion or another.

## Constantine Put the "Roman" in Roman Catholic

But this dynamic changed in the 4th century, when Constantine the Great became emperor (AD 306 to 337) and embraced Christianity. In wedding Christianity to Roman political power, Constantine created the Holy Roman Empire. Some historians say that Constantine co-opted the Christian movement and changed its course by taking it from a popular movement to making it essentially a state religion.

When the Roman Emperor embraced monotheism, Constantine transferred his former pagan intolerance of Christianity to a Christian intolerance of paganism. Monotheism does not tolerate other gods and divination and so now it was the pagans who

## Thomas Jefferson and Religion

Throughout history when religion and government power are closely aligned in governance, problems often ensue. American founders saw the role of organized religion as being in conflict with freedom and liberty. They felt this was particularly true when religion had close ties to the state government apparatus.

**"In every country in every age, the priest has been hostile to liberty. He is always in alliance with the despot, abetting his abuses in return for protection to his own.** [16]

**Thomas Jefferson**
Founding Father
and President of the United States, 1801-09

The term "god" has many definitions, ranging from nature to supernatural. Jefferson believed in a Creator, but his term was "Nature's God," the term used by Deists of the time. He believed that Christianity changed after the Romans stuck their oar in the water because the Roman government destroyed much of the gospels and incorporated pagan holidays into Christianity. Jefferson rejected what he deemed as the superstitions and mysticism of Christianity, much of which he saw as insinuate by the Roman government by a scheming Roman priesthood.

Jefferson saw Jesus as a genuine moral philosopher. Jefferson edited the gospels, keeping the parables that had ethical value and removing the writings of Paul, the miracles and mysticism of Jesus; what remained became *The Jefferson Bible*. [17]

Jefferson was a deist, as were all six of the first American presidents. [18.19] The fundamentalist position that they were standard-issue Christians is not supported by history.

The religion historian William Edelen notes that the *Bible* was used to create religious mythology. He specifically documents that it contains many elements of Zorastrism and Egyptian belief. He points out logical inconsistencies. For instance, even if the Bible were infallible, it would take an infallible reader to infallibly interpret its meaning.

Edelen makes the point that Biblical illiteracy is a problem. He argues that this illiteracy causes fear, superstition, and misunderstanding. He points out the fact that many pick and choose from the Bible. As an example, he notes that King James of the *King James Bible* was gay.

were marginalized. With Constantine's adoption of Catholicism/Christianity as the state religion of Rome, Christianity became an effective tool for expanding the Empire. In the hands of the Emperor, Christianity was another lever of power for the state.

In an effort to attract heathens (literally those from the heath) and pagans, many pagan celebrations and rituals were co-opted by the statist Church of Rome. There is little controversy that pagan rites were the foundations of such contemporary holidays as Christmas (Winter Solstice/Saturnalia), Easter (the Spring Equinox), and Halloween (All Hallows Eve/Samhain).

## Entheogens & Christianity: The Soma

As noted in Chapter II, Soma was a generic name given to many psychoactive drugs used for spiritual purposes in many historical spiritual activities. According to *The Encyclopedia of Psychoactive Substances*, cannabis, opium, ephedra, Syrian Rue, magic mushrooms (psilocybin), *Amanita muscaria* mushrooms (fly agaric), peyote (mescaline) and even rhubarb, have been identified as the Soma. Other Soma candidates include ergot, chicory, and morning glory seeds. [20] Soma differed depending upon the culture or religion, climate, geography and/or the speculations of various historians. [21]

The ancients in Paleolithic, Neolithic and Bronze Age cultures relied on mind-altering plants to

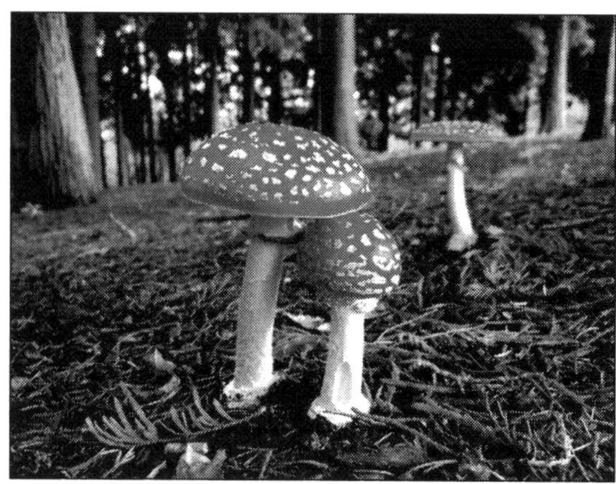

*Although disputed, the* Amanita muscaria *mushroom is probably the legendary psychoactive Soma extant in many ancient cultures.*

communicate with the mystical spirits. This period preceded the dawn of Judaism and was well before the emergence of Christianity and Islam. The role of entheogens in religion and spiritual thought is well known. Ritual use of plant-based entheogens by priests and in some cases the laity were the basis for many of human kind's first spiritual endeavors. Visions, ecstasy, and spiritual insights from ingestion of Soma helped form the ancient naturalistic religions which form the foundations of contemporary faiths.

In *Shamanism and the Drug Propaganda: The Birth of Patriarchy and the Drug War* (1998), Dan Russel points out that herbal metaphors are at the heart of many religious mythologies. These stories are familiar to all of us. They include the Burning Bush, the Tree of Life, the Golden Bough, the Forbidden Fruit, the Blood of Christ, the Blood of Dionysus, the Holy Grail (or rather its contents), the Chalice (Kalyx: 'flower cup'), the Golden Flower (Chrysanthemum), Ambrosia (Ambrotos: 'immortal'), Nectar (Nektar: 'overcomes death'), the Sacred Lotus, the Golden Apples, the Mystic Mandrake, the Mystic Rose, the Divine Mushroom (teonanactl), the Divine Water Lily, Soma, Ayahuasca ('Vine of the Soul'), Kava, Iboga, Mama Coca and Peyote Woman. [22]

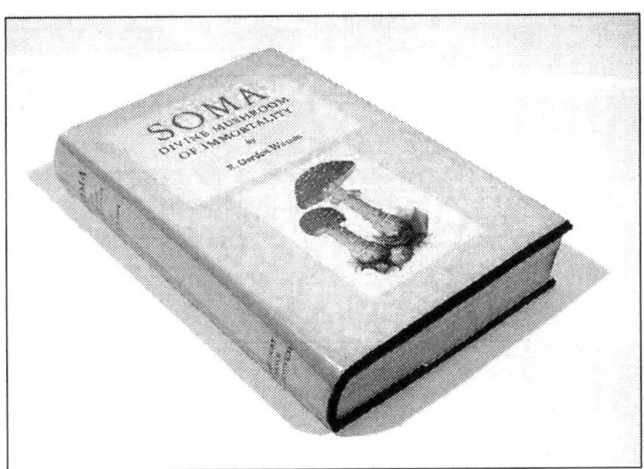


*In* The Sacred Mushroom and the Cross *(1970), author John Allegro equated the mushroom* Amanita muscaria *with Jesus Christ.*

John Allegro's controversial 1970 book, *The Sacred Mushroom and the Cross*, carries the divination of Soma to its logical extreme. His analysis gives *Amanita muscaria* iconic stature by equating Soma with Christ/Christianity. Allegro sees the spiritual insights gained from the mushroom generated hallucinogenic altered states as woven into the Book of Genesis and the Christ story. He sees this entheogenic fungi as more than just a spiritual gift but as a spiritual messenger. The fungi was perceived as borne from "Mother Earth" after being impregnated by God with rain or dew (i.e., semen). Ancient peoples considered the emerging of this mushroom from the ground without any visible seed to be a "virgin birth" and the result of the morning dew. The dew was thought to be the semen of the deity. Using this iconology, Allegro interprets *A. muscaria* as the Son of God or Jesus. [23]

Allegro writes that equating this sacred mushroom to bread gives an entirely different meaning to statements attributed to Jesus in the book of John. Biblical references to bread (dried mushroom) and flesh (fresh mushroom) and blood (mushroom tea) gives a much different meaning than when taking these references literally.

Some ethnomycologists see the virgin birth as symbolic of the seedless germination of the mushroom. Microscopic spores cannot be seen with the naked eye, so the appearance of mushrooms, apparently from nothing, was considered by ancient people as miraculous. [24] For many ancient people, *Amanita muscaria* was literally "the fruit of the tree." This heretical analysis of the origins of the Christ saga is yet another possible source of energy for the enthusiasm for today's drug laws.

## *A. muscaria* and Biblical Icons

In Medieval Europe, several images of Jesus Christ and other Christian icons appeared with psychedelic mushrooms in many paintings, murals and stained-glass windows in Roman Catholic edifices. Some ethno-mycologists believe Soma may have been the forbidden fruit in the *Bible*'s Garden of Eden. For examples, see the illustrations on the next page.

## Zoroastrian Roots

Many of the beliefs, rituals and holidays of modern day Christianity, Judaism and Islam trace their origins to more ancient re-ligions, including Zoroastrians, and possibly Mithraism. These in turn are based on pagan religions that came before them. Zoroa-strians concept-ualized heaven and hell, the devil, angels, resurrection, the final judgment. The story of Zoroaster has many elements that are similar to the story of Jesus Christ in the *Bible*.

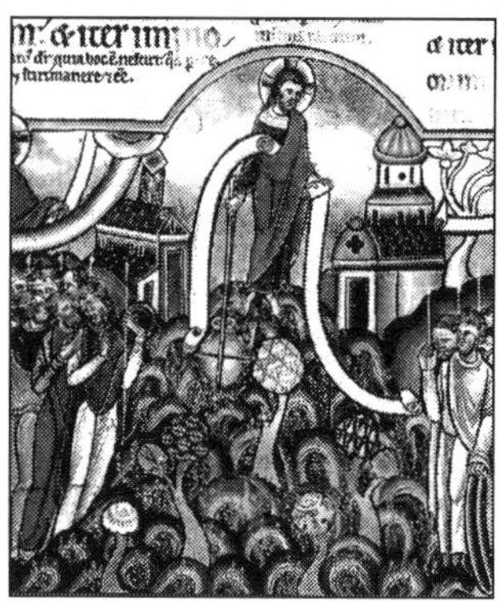

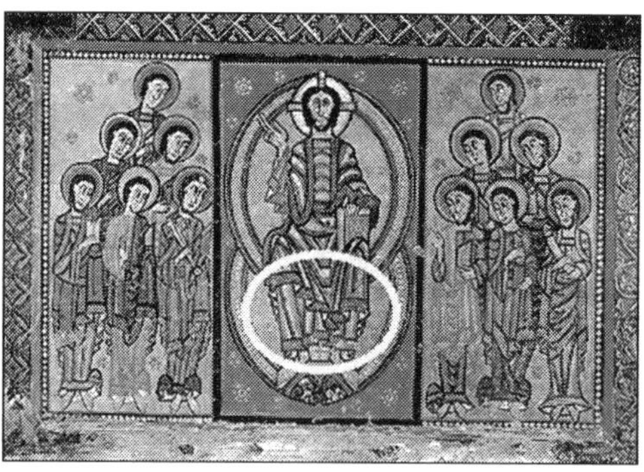

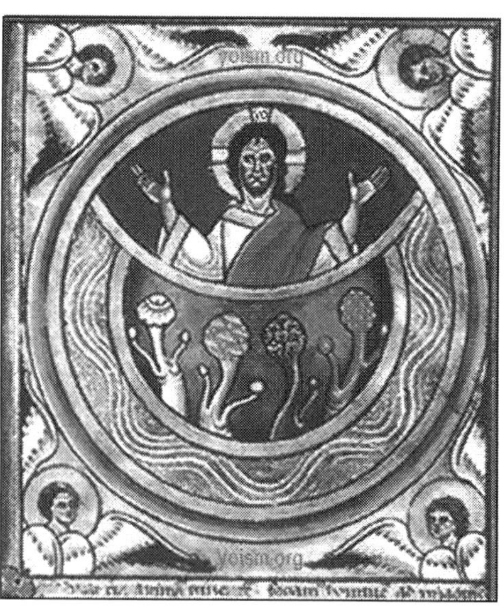

*Left: Jesus on a mountain of psychoactive mushrooms, a panel in the Paris Eadwine Psalter. Made in Canterbury in about 1180, it is a copy of the Utrecht Psalter made at the Benedictine abbey in Germany in the 9th century. Center: This 12th-century mural is now in the Museu Nacional d'Art, Barcelona.* Amanita muscaria *mushrooms are shown in Jesus' pant leggings. Right: An image in a 12th century sbook howing Jesus with several "magic mushrooms."*

Some religious historians see these themes as related to Soma and/or mushrooms. Indian and Iranian pagan religion precursors to Zoroastrian may be the ground from which grew some of Christianity and Judaism's core concepts. The Jews came into close contact with Zoroastrianism after 563 BC when the Babylonians, under King Nebuchadnezzar, took many Jews into exile for over 50 years.

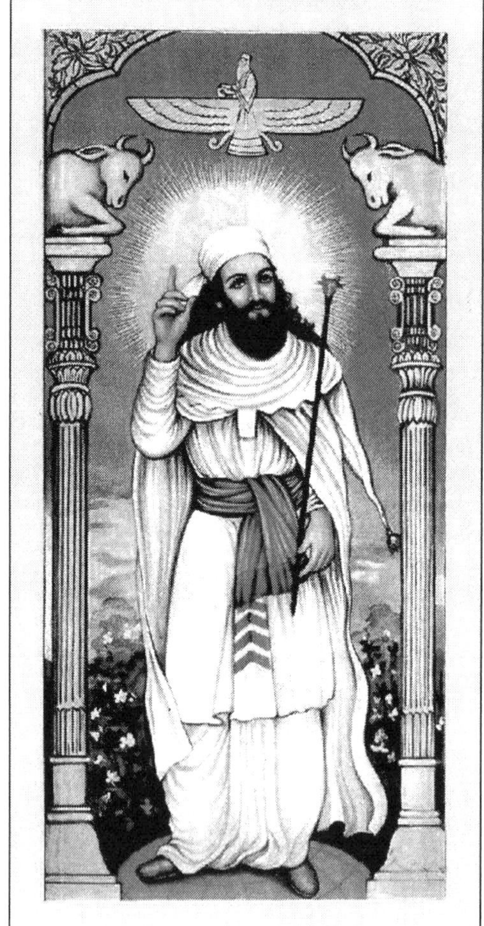

*Zoroastrianism is the first known monotheistic religion. The winged Faravahar above his head in this painting of Zoraster is employed as the modern symbol of the Zoroastrian faith.*

Many changes occurred in the Jewish religion during their Babylonian exile. It was during that period that one god, Jehovah, entered Jewish liturgy. This appears to have been influenced by Zoroastrianism beliefs. Zoroastrians believe in one God that was the creator of all things and the source of all that is good. The Zoroastrians also believe that all mortals are equal before God, differing only in their degree of righteousness, and that each individual is responsible for his or her own fate. Several other Zorastrian concepts influenced the Jews during their forced sixty year stay in Babylon. These Zorastrian concepts included Monotheism, Heaven and Hell, Satan, the Resurrection, the coming of the Messiah, and the Last Judgment. Many of these concepts later reappear in both Christianity and Islam.

Laurence Gardner, author of *Bloodline of the Holy Grail* (1966) and *Realm of the Ring Lords* (2003), has noted that outside Biblical references, "there is no documented reference to the 'one' Jehovah god, as such, before" 600 BC. He writes that:

> "Onwards from c.586 BC, when the Israelites were captive in Babylonia, they began to compile the Old Testament. The new Jewish One God concept (which did not exist before their return to Judah after the captivity) was applied retr-spectively to all their ancestral accounts. In reality, the beliefs of those such as Noah, Abraham, Moses and co. were based on the old notions of the plurality of gods, with the only monotheistic concept being the Aten culture of Amarna (c. 1360 BC). This was ready-made for the Israelite

writers, who converted the word to Adon (Lord) and applied the principle back to the beginning of time."

## Mythic Hero Archetype

The major religions in the Far East – Buddhism, Shintoism, Taoism and Confucianism – as well as Islam, usually consider Jesus to be either a prophet or just another character in Western religious mythology, on a par with Thor, Zeus and Osiris. Most Hindus do not believe in Jesus. Those that do, consider him to be one of the many avatars (an avatar is a human incarnation of an immortal or divine being) of the Hindu god Vishnu. Muslims believe in the historical Jesus but they consider him to be a prophet who announced the coming of Muhammad. They explicitly deny that he was ever crucified. Hayyim ben Yehoshua sums up this diversity of belief regarding Jesus of Nazareth, writing, "there is no story of Jesus which is uniformly accepted worldwide." [25]

Why would those in the Far East conclude that Jesus was a mere prophet? Possibly because there is so much similarity between the life of Jesus, as portrayed in the gospels, compared to the Mythic Hero Archetype. This widespread Hero Archetype mythology predates the birth of Christ by a thousand years. The details have a familiar ring – a divine hero is supernaturally conceived, and his birth supernaturally predicted, as an infant the hero escapes attempts to kill him, even as a child he demonstrates precocious wisdom, receives a divine commission, defeats demons, wins acclaim, is hailed as king, then betrayed, losing popular favor, executed, often on a hilltop, and is vindicated and taken up to heaven.

These archetypical features are not unique and are found in heroic myths and epics world wide. Joseph H. Fussell in "The Significance of Easter, A Masonic Interpretation" (1917), said that, "In very truth, then, the story given in the Gospels of the passion, death, and resurrection of the Nazarene teacher is the same in essentials as that told ages earlier of other saviors: the same teachings, the same rites and sacraments, the same crucifixion of self, the same hope of resurrection, that are celebrated today in Christendom. This formed the core of the wisdom-teachings of antiquity which are among the greatest heirlooms that have come down to us, brought to each race and age by its divine savior who gave his life, not merely for his own people, but for all humanity." [26]

The more closely a supposed biography – say that of Hercules, Appollonius of Tyana, Dionysus, Oden Padma Sambhava, or Gautama Buddha – corresponds to this plot formula, the more likely a historian is to conclude that a historical figure has been transfigured by myth. [27] In many of the stories, a role for the mythical Satan is involved. The concept of Satan also precedes Christianity. The Satan concept traces to the Zoroastrians.

The framework of our social assumptions and ideas is laden with myths and legends, both historic and contemporary. *The Da Vinci Code*, written in the early twenty-first century, created a popular stew of fact and fiction that very likely will become grist for the mill of future cultural "facts." People take these stories, myths, archetypes, facts, fiction and history and uncritically incorporate them into their cultural assumptions.

This is not to state that there is no historical Jesus; numerous historians and other cultures and religions have made that case. It's just likely that stories written about Jesus over 300 years after his birth may include myth or a mixture of fact and fiction.

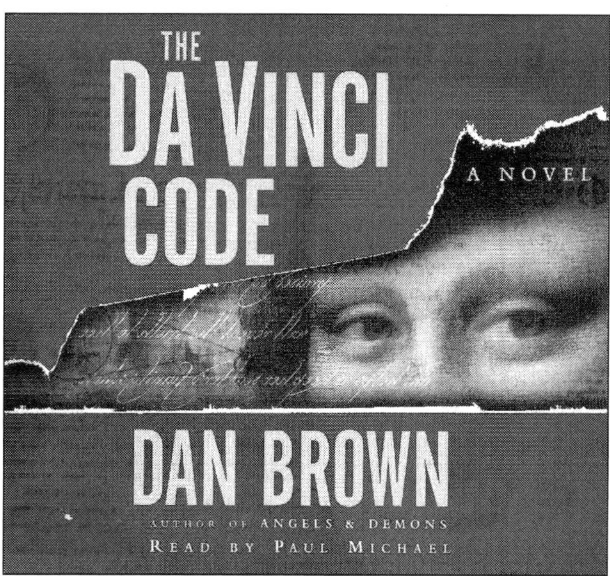


*Dan Brown's 2003 book was called "a gleefully erudite suspense novel" by the* New York Times. *It sold millions and was made into a popular movie starring Tom Hanks. Some people found it hard to accept that it was fiction.*

Biologist Richard Dawkins coined the word "memes" (a unit of cultural transmission) to describe how cultural ideas are transmitted from generation to generation. He makes the analogy that ideas replicate rather like genes do.[28] That seems a little too Lamarckian and contrived to this writer. But the explanation of intellectual vehicles passing on cultural ideas from one generation to the next makes sense. Over time, these factoids or memes become culturally accepted "facts" that aren't questioned, even though, as with *The Da Vinci Code*, some of these so-called facts are fiction.

## Origins of Modern Holidays

Most modern religious holidays have their origins in pagan rituals and commemorations of pre-historic events in the natural world.

### The Winter Solstice and Christmas

Commemorating the winter solstice, long before the mythological birth date of Jesus, humans worshipped the sun as a god. Early humans were terribly aware that their very survival depended upon the return of the sun. In fact, almost all cultures and religions have a festival of lights at or very near the winter solstice. According to religion scholar William Edelen,

> "The Greeks and Romans, barbarians in the Germanic forests, northern worshippers of Thor, and Egyptians, Jews, Persians in the Middle East and Native Americans have all worshipped the sun. It is no wonder that human beings have had celebration of the date of Winter Solstice."[29]

And so it is that the birth of the gods in almost all religious traditions were said to have taken place during the winter solstice. "Major birthdays celebrated on Dec. 25 included those of the gods Marduk, Osiris, Horus, Isis, Mithra, Saturn, Sol, Apollo, Serapis and Huitzilopochtli. In 350, Pope Julius I decreed that the birth of Jesus would be celebrated on the same date as all of the other solstice gods on December 25."[30]

Not at all surprisingly, Christian thought was influenced by the cultural ideas existing in the era of Jesus' life. Christianity incorporates many concepts of the Zoroastrians, a major religion at the time of Christ. Mithra was the Zoroastrian's savior. The myth of Mithra bears an uncanny resemblance to the story of Christ and the Christmas story. Mithra was considered a savior for all of mankind. When Mithra, the Son of Righteousness, was born, a star fell from the sky. Shepherds witnessed the birth and Zoroastrian priests called "Magi" followed the star to worship Mithra. They brought golden crowns to their newborn "king of kings". His birth was celebrated on December 25 and was called the Mithrakana.[31,32]

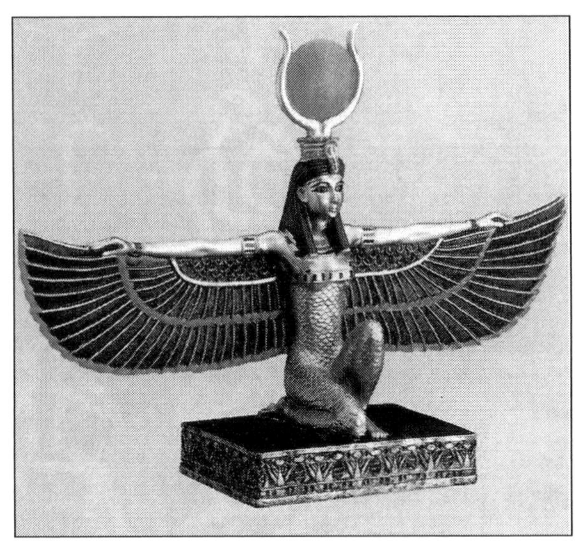

*Isis, the Egyptian goddess of motherhood, magic and fertility, was adopted by the Greeks and Romans. Her birthday was one of many gods and goddesses celebrated on December 25.*

The Romans frequently absorbed concepts and rituals from faiths practiced throughout their expansive empire and incorporated them into their own pagan religious beliefs. The Zoroastrian's Mithra celebration got folded into the Romans' celebration of the sun god, Saturn, and the sun's rebirth during the Winter Solstice. This Roman holiday, starting the week prior to December 25th, was called Saturnalia. Saturnalia was a festive holiday marked by gift giving, singing, and feasting; with plenty of debauchery thrown in. The Roman priests carried wreaths of evergreen in processions through the Roman temples.[33]

Early Christian leaders/propagandists were trying to create a religion that would appeal to both the existing pagan and Jewish populous. These Judeo-Christian proselytizers were part of the culture too, and their culture was the product of those pre-existing pagan ideas. Weaving existing myth and belief into the Christ story was a reasonable, logical way of reaching out beyond their Jewish base. Incorporating the pagans' accepted cultural worldview into this new and evolving religion, ostensibly based on the teachings of Jesus of Nazareth, made it easier for nonbelievers to convert to and/or accept Christianity as their faith.

## Here Comes Santa Claus, Here Comes Santa Claus

Most religious scholars concur that the modern secular Christmas has ancient pagan origins. Christmas owes much to pagan holidays like the Roman Saturnalia honoring Saturnus, the God of Agriculture, and to various Yule festivals, celebrating the return of the sun following the winter solstice. The Saturnalia celebration included drinking, banquets and exchanging of presents. [34] Saturnalia was a wild week-long celebration of feasting, sex, and gambling. Men dressed as women; women dressed as men. It was a raucous time.

The connection between Saturnalia and Jesus' birth was a clerical religious/political decision made in the 4th century to introduce religious elements into the exchanging of gifts and the more carnal festivities that the early Christian laity was already indulging in during winter solstice. According to a Roman almanac, the festival of Christmas was celebrated in Rome as early as 336 AD. [35,36]

The Christianization of pagan holidays started in earnest in the 4th century AD, when the Roman Emperor Constantine became, or some say feigned becoming, a Christian. Cynics see this as a successful effort to consolidate his rule. To attract more pagans, he incorporated the pagan holidays and festivals into the church ritual. The old pagan holidays and festivals just got a little remodeling, with some new "Christian" names and identities. [37] The theme of the existing pagan winter solstice holidays was rebirth – rebirth of the sun, rebirth of the earth. Church officials were comfortable incorporating Christ's birth into this season of feasting, decoration and rebirth. [38]

> "No such festival as Christmas was ever heard of until the THIRD century, and not until the FOURTH century was far advanced did it gain much observance. Long before the fourth century, and long before the Christian era itself, a festival was celebrated among the HEATHEN, at that precise time of the year, in honor of the birth of the son of the Babylonian queen of heaven; and it may fairly be presumed that, in order to conciliate the heathen, and to swell the number of the nominal adherents of Christianity, the same festival was adopted by the Roman Church, giving it only the name of Christ. This tendency on the part of Christians to meet Paganism half-way was very early developed." [39]

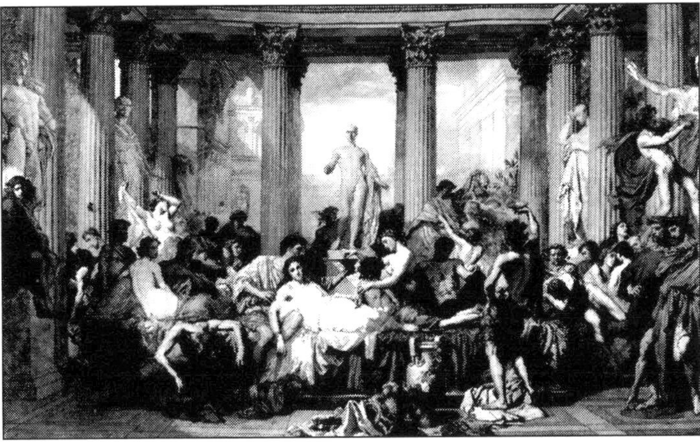

*This painting by the French artist Thomas Couture (1815-1879) portrays the debauchery associated with the celebration of the winter solstice in Ancient Rome.*

## Is Christmas All About a Mushroom?

Ethnobotanists make the case that drugs for recreational and spiritual use were incorporated into these pagan winter solstice time celebrations which predated Christmas. Today, many fundamentalist Christians find the celebration of Christmas with all its non-Christian aspects as very objectionable. They clearly recognize the pagan roots of today's Santa Claus-centered Christmas. They believe the focus should be on a contemporary conservative, Protestant view of the New Testament and the Old Testament. [40]

Ethnobotanists, led by James Arthur, make an intriguing case that Christmas traditions owe a lot to the red and white mushroom, fly agaric (*Amanita muscaria*).

Symbols like presents, Christmas trees, Santa's suit and ho ho ho are all potentially related to *A. muscaria.* Santa's suit is red and white; the colors of *A. muscaria.*

In this view, a Christmas tree with presents under the tree symbolizes both the celestial and spiritual present of *A. muscaria*, which grows mostly under pine trees. [41] Santa comes down the chimney, the same as the mushroom-eating Siberian Shamans entered the Medieval peasants' Siberian yurts. (At that time and place, the yurt door and chimney were the same opening.) Santa's "ho ho ho" is recognized by ethnobotanists as the ecstatic laugh of one who is under the influence of a euphoriant. [42] Even Santa's ruddy complexion can be attributed to consuming the mushroom because it causes the skin to be flushed and glowing.

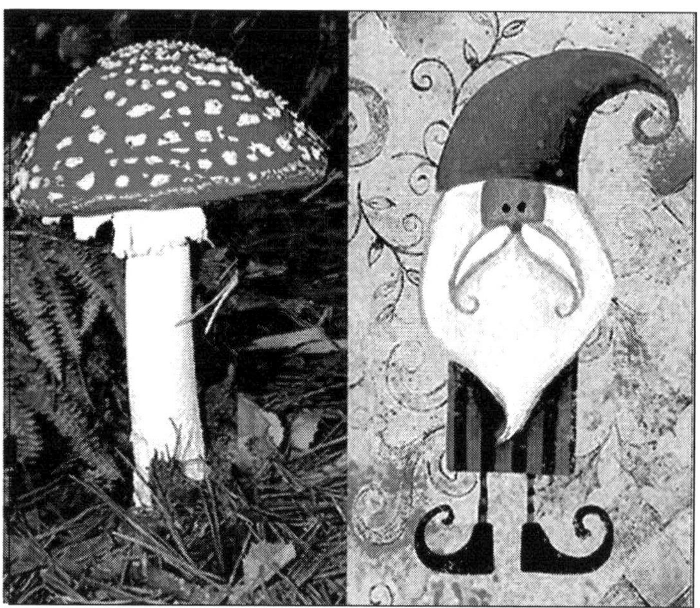

*The similarity of the coloration of the psychoactive mushroom, Amanita muscaria, and the conventional Santa Claus has led many historians to conjecture that they are related.*

R. Gordon Wasson observed that "Reindeer have a passion for mushrooms and specifically fly agaric..." [43] When reindeer eat the red with white flecked mushrooms or drink the urine of humans or other reindeer that have consumed the *A. muscaria* mushroom, they act unusual, at least for reindeer. It's suggested that the story that reindeer pull Santa's sleigh comes from the reindeer's fondness of browsing on these hallucinogenic mushrooms and their behavior after partaking of this hallucinogen. Indeed, reindeer dance, prance, "fly around" and act strange after eating the *A. muscaria* mushroom. [44]

"Reindeer were the sacred animals of these semi-nomadic people, as the reindeer provided food, shelter, clothing and other necessities. Reindeer are also fond of eating the *amanita* mushrooms; they will seek them out, then prance about while under their influence. Often the urine of tripped-out reindeer would be consumed for its psychedelic effects." [45]

Some of the connections attributed to the pagan origins of Christmas are a bit of a logical stretch, others pure supposition, others at least give pause for thought.

Santa's eight reindeer may symbolize the pagan stag god and eight is the number for a new beginning. [46] Thor, the Norse god, rode through the sky in a magic chariot pulled by reindeer. The names of the reindeer mirror reindeer behavior post mushroom eating, and suggest pagan gods and nature. That may just be coincidental, but then again ... Donner and Blitzen, are Dutch for thunder and lightning (actually Donner was changed from Dunder) and Cupid is a messenger of Eros, an ancient pagan god of love. This might reflect the use of the Shamanistic mushroom to enhance the ecstasy of sexual orgasm. [47] Dance and Prance are what reindeer do after eating the mushroom. Comet is a celestial body in flight. Vixen may just be there for poetry or may represent witches' (a vixen) magic. [48]

This line of thinking traces the origin of our contemporary flying Santa Claus and his sleigh to the hallucination of flight caused when humans ingest the colorful red and white topped *A. muscaria* (fly agaric) mushroom. Expositions of this thesis continue that the Santa flying myth relates to the experience of Koryak shamans of Siberia. To the Koryak people, *A. muscaria* was a spirit that they called "wapaq." They believed that these spirits would tell any person who ate them, even a layman, what ailed him if he was sick, explain a dream, foretell the future and/or show the person the upper or lower world. [49]

Taken in small doses, fly agaric is a powerful hallucinogen. Its active ingredients are ibotenic acid and muscimole. In order to be safely consumed, it must be properly prepared. When the mushroom

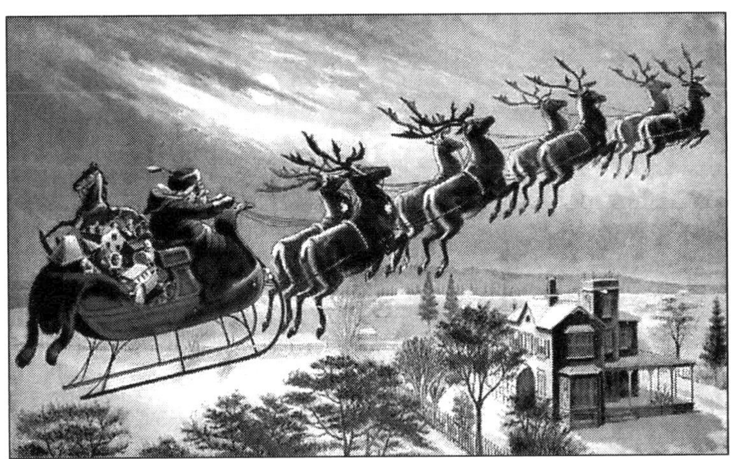

*"On Dasher, On Dancer, Now Prancer and Vixen, On Comet and Cupid. On Donner and Blitzen." Some historians contend that Amanita mushrooms are why we have the mythology of Santa's flying reindeer. These same historians suggest that these mushrooms are why we put pretty presents under pine trees. They say this is because this colorful mushroom can be found growing under pine trees.*

is dried, the ibotenic acid is converted to muscimole, the mushroom's most active entheogenic constituent.[51] Muscimole is said to be ten times more potent than ibotenic acid.

The Koryak shaman knew how to prepare the mushroom to remove its more toxic components. They would bring prepared fly agaric to spiritual ceremonies in a sack, like Santa's bag of toys, and enter the yurt (a portable circular-domed dwelling) through the smoke hole (like a chimney).[52]

These shamans used *Amanita muscaria* to put themselves into an ecstatic trance. During this mushroom-induced trance, the shaman would start to twitch and sweat. His soul was thought to leave his body in the form of an animal, ascend through the smoke hole in the yurt and fly to the spirit world to communicate with the spirits. The shaman would seek the spirits' help for him to deal with pressing problems of the village.

Historian Ronald Hutton said in a *National Public Radio* story that "If you look at the evidence of Siberian shamanism, which I've done, you will find that shamans didn't travel by sleigh, didn't usually

### Argument for the Mushroom & Christmas Connection

• Saint Nicholas is the patron Saint of children in Siberia (Russia). He supplanted the indigenous Shamans who used the Amanita mushroom
• Reindeer eat fly agaric mushrooms and dance and prance. These actions are the basis for their presumed flight
• Santa brings presents in his white bag/ sack.
(a) Mushrooms are gathered in bags and
(b) Amanita muscaria sprouts out of a white oval sack
• The mushrooms are red and white and grow under a green tree.
• Typically, the red and white mushrooms are dried by stringing them on the hearth of the fireplace. Christmas stockings are red and white, hung in the same way, and shaped similar
• The Virgin Birth is symbolic for the "seedless" growth/germination pattern of the mushroom. To the ancient mind, with no microscope to see the spores, it's appearance was said to be miraculous."[50]

**James Arthur**
*Mushrooms and Mankind* (2000)

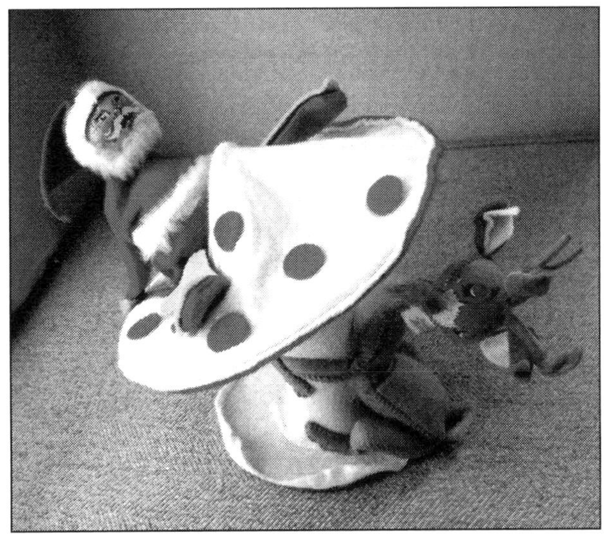

*Those who believe modern Christmas icons are found in the* Amanita muscaria *mushroom equate Santa's ho, ho, ho to the euphoric laughter found in one who has consumed the red and white mystical mushroom.*[53] *Well, "ho, ho, ho" to you, too.*

deal with reindeer spirits, very rarely took the mushrooms to get trances, didn't have red-and-white clothes." But authors Rush and Ruck claim that shamans did deal with reindeer spirits. As for sleighs, the point isn't the exact mode of travel, but that the "trip" involves transportation to a different, celestial realm, Rush said.

"People who knew about shamanism accept this story," Ruck said. "Is there any other reason that Santa lives in the North Pole? It is a tradition that can be traced back to Siberia."

## The Evolution of Christmas

The celebration of Christmas has definitely changed over time. Christmas didn't exist prior to at least the 3rd century and possibly not until 336 AD. In certain historical epochs, many Christians didn't see Christmas as a holiday worthy of celebration. In the 16th century, some English churches even tried to ban Christmas because of its pagan origins and trappings. [54] The Puritans that came to America were from that No-Christmas tradition. Thus, the pilgrims to America weren't into celebrating either the secular or religious Christmas. Since the early New Englanders didn't celebrate Christmas, their major late fall holiday was Thanksgiving.

The modern secular Christmas and yuletide customs and traditions owe more to 19th-century literature than to either Christian liturgy or the pagans' winter solstice celebrations of light that preceded Christmas by thousands of years. Washington Irving (1783-1859) may have introduced Santa to U.S. audiences in 1809 when he first wrote of Sinterklaas, the Dutch version of Santa Claus. [55] Santa Claus appeared in Irving's satirical book *A Knickerbocker's History of New York From the Beginning of the World to the End of the Dutch Dynasty* (1809) by Diedrich Knickerbocker, one of Irving's many pen names. It was Irving's satiric use of the name Knickerbocker that resulted in the term being synonymous with all things Dutch in 18th-century New York.

Irving is best remembered for his famous short stories, *Rip van Winkle* (1819) and *The Legend of Sleepy Hollow* (1820). But Irving was also familiar with the plight of the Native Americans. In the 1830s, he traveled to the Western frontier and wrote of his observation of the western tribes in *A Tour on the Prairies* (1835). He was outspoken about European and American mishandling of the religions of Native American tribes.

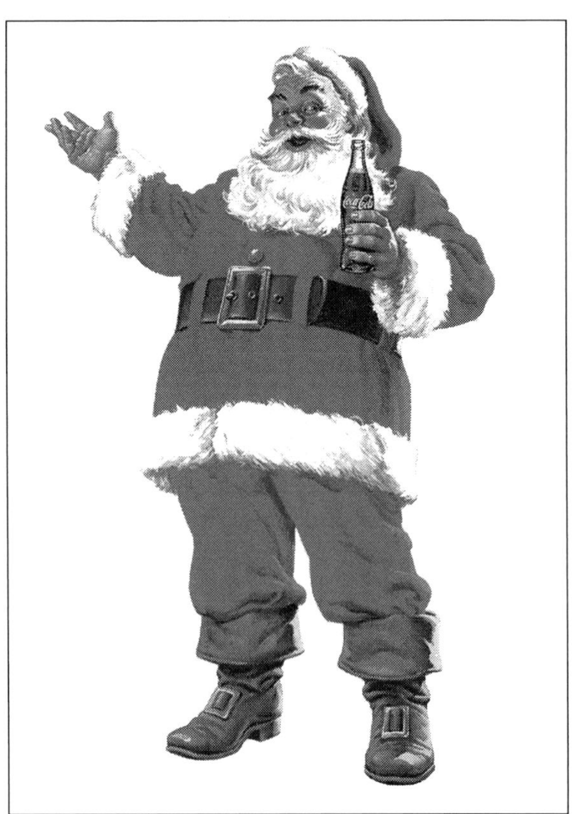

*The final touch to the modern Christmas was the institutionalization of Santa's visage as portrayed in 1930s-era Coca Cola advertising. Previous Santas had sometimes been short or thin and wearing green or brown outfits. Today, thanks to Coke's advertising acumen, it's clear that Santa is the jolly fat man in a red suit.*

> "It has been the lot of the unfortunate aborigines of America, in the early periods of colonization, to be doubly wronged by the white men. They have been dispossessed of their hereditary possessions by mercenary and frequently wanton warfare, and their characters have been traduced by bigoted and interested writers." [56]

Our modern Christmas was more obviously influenced by the poem, *'Twas the Night Before Christmas*, written by Clement Moore in 1823. Historians Rush and Ruck believe that Moore drew his material from northern European themes that derive from Siberian or Arctic shaman motifs and traditions. While the descendants of one Major

## What About Fly Agaric and Drinking Urine (yuk!)

"In Victorian times, travelers returned with intriguing tales of the use of fly agaric by people in Siberia, Lapland, and other areas in the northern latitudes. One of the first such stories was reported by the mycologist Mordecai Cooke, who mentioned the recycling of urine rich in muscimol in his *A Plain and Easy Account of British Fungi* (1862)." [57]

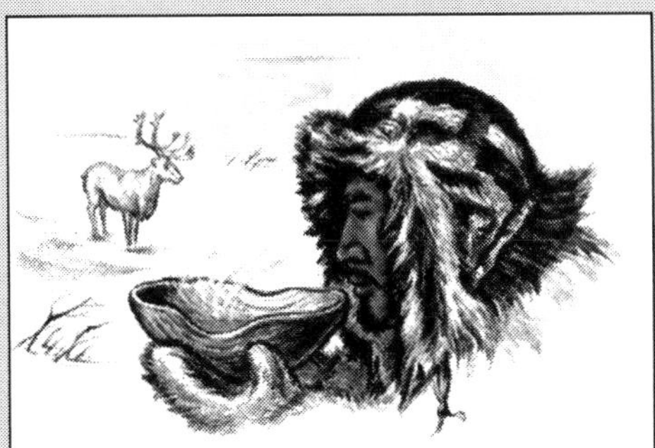

References to fly agaric and flight can be found in books about St. Catherine of Genoa (1447-1510). According to Dr. Daniele Piomelli, formerly of the Unite de Neurobiologie et Pharmacologie de l'Inserm in Paris and later at UC Irvine School of Medicine, St. Catherine used fly agaric to achieve heights of religious ecstasy. One account of St. Catherine's use of ground agaric, describes God as having "infused such suavity and divine sweetness in her heart that both soul and body were so full as to make her unable to stand." [58]

The hallucinogenic chemicals in the *Amanita* mushrooms go through the body without being metabolized, so these substances remain active in the urine. The mushroom's entheogenic ingredients remain unmetabolized even after six passes through the human body. For those so inclined, it is safer to drink the urine of one who has consumed the mushrooms than to eat the mushrooms directly, as many of the toxic compounds are processed and eliminated on the first pass through the body.

It was common practice among ancient people to recycle the potent effects of the mushroom by drinking each other's urine. Some scholars argue that this is the origin of the phrase "to get pissed," since this urine-drinking activity preceded alcohol by thousands of years." [59]

Henry Livingston, Jr. say Livingston wrote it in 1808, this interesting claim has no historical data backing it.[60]

Charles Dickens' novel *A Christmas Carol* (1843) featuring Tiny Tim, Victorian carolers and 19th-century political cartoonist Thomas Nast's drawings of Santa, also heavily influenced the contemporary celebration rituals of what is called Christmas.

Again, Richard Dawkins' term "memes" comes to mind. One doesn't have to study history to make cultural assumptions. They are passed on in many ways — the making of pots or building arches, clothes, fashions, stories, songs, catch phrases, plays, movies, religion, and holidays. It seems pretty clear that this is how the current persona of Santa Claus/Father Christmas developed and most of the rest of the trappings of the modern American Christmas. [61]

## Easter

The pagan festivals heralding springtime existed thousands of years before Christ and the advent of Easter. Annual spring equinox festivals, which celebrated the fertility of plants, animals and humans, were the precursor to Easter. These holiday celebrations usually expressed veneration for the love goddess and/or fertility goddess. This goddess was known under different names in many cultures, including: Eostre, Esthe, Oeistern Ishtar, Ostara, Astarte, Esthler, Istace and Eastra. [62,63] It is from this name, the words Easter and estrus are derived.[64] And rabbits (i.e., the Easter bunny) are the oldest pagan symbol of fertility. [65]

These pagan spring festivals were celebrated until at least 1,000 AD. The celebrations were bacchanalian orgies, complete with fertility rites to the various love goddesses of the pagan sects. And until about 1,000 AD, cannabis was often part of these spring fertility rites and made as an offering to Ostara and the love goddesses Freya and Venus. [66]

Spring equinox celebrations often included the sacrifice and eating of Eostra's sacred rabbits (the origin of modern chocolate bunnies). The pagans usually washed this down with a good hemp beer. But, as Dr. Christian Rätsch says in his book *Marijuana Medicine* (2001), these pagan festivities "fell victim to the Christian liturgy."[67] Contemporary Easter incorporates traditions from ancient spring festivals that occurred in Sumer, Babylon, Egypt, Greece, Europe and both pagan and Christian Rome. [68]

## Eleusinian Mysteries

The celebration of the Eleusinian Mysteries was an important pagan holiday that did not survive to modern times. This was another wild, bacchanal festival. The activities were an initiation rite held in Eleusis, Greece. The festivities celebrated Demeter, the goddess of life, agriculture and fertility (aka, the Earth Goddess), who was said to have taught mankind the art of wheat and barley cultivation, and her daughter, Persephone, the goddess of the underworld.

The Eleusinian Mysteries holiday was based on the Greek myth of Demeter, Persephone and Hades. In this legend, Demeter's only daughter, Persephone, is abducted by Hades, the Lord of the Underworld. Hades grabbed up Persephone while she was picking flowers and playing with her friends amongst the poppies. Suddenly, a deep chasm opened up in the earth, Hades emerged, took Persephone, and they both disappeared into the abyss. This sent Demeter into a depression as she searched for her daughter. During this long search, Demeter found relief from her emotional pain in "taking the Poppy." [69]

This myth explained the origin of the seasons: the death of the plants in the winter and their rebirth in the spring. It celebrated Persephone's return and with it the return of plants and life on earth. This celebration appears to be another honoring of the mystery of the eternally changing seasons.

The celebration of the Eleusinian Mysteries was the most revered and sacred ritual in ancient Greece.[70] These ancient initiatory harvest rites began about 1500 BC [71] and were held every five years for almost two millennia. What the celebration actually consisted of remains a mystery. Participants took an oath of secrecy in the Temple of Demeter. They were quite effective at keeping the mysteries mysterious so there is still only a vague idea of what the festivities entailed. It is known that it occurred in autumn and a sacred drink, kykeon, was consumed in a ritual setting.

This nine-day celebration was held each September. The ritual began with a procession to Eleusis from

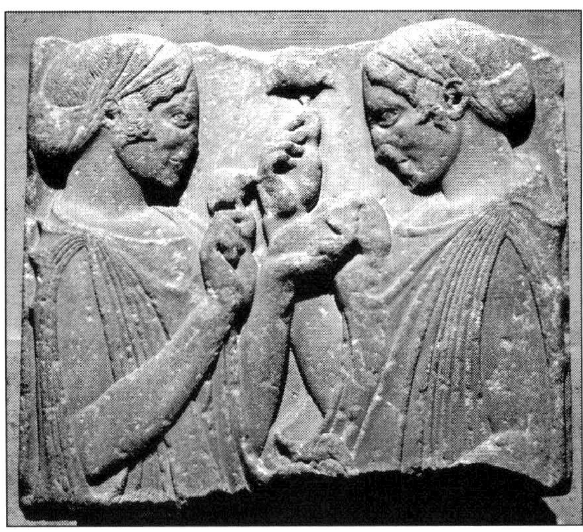

*This stone carving depicts Demeter passing the central sacrament of the Eleusinian mystery to Persephone. The mushroom has a distinctive liberty bell appearance, similar to the Psilocybe semilanceata mushroom.* [72]

Kerameikos (the Athenian cemetery), followed by a day-long fast. The fast was broken the following day by drinking the special drink, kykeon. [73] The initiates entered a great hall called Telesterion. Here the initiates were shown Demeter's sacred relics. This was the most secretive part of the Mysteries. Those who had been initiated were forbidden to ever speak of the events that took place in a great hall called Telesterion. The penalty was death.

Kykeon fueled these orgiastic rituals. [74] What's important for our story is that kykeon was definitely a psychoactive brew of some sort. Consuming kykeon represented either a communion with or the drinking in of the spirit of the deity or an act of religious rembrance. [75] It was likely made with ergot, opium, barley and penny royal. Ergot is a psychotropic fungus that grows on rye and barley. It contains lysergic acid, which can trigger hallucinations. Kykeon probably also contained opium.

Because the Eleusinian Mysteries celebrated fertility, it is speculated that there was a large sexual content to the festivities. [76,77] It has been postulated that the participants believed that by venerating Demeter and being her subject, they would fare better in Hades (the underworld or hell). The use of the opium poppy added bliss to these sacred rites. [78] The poppy, with its prominent, rounded seed pouch, was considered a fertility symbol. Furthermore, in those times opium was often used as an aphrodisiac, which was perfect for the fertility festivities.

These Eleusinian revelries went on for over two thousand years. In 392 AD, the emperor of Rome, Theodosius I, issued a decree that ended the Eleusinian Mysteries. This decree was part of his effort to suppress Hellenistic resistance to the imposition of Christianity as a state religion. The Mysteries' last remnants disappeared in 396, when Alaric, King of the Goths, and the Christians invaded and desecrated the pagan sacred sites, as reported by Eunapius, a historian and biographer of the Greek philosophers in his 4th-century work *Lives of the Sophists*. Still, the Eleusinian Mysteries had an influence on early Christian practices and teaching. [79]

## The Festival of Drunkenness

Celebrations of other ancient civilizations have also slipped into historical oblivion.

### An Egyptian Celebration of Sex, Drugs & Rock 'n' Roll

It seems only reasonable that booze should figure into an Egyptian celebration, what with the Code of Hammurabi (1772 BC) containing the first known drug law, a tax on beer.

Sex as well as booze figured into an ancient Egyptian religious rite. The festival was held during the first month of the year, just after the first flooding of the Nile and re-enacted the myth of Sekhmet. According to the myth, the bloodthirsty Sekhmet, a lion-headed war goddess, nearly destroyed all humans, but the sun god Re tricked her by providing her with ochre-colored beer. Thinking it was blood, she drank very large amounts. Once Sekhmet passed out, she was transformed into a kinder, gentler goddess named Hathor, and humanity was saved. This festival of drunkenness was justified as celebrating the salvation of humanity. [80]

Some archaeologists have dubbed this holiday "The Festival of Drunkenness." Archaeological evidence found in the ruins of a Luxor temple described these annual raucous rituals that included sex, drugs and, would you believe, the ancient Egyptian equivalent of rock 'n' roll.

Betsy Bryan of Johns Hopkins University, the lead archaeologist since 2001 in the Temple of Mut excavation, presented her team's findings in October 2006 at the annual New Horizons in Science Conference. She is quoted by *MSNBC* that, "We are talking about a festival in which people come together in a community to get drunk. Not high, not socially fun, but drunk – knee-walking, absolutely passed-out drunk."

**Figure 3.5: Top Ten Drugs Used in Ancient Rome**

| Drug/Plant | Effect |
|---|---|
| • **Opium** | pain relief, poison, suicide, pleasure. |
| • **Mandragora** or **Mandrake** | delirium, soporific, anesthetic. |
| • **Belladonna** or **Deadly Nightshade** | delirium, sedation, paralysis. |
| • **Henbane** | sedative, hallucinogenic. |
| • **Thorn Apple** | delirium. |
| • **Hemlock** | sedative, narcotic, poison. |
| • **Aconite** | painkiller, slows heart rate. |
| • **Alcohol** | social lubricant |
| • **Mushrooms** | food, poison, spiritual aid. |

*Note: Opium was openly on sale in the shops of Ancient Rome.* [81,82]

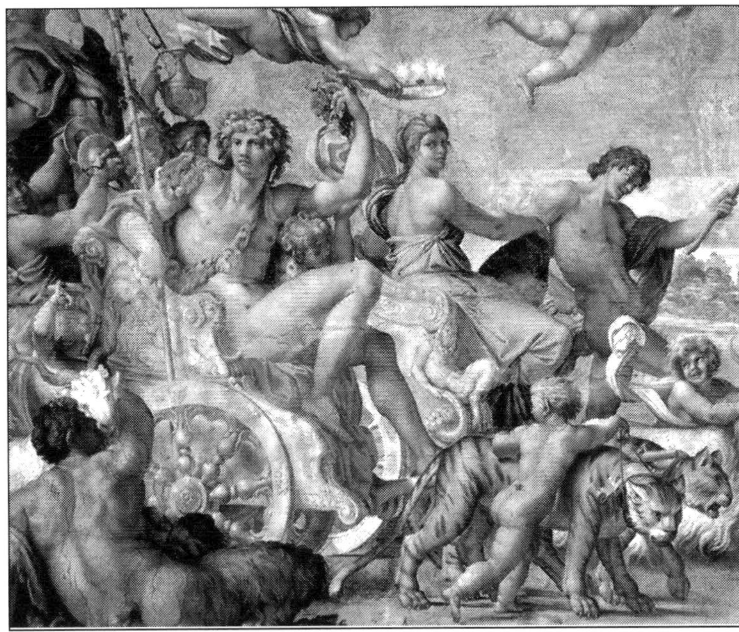

*Here is Bacchus, the Greek and Roman God of Wine and revelry.*

The temple had what's been called a "porch of drunkenness." It was associated with Hatshepsut, the wife and half-sister of Thutmose II. After Thutmose II died in 1479 BC, Hatshepsut ruled New Kingdom Egypt for about 20 years as a female pharaoh. The porch was erected at the height of her reign.

Inscriptions at the temple link the drunkenness festival with "traveling through the marshes," Bryan said this was an ancient Egyptian euphemism for having sex. Graffiti depicting men and women in various suggestive positions worthy of modern-day tut-tutting, reinforce the sexual connection of this celebration.

## Flying Witches

Witches were herbologists. They were aware of both the healing quality of some plants and the ability of plant materials to create spiritual, hallucinogenic visions. Tradition says witches would collect plants at night in the full of the moon. This was done not as part of some obscure ritual, but is based on plant biology. Many plants farmed by witches have their highest active drug content in the evening. [83]

Many modern drugs come from plants or are based on plant molecules. Numerous medicinal plants were known to witches. For instance, Dr. William Withering is credited with discovering foxglove's medicinal benefits. In his 1785 book, *An Account of Foxglove and its Uses*, Withering acknowledged the importance of witchcraft's herbal lore in leading him to the use of foxglove (aka fairy's glove), the natural source of digitalis. The digitalis in foxglove assists the heart function of those with conditions that can cause congestive heart failure.

As Cathy Peterson puts it in *Witchcraft Herbal Lore and Flying Ointments* (1998): "Our society, modern medicine and the multimillion dollar pharmaceutical industry, owe much to the traditions of Witchcraft and the knowledge passed through the centuries by these practitioners of an ancient, persecuted art." [84]

The use of plants to promote a sense of flying, "out of body experience" and the ability to convene with the spiritual world, is a recurrent theme in ancient religious practices. The shamans, priests and priestesses of religions throughout the world, as well

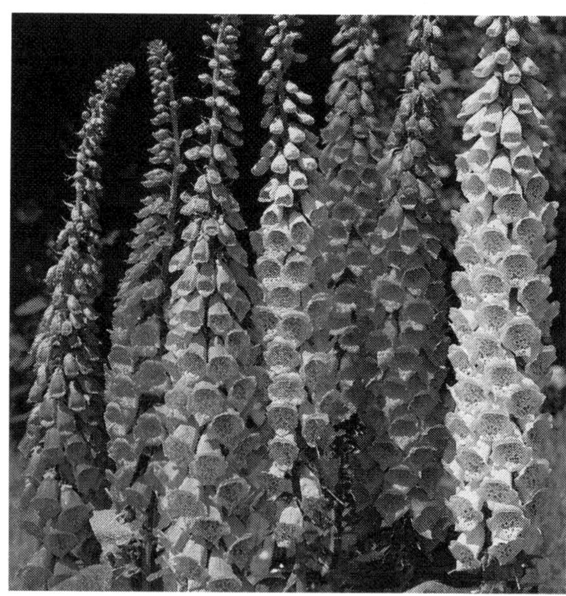

*The group of medicines created from foxglove plants for the treatment of heart conditions was first developed by William Withering in 1785.*

as the witches of the Middle Ages, used specific plants to extend the normal boundaries of human experience, to further a spiritual connection with a force greater than ourselves.

The Datura plants henbane, mandrake, monkshead and belladonna were common ingredients in flying ointments. They are all natural sources of atropine and other atropine-like drugs. McKenna describes the use of Datura "...flying ointments and magical salves were compounded out of Datura roots and seeds, parts of the plant rich in delirium and delusion-producing tropane alkaloids. When this material was applied to the witch's body, it produced states of extraordinary derangement and delusion."[85]

In the right dosage, these plant chemicals can cause hallucinations. In addition to their use from India to Rome for spiritual communion, these alkaloids were commonly used as both poisons and in cosmetics. They can also block parasympathetic functions, our vegetative functions. It should be little surprise that atropine-like drugs, in appropriate therapeutic doses, are found in many modern common cold remedies to decrease runny nose and post nasal drip.

These atropine containing drugs were used in naturalistic (e.g., pagan) religions in Europe to induce hallucinations that were interpreted as spiritual flight.

Witches used hallucinogenic plants to perform rituals linked to the cycle of the seasons. The Church did not approve. Knowledge of Datura was suppressed during the witch burning times by the church. The Church associated Datura and other related, similar atropine containing plants, such as deadly nightshade and monkshood, with the devil.[86]

In addition to the atropine found in Datura plants, it is postulated that opium was an important ingredient in the witches' ointment. It was certainly used in magic and witchcraft in the Middle Ages.

Because midwives were familiar with ergot's hallucinatory effects, ergot may also have gotten in some flying-potion formulas. Powdered calamus root was an ingredient in several of the ancient, psychoactive witches flying ointments. Calamus can have euphoric mind-altering and hallucinogenic effects, depending on the amount taken. It also positively affects the sex drive. [87]

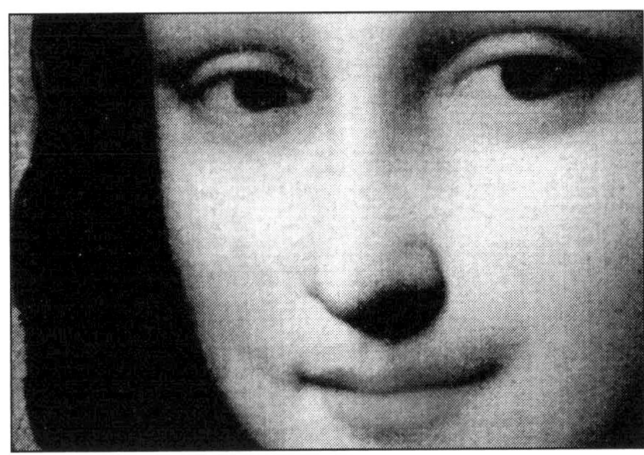

*A weak solution of atropine in the eyes dilates the pupil. In the Middle Ages, large pupils were considered a sign of beauty so, Italian courtesans dissolved* Atropa belladonna *(atropine) in water and placed the fluid in the eye. Belladonna means beautiful woman. Medical historians agree that the wide-eyed Mona Lisa had certainly used belladonna to dilate her pupils.*

## Halloween

Halloween began as an important pagan holiday. It was called Samhain (pronounced sow-een) and means "summer's end". Like most naturalist holidays and celebrations of ancient religions, it was tied to the cycles of the seasons. Samhain was held in late fall in Ireland, England and many parts of Europe. It was a celebration before winter's gloom, a combination of the end of the harvest and a New Year's festival. The harvest signaled the end of the growing season, the end of one year, the beginning of the next. It was celebrated from sunset October 31st to sunset November 1st.

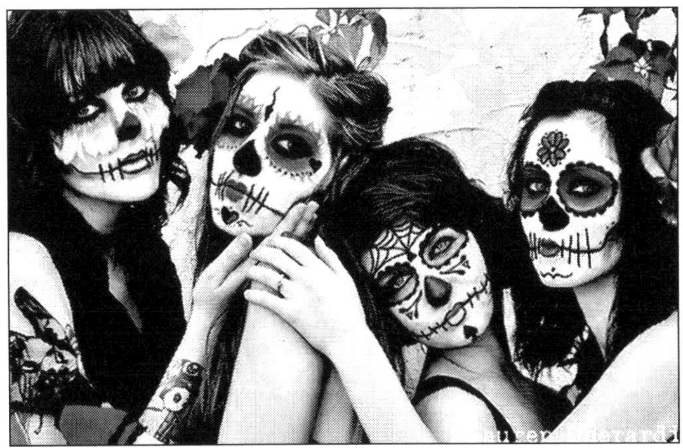

*Halloween was also a special time when the dead could return and their spirits walk the earth. In this way it bears a similarity to Dia de los Muertos, the Mexican "Day of the Dead" in which death masks play an important role. It celebrates the unity between life and death and accepts death as part of the life cycle.*

The Church worked hard over several hundred years to eradicate this popular pagan holiday, but finally settled on co-opting it. In the 7th century, Pope Boniface IV designated November 1 as All Saint's Day, a day to honor saints and martyrs. Then in 1,000 AD, the church made November 2nd All Souls' Day, a day to remember the departed and to pray for their souls. Even still, people continued to celebrate Samhain. The three celebrations (All Saints' Eve, All Saints' Day and All Souls' Day) taken together were called Hallowmas and people costumed as angels and devils, celebrating with bonfires and parades. The night before November 1st, came to be called All Hallows Evening, which was eventually shortened to Halloween. [88]

### Witches, Broomsticks and Halloween

Witches and broomsticks are icons of Halloween. Most ethnohistorians believe that riding broomsticks became associated with witches because sticks and/ or other phallic-shaped objects were used to apply hallucinogenic ointments and salves upon the vagina's very absorbent mucosa. [89,90,91] Topical mucosal application of the "flying" ointment is both a faster and safer route of administration for these emoluments than oral ingestion. But these witches' brews were also absorbed orally.

Writers from the Middle Ages documented this association of witches and broomsticks. A 1324 witchcraft investigation mentioned in Michael J. Harner's article, "The Role of Hallucinogenic Plants in European Witchcraft" in the book he edited, *Hallucinogens and Shamanism* (1973), supports this contention of applying the hallucinogenic "flying" ointments with a staff to the vaginal mucosa. "In rifleing the closet of the ladie, they found a Pipe of ointment, wherewith she greased a staffe, upon which she ambled and galloped through thick and thin."[92] And we find in a 1470 reference: "But the vulgar believe, and the witches confess, that on certain days or nights they anoint a staff and ride on it to the appointed place or anoint themselves under the arms and in other hairy places." [93]

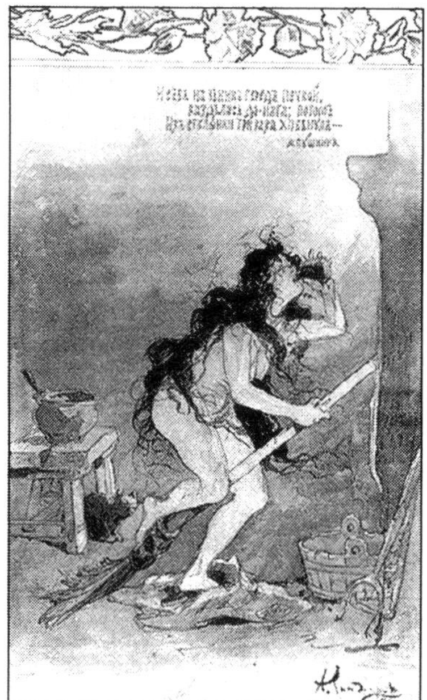

*Witches' flying ointments were made from plants high in the tropane alkaloids; atropine, scopolamine, hyoscyamine, and hyoscine, plus a dollop of animal fat. The fat was employed to provide an oily base for the crushed plants, enable its application on the skin and mucous membranes, and as a medium to prevent the rapid evaporation of the volatile plant alkaloids.*

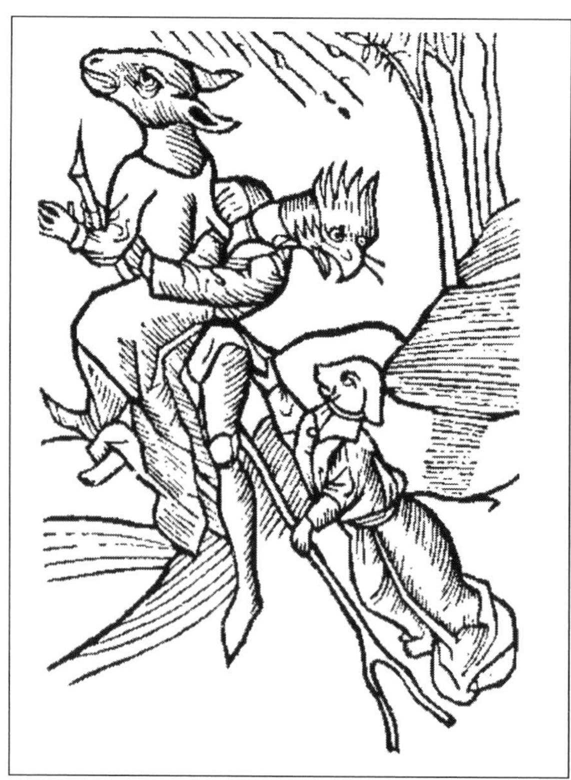

*The earliest image of a witch flying on a broomstick dates to 1440 in Martin LeFranc's manuscript,* Le Champion de Dames. *Ulrich Molitor's,* "Of Witches and Diviner Women" *in 1489, has the first printed picture of witches – three half-human/half-animal characters, each riding a broom.* [94]

The first stage of seduction into witchcraft was related to a woman's state of mind. Someone who was in a receptive psychological state would be a target for the devil. Examples of a "receptive state of mind" are someone feeling: anger against someone else, despair caused by poverty or hunger or, anxiety over being called a witch. Persons in those states of mind were popularly believed to be easy targets for the Devil to seduce.

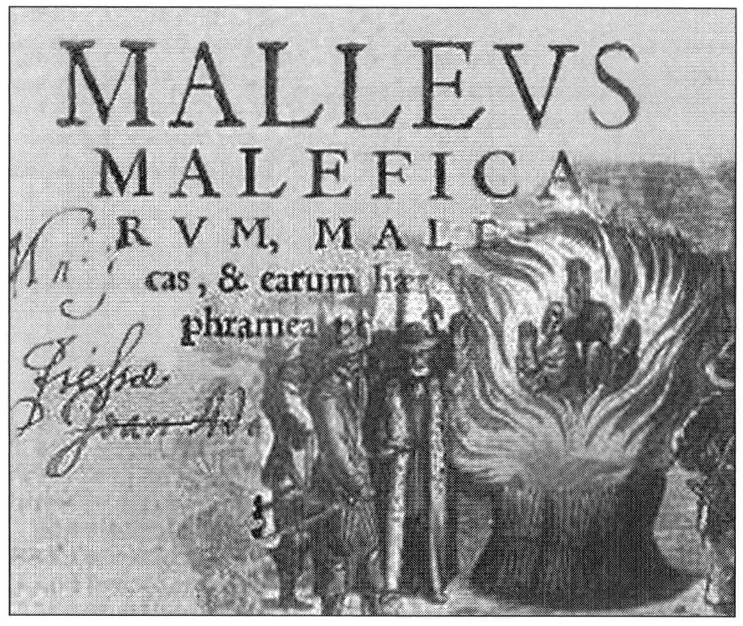


*In 1484, the Germans Heinrich Kramer and Jakob Sprenger requested a papal bull, or Hammer of the Witches, which codified the Catholic Church's teachings on witches. They published this in 1487 as* Malleus Maleficarum. *This is the cover of an early edition of this handbook, which was widely distributed throughout Europe and used to prosecute witches during the late Middle Ages.*

# CHAPTER IV
# 1300-1700: Bring on the Witches

## The Inscrutabilities of Changing Times Need a Scapegoat

What do witches and their potions have to do with today's drug laws? The witch hunts of the middle ages demonstrate how an anti-science, illogical, hysterical approach can occur in an environment of change and fear. Casting blame on scapegoats seems to occur more frequently in times of change. The demonization of some men and women as witches is analogous to drugs being demonized. With demons, witches or drugs, there is a simplistic way to detect who is evil and place the blame, whether warranted or not, on things and events happening in human experience that are not readily understood and over which humans have little or no control.

The witch hunts of the Middle Ages demonstrate the length to which humans will go in hurting other humans in the name of "all that is right and good." The witch hunts represent a historical antecedent, a veritable training manual for an inappropriate, ineffective, wrong-headed, over-the-top, hysterical, and morally dubious (at best) response to a problem perceived demonic. This hysterical mindset then creates its own set of problems. A powerful tactic of the witch hunts was equating an opponent's behavior to demonic activity. Demonic characterization apparently gives a culture permission to take drastic, draconian action.

Over the past 30 years, the motivation for the medieval witch-hunting era has been distorted and relative blame misplaced. Conventional wisdom points to the Roman Catholic Church and/or misogyny as motivation for the witch hunts. In some sense these causes are accurate, but closer scrutiny of the historical record reveals that this is an oversimplification and many historians have largely discounted these as the major influences.

### Satan and the Zoroastrians

The Roman Catholic Church did make a strong effort to snuff out the naturalistic beliefs of pagan religions. Witches were healers. They knew of the therapeutic value of many plants. The Church viewed using plants to heal as being in conflict with the purview of priests who used faith to heal. The Church associated certain plants and animals with pagan religions and labeled them satanic. This represents an early association of the "devil" with anti-drug propaganda.

In fact, the pagans were worshippers of nature not the devil. Pagans often had many gods and goddesses but the devil or Satan was not among them. The concept of Satan, the ultimate demon, sprang from the Zoroastrians, a Persian religion whose origin is traced to the prophet Zoroaster (Greek for the Iranian Zarathustra). Zarathustra is thought to have lived between 1500 and 1000 BCE in northeastern Iran. Zarathustra/Zoroaster's teachings are found in the *Avesta*, the sacred text of Zoroastrianism. Zoroaster saw humanity confronted by a choice between good (god), represented by Ahura Mazda (what we may call God), and evil (devil). What we refer to as the devil and other false gods or daevas, Zoroaster called Angra Mainyu.

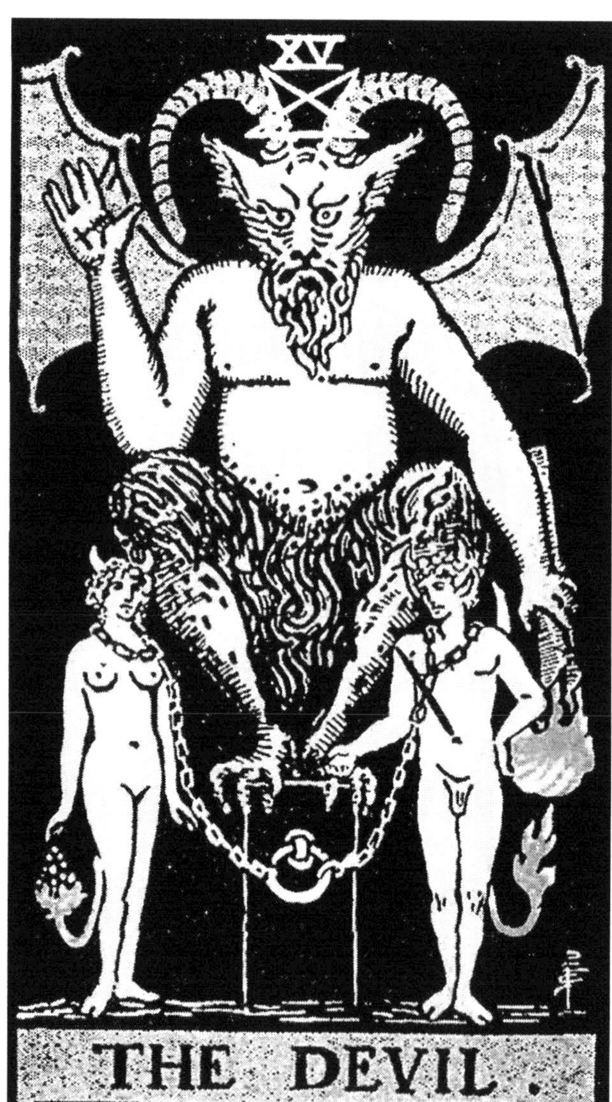

*A fairly typical depiction of the devil and his relationship to sex and lust.*

In some ways Zoroastrianism was a bridge between ancient multi-god pagan religions and monotheism. Zoroastrianism retained the pre-Zoroastrian gods and divinities but they were under the uncreated Creator, Ahura Mazda (or Mazda Ahura), the Wise God.

Zoroastrianism and Vedic Hinduism both sprung from a common background, the ancient Indo-Iranian religious culture. [1,2,3] Zoroastrianism also inherited ideas from other belief systems and, like other practiced religions, accommodates some degree of syncretism (i.e., the attempt to combine or reconcile different beliefs). Both Judaism and Christianity owe much to the Zoroastrians in terms of their core beliefs.

The *Avesta*, the Zoroastrian bible, has an insistence on the presence of God in human lives and saw human history as a grandly devised plan. The combat between good (god) and evil (the devil) comes from Zoroastrianism. The Zoroastrians not only invented the concept of Heaven, Hell and the devil but also the concept of a messiah as a universal savior, being inscribed in the concepts of the Resurrection and the last Judgment.[4] The abstract concepts of heaven, hell, personal and final judgment were developed in the period of the Achaemenid Empire (550-330 BCE).

Extended contact between exiled Jews and Zoroastrians occurred for fifty years in that era. In 563 BCE, thousands of Jews were taken into exile by the Babylonians. By the necessity of exile, some things had to change in the Jewish ritual. There being no access to the temple in Jerusalem, the Jews moved away from reliance on animal sacrifice, which had traditionally taken place at that temple. In addition, Zoroastrian concepts made their way into Jewish thought. Some of what these Jews learned from the Zoroastrians in their 50 years in exile was incorporated into the Old Testament.

The devil concept was adopted by apocalyptic Jews, who incorporated it into the classic conflict between good and evil. Still later the concept of Satan was embraced and embellished by Christianity. The

Christians were in conflict with the pagans for the hearts and souls of the populace. The Christians perceived the pagans' efforts to collectively preserve their own naturalistic spirituality as "doing the devil's work" by thwarting the spread of Christianity. Once a belief system is developed, it will uphold all kinds of rationale to defend favored religious concepts.

## The Church's Preoccupation with Sex = Satan

The Middle Ages were not happy times. They were filled with depression, fear, despair and oppression. For 1,000 years, from 500-1500 AD, daily life for the peasantry was miserable. In addition to minimal shelter, lack of sanitation and omnipresent disease, the Church removed all the joy from sex.

The Church of medieval time had strict and foreboding sexual codes. Their premise was that the act of sexual intercourse was to be performed as seldom as possible and forget about love in marriage. To love, or even desire, one's lawful marriage partner was considered sinful. Intercourse was to be done sparingly, then only for procreation and shouldn't be enjoyed. The Church saw only desire, not love.

G. Rattray Taylor, in *Sex in History* (1954), summarized the strict system of Church morality. "The Church was obsessed with sex. Every imaginable misdeed and every conceivable sin is discussed and analyzed at great length and appropriate penalties are set forth for each sexual misstep."[5]

Kurt Seligman in *The History of Magic* (1948) gave this analysis:

> "... the ancient survivals, the amusements of serfs, the most innocent stories, were henceforth Satanic, and the women who know about the old legends and magic traditions were transformed into witches. . . the traditional gatherings, the Druid's Festival on the eve of May Day, the Bacchanals, the Diana feasts, because the witches' Sabbath . . .the broom, symbol of the sacred hearth . .. became an evil too. The sexual rites of old, destined to simulate the fertility of nature, were now the manifestations of a forbidden carnal lust. Mating at random, a survival of communal customs . . .now [were] an infringement of the most sacred laws.[6]

This extreme sexual asceticism was not preached by Christ. The Church's medieval sex code is not supported by either the Old or New Testaments.

Sex has also become part of the mix of demonizing people who use drugs. Throughout history, an association between drug use and sex has been seen as being a tool of the devil. This theme has been played out over and over. Be it alcohol, opiates, cocaine or marijuana, each has supposedly lead good girls to go bad and somehow causes "our" women to love sex with "them".

Many scholars point to the Church itself and its extreme, intrusive doctrines and dogmas as causing a rebirth of paganism. The extreme regulation and repression of the private lives of common folk allowed for the seeds of the old pagan practice to once again take root and flourish. The Church's obsession with sex and equating it with sin and their attempt to eradicate this sin, inadvertently created fertile ground for the rebirth of the dormant Old Religion. The stories of the old pagan ways, and customs, with their emphasis on fertility and community sex rites became appealing to the common folks.

SENSATION! . . .
ALWAYS ENTERTAINING, ALWAYS Revealing!
"DEVIL'S HARVEST"
MARIJUANA
THE SMOKE OF HELL!
A FIFTH COLUMN SOWING DESTRUCTION IN THE YOUTH OF AMERICA....

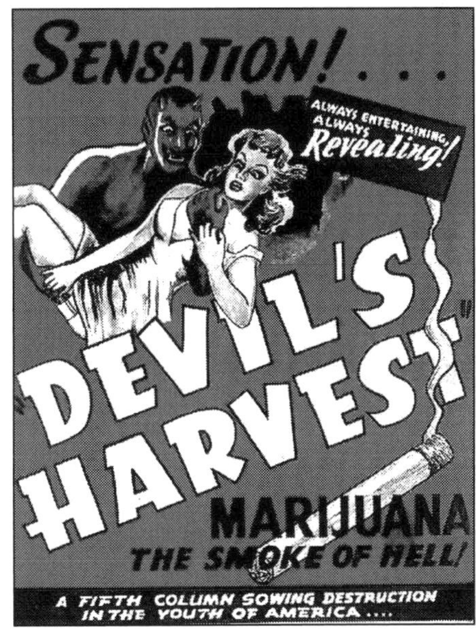

*Marijuana as a tool of the devil was a common theme in 1930's anti-marijuana propaganda. The more familiar term, cannabis, was almost never used in these negative campaigns.*

There was basically a way between Christianity and paganism. The Medieval Church characterized paganism as demonic witchcraft that worshipped Satan and sought to destroy Christendom. "The

Church saw the nature-worshipping rituals of the common people as a threat to its authority and condemned these men and women as being practitioners of an organized satanic religion. This demonic pagan religion never existed. The only historical problem is that this was a propaganda move on the part of the Church to marginalize paganism of the Dark Ages." [7]

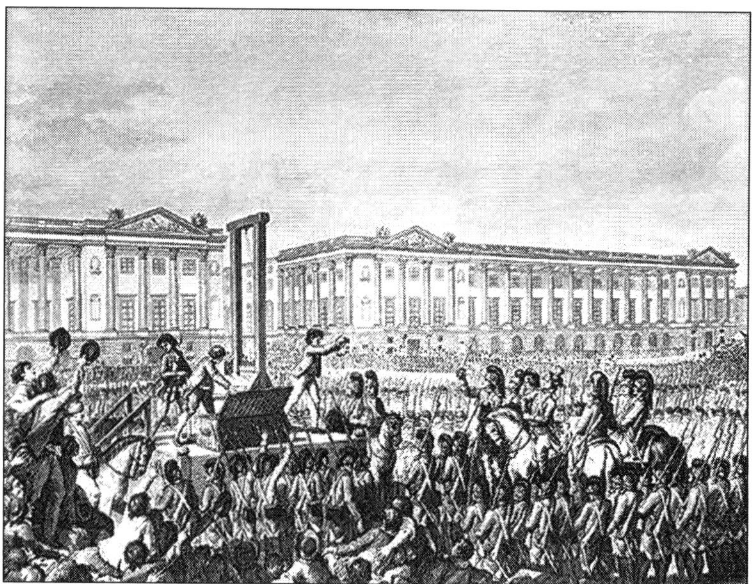

*A long cold spell in France led to a shortage of bread and the execution by guillotine of Marie Antoinette in 1793.*

## The Devil Made Them Do It

By the 9th century AD, the Roman Catholic Church had consolidated its power over much of Europe and the pagans residing there. This control is credited with bringing scientific development and social enlightenment to a grinding halt.

However, the so-called Dark Ages were not all that "dark". While later voices worked at painting the previous period as darker than it actually was, the prime era of witch burning was from 1450 to 1750 — the height of the Renaissance and the early years of the so-called "Age of Enlightenment."

## The Little Ice Age

### Global Cooling Was as Bad as Global Warming

Several phenomena came together in the late Middle Ages and the Renaissance era that supported the institution of witch hunting. This was a time when religious boundaries were becoming blurred and private beliefs and practices were being scrutinized with increasing consternation. Much of these phenomena occurred during the "Little Ice Age," a climatological phenomenon that lasted from the 13th century to the early 19th century.

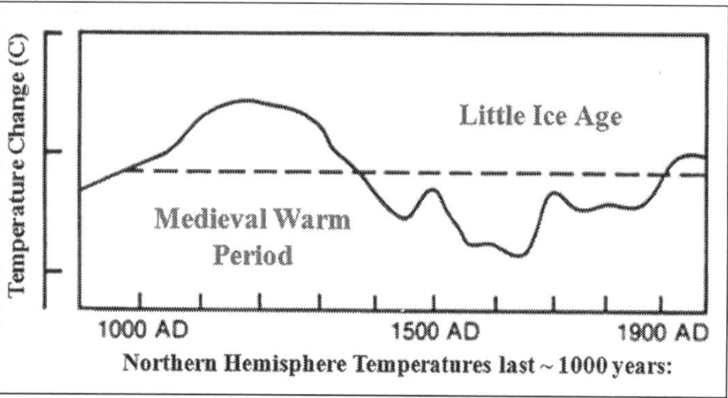


While it represented only an average decrease of one degree in temperature, this change caused substantial social and economic dislocations. [8] It had a profound, adverse effect on normal life. [9,10,11] It contributed to poor crops, which led to weakened human resistance to the Black Plague and the increased need or willingness to use ergot-tainted grain to make bread.

The fallout of this climatic change created economic and cultural stress that led to substantial social unrest. [12] One illustration of this social unrest occurred in 1740. A particularly bad winter was followed by a very short spring and a damp, cool summer, which spoiled the annual wheat harvest. There was literally no bread to eat. The poor rebelled in many parts of Europe. The governor of Liege, in what is now Belgium, told the rich to "fire into the middle of them. That's the only way to disperse this riffraff, who want nothing but bread and loot." [13]

Some historians attribute French Queen Marie Antoinette's infamous "Let them eat cake" remark to incredibly bad weather combinations in France leading to several famines during the reign of her husband, Louis XVI. A cool winter was often followed by drought and heat, which made for adverse agricultural conditions. These weather conditions were bad enough for growing grain, but things often got worse. When the grain finally came in, what remained of the crop was decimated by hail. This left a limited supply of wheat for the harvest, creating a great scarcity of bread. This crop failure was a major contributor to the rebellion that led to the overthrow of the monarchy, the hanging of the king in 1792 and the beheading of his queen in 1793.

## The Black Plague

The temperature change during the Little Ice Age contributed to the high incidence of the bubonic plague in the Middle Ages. Starting in the 14th century, the bubonic plague — the Black Plague — was killing people like flies. It first appeared in 1313 and ravaged Europe until 1375, during which it killed fully one-third of the population. But the lengthy period of poor weather devastated food production, causing starvation and weakening of the human immune system. Thus, there continued to be outbreaks of the plague over the next 300 years.

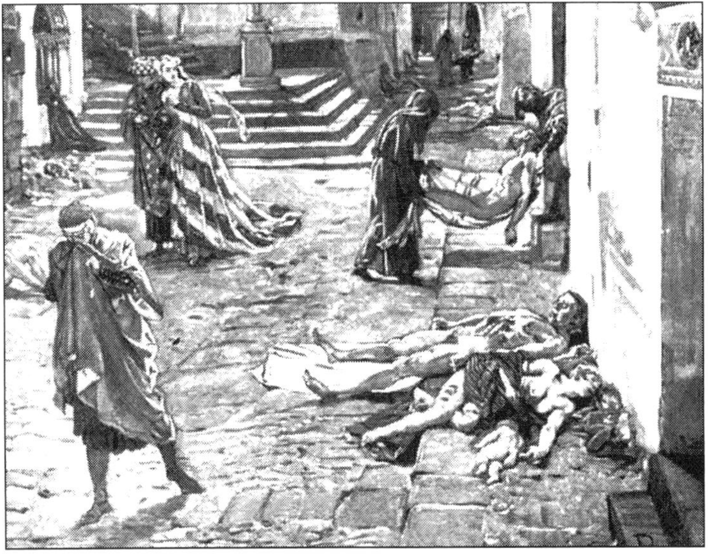

*Imagine a third of the population dying within a few months. The dead and dying, previously vibrant and healthy, were now oozing pus from large infected lymph nodes. This scene and hard fact had a profound impact on the psyches of the survivors. Clearly, many thought, this terrible carnage is the work of the devil and his minions.*

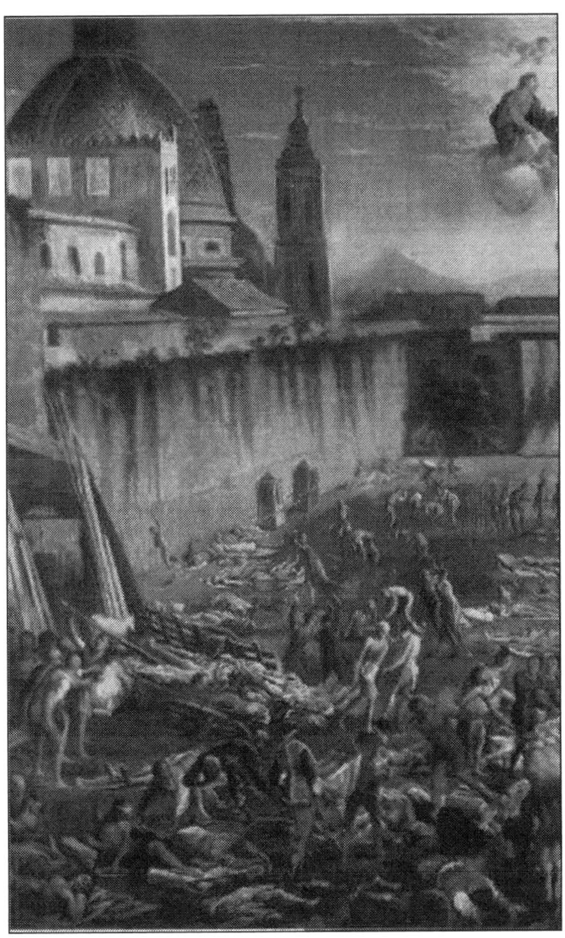

*Many painters were motivated by the specter of the Black Plague to paint ghastly landscapes. The times must have been frightening. Knowledge about what caused diseases was still primitive. For the average person, witches were as good an explanation as any for calamities.*

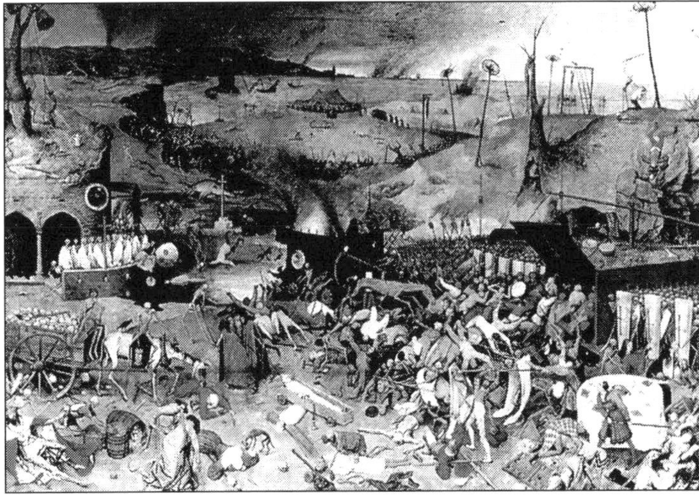

*The "dance of death" was a pervasive theme in medieval iconography. This painting, entitled "The Triumph of Death", is by Pieter Bruegel the Elder (1525-69). It depicts marching skeletons over a land devoid of life.*

This deadly disease was caused by rats that carried the organism causing this painful and deadly condition. Bubonic plague is marked by large, black painful pus-filled masses called buboes often found in the groin or arm pits. These buboes were actually enormously swollen lymph nodes. These inflamed lymph nodes were most painful and could break through the skin and become an oozing, superative mass. Death commonly occurred in three days.

Giovanni Boccaccio, a Florentine writer writing in 1351, provides a vivid description of the plague's symptoms. They included black spots and discoloration over the entire body:

> "In men and women alike it first betrayed itself by the emergence of certain tumors in the groin or the armpits, some of which grew as large as a common apple, others as an egg, some more, some less, which the common folk called gavoccioli." [14]

With these kinds of symptoms, it's no wonder the populace was desperate to find out the cause, to try and prevent and/or cure the Black Plague.

## Ergot Poisoning

The cooler climate of the Little Ice Age both decreased the amount of the grain harvest and promoted fungal growth or ergot. Ergot is a fungus that affects rye, barley and other grains. Grain stored under cool, damp conditions can develop a fungus known as ergot blight. The ergot alkaloids vary in kind and amount depending on the climate and location where the grain is grown.

Because of their vasoconstrictor properties, ergot alkaloids were used by midwives of the Middle Ages to stem postpartum bleeding. The midwives were wise to using the proper dosage to avoid the potentially dangerous side effects associated with ergot poisoning.

This ergot fungus also contains chemicals very similar to lysergic acid diethylamide (LSD), the psychedelic drug. When these psychotropic fungi were unknowingly consumed, such as by eating bread tainted with the ergot fungus, it caused wild and unsettling hallucinations.

The cool, wet summers of the Little Ice Age contributed to numerous outbreaks of ergot poisoning throughout Europe. In those times, small villages were often served by one or two bakeries. Eating bread accidentally, or in some cases

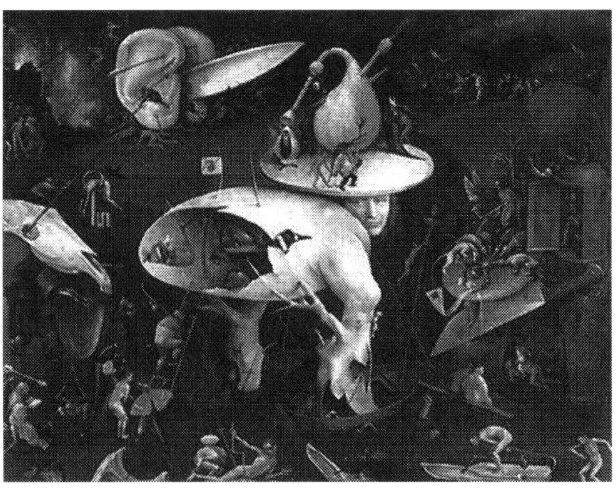

*This is a detail from a triptych of "The Garden of Earthly Delights" by Flemish artist Hieronymus Bosch (1475-1516). It depicts the social cacophony of the late Middle Ages. The odd vegetable creature is painted in the shape of a mandrake root. Mandrake was the herb used to stanch the feverish pains of St. Anthony's Fire. The egg-shaped building is exactly the shape of an apothecary's retort – the distillery used to condense medicinal herbs. The meaning of his emotional paintings is a metaphor of the medical knowledge of his day.*

purposely, made with ergot-afflicted rye (due to shortage of grain caused by the cooler weather), could cause ergot poisoning throughout a small community. This caused many who ate the bread to have hallucinations with no idea of the source of these visions.

Not only could those afflicted with ergot poisoning suffer troubling hallucinations, but because ergot is a vasoconstrictor (temporarily decreases the diameter of blood vessels). This decreased blood flow and lack of oxygen to tissue can cause fiery pain. Ergot poisoning can also cause extreme muscle spasms, which can result in uncontrollable movements called St. Vitus's Dance. In some cases, blood flow was so compromised for so long that the prolonged lack of oxygen caused arms and legs to become gangrenous. The gangrene could require amputations, and even cause death. These were all symptoms of what was called "St. Anthony's Fire". St. Anthony was appealed to because he had allegedly vanquished the devil so it was felt this was something he could handle.

## Someone or Something Must be Responsible: Witches

The denizens of the Middle Ages were faced with several concurrent negative phenomena: enormous

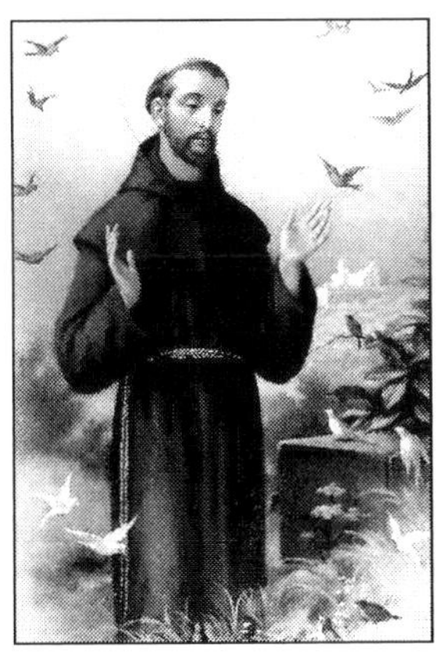

*Ergotism results from ingesting the toxic grain fungus, ergot. St. Anthony was the patron saint of persons afflicted with "St. Anthony's Fire" (ergotism).* [15] *Because of his presumed powers (he had vanquished the devil), victims of ergotism prayed to him for protection.* [16]

weather changes, rapidly spreading illnesses among previously healthy people, the stress of starvation, and inexplicable hallucinations – none of which had "rational" explanations. These forces had enormous psychological consequences, including great pessimism, fear, gross sensuality, flagellantism, divisiveness, and religious fervor. [17]

There needed to be an explanation. Ignorance and fear provided motivation to find someone or some force to blame. Many blamed the Jews. Thousands of Jews were murdered in medieval times for their presumed role in causing the Black Plague. [18] Ah, but weather-making was an ability traditionally ascribed to witches, so much of the blame was laid on the devil and his cohorts — the women accused of being witches.

So in the late 14th and 15th centuries, it came to pass that many inhabitants of what is now Europe believed the poor weather was caused by a great witch conspiracy. Extensive witch hunts took place during the most severe years of the Little Ice Age, as people looked for scapegoats to blame for their suffering. [19]

During the midst of a seven-year drought in 15th-century England, a large conclave composed of the landed gentry, clergy and the nobility met to decide what to do about the declining food supply. [20] Should they irrigate; should they ration food? They concluded that a plague should be called down upon the poor. Their prayers were answered. The plague being what it is, within a year more than one-third of the attendees were dead from the plague. [21]

The search for scapegoats to explain these disturbing social changes and inexplicable and equally disturbing weather, health and perceptual distortion phenomena was an important factor leading to the rise in accusations of sorcery. Because of torture and other tactics, these accusations inevitably led to persecution and prosecution. To be accused of being a witch became a self-fulfilling prophecy that a person was a witch.

## The Witch Hunts

In 1484, Pope Innocent VIII issued his infamous Witches' Bull, [22] a proclamation that condemned witchcraft and ordered the punishment of witches. His Bull declared the absolute reality of witches. After this papal pronouncement, it became a heresy to even doubt the existence of witches. This Bull became the law for all of Europe and was the legal basis for the Inquisition and to punish and/or exterminate witches.

---

**"Science is an attempt, largely successful, to understand the world, to get a grip on things, to get hold of ourselves, to steer a safe course. Microbiology and meteorology now explain what only a few centuries ago was considered sufficient cause to burn women to death."** [23]

**Carl Sagan**

astronomer, philosopher, author, 1934-1996

---

The papal condemnation of witchcraft explicitly cited cannabis as an "anti-sacrament" used in non-Catholic worship. At the time, any non-sanctioned religious ceremonies were by definition considered satanic masses. This condemnation also helped taint cannabis' reputation.

## Malleus Maleficarum: Nasty Stuff

To ensure that his bull was properly implemented, the Pope appointed two German Dominican monks as inquisitors, Jakob Sprenger and Heinrich Kramer. Three years later, these two monks published a legal commentary on the Bull, the *Malleus Maleficarum* (or *Hammer of the Witches*). It was an instruction for the authorities — magistrates and inquisitors — on how to deal with witches. They wrote about how witches were to be detected, tortured, made to confess, tried and executed. The torture described is almost unspeakable.

Their misogynist statements sound outrageous today. Unfortunately, they apparently didn't seem so

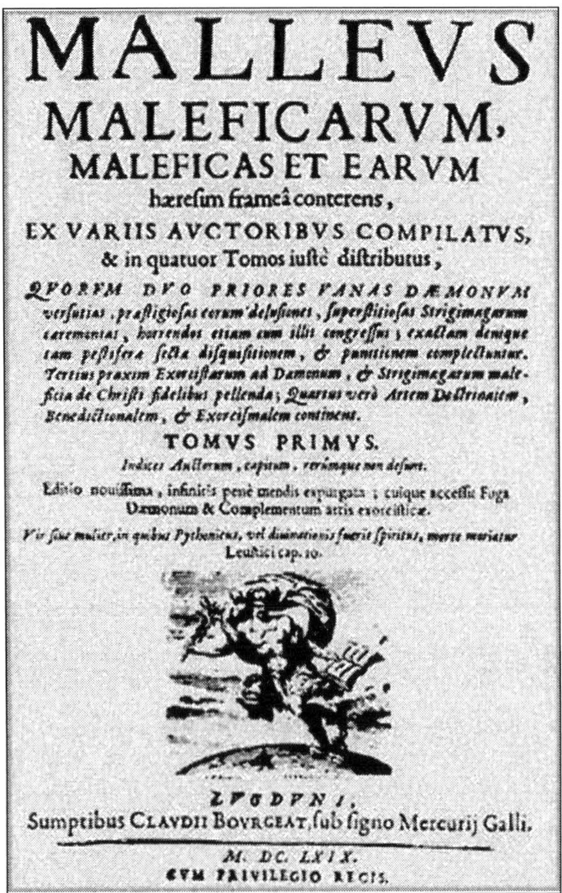

MALLEVS
MALEFICARVM,
MALEFICAS ET EARVM
hæresim frameâ conterens,
EX VARIIS AVCTORIBVS COMPILATVS,
& in quatuor Tomos iustè distributus,
QVORVM DVO PRIORES VANAS DÆMONVM versutias, præstigiosas eorum delusiones, superstitiosas Strigimagarum cæremonias, horrendos etiam cum illis congressus; exactam denique tam pestiferæ sectæ disquisitionem, & punitionem complectuntur. Tertius praxim Exorcistarum ad Dæmonum, & Strigimagarum maleficia de Christi fidelibus pellenda; Quartus verò Artem Doctrinalem, Benedictionalem, & Exorcismalem continent.
TOMVS PRIMVS.
Indices Auctorum, capitum, rerùmque non desunt.
Editio nouissima, infinitis penè mendis expurgata; cuique accessit Fuga Dæmonum & Complementum artis exorcisticæ.
Vir siue mulier, in quibus Pythonicus, vel diuinationis fuerit spiritus, morte moriatur Leuitici cap. 10.
LVGDVNI,
Sumptibus CLAVDII BOVRGEAT, sub signo Mercurij Galli.
M. DC. LXIX.
CVM PRIVILEGIO REGIS.

*The* Malleus Maleficarum *(aka, the Hammer of the Witches) was a legal commentary on the Witches Bull, a handbook for torturing witches published in 1487. Penned by two German Dominican monks, it was based on a bull released in 1484 by Pope Innocent VIII, and played a central role in the witch hunts of the late Inquisition.*

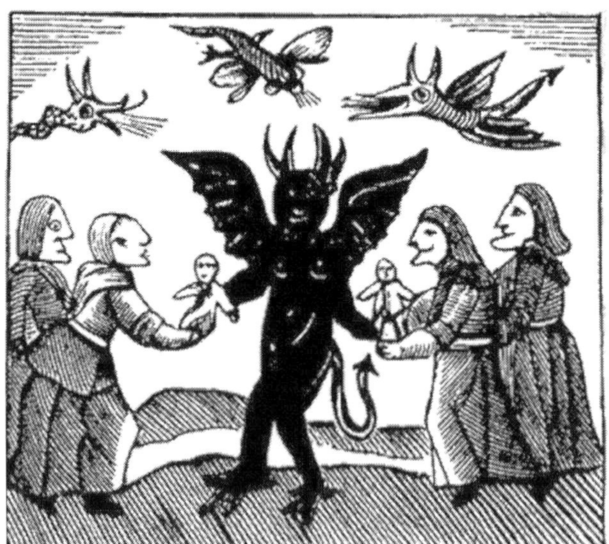

*A graphic depiction of a widespread superstition in the 15th century that witches were in cahoots with the Christian devil. This woodcut is from a later edition of the* Malleus Maleficarum.

outrageous in medieval times. They wrote: "All witchcraft comes from carnal lust, which is in women insatiable." [24] Here is an effort to control women through the threat of being declared a witch if she enjoyed her orgasm or desired sexual activity more than once in a blue moon. This seems to reflect a lot of male sexual insecurity.

The pagan spring fertility rites were sometimes mischaracterized by the Christians as "orgies with the devil," [25] Witches, they asserted, were guilty of copulation with the devil, assembling at sabbats (annual festivals based around the solstices and equinoxes). In the ancient world, only the Zoroastrians, Jews and Christians believed in the devil. The satanic witchcraft of Christian invention conceived of witches as tools of the devil. The Christians of the Middle Ages believed that the deal between witches and the devil was that witches served the devil in return for receiving certain powers. These powers included causing practically every conceivable misfortune, from the prevention of the conception of babies, the loss of cattle and crops, to illness and insanity and the ability to affect the weather – make it storm, rain, snow, and cause heat, cold and drought. [26]

The *Malleus Maleficarum* devoted several chapters to describing how the devil copulates with witches and how witches can make men impotent or their penises disappear. It explains the lascivious and immoral pleasure witches got from performing sexual acts with the devil. Proverbs 30:16 says: "there are three things that are never satisfied; yea a fourth thing which says not 'it is enough': that is the mouth of the womb. Wherefore for the sake of fulfilling their lusts they consort even with devils."

Well, who wouldn't be concerned about that? And the "witches" both used and dispensed drugs. Wow!

## Healers, Drugs and the Medieval Church

In 1484, the Catholic Church put a stamp of approval, of sorts, on alcohol when they adopted wine as a sacrament. At the same time, the Pope put the taint of the devil on cannabis. Pope Innocent VIII singled out cannabis as an unholy sacrament of the Satanic mass and the Inquisition outlawed cannabis ingestion. So during the Middle Ages, anyone found using the herb to communicate with God or heal others with it would be branded a witch. [27] Presumably this was to undermine paganism and encourage contact with God through the church hierarchy rather than endorsing an individual, drug-induced spiritual connection with the life force.

In Medieval times, studying and believing in the laws of nature were considered an offense against the authority of the Church. (Shades of today's evolution/creationism imbroglio.) Thus, in Medieval Europe the Church had most of the books on medicine tucked away in monasteries. The Church kept alive the ancient medical wisdom left from Greece and Rome and championed the status quo that that knowledge represented. Some priests in the Middle Ages interpreted efforts on the part of any man (or worse, woman) to heal the sick as being presumptuous, placing oneself as an equal with the Christian God. Prayers and fastings were the only Church-sanctioned remedies for ministering to the ill.

The policy of the Church of the Middle Ages toward pharmacy, medicine and healers was a form of substance control. Life and death were considered God's will and within the purview of the church, not "healers", who were often referred to as witches. Such healers were seen as having magical powers to heal people or make them ill. Some theologians of the day saw healers as tampering with God's will and acting against God. [28] Author Hellen Ellerbe writes in *The Dark Side of Christian History* (1995) that, "The Church included in its definition of witchcraft anyone with knowledge of herbs for 'those who used herbs for cures did so only through a pact with the Devil, either explicit or implicit.'" [29]

For two hundred years (1300-1500), opium is absent from European records. An explanation is that it was man's medicine, not God's, and the availability of an effective man-created medicine was declared by the Church to undermine faith. Even worse, opium was from the East. Things from the East being different — not from here — were considered a possible challenge to the established order and thus were often demonized. [30]

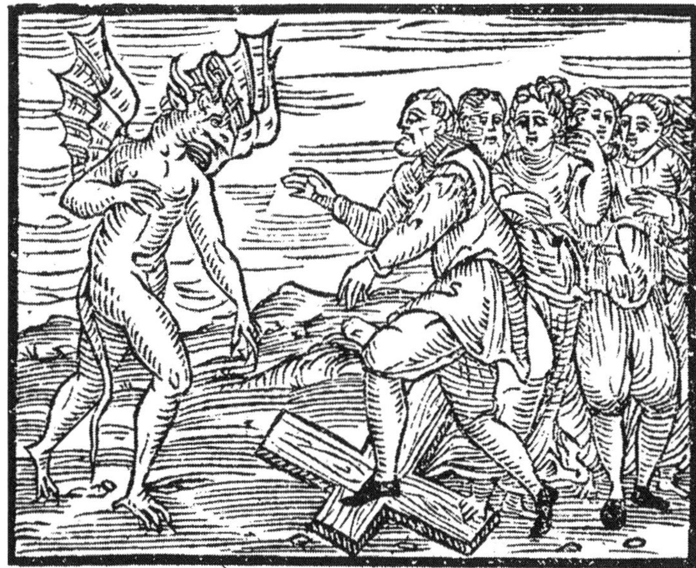

*There are numerous woodcuts that depict the imaginary sexual goings on between that fallen angel, the devil, and flesh-and-blood women. This one is from a later edition of the* Malleus Maleficarum, *which was first published in 1487.*

"The Holy Roman Empire was not holy, not Roman and was not an Empire."

**Voltaire**

French philosopher and writer, 1694-1778

The traditional medical treatments and natural remedies of healers in the Middle Ages were considered pagan. The influential *Malleus Maleficarum* created problems for some healers. It is debatable as to the actual percentage of healers targeted as witches. Not all accused witches were healers, neither were all healers accused of witchcraft. In fact, sometimes being a midwife was protective against being accused as a witch. Also in some countries, up to 25% of the accused were men, in others less. [31]

## The Progenitor of the Witch Hunts

The one-two punch of the Witches Bull and Witches Hammer was a powerful combination for social control. It coupled a dictum or law from the highest governmental level with unscrupulous, vicious, coercive enforcement in the field. There was little or no regard for truth or fairness. The actions surrounding the witch hunts were considered justified as part of the zealous no-holds-barred fight by the so-called "forces of good" against pure evil.

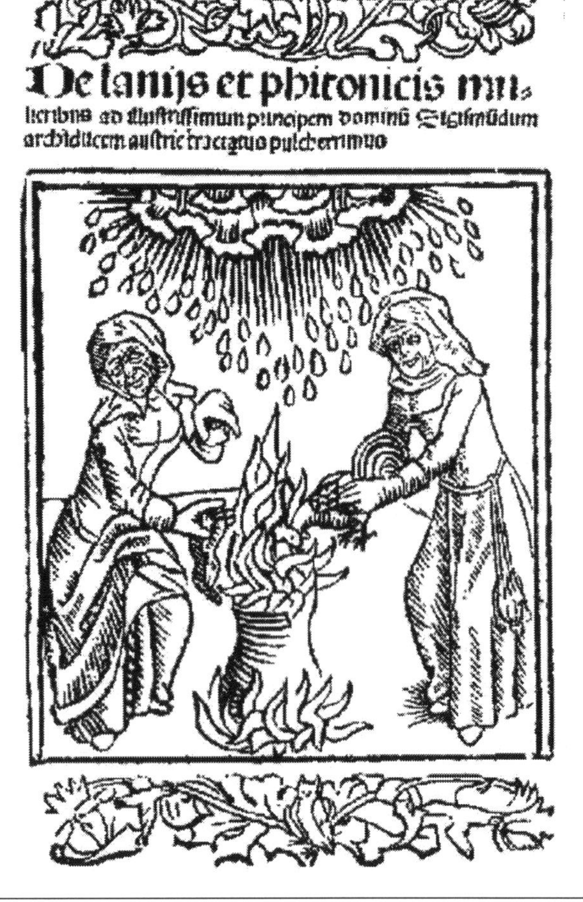


*A woodcut by J. Otmar Reutlingen in Ulrich Molitor's 1489 book,* Of Witches and Diviner Women, *that purportedly shows witches brewing up an ointment that gave them the ability to fly.*

The Witches Bull/*Malleus Maleficarum* and its policy fallout gave the Catholic Church its historical high profile for witch hunting responsibility. But the witchcraft hunting craze afflicted both Catholic and Protestant countries. Hysteria over witchcraft affected the lives of many Europeans in the 16th and 17th centuries, regardless of religious orientation.

Protestant reformers such as Martin Luther (1483-1546) and John Calvin (1509-1564) wanted to see all witches "burned" (Luther) or "exterminated" (Calvin). [32] Many witchcraft trials occurred in areas where Protestantism had recently prevailed or in other regions like Southwestern Germany, where Protestant-Catholic controversies persisted. Witchcraft trials were prevalent in England, Scotland, Switzerland, Germany, some parts of France, in the Low Countries, and even in America. Unquestionably in locals where religious passions were inflamed, accusations of being in league with the devil were more commonplace.

## Getting the Word Out on Witches

*Malleus Maleficarum* was not translated from Latin into English until the 18th century. A more accessible book, *The Witches and Diviner Women,* written by Ulrich Molitor, a professor at the University Constance, had a wider reach. In 1489, it was published in both Latin and German and was therefore accessible to those not learned in Latin. It was often reprinted, with thirteen Latin and three German editions. The early copies are usually illustrated with six or seven woodcuts depicting witches and witchcraft. [33]

These early pictures carried a graphic message of witches' demonic connection. The 4th edition of Molitor's book included a woodcut of two witches being taken by a demon to a sabbat, a pagan festival based around the solstices and equinoxes. All three are mounted on a cleft stick and the witches' heads have taken on animal form. This edition also included illustrations of so-called witches brewing up a potion to enable them to fly and another of a witch inflicting disease with a bow and arrow. [34]

Secular authorities and politicians published various witch-hunting manuals. For example, the French scholar Jean Bodin wrote *De la démonomanie des sorciers* (*Of the Demon-mania of the Sorcerers*), originally printed in 1580. By 1603, 17 editions had been printed. Secular law codes, such as the famous Constitutio Criminalis Carolina of Emperor Charles V of 1532, included laws against witchcraft, most of them prescribing the death penalty. [35]

Anglican King James ruled England during the height of the witch hunts. He fanned the flames of hysteria. *Demonology* was written by King James in 1597. But more importantly, his version — the King James Version -- of the New Testament included a method for dealing with witches: "Exodus 22:18 *Thou shall not suffer a witch to live."*

King James did not do Christianity any favor with that sentence. *A Skeptic's Guide to Christianity* claims that "this verse is a strong candidate for the passage in the Bible that has caused the most misery." This passage was telling Christians that witches should not be allowed to live. [36]

**"Those who crusade, not for God in themselves, but against the devil in others, never succeed in making the world better, but leave it either as it was, or sometimes even perceptibly worse than it was, before the crusade began. By thinking primarily of evil we tend, however excellent our intentions, to create occasions for evil to manifest itself.... [During the Inquisition] by paying so much attention to the devil and by treating witchcraft as the most heinous of crimes, the theologians and the inquisitors actually spread the beliefs and fostered the practices which they were trying hard to repress...."** [37]

**Aldous Huxley**
author, 1894-1963

Right along with witchcraft trials went the demonization of drugs.

## Blaming the Witches

But by far the biggest propagators of the witch craze were the friends and neighbors of the witches, be they Catholic, Protestant or who knows, maybe even a closet pagan or two. Money, power, greed, scapegoating and petty jealousy fueled the witch hunts. If a person coveted their neighbor's property, they could simply accuse them of being a witch. Your wife cheated on you? Someone's a witch. Your crops failed? Must be a witch. The social structure is changing? It's a witch. And hey, it's a great way to quash dissent.

## The Salem Witch Trials

In 1692, 19 women and men in Salem were found guilty of being witches and hanged. In addition, an eighty-year-old man was pressed to death, crushed under heavy stones for refusing to be tried. There were an additional four more accused Salem witches, who either died in prison or from torture. This outrage in the name of combating witchcraft was ostensibly triggered by the testimony of several teenage girls. [38] It is suggested that ergot poisoning may have played a role in the hallucinations the teenage girls in Salem claimed to suffer from. But many historians conclude that the Salem Witch Trials in 1692 in the United States are a good example of the role of ulterior motives in calling a person a witch.

There was a dispute among the denizens of Salem Village as to whether to have their own church, or walk the five miles to the existing church in Salem Town. Having a church of their own would require raising taxes. One faction of the village – the Putnams, a large, successful local family that had the most power in Salem Village, wanted to keep down taxes. They opposed building a church in the village, and favored the practice of going to the established church in Salem. The pro local church faction was led by less influential parties. [39]

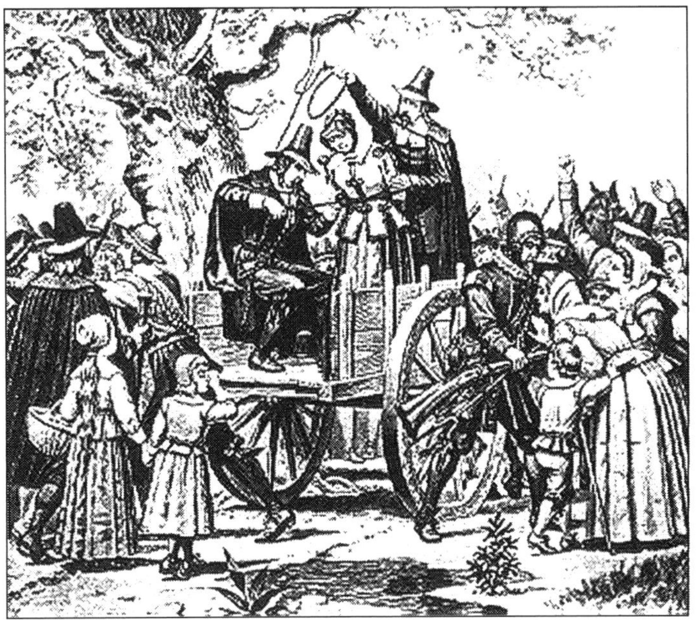

*On May 28, 1692 Martha Carrier and several members of her family were arrested and charged with witchcraft in Salem, Mass. She was pronounced guilty on August 2nd and hanged on August 19. Salem lives on in infamy as the place where 19 accused witches were put to death.*

The Putnam faction was responsible for almost all the accusations made. They only charged those in the other faction with witchcraft. All but two of the accused lived on the other side of town, the east side, while thirty of the thirty-two accusers lived on the west side. [40] From a historical vantage point, the Salem witch rhetoric was a way of settling old scores about power and social control. Who knows, some may have even believed in witches. At its core, this was most likely about two feuding community factions, with the more powerful group prevailing. [41]

**"If the merits of Christianity as a civilizing force are to be in any way determined by its influence in avoiding bloodshed; its record in the matter of witch-slaying alone serves to place it, in that regard, lower than any other creed."** [42]

**J.M. Robertson**
author, 1856-1933

Brian Fagan notes in his 2001 book, *The Little Ice Age: How Climate Made History 1300-1850*, that "As scientists began to seek natural explanations for climatic phenomena, witchcraft receded slowly into the background." Resorting to supernatural explanation of the natural world recede with increasing scientific understanding. But superstition is still rampant.

Fagan is not optimistic that science inoculates us against supernatural explanation for natural phenomena. He notes that most people still believe in horoscopes and that most Americans have only rudimentary science literacy. He states that "The rational aspects of civilization are a thin veneer and scapegoating, perhaps escalating to genocide, could still happen in future climatic crises."[43] Hmmm. Is global warming the next climate crisis?

## Identifying a Witch

It was clear to the witch hunters what must be done to curtail all this imagined harm done by witches in the service of evil. The problem was, at least superficially a suspected witch looked much like anyone else. The *Malleus Maleficarum* recommended stripping the accused naked and shaving off all of the victims' body hair. This was allegedly to facilitate looking for the alleged telltale signs of being a witch — the "Devil's mark" and the "witches tit."

### The Devil's Mark and Witch's Tit

Some think that the phrase "colder than a witch's tit" is just a vivid metaphor like "hotter than hell fire." But it's more than that. The witch's tit is an alleged specific anatomical structure that medieval witch hunters looked for on the body of the accused. The witch hunters were seeking a third teat with which a witch suckled her "familiars" (e.g., devilish animals that witches cavorted with, such as black

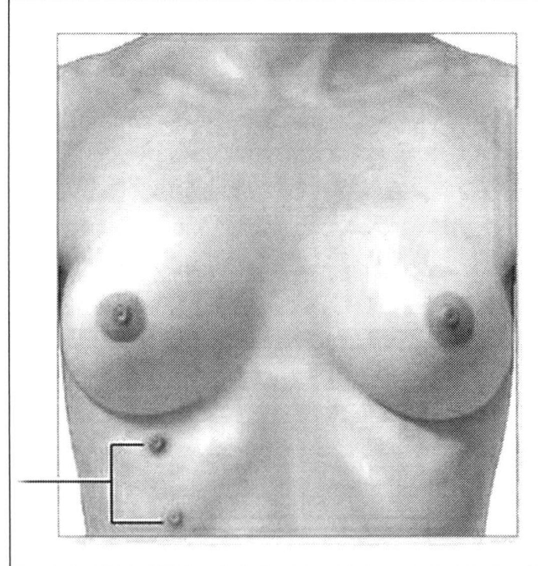

*These extra (supernumerary) nipples are residues of embryological development when humans initially have two vertical milk lines, each having eight or so nipples going from chest to groin. In most people, they consolidate in utero to the more conventional two nipples. Anne Boleyn, second wife to King Henry VIII of England and mother of Queen Elizabeth I, was rumored to have three breasts. This may well have been a slanderous rumor because such additional breasts were considered a sign of being a witch.* [44]

cats) or the devil himself. Some church authorities felt that those so-called familiars were the devil, and that the devil turned himself into one of these animals.

There are some not uncommon anatomical structures that a witch hunter might feel justified in labeling a witches tit. The best fit is a supernumerary nipple. Supernumerary nipples are an extra nipple or nipples left over from a human's embryological development. As embryos humans have a whole line of nipples that generally, but not always, consolidate into the usual two.

Extra nipples and also misplaced breast tissue, are actually fairly common. Two to seven percent of women (less in men) actually have supernumerary nipples.[45] This was fortunate for the witch hunters' thesis but they didn't even need to find a real supernumerary nipple. The hunters simply used their imagination much of the time.

**According to folklore and superstition, a witch's tit was a hidden "teat from which the**

**devil himself would suckle" and such suckling would drive the witch into a frenzy.** [46]

Historians have surmised that some inquisitors identified the clitoris as the witch's tit. This guess is based on the historical record that interrogations: (1) were sometimes conducted on women suspected of being overly passionate, loose or those branded as harlots; (2) consisted of searches of the most intimate body parts; and (3) were conducted by men. This suggests to some who speculate on this ghoulish sort of thing, that the interrogators would most likely test any witch's tit they found for the predicted frenzied response. Hence the clitoris was sometimes proclaimed a witch's tit.

The devil's mark was even more vaguely defined. This mark, sometimes called the devil's seal (sigillum diaboli) was allegedly caused by a bite of the devil's teeth or a mark left by the devil's claws. These imaginary things — the tit and the mark — could be just about any protuberance on the human body. Finding such "evidence" was proof of the accused's wickedness.

Familiars, the devil's mark and the witches tit were all described by contemporary 15th, 16th, and 17th-century writers. One such writer was Michael Dalton who wrote in his *Country Justice* (London 1618, 1630, 1647): "Their said familiars hath some bigg, or little teat, borne by the witch upon their body, and in some secret place, where he sucketh there". Of the devil's mark he wrote: "being pricked it will not bleed, and be often in their secretest parts, and therefore require diligent and careful search." [47]

The witch hunters would scrutinize the victim's body most sensitive body parts, such as the anus or the genitalia. The dermatologist Lambert Daneau in his *A Dialogue of Witches* wrote: "Judges should always, when suspects are presented to them, pull out hair and shave, where occasion shall serve, all the body over, lest haply the mark may lurk ender the hair in any place." [48]

The witch hunters had fertile imaginations. Pretty much any bump or mark might be called a witches tit or devil's mark; a skin tag, a mole, a blemish, scars, birthmarks, a corn, a wart, cancer, or really any mark. In some cases no mark at all. If a telltale blemish couldn't be found, the inquisitors just made it up. [49]

---

> **"Nothing is more terrible than to see ignorance in action."**
>
> **Johann Wolfgang von Goethe**
>
> *Proverbs in Prose* (1819)
>
> German philosopher, 1749-1832

---

In some ways the demonization of some men and women as witches is analogous to demonization of drugs. With demons, witches or drugs, it was a simplistic way to detect something evil was happening and place blame, whether warranted or not, on some unconventional occurrences or something over which humans had little or no control.

## The Bodkin

As their names suggest, both the witches tit and devil's mark were considered telltale signs of evil. These signs of the devil were believed to feel no pain and not to bleed. The witch hunters would go over the innocent victim's (the accused witch) entire nude body, not with a fine-tooth comb, but with a three-inch-long needle called a bodkin. They would plunge the bodkin into about every inch of the victim's skin to find the spot that neither felt pain nor bled. [50]

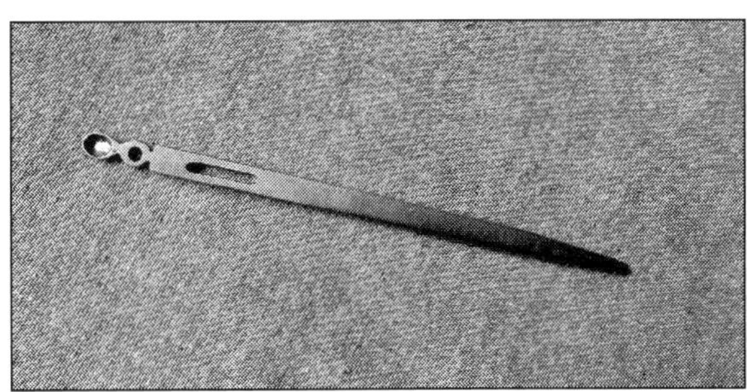

*A duplicate of a 17th-century bodkin, which is five inches long, 1/4 inches wide and 1/8 inches thick. Imagine this being pushed into your body to determine if there is a spot where you don't have pain. The bodkin was an effective instrument of torture for the accused witches.*

---

Often the victim was stripped naked in the public square for this inspection. This stripping and public inspection was not only the better to check the entire body around the victim's most private parts, the genitalia and the anus, [51] for the telltale signs, but was also a great way to intimidate. Oh, our ancestors knew how to entertain and scare the populous all at once.

**"Here it is!
The bodkin (or perhaps a false bodkin) has found the bloodless, painless spot."**

The lack of pain from inserting this three-inch needle in the body might be caused by disease, as from peripheral neuropathy caused by diabetes. The lack of scream could just as well be that after hours of being poked with a long needle over every inch of their naked body, the victim was just too exhausted to express pain.

If the victim didn't have such a bloodless, pain-free spot, that could be dealt with; one could be fabricated. Some witch examiners used a "false bodkin" to prove the person had the telltale painless, bloodless devil's mark and thus prove that this person was indeed a witch. A false bodkin was much like a stage knife. The tip of the needle or the false bodkin would recede into the hilt when pushed on the skin. This normally innocent stage prop would give the appearance of a needle going three inches into the skin, drawing no blood nor causing pain. [52,53] "We have another witch here."

The false bodkin is very much akin to planting drugs on people or relying on the testimony of snitches. Relying on snitches is similar to the weight given to the accusations of witchcraft made in Salem by teenage girls. Snitches and undercover agents (often acting as agent provocateurs) further undermine our right to be left alone. Planting drugs is a charge leveled at police that law enforcement invariably denies. Law enforcement also says they never lie on the stand. These blanket denials are not always credible.

A fairly recent U.S. Supreme Court ruling allows police to enter anyone's house without knocking or announcing themselves. [54,55] Notwithstanding the Fourth and Fifth Amendments, it's now constitutionally okay for the government, schools, prospective employers and employees to scrutinize another human's bodily fluids (e.g., urine and blood) at random, even if that someone does not stand accused of anything.

Hysteria, some led by former Yale cheerleader George W. Bush, an admitted alcoholic, has driven citizens to give up the values of the founders of the United States. The invasion of homes and bodies – guilty and innocent alike – is what the Founding Fathers tried to prevent through the Bill of Rights. Libertarians and some conservative Republicans are particularly horrified at our present day drug laws and the power they cede to the government to intrude into the lives of everyday citizens, law-abiding and law-breaker alike.

## Suspected Witches Faced Unbelievable Torture

Once the devilish mark and/or tit was found, proving that the accused were indeed a witch, the victim must, of course, confess. So, those accused of witchcraft and already "proven" to be witches by use of the bodkin, were asked to confess to the crime. Should they refuse to confess (it didn't seem to occur to the inquisitors that an innocent person having nothing to confess would refuse to confess), the suspect was further relentlessly and brutally tortured until a confession was extracted.

The means of torture of suspected witches included, but were not limited to, being hung by the arms with the arms tied behind the back and then weights being added to pull the victim down, thumb screws, the rack, beating the bare feet, and burning the body with a hot poker. Not too surprisingly, after being exposed to this level of torture, innocence didn't stop one from confessing.

Medieval witch torturing methods were unparalleled in their cruelty. One eyewitness of the tortures, a

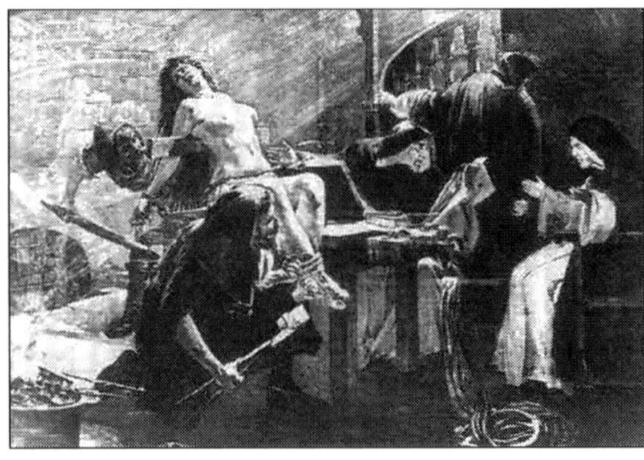

*Witch torture was brutal. Usually the victim was tortured nude. They were stretched with weights and winches, burned with hot metal, their genitals abused, and subjected to that "enhanced interrogation technique" of waterboarding.*

Johann Matthaus Meyfarth, wrote this sadly typical account of the barbarism he saw in the torture chambers:

> **"I have seen limbs torn asunder, the eyes driven out of the head, the feet torn from the legs, the sinews twisted from the joints, the shoulder blades wrung from their place, the deep vein swollen, the superficial veins driven in, the victim hoisted aloft and now dropped, now revolved around, head undermost and feet uppermost. I have seen the executioner flog with the scourge, and smite with rods, and crush with screws and load down with weights, and stick with needles, and bind around with cords, and burn with brimstone, and baste with oil and singe with tortures. In short, I can bear witness, I can describe, I can deplore how the human body is violated."** [56]

That was not enough. After the confession, the victim was further tortured to name other witches. If the victim recanted the original confession, he or she was tortured all the more until the earlier confession was reaffirmed. Having confessed and named other witches, the accused was then burnt at the stake. If a person accused of witchcraft withstood these unspeakable assaults and refused to confess to the crime after repeated tortures, he or she was still usually burnt at the stake anyway; if not for the crime of witchcraft, then for their stubbornness!

"The confession was frequently used to justify the imposition of ghastly punishments in the guise of preparing the accused to receive religious absolution thought necessary for entry into heaven following execution. Thus, crimes were confused with sins and punishment confused with blessings." [57]

## We Don't Believe in Witches So We Don't Have Witch Hunts and We Don't Torture ... Right?

Today most people do not believe in witches and are shocked at the inhumanity that ran wild in the so-called "Burning Times." The people of the Middle Ages were relentless in ferreting out and

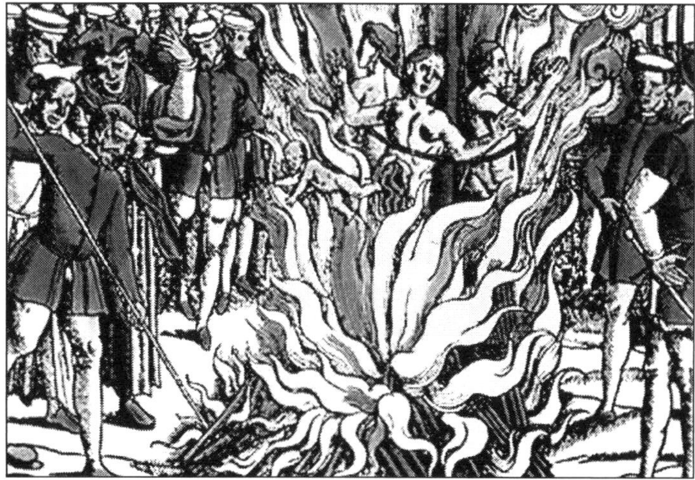

*Many declared witches were burned alive, and again, often nude.*

brutally punishing witches. Does this differ much from modern-day drug-related witch hunts?

It appears that fear can still make people do strange things in the name of goodness and all that is right. The same twisted thinking is evident in incarcerating those who suffer from the malady of substance abuse. Most everyone has been willing to give up their constitutional rights of free speech and privacy and permit our words, our bank accounts, and our property to be closely scrutinized. One has to ask whether humans have progressed much beyond the thinking of medieval times.

Based on today's reality that witches don't exist, the intense, terrible, illogical, anatomical searching by witch hunters for imagined clues to demons, was based on a combination of faith, greed, and/or hysteria. It bears a disturbing similarity to the U.S. government's reasons for abrogating the historical protection afforded all Americans against illegal search and seizure and self-incrimination provided by the Fourth and Fifth Amendments to the Constitution.

Torture, once thought to be either a relic of history or not acceptable to Americans, has once again appeared on the American scene. Toward the end of his presidency (2001-09), George W. Bush admitted he had approved what has historically been called torture, or what he called "enhanced interrogation techniques". This term hints of "newspeak" in George Orwell's book *1984*. In a performance that many deplore in the supposed civilized time of the early 21st century, an appointee for U.S. Attorney General, Michael Mulkasey, was

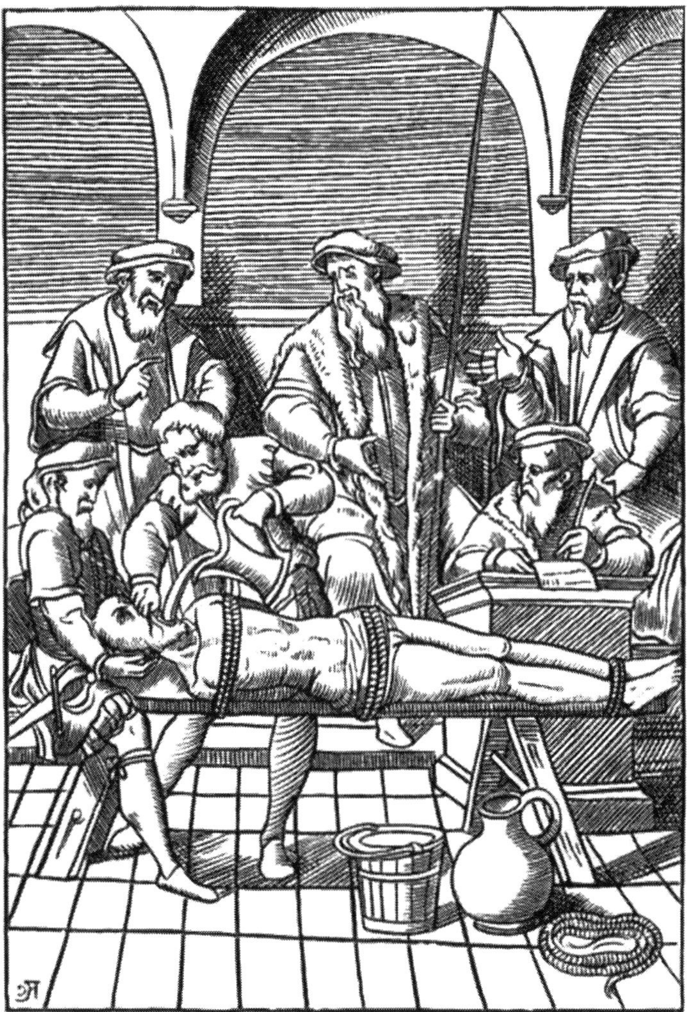

*This facsimile of a woodcut from a book published in 1556, depicts waterboarding taking place during the Inquisition. For centuries, water boarding was considered torture. However, the administration of George W. Bush used it during the U.S. military involvement in Iraq (2003-2011), labeling it an "enhanced interrogation." From the Inquisition through the first Iraq war, it was unequivocally defined as torture.*

confirmed by the U.S. Congress even though he could not define torture and refused to condemn waterboarding as torture. This torture technique, which simulates drowning, was used in the Spanish Inquisition.

Medieval tortures clearly surpassed contemporary U.S. torture efforts at Abu Grad and Guantanamo Bay. Whether "enemy combatants" we have sent to other countries to be interrogated faced worse torture than witches is as yet unknown. The value of the information gained from torture, be it from witches or prisoners of war, appears to be of dubious value. Senator John McCain, the 2008 Republican presidential candidate and a prisoner of war for five years during the Vietnam War, said that his torture in Vietnam produced no useful information. [58]

McCain also said in a 2005 Senate debate that the United States should ban cruel, inhuman and degrading treatment of detainees, "...because we're American and because we hold ourselves to humane standards of treatment no matter how evil or terrible they (the enemy) may be." [59]

Labeling one as bad, as in the case of a witch, based on hysterical, nonscientific thinking bears an uncanny resemblance to our present day approach to drug policy. How different is medieval torture from saying, "Well you can go to trial and face life in prison, but if you plead guilty we'll 'only' give you ten years?"

The suggestion that parents have little effect on whether children abuse drugs smacks of what Sigmund Freud called magical thinking: Something is being done, although not necessarily because it has been proven to be effective (e.g., treating drugs criminally as opposed to medically or parental), but because it's generally believed it will work.

In my over 40 years of experience providing drug-abuse treatment and prevention services, it is far more likely that a substance abuser will have grown up in a dysfunctional family or feels unloved or ignored than someone who has self-esteem and feels valued. I have noticed that people that have experienced real psychological trauma often suffer from obsessive-compulsive disorder, bipolar disorder, post-traumatic stress disorder (PTSD) and/or attention deficit/hyperactivity disorder.

Sadly the American people, by putting our men and women in harm's way in Desert Storm, the subsequent Iraq War, and the war in Afghanistan, are generating large numbers of veterans with PTSD. The Veterans Administration (VA) has made some helpful responses but must do much more. One of the reasons medical cannabis has been approved in over twenty states is that more and more people recognize that cannabis has proved helpful to the tens of thousands of Vietnam, Desert Storm, and Iraq veterans with PTSD in controlling symptoms of exaggerated startle response, hyper-alertness, excessive diffuse anger, and nightmares.

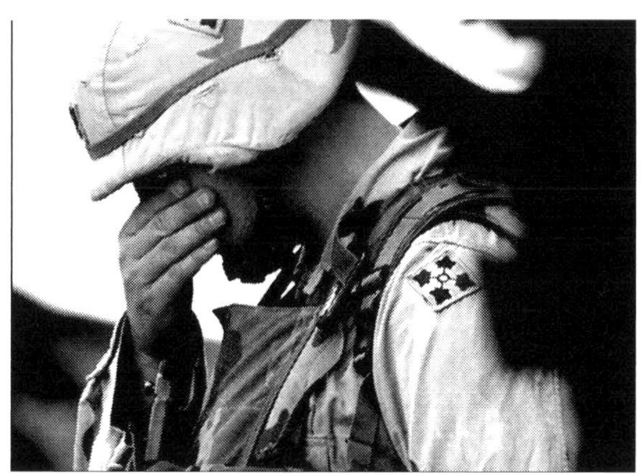

*Traumatic experiences may affect brain chemistry by increasing a neuro-chemical called dopamine transporter. While the exact neurological changes aren't currently determined, it's known that the symptoms of post-traumatic stress disorder include easy startle response, hyper-alertness, nightmares and anger. Patients and physicians have seen that cannabis and canabinoids have been helpful in treating these symptoms.*

Incarcerating people suffering from the medical problem of substance abuse and related mental health ills rather than treating them is counter-productive and strongly resembles medieval torture. At the very least, it is an illogical response to a mental health problem. Criminalization of mental health issues is a recipe for failure. There are other options. We know that drug-abuse treatment is both more efficacious and cost-effective than incarceration. Are today's prisons really our new "mental hospitals"?

## Mixing in a Little Greed

The hysteria motivating the witch examiners contributed to the witch-fearing populous' selective apperception. They often saw what they wanted, rather than what was in front of their eyes. When people have a largely unsupported bias or prejudice, in order to maintain it in the face of reality, they exclude contrary data through selective apperception. This psychological mechanism of selective apperception helps reinforce one's preconceived notions. Either a person doesn't see the thing contrary to the preconceived notion, or they say, "Oh that's an exception, so it doesn't count."

There was pressure to find witches. In certain locales in Medieval Europe, priests were considered derelict in their duty if they didn't reach a monthly witch quota. [61] They might themselves be accused of being a witch if they were derelict in identifying sufficient witches in their villages. There's no doubt that many witch hunters' judgment was clouded by the fact that in some places either the accuser, the prosecutor and/or the witch examiner got part of the property of a convicted witch. But the clergy actually played a minor role in all of this; the vast majority of witches were condemned by secular courts. [62]

These dynamics are addressed in Carl Sagan's *The Demon-Haunted World: Science as a Candle in the Dark* (1995). Sagan concluded that the witch hunts quickly became an expense-account scam. Sagan went on to point out the self-fulfilling prophecy of all this. As more people confessed under torture to witchcraft, it became harder to maintain that the whole business was mere fantasy. Since each "witch"

**"All costs of the investigation, trial and execution were borne by the accused or her relatives, down to per diem for the private detectives hired to spy on her, wine for her guards, banquets for her judges, the travel expenses of a messenger sent to fetch a more experienced torturer from another city, and the faggots, tar and hangman's rope. Then there was a bonus to the members of the tribunal for each witch burned. The convicted witch's remaining property, if any, was divided between Church and State. As this legally and morally sanctioned mass murder and theft became institutionalized, a vast bureaucracy arose to serve it, and attention was turned from poor hags and crones to the middle class and well-to-do of both sexes."** [60]

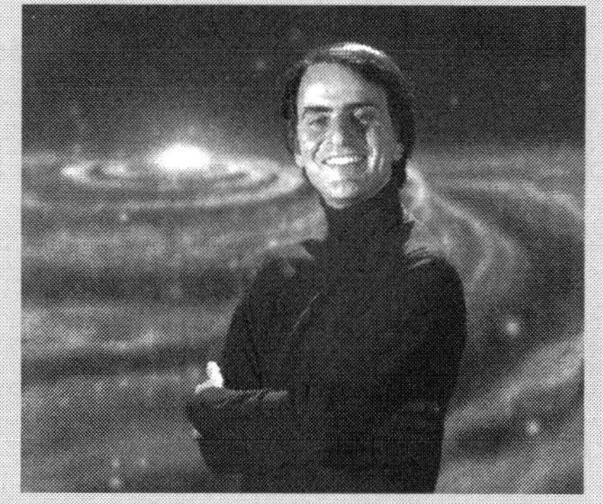

**Carl Sagan**
astronomer, philosopher, author, 1934-96

was made to implicate others, the numbers grew exponentially." [63] The whole system tended to support the existing cultural assumptions.

## Modern Madness

Today, society is more sophisticated. But, as many have noticed, U.S. drug policy enforcement methods are suspect and the results of American drug laws are cruel.

In medieval times, witch accusers could get some of the assets of the accused, which is similar to modern day forfeiture laws. The possibility of financial gain for the government through forfeiture is as seductive an inducement to stretch the truth today as it was in the witch hunting days of yore.

Such forfeiture laws are draconian and should shake all fair-minded Americans to their core. So too, should the appalling horror stories of ten years in jail for possession of one joint.

Forfeiture and extreme sentences have been applied against ordinary citizens. This is a form of modern madness, just as the witch hunts of the 15th through the 18th centuries are a testament to humankind gone mad. The witch hunters of medieval times had an excuse. Starvation, rampant disease, changes in weather can do that to people.

This motivates law enforcement to find real or maybe ersatz drug kingpins, modern witches, right here in River City. And Christianity, with its world view, was a significant contributory cause of this bloodbath. Approbation of witches is clear in the Bible. The New Testament has Paul's denunciation of witchcraft and, of course, King James added his "get the witch" touch in the King James Bible.

In 1484, the Pope labeled cannabis "an unholy sacrament" of satanic masses. He banned its use as a medicine. In his 2002 essay, "Witch Hunt and the War on Weed", Reverend Damuzi states that "what was once a religious war against plant-using pagans (has) evolved into the secular drug war of our current age." Damuzi continued that this demonization is "still fulfilling all of the same social functions as its predecessor, but now justified by "logic" instead of "religion." [64]

Make no mistake, the *Malleus Maleficarum* was a misogynist document. It condemned women as being imperfect humans and responsible for original sin. This was offered to explain why "a greater number of witches is found in the fragile feminine sex than among men." [65] And it certainly fingered women healers and midwives as being in the company of witches. In some locales, witches were accused of not healing people, "but only seem to do so by ceasing to injure them." [66]

The *Malleus Maleficarum* stated that: "No one does more harm to the Catholic faith than midwives. For when they do not kill children, then as if for some other purpose, they take them out of the room and, raising them up in the air, offer them to devils." [67] Midwives' traditional practices were in conflict with teachings of the Catholic Church. Midwives used herbs, provided contraception, procured abortions, and gave pain relief during childbirth. So some, but by no means all, that were accused of being witches were midwives.

There are many theories about why certain people were accused of witchcraft, including the view that the witch hunts were just the ultimate power play by men. On balance it appears modern feminist interpretations may emphasize only one aspect of historical accounts, but they certainly catch the mean, irrational spirit of those literal witch-hunting times.

Today's substance policy is often called a witch hunt. This contemporary witch hunt shares with its medieval predecessor a lack of respect for science or truth, irrationality, demonization, and focus on "them". The effort of modern drug-policy warriors to avoid responsibility and change the topic, very closely resembles the witch-hunting mentality of the Middle Ages.

## The Times They Were a Changin': "More Scapegoats"

As the Middle Ages were drawing to a close, roughly from the 14th century onward, change was in the air. A new medical hierarchy was taking hold and gaining in power. Simultaneously, the Church was suffering a decline in faith. Allowing women to practice medicine was in conflict with these medieval social and religious changes. These female medieval medical practitioners were one of the scapegoats for the times.

Other significant changes were also occurring. Important economic changes were causing social turmoil. The old communal values that stressed working together for the good of the community were being replaced. The new economic ethic taking hold emphasized that each person look out for him or herself. The changing social-economic structure favored the landed, the rich, and a professional class. If people were opposed to these changes, just label them a witch and hang 'em. Don't forget to torture them first.

---

**Today's substance policy is often called a witch hunt. This contemporary witch hunt shares with its medieval predecessor a lack of respect for science or truth, and an irrationality, demonization, and focus on "them".**

---

Some historians speculate that property owners were fearful of the growing numbers of poor in their midst. They started to paint them as agents of the devil. This period of change and transition contributed to the witchcraft hysteria. When problems arose, it was helpful to have scapegoats at hand. "Witches" were a handy tool, not so much of the devil but of the powerful, to avoid dealing logically and rationally with change.

## Wars on People

The witch hunts are not one of mankind's crowning achievements. In fact, they are a tribute to ignorance and evil, a triumph of superstitions and hysteria over science, reason and common sense. The same can be said of today's "war on people", misnamed the "War on Drugs." Authorities need to create fiends, demons, evil doers and drug abusers to justify what is done to its victims. Aldous Huxley wrote that humans have an unhappy pattern of "turning their theories into dogmas, their bylaws into first principles, their political bosses into gods, and all those who disagree with them into incarnate devils." [68]

Future historians will look back on the demonization of drugs, marijuana in particular, and wonder what rationalization was employed.

Some people with the most intractable substance abuse problems come from very dysfunctional families. They may have suffered mental, physical and/or sexual abuse. Yet, substance abusers that are so afflicted, are seldom treated as if they have a medical problem.

Criminalizing the medical problem of drug abuse (not to be confused here with drug use) has destroyed lives, broken up families, and punished the innocent. The book *Shattered Lives* by Mikki Norris, Chris Conrad and Virginia Resner, chronicles the obscene penalties meted out to average American citizens for little or no involvement with illicit drugs. [69]

Too often the significant others, who are frequently innocent or near innocent bystanders, of real and imagined drug dealers are punished more harshly than the dealer themselves. Those who are only peripherally or unknowingly involved in the drug trade get these stiffer sentences because, unlike their significant-other dealer, they have little or no useful information to trade to the police. These are more or less inadvertent bystanders that have chosen the wrong lover. Often, they don't know details of their significant other's illicit drug business and, therefore, are in no position to cut a deal with legal authorities in order to obtain a lighter sentence.

As Carl Sagan said:

> "If we can't think for ourselves, if we're unwilling to question authority, then we're just putty in the hands of those in power. But if the citizens are educated and form their own opinions, then those in power work for us.
>
> In every country, we should be teaching our children the scientific method and the reasons for a Bill of Rights. With it comes a certain decency, humility and community spirit. In the demon-haunted world that we inhabit by virtue of being human, this may be all that

stands between us and the enveloping darkness." [70]

## Drug War Justice: Tulia, Texas

A frequent criticism of the American criminal justice system is the uneven application of justice. The famous and the wealthy usually do much better than the poor. Mounting a good defense can be expensive. One wag has said, in explaining the economic impact of defending oneself, a person is innocent until proven broke.

In today's environment, whole towns like Tulia, Texas, a poor hamlet, can be torn asunder by one corrupt lawman. In this instance, with no evidence whatsoever, a single rogue law enforcement agent with a checkered past, Tom Coleman, falsified evidence and plain lied. This led to the local district attorney charging at least 46 impoverished people, mainly Black and a few who were significant others of Blacks, with being drug king pins.

It has to be admitted that living in abject poverty, in homes with no heat or electricity is a great cover for a community of big drug dealers. The absurdity of this obvious financial disconnect should have been the first clue something was amiss. [71,72]

After the first few innocent people were convicted, the remainder of those wrongly charged pled guilty to avoid the draconian prison sentences meted out to those already tried. It took almost a decade of intense publicity exposing the legal corruption that led to this travesty, before this miscarriage of justice was finally rectified. Texas Governor Rick Perry pardoned the Tulia inmates in 2003.

The pardon came after judicial review in which a judge accused Coleman (the criminal justice officer responsible) of being a liar, thief and a racist. *CBS News* reported this episode as "one of the worst miscarriages of justice in recent memory." [73]

## America Pays a High Cost

The toll from contemporary U.S. drug policy is high and climbing higher. The United States holds the abysmal record of having a higher rate of incarceration than South Africa did during the height of Apartheid [74] or the U.S.S.R. during its heyday.

Government resources are wasted, respect for law enforcement drops, police and government officials are corrupted, dealers have lethal fights over drug territory, and drug profits purchase semi-automatic weapons for these drug territory fights.

Young men are sent to prison for possession of marijuana where they can then be raped and contract AIDS. Add this to the toll of misplaced priorities, such as our under-funded drug-treatment programs, and all but ignoring prevention and early intervention.

These ingredients contribute to America's abysmal record of dealing with substance abuse. In order to effectively and wisely address drug abuse, much more emphasis must be placed on treatment, prevention and healthy nurturing families.

The death toll in Medieval Europe due to the witch-hunts is hard to quantify. Phyllis Graham, a Carmelite nun who later became an atheist, said "bearing in mind the small population of those times [the number of deaths from the witch-hunts] ... is well in proportion to Hitler's six million Jews." [75]

This far exceeds that related to the present very constitutionally shaky, ineffective and expensive approach to substance use and abuse. Of course, the witch hunts went on for over 300 years. While the modern witch hunt has been shorter, it has cost American's principle, freedom, and constitutional protection and it has slowed scientific advancement.

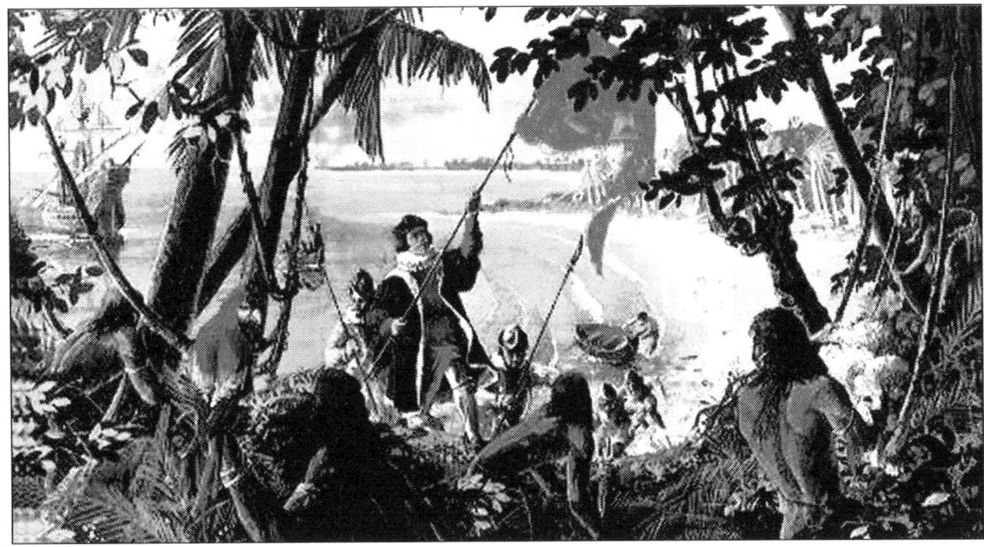

*The European explorer Christopher Columbus "discovered" America in 1492 and named the indigenous people he found there "Indians."*

# CHAPTER V
# 600 BC – 1776 AD:
# Spices, Colonialism, Genocide

## Spices

Spices are an important ingredient in our drug policy saga. The history of the spice trade is filled with unbelievable savagery and wealth, tall tales and discrimination. Spices fall into several categories. They are a seasoning, a food, an erotic stimulant, and spices have been and can be used medicinally. By most definitions of what a drug is, spices are drugs. Lies, duplicity and commerce are all part of the history of spices, not unlike current tall-tales about what are contemporaneously called drugs.

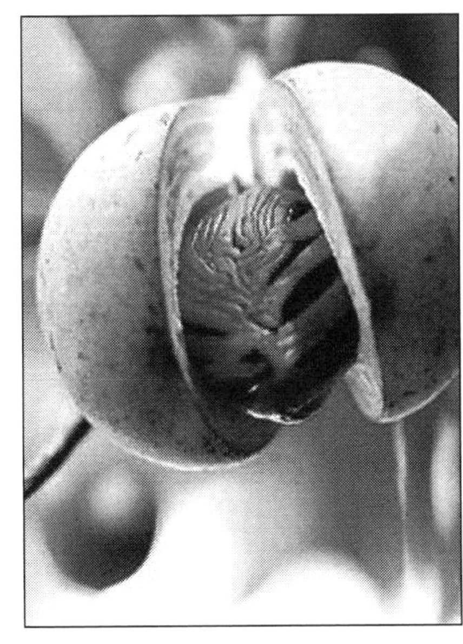

*Nutmeg was one of many exotic spices used as a seasoning. It was also considered a medicine. In higher doses it can cause hallucinations. In very high doses it may cause cerebral edema and death.*

Europe imported spices from mystical lands since before Rome was founded. From at least 950 B.C. until the end of the 15th century, spice caravans traveled across trade routes stretching from the Far East to the Mediterranean. Spices were much sought after by Europeans. This made the spice trade big business during the Middle Ages. Arabs controlled the lucrative spice trade. Of course, spices were instrumental in the European rediscovery of the Americas, which Columbus ran into looking for the short route to India in order to cut out the Arab middlemen.

The spread of Islam owes much to the spice trade. Mohammad (570-632 AD), the great prophet of Islam, was a spice dealer. He plied his trade between the Indian Ocean and the Mediterranean Sea in the 7th century, spreading his gospel along the way as he traded his wares. As he plied the spice trade, he spread Islam throughout the Middle East, particularly in Southeast and Central Asia as well as Sub-Saharan Africa. [1]

In this era, spices were principally for the benefit of the upper classes. Spices were considered exotic and the wealthy admired the exotic. In the era of exploration, the rich dressed in "new" materials from the Orient such as silk, and refurbished their residential quarters in the new Eastern style. Oriental seasonings were used to "disguise" native foods. [2]

Spices traded by Arab spice merchants included long pepper, black pepper, cinnamon, silver fir tree, frankincense, myrrh, nutmeg, balsam, cardamom, cassia and dill. The spice merchants' stock-in-trade was spices from plants indigenous to Arab lands. Spices were put into food or drinks to improve their taste, preserve them, or endow them with medicinal or magical power. [3]

Patrick Crose writes in *The Meccan Trade and the Rise of Spices* (2004) that the term "spices" meant more than just seasoning. Spices were also used to produce "aromatic resin, oleo-resins and gums" which were the bases of perfumes, incense and aromatic oils. [4] These pleasant olfactory uses for spices included not only incense, but also perfumes, ointments, and other sweet-smelling substances with which one dabbed, smeared, or sprinkled on oneself or one's clothes.

Besides making food taste more interesting and flavorful and creating pleasant aromas; exotic spices like pepper, cinnamon, cloves, nutmeg, ginger and saffron had one other thing in common, their non-European origin. They all came from the Far East. India and the Moluccas Islands (in present-day Indonesia) were the main source of these storied spices.

The consumers of spices in the Middle Ages imagined their source to be more fantastic than their subtropical and tropical reality. Spices triggered even more exotic imagery. Spices were emissaries from fabled, fantastic, far-off lands. Pepper was imagined to grow like a bamboo forest, on a plain near Paradise. It was said that Egyptian fishermen hauled in ginger by casting nets into the floodwaters of the Nile. [5] And cinnamon was thought to be gathered from nests allegedly made from cinnamon by vicious birds. [6]

In reality, ships and caravans brought these spices, tea, silk and other profitable merchandise from the East. Pepper and cloves came from India, cinnamon and nutmeg from the Spice Islands, and ginger and tea from China. The caravans came from Goa, Calcutta and the Orient to the spice markets in Babylon, Carthage, Alexandria and Rome.

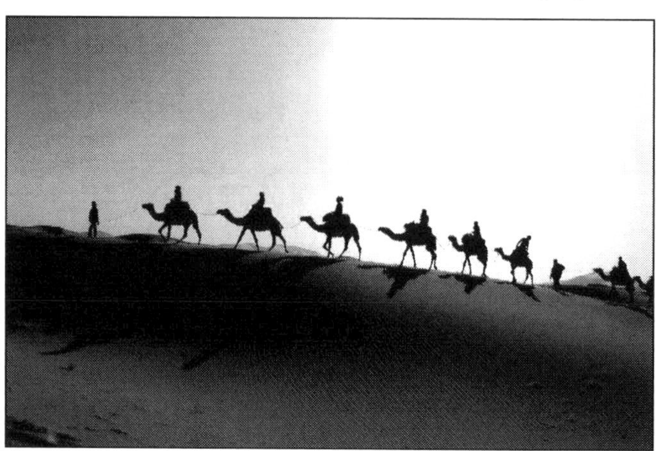

*Caravans came to the Mediterranean from Goa, Calcutta and the orient. Some caravans had up to 4,000 camels carrying tea, silk and spices and other treasures of the East.*

The theory that in the days before refrigeration spices were used to cover the taste of rotting meat has been largely discredited. For one, spices fell out of fashion by the 17th century, three hundred years before refrigeration was invented. Further, rotten meat causes illness. Someone wealthy enough to afford spices could toss out the spoiled meat. Finally, in the Middle Ages there were laws requiring that butchers sell only fresh meat but spices did play some role in preserving meat (e.g., peppered beef, salt pork). [7]

Spices were used as a physical symbol of wealth, happiness and fertility. They were prized as a sign of status, as well as for their exotic and erotic aura. Of course they made food taste more interesting but better yet they came from the mysterious Far East. A thousand years ago Arab traders kept the source of spices a closely guarded secret from the West.

For hundreds of years, myth, fable and fear were used by Arab merchants to try to conceal the East

Indian source of these profitable, highly sought-after herbs and spices from Europeans and other competitors. This tactic made it so much easier to maximize profit by using fear of the unknown to deny access to European merchants, keeping them and other potential competitors in the dark and at bay, as much as possible.

## Arabs and the Spice Trade

This exotic status symbol came to Egypt, Syria, Turkey and Genoa by both sea and land trade routes. Spices came in fragile ships to Egypt from the Spice Islands in and around present day Indonesia, or they came overland by caravan to Egypt. The ancient trade routes that caravans traveled were kept very mysterious in order to limit the competition and maximize profits. When these wares came by land based spice caravans, they could be transported by as many as 4,000 camels. By the 9th century, the Indian Ocean was "a sort of Muslim lake," [8] with regular trading routes between China and Arabia.

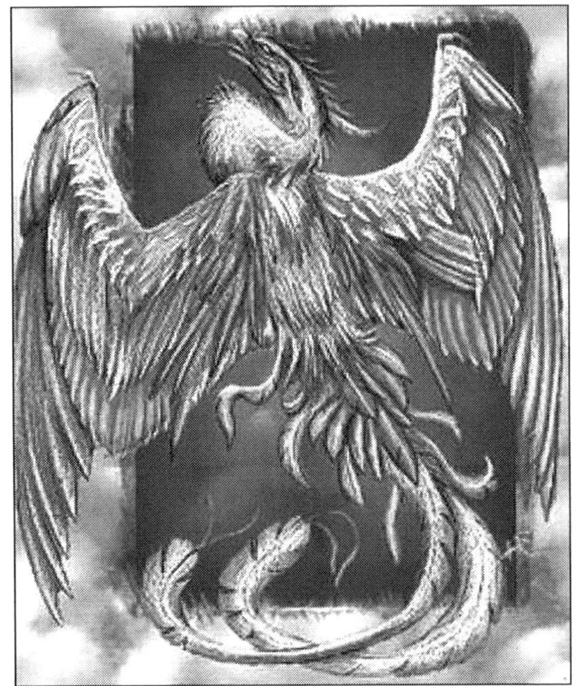

*Herodotus, fifth century Greek historian, reported as fact, the Arab myth of cinnamon coming from the nests of fierce birds such as the one shown above.*

Natural phenomena were poorly understood in ancient times. Fantasies helped explain the mystery surrounding certain seemingly-miraculous events. The mysterious exotic aura surrounding spices was perpetuated by fantasy. In ancient times it was common for people to believe in places that never existed. Spices were given exotic and incredible backgrounds.

This making up of fantastic tales has always been a part of the drug story. If the stories generated around the spice trade weren't the start of fabricated drug stories, the spice trade certainly didn't diminish or discourage story-telling about drugs.

An ancient Arab cover story fooled 5th-century BC Greek historian Herodotus into believing that cinnamon was found only on a mountain range somewhere in Arabia. Herodotus recorded the Arab tale that cinnamon was found in nests guarded by vicious birds of prey. These mythical, dangerous birds allegedly made their nests from scraggly cinnamon vegetation found on steep mountain slopes. [9]

The tale continues that in order to obtain the cinnamon nests, brave Arab spice gatherers would put out large chunks of fresh donkey meat for the birds to take back to their spicy nests. When these vicious flying carnivores deposited the heavy piece of meat in the cinnamon nests, the nests, under the weight of the meat, would crash to the ground. Then the brave Arabs grabbed the nests, taking the cinnamon from under the talons of their previous owners. The Arab story not only extolled this bravery, but justified the price of this rare commodity. [10]

By the end of the 10th century, there existed an Islamic world united by a common religious culture expressed in the Arabic language. The Islamic culture was made up of human links forged by trade, migration and pilgrimage. The Muslims had the perfect mechanism to further propagate the word of God (as they saw it) – the spice trade, over which Muslims had firm control. And by the 10th century, Muslims saw the world as dichotomous; either one lived in Dar al-Islam (the House of Islam or Submission) or Dar al-Harb (the House of War). [11]

## The Old Man in the Mountain and Islamic Extremism

The dangers of the spice trade were not mere fantasy. There were real pirates and thieves on land and sea. This is reflected in an old shibboleth that hashish means assassin. This comes from the tale of Hasan-Ibu-Sabah, the *Old Man of the Mountain*, and his band of Islamic fanatics and caravan pirates.

His religious enemies alleged he led a band of hashish-hopped up caravan robbers. This fanciful story, which was spread by Hasan's sectarian Islamic enemies, implicated hashish as playing a part in murderous caravan-robbing activities. The tale was believed by gullible Western Crusaders and passed on not only by them, but by the famous 14th-century traveler, Marco Polo. In truth, Hasan-ibu-Sabah was a religious fanatic. Any caravan robbery, if there was any, helped to fund efforts to spread his religious beliefs.

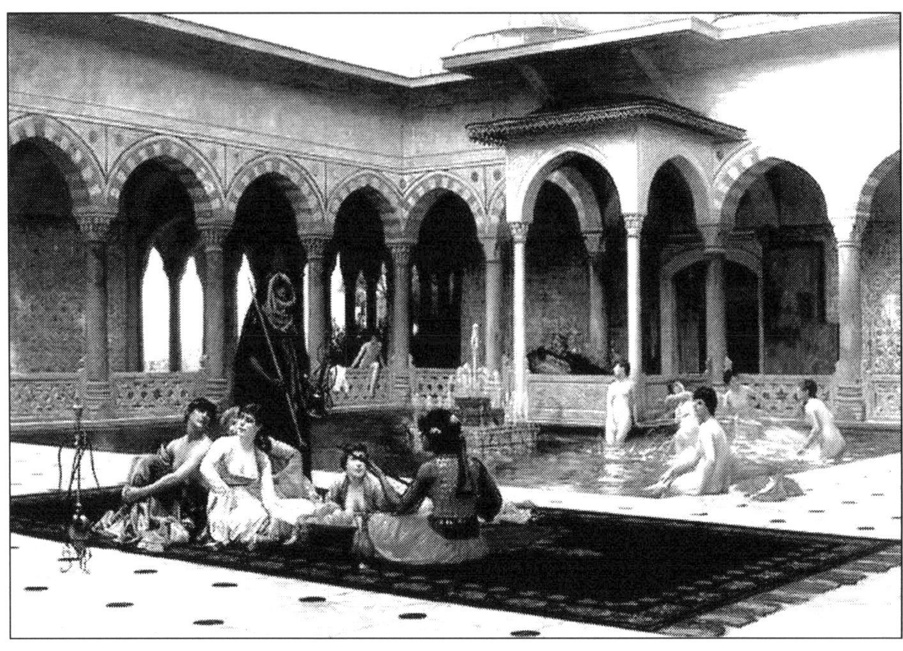

*This exotic courtyard is a depiction of what the earthly delights provided by The Old Man in the Mountain for his Islamic terrorists, might have looked like. It represents a picture of elegant living in the Spice Age.*

The fabricated story went something like this. Hasan-Ibu-Sabah was a caravan robber with a band of vicious henchmen who plied their barbarous and murderous ways circa 1090 AD. Hasan-Ibu-Sabah's Islamic religious enemies promoted the bogus story that he allegedly worked his men into a murderous rage with hashish prior to initiating a ruthless caravan robbery. The robbers' goal was to get a share of the wealth associated with the spice trade.

According to one version of this legend, Hasan promised his band of men paradise on earth or in some tellings of the tale, paradise in the after life. Instead of wine, women and song, it was more like hashish, harem girls and hedonism. The story goes on that Hasan had opulent gardens at his hideout where his band of spice caravan robbers would party. The party was either (1) to celebrate a successful caravan robbery or (2) to give the men a foreshadowing of what awaited them in the afterlife. one and three are bogus. We'll take door number two.

It would be most charitable to say that the true version bears only the most superficial relationship to the caravan robber story. Hasan was a religious zealot promoting his particular brand of Islam. He used his team of fanatic assassins to dispatch his religious adversaries. Hasan very likely did have opulent gardens, which may or may not have been staffed by lovely women and had fountains flowing with milk and honey. Hasan's band of Islamic zealots were exposed to this garden experience as a taste of what awaited them in the afterlife should they die in the service of Hasan and his Islamic cult (sounds like a foreshadowing of the present-day tale of a 72-virgin-reward waiting in the hereafter for any murderous Muslim suicide bomber).

The basis for today's conventional wisdom regarding hashish and the origin of the word "assassin" comes not from an accurate history of the time, but from these stories spun by Hasan's Islamic opponents.

Islamic zealotry in the 11th and 12th centuries, then, just as today, was not well-understood by Westerners. At that time the caravan robbers- hashish-assassin stories passed off as truth by other competing Islamic sects were believed by the gullible English, French and German crusaders. It was easier for the Europeans to ascribe the motivation behind assassinations to a drug rather than to religion. [12] A

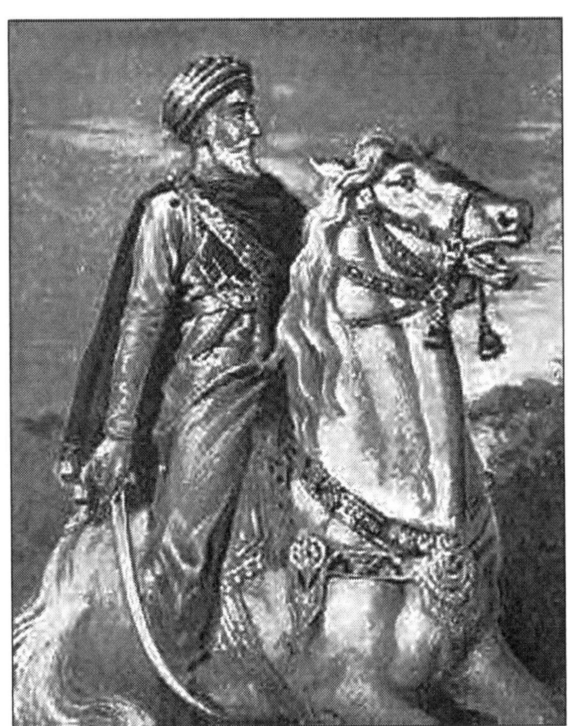

*Hasan-Ibu-Sabah's group was just another sect of Islamic terrorists but with a twist. He gave his warriors a preview of the afterlife and a bit of heaven on earth as encouragement to participate in his brand of religious mayhem.*

version of this fable was brought back by Marco Polo after his 14th-century journey to the Far East.[13] Polo's popularized account of his journey helped spread this bogus historical tale.

Martin Booth's book *Cannabis* (2007) provides a more historically accurate story of the Old Man in the Mountain. Today, it's understood very clearly the lengths to which Islamic extremists and terrorists will go. It is easy to comprehend the demonization of Hasan-Ibu-Sabah's Nizari Ismailli Islamic sect by his religious enemies. His opponents falsely associated cannabis intoxication with the religious assassinations. Booth writes:

***"The truth is somewhat different. Within a century of the foundation of Islam by Mohammed in 622 AD, the religion had divided into two branches, the Sunni and the Shiite. Each contained a number of sects, which were often at theological or ideological logger-heads with each other. One such sect, a schism of the Shiite branch of Islam, was known as the Nizari Ismailli. It was founded around 1090 by Hasan-ibn-Sabah, a famous Islamic dissident who was born in 1050 in the city of Qom, just south of Tehran, and educated in the orthodox thinking of Islam. Tradition has it he shared the same teacher as the famous Islamic writer Omar Khayyam….***

***"With his sect, Hasan-ibn-Sabah intended to politically promote the Ismailli cause across the Arabic world, which meant giving support to the Ismailli Fatimid rulers of North Africa.***

***"His politico-religious stand put Hasan ibn-Sabah at odds with the rest of Islam. He was vilified and regarded as a danger or a renegade, cunning, ambitious, determined and exceedingly cruel. He allegedly had two of his own sons put to death, one for drinking wine and one for alleged murder."***[14]

Booth continues: "Even if they did use hashish, it cannot—as was believed in their time (note: the time of the 12th & 13th-century crusaders) and as has been perpetuated ever since—have been in order to raise their courage and excite their battle rage. Hashish does not produce any mental state that would incite either violence or brutal murder."[15] The same disclaimer could be applied to the caravan robber myth.[16] It's hard to imagine an effective,

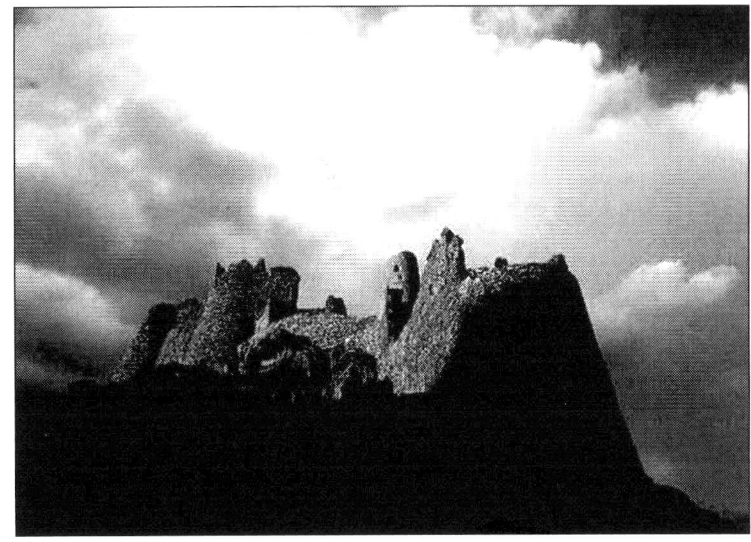

*Here is where the forces of Ibu-Sahab holed up. It is where there were said to be lovely women, fountains flowing milk and honey, and plenty of hashish. Maybe a tall tale, maybe not.*

## Well, Where Was the Hashish?

The story of The Old Man in the Mountain is a classic example of cobbling together a story based on a mixture of fiction, fact and wild imagination. Hasan certainly promoted the assassination of his political-religious enemies, but the fundamental association of hashish in carrying out these murderous acts, is historic hogwash.

Booth writes: "The Assassins were highly motivated, trained merciless political killers. Yet there is one fundamental puzzle about them that has never been satisfactorily answered and is of considerable importance to the history of cannabis." Despite the acceptance of the association of Hasan with the origins of the word hashish, Booth continues that "it is by no means certain if they (e.g. Hasan and his men) ever used hashish at all." Booth stated that there has "yet to be found any Islamic texts contemporary to that historical time stating that the Nazari Ismailli categorically used hashish." [17]

The most commonly accepted explanation of a possible role for hashish is that Hasan was trying to give his followers a taste of what their reward, either here on earth or in the afterlife, might be should they join his sect and do his bidding. In the *Botany of Desire* (2001), Michael Pollard writes that Hasan would give his new recruits so much hashish that they would pass out. When they awoke they would be in the midst of a beautiful garden, resplendent with sumptuous delicacies and staffed by gorgeous young women who would gratify your every desire.

Here is where a bit of stagecraft came in. Scattered in this veritable paradise were several apparently severed heads lying in ersatz pools of blood. The severed heads speak and tell the men of the afterlife and what they will need to do to return to this paradise. In truth the heads were connected to the fully intact bodies of actors buried up to their necks. So there you have it – sex, drugs, religion. This is a recurring combination to generate fearful scenarios and thus justify outrageous public policy regarding psychoactive substance.

stoned caravan robber. What would they do? Stare blankly and say, "Wow, dude, a camel."

Jerry Mandel was close to the mark when he wrote in a 1966 article entitled "Hashish, Assassins and the Love of God", that "Religion leads to assassinations, not hashish. The supposed hashish-induced 'visions of paradise' are as responsible for assassinations as the religiously fortifying drinking of wine and eating of wafers are responsible for the bloody crusades." [18]

## Anslinger's Tale

Booth wraps up his observation on this attempt to link the use of hashish use to assassination with the comment that "[W]hatever misinformation was promulgated by Sunni propagandists was embellished by Western chroniclers who did not appreciate the fact that the Assassins' name was abusive; nor did they understand the position of the Nazari Ismailli sect in the political structure of Islam. Being largely ignorant of the Muslim religion, and always eager to tell a good tale, they came to present a grossly inaccurate picture. The truth is, the Assassins have been given a reputation they did not really deserve and, through them, so has hashish." [19]

Harry J. Anslinger, appointed director of the Federal Bureau of Narcotics in 1930, was never one to let the truth get in the way of a good propaganda piece. In his 1930s efforts to gain support for the Marijuana Tax Act, Anslinger apparently bought the tale cooked up by the 11th-century fundamental Islamists about hashish and Hasan-Ibu-Sabah's alleged band of caravan robber assassins. The Anslinger-style assassin story has been refuted by many researchers, historians and sociopsychiatrists. [20]

In Anslinger's embellishment of the tale, hashish was trumpeted as being used before the caravan robbing, directly inciting the mayhem and murder which accompanied this marauding. In Anslinger's version of Islamic history, hashish was not part of internecine religious warfare; hashish was used to work the robbers up to a murderous froth and incite greater, even more fiendish mayhem. No mention whatsoever from Anslinger of Hasan's efforts to use assassination to create his vision of Islam. [21]

“Reefer makes darkies think they’re as good as white men.”

Harry J. Anslinger

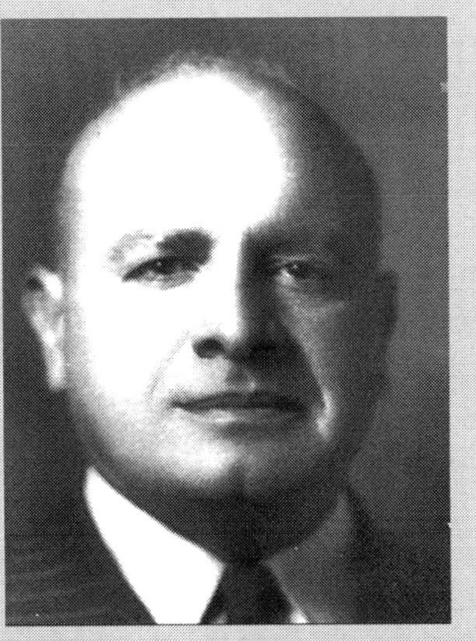

*Harry Anslinger initially headed up the nation’s Prohibition Department. As Prohibition drew to a close, his fiefdom shrank. Being a consummate bureaucrat, he created a problem where none existed and became the first director of the Federal Bureau of Narcotics in 1930. The Marijuana Tax Act of 1937 soon followed.*

Anslinger’s premise is not only historically false, but so too is its base assumption that cannabis leads to madness, mayhem, marauding and murder. It’s hard to imagine the use of this muscle relaxant and axiolytic (tranquilizer) being of much help in attacking a caravan.

On the other hand, from what has been demonstrated in recent times about Islamic extremism -- from 9/11, the Iran-Iraq war and the factional violence in Iraq -- it is quite understandable that Hasan’s enemies could make up stories to demonize him and his religious movement.

The idea of hashish-besotted, camel-riding, land pirates negotiating a successful attack on an 11th-century caravan stretches credulity to the breaking point. In fact, this picture of bloody veins and intestines dripping from the teeth of hashish-intoxicated caravan robbers is even inconsistent with the Anslinger position of the late 1940s. At government hearings in 1948, Anslinger’s tune was that cannabis made a person a passive dupe, ripe to believe in communism and/or lose their will to fight. He testified that “marijuana leads to Pacifism and Communist brain washing.”[22]

The name hashish was in the past sometimes spelt “hasheesh” or “haschisch.” It most likely comes from the Arabic word for dry fodder or herbage not from the Arabic word for assassin or from a corruption of Hasan’s name.

## The Sufis’ Use of Hashish for Religious Ecstasy Alienated the Rest of Islam

There was an ambiguity in Islam over the role cannabis could play, if any, in the life of a devout Muslim. This controversy went on for many centuries after the founding of Islam in the 7th century. The prophet Mohammad was clear that alcohol was forbidden. He taught that “there is a devil in every berry of the grape.” The Qu’ran or Koran teaches that one should not talk to Allah when drunk. While there was some ambiguity about cannabis, most Muslims see it as a forbidden intoxicant. There is a role, however, for cannabis in at least one Islamic sect, the Sufis. They used cannabis for assistance in achieving religious ecstasy. This did not sit well with the more orthodox elements of the faith.

The Qu’ran actually makes no special reference to hashish. Booth wrote of the use of cannabis in Islam, “The *imams* justifiably dreaded the thought that prayers might be offered to Allah while the supplicant was intoxicated. The upper classes supported the ban not only on the grounds that it was sinful but also because it threatened to undermine the labor force.”[23]

The issue was what the prophet Muhammad intended by forbidding wine? Some saw the Prophet’s admonition in forbidding consumption of wine as intending to stop the faithful from resorting to a substance (alcohol) that promoted violence. Supporters of cannabis said that (1) hashish induced pacificity and (2) it did not truly intoxicate, so therefore it was outside the Prophet’s restriction. (3) Furthermore, doctors declared it was a valuable analgesic, which was much less dangerous than opium. To comply with the Prophet's wishes, Muslim doctors attempted to establish a dose of hashish that killed pain but did not intoxicate. In that vein, 14th-century Muslim texts mention hashish as a digestive aid.[24]

The mystical Sufi Muslim sect, which started in the 13th century, is an Islamic hashish holdout. The Sufis believe that one attains spiritual enlightenment through a state of ecstasy or altered consciousness. They used hashish to attain that ecstatic state. They believed that hashish was a sacrament, a portal through which to commune directly with Allah.[25]

Haydar (1155-1221), the Persian founder of the Sufis, is credited with discovering the spiritual benefits of hashish.[26] He warned his Sufi disciples to keep this spiritual discovery from the ignorant because he feared they would abuse it. But the secret got out. This could be because Haydar requested that cannabis be planted around his grave. So when pilgrims came to visit his final resting spot, they began spreading the spiritual word on cannabis in the Islamic world.

Sufi poets wrote mystical didactic verses (which are apparently central to Islamic literature). This poetry referred to cannabis ingestion, probably in the form of tea, as a "cup of Haydar."[27] Eating hashish was an act of worship for the Sufi. They believed that using hashish would give them insights into life and spirituality, which were otherwise inaccessible.

Class distinctions influence Islamic thinking, just as it has Western thought. Sufis usually come from the lower, working-class part of society. In most any society, a religion that caters specifically to the poor can be denounced as a problem rather than seen as a denouement of the greater society. Here we had a religion of the poor that used hashish in their religion for heretical purposes. For these reasons, Sufis were not looked upon kindly by mainstream Islam.[28]

Amongst other Muslim sects (e.g., Sunnis, Shias, etc.), Sufism was regarded as a deviant religious movement of the lower class. "They were seen as dissidents and subversives, challenging orthodox theology." Does this criticism sound familiar?, claiming a direct communication with Allah. For this, they were, and in some places still are, reviled within Islam. Sufis are thought by orthodox Islam as being of lower moral standards and classed as heretics."[29] Sufism increasingly came under attack from orthodox Islam, even though their sect spread throughout the Arabic world, taking along with them their religious use of hashish.

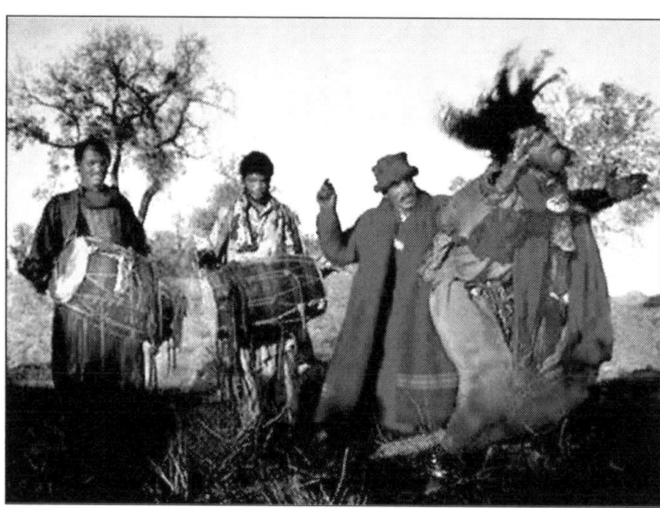

*The Sufi's used hashish to attain a spiritual state and enlightenment This may have once been acceptable in Islam but for centuries it has been looked upon by Islam with disdain.*

## Sikh

The Sikh religion developed in the Punjab region of India. The common use of bhang, a kind of cannabis tea, in religious festivals by Hindus carried over into Sikh practice. Sikhs were required to observe the commemoration of the founder of the Sikh religion, Guru Nanak, with bhang.

The traditional use of cannabis in the Sikh religion is described in the 1894 Indian Hemp Drugs Commission Report. The Commission states that the use of cannabis by the Sikhs appeared to be an essential part of their religious rites.

Today most Sikhs consider bhang, as well as liquor, to be against their religious teachings. Similarly to the stories of Muslim cannabis use, most modern day Sikhs feel the religious justification of the role of cannabis are just rationalizations made by "wayward" Sikhs who wish to partake in drugs, rather than proper religious teachings.[30]

As was shown in chapter two, cannabis has a long history of association with spirituality as well as religion. Neil Montgomery has observed that, "Many users of cannabis today recount feelings of 'oneness with God,' 'peace and tranquility,' 'reduced anxiety,' 'a greater understanding of life' and a 'greater appreciation of music and art.'"

Both spirituality and music seem inextricably linked to the cannabis culture – from ancient Scythian partying, to black soul and jazz, Sixties' rock'n'roll, and the Rasta influences of today. The Sufis, African dagga cults, the Cuna Indians of Panama, the Cora Indians of Mexico, Ethiopian Copts, Taoists, Scythians, Buddhists, Essenes, Hindus, Zoroastrians and the Rastafarians have all used cannabis in religious ceremonies, many regarding it as part of their culture and an important sacrament." [31] There are even claims that Jesus used sacramental oils made from cannabis for anointing people. [32]

## Europe Wrests Control of the Spice Trade from the Arabs

For centuries, Arab nations controlled the overland trade routes from the East transporting the spices wildly desired by Europe. The veil of mystery over the origin of spices had been pierced as early as the 13th-century by adventurers like Marco Polo. By the late 15th century, Europeans were well aware that the East Indies was the source of these exotic drugs. They were eager to eliminate the Arab middleman from the lucrative spice trade. Seafaring explorers set out to find a water route to these agricultural riches.

In 1503, Italian explorer Ludovico de Varthema, landed on Banda, one of the Spice Islands, in what is now Indonesia, and found the source of nutmeg. He shared his information with the Portuguese. Soon the Portuguese, the Spanish, the Dutch and the English sailed to Banda and the other Spice Islands to trade for nutmeg and other spices.

By 1513, the Portuguese were trading with much of the East Indies, including the Spice Islands. By 1520, Portuguese traders were importing 6,000 tons of pepper and loads of other spices to Lisbon. [33] The price of pepper in Lisbon fell to one-fifth the price in Venice, knocking the economic pins out from under the Venetians and the Egyptians. [34]

The exotic spice illusion was gone. The curtain of mystery and fantasy regarding the origin of spices pulled back, the "Wizard of Oz" revealed – it was business now. European merchants knew that what had been exotic, magical, fantastical places were real

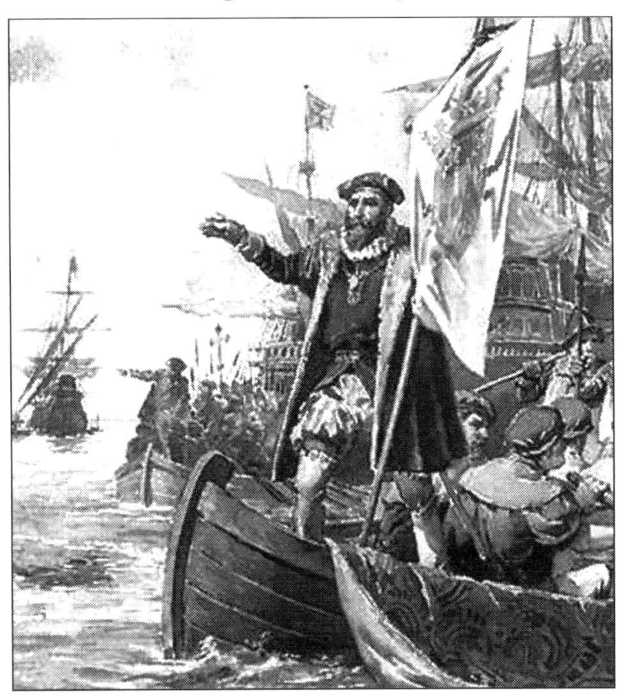

*In 1498, Vasco da Gama rounded Africa's Cape of Good Hope and reached India. His exploration allowed the Portuguese to establish colonies in Angola and East Africa and open new trade routes to the East.*

and reachable by sea. The gloves came off. Portugal claimed Ceylon, the East Indies and finally the Spice Islands themselves and for a time became one of the richest nations in Europe. A long competition for the spice trade ensued, involving first Portugal, then Spain, followed by England and Holland.

The commercial aspect of spices as a commodity set off intense and ruthless competition. There was money to be made! By most definitions, spices are drugs and the economic aspect of drugs has had and continues to have an important impact on American and international drug policy. Discrimination and "demonization" have also been used to gain commercial and economic advantage.

## Nutmeg – You Take the Nutmeg, I'll Take Manhattan

Pepper was the major spice in the spice trade, but nutmeg was also a much sought-after and profitable flavoring ingredient. Elizabeth David wrote in *Spices,*

*Salts and Aromatics in the English Kitchen* (1970) that during the Middle Ages nutmeg was extensively used as a fumigant against the plague. [35] The story of nutmeg reveals the violence associated with even prosaic spices and how the profit motive can lead humans to discount, marginalize and even kill people.

The Island of Run in Southeast Asia was an important source of nutmeg. Run was about as close to paradise as one could get; a tropical isle with a forest of nutmeg trees and other fragrant vegetation set in the middle of an azure sea. Even in modern times, arriving on a ship is described as a magical experience; dolphins splashing about the boat, afloat in the clear blue sea as you land on this aromatic, tropical paradise. [36] No doubt the English adventurers that first claimed the place felt the magic.

Run was England's first colony anywhere. The island was a small but important English colony. It is so tiny that even a smallish fishing vessel can come ashore only at high tide. But this small island was one of the famous Spice Islands, the epicenter of the spice trade.

The Dutch were one of the aggressive participants in the race for spice trade riches. The Dutch monarch established the Dutch East India Company (Vereenigde Nederlandche Oost-Indiche Campagine or VOC) in 1602. In order to protect their nutmeg monopoly, the Dutch colonized Indonesia in the 17th century. The nutmeg-rich island of Run was traded off by England to the Dutch for the island of New Amsterdam (Manhattan today).

The Dutch sent a governor general, the military, and military and merchant fleets to control some of the riches of the East and to establish permanent residences in Batavia, on Java (now part of Indonesia). The Dutch monarch was the major shareholder in VOC. This gave the VOC's governor general the sovereign authority to declare war or make peace, to rule colonies or cede territory in the Far East. This power was often used brutally to the advantage of the colonialists. What stands out in the VOC effort to control nutmeg is the company's cruelty -- usually, but not exclusively, meted out to non-Europeans. [37]

## Nutmeg High

Yes, a person can get high on nutmeg and even die of a nutmeg overdose. Both the kernel and its covering contain psychedelic oils including myristicin, satrole and elemicin. These can alter consciousness. The mind-altering effects of nutmeg can last up to 24 hours. Nutmeg's mind-altering effects became known in the West shortly after its 16th-century introduction to Europe.

Dr. Andrew Weil, author of *From Chocolate to Morphine* (1983), notes that in the right setting, nutmeg brings about pleasant sensations. In most cases, the use of nutmeg as a psychotropic agent does little more than make a person dizzy, but nutmeg in higher doses can also cause alarming symptoms.

The unpleasant effects of nutmeg can include nausea, vomiting, diarrhea and dry mouth. [38] Ingest too much, however, as one would from eating a whole nutmeg, and a person would get serious side effects of stupor, delirium and even death. The most likely cause of these symptoms is swelling (edema) of the brain. Some texts suggest the cause is hyper-sensitivity, as this too could be the cause of cerebral edema. [39]

Trade between the Dutch and the Bandanese was initially amicable. This all changed with the arrival of Jan Pieterszoon Coen as the Dutch East India Company's governor in the 17th century. Coen convinced the reluctant Bandanese of his firm's God-given right to monopolize the nutmeg trade. He did so in an all too typical European style: he butchered every single male over the age of fifteen that he could get his hands on. [40] Coen also brought in Japanese mercenaries to torture, quarter and decapitate village leaders and displayed their heads on long poles. The indigenous population of the

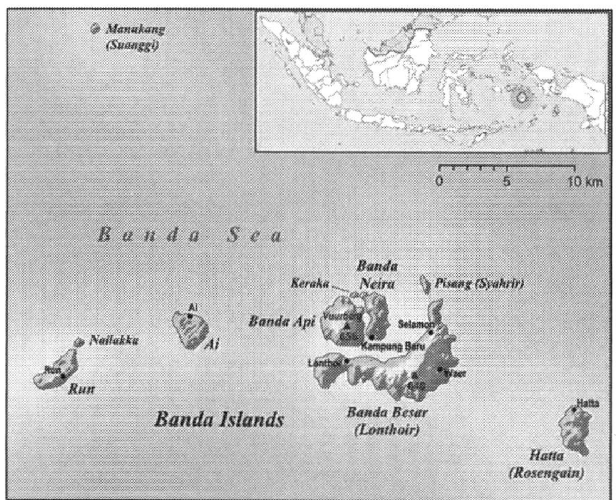


*The origin of nutmeg is the island paradise, Run, which today one of the Banda Islands, Indonesia. After the arrival of Jan Pieter zoon Coen in the 17th century, the island, home to the Bandu, became a living hell.*

isles was 15,000 before the VOC arrived; 15 years later the native population numbered 600. [41]

## The Colonial Years / Spain's Influence

Columbus' trip to America was part of the European effort to cut the Arabs out of the spice trade. Europeans were competing to corner the spice trade not only with the Arabs but with each other. Columbus left Spain in 1491, searching for the mythical short route to the East. Had he found such a route, presumably it would have given the Spanish an edge in the spice trade.

When Columbus set sail, the Spanish Inquisition was in full bloom. The mind-set of the Inquisitors was: if you're Muslim, Jewish or heathen, convert to Catholicism or perish. Columbus and his men landed in the New World in 1492, bringing the cultural baggage of Europe with them. They and the Spanish, who followed them, unpacked and set up shop accordingly. If those they met weren't Catholic, their blood wasn't "clean" and such people were in big trouble. If a people's religion relied on entheogens, then they were almost certain to be enslaved or eliminated.

### Columbus "Discovers" America and Tobacco

In San Salvador, Columbus and his men were confronted not only with heathens, but heathens that smoked tobacco. Europeans smoked other plants

**(Oh, ok, you got me. The people who were already there to greet Columbus, the ones Columbus misidentified, the so-called Indians, "discovered" both tobacco and America thousands of years earlier.)**

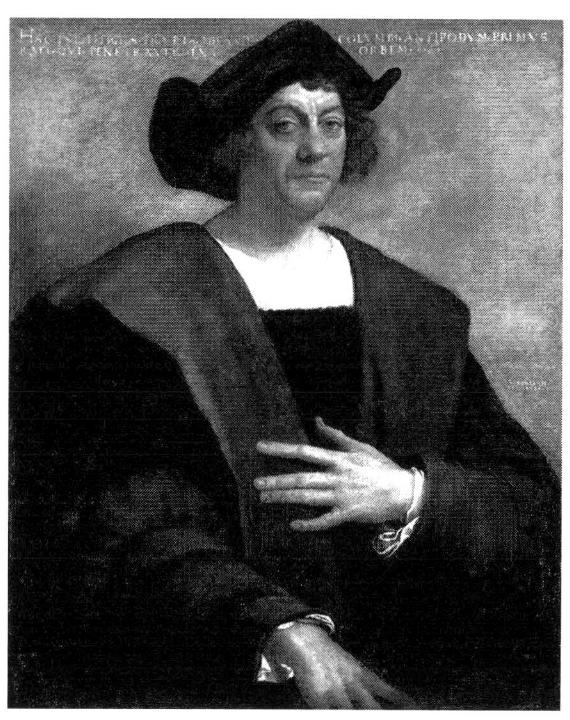

*Christophorus Columbus / Cristobal Colon, painting by Sebastiano del Piombo from the 16th century.*

> **"They do not bear arms ... They have no iron ... With 50 men we could subjugate them all and make them do whatever we want."** [42]
>
> **Christopher Columbus**
>
> in his diary

but tobacco smoking was a custom heretofore unknown to Europeans. So it should come as no surprise that Columbus and the other early explorers that followed him were amazed to meet Indians who carried rolls of dried leaves that they set afire – and who then "drank the smoke" [43] that emerged from the rolls. Other Indians carried pipes in which they burned the same leaves, and from which they similarly "drank the smoke".

The law of *limpieza de sangre*, the cleanliness of blood, was perhaps the most important cargo on the 1492 voyage of Christopher Columbus, sailing under the flag of Spain.

The native custom was to stick a rolled up tobacco leaf in their mouth and in some cases their nose and light it. Two of Columbus' crew, Rodrigo de Jerez and Luis de Torres, were the first Europeans to observe tobacco smoking in the New World. They reported that the natives wrapped dried tobacco in leaves of maize "in a manner of a musket formed of paper." They lit one end and "drank" smoke through the other. [44] Here these God-fearing Europeans were face-to-face with heathens breathing fire and smoke. So now, the first white men to see the Americas since Leif Erickson in the year 1000, could demonize a people, not only because they were a different religion, but because they used what was characterized by some as a satanic drug.

## Tobacco for Spiritual, Medical and Recreational Use

Tobacco has existed in the Americas for over 10,000 years. It was cultivated by the actual discoverers of America, the "so-called" Paleo Indians. The Paleo Indians grew tobacco in the Patagonia lowlands of South America. In many Indian cultures, tobacco was used by Shamans to induce visions, and hallucinations. Rudgley states that the South American shamans saw the spirits as being hungry for tobacco in much the same way as humans hunger for food. "By taking tobacco in various forms (drinking, smoking, snuff, eating) the shaman was thought to be "making direct and intimate contact with the spirits." [45] Rudgeley speculated that tobacco spread northward from its original South American beginnings.

When Columbus arrived, tobacco was used throughout North and South America, mainly for religious purposes but also for political and hedonistic reasons. Louis Seig quotes F.G. Speck who wrote of the Iroquois Indians, "...tobacco is a sacred plant esteemed ... as one of the blessings bestowed on them by the Creator. Smoking and

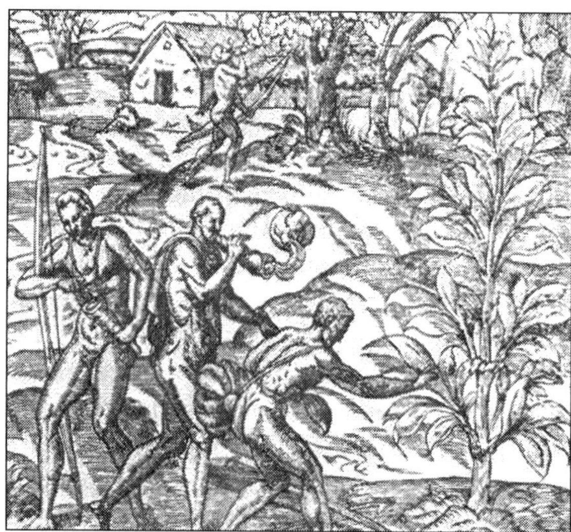

*Native Americans "drinking" tobacco smoke.*

burning it in the fire as a 'sacrifice offering' is another form of pledging sincerity of mind and heart..." [46] In the late 1500s, Spanish physician Nicolas Monardes described the role tobacco played in the priestly duties of "Indian" priests. Monardes' journal recorded that Indian priests used tobacco to aide in answering questions put to them by their patients. The patients expected the shaman to be able to find the answer from a tobacco-induced trance. After inhaling tobacco, the priest "fell downe upon the grounde, as a dedde manne, and remaining so, accordying to the quantitie of the smoke that he had taken, and when the hearbe had doen his woorke, he did revive and awake, and gave theim their answeres, according to the visions, and illusions whiche he sawe." [47]

Many native tribes in addition to the Iroquois venerated tobacco. They generally reserved tobacco for ceremonial purposes. It was widely used among the Plains Indians, who smoked tobacco in a ceremonial pipe, the Calumet. "Tobacco was used in the ratification of treaties and alliances; in the friendly reception of strangers; as a symbol in declaring war or peace; and it afforded its bearer safe transport among savage tribes. Its acceptance sacredly sealed the terms of peace and its refusal was regarded as a rejection of the same." [48]

Monardes reported in 1571 that tobacco was a popular treatment prescribed by Spanish doctors. He listed 36 conditions that tobacco was thought to cure. Monardes also informs us that early African slaves in America were banned from drinking wine.

Monardes states that these slaves used tobacco for intoxication and trance status.[49]

> "All along the sea routes … wherever they had trading ports, the Portuguese began the limited planting of tobacco. Before the end of the sixteenth century they had developed these small farms to a point where they could be assured of enough tobacco to meet their personal needs, for gifts, and for barter. By the beginning of the seventeenth century these farms had, in many places, become plantations, often under native control."[50]

**Jerome Edmund Brooks**
*The Mighty Leaf: Tobacco Through the Centuries*, 1952

## Look, the Inhabitants Aren't Christian

From the beginning, Columbus' party exploited the American native inhabitants and treated them with contempt. Columbus' journal records that the natives "invite you to share anything that they possess, and show as much love as if their hearts went into it." He was quick to add, "They should be good servants and intelligent, for I observed that they quickly took in what was said to them." He took six of them as prisoners.[51]

Joseph J. Fahey has noted the irony of Jesus Christ, the Prince of Peace, being used to promote war.

> "Before his crucifixion at the hands of the Romans, Jesus bestowed "peace" upon his followers, but the supreme irony is that the peace of Jesus has consistently been invoked by the followers of Jesus to justify the slaughter of innocents for the past seventeen hundred years. What brutal wars, pogroms, crusades, and inquisitions have been carried on in his name? Missions of soldiers, as they died of war wounds, devoted their last words to a prayer to this simple Hebrew pacifist, asking God's blessing on the butchery of spiritual brothers and sisters. Slavery, torture, rape, and pillage have been committed in his name. When Christians fought each other – as they frequently have – both sides claimed that Jesus had blessed their cause."[52]

**Joseph J. Fahey**
in *The Peace Review*, 1992

So in 1492, the Arawak people, who warmly greeted the Spanish ships, not only met Christopher Columbus, but also the mindset of the crusades. The militancy injected by the Romans into Christ's teaching has led to the belief that spreading Christianity by whatever means was God's work. The Columbian invasion of the Western Hemisphere was a combination of apocalyptic vision, messianic imperative, financial reward, and territorial expansion.[53] These beliefs were an integral part of the Europeans' worldview in the age of Columbus. These concepts were the frame that characterized Medieval Christian thinking. Speading Christianity and eliminating non-believers was the foundation for the Crusades and the Inquisition.

The Spanish treated the inhabitants of the New World barbarously. They slaughtered the indigenous population, appropriated their mineral riches and destroyed the indigenous population's religious system. The Natives' religion, the veneration of the vision-inducing, spirituality related hallucinogenic plants ololiuqui, peyote and psilocybin mushrooms was heresy to the Spanish.

## The Sweetness of Chocolate Cannot Hide the Bitter Savaging of Mesoamerica

The Spanish found a drug in the Americas that was more to their liking than tobacco -- chocolate.

Chocolate is part of this story for several reasons. Cacao trees (*Theobroma cacao*) became yet another plantation crop using slave labor and their dried cocoa beans were one of the trade stuffs of mercantilism. The Spanish were ruthless in their treatment of the people that had shown them hospitality by sharing this drink of the elite. Soon the native population was enslaved or near slavery.

Historians speculate as to how far back the cultivation of cacao goes. Various pre-parations from the

Mexican beans have been consumed for at least 2,500 years. Cocoa most likely originated in Mesoamerica, those parts of Mexico and Central America where great Native American civilizations developed. Ceremonial bowls for drinking chocolate found in western Honduras date back to 1600 BC. Most sources credit the Mayans, who thrived between 250 and 900 AD, with establishing the first cacao plantation in Mexico's Yucatan peninsula about 600 AD. Some experts, such as Sophie and Michael Coe, support the idea that the cacao tree's domestication goes back even centuries earlier to the Olmec. [54]

When the Spanish arrived, they found cocoa beans were highly prized and used like money throughout Mesoamerica. Other commodities were also used as money by the inhabitants of Mesoamerica – particularly the Mayans. These commodities included red spiny oyster shell, obsidian, jade, salt, and cloth. The use of cocoa beans as a kind of money did not end with the Spanish conquest of Mesoamerica. These "chocolate" beans were considered such a valuable commodity that in the 1540s, Nicaraguan prostitutes charged ten cocoa beans for their services. [55]

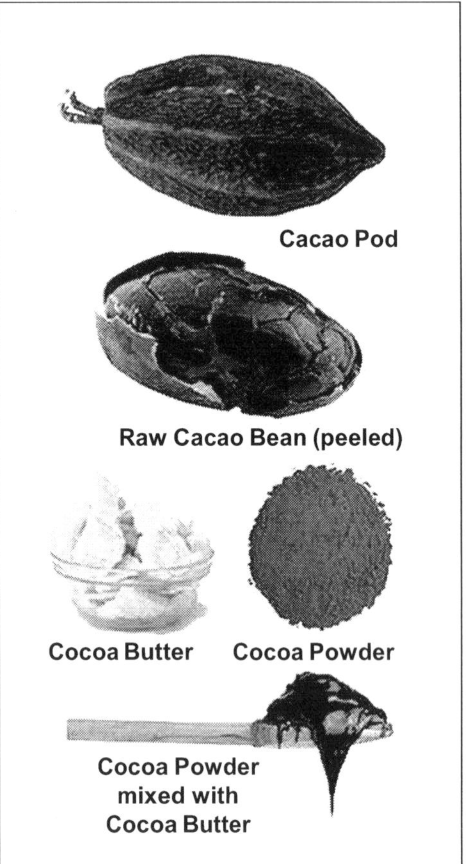


## The Chemistry of Chocolate

It has been said that "Chocolate is by far the most craved substance in our culture." [56] Some might even say that chocolate is "addictive." Forty percent of women and 15 percent of men admit to chocolate cravings on a regular basis. [57]

The chemical composition of chocolate helps explain its popularity. There are a number of chemical substances in chocolate that affect our brain chemistry. Like most plant material, chocolate is complex, containing over 400 different chemical com-pounds, several that affect human neuro-chemistry. A couple of these com-pounds, which are called biogenic amines, are chemically related to adrenaline and amphetamine. They show an ability to regulate mood and depression.

Chocolate also releases phenylethylamine and serotonin into the blood stream, both of which have euphoriant effects. At least one study showed that people that stop using the drug "ecstasy" (MDMA) have developed strong chocolate cravings. [58]

Chocolate has been said to be an aphrodisiac. This is one reason why Montezuma drank 50 cups of chocolate every day. When Cortez took chocolate back to Spain, its aphrodisiac reputation went along. In some places, nuns were prohibited from eating or drinking chocolate because of its reputation as a sexual stimulant. [59] This didn't change until 1867.

Indeed, chocolate's chemical makeup provides some basis for these allegations.

## Anandamide

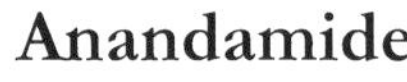

There has been recent speculation that chocolate might affect the brain similarly to tetrahydrocannabinol (THC). Chocolate contains certain fats that closely mimic anandamide, a neurotransmitter produced in the brain (an endocannabinoid). Marijuana activates the same chemical receptors in the brain that anandamine does. But don't rush out and buy a Whitman's sampler. It would likely take 25 pounds of chocolate to produce an actual "high". Researchers have concluded that an average serving of chocolate may produce a mild sense of well-being and might stimulate the senses that regulate craving. [60]

According to endocannabinologist Dr. Danielle Piomelli, a neuropharmacologist and researcher at the UC Irvine School of Medicine, chocolate seems

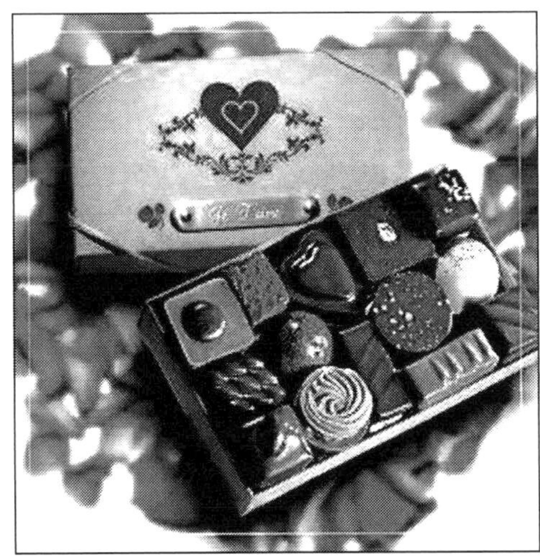

*Chocolate slows destruction of anandamide. Anandamide is one of the naturally occurring cannabinoids in humans. It is probably associated with a feeling of well-being. But hold on, don't run out and buy a Hershey bar expecting to get high. A person would need to eat about 25 pounds of chocolate in order to get euphoric.*

to interfere with the internal metabolism of the endocannabinoid neurotransmitter anandamide (named after the Sanskrit word for "bliss"). Anandamide, like other neurotransmitters, is broken down soon after it's produced. Piomelli's study indicated that two chemicals in chocolate inhibit the natural metabolic breakdown of anandamide. [61] When chocolate generates a pleasant feeling it could be caused by the natural release and slightly prolonged presence of the endocannabinoid, anandamide.

## The Spanish Destroy Mayan and Aztec Cultures

In short order, the Spanish killed or enslaved the people of the Caribbean, Mexico, and South America. When the Arawaks organized an army of resistance, they were burned at the stake, hanged, and tortured in inquisitional fashion. Mass suicides began among the Arawaks and they killed their own infants rather than let them grow up to face the Spaniards.

Columbus founded the "encomiendas", which were huge Spanish-run estates worked by the slave labor of the indigenous people and the African slaves that began arriving during Columbus' lifetime. Because disease killed such a large percentage of the native population, it wasn't long before the plantations were worked largely by Irish and African-American slaves. The encomiendas survived well beyond Columbus' lifetime. For centuries, they were a major source of exploitation of people and land in Latin America.

The Spanish systematically destroyed the Mayan culture. The Mayans were a literate civilization but after the Spanish occupation, only four of their books remain. Because the Spanish destroyed almost all the Mayan books, the role of chocolate in the Mayan culture can only be speculated. The Mayan's chocolate consumption patterns are documented in the few books that survived the destruction of the Mayan libraries. Two of the four books mention cocoa often. Cocoa is also mentioned in the sacred book of the Quiché Maya of Guatemala, *Popol Vuh*. [62]

Mayan artifacts suggest a pattern of chocolate consumption that persisted for hundreds of years. Pottery containers found in the tombs of Mayan nobility bear the hieroglyph for cocoa and depict the preparation process. These containers were analyzed. This analysis of trace contents suggests that these vessels once held chocolate beverage. The consumption of chocolate was, in all likelihood, restricted to the Mayan society elite. This was also initially true when chocolate was introduced in Europe.

### Chocolate: Food of the Gods

Chocolate was also a part of the Aztec's spiritual culture of central Mexico. The Aztecs believed that cocoa beans had been brought from paradise on a beam of the Morning Star by the god Quetzalcoatl. For the Aztecs, wisdom and power came from eating the fruit of the cacao tree. This ancient native Central American delicacy was considered by the Mayas, Incas and Aztecs as a "gift of the gods" and they extolled its stimulantive and aphrodisiac qualities. The name given cacao tree by the Swedish botanist Lineas — "theobroma" — means "gift of the gods".

## Cortez Confused for a God

Columbus was only the beginning of the European invasion of the Americas. In 1504, twelve years after Columbus' first voyage, Spanish navigator Hernan Cortez sailed to the New World and landed

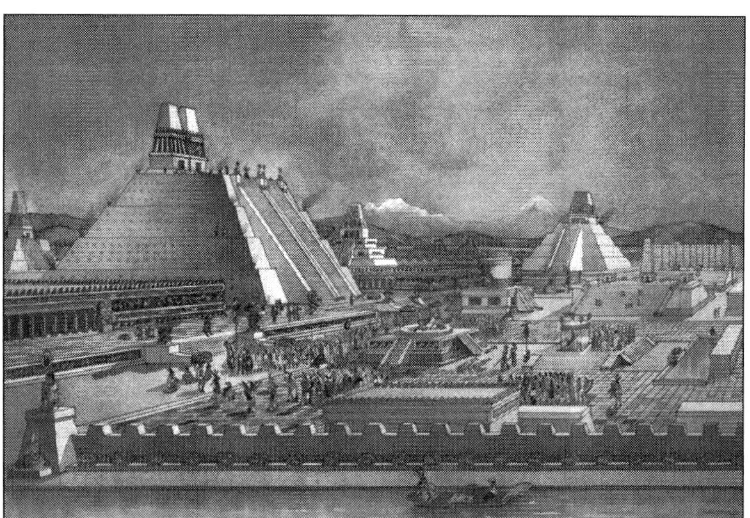

*When Cortez came to Mexico City in 1519, it was the largest, cleanest and most architecturally advanced city in the world.*

in the West Indies. In 1518, Cortez led an expedition to Mexico where he found a very advanced Aztec civilization. The Aztecs had governmental leaders, a religious belief system, and agriculture and were well ahead of the Europeans in many material ways.

The Aztec's pyramids, overall building design, urban layout and cleanliness of their cities held the Spanish in awe. Clearly in architecture and civic design, and cleanliness of public places, the Aztecs were decades, if not a century or two, ahead of the Europeans. Nevertheless, as a result of luck, aggression, disease and superior weaponry, within a short period of time, the Spanish, under Cortez, attacked, defeated and enslaved the Aztecs and destroyed their culture.

Cortez was mistaken for a mythical, fair-skinned Aztec god who, according to legend, would some day return. The Aztecs were awed by the possible prophesized return of their Aztec god. They were impressed by Cortez's armored horses and terrified by his attack dogs. Cortez was greeted enthusiastically and given a warm welcome. This included a cup of the Aztec's chocolate beverage, offered to Cortez by Montezuma. What Cortez got was a bitter tasting, spicy mixture quite different from today's chocolate drinks. [63]

Cortez destroyed the Aztec civilization. He did, however, recognize that chocolate had potential value. At the time, Cortez was much more interested in the first gifts he received from Montezuma; a huge silver plate and an equally huge gold plate representing the moon and sun respectively. Soon, all hell broke loose.

**The Spanish subjugated the Aztecs and destroyed their entheogen-based religion**

### But Wait ... Just Add Sugar

The Spanish appropriated the chocolate of Aztec culture, albeit after chocolate was sweetened to appeal to European tastes. Almost a quarter century after his first trip to Mexico, Hernan Cortez introduced a sweetened chocolate drink to Spain. Cortez's chocolate drink contained sugar and two newly discovered spices, cinnamon and vanilla, although a few sources give credit for the sugar idea to the King of Spain. It is suggested that he added it to the mix only after Cortez took chocolate back to Spain in 1528. [64] Sugar and spices eliminated the bitter taste of the original Aztec frothy drink. This sweetening made the Natives' chocolate beverage more pleasing to the European palate. The final improvement was that ultimately, someone decided the drink would taste even better if served hot.

The new improved chocolate drink quickly won favor amongst the Spanish aristocracy. In the spirit of Mercantilism, Spain planted cocoa in their overseas colonies. Through the 16th century, there was much trade and travel between Spain and its New World possessions. Amazingly, the Spanish were successful in keeping the art of the cocoa industry a secret from the rest of Europe for nearly a hundred years. To help keep that secret, only monks in monasteries were allowed to process cocoa beans into chocolate. Chocolate largely remained Spain's secret until 1606. [65]

The knowledge of chocolate was probably disseminated through the rest of Europe in two ways. One was via the network of monasteries and convents that by then linked Europe with Latin America. The other was through the independent discovery by sugar planters in the New World colonies. Finally, with the decline of Spain's power in the early 1600s, the secret leaked out. In 1606, an Italian traveler in Spain, Antonio Carletti, discovered the secret of chocolate and brought it to other European nations.

The cacao trade became a very profitable business. This being the heyday of mercantilism, many countries followed Spain in the cocoa trade. As chocolate's popularity in Europe grew, other European nations began growing the beans in their own tropical colonies. These were grown and harvested in the plantation system. Native Americans, African, and Irish slaves provided the labor on the plantations.

By the beginning of the 17th century, hot chocolate had become quite the rage and was popular among wealthy Europeans. In 1657, the first chocolate house opened in London. [66] Europeans valued chocolate for its nutritional and stimulative qualities. People believed it was a cure for a variety of physical and mental disorders. [67] Still, not everyone was pleased and some felt that anytime something was enjoyable, the devil may be lurking. In 1706, a doctor wrote "Satan makes us believe that ... chocolate will do us no hurt ... (but it actually) weakens the spirit, causes disorders of breath." [68]

By the early 18th century, the price of chocolate had dropped substantially so that many beyond the wealthy were able to afford and enjoy it. During this era, chocolate houses became as popular in England as coffee houses. In fact, there were chocolate houses that catered to only certain types of clientele such as politicians, gamblers, and the literati. [69]

## Peru, Pizzaro and the Devine Plants

The Incas were the indigenous inhabitants of Peru. Against enormous numerical odds, Pizzaro conquered the Incas in 1532. He was outnumbered 40,000 to 168. His success was due to trickery, surprise, superior weaponry, recent changes in Inca leadership, smallpox decimating the population and the Incas being more than a little too trusting. The Spanish attitude toward the Incas is well-illustrated in Jared Diamond's *Guns, Germs and Steel* (1999). The following passage is a distillation derived from the accounts of six of Pizarro's companions, including his brothers Hernando and Pedro.

> "The prudence, fortitude, military discipline, labors, perilous navigations and battles of the Spaniards – vassals of the most invincible Emperor of the Roman Catholic Empire, our natural King and Lord – will cause joy to the faithful and terror to the infidels. For this reason, and for the glory of God our Lord and for the service of the Catholic Imperial Majesty, it has seemed good to me to write this narrative, and to send it to Your Majesty, that all may have a knowledge of what is here related. It will be to the glory of God, because they have conquered and brought to our holy Catholic Faith so vast a number of heathens, aided by His holy guidance. It will be to the honor of our Emperor because, by reason of his great power and good fortune, such events happened in his time. It will given joy to the faithful that such battles have been won, such provinces discovered and conquered, such riches brought home for the King and for themselves; and that such terror has been spread among the infidels, such admiration excited in all mankind." [70]

The native peoples encountered by the Spanish ascribed supernatural power to several psychotropic plants – mushrooms, morning-glory seeds, peyote, datura, psilocybin mushrooms, salvia divinorem, various snuffs, tobacco, and other "magical" (that is, consciousness-transforming) plants. These plants caused ecstatic intoxication, which contributed to the spiritual life of the native population. The missionary clergy correctly perceived these intoxicants as obstacles to the eventual conversion of the natives to Catholicism.

For the Spaniards, there was a clear association between the spiritual use of these euphoriant plants and the Devil's attempts to prevent the victory of Christianity over the traditional naturalistic religion of the New World's indigenous people. The Spanish saw these entheogens as agents of the devil designed to prevent the native's acceptance of Catholicism.

The Devil's hand in all this was apparent to the Christian conquistadors. The Spanish reasoned that if this were not the work of the devil, the native population would not continue to secretly use these entheogens in the face of the constant threat of extreme punishment from the Spanish, ranging from public flogging to being burned at the stake alive.

So, to the Spanish these drugs were the Devil, or tools of the devil. This was neither the first nor the last time that drugs would be so characterized. Modern 20th-century posters from the drug wars use that imagery.

> "The early missionary fathers were generally willing to accept as true the reports from the Indians of the wondrous effects of the magical plants, especially in connection with divination and curing, the two areas in which the native hallucinogens played their most important role. What they primarily objected to – apart from aversion to any kind of intoxication among their Indian charges – was that Christ was missing from the system, so the supernatural effects could only be explained in terms of the Devil, who was trying to maintain and enlarge his ancient hold on the native souls whose salvation the Spanish were convinced was their divine mission." [71]
>
> **Peter T. Furst**
>
> *Hallucogens And Culture* (1976)

Drugs are given a persona, human attributes. They are depicted as seductive or demonic. We infuse certain drugs with evil. The practice of giving drugs personalities and human characteristics continues up to the present day. The cartoon strip "Doonesbury", by Gary Trudeau, lampoons drug policy with his discussion between his cartoon depiction of Buttsy, the tobacco cigarette and Mr. Jay, the joint (marijuana cigarette).

## Coca

During the height of the Incan Empire, coca leaves were reserved for the nobility and for religious ceremonies. [72] In *Narcotics: Nature's Dangerous Gifts* (1966), Norman Taylor states that, "However when Pizarro arrived he found everyone chewing it; and it is chewed by over fifteen million people today. Its veneration stretches back for centuries before Pizarro found the Peruvians chewing it. It provided energy and hope, sustained one through hunger and provided spiritual insight." [73]

The Spanish had come looking for treasure and they found it in the mineral riches; the silver and gold of Mexico, Central America, and Peru. These mines were worked by native workers who were technically not slaves. Nevertheless the working conditions were deplorable, the work hard, the hours long, and food scarce. The workers chewed coca leaves to help them endure working under those oppressive circumstances.

The Spanish believed coca was an agent of the Devil. [74] After their conquest of the Incan Empire, the Spanish initially banned the use of coca. They quickly changed that attitude when they found that without coca there was a dramatic decrease in the natives' productivity in performing the back-breaking work in the fields and mines, demanded by the Spanish. It was clear to the conquistadors that their near-slave Native American workers worked harder and required less food when allowed to chew coca. [75]

Very pragmatically, the church legalized and taxed the coca leaf, charging ten percent of the value of the crop as tax. For some time these taxes were the main support of the Catholic Church in the

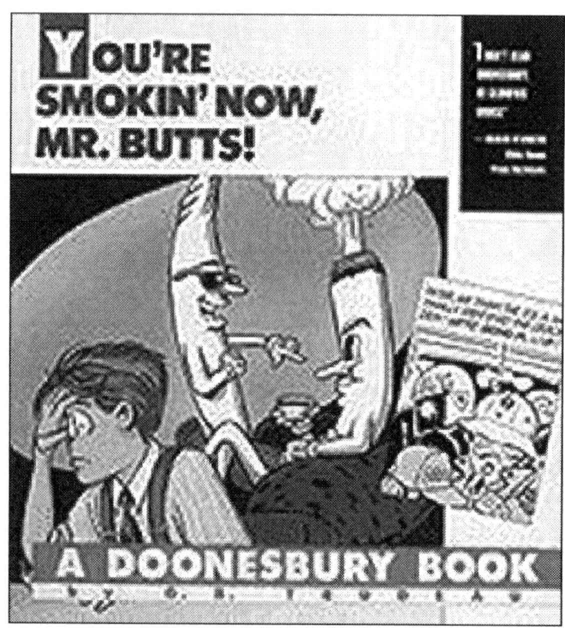


*In his "Doonesbury" comic strip, Gary Trudeau uses humor to compare the adverse effects of tobacco with the relatively benign effects of cannabis.*

coca-growing region of South America. [76] The Catholic church began to cultivate coca plants and many times paid the Indians in coca leaves. [77] In fact, some Spanish clergy extolled the medical virtues of cocaine. In 1609, Padre Blas Valera wrote:

> "Coca protects the body from many ailments, and our doctors use it in powdered form to reduce the swelling of wounds, strengthen broken bones, to expel cold from the body or prevent it from entering, and to cure rotten wounds or sores that are full of maggots. And if it does so much for outward ailments, will not its singular virtue have even greater effect in the mind of those who eat it?" [78]

Spain had a very successful colonial enterprise. They took silver, gold, cocoa and indigo from the New World to Spain. In return, traders sold high-priced manufactured items to the inhabitants of the Americas. The Spanish accrued enormous mineral wealth from America. From 1503 to 1660, over 7,000,000 pounds of silver were taken to Spain from America. This enriched the crown's wealth, as it got forty percent of the take. The government needed these funds from the New World to pay for their military efforts in Europe. They were so over-extended that even with this infusion of wealth, the Spanish Crown was bankrupt. [79]

In spite of the church's initially hostile position and later reluctant approval, coca continues to be held in an almost mystical reverence in South America. The mysticism and the reverence for coca are a legacy of Inca mythology, mixed with coca's practical value in helping one to work and survive under the harsh conditions of living and working at higher altitudes with sparse food supplies.

Almost all cocaine is still produced in northern South America. However, consumption of cocaine has gone worldwide. Although it is considered illegal by almost all governments, it is estimated that the black market in annual sales is roughly $100 billion. In the past decade, over 60,000 people have been killed in Mexico alone in heavily armed battles among numerous cartels for access to the lucrative United States' black market. Perhaps as many have died along the routes through Central America.

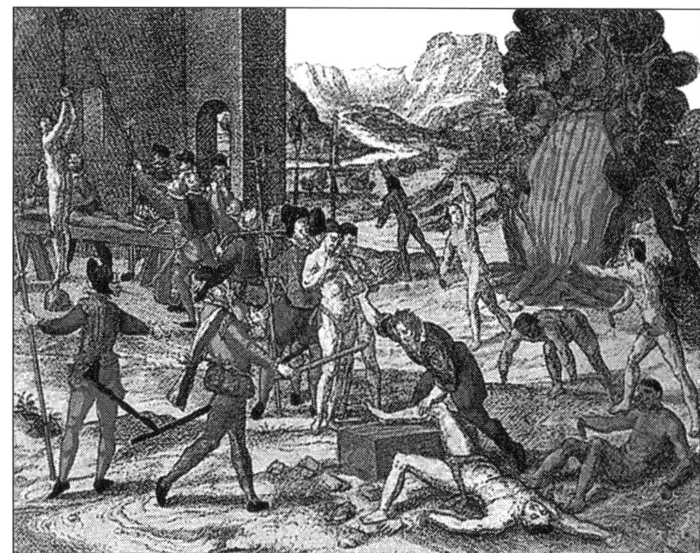

*Pizzaro defeated the Incas with superior weapons, trickery and some luck. He was aided by several recent changes in the Inca leadership and the Incan population being weakened by smallpox and other European diseases.*

Today in South America, coca is either chewed or a wad is stuck in the cheek and gum and is sucked on. This is not as concentrated or as potent as the more processed coca used in the United States. A popular South American tea, *mate de coca*, is made from the leaves of the coca shrub. Coca paste, also known as basuco, is a smokable form made from the leaves and used primarily in countries where the plant grows.

In Britain and America, cocaine is commonly consumed as a white powder. Most users sniff it up the nose, often through a rolled banknote or straw.

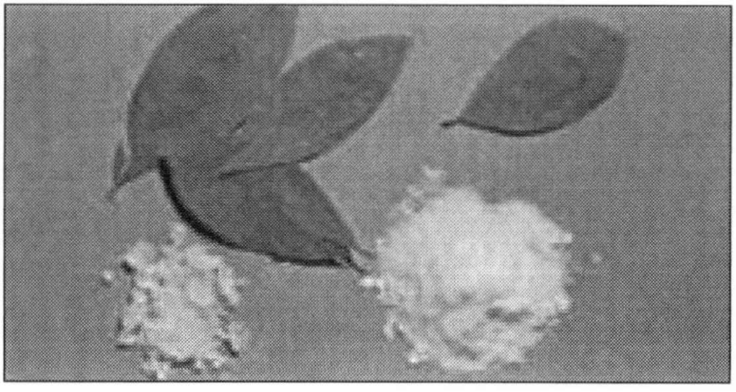

*Powdered coca and cocoa leaves.*

Crack cocaine is made up of small lumps or "rocks" of coca. It is usually smoked in a pipe, glass tube, plastic bottle, or in foil. It gets its name from the cracking sound it makes when being burnt. Free-basing is made by dissolving powder cocaine hydrochloride in water, heating with a base chemical reagent, such as baking soda or ammonia, to "free" the cocaine alkaloid "base" from the salt.[80]

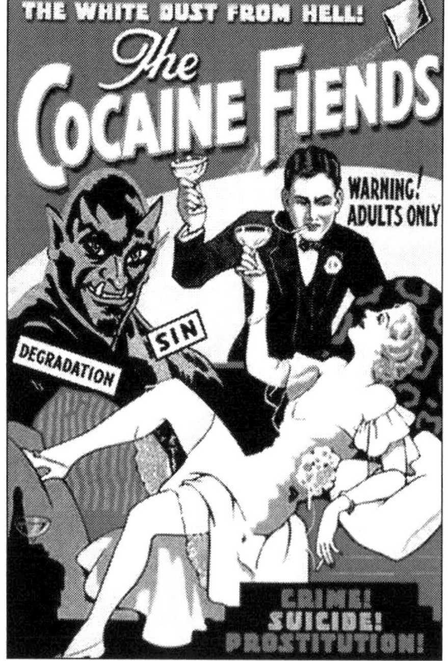


*This movie poster from the 1930s carries a recurring theme of demonized drugs, in this case cocaine, as being a tool of the devil.*

## Many Entheogens Discovered

As the Spanish conquistadors moved outward from the center of Mexico, they discovered many other hallucinogens that were sacred to the indigenous populations. Among them were the peyote cactus, ololiuqui and other morning glory seeds, psilocybin mushrooms (called teonanactl), salvia divinorum, the San Pedro cactus, and several kinds of datura.[81] It turned out that the Americas were a veritable treasure trove of spiritual, shamanistic, psychedelic drugs.

## Peyote

Many North American tribes considered peyote divine. It was used as a sacrament to facilitate direct communication with God without the need for a priestly intermediary.

The spiritual use of peyote was arguably an even worse affront to the Catholic Church than coca and natives could be killed for its use. In many ways, the symbolism of peyote in the native population's spiritual life was analogous to the use of the Host in Catholicism. Much as the host represents ingesting the body of Christ, peyote is seen as a taking in of the godhead and thereby obtaining insight into the spiritual aspects of life. Here was further justification, if any was needed, for annihilation of the original Americans. But it was much more complicated than that.

Peyote use was a part of rituals designed for seeing visions and contacting the spirit world. Mexico's Spanish conquerors and missionaries felt divinely inspired to "civilize and evangelize" the indigenous peoples of the New World. After the Spanish conquered Mexico and the Aztecs in 1521, the victors made a concerted attempt to erase all things related to the native culture. The Spanish carried on battles to annihilate, subjugate, and/or assimilate the Aztecs. In forcing the Aztecs to accept Catholicism, the religion of the Aztecs took on the trappings of Catholicism.

The Aztecs' use of peyote was demonized by the Spanish. The Spanish reasoned that if the indigenous people continued to worship with peyote, as they had for centuries, in the face of their extreme efforts to stop this practice, peyote must be a tool of the Devil used to thwart the acceptance of Catholicism. Native Americans who used peyote for religious purposes were tortured and subjected to barbarous acts by the Spanish. These included beatings, flogging, extended torture and even death. This was consistent with the Inquisitional mindset. The witchcraft hysteria of Europe easily transferred to the New World.

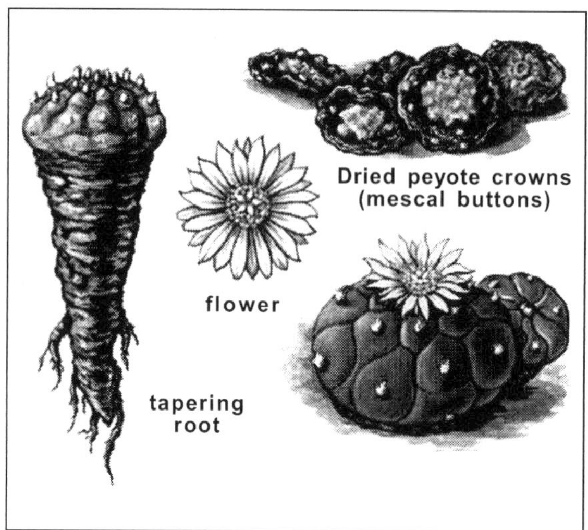


*Peyote was sacred to many Mesoamerican Indians. It promised a spiritual flight.*

The first drug law in the New World was imposed by the Holy Office of the Inquisition [82] in June 1620. Peyote use was castigated as an act of superstition and a source of visions and foretelling the future:

> "The use of the Herb or Root called Peyote… is a superstitious action and reproved as opposed to the purity and sincerity of our Holy Catholic Faith,

> being so that this said herb, nor any other cannot possess the virtue and natural efficacy attributed to it for said effects, nor to cause the images, phantasms and representations on which are founded said divinations, and that in these one sees notoriously the suggestion and assistance of the devil. Inquisitors against heresy, depravity and apostasy – June 19, 1620, Mexico City." [83]

The Spanish were not successful in extinguishing this spiritual veneration of peyote. To this day, the Huichol in the states of Jalisco and Nayarit in Mexico, continue to have the peyote cactus as the centerpiece of their religion and art. The principal psychoactive constituent of peyote is mescaline.

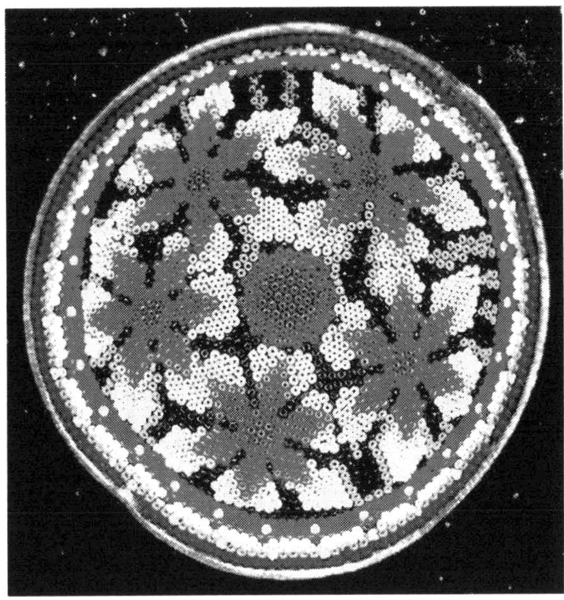

*Gourd bowls called onierikao in Huichol are completely covered with beeswax and beads usually in mandala designs. These mandalas represent the doorway to the other world. The Huichol bead work and yarn paintings convey the Huichal religion. The deer, the hexagon, and the wolf are also some of the symbols they use. The deer is the spirit guide that teaches the shamans. The hexagon represents the peyote that enlightens and wolves are the spirit bearers from whom the Huichal believe they are descended.*

## Ololiuqui

The Aztec religion worshipped the Sun God. The Aztecs believed that in order for the sun to continue to reappear, the Sun God must be regularly appeased with blood sacrifices. Their pyramids served several functions, including the altar upon which these human sacrifices were made. Both the priests and the sycophants prepared for the brutal ceremony on the pyramid, the removal of the heart while it was still beating, by partaking of various psychoactive drugs. These usually included psychedelic mushrooms and ololiuqui.

The Aztecs used ololiuqui, "the magic plant," a member of the morning glory family, in their religious ceremonies. It, too, is a hallucinogen.

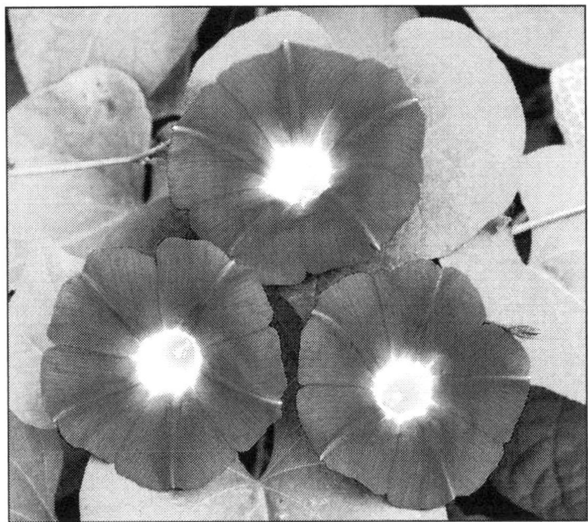

*The Aztecs had several psychoactive plants that they used in their religious ceremonies. One was the seeds of the morning glory plant or ololiuqui, which contain lysergic acid (LSD) derivatives.*

Before performing the human sacrifices, the Aztec priests covered themselves with a liquid mixture containing ololiuqui seeds, allegedly to numb their skin and remove all fear. [84] The shamans and priests also used ololiuqui to generate visions and commune

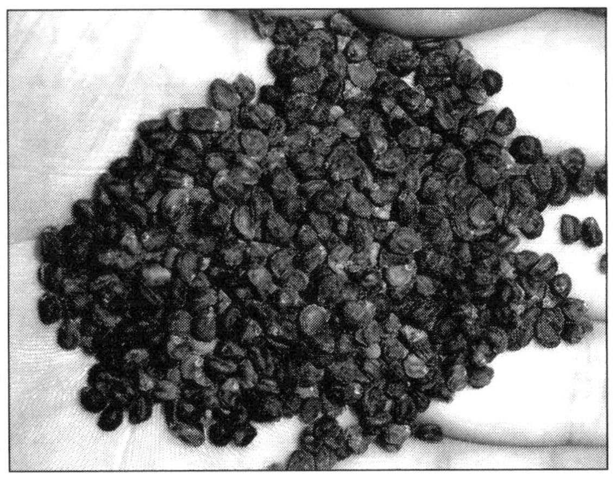

*Ololiuqui is a small, reddish-brown morning glory seed.*

with the spirits. The sacred seeds were kept in secret boxes or on the altar.[85]

Priest chroniclers, traveling with the conquistadors, provide the first western record of ololiuqui. These clerics were very disturbed by the Aztecs' ritual use of ololiuqui. The problem, in their view, was that the Aztecs venerated ololiuqui as a god one could pray to for miracles.

At least two Spaniards have left descriptions of the role of ololiuqui in Aztec culture. Francisco Salverio Clavigero, one of the Spanish chroniclers with the conquistadors, wrote this of ololiuqui seeds:

> "Besides the usual unction with ink another extraordinary and more abominable one was practiced every time they [the Aztec priests] went to make sacrifices on the tops of the mountains, or in the dark caverns of the earth. They took a large quantity of poisonous insects . . . burned them over some stove of the temple, and beat their ashes in a mortar together with the foot of the ocotl, tobacco, the herb Ololiuqui, and some live insects. They presented this diabolical mixture in small vessels to their gods, and afterwards rubbed their bodies with it. When thus anointed, they became fearless to every danger . . . . They called it Teopatli, or divine medicament, and imagined it to be a powerful remedy for several disorders; on which account those who were sick, and young children, went frequently to the priests to be anointed with it."[86]

In 1590, Joseph Acosta wrote this about ololiuqui:

> "By means of this ointment, they become witches and did see and speak the devil. The priests [meaning the Aztec priests] being slobbered with this ointment lost all fear."[87]

The Aztecs saw ololiuqui as a substance that confers special powers to mere mortals. One chronicler said, "They consult it as an oracle in order to learn many things . . . especially those things which are beyond the power of the human mind to penetrate."

Ololiuqui is described by Norman Taylor as inducing "a kind of hypnotic sleep or coma." The experience first begins with "hallucinations, sometimes preceded or punctuated by giddiness, but always leading to a kind of euphoric bliss."[88] Most Native Americans who have used ololiuqui and peyote admit that subsequent visions from both plants are pretty much the same.

Ololiuqui is still used today for both sacramental and medical purposes. Native Central Americans value the seeds as a painkiller. Whether or not ololiuqui's painkilling properties are real or imagined, Dr. Richard Evans Schultes, Harvard professor of ethnobiology, suggested that additional investigation was warranted. Be that as it may, many Native Americans believe that ololiuqui is not only curative, but provides spiritual insight, reveal life's meaning and other things "beyond the power of the human mind to penetrate."

The "curandero", a Central American and Southern Mexican neighborhood lay native healer, is similar to the Russian felcher but with strong mystical overtones. The curandero's healing power, much like shamans, relies on a belief system in his/her healing efforts. Because the ololiuqui seeds come from the curandero, there is the power of suggestion, which invests the seeds with a magic power. This combination of spirituality and placebo effect gives a healing affect which surely adds to any inherent medical benefit in the seeds.

As recent Western research has shown, incorporating spirituality, visualization and hope into treatment regimes can be beneficial.

## Mushrooms as Pagan Gods

The Psilocybe mushroom, *P. mexicana,* has been around as long as humanity. It was esteemed by the Mayans of eastern and southern Mexico as a holy sacrament. The Aztecs of central Mexico called the mushrooms *teonanactl*, "flesh of the gods" or "god's flesh". They considered these mushrooms divine and referred to their hallucinogenic trip as "the flowery dream."

Both the Mixtec of southwestern Mexico and Aztec cultures worshipped a god of psychoactive mushrooms. The Mixtec god was named Piltzintecuhtli (meaning Seven Flowers). The comparable Aztec god was Xochipilli, the Prince of Flowers, patron of "the flowery dream". Mushrooms were served with chocolate or honey during religious services. [89]

The Franciscan friar Bernardino de Sahagun reported the use of *teonanacatl* by the Aztecs. [90] De Sahagun had traveled to the New World in the mid-16th century and wrote about the Aztecs' use of hallucinogenic mushrooms in his *Florentine Codex*:

> **"The first thing to be eaten at the feast were small black mushrooms that they called *nanacatl* to bring on drunkenness, hallucinations and even lechery; they ate these before the dawn ... with honey; and when they began to feel the effects, they began to dance, some sang and others wept .... When the drunkenness of the mushrooms had passed, they spoke with one another of the visions they had seen."** [91, 92]

The Spanish clergy viewed the Aztec's claim that psilocybin-containing mushrooms were "God's flesh", as a blasphemous unholy communion. The Roman Catholicism of the invading conquistadors did not base its communion with the divine, or the spiritual, upon personally revealed knowledge or gnosis. Such spiritual communication was to be made through the rituals and structure of the Church.

R. Gordon Wasson, one of the first 20th-century ethno-botanists, cited 16th-century writers describing the divine role mushrooms played in the religion of the natives at the time the Spanish conquered Mexico. He wrote of the Catholic Church's systematic efforts to remove mushrooms' influence on everyday worship and spirituality. He coined the term "bemushroomed". This describes both the altered state induced by consuming these hallucinogenic mushrooms and their central role in the religion of the native peoples in the 16th century.

Wasson validated this religious experience of the Aztecs and others with a description of his own ingestion of spiritual mushrooms: [93]

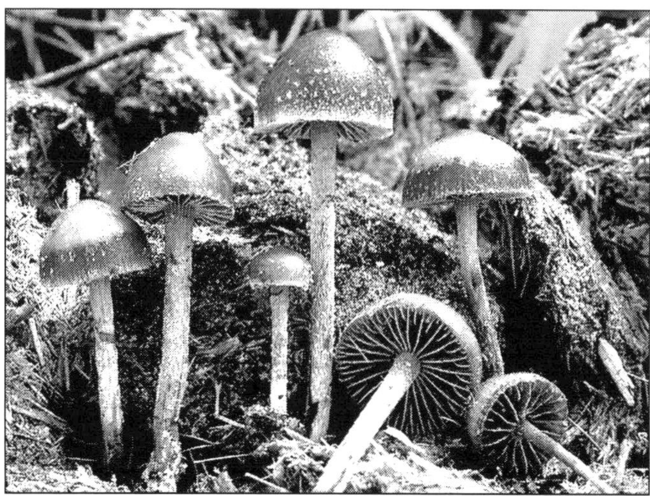

*Forty species of psilocybin mushrooms have been identified. They are found throughout Mesoamerica and beyond. They were one of several psychoactive ethnogens used in Aztec spiritual ceremonies.*

> "And all the time you are seeing these things, the priestess sings, not loud but with authority. Your body lies in the darkness, heavy as lead, but your spirit seems to soar and leave the hut, and with the speed of thought to travel where it wishes in time and space, accompanied by the shaman's singing and by the ejaculations of her percussive chant." [94]

Wasson's description of the effect of being bemushroomed continues:

> "The bemushroomed person is poised in space, a disembodied eye, invisible, incorporeal, seeing but not seen. In truth, he is the five senses disembodied, all of them keyed to the height of sensitivity and awareness, all of them blending into one another most strangely, until the person, utterly passive, becomes a pure receptor, infinitely delicate, of sensations. As your body lies there in its sleeping bag, your soul is free, loses all sense of time, alert as it never was before, living an eternity in a night, seeing infinity in a grain of sand. What you have seen and heard is cut as with a burn into your memory, never to be effaced." [95]

As recently as July 26, 2007, according to an on-line article in the *Wall Street Journal* and on *FoxNews*, mushrooms are still working their magic. In the reported study, researchers gave participants psilocybin cubensis. The patients reported such things as a sense of pure awareness and a merging with ultimate reality, a transcendence of time and space, a feeling of sacredness or awe, and deeply felt positive moods like joy, peace and love. People say, "they can't possibly put it into words," Dr. Griffiths, the head researcher, said: [96]

> **"Two months later, 24 of the participants filled out a questionnaire. Two-thirds called their reaction to psilocybin one of the five top most meaningful experiences of their lives. On another measure, one-third called it the most spiritually significant experience of their lives, with another 40 percent ranking it in the top five. About 80 percent said that because of the psilocybin experience, their sense of well-being or life satisfaction was raised either "moderately" or "very much."** [97]

These results are quite similar to what Timothy Leary, Ph.D., found in his psilocybin studies at Harvard in the 1960s.

Mushroom motifs and mushroom stones found on Mayan temple ruins document the important role mushrooms played in Mayan culture. The mushroom stone art objects were the *symbol of a religion*, like the cross in the Christian religion, the star of Judea for Judaism, or the crescent of the Muslims.

Catholic missionaries in their campaign against "pagan idolatry," soon forced mushroom ceremonies into secrecy by persecuting those who were caught using them. These mushroom stones and other motifs were viewed by the conquering Catholics as idols to pagan gods and they systematically destroyed them. The Spanish efforts to wipe out all aspects of Aztec religion included the use of the psilocybin mushroom. The mushroom gods were condemned by the Spanish as a devilish heresy.

Wasson points out that the religious use of the divine mushroom has "disquieting parallels" to elements of the Eucharist.[98] In the Eucharist, "Take, eat, this is my body...", and again "Grant us therefore, gracious Lord, so to eat the flesh of Thy dear son..." The orthodox Christian must accept, by faith, the miracle of the conversion of the bread into God's flesh: That is what is meant by the Doctrine of Transubstantiation. By contrast, the mushroom of the Aztecs carries its own conviction; every communicant will testify to the miracle that he has experienced."[99] This parallel was also true of some ritual use of peyote.

The Aztecs used psilocybin mushrooms, morning glory seeds and peyote to achieve altered states of spiritual awareness. The witches of the Middle Ages achieved similar mystical spiritual states using atropine-containing plants like datura, mandrake, henbane and belladonna, which contained deadly nightshade. The Spanish clerics had the same intense disgust toward the Aztecs' and their religious beliefs as they did toward those they accused of being satanic witches in medieval Europe.

The conquerors were eager to perpetuate their own ideology. The use of plants and fungi by the indigenous population of the New World to achieve spiritual oneness led to unremitting persecution by the dominant Spanish culture. And why not? This is the same response the pagans of Europe got for their heretical use of botanicals. The Aztec religion succumbed to this fate.

## Native Population Devastated by Europeans/American Genocide

The rediscovery of the Americans by the Europeans was bad news for the survival of the indigenous inhabitants. From Columbus' landing in 1492 until 1520, the population of Espanola (Santo Domingo) fell from approximately one million to only a scattered few.[100] At the time of Columbus' arrival, the Arawak/Taino population is variously estimated at anywhere from 100,000 to 4,000,000. A Catholic priest contemporary of the time estimated that 3,000,000 "Indians" died between 1494-1508.[101] It is documented that by 1507, when the Spanish did a census, the population of the native inhabitants was 60,000 and by 1531, the population was 600.[102]

Barbaric savagery contributed to the demise of the native population in Hispanola and elsewhere under Spanish rule. The Spanish enslaved hundreds of thousands of the native population. The conditions in servitude were abysmal. Torture was commonplace.

However, far and away the principle causes of death for the native inhabitants of the Americas were the European illnesses like smallpox, measles and malaria.

As Charles C. Mann documents in his 2005 book, *1491: New Revelations of the Americas Before Columbus*, the Americas had never before encountered these European diseases. Therefore, the Native Americans' immune system had not developed any resistance/immunity to these conditions. Decimation of the indigenous population played a major role in the European conquest of the New World. In some areas of the New World, up to 95% of the population died from infectious diseases heretofore unknown on the continents of North and South America.

Nevertheless, the sheer brutality and inhumanity of the Spanish toward the Native inhabitants was impressive. Some inhabitants of the Americas were killed in battle, others by the deceit of the European adventurers. One illustrative incident was when the Spanish threw a feast for the local indigenous leadership. When several hundred of the natives were in the wooden structure where the feast was ostensibly to be held, the armed Spanish left the hall, closed the doors behind them, surrounded the building with soldiers, set the place on fire, and burned the heathens alive.

The Spaniards believed that their behavior was justified by (1) their religious beliefs, (2) having the power to impose their will, and (3) the benefits of the riches to be had by exploiting the mineral and agricultural riches of the New World.

> "The discovery of precious-ore deposits led to further exploitation of the natives. War, disease, overwork, and suicide caused the population of the Antilles to sink like a rock in deep water. Historians have estimated the decline as proceeding from 300,000 in 1492 to 60,000 in 1508, 46,000 in 1510, 20,000 in 1512, and 14,000 in 1514; a Catholic priest who lived through it figured that fully three million Indians had died between 1494 and 1508, comprising one of the worst genocides in recorded history." [103]
>
> **Scott Christianson**
> *With Liberty For Some: 500 Years of Imprisonment in America,* 1998

At least one Spaniard, Bartolomé de las Casas (1484-1566), was appalled by what was happening to the indigenous population. A Dominican priest, he had been appointed by the king to be the Bishop of Chiapas. He vowed to secure "the justice for those Indian peoples, and to condemn the robbery, evil and injustice committed against them".

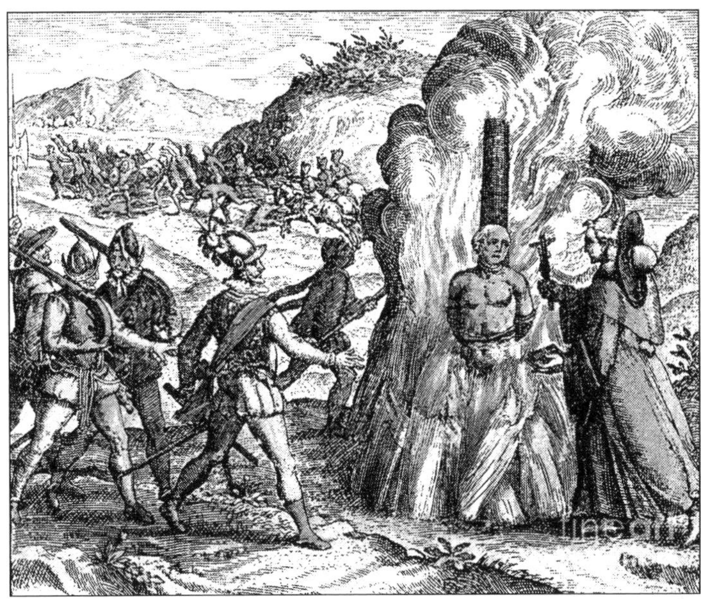

*Many indigenous Americans died by fire. Bartolomé de las Casas, a Dominican priest, is shown here blessing the soul of one unlucky Indian.*

His solution was the usual illogic of the Europeans. He implored his King to introduce Negroes from Guinea as slaves to replace the native workers. He argued that "the labour of one Negro was more valuable than that of four Indians." His argument persuaded the King. Slaves from Africa began arriving a few months later with the King's blessing. Starting in 1517, four thousand Negroes were imported to the West Indies over the next eight years. [104]

The Spanish applied the same rigid, Inquisition-attitude toward religion to the Americas that prevailed at that time in Spain. The inhabitants of the New World weren't Christian and so this made them less worthy, less human, less valued. This was no different than in Spain of that time. There the choice was between retaining your religion and being put to death, or converting to Catholicism and living. In many instances, the Native populations of the Americas weren't given that choice.

## Did Our American Forebears Commit Genocide?

Native American labor was used by the Spanish to search for and mine gold and silver. The New World had significant slave raiding and slavery. Nicaragua lost 200,000 native Americans to slave traders in the first half of the 16th century. The slavers sold their human merchandise in the islands of the Caribbean, Panama and Peru. In 1560, there were 40,000 Native American slaves in northeastern Brazil alone. In all, at least 350,000 Native Americans were slaves in Brazil during the period of Brazilian slavery. [105]

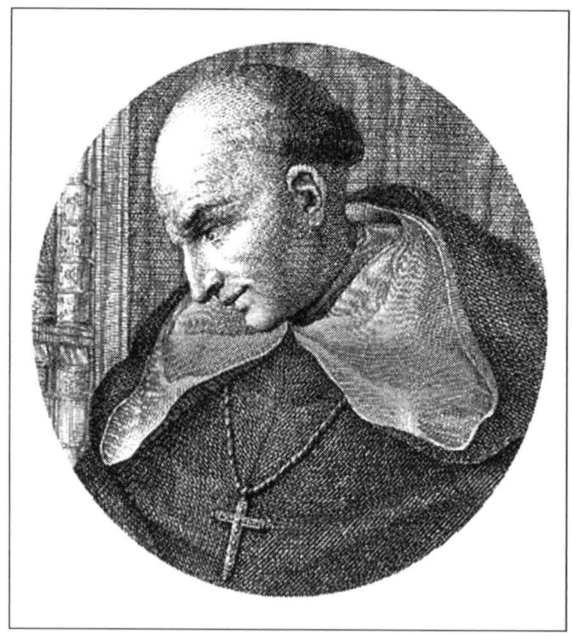

*Spanish Bishop Bartolomé de las Casas showed great sympathy toward the indigenous Americans but became partially responsible for the origin of the slave trade from Africa to the New World.*

The Natives fared little better under the British and other European colonists than they did under the Spanish. The genocide of the original Americans initiated by the Spanish continued unabated under the English. In *American Colonies: The Settling of North America* (2002), Alan Taylor demythologizes colonial history. [106] He shreds the view that English colonialism in North America was some "exceptional" moral exercise. On the contrary, one reviewer of his book called the English colonial experience in America an "uncanny artifact of moral, political and intellectual decay."

Taylor endorses John Murrin's claim that "most American colonies were founded by terrorists." [107] By this reference, he means the barbaric tactics Europeans used to conquer the people that they had found upon their arrival. Taylor puts death, disease and violence to Indians at the center of what early America was all about. [108]

When the Europeans arrived, North, South and Central America had a combined population of over 50 million people. North America alone had more than eight million Native Americans, possibly as many as 12 million. [109] This demise of the indigenous people of the Americas hastened the "need" to import slaves and indentured servants.

By the 19th century, Americans of European descent had a vision of Manifest Destiny. Manifest Destiny was the idea that the Europeans who populated America were destined to occupy all the land "from sea to shining sea." The Indians of the Great Plains were just in the way. The last quarter of the 19th century was pretty much open season on the "Red Man". By the late 1890s, there were fewer than 900,000 indigenous people left in North America. [110]

The carnage wrought on native peoples in South and Central America was similar if not greater than in North America. In lower and upper Peru, the population from the 16th century to the late 18th century declined from five million to 300,000. [111] The native populations of Mesoamerica and South American had 25-35 million people when the Spanish arrived. By its low point of 1650, the population of Mesoamerica had fallen to 1.5 million. [112]

Through disease, "demonization", iron weaponry, horses, and dumb luck, the Europeans wreaked havoc on the American native population. The Europeans prevailed even though in many ways the indigenous populations of the Americas were more advanced than the invaders. Nevertheless, these great indigenous American civilizations were soon obliterated.

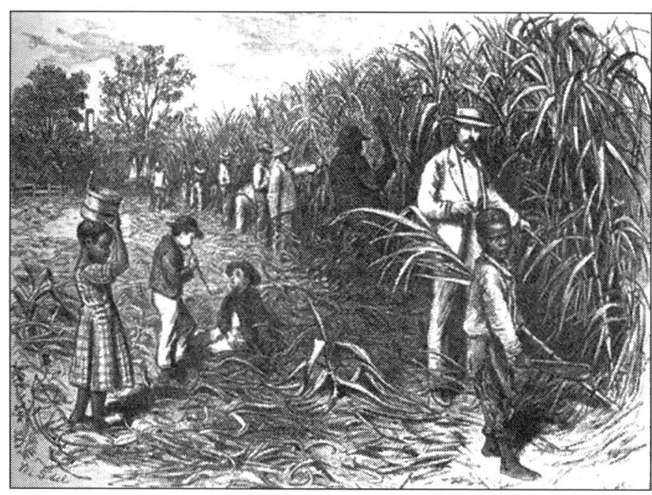

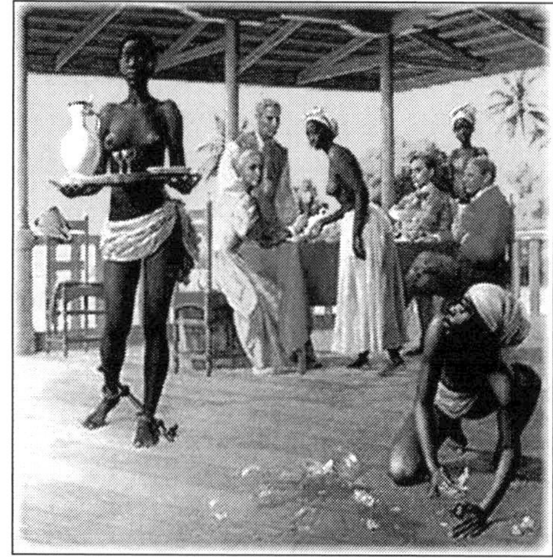

*From the cane fields to serving the rum, slaves were the energy fueling the economic engine of the New World.*

# CHAPTER VI
# 1500-1863:
# Mercantilism, Triangular Trade, Slavery

## Mercantilism

During the 16th, 17th, and 18th centuries, Mercantilism was the European world's accepted economic philosophy or policy. Mercantilism contained many rather disparate elements, but it boiled down to this: the value of a nation's exports must exceed the value of its imports, and you must get paid in – and accumulate – gold and silver. Mercantilists believed that a nation's wealth was determined by the amount of bullion it had, so a positive balance of trade was very important. Having colonies whose wealth you could appropriate made you a mercantilism "winner."

Jean Bodin, the 16th-century author of a secular witch-hunting manual, was also a politician, scholar and advisor to the French King. He was apparently more interested in advocating Mercantilism rather than in furthering Christianity. Bodin promoted Mercantilism and developed the economic theories of inflation and political economy.[1] Ironically, his writing was a forerunner to Adam Smith's anti-Mercantilist economic theories.

Under Mercantilism, exploitation of colonies was considered a legitimate method of increasing the wealth of the parent country. This exploitation called for having a ready source of resources and cheap labor. Raw materials were to be exported by the colonists and finished goods were to be imported from the mother country. Local colonial manufacture of finished goods was discouraged. The colonies were getting the short end of the economic stick. When colonies built up industries the parent country tried to hobble them to stifle any manufacturing competition which might arise. With that arrangement, it's not surprising colonial opposition developed to mercantilist practices.

American colonial dissatisfaction with the mercantilist practices of England contributed to fomenting the American Revolution. After the Revolution, the United States adopted a new economic policy called *laissez-faire*. Laissez-faire economics favored limited government control and promoted a philosophy of free trade, allowing those involved in industry and trade to determine what was best for the economy. This philosophy was first defined in the 1776 book, *The Wealth of Nations*, by Adam Smith, considered by many to be the first great economist. His chief objective was showing that mercantilism is a bad idea. He believed that the real wealth of a nation is in its ability to produce goods and services.

## Tobacco, Slavery, Alcohol and Triangular Trade

America was literally founded on drugs. By the late 16th century, tobacco, a plant native to the Western hemisphere, was a part of the Mercantile trade. It quickly joined a host of other agricultural commodities exported to Europe. Tobacco was well known to the Native Americas. Its use in the Americas goes back at least to the time of Christ. [2] It has been consumed through drinking, chewing, snuffing, licking and smoking. Tobacco has a central role in Indian mythology, religion and medicine. It was used to contact the spirits as part of purification ceremonies and medicinally as an emetic and poltice. [3] The Aztecs used it in their human sacrifice ceremonies.

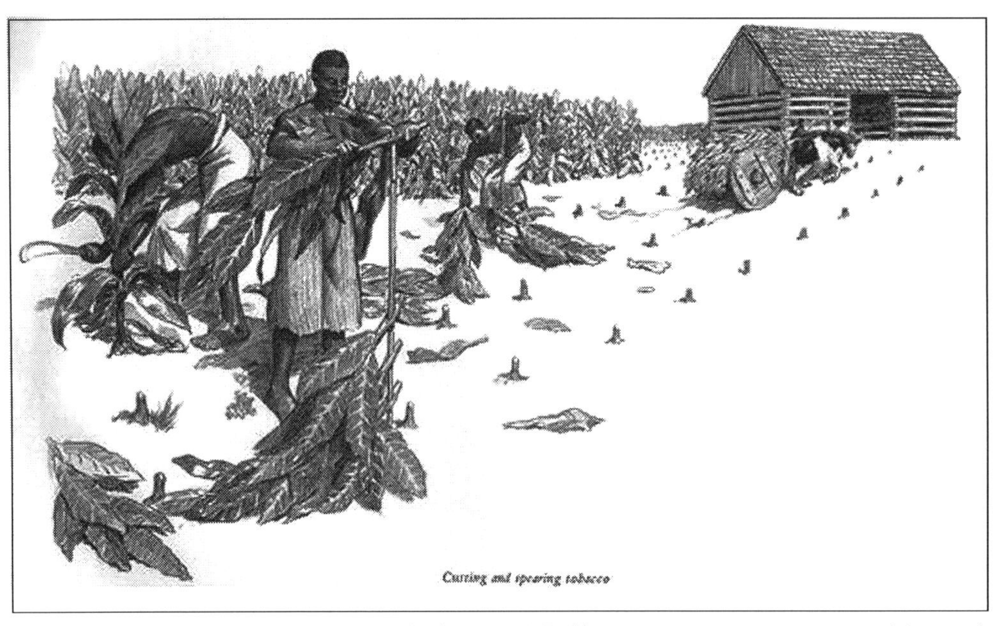


*As a result of slavery tobacco, sugar and other New World crops were economic winners in Mercantilism. Slaves were the fuel that ran America's economic engine. In the early years of colonization, slaves came from the indigenous population, Ireland or Africa.*

Andre Thevet is credited with being the first to bring tobacco seeds from the New World to Europe, transporting the seeds from Brazil to France in 1556. But, it was the much better connected Jean Nicot de Villeau I, who introduced tobacco to the French court a few years later, for whom nicotine is named. [4] To be clear, Europeans had smoked other plant material before tobacco. Tobacco, a New World plant, was something new and different.

Tobacco was introduced into England in 1586 and, notwithstanding the harsh opposition of King James I, quickly became popular. In "A Counterblast to Tobacco" written in 1597, King James described tobacco as "a custome lathsome to the eye, hateful to the nose, harmeful to the braine, dangerous to the lungs, and the blacke stinking fume thereof, nearest resembling the horrible stygian come of the pit that is bottomlesse." [5] The King managed to find some comfort by putting heavy taxes on tobacco and generating substantial funds for the Royal coffers.

Tobacco soon hit the big time. By 1614, there were 7,000 tobacco shops and outlets in London alone. [6]

Tobacco earned its popularity in part, due to the belief that smoking it could effectively prevent the plague. [7] With those 6000 to 7000 tobacco shops in London, it naturally seemed like a profitable idea to get over to the Colonies and plant some more tobacco. By 1619, Virginia was exporting 40,000 pounds of tobacco to England. [8] Tobacco was so valuable that 40 pounds of tobacco bought you a bride from England.

In 1619, the first African slaves were sold in Virginia. John Rolf wrote in his diary, "About the last of August came a Dutch man of ware that sold us twenty Negars (sic)." [9] Tobacco, hemp, and alcohol all played key economic roles in the colonies. Soon the economy was heavily reliant on slavery.

History has proven King James and many other critics of tobacco correct. Tobacco kills over 400,000 people each year in the United States alone. The British medical journal, *Lancet*, estimates that tobacco is the cause of death for twenty percent of the people in the developed world. [10] Yale law professor Steven B. Duke, who wrote *America's Longest War: Rethinking Our Tragic Crusade Against*

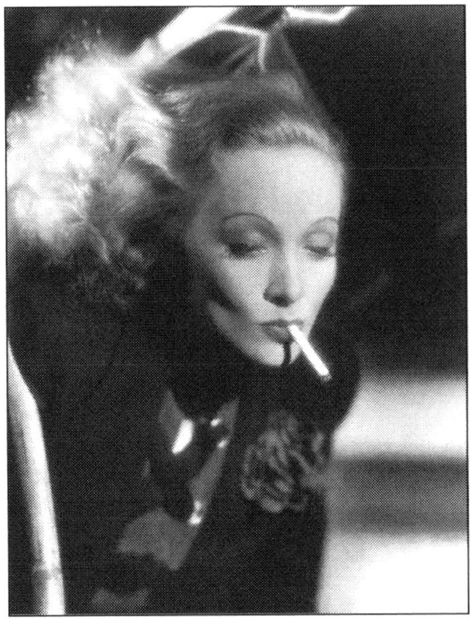

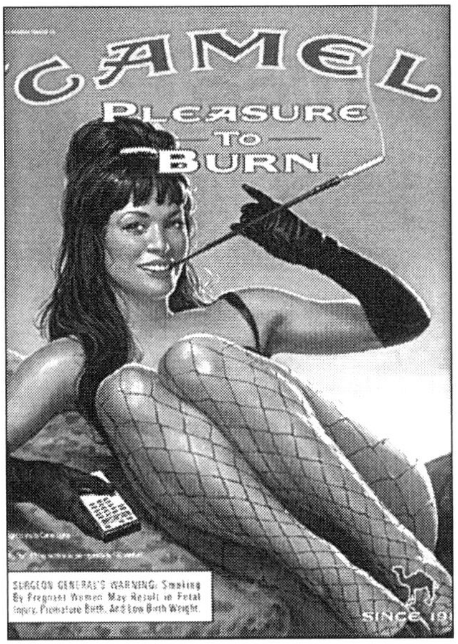


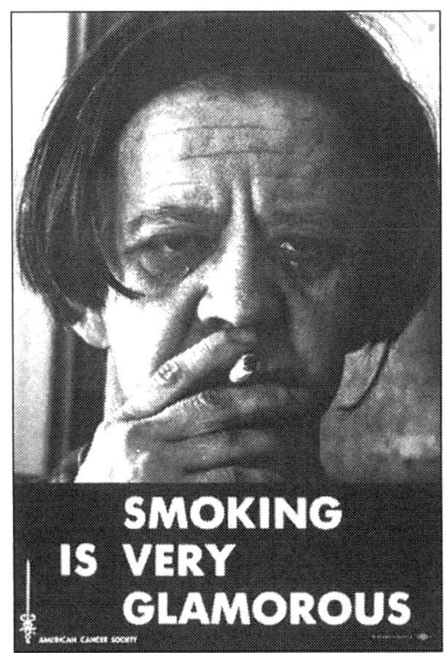


*A woman was considered a lot sexier in the '50s if a cigarette was in her hand or dangling from her lip. The "Smoking is Very Glamorous" poster at the far right was used in the 1980s as a clever bit of counter-advertising.*

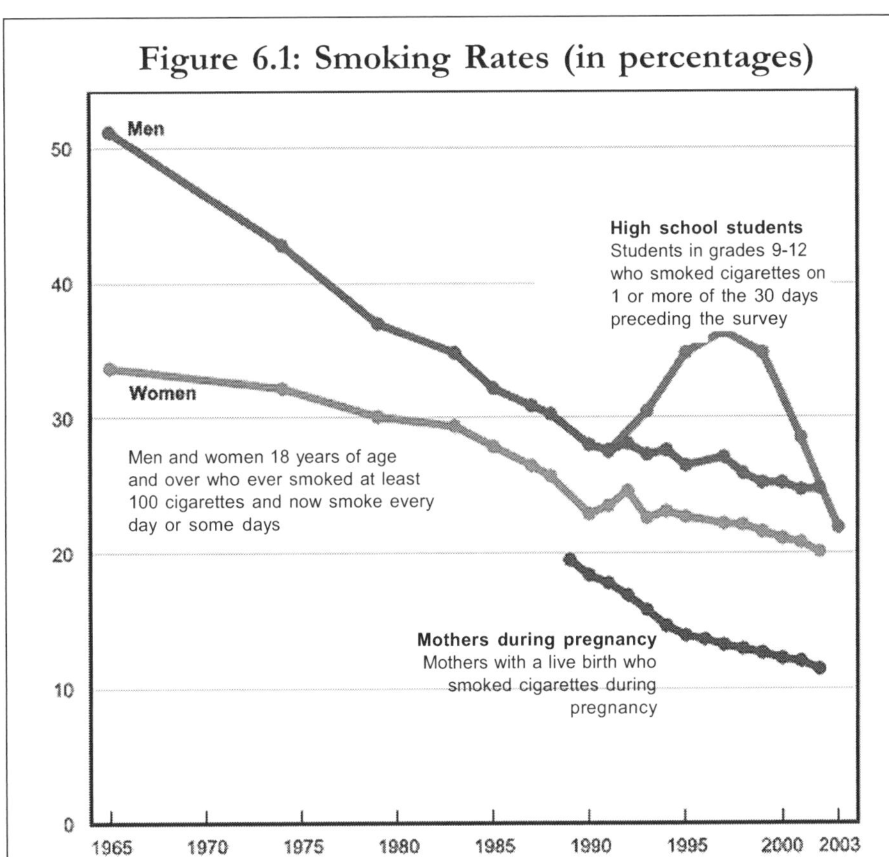


*Big tobacco was undercut by the 1964 Surgeon General's report linking tobacco smoking to lung cancer. This chart shows the effect of explaining the facts and respecting people's judgment. Motivating people to get treatment, having treatment readily available and having a tax (a tax, by the way, that may be a deterrent to starting smoking but is not an excuse to criminalize the drug), has had a noticeable effect on decreasing tobacco use in the United States in the past fifty years.* [12]

*Drugs* (1993), believes, "Our biggest, worst drug problem is the tobacco problem." [11]

The contemporary approach to the scientifically proven health menace of tobacco is instructive. Effective ways to deal with this most addicting drug have been developed. The United States has increased taxes, which discourages the young from starting to smoke by making cigarettes expensive to buy. Research clearly and unequivocally demonstrates the adverse health effects of tobacco smoking, and the government has widely disseminated that information.

Federal law requires tobacco product packaging to carry warnings of the health consequences of tobacco. Local and state health departments in the United States use the media to warn people of tobacco's proven health dangers. Believable, scientifically accurate counter-advertising has proven particularly effective in decreasing tobacco use. Also, there are a variety of treatment methods for tobacco addiction which are readily available and widely advertised. Some are even subsidized by taxes and lawsuit settlement dollars from cigarette companies.

For many years alcohol abuse policy has been transitioning from a criminal to a medical approach. Presently the alcohol policy of the United States is a hybrid of medical and criminal approaches. Even now funding still tilts toward a criminal justice approach.

U.S. governmental policies have created daunting barriers to providing adequate treatment modalities and opportunities for those whose substance problems include consumption of opiates, cocaine, and other illicit drugs.

---

**"The Drug War has arguably been the single most devastating, dysfunctional social policy since slavery."** [13]

**Norm Stamper**

Seattle Police Chief (ret.), Spring 2006

---

The United States needs to learn from its relatively successful approach to decreasing tobacco use. Mostly truthful education, high taxes and removing the glamour of smoking has had some positive effect at lowering rates of tobacco use. The government has not arrested and jailed hundreds of thousands of tobacco "addicts" in an effort to address this very serious and costly public health problem. But there are cities where one may not smoke in public.

## The Invention of the White Race

Prior to the 18th century, the English mainly enslaved non-Christians or the Irish. They did not particularly target Africans. Slaves came from the ranks of the conquered and the poor. This is not to say that Europeans did not have African slaves prior to the colonization of the Americas. They did, but prior to slavery here in the New World the status of slave was not necessarily one that was life-long. In most cases, a slave could become free by converting to Christianity.

The first Virginia colonists did not even think of themselves as "white" or use that word to describe themselves. They saw themselves as Christian or Englishmen, or in terms of their social class. They were nobility, gentry, artisans, or servants. **Race was a concept introduced in the 17th and 18th century to justify slavery.** [14]

Most scholars agree that "whiteness" is a historical rather than a biological category. In Theodore W. Allen's *The Invention of the White Race* (1998), he makes the case that the concept of race is not biological, nor a concept born of biology, but a concept related to power and economic control. He says:

> ***"...eminent authorities in the fields of physical anthropology, genetics and biology, such as Stanley M. Garn and Theodosius Dobzhansky, state that the study of evolution has nothing but disclaimers to contribute to the understanding of 'racism' as a historical phenomenon. As Dobzhansky puts it: 'The mighty vision of human equality belongs to the realm of ethics and politics, not to that of biology.'*** [15] ***With greater particularity, Garn writes that Race 'has nothing to do with racism, which is simply the attempt to deny some people deserved opportunities simply because of their origin, or to accord other people certain undeserved opportunities only because of their origin."*** [16, 17]

Professor George M. Frederickson of Stanford University, a noted teacher and writer on the history of relations between Blacks and Europeans, says that "the proposition that race is 'a social and cultural construction,' has become an academic cliché." [18]

Allen states that "the "white race" must be understood, not simply as a social construct, but as a *ruling class, social control formation* and an exercise of power. He quotes socio-biologist and historian Carl N. Degler, "...blacks will be discriminated against whenever nonblacks have the power and incentive to do so, because it is human to have prejudice against those who are different."[19] And so it appears to be with the Drug War.

Allen lays out his view of essential social structure in class societies. He defines the ruling class as that part of society which has "control of the organs of state power, and has maintained domination of the national economy through successive generations and social crises." He sees this class as being "able to limit the options of social policy in such a way as to perpetuate its hegemony over the society as a whole."[20]

## Race

The notion that humans are divided into biologically well-defined groups associated with skin color – is a relatively modern historical concept. It is a concept with no scientific basis. The idea was developed for economic and philosophical reasons to justify the slavery in the New World and more specifically the U.S., where "all men are created equal." Previous to the major reliance on black slaves, we humans had slavery but slaves' status was not based on race. Even Jesus said, "Treat your slaves well."

Prior to the origin of race as a concept, there were several principle categories for division within humanity: civilization and barbarism, or Christianity and heathenism, or English and non-English, upper and lower class to name the most common. Race meant language, custom and law, not skin color or other biological, anthropological differences.

The English disdained all alien peoples, but this does not mean they saw all English people as equal to one another. England was a hierarchical society. It was generally believed (certainly by the upper classes), that the English were justly and naturally separated into superior and inferior levels and that members of different statuses enjoyed varying degrees of freedom. When it came to the Irish the British practiced extreme racial and religious discrimination.[21] To the British, the Irish were of a lower echelon of evolutionary development.

Eric Foner claims that it was only after the American Revolution that the concept of race needed to emerge. There had to be "an explanation for the existence of slavery in a land that proclaimed that all men were created equal." A democratic republic required justification for slavery, and racism was it."[22] So at bottom it was the demand for cheap labor that led to slavery. According to Barbara J. Fields, the founders of the United States needed to justify the incongruity, illogic and cognitive dissonance between our Declaration of Independence proclaiming all men are created equal and our laws ensuring property rights, which said it's okay to own Black slaves. Racism and the invention of the white race was an effort to make the incompatible, compatible. In "Slavery, Race and Ideology in the United States of America" (1990), Fields wrote, "Whatever truths have appeared self-evident in those days, neither an inalienable right to life and liberty nor the founding government on the consent of the governed was among them ... Neither white skin nor English nationality protected servants from the grossest forms of brutality and exploitation."[23]

Fields states that the ideology of race came at a "discernable historical moment for rationally understandable historical reasons."[24] She also sees the American Revolution as this moment of the invention of race: "American racial ideology is as original an invention as is the United States itself. Those holding liberty to be inalienable and holding Afro-Americans as slaves were bound to end by holding race to be a self-evident truth."[25]

This illogical "logic" required lots of buttressing. The concept of so-called "inferior races" was a significant buttress. Herein is the very essentials of "demonization" of the human existence: cleanliness, organizational and leadership skills, work habits, sexual lust, religion, recreational drugs -- what have you. This "demonization" became a necessary part of American thinking. It helped justify the unjustifiable.

## Indentured Servants Can Be Troublemakers

Many of the colonists who came to the Americas from Europe were dirt poor. Those immigrants who could not pay for the long, treacherous journey to America, indentured themselves to wealthier colonists – selling their services usually for a period of years, in return for the price of the passage. When their ships landed after the trans-Atlantic voyage, those who had paid for their passage or gave good security could leave. Those without the means to pay remained on board the ships. They stayed until they were purchased, and then were released to their purchasers. [26]

The institution of slavery, and more specifically racial slavery, in colonial America did not happen all at once. The American colonial world moved from indentured servitude to slavery to racial slavery over at least a century. In the early years of the colonies, many Africans and poor whites – most of the laborers came from the English working class – were equal as indentured servants. During their time as servants, they were fed and housed. After the indentureship they got a piece of land, supplies, a gun, and were free.

The moneyed classes soon found that indentured servants were costly and potentially dangerous. First indentured servants moved on to be unindentured. This created an obvious need for costly replacements. Secondly, former indentured servants could become unruly. In 1676 during Bacon's Rebellion, working class men, many former indentured servants, burned down Jamestown. This rebellion made having work performed through indentured servitude look decidedly less attractive to Virginia leaders than having slaves do the work. Slaves, especially ones you could identify by skin color, could not move on to become free and competitors could not rise up against you politically or militarily, at least not very easily.

## The Negro Child of an Englishmen is Not a Slave. What?

The institution of "Negro" slavery was threatened in 1656 by the Elizabeth Key decision in Virginia. Key was the child of an African-American bond servant mother and an English-American father. When Key's father left for England, the arrangement was that her godfather was to *possess* her for nine years and then she was to be freed. Both her father and godfather died and the executors of her godfather's estate ruled that because her mother was a lifetime bond servant, Key was too. [27]

This decision was overturned by the Virginia General Assembly who applied traditional English Common Law. In English Common Law, your condition -- free or slave -- depends upon the status of your father, not your mother. Furthermore, Key was a Christian. It was therefore illegal to hold her for life since obviously this would make her a slave and a Christian could not be a slave. Had the principles established in this case prevailed, racial slavery would not have gotten a foothold in the United States. [28]

So, here was a conflict as to whether Christian principles and English Common Law trumped the profitability of agriculture. They didn't. A few years later the Virginia General Assembly responded to the decision in the Key's case by passing a law that stated that whether a person was a Christian or not did not alter the person's condition as it related to bondage. Allen says, "the solution was to establish a new birthright not only for Anglos but for every Euro-American, the white identity that 'set them apart at a distance....'" [29]

The 1705 declaration passed by the Virginia Assembly stated:

> **"All servants imported and brought into the Country ... who were not Christians in their native Country ... shall be accounted and be slaves. All Negro, mulatto and Indian slaves within this dominion ... shall be held to be real estate. If any slave resists his master ... correcting such slave, and shall happen to be killed in such correction ... the master shall be free of all punishment ... as if such accident never happened."** [30]

This action was important. It addressed the problem exposed by Bacon's Rebellion. Bacon's insurrection demonstrated that when you had poor European-Americans workers who were not in lifetime bonded servitude, you could create a disgruntled, easily aroused underclass. The financial and class status of those freed from their indentured servitude was indeed humble. This created a skewed playing field which made it difficult for former indentured servants to compete with the gentry class. Recognition of this competitive disadvantage naturally caused many former indentured servants to align themselves with the lifetime bond servants regardless of so-called race.

This was potentially dangerous to the colonial power elite. If this alliance were allowed to occur it could undermine the economic advantage and power of the colonial agriculture and power elite. But by denying all African-Americans of their liberties, the plantation power structure was able to say to the poorest European-American in Virginia that although they did not own bond-laborers, they were still part of the elite in that they "*enjoyed*" privileges that were denied to African-Americans, *free or slave.*

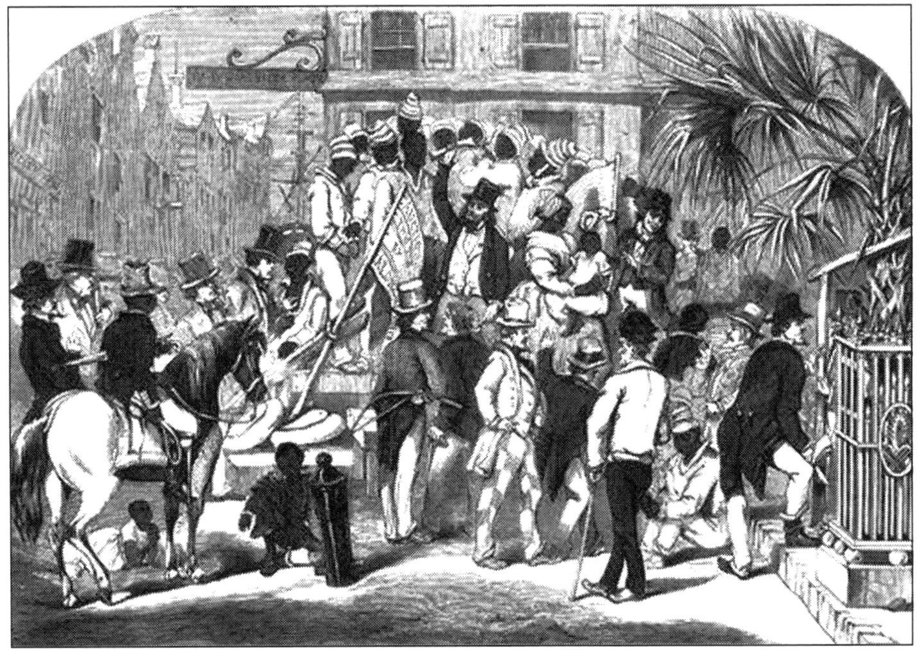

*Here is a drawing of a typical slave sale of our fellow humans.*

> **"With racial slavery, you now had a permanent dependent labor force, who could be defined as a people set apart. They were racially set apart. They were outsiders. They were strangers and in many ways throughout the world, slavery has taken root, especially where people are considered outsiders and can be put in a permanent status of slavery.** [31]
>
> **David Blight**
> Historian

## How to Determine Who's Black?

It took awhile to figure out who was Black and who wasn't. Until the 1830s, 19th century accounts of slavery in Journals and Diaries invariably included references to "white" slaves in the South. These were not the Irish we referred to earlier, but were people who were of mixed European and African ancestry who had light complexions.

The case of one Polly Gray, a fair-complexioned biracial woman from Hamilton County, Ohio, illustrates the early 19th-century practice of using appearance as *THE* factor in assigning race. [32] In the fall of 1829, Gray was convicted of robbery based on the testimony of a dark-complexioned, admittedly Negro, witness. At that time Ohio statutes forbade Blacks from testifying against Whites. So, the rather aptly named Ms. Gray understandably appealed to the Supreme Court of Ohio on the grounds that she was White.

The prevailing legal rule was that physical appearance decided which side of the color line someone was on. Jurists of the day reasoned that appearance was the only legal way to decide. Her attorney argued that, despite Ms. Gray's having some small bit of African ancestry, it was irrelevant since she clearly looked more European than African. So, her attorney argued that the rule in effect in Ohio at the time, the rule of physical appearance, meant that the African/European Gray was legally White. Demonstrating that this was indeed the standard of the day, the prosecutor, a Mr. Wade, agreed with the defense attorney on that standard. [33]

But the prosecutor argued that Mulattos were a separate case. He argued that "White" in the law, did not apply to Mulattos. He noted that Ms. Gray was "a shade of color between the mulatto and white". Therefore Ms. Gray was too "cafe au lait" complexioned to be considered White. [34]

The Ohio Supreme Court agreed with the defense that the rule of physical appearance was the only criterion for determining a person's racial identity in Ohio. They wrote "We are unable to set out any different races. Color alone is sufficient." [35]

**In January of 1831, the court ruled that: "We believe a man, of a race nearer white than a mulatto ... should partake in the privileges**

**of whites. We are of opinion that a party of such a blood is entitled to the privileges of whites, partly because we are unwilling to extend the disabilities of the statute further than its letter requires, and partly from the difficulty of defining and of ascertaining the degree of duskiness which renders a person liable to such disabilities."** [36]

So now the question was where to draw the line. How white was white enough to be considered White. But that was it. It is the last appeals case in the free states where either side argued that an invisible trace of African blood should be taken into account. After 1831, it was pretty much one drop of African ancestry and you were considered a Negro.

### It Became OK to Convert Non-Christian Slaves to Christianity

European slaveholders in North America were not originally motivated to convert non-Christian slaves to Christianity. "The fact that the slaves were 'pagans' was moral justification enough for slavery. They were not 'Christians', and in those days 'Christian' meant 'human'. People who were not 'Christian' were inferior beings." [37]

But a Methodist and Baptist revival -- the "Great Awakening" -- starting in 1734 in Massachusetts, generated a creative new justification for slavery: slavery was justified because it was a means to save the pagans from certain damnation. Now "the conversion of pagans ... became not only welcomed but later even mandatory." [38]

## Coffee – Just Add Plantations, Slaves, Sugar and Stir

That Starbucks favorite, coffee, has accounted for imperialism, warfare, colonial subjugation, and terrible slavery. The economic success of coffee, like so many New World commodities, revolved around the plantation system.

The stimulatory properties of the coffee bean are thought to have been discovered in Ethiopia around 1000 AD. One story has it that a goat herder named Kahli noted his goats were energized after eating the red berries of the coffee bush. Soon he was brewing the beans up in hot water, drinking it and feeling the stimulating affects of caffeine himself.

By about 1100 AD, Arabs were roasting and boiling coffee beans making "qahwa" what we now call coffee. Coffee took the place of Khat, a stimulant herb that is chewed. Soon, coffee was available in monasteries and inns. By the 1200s, there were public coffee houses, known as "Qahueh khanen" on the Arabian peninsula. Another story tells of Sheik Omar buying coffee seedlings from Ethopia [39] and bringing them to Mocha in Arabia in 1258. Soon coffee houses flourished in Arabia.

These coffeehouses soon became social centers. Much as today, people would sit and gossip over a cup of coffee. Sultan Amurat III had murdered all his brothers to gain power. He noted there was too much talk at coffeehouses about his accession to the throne. He handled that by closing down the coffeehouses and having the proprietors tortured.

His successor, Mahomet IV, reopened the coffeehouses, although he wasn't crazy about the conversation at the coffeehouses either. Customers whose conversation Mahomet had a particular distaste for were thrown into the Bosporus after he had them sewn into leather sacks. It did not deter coffee drinking, but the conversation was apparently a little less political. [40]

The first known coffee shop outside Arabia opened in Turkey in July of 1475. It wasn't until 1600, that Italian traders introduced coffee to the West. It took a while for coffee to catch on in Europe. Concern about the devil caused some hesitation. Early Christians claimed coffee was the drink of the devil. Pope Vincent III had the presence of mind to drink the stuff before banishing it. He allegedly stated that "coffee is so delicious it would be a pity to let the infidels have exclusive use of it." To make coffee an acceptable Christian beverage, Pope Vincent III baptized it. [41]

Coffee joined other exotic imported commodities. It, too, contributed to the expansion of trade across the globe. [42] From the 16th to the 19th century, coffee's popularity continued to expand in the West. In 1607, John Smith introduced coffee to Jamestown. [43] By the late 1700s, over 19 million coffee trees grew on the Island of Montserrat. Eventually the rest of tropical Central and South America became home to coffee plantations. [44]

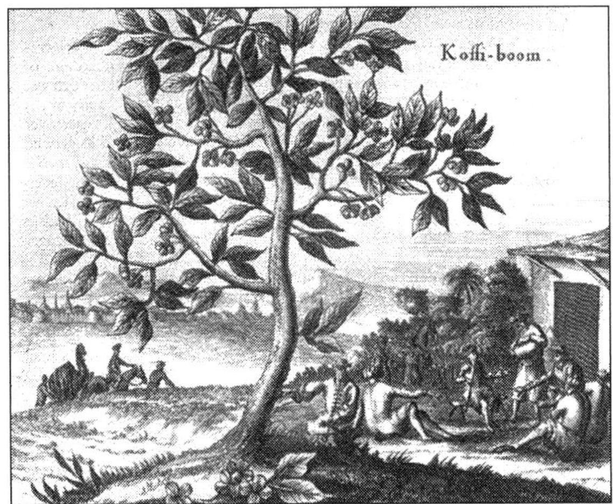


*Coffee was another drug crop that was part of the mercantile system of trade.*

## With Cheap, Forced or Slave Labor, European Nations Made a Profit Off the Commodities from the Colonies

By the 19th century, coffee, like tea, spices and chocolate, was an important part of the colonial systems' coercive labor, exploitive land use, resource extraction, and commodity trade. [45] By 1835, 217 million pounds of coffee came from far-flung colonies like Yemen, Abyssinia, Haiti, Brazil, and Java, into the imperial ports of Europe, from Amsterdam to Marseilles, and including London to Genoa and Trieste. And, to sweeten the coffee, nearly one billion pounds of sugar was imported. [46]

Much of Europe was involved in the intercontinental commodities trade. Italy and France dominated the trans-European trade in coffee. The British monarchs chartered companies to import tea from India, Ceylon, and China. Spain dominated the importation of maize and chocolate from Mexico. The Dutch employed forced labor in Sumatra and Java to produce spices and coffee. [47] Omani Sultans and later Portuguese, German, and the British military occupations, converted the Swahili coastal city-state Zanzibar, into a massive slave plantation for the production of highly prized spices.

Slaves were the low cost, muscle energy that produced the crops for the America's booming commodity export trade. Slaves grew, harvested and loaded the cocoa, coffee, tobacco and the versatile hemp. They were "required" to meet the need created by increased European consumption of these products. They helped to slake the Europeans' thirst for coffee. As European demand for coffee rose, the slaves grew even more coffee to help meet that demand.

Commodity exports from the New World to Europe increased dramatically in the 18th century. Coffee exports went from 2 million to 120 million pounds, chocolate exports went from 2 million to 13 million pounds and tobacco went from 50 million to 125 million pounds. [48] Hemp was so necessary to England that it was mandated to be grown in the colonies. [49]

## Sugar: Not Only Fattening but ...

The history of sugar's popularity, production and consumption provides insight into the inter-related issues of economics, human rights, slavery, environmental degradation, health, alcohol consumption, drug policy, and consumerism. While tobacco may have initiated slavery in the United States., it wasn't tobacco, or even indigo or cotton, that was the main engine driving slavery in the Americas. No, it was sugar cane, the sugar refining and the plantation system that shaped the economy and society in Brazil, the West Indies and later the United States. [50]

These choices of commercial enterprise have hidden costs and impacts on society. The moral opprobrium of slavery and the racism that followed (which remains evident to this day), were the hidden costs of U.S. reliance on slavery to propel the colonial and post American Revolution economic engine. Similarly, today it is clear that the choice of fuel to run the internal combustion engine had significant hidden costs. Had ethanol (which can be made more efficiently from sugar cane or hemp hurds than from corn) been the fuel of choice, as Henry Ford and other Detroit moguls of the 1920s expected, or biodiesel as Rudolph Diesel had designed his diesel engine to run on, it is unlikely the United States would have become enmeshed in a military intervention in Iraq in the early 21st century.

Between 1663 and 1775, the consumption of muscovado sugar (i.e., unrefined, brown sugar) in England and Wales increased twenty-fold. The commercial demand for sugar came not only from its uses as a sweetener, but also to ferment it into alcohol. British rum consumption rose from the 207 gallons imported in 1698 to an annual average of two million gallons in the years 1771 to 1775, [51] thus contributing to the "need" for greater sugar production.

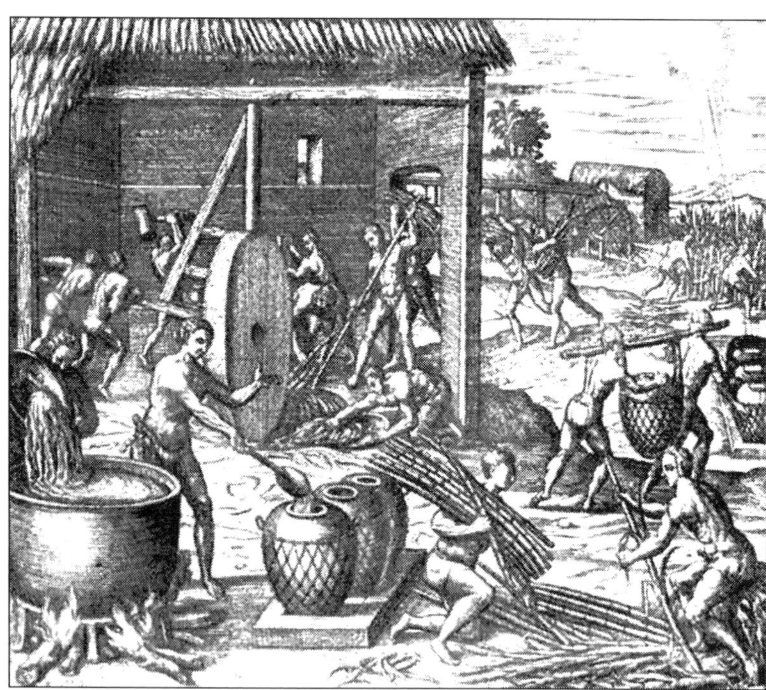

*Sugar was the crop that was inextricably involved in establishing slavery in the Americas. By any definition, sugar is a drug and also a principal raw material in the making of rum.*

The American plantation agricultural system was built on the model developed in Madeira and the Canary Islands. These islands were colonized during the last half of the fifteenth century, and sugar cane and the resultant plantations were introduced to Madeira and the Canaries. The plantation system and colonial governments implemented on these islands became models for the sugar plantations of the New World. [52] The techniques of sugar production, exploitation of labor, and economic organization were developed on these islands. These practices were easily exported to the New World. [53]

Well over ninety-five percent of the sugar carried from the Americas "during the slave era, well over ninety percent of the slaves ever carried across the Atlantic, most of whom were intended to make that sugar, sailed after 1650. After 1650, when sugar and increasingly slaves, moved out of the Mediterranean and into first the 'Mediterranean Atlantic,' then into the Gulf of Guinea, and finally to Brazil and the Caribbean, sugar shaped the evolution of the heartlands of the Americas in almost every sense." [54]

> ***"The first sweetened cup of hot tea to be drunk by an English worker was a significant historical event, because it prefigured the transformation of an entire society, a total remaking of its economic and social basis. We must struggle to understand fully the consequences of that and kindred events for upon them was erected an entirely different conception of the relationship between producers and consumers, of the meaning of work, of the definition of self, of the nature of things."***
>
> **Sidney W. Mintz**
>
> *Sweetness and Power: the place of sugar in modern history*, 1985

## Triangular Trade

Tobacco and other field crops like cotton, coffee, cocoa, rice, indigo and hemp were all labor intensive. Unfortunately for America, we opted for slavery and indentured servants to provide that labor and make plantation agriculture profitable. Slaves came here as part of the alcohol-molasses-slave trade involving the United States, the Caribbean and Africa, dubbed "The Triangular Trade."

"Triangular trade is a simplified term for the trading patterns that developed among the American colonies, the West Indies, the coast of Africa, and the British Isles during the eighteenth century. The patterns of commerce were more complex than the term triangular trade suggests. Many trading voyages involved more than three exchanges of goods, and others were limited to two ports." [55]

## Sugar is a Drug

"Some of you might ask what is sugar doing in a book about drugs? You say 'Sugar isn't a drug.' I beg to differ. Not only is sugar a key ingredient in the production of alcohol, but by most definitions it's a drug in its own right. As Dr. Andrew Weil points out in *From Chocolate to Morphine,* the distinction between food, spice, poison, medicine, good drug, bad drug is often quite arbitrary."[56]

"These categories are sometimes conflicting and dependent upon dose and, preparation. Tapioca, for instance, is a poison until you pound it thoroughly. Then, it becomes a tasty dessert. A substance may also change over time from one category to another depending upon who holds the cultural power.

Webster defines drug as, '...any substance used as a medicine or an ingredient in a medicine'. More importantly, Webster's Dictionary defines medicine as 'any drug or other substance used in treating disease, healing, or relieving pain."'[57]

"Some would say a drug is something you buy in a drug store, a pharmacy. Others would say a drug is what a doctor gives you. By that definition, sugar is a drug because it is used for medicinal purposes. Your hospital IV is almost always a 5% solution of dextrose (sugar) and water. Others may say, 'No, a drug must be used to treat a medical condition.' An overdose of insulin can create life-threatening hypoglycemia. The treatment? Sugar!"'[58]

**Syndney W. Mintz**
*Sweetness and Power*, 1985

The classical definition of Triangular Trade describes a three-point trading arrangement. It starts with rum from the Americas being traded for slaves from West Africa. The slaves in turn were traded in the West Indies for more molasses and the molasses was then used in the Caribbean and the United States to be made into more rum.[59] The United States made lots of rum. Rum distilleries were ubiquitous. Just about any town of any consequence from Massachusetts to the Carolinas had a rum distillery.

The so-called triangular trade was an integral part of mercantilism and a most important component of colonial American trade, communal life and economy. The slavery business involved not only sugar, molasses, alcohol and slaves, but trade in those "commodities" essential for shipbuilding, rigging manufacturing (and therefore hemp), and other industries necessary to promote maritime commerce. While the triangular trade is closely associated with slavery, it was part and parcel of the colonial American economy of the Northeast as well as the South.

By the heyday of triangular trade, the institution of slavery and the slaughter of Native Americans were old hat in the New World. Slavery was first instituted in the Caribbean and Brazil, then introduced to South Carolina, Virginia, and other states where plantation crops flourished. Slavery occurred with religious justification. After all, the enslaved were heathen, non-Christians.

## Irish Slaves

The English colonists brought plenty of cultural detritus that fouled the American ideological stream. One of the British most odious acts is their centuries long ill treatment of Irish Catholics. The British were brutal toward the Irish. Why? They were Irish and Papists. The sixteen hundreds were not a good time to be Irish. It could get you killed, captured and enslaved, made a virtual slave as an indentured servant, or a breeding mare to produce slaves. British hostility toward the Irish did not go away once they both arrived in America. After the potato famine of the early 1840s, the Irish started coming to America in large numbers, this long standing British animosity translated into enthusiastic support for "Temperance".

This ill-treatment of the Irish by the British was not just a 17th-century phenomenon. In 1317, the Irish, under Donal O'Neill, the King of Tyrone, petitioned Pope John XX regarding atrocities perpetrated upon the Irish by the British. In this manifesto, the Irish charged that the Kings of England had practiced genocide against the Irish "enacting for the extermination of our race most pernicious laws."[60]

In her book *Criminalizing A Race: Free Blacks During Slavery* (1993), Charshee McIntyre makes the case that the English perfected the institution of slavery after conquering the Irish. The English claimed that their slavery of the Irish was preferable to the freedom the Irish had held under their own barbarous customs. She goes on to state that "Later, the English used the same justification to commit genocide on the Native Americans, to destroy their culture, and to enslave Africans everywhere."[61]

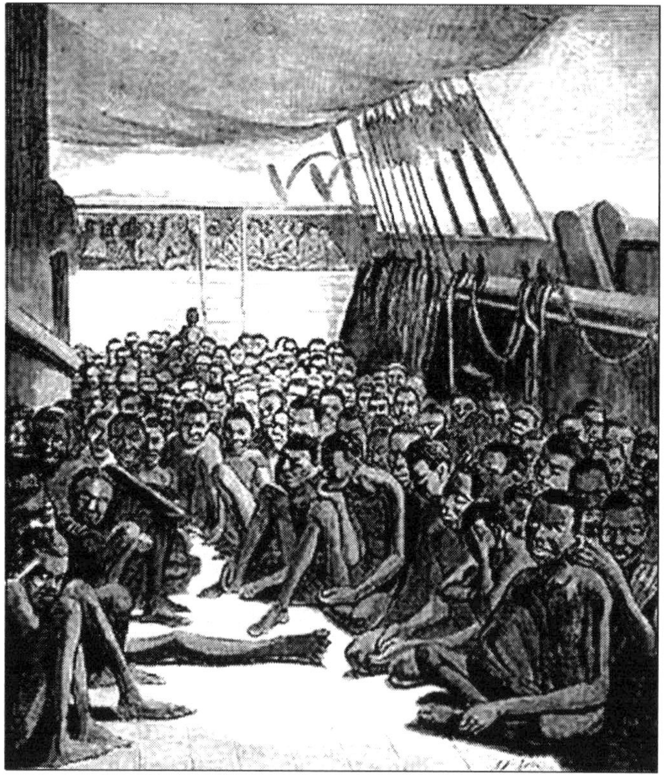

*Slaves were forced to travel in cramped quarters with few sanitary conveniences. Many died on the voyage from Africa to the New World.*

British law forms much of the foundation of American jurisprudence. The early colonists retained parts of English law and revised other parts. The colonists "continued many English patterns and adapted them to the new world."[62] McIntyre makes a very interesting observation. "The rigidity of the English outlook perceived any variations of lifestyle as hostile and threatening. The Irish lifestyle offered much pleasanter rewards to the masses than Anglo-Norman feudalism."

McIntyre states that the usage (meaning subjugation) of the Irish by the English predated the development of the New World colonies. He continues that the English relied on the experiences of colonizing Ireland and adjusted their Tudor approach to the conditions in America. The colonists were no strangers to discrimination, exploitation and subjugation of *the others*. McIntyre notes that "more than forty members of the Virginia Company at Jamestown had an interest in Irish conquest and the colonization by Englishmen of Ireland."[63]

The Irish saw themselves as virtual slaves in Ireland. The English viewed the Irish as savages: "lazy, 'naturally' given to 'idleness' and unwilling to work for 'their own bread.'"[64] Americans, of course, used similar disparaging terms toward the African slaves. George Fitzhugh, in a justification and defense of slavery, described a slave as one who has "neither energy nor enterprise" and if the slave had liberty, he would be "a curse to himself and a greater curse to the society around him."[65]

## Negroes* Were Treated Horribly. But It's Possible That For a Century or Two, the Irish Were Treated Even Worse

A British Proclamation of 1625 ordered Irish political prisoners to be transported to the West Indies and sold to English planters as laborers. It made many Irish literal slaves. This official policy continued for TWO CENTURIES! In 1629, a large group of Irish men and women were sent to Guiana. By 1632, Irish were the main slaves sold to Antigua and Montserrat in the West Indies. A 1637 census showed that 69% of the total population of Montserrat were Irish slaves. In 1650, 25,000 Irish were sold to planters in St. Kitt. In the 12-year period from 1641 to 1652 following the Confederate revolt, over 550,000 Irish were killed by the English and 300,000 were sold as slaves. During that period, the Irish population in Ireland fell from 1,466,000 to 616,000.[66]

In the mid-17th century, Irish soldiers were banished from Ireland by the British. Neither banished soldiers, nor the Irish sold into slavery, were allowed to take their wives and children with them. This resulted in a growing population of homeless

** The word "Negroes" is used here because that was the more polite term used to describe Black Africans from the 16th century through the mid-20th century.*

women and children who were seen as a public nuisance. They were, of course, rounded up and sold into slavery. But, the worst was yet to come.[67]

Oliver Cromwell began his Ethnic Cleansing of Ireland on August 14, 1652. He ordered the Irish to be transported overseas and 12,000 Irish prisoners were promptly sold to Barbados. "In the decade of the 1650s during Cromwell's Reign of Terror, over 100,000 Irish children, most of them between the ages of 10 and 14, were taken from their Catholic parents and sold as slaves in the West Indies, Virginia and New England. More Irish were sold as slaves to the American colonies and plantations from 1651 to 1660 than the total existing *free* population of the Americas!"[68]

The plantation owners were aware that Negroes were better suited than the Irish to work in the semi-tropical climates of the Caribbean, but they had to be purchased. The Irish, on the other hand, were basically free for the catching and didn't require having to sail all the way to Africa to get them. It should come as no surprise then that in 17th-century slaving, Ireland was the biggest source of "livestock" (as slaves were considered) for the English slave trade.[69]

The Africans and Irish were housed together and both were the property of the planter owners, but the Africans received much better treatment, food and housing. This was not out of Christian charity. Black slaves had more property value than Irish slaves. In the British West Indies, the planters routinely tortured white slaves for any infraction. Owners would hang Irish slaves by their hands and set their hands or feet on fire as a means of punishment.

The British were equally bigoted in their racist stereotypes of the Irish and Negroes. They used a little perverse Darwinism to claim that both were more closely related to the apes than Anglo-Teutonic types. A 19th-century issue of *Harper's Weekly* carried an illustration showing the alleged similarity of the Irish and Negro as they compared to the allegedly more highly evolved Anglo-Saxon. No wonder Irish immigrants to America were referred to as "White Niggers."[70]

## The "Compassion" of Slavery: Breed the Indentured Irish with Negroe Slaves. *(It's the only decent thing to do, right?)*

In 1656, as a way to end this barbarous treatment of Irish Slaves, Colonel William Brayne wrote to English authorities with his idea, which at the time apparently seemed less barbaric. He urged the importation of only Negro slaves because "as the planters would have to pay much more for them, they would have an interest in preserving their lives, which was wanting in the case of (Irish)..." many of whom, he charged, were killed by overwork and cruel treatment.[71]

His position was based on the existing financial and political reality. African/Negro slaves generally cost about 20 to 50 pounds Sterling, which was four to ten times the value of the 900 pounds of cotton (about 5 pounds Sterling) paid for an Irish slave.[72]

Due to this larger "investment", Negro slaves were not as disposable as Irish slaves. Africans were also more durable in the hot climate, and caused fewer problems. The biggest bonus with the Africans though, was they were NOT Catholic, and to the British any heathen pagan was better than an Irish Papist.

Soon, planters began to breed indentured servant Irish women, (most of whom were technically and legally not slaves), with African men, who were slaves, to produce more slaves since children of

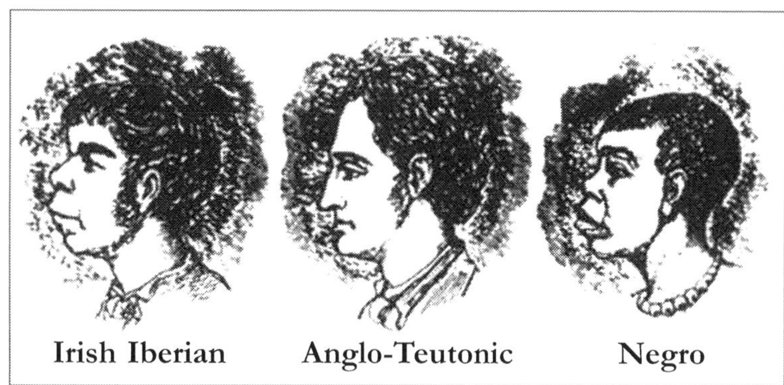


*An illustration from the influential American magazine* Harper's Weekly *(whose subtitle "Journal of Civilization" sounds ironic a century later) shows an alleged similarity between "Irish Iberian" and "Negro" features in contrast to the higher "Anglo-Teutonic." The accompanying caption indicated that the so-called Iberians were "believed to have been" an African race that invaded first in Spain.*[73]

slaves were themselves slaves. So, although the indentured servant Irish woman could eventually become free, her children by Negro slaves could not. The planters bred the comely Irish women, because their offspring were both slaves and attractive, which made them quite profitable. These lighter skin children of slaves brought a higher price than slaves brought directly from Africa.

This forced mating practice became so widespread that in 1681 legislation was passed "forbidding the practice of mating Irish slave women to African slave men for the purpose of producing slaves for sale." This legislation was not the result of any moral or ethical consideration. The law was passed because the practice was interfering with the profits from slavery of the politically well connected British Royal African Company.[74]

## History of Marginalizing "Them" Repeats Itself … Over and Over and Over

This ready willingness to brutalize, demean and dehumanize *"them"* resurfaces in our absurd, harsh, criminal justice approach to drugs. This is apparent in the U.S. approach to opiate use. While opiates had been readily available before 1906, after the Harrison Narcotic Tax Act the U.S. quickly made sure there was no medical gray areas. Heroin maintenance clinics were outlawed in 1924 by the Heroin Act, the last one closing in 1925 in Knoxville.

Doctors were intimidated and harassed so as not to treat habitual opiate users medicinally. From 1920-1938, over 30,000 doctors were arrested for treating opiate abusers.[75] This simply reflects the fact that if one were treating the marginalized and demonized, that the treatment itself can become marginalized and/or underfunded.

Treatment and prevention is clearly an afterthought in our present day drug policy. Providing plenty of funding for jails, and comparatively little for drug abuse treatment, seems an odd way to approach an obvious medical problem. This is particularly appalling in view of a study done by the State of California that demonstrated that for every taxpayer dollar spent on treatment, seven taxpayer dollars were saved.[76]

For years in the United Staes, penalties for crack cocaine, used largely by Blacks, is substantially higher than the penalties for the powdered cocaine preferred mostly by Caucasians. Putting people in jail for minor drug crimes longer than for murder, rape and mayhem; as well as disproportionately arresting, trying and punishing Blacks and Hispanics is not only not reasonable or fair, but also at odds with American Constitutional values and just plain doesn't work.

The confiscatory U.S. forfeiture laws, where the property is put on trial by the government, is contrary to the basic American value of fairness. These laws are so repugnant that conservative Republican and former Speaker of the U.S. House of Representatives, Henry Hyde, made efforts before he left Congress to modify U.S. forfeiture laws. Sadly these laws are still repugnant to any Constitution-loving American. The forfeiture laws say the government can take the property of an alleged perpetrator of a drug crime, even if the accused has not been tried or found guilty of committing any crime. This is all too reminiscent of the outrageous policies of the colonial British and the witch trials before that.

The list of abuses generated by U.S. drug policy goes on and on. How else to explain these seemingly illogical, arbitrary and un-American acts, other than that they are accepted as being part and parcel of our long sad history of demonization and discrimination against the *other*.

## The Tea Tax: the Trigger for the Revolutionary War

Tea gained popularity in England in the 17th and 18th centuries. Tea was first sold in London in 1657, at Garway's Coffee House where it was sold as a health drink. Charles II's 1662 marriage to Catherine Braganza of Portugal helped jump-start the popularity of tea in England. Catherine was a fan of tea, so tea became chic in England. In 1664, the powerful English East India Company brought the king and queen, Charles II and Catherine, the gift of tea. By 1669, the English East India Company monopolized British tea imports.[77]

Tea was increasingly popular in the New World, including the United States. In 1650, the Dutch introduced several teas and tea traditions to New Amsterdam, which later becomes New York. When the British purchased and took over New Amsterdam from the Dutch, the British tea tradition took hold. It wasn't until 1690, that the first tea was publicly sold in Massachusetts. But don't let the slow start fool you. By 1765, tea ranked as the most popular non-alcoholic beverage in the American colonies.[78]

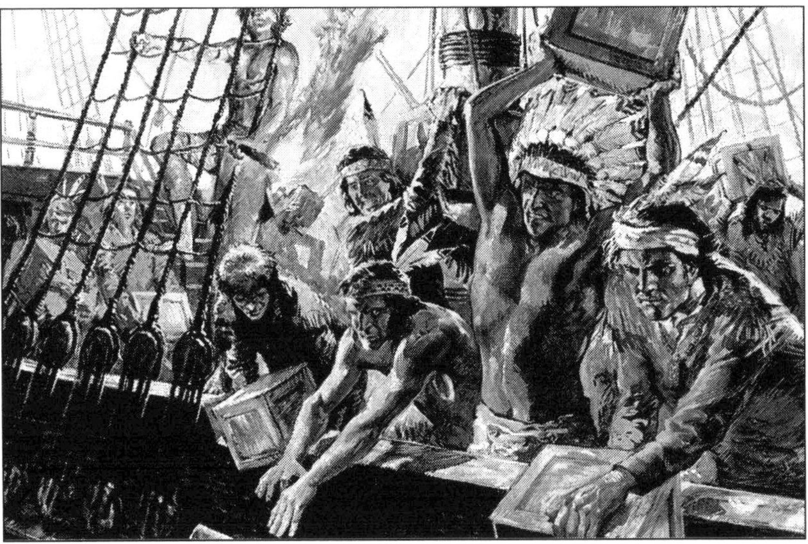

*The colonists were mad as hell and they weren't going to take it any more. The "It" being the exploitation of the colonies and taxation without representation.*

Mercantilism and squeezing taxes from the colonies led the British to become very over-bearing with their tea tax. This offended America sensibilities to such an extent that the American Revolution was ignited. The chain of events is familiar to most American school children. In 1767, British parliament passed the Townshend Revenue Act. This Act imposed a duty tax on tea and other goods imported into the British American colonies. A town meeting was held in Boston to protest the Townshend Revenue Act which led to an American boycott of British imports and a smuggling in of Dutch teas. This was much more than a tempest in a teapot. Soon the Continental Congress declared coffee the national drink of the then-colonized United States.[79] (That'll show 'em!) Compared with what was to come, this was a mild protest against the tea tax levied by the British.

In 1770, the British Parliament partially rescinded the Townshend Revenue Act, eliminating all import taxes except those on teas. In 1773, to add insult to injury, a new Tea Act not only retained the duty on tea but gave the East India Company a virtual monopoly on importation of tea to the colonies.[80]

This British law is what led to the December 16, 1773 protest of British tea taxes known as "The Boston Tea Party". The colonists were thinly disguised as Native Americans. They boarded the East India Company ships anchored in Boston and tossed hundreds of chests of tea into Boston Harbor. Throughout 1774, such "tea parties" were repeated in Philadelphia, New York, Maine, North Carolina, and Maryland.

Well, the British were furious. In 1774, in response to the American "tea party" rebellions, the British Parliament compounded their folly by passing the so-called "Coercive Acts". King George III also agreed to the Boston Port Bill, which closed the Boston Harbor until the East India Company was reimbursed for its tea. The East India Company is still waiting for the check. And in 1775, after several British attempts to end the taxation protests, the American Revolution began.[81]

## Hemp

Indispensable to this entire Triangular Trade, Mercantilism, and slaving operation was hemp. During this time hemp was to colonial trade and transportation, as oil is to commerce in present times. Hemp was the essential lubricant of colonial trade.

A sea-going vessel could not function without tons of hemp. Thousands of yards of canvas sail, and the miles of rope and rigging necessary to move a great sailing ship, were made from hemp. Hemp sails and rigging withstood the rot from salt water better than any other fiber. Hemp was a must.[81]

Thomas Jefferson – also a slave holder – championed hemp as a far superior crop compared to tobacco, because it wasn't as hard on the land and was more profitable.

**Tobacco is a culture productive of infinite wretchedness.**

**Thomas Jefferson**

*Notes on the State of Virginia*, 1787

Hemp was necessary for the manufacture of the over 60 tons of rope, rigging and canvas required to outfit each of the colonial sailing vessels; the vessels necessary for trade in that mercantile society. And in most colonies it was mandatory to plant hemp.

During the Revolutionary War, the patriots' wives and mothers organized "spinning bees" to make clothes for Washington's troops, spinning the thread from hemp fibers. The Continental Army would have frozen to death at Valley Forge without hemp. Thomas Payne, famous Revolutionary pamphleteer, author of *Common Sense*, written in 1776, listed cordage, iron, timber and tar as America's four essential natural resources. He wrote that "Hemp flourishes even to rankness, we do not want for cordage." [82]

## Hemp is Not Intoxicating, Nor is it What is Usually Referred to as "Marijuana"

Hemp is basically the male Cannabis Sativa plant. It is tall and reedy, low in the euphorogenic THC and high in cannabidiols (CBDs). THC (delta 9 tetrahydrocannabinol) is commonly credited [83] as being the most pharmacologically active chemical and principle intoxicant of the 483 chemicals in cannabis. (This is not an exceptional number of chemicals for a plant; coffee has about 880, a tomato 380.)

It's easy to grasp why hemp won't get anyone high; it's very low in the principal euphoriant in the hemp/ cannabis plant, delta 9 THC. Hemp is about 0.3-1.0% THC, whereas cannabis/marijuana has 4-20% THC (usually in the 5-8% range). Hemp is high in CBD, an anti-euphoriant, to boot.

The title of the 1937 Marijuana Tax Act is a curious one. Given the lingo of the time the obscure name appears calculated to mislead the very industries that might oppose a law that marginalized hemp and cannabis. "Marijuana," the American Medical Association (AMA) said in their 1937 Congressional testimony on the Marijuana Tax Act, is slang for cannabis and hemp, employed as a mongrel word to confuse people about what was really being discussed.

At the time of the Marijuana Tax Act passage in 1937, marijuana was a word that was not familiar to mainstream America. It was used mainly by poor Mexicans (then a much smaller, even more marginalized part of the U.S. population than today) as their name for cannabis. Blacks (then known as Negroes) were likely to use other names – "Gage", "Mary Jane", "muggles", "Reefer", etc. Only a fraction of urban whites were familiar with the smoking of cannabis and fewer still with the slang terms marijuana, "gage", "muggles" or the like.

It has been speculated that this misleading title was no accident. In 1937, even most of those professionals and industrialists who would be affected by the proposed Tax Act, did not realize, until it was too late, that the marijuana in the Marijuana Tax was referring to both medicinal cannabis and industrial hemp. Because the legislation went to the U.S. House Ways & Means Committee, it would go to the full House without being heard by any other committees. This stealth legislation was flying almost below the radar. It was only at the last minute that the AMA became aware that this tax was indeed about cannabis.

"Hemp" is a rather general term. It encompasses many different fibers. The hemp name is applied to more than just fiber derived from the cannabis plant. Other sources of hemp include Manila hemp (*abaca*), a plant in the banana genus from the Philippines, and sisal hemp made from the sisal cactus. Then there is New Zealand hemp which comes from the harakeke plant, also Deccan hemp from a hibiscus species, and jute, also known as Indian hemp, from the jute shrub. The real thing, what is usually called hemp, comes from cannabis.

From 1000 B.C. until a generation after the American Civil War (1883), hemp was the world's LARGEST agricultural crop. For much of that time, it provided over 80% of the world's textiles including 50% of the fabric called linen. [84,85] Flax was one of the earliest domesticated fiber crops dating to about 7000 B.C. [86] Artifacts found in China, Taiwan and India indicate hemp rope or fiber existed at least 1000 years before that. Hemp rope imprints were found on pottery shards which were likely 10,000 years old. [87,88] This is consistent with a recent find in China of a shaman's 2,800-year-old medicine bag containing cannabis. [89]

Hemp is a very versatile plant. Hemp was used to make fabric, lighting oil, fuel oil, incense, medicine and paper; all the drafts of the Constitution were written on hemp paper.. Hemp is a food rich in Omega 3 fatty acids and an important source of protein for human and animal consumption.

The high THC-producing female cannabis Sativa, looks very little like the low THC content hemp. The high resin cannabis plants are short and bushy, containing many resin-laden flowers, and have short fibers. Hemp is tall and spindly with few flowers and has longer fibers, the better to make rope, canvas and textiles. From 1000 B.C. to 1900, cannabis extracts were either the first, second or third most frequently used medicine for two-thirds of the world's people. [90]

## Washington and Jefferson Grew Hemp

Two of America's earliest presidents – George Washington and Thomas Jefferson – were hemp growers. [91]

There has been some speculation that Washington may have used cannabis medicinally or recreationally (1) because he separated the male from the female plants and (2) because he once wrote in his diary he hoped he got home in time for the hemp harvest because he so enjoyed the burning of the slag. [92] Another entry in Washington's diary is frequently cited as the evidence that he separated the males and the females and therefore used hemp recreationally.

The argument depends on a tradition that the quality or quantity of marijuana resin (hashish) is enhanced if the male and female plants are separated before the females are pollinated. There can be no doubt that Washington separated the males and the females. Two entries in his diary supply the evidence: May 12-13, 1765: "Sowed Hemp at Muddy hole by Swamp." August 7, 1765: "...began to separate (sic) the Male from the Female Hemp at Do – rather too late." [93]

### What Did George Mean?

Most likely Washington separated the male from a female plant to improve the quality of the yield from the male plants so as to make better rope not stronger dope. George Andrews argues the opposite. In *The Book of Grass: An Anthology of Indian Hemp*, Andrews concludes that Washington's August 7 diary entry "clearly indicates that he was cultivating the plant for medicinal purposes as well for its fiber." Andrews agrees that Washington might have separated the males from the females to get better fiber—but he argues that the phrase "rather too late" suggests that Washington wanted to complete the separation before the female plants were fertilized—and this was a practice related to drug potency rather than to fiber culture. [95] Nevertheless, without additional historical data, this is conjecture on the part of Andrews and many others. But, you never know.

### Thomas Jefferson & Hemp

Jefferson was a fan of hemp and a critic of the tobacco plant. He said tobacco "greatly exhausts the soil" and "requires much manure."

The fact well established in the system of agriculture is that the best hemp and the best tobacco grow on the same kind of soil. The former article is of first necessity to the commerce and marine, in other words to the wealth and protection of the country. The latter, never useful and sometimes pernicious, derives its estimation from caprice, and its value from the taxes to which it was formerly exposed.

The preference to be given will result from a comparison of them: Hemp employs in its rudest state more labor than tobacco, but being a material for manufacturers of various sorts, becomes afterwards the means of support to numbers of people, hence it is to be preferred in a populous country." [94]

---

**"began to separate the Male from the Female Hemp at Do—rather too late."**

**George Washington**
Entry in his Diary
August 7, 1765

---

The cannabis plant of colonial America was industrial hemp. Washington and Jefferson, and the other hemp planters, grew the tall, spindly, high-fiber, low-THC plant. They knew the difference between the tall sparsely festooned hemp and the squat bushy, leafy budding marijuana.

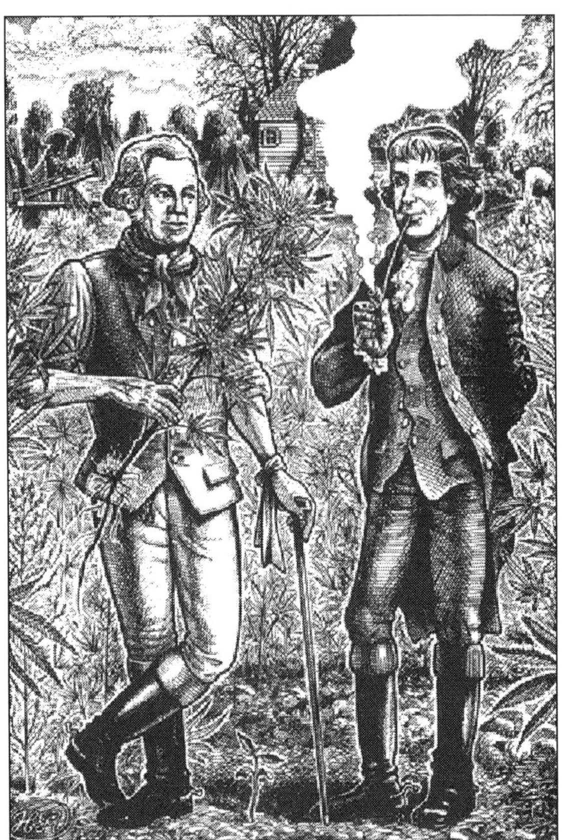

*Both Washington and Jefferson grew hemp on their plantations. As it was a very profitable and important colonial crop, this was not at all unusual.*

It is easy to tell the difference between cannabis and hemp. If one can distinguish a tall, thin basketball player from an overweight midget, they can distinguish hemp from marijuana.

In the United States, law enforcement spokespeople have argued that our police can't tell the difference between the male and female cannabis plant. This seems a mean, false condemnation of the observational and plant discrimination abilities of American law enforcement personnel.

Surely, they can make the distinction between these two rather different plants, as well or better, than law enforcement officers in other countries. This well-known fact, that it's easy to tell the difference between hemp and cannabis is why, in over 30 countries in the world today, the growing of industrial hemp is legal. Certainly our neighbors to the north in Canada have had no such problems distinuishing hemp from cannabis.

In the colonies as elsewhere, the hemp fibers extracted from the hemp cannabis plant were used mainly for textiles, rope, canvas, and paper. Hemp was also used in the manufacture of hemp food, hemp seed oil and other industrial products. Hemp seed oil fueled many of the colonists' lamps. Hemp based products – clothing, books, lamp oil, etc. – were an integral part of American life for hundreds of years. During the 17th, 18th and 19th centuries in many parts of the United States., it is against the law to refuse to grow hemp. [96] The first Bibles, maps, charts, the Betsy Ross flag, the first drafts of the Declaration of Independence and the Constitution were all made from hemp. [97]

For at least 200 years (1620-1820), hemp was the most important agricultural crop produced in America. [98] It is also why there are towns all along the Atlantic coast, and into the Midwest, with the name Hempstead, Hemp Hill, Hampton or something similar.

For millennia, the hemp fiber extraction process was extremely labor-intensive. The results were considered worth the effort. Hemp is softer, warmer and more water-resistant than cotton, and has three times as much tensile strength. In the 1820s, Eli Whitney's legendary cotton gin launched cotton as America's number one textile, but hemp remained the second most popular natural fiber until after the Civil War. As late as 1850, U.S. census records document 8,327 cannabis plantations of over 7,000 acres each. [99]

Competition from the less labor-intensive cotton, the loss of slave labor and the rise of the steam driven boat sent the hemp business into steep decline after the Civil War. The hemp business struggled on in America until the last legal crop of hemp was harvested in Wisconsin in 1957. [100]

The hemp industry had been introduced into Wisconsin at the turn of the 19th century by former Wisconsin Governor Henry Dodge, who in 1890, had become the first U.S. Secretary of Agriculture.

But, Kentucky is a state where the economy was not closely associated to hemp. Today, a marker placed by the state of Kentucky stands outside Leafland, Kentucky proclaiming hemp as the "State's Largest Cash Crop Till 1915." [101]

## U.S. Fought a War Over Hemp

The British needed hemp for their maritime activities. This need for hemp was a motivator for Britain to settle North America and grow more hemp. This need for hemp gave the British a strong reason to staunchly defend the colonies from infringement by the French and Spanish. Laws were passed in many colonies making it mandatory to grow hemp. At one of the first, if not the first English-speaking, rule-making assemblage in Virginia – July 31, 1619 – one of the brand new laws was that every family must grow at least a patch of hemp. [102]

Since hemp was the most profitable agricultural crop in the world for almost a thousand years, it's hardly surprising that the British tax on the colonial production of hemp (e.g., the Navigation Act, one of the "Acts of Intolerance"), helped fuel support for the Revolutionary War.

### The War of 1812

American school children learn that the War of 1812 was something vaguely about the British impressment of U.S. seamen (e.g., U.S. merchant marine sailors being pressed into the service of the British). That is only the tip of the iceberg. The rest of the story involves European treaties, conflicts and mil-itary pow-er. This is what was behind the British impress-ments of U.S. sailors that pro-voked the Americans to go to war.

From 1740 until well into the 1800s, Russia produced 80% of the West-ern world's cannabis hemp. [*Note: This is as opposed to other products called hemp; sisal hemp, New Zealand hemp, jute (also known as Indian hemp), manila hemp, and Decca hemp.*] Russian hemp was the world's best-quality cannabis hemp for sails, rope, rigging and nets used on the high seas. This is because Russia had the best retting process. Retting is the process of curing the rope. The retting process slows the rotting of hemp by sea water and Russia had the most effective retting process. Hemp, not surprisingly, was Russia's number one trading commodity – ahead of furs, timber and iron. [103]

THIS HEMPCROP IS FO
INDUSTRIAL FIBRE
T.H.C. CONTENT NIL
PLEASE LEAVE ALON
www.hemcore.com

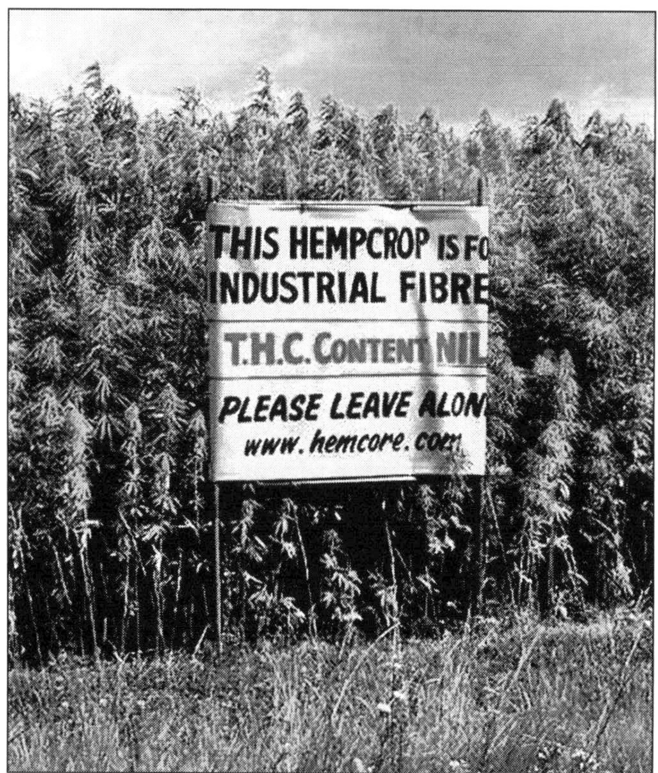

*Here is the tall woody hemp plant grown by the colonists. It was crucial to making rope rigging and sail and used for making paper. For over 1,000 years, it was the world's largest agricultural crop.*

### Rule Britannia

In the late 18th and early 19th century, Britain controlled the seas and world sea trade through its navy and merchant fleet. Britain's sea power ran on Russian hemp. More than 90% of Britain's marine hemp came from Russia. There was no substitute; for example, flax sails, unlike hemp sails, would start rotting from ocean salt and spray in three months or less. Each British ship had to replace 50 to 100 tons of hemp sails every year or two. Clearly hemp – Russian hemp – was a key ingredient to British military sea power.

As the 18th century came to a close, the British ruling classes were afraid that the French Revolution (1789-93) could spread across the Channel. The British nobility was hostile toward the new French gover-nment, understanding that if the French invaded England, the consequences could be dire, up to and including the loss of the nobility's collective heads.

America probably should have thanked the British for putting pressure on France and Napoleon. Napoleon had a desire for conquest and Empire. But Napoleon's efforts to fight the British and gain control of Europe were costly, draining the French treasury. And by 1803, France was running out of money. This allowed Jefferson to make one of his greatest moves. He bought the Louisiana Territory from France at the bargain price of $15 million, roughly two-and-a-half cents per acre. At the time, many of Jefferson's political opponents thought him a fool for making this purchase.[104]

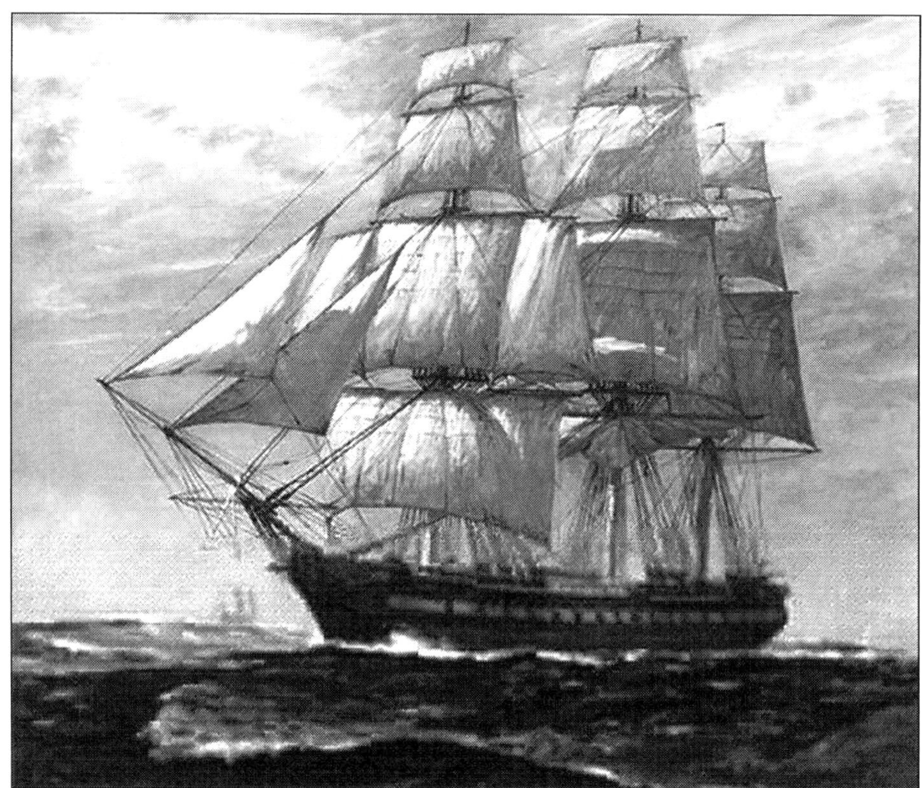

*Hemp was critical for seafaring. It was made into rigging, rope and sails. A great ship of the mercantile era, like the USS Constitution, required over 60 tons of hemp to manufacture these rugged fiber products necessary for travel on the high seas.*

Cutting to the chase, sea power was important in this Anglo-Franco confrontation. The British blockaded France from 1803 to 1814, closing French ports on the English Channel and the Atlantic Bay of Biscay. Anything that weakened British sea power was helpful to the French. In 1807, Napoleon and Czar Alexander of Russia signed the Treaty of Tilsit, cutting off all legal Russian trade with Great Britain, its allies, or any other neutral nation acting as agents for Great Britain in Russia. Its goal: stop Russian hemp from reaching England.

Napoleon believed that without Russian hemp to meet the British naval needs for canvas and rope, the might of the British Navy would be diminished. Napoleon reasoned that the British would be forced to cannibalize sails, ropes and rigging as their existing sail and rigging rotted from the salty sea. This would decrease British vessels at sail and Napoleon reckoned would end Britain's blockade of France and the Continent.

## English Impressed U.S. Sailors by Blackmail

Britain's strategy to circumvent the Treaty of Tilsit's desired effect of eliminating British access to Russian hemp, was to impress (e.i., force) American sailors into getting that good, old Russian hemp. After the British "overhauled" – boarded and confiscated – an American ship and brought it into an English port, the British secretly offered the captured American traders a "deal" (actually a blackmail proposition).

The deal: Either lose your ship and cargos forever, or go to Russia and *secretly* buy hemp for Britain. The British would pay the American traders with gold in advance, and more gold when the hemp was delivered back to England. At the same time, the Americans could keep and trade their own goods (rum, sugar, spices, cotton, coffee, and tobacco) to the Czar for the hemp – a double profit for the Americans.

This was not such a bad deal and many Americans were not that upset. When the United States finally did declare war on Britain, not one senator from a maritime state voted for the war, nearly every western senator voted for it. It was calculated that such a war would allow the United States to expand into Canada and fulfill the American dream of "Manifest

Destiny" (e.i., it was U.S. destiny to occupy all of North America above Mexico). The War of 1812 was on.

After the war ended in 1814, the seas were once again safe. The United States saw the beginning of a great influx of immigrants, first a trickle and then a deluge. This massive immigration of people from Ireland, Germany, China and beyond had a profound effect on shaping American drug laws.

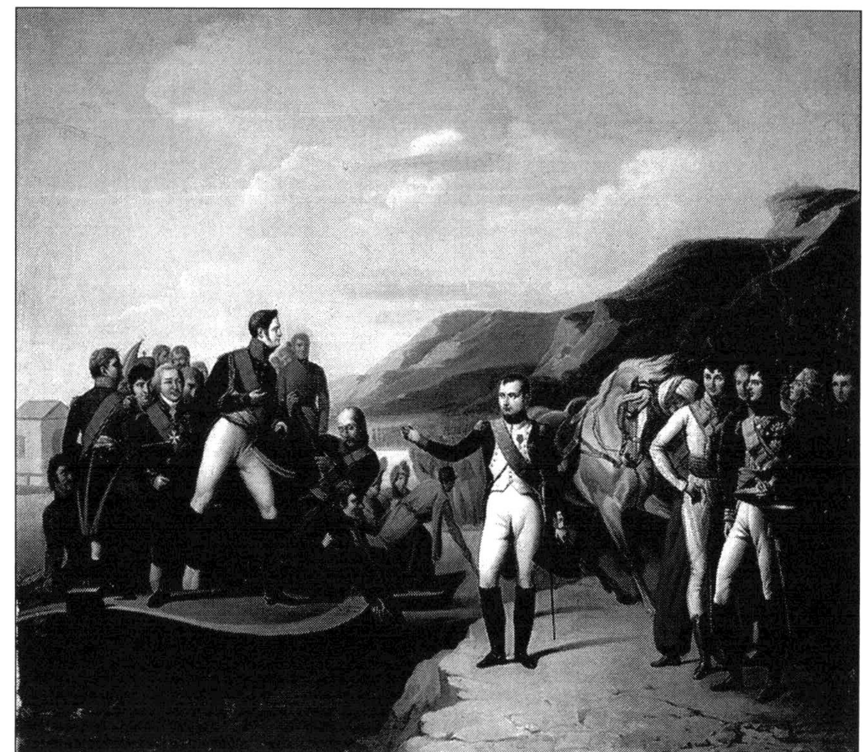

*The Treaty of Tilsit entered into by Czar Alexander of Russia and Napoleon of France, was an attempt to cut off Britain's legal supply of hemp sails from Russia. This led the British to impress American merchant ships and sailors to secure Russian hemp for them. This impressment of U.S. sailors and vessels led to the War of 1812.*

## Booze, America's First National Pastime

Alcohol, a drug by any definition, was very popular in colonial times. After all, it was safer than the polluted water of the time. Alcohol was preferred on long ocean voyages. Before casting off for the New World, the Puritans loaded more beer onto the Mayflower than water, packing 42 tons of beer on the Mayflower and only 14 tons of water. In fact, one reason the ship landed at Plymouth Rock is that the settlers had used up their ration of beer. Bradford, the diarist and later Plymouth's governor wrote, "The settlers were hastened ashore and made to drink water," he lamented, "so that the seamen might have the more beer." [105]

The Puritans and other Protestants may have had different attitudes than Catholics about drinking patterns but they were not teetotalers. No. "They saw alcohol as a natural and normal part of life. Their religious tradition taught them that alcohol was created by God and inherently good. Jesus had used wine and approved of its moderate consumption." [106]

### Don't Drink the Water

The colonists were afraid of drinking the water – a fear they rightly had from centuries of experience drinking Europe's polluted waters. This was before a clear understanding of the relationship between microbes and communicable disease. Fundamental rules of sanitation weren't in place. Villages, first in Europe and later in the New World, often violated the first rule of public health – do not contaminate your water supply. Communities frequently contaminated their water supply by taking water from streams and wells downhill or down-stream from privies. This arrangement often created sewage-contaminated waters. Germ-free alcohol was much safer to drink than potentially polluted waters from wells and streams.

The New England colonists rather quickly changed from drinking beer to drinking hard cider (the fermented variety of apple cider). English grains did not grow well in New England, and were expensive to import. Apple crops, however, grew well in the New England climate. Apple orchards were found on most every farm. The easy supply of apples stimulated demand for hard cider. Cider was a good fit for facing the sharp New England air and certainly tasted better hot than ale, and was a good bracer for the brisk weather. [107]

At least until Prohibition, apples were much more frequently consumed in the form of cider (hard cider: there was no soft cider) than eaten. With that in mind, it's interesting to take a new look at the life of John Chapman, better known as Johnny Appleseed. He was real, an American folk hero and deservedly so. He was one of the great real estate developers in early America.

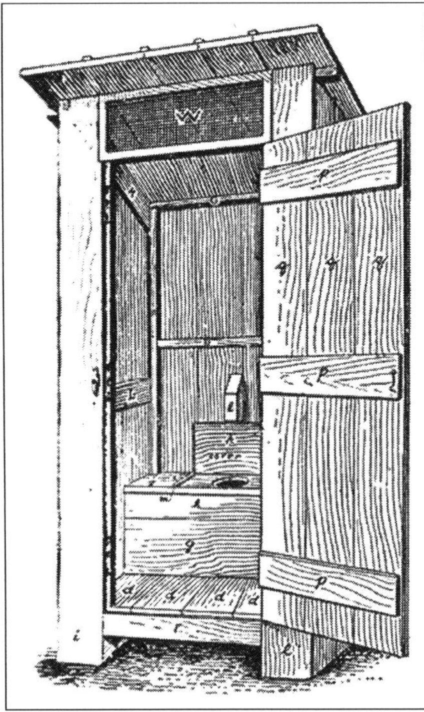

*Putting the outhouse higher than the water supply. Putting sewage into streams from which water was used for drinking exposed people to high doses of pathological bacteria.*

Chapman went into the wilderness and planted apple orchards where he felt new settlements would arrive. [108] He was almost always right. In a few years settlers would come.

The apple orchard was a sign of pioneers conquering the forest. Soon, the new arrivals would buy his young apple trees. These apples were for drinking, not eating. Then Appleseed would move on into the wilderness, sometimes selling the entire orchard, sometimes holding on to a pice of the real estate.

Historian Ken Burns dubbed drinking alcohol "America's first national pastime." By all accounts this is an accurate characterization. "All the colonists drank cider, old and young, and in all places – funerals, weddings, ordainings, vestry-meetings, church-raisings, etc. Infants in arms drank mulled hard cider at night. It was supplied to students at Harvard and Yale colleges at dinner, being passed in two quart tankards from hand to hand down the commons table. Old men began the day with a quart or more of hard cider before breakfast." [109]

Benjamin Franklin has been credited with a variation on this love of alcohol. He is often quoted as saying that "Beer is God's Way of Saying He Loves Us." It sounds pithy but this is probably not a real Franklin quote. Bob Skilnick, author of the book *Beer and Food: An American History* (2006), searched for the source of this alleged Benjamin Franklin homage to beer. Skilnick did not find the quote in any of Franklin's writings. [110] His search found several comments in Franklin's writings praising wine but none in praise of beer.

The consumption of alcohol was an integral part of colonial life and usually seen as beneficial to a good life. Famed colonial preacher Increase Mather praised alcohol. He said "Drink is in itself a creature of God and to be received with thankfulness." Drinking per se was not frowned upon. Colonists did have some concerns about drinking to a point of excess. They believed alcohol was dangerous for Indians to drink and worried that too much drink could produce unseemly behavior in ministers. [111]

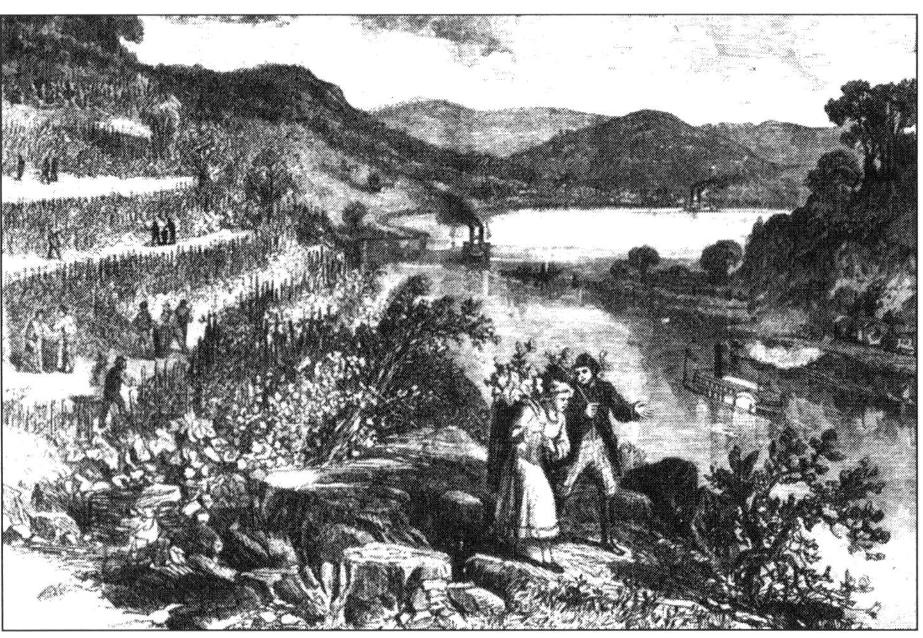

*Johnny Appleseed, whose true name was John Chapman, was one of the first real estate developers in America's frontier. By planting apples along inland waterways, he encouraged colonists to settle on land he owned. Apples were commonly used to make hard cider.*

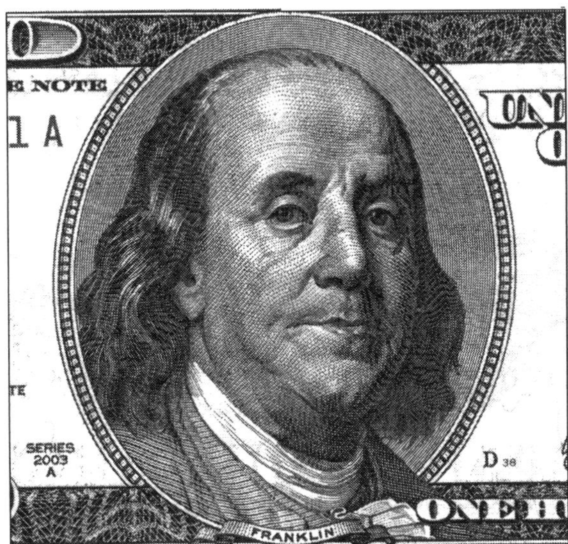


*Benjamin Franklin eloquently expressed colonial approval of alcoholic beverages, "Behold the Rain which descends from the heaven upon our vineyards; there it enters the roots of the vines, to be changed into wine, a constant proof that God loves us and loves to see us happy.* [110] *Letter from Ben Franklin to Andre Morellet (a French economist) c. 1779 .*

---

The culture of the English encouraged alcohol use. Colonial people drank alcohol at every meal, while at work and at every social and public get-together. Historian W.J. Rorabaugh wrote in 1979:

> "Alcohol was pervasive in American society; it crossed regional, sexual, racial, and class lines. Americans drank at home and abroad, alone and together, at work and at play, in fun and in earnest. They drank from the crack of dawn to the crack of dawn." [112]
>
> **W.J. Rorabaugh**
> *The Alcoholic Republic: An American Tradition* (1981)

Alcohol didn't spoil like the grain it was made from. It was easier to transport grain as alcohol. During the colonial period, alcohol was considered an aide to healthy living. Therefore, alcohol abstainers paid ten percent higherrates to life insurance companies than drinkers. And, because of the water quality problem alluded to above, those companies may have had a point.

The tavern was the colonial court house, town meeting hall, the local trading post, post office, auction house, courtroom, polling place, recruiting and militia office, stage coach depot, and liquor retailer. As community gathering spots, they encouraged patrons to drink and smoke – often and in great quantities. Many colonies mandated that each town have an "ordinary" (a tavern). Taverns were everywhere in the colonies. They were far more common than any other type of building except for dwellings.

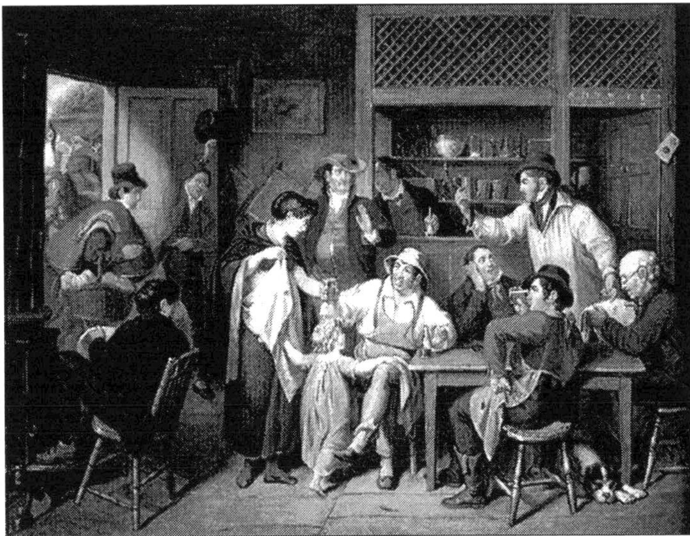

*Taverns were the center of activity in colonial communities. Not only were they inns for weary travelers, but meeting halls, courthouses, post offices and a place to plot revolution.*

---

There were laws in many locales that denied tavern access to several groups: Sailors, apprentices, servants, African-Americans, slaves, and Indians.

In his review of *Taverns and Drinking in Early America*, (2002), John Crowley says, "As with most such regulatory wars against drugs – think of the Volstead Act or the War on Drugs – these efforts largely failed, though not for want of legislative persistence." [113]

Alcohol was ubiquitous in the colonies. Rum and whiskey were legal tender. People bartered with whiskey, paid their taxes with whiskey, and on some occasions, paid their ministers' salaries with whiskey. The Colonial Army supplied its troops with a daily ration of four ounces of either rum or whiskey. A common treat for colonial kids after school was a little bread soaked in beer. Harvard's first master was canned because Harvard students were "wanting beer betwixt brewings a week and a week and a half together." [114]

## Whiskey Rebellion – 1794

Drugs played a major role in the U.S. federal government's first significant crisis. The problem was caused when the federal government imposed an excise tax on whiskey. This tax was not well accepted in the young America.

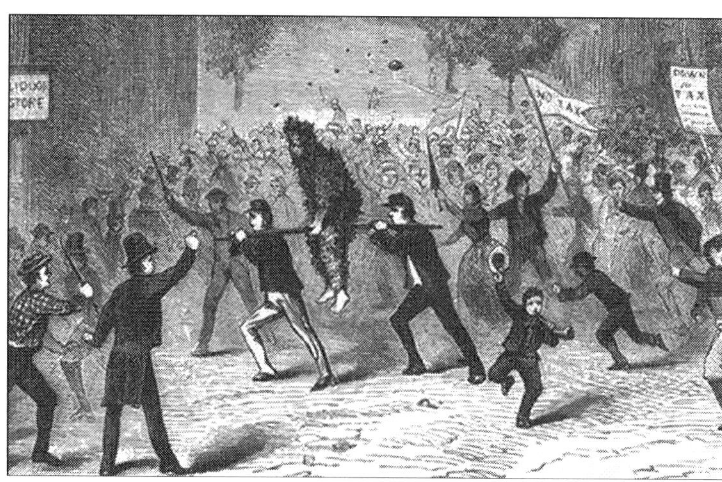

*A tax collector being tarred and feathered by an angry mob during the Whiskey Rebellion of 1794, which President Washington had to forcefully put down.*

Colonists had historically opposed British excise taxes such as the 1765 Stamp Act. The Stamp Act taxed all internal documents and transactions. It was very unpopular and was soon repealed. Had the Stamp Act not been repealed, the Revolutionary War could have started ten years earlier than it did.

The new federal government's excise tax on whiskey was widely unpopular. The average American saw the new federal government's assuming this power to impose excise taxes as little different from the old levies of the British crown. No one paid the tax on whiskey in the American "back-country" (the state of Kentucky and the frontier areas of Maryland, Virginia, North and South Carolina, and Georgia).

However, numerous wealthy officials in western Pennsylvania were foolishly willing to try and collect the whiskey tax. When they attempted, these tax collectors were tarred and feathered. The whiskey tax provoked riots and demonstrations in Pennsylvania. The demonstrators' slogan was, "liberty, property, and no excise!" There were no attacks on tax collectors in Kentucky and the rest of the frontier because no one there was willing to be a tax collector.

President Washington and Secretary of the Treasury Alexander Hamilton made their excise tax stand in Pennsylvania. It took 15,000 militia men to bring an end to this first governmental crisis in the United States of America.[114] These taxes remained through the Washington administration but they didn't last long. Opposition to the program was a cause championed by the emerging Democrat-Republican Party. It was part of the Jeffersonian "Revolution" of 1800. In Jefferson's first term, the entire Federalist excise tax program was repealed.

## Nitrous Oxide & Ether

Sir Joseph Priestly made the ground breaking discovery of nitrous oxide gas in 1776.[115] In 1799, English scientist Humphry Davy (later Sir Humphry) recommended nitrous oxide, or laughing gas, as a form of anesthesia. Unfortunately most of Davy's colleagues refused to take this claim very seriously.[116] Many, however, embraced the recreational use of nitrous oxide.

During this time it was common practice by men of science to test out these new drugs on one's self. Poets Coleridge, Southey and Wordsworth were among Davy's friends. They all were fascinated with Davy's chemistry. With Davy's encouragement, they were happy to follow his example and sample nitrous oxide. Afterward Southey wrote: "Davy has actually invented a pleasure for which language has no name…"[117]

Not all of Davy's friends were enamored with nitrous. Peter Mark Roget, the compiler of the 1852 Thesaurus bearing his name, was a member of Davy's circle, but he did not share Southey's conclusion. He said that nitrous oxide didn't give him any pleasant feelings whatsoever.[118] This is not surprising. It's known in medicine that the same chemical can have different effects on different people and even the same person at different times.

Nitrous oxide was largely known as a gas used by show men of the day who gave "scientific" demonstrations. Nitrous and Davy's other anesthetic

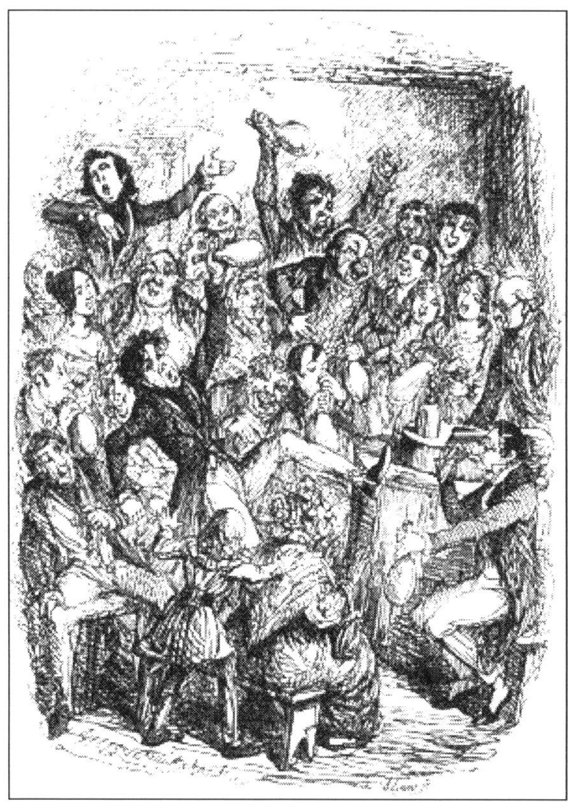

*In the early 1800s, ether and nitrous oxide were not just of scientific interest. They were used both for partying by medical students and in demonstrations at carnivals or chataqua. It wasn't until the 1820s, that dentistry used nitrous oxide as a pain killer. Physicians first used inhaled anesthetics in the 1840s.*

agents were a source of considerable amusement to the general public. By the early 19th century, a little more than 40 years after Priestly discovered it, nitrous oxide had become the most popular "experiment" at scientific exhibits and public chemistry demonstrations in the United States, and was commonly called laughing gas.

These popular public experiments led to medical students entertaining themselves with nitrous oxide outside of class. Many found nitrous oxide gas euphoric properties appealing. It was frequently incorporated into partying and personal entertainment. Social events called ether and/or nitrous oxide parties were held by medical and dental students and many others. The attendees became intox-icated at these functions by inhaling ether or nitrous oxide. These parties were common all over the country.[120] Some have likened these collegiate escapades, these "laughing gas frolics", to the use of marijuana on college campuses in the 1960s.

## The Holy Grail of Analgesia and Anesthesia

Pain is among humankind's greatest fears. Through the ages we have sought control of that pain. Opium and alcohol have the longest history as pain relievers. Until the end of the 19th century, opium was revered by physicians as God's Own Medicine, abbreviated G.O.M. In performing surgery, they were soon to be replaced by the far more effective gaseous anesthesia. It turned out Davy was correct about the analgesic potential of nitrous oxide. Nitrous oxide and ether were a 19th-century answer to man's quest for freedom from pain.

As early as 1824, "painless" dentists used $NO_2$ (nitrous oxide) as an anesthetic. It took another 30 years before allopathic physicians embraced nitrous oxide as an analgesic. As analgesics, both nitrous oxide and ether were more effective than alcohol and opium. These gases heralded our modern era of surgery under effective, controlled anesthesia.

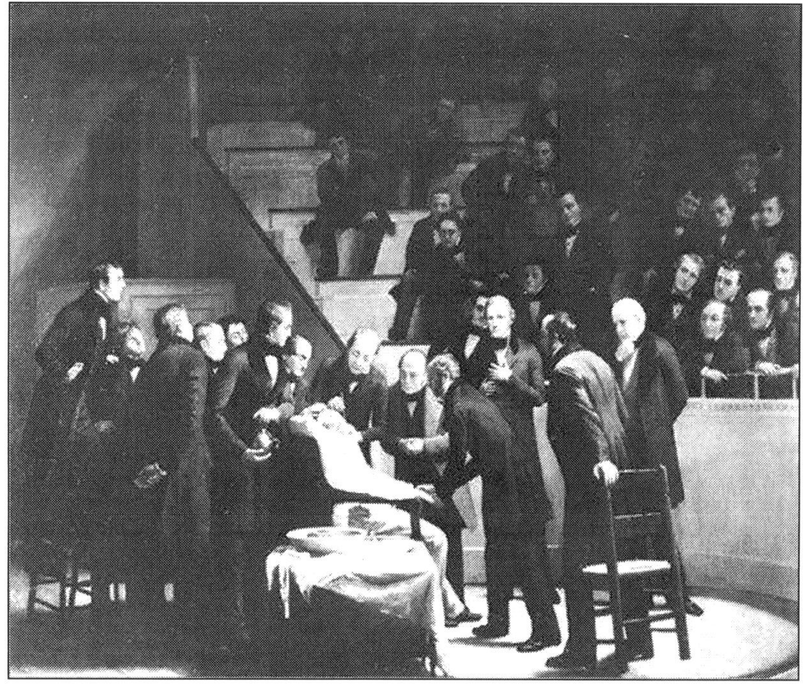

*The famous ether dome operation at Harvard in 1848. With Harvard's seal of approval, ether and other gas anesthetics became more widely accepted in medicine.*

Chloroform was another 19th-century gas that doctors partied with which gained acceptance as a gaseous anesthetic. In the mid-19th century, obstetrician James Young Simpson, MD, participated in a "chloroform party" where he discovered the analgesic effects of chloroform. The story goes that after all the party participants had awakened from their drug-induced revelry, they composed themselves and related the chloroform intoxicated dreams and visions that they had had.

When it was his turn, Dr. Simpson allegedly said "This, my dear friends, will give my poor women at the hospital the (pain) alleviation they need. A rather larger dose will produce profound narcotic slumber."[119] Simpson had stumbled on a method to control the pain of childbirth.

In 1847, he introduced chloroform into obstetrics but not without having to overcome some religious obstacles. Rather than acclaim, he was initially criticized for easing the pain of childbirth. The use of chloroform to ease the pain of childbirth (punishment for Eve's sin), was called "a satanic invention." He was called a "shameless heretic" and some of his fellow physicians snubbed him and called him an "irresponsible charlatan."[120]

Fortunately for him, and anesthesia, he was a religious man, and so was equipped to deal with his critics. "Simpson became a biblical scholar and met each pseudo-religious condemnation with skilled theological refutation. During four years of vigorous debate, his reputation grew; and gradually the wives of the clergy and his fellow physicians began seeking his obstetrical services. After Queen Victoria commanded her physician to give her chloroform during the birth of her eighth child, "the opposition to the obstetrical use of chloroform evaporated. Simpson was eventually given great honors and fame."[121]

## The Opium Trade

Opium's use as an analgesic goes back thousands of years. Opiates were and still are widely used to control pain. But, the influence of opiates on drug policy is related to their recreational use – particularly by the Chinese – rather than to the well known medical uses of opiates.

While the use of opium for medicinal purposes had long been known to the Chinese, the practice of smoking opium was not originated by the Chinese. In the late 1500s, within 30 years of tobacco being introduced into Europe from the New World by deNicotine and Thevet, tobacco laced with opium was introduced into China by Spanish, Portuguese and Dutch sailors. They ostensibly used it to ward off and/or treat malaria. Indeed because opium slows peristalsis it helps treat the accompanying diarrhea.[122]

The Europeans desired Chinese tea, spices and silk. But there was no commodity the Chinese would accept since they held the Europeans in great disdain. The Chinese saw Europeans as nothing more than "monkeys in opera suits" and certainly did not want what they deemed inferior European manufactured goods in trade for their coveted spices. They wanted to be paid in hard currency – gold, silver, jewels – and the Chinese got them. That is, until smoking opium was introduced into China by Europeans in the very late 1600s.

Under the mercantilism philosophy, it was imperative to have a positive balance of trade. In order for the Europeans to stop the hemorrhaging of hard currency going to China for silk, tea and spices, a satisfactory trading commodity needed to be found. With opium grown in the Mediterranean or India, the Europeans eventually had found a commodity to trade for China's valued tea, silk and spices.

The Emperor of China, concerned about the scourge of opium use, outlawed opium growing in China in 1729. The illicit opium trade flourished throughout the 18th century. However, the Chinese resolve grew and, in 1799, possession and cultivation of opium became banned completely. As has been the case with any desired forbidden commodity, the prohibition backfired. There was money to be made in the illicit market.

Opium was a good choice of a trading product. It's easy to transport, doesn't spoil easily, and there was a ready market in China. In addition to opium's real medical utility, demand exists from people who develop a physical and/or psychological dependency on opium.

Many a Chinese viceroy (roughly equivalent to a governor), became rich through bribes from European merchant traders. [123] To this day, when a desired, sought-after commodity is prohibited, there are enormous profits to be made on sale of the forbidden product. Since it is impossible to stop a plant from growing when there is a demand for a forbidden plant, humans can easily design ways to get it and to make money trading it.

The British were not the first to get into the opium trade with China, but the British East India Company (started by Queen Elizabeth in 1604) got in pretty early and by the mid-1700s, the British had control of the opium trade with China. In 1764, the British won control of Bengal where poppies flourished. British opium exports were 15 tons in 1720, 75 tons in 1773 and by 1820, 900 tons of opium/year were going from Bengal to China. [124]

Come the early 19th century, after trading opium with China since the early 1600s, some of the British people, particularly Quakers, were beginning to feel such trade was immoral and applied political heat at home. So in the 1820s, the British brought in a few U.S. middlemen, to assuage the moral sensibilities of their home grown critics. These U.S. businessmen included such prominent American families as the Forbes (John Kerry's forbearers), the Russells, who were cousins to the Bush family, and the ancestors of U.S. Presidents George H.W. Bush and George W. Bush. [125]

The British sold the opium to accommodating Americans, like Charles Russell & Company of Boston, who then put it on those classic tall-masted China Clipper sailing ships and sold it to the Chinese. The Charles Russell Company traded opium with the Chinese for silk, tea and spices, and then traded much of that to the British. The United States was basically laundering the drug trade for the British. Russell helped found "Skull and Bones", a secret society at Yale. (Both President George W. Bush and his 2004 Democratic opponent, John Forbes Kerry, were members.) Both the Forbes and Bush families' ancestors prospered from 19th century drug trade.

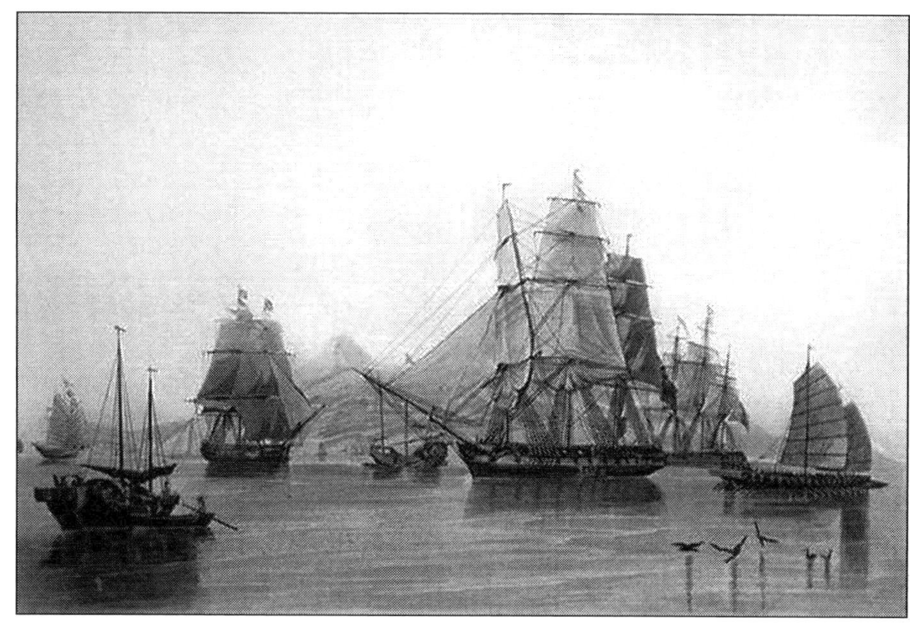

*The United States engaged in the opium trade with China. Due to increasing moral concerns in Britain in the early 19th century, the Americans were "cut" in on the opium trade. The British sold the opium to the Americans who sold it to the Chinese. The British hands were clean and along the way fortunes were made by such as John Jacob Astor, the Bushes and the Forbes. This drug dealing was all legal by the way.*

For over 150 years, "Skull and Bones" members have been implicated in the drug trade. [126] Other families of wealth can point to drugs as one source of their fortune. Joe Kennedy was a bootlegger and John Jacob Astor, the first U.S. multi-millionaire, was an opium shipper.

## Europeans Instigated Wars to Force Importation of Foreign Opium to China

All the European trading nations played a role in the growth of the modern drug trade but for almost two centuries the British were dominant. There was substantial money to be made in opium. The East India Company provided "massive profit for London companies and substantial revenues for the state." [127] At that time Britain was selling 1400 tons of opium to the Chinese, generating an enormous amount of revenue. The British East Indies Company continued to trade opium against the Chinese Emperor's dictate.

The first Opium War (1839-42) was fought because the British continued to force the opium trade upon China, even after stronger enforcement of the Emperor of China's opium ban. It wasn't long until this escalated into a clash. The financial, not to mention the moral stakes, were high. Only a relatively small percentage of the Chinese populous were smoking opium, nevertheless this still amounted to millions of consumers. By 1839, opium had become the world's most valuable single commodity of trade and remains so to this day. [128]

In 1838, the port of Canton got a new commissioner. Unlike his predecessor, who ignored the opium ban, he enforced the emperor's orders. The British government supported the British merchants who were supplying opium to China against the Chinese emperor's wishes and Chinese law. This led the British to fight the two Opium Wars to maintain access to Chinese markets and undermine Chinese law. [129]

In 1839, the Canton provincial government seized and burned British opium stores. The English responded in 1840 with war; attacking Chinese ships. The Chinese were subsequently defeated by the technologically superior British. In 1842, China signed the Treaty of Nanking, which gave the British the ability to trade opium and as an added bonus, control of Hong Kong for 150 years. The Second Opium War was fought in 1856 with China again losing. As a result of these losses, China was forced to accept increased opium imports. The Nanking Treaty (1842) and the Treaty of Tientsin (1858) brought the British government territory in China and the legalization of the opium trade. [130]

Not surprisingly, the opium trade and the Opium Wars with Europe created hostile feelings in China toward the West. China emerged from its long control by the Manchu Dynasty in 1910 as a result of a revolution led by Sun Yat-Sen.

By that time, the West was eager to increase trade with China. Only the United States was enthusiastic about worldwide control of opium but Europe was willing to attend conferences to mollify America and make a show of making amends to the Chinese.

Mid-19th century Oriental immigrants brought smoking opium to America, or at least made it more widely used. [131] Less than a decade after the end of the First Opium War, a disastrous flood wiped out a million acres of prime Chinese farmland. This created an economic crisis for that part of China and brought Chinese immigrants to American shores in large numbers. They worked hard and cheap and found work in the gold fields or supplying services and goods, such as doing laundry and selling groceries to the mining camps. A decade later, the Chinese and Irish provided much of the labor for building the Intercontinental Railroad.

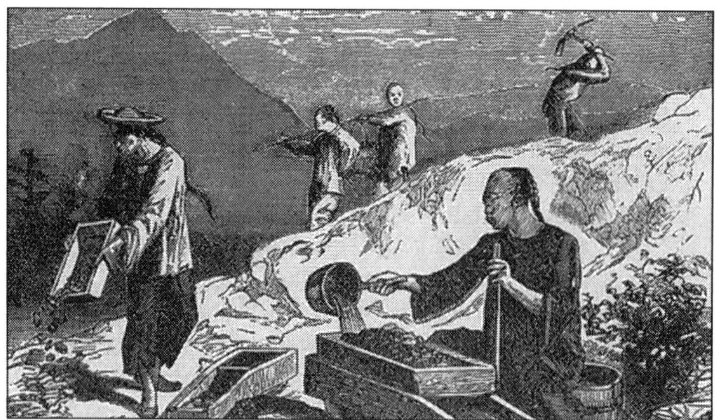

*Plagued by civil war, floods, droughts, typhoons and other disasters at home, many young Chinese boarded ships to California following the 1849 gold strike. By 1852, 25,000 Chinese were working in California's gold fields.* [132]

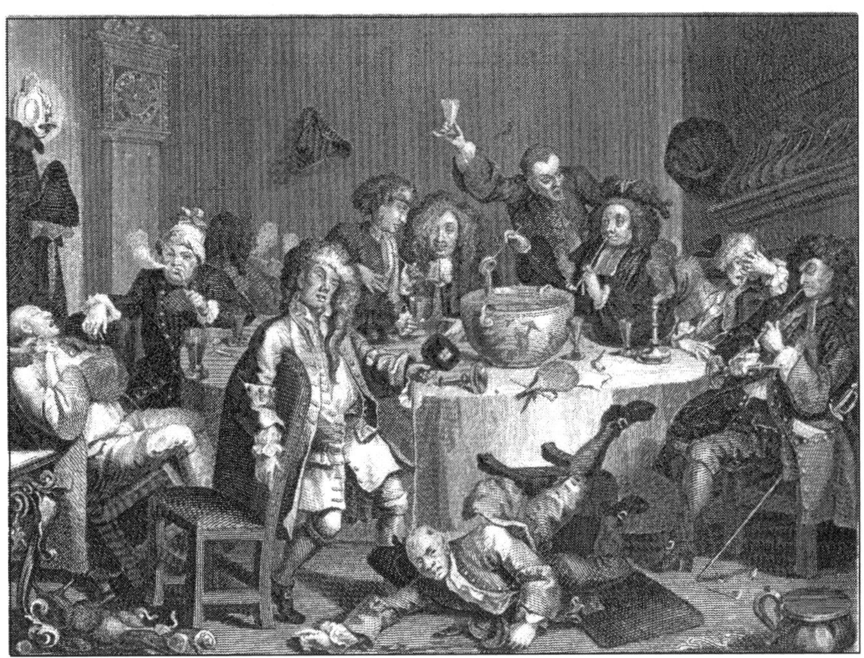

*"A Modern Midnight's Conversation" is a drawing by William Hogarth (1697-1764), an English painter, satirist and editorial cartoonist. It depicts a group of well-to-do men in various degrees of drunkenness at a late-night drinking party.*

# CHAPTER VII
# 1650-1900: Booze, Temperance & Abolition

## The Road from Booze

How did the United States go from a Colonial America founded on tobacco, mandating the growing of hemp, trading opium, frolicking with ether, and drinking beer and ale pretty much morning, noon and night – to Prohibition? The cultural attitude toward intoxicants started to change dramatically with the end of the Revolutionary War.

In the mid-18th century, well before the Revolutionary War, drinking habits in England changed from consuming alcohol drinks relatively low in alcohol content such as beer and wine with 3.5 to 8-percent alcohol content, to drinking fortified wine (port, etc. at 18-22 percent) and distilled spirits (gin at 35-40 percent). This led to more drunkenness and social disorder from alcohol consumption than had heretofore been the case.

The fortified wine came about as a result of England's traditional friction with the French. This led the British to impose high tariffs on French wine. Soon the British were drinking more fortified (e.i., alcohol-added) Portuguese wine. Replacing some beer and wine drinking with gin largely came about because the British started producing cheap gin.

## Drinking Gin

Gin, likely gets its name from the Arabic word *gin* meaning spirit or genie, and was first distilled in the East. England started producing gin -- hard liquor -- in the 18th century. Gin was cheap, readily available and heavily used. It was the "new urban drug." [1] Gin was popular with both the landed gentry and the poor.

The poor were fans because gin was both cheap and provided an escape from the misery and squalor of poverty in 18th-century England (think Charles Dickens'1838 novel *Oliver Twist*). Gin helped London's poor deal with their wretchedness. The landowners that produced grain favored gin for economic reasons and the governors didn't mind collecting the alcohol taxes. This increase in alcohol intake increased the incidence of real drinking problems. The British began to look more negatively upon drinking. This attitude soon crossed the pond.

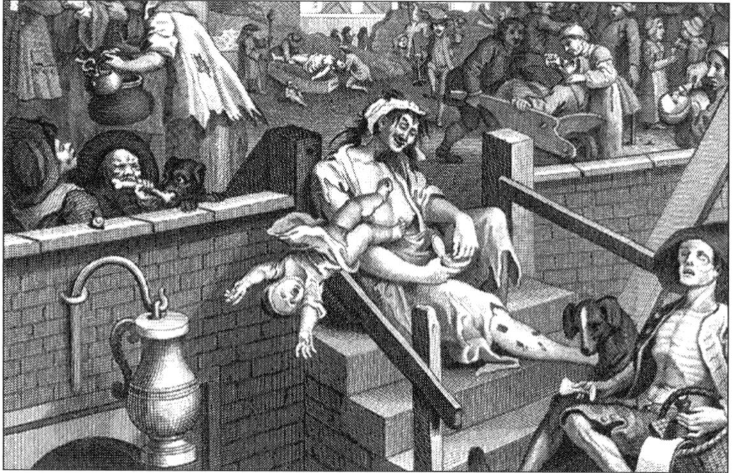

*Gin was popular among the lower classes. Gin was equated with back-alley shops where thieves met. It was associated with squalor, debauchery and crime. This all helped change the British attitude about drinking. Gin Lane is a famous painting depicting a demonic drink creating a nightmarish scene.*

These social attitudes were reflected in actions by the body politic. In the 1730s, the British Parliament passed a series of laws called the Gin Acts aimed at curbing the use of gin amongst the poor. These were an utter failure. Gin use actually increased, and there was "open contempt for the law and its agents." [2] As with today's war on drugs, there were paid informants, who only made matters worse. In, *Gin and Debauchery in the Age of Reason*, author Jessica Warner opines that the practice of using informers did more to undermine society than gin ever could. [3]

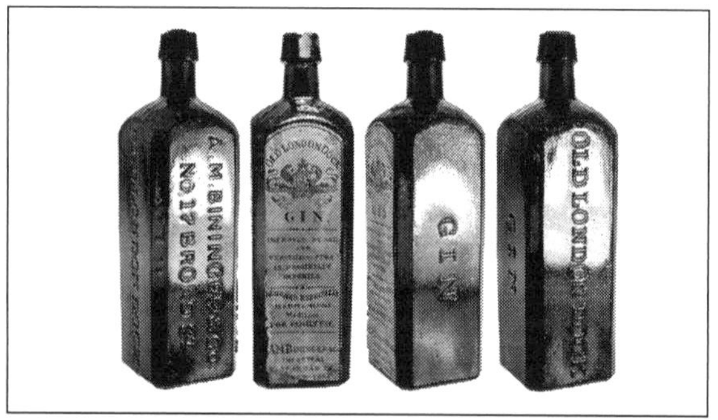


*Old Gin Bottles. Cheap gin helped fuel 18th-century British drunkenness.*

There had always been some colonists who had railed against drinking to excess. But the idea that alcohol is truly evil really took root in the United States some 175-225 years ago. [4] The writings of surgeon general of the Revolutionary Army and signer of the Constitution, Dr. Benjamin Rush (*An Inquiry into the Effects of Ardent Spirits on the Human Mind and Body* (1784), which pointed out the problems of drunk soldiers, plus the changing British attitude toward drink, helped turn the tide against the heretofore wide acceptance of the colonial drinking culture. Rush described the drinker's symptoms thusly: "...unusual garrulity, unusual silence, captiousness ... an insipid simpering ... profane swearing ... certain immodest actions" and "certain extravagant acts which indicate a temporary fit of madness." [5]

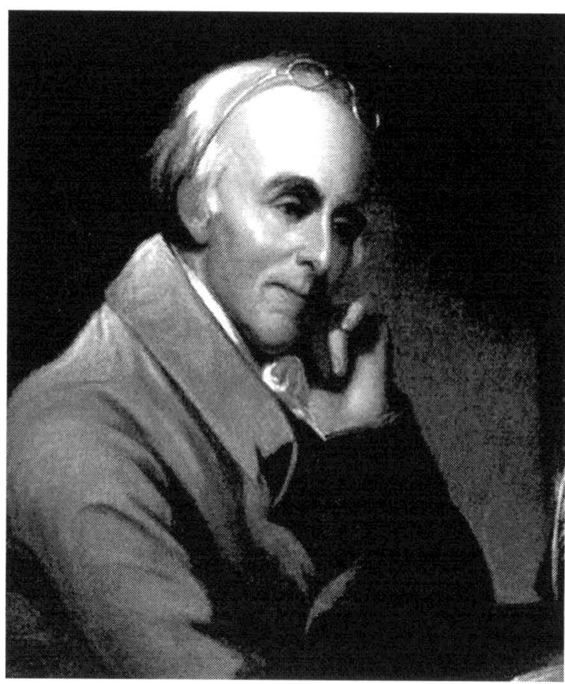

*Benjamin Rush was the surgeon general of the American Revolutionary Army. He was the only physician who was a signatory of the Declaration of Independence and the author of* An Inquiry into the Effects of Ardent Spirits on the Human Mind and Body. *His assessment of the adverse affects of alcoholic drink was promptly incorporated into the Temperance Movement's lexicon.*

Rush was neither a prohibitionist nor a temperance supporter. He was for moderation in drinking. Nevertheless, Rush's work was quickly incorporated into the campaign against the evils of alcohol, which was championed by some Protestant religious leaders. In 1789, the Methodist Church opposed the sale or drinking of "ardent spirits", the term for distilled liquor. The Presbyterian Synod of Pennsylvania and the yearly meeting of Friends of New England took the same position. [6] As the United States entered the 19th century, the Temperance flame was fanned by religious leaders including Cotton Mather, Dr. Lyman Beecham and John Wesley. [7] Thus were sown some of the earliest seeds of the Temperance Movement.

The American Temperance Society was formed in 1826. It was supported by religious groups that ran revival-style meetings. [8] This was "the new Protestant sects trying to impose a muscular Christianity on the denial of pleasure." [9] The Temperance Movement saw physical health and morality as closely aligned. Excessive use of alcohol (and later other drugs) was seen as a lack of self-discipline. In the Temperance Movement, first drug abuse and then, with Prohibition, mere drug use, came to be defined as a disease of moral weakness. [10]

In fairness to the Temperance promoters, after the Revolutionary War there was a significant increase in the already heavy consumption of alcohol. This increase in booze intake largely preceded the immigration influx. Figures vary, but it's agreed that the consumption of alcohol increased in the early 1800s as supply increased and the price of alcohol fell. [11]

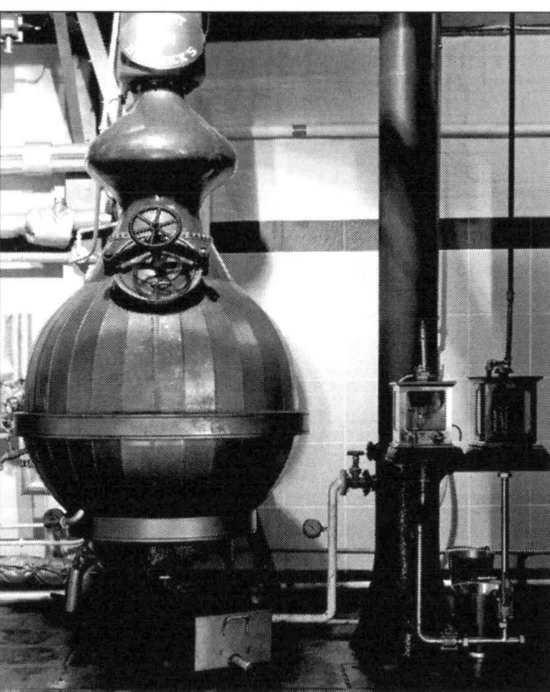

*A Bennet copper-pot still made in 1860. Distilled spirits usually contain 25-50% alcohol. Beer 3-6%, wine 9-12% and fortified wine 15-20%.*

By some accounts, the average American in the 1830s aged 15 or older consumed over seven gallons of absolute alcohol. This is based on an average yearly consumption of 4.3 gallons of distilled spirits, and 2.8 gallons of beer, wine and cider, which is several times the current rate of consumption. [12] W.J. Rorabaugh estimated the per capita consumption of distilled spirits was only five gallons annually, but this is still about five times the current rate. [13]

Rorabaugh noted that with this increase in drinking, there was a marked increase in drunkenness, causing widespread community complaint and commentary. Family violence became more visible. Stories of domestic violence, wife and child beating increased and there were more accounts of drunken mothers neglecting their children.

## Irish Immigration to America During the Potato Famine Changed the Discussion

Even with the increase in drinking and Rush's writings, influential as he was, it's unlikely this would have triggered prohibition as a legal, not a medical approach, to problems associated with alcohol abuse. Were it not for the influx of immigrants, particularly Irish Catholics, in the second and third quarters of the 19th century, Temperance and Prohibition would not have had the immigrants to use as a handy whipping boy. The Irish Catholics in the 1840s were only the first large wave of new, different immigrants to arrive in the United States in the 19th century. They were soon followed by German Catholics, the Chinese and, from 1880 to 1924, a virtual tsunami of immigration from Italy and Eastern Europe.

By the mid-19th century, immigrants were coming to the United States in large numbers. This large infusion of foreigners from different countries with different religions than the existing European inhabitants of the United States, coupled with economic concerns, fanned the flames of nativism. Americans found ample things to criticize these newcomers for – their food, their smell, their drink, their partying, their desire for "our" women and "our" jobs.

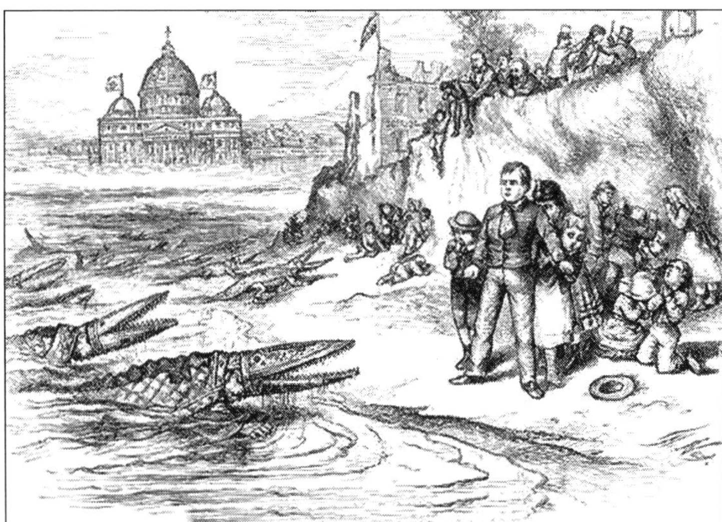

*An editorial cartoon by the famous Thomas Nast demonstrates the anti-Catholic attitude of the time portraying bishops as alligators.*

In the mid-19th century, the arrival of large numbers of Irish into the United States supercharged the Temperance Movement. It is no exaggeration to speculate that without the massive immigration of Irish Catholics, we would NOT have the drug laws we have today.

In certain parts of the Northeast, Irish immigrants arriving in mid-19th-century America had lower social status than freed slaves. [14] This reception was different than what 18th-century Irish immigrants had faced. The earlier Irish Immigrants were largely Protestant. Further, many were Scotch-Irish. They traced their ancestors to those Scots that had been transported from Scotland to Ireland by the English in the 1600s in a British effort to blunt the political power of the original, indigenous Irish.

THE HOME OF AN INDULGENT MOTHER
PLENTY OF PICKLES AND PORK
MEXICANIZED DISHES AND PEPPER SAUCES
CANDIES AND RICH PASRIES
TEA, COFFEE AND COCA
SODAS, POP AND GINGERALE
TOBACCO AND CIGARETTES
CARDS, DICE AND POOL
LIQUOR AND STRONG DRINK
A DRUNKARD'S GRAVE

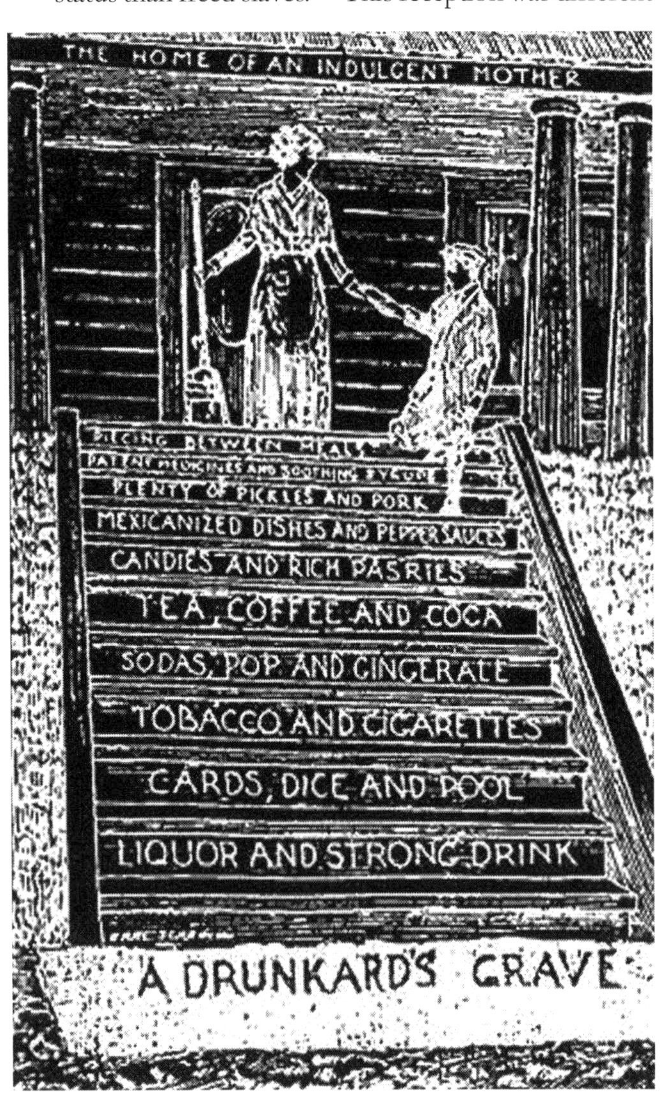

"Starting Her Son Toward a Drunkard's Grave." *The concept that one thing leads to another goes back to the 19th century.*

Many of the relatively small number of Irish Catholic immigrants that arrived before 1815 quickly adopted Protestantism, in part because in most of the United States Catholics were a decided minority. The Irish also were fierce fighters in the Revolutionary War. So the early, largely Scotch-Irish immigrants were better accepted by the English colonists, than their 19th-century immigrant Catholic cousins.

After the great potato famine of the 1840s, there was a deluge upon U.S. shores of millions of Irish Catholic immigrants. The Protestant English, particularly in the Northeast, often stereotyped these newcomers as nothing more than a collection of drunken bums that coveted their pure Protestant women.

It has been derided by many historians as hyperbole, but Irish-Americans insist that in the first half of the 19th century, "Help Wanted" signs could be seen in Boston reading "Help Wanted – No Irish Need Apply." True or not, it accurately reflects the animosity directed by

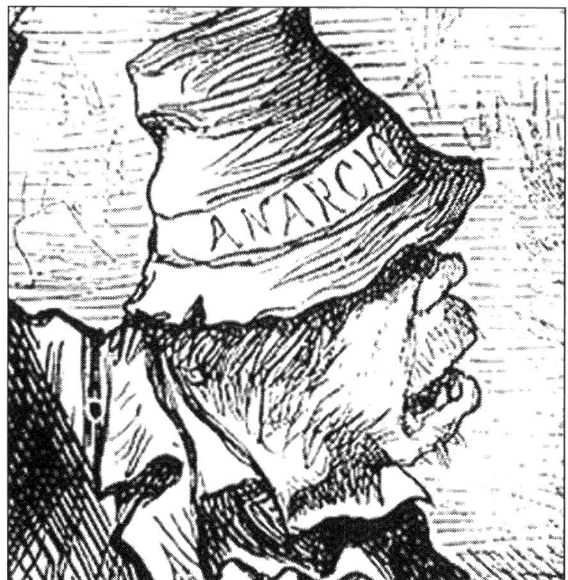


*Cartoons in* Punch, *a British weekly magazine of humor and satire, portrayed the Irish as having "bestial or demonic features, and the Irishman (especially the political radical) was invariably given a long, protruding or prognathous jaw.*

the so-called "native" Americans (Americans of European descent born on the North American continent) toward the Irish in 19th-century America.

With this flood of Irish immigration, the Temperance Movement in mid-19th-century America was being whipped up to a full gallop. As later waves of immigrants arrived, each was marginalized and discriminated against. This was certainly true for Chinese and Germans starting in the late 19th century and Jews, Eastern Europeans and Southern Italians in the early 20th.

There was enormous anti-Irish prejudice in 19th-century England and this attitude had acceptance by many in America. Professor Anthony Wohl of Vassar describes it this way:

> **"During the 19th century, theories of race were advanced both by the scientific community and in the popular daily and periodical press. Even before Charles Darwin published *On the Origin of Species* in 1859, the old concept of the great chain of being, marking the gradations of mankind, was being subjected to a new scientific racism. The 'science' of phrenology purported to demonstrate that the structure of the skull, especially the jaw formation and facial angles, revealed the position of various races on the evolutionary scale, and a debate raged on whether there had been one creation for all mankind (monogenism) or several (polygenism)."** [15]

Dehumanizing, demeaning and demonizing have always been used to marginalize the others. The most extreme example is the Nazi anti-Jewish propaganda but the British give the great WW II German propagandist a run for their money in their relentless multi century efforts to dehumanize the Irish.

The pseudo-scientific literature of the day held the Irish to be inferior. "The Irish were understood to be an example of a lower evolutionary form, closer to the apes than their 'superiors,' the Anglo-Saxons. The phrenologists of that day saw this (e.g., physiognomy) as the mark of a lower evolutionary order, degeneracy or criminality." [16] This attitude justified, for the British, their greater concern about drinking in the Irish than in their own alcoholic consumption.

Nineteenth-century Irish immigrants arriving in America quickly saw the parallels between their former lives back in Ireland under the British and that of the African slaves in America. Instead of sympathizing with the slaves of African origin and working for their emancipation, the Irish immigrants seized the opportunity to climb from the bottom rung of society by stepping on the African slaves. "The Irish learned this lesson through hardship. As one Southern planter explained to his Northern visitor, the planter had hired an Irish gang to drain a swamp because "It's dangerous work and a Negro's life is too valuable to be risked." [17]

Many Irish crowded near the ports where they landed. They were uneducated and poor, and lived in slums of horrible filth, like Manhattan's Five Points slum. (Think of the Martin Scorsese directed movie *Gangs of New York*.) The Irish were denigrated by society, discriminated against in employment and competed with freed blacks for the same jobs. The Irish did what they could to promote themselves by using their "whiteness."

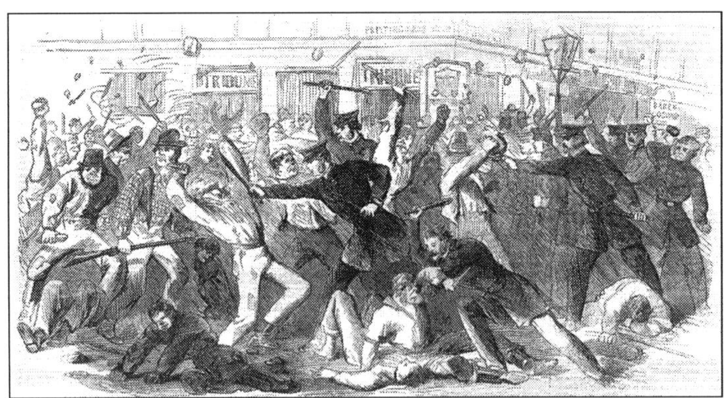

*The New York Draft Riots of July 13-16, 1863 were the second largest civil insurrection in U.S. history. A Black sailor, William Williams, was beaten and lynched. Afterward a member of the mob swore "vengeance on every Nigger in New York."* [18]

between Irish immigrants and free Negroes. The riots saw 11 blacks murdered and many more beaten. Fifty buildings including two churches and an orphanage for Black children were burned. One consequence was that Negroes left New York proper and moved to Harlem, which in time became a center of Black society. [19]

## The Rise of Nativism — "Them Immigrants Is Different"

The 1840s and 1850s saw more and different immigrants coming to America's shores. There was general concern amongst the citizenry about the immigrants' real and imagined differentness and this extended to their use of recreational drugs. First there were Irish Catholics who the British said couldn't hold their whisky, then the German Catholics, with their beer drinking and hearty partying. The California Gold Rush and the railroads' need for cheap labor, coupled with a devastating flood in China, saw an influx of Chinese immigrants, often vilified as "non-Christian" opium "addicts".

This increased rate of immigration of "them", stoked American nativism, the idea that America was only for the native born, preferably of English or Dutch descent and definitely Protestant. These new immigration patterns of the mid-19th century, stimulated a strong strain of nativism.

Nativisms' ugly stereotypes and prejudices against new immigrants soon had a strong impact on American drug policy. Allegations included such ideas as: the Irish couldn't hold their liquor; they came to work drunk; and besides that, they were Irish and they were Catholic. The Germans drank beer and too much of it and had a good time. They were Catholic, too. The Chinese were sneaky: they lured innocent white women into opium dens and, they weren't even Christians.

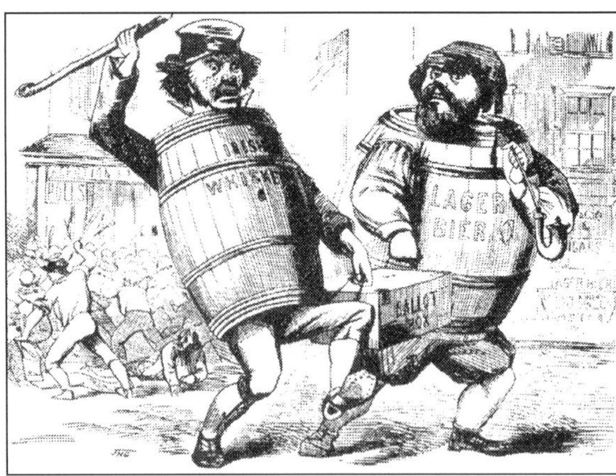

*19th-century Nativism sentiment is reflected in the cartoons of Thomas Nast. The barrel of the man with the club, reads "Irish Whisky." The other barrel reads "Lager", a German beer. They're shown fighting over a stolen ballot box.*

Roman Catholic immigrants concentrated in Eastern cities where they added to the political strength of the Democrats. Local nativistic societies formed to combat these "foreign" influences and to champion the "American" view. In the 1850s, these nativist societies were anti-Catholic organizations. Only after the Civil War (1861-65) and the end of slavery was it "necessary" for them to be anti-Black as well. It wasn't until 1865, in Pulaski, Tennessee that the Ku Klux Klan was founded.

While the movie *Gangs of New York* compressed and rearranged history, it did accurately depict the

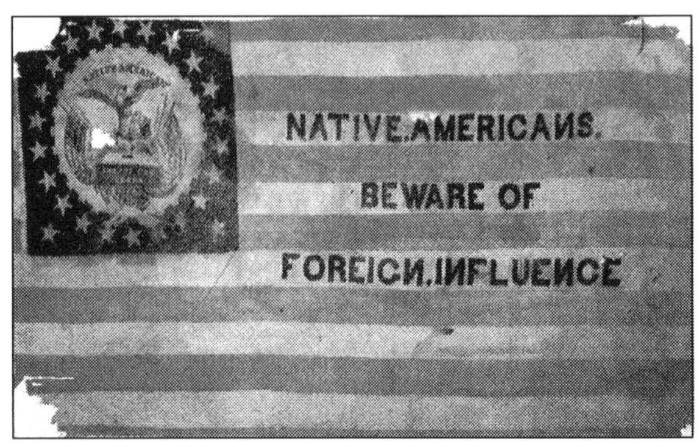


*Emerging in the 1850s as part of the anti-Catholic movement of the era, the Know Nothing Party somehow was able to graft itself onto the new anti-slavery Republican Party, although Abraham Lincoln disavowed it.*

brutality of the New York Draft Riots of 1863. These riots occurred during the Civil War and represent the largest U.S. civil insurrection except for the Civil War itself.

The riots started as objections to new draft laws. which allowed the rich to hire someone to take their place. They soon took on an ugly racial overture, ostensibly blaming Negroes for the war but also triggered in part by job competition.

The Republican Party was formed in 1854 in Ripon, Wisconsin and held its first convention later that same year in Jackson, Michigan. Another nativist group, the so-called Know Nothing Party of the 1850s, got its informal name from its members replying, when asked about their role, "I know nothing." The party was anti-Catholic and anti-immigrant. It grew out of the Order of the Star-Spangled Banner, a secret society founded in New York City in 1849.[20,21] The increasing popularity of the Temperance Movement was aided by these nativistic fears, stereotypes and bigotry.

Elements of the Know Nothings merged with Whig factions to form the Republican Party. Even so, Lincoln, a Republican, was no fan of the Know Nothings. In an August 24, 1855 letter to Joshua F. Speed, he wrote:

> "I am not a Know-Nothing. That is certain. How could I be? How can anyone who abhors the oppression of Negroes be in favor of degrading classes of white people? Our progress in degeneracy appears to me to be pretty rapid. As a nation, we begin by declaring that 'all men are created equal.' We now practically read it 'all men are created equal, except negroes.' When the Know-Nothings get control, it will read, 'all men are created equal, except negroes, and foreigners, and Catholics.' When it comes to this I should prefer emigrating to some country where they make no pretense of loving liberty – to Russia, for instance, where despotism can be taken pure, and without the base alloy of hypocrisy."[22]
>
> **Abraham Lincoln**
> U.S. President, 1861-1865

## Nativism: A Motivation for Drug Laws

Notwithstanding Lincoln's condemnation, this kind of Nativistic thinking was part and parcel of the forces motivating the demonization and discrimination of "them". There was a litany of concerns expressed about those who weren't "us". This fear of those who were different — used different drugs, or familiar drugs in different ways — eventually helped lead to the Harrison Narcotics Tax Act of 1914. The Harrison Act targeted Chinese and Negroes and presumably the low-life criminal element for their opium and cocaine use. Then as now, the widespread use of these substances by white society was overlooked or minimized.

Prohibition was put over the top by anti-German feelings in the World War I-era . These anti-German sentiments extended to the use of grain to make beer (the vast majority of U.S. breweries being owned by Germans), which, it was said, could have gone to make bread for the troops. It was like throwing gas on the fire of support for alcohol prohibition, a fire that was already fueled by anti-Irish and anti-immigrant hostility.

Similarly, the 1937 Marijuana Tax Act was largely driven by fears and demonization of Mexicans, Puerto Ricans, Negroes and jazz musicians. Although, the real behind-the-scenes momentum was probably Big Business lining up against the potential economic impact of hemp on the petrochemical, munitions and paper industries.

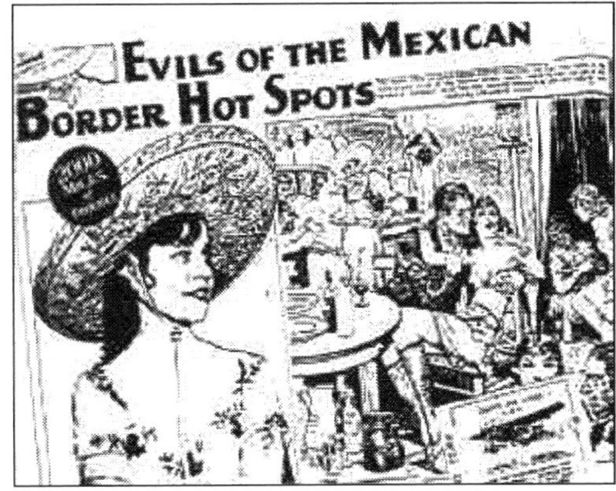

*Anti-Mexican propaganda of the 1930s, showing drunken partying with Mexicans of low morals at border "hot spots".*

By the time of the Controlled Substances Act of 1970, the U.S. government was targeting not just minorities, but the poor, the young, hippies, anti-war activists and the occasional liberal. These anti-drug laws have eroded civil rights like the sea lapping against a high cliff, which over time gets undermined and crumbles.

## What about those (indigenous) Redskins?

The 1860s through the 1950s were the height of American hostility – hostility is way too mild a word – toward those who were "different". Animosity toward the Chinese was huge during this period, but it merely resulted in discriminatory laws against smoking opium, stopped immigration from China and vilified the Chinese and their traditions. Blacks were still being lynched, Italians judicially railroaded, Japanese interned, the Jews rounded up and gassed in Europe while for several years the United States looked the other way, and Mexican workers were exploited and marginalized in the United States.

Still, Native Americans received by far the worst of it. They were forced off their land, women and children murdered, entire villages decimated, their way of life, culture, and religion destroyed. The reasons for this holocaust are many and varied. The Native Americans were definitely "different". Worse yet, the Native Americans, so-called Indians, venerated the land and some tribes used tobacco or peyote to enhance or generate spiritual visions. They slowed American expansion westward.

The Native Americans had the audacity to suggest that the lands they had roamed for thousands of years were theirs, and should be preserved and held in perpetual trust for future generations. The Indian belief is that no one owns the land, the land owns people. The land is here when a person is born and when the person dies the land is still here. The land is perpetual. Humans are merely the interim caretakers.

---

"Sell your country! Why not sell the air, the clouds, and the great sea?"

**Tecumseh**

Indian warrior chief, 1768-1813
in resisting suggestions that the Indians cede their lands in the Ohio country to the United States, 1810.

---

## It was Genocide for the Real Native Americans

It's a close call as to whether indigenous peoples or Blacks have fared the worst over the full span of American history, but between the 1860s to the 1890s, clearly the heinous brutalization of Native Americans was genocide.

In the early 1600s, disease effectively killed 95% of the Native Americans, thereby easing the way for the Pilgrims to succeed in the New World. [23] The remnants of these coastal tribes moved inland, vacating their villages and cleared land. There they joined other clans and tribes in the interior who had yet to encounter the European germs to which they had little resistance.

As a result of this exodus of Native Americans, there was little opposition to the European newcomers. The early colonists could till land already cleared by the native population, now abandoned due to pervasive death from infectious disease. [24]

The lot of the true discoverers of America only got worse. In 1823, John Ridge, a Cherokee leader and a man of some considerable wealth, described the racial oppression of the 19th-century American Indian:

> **"An Indian ... is frowned upon by the meanest peasant, and the scum of the earth are considered sacred in comparison to the son of nature. If an Indian is educated in the sciences, has a good knowledge of the classics, astronomy, mathematics, moral and natural philosophy, and his conduct equally modest and polite, yet he is an Indian, and the most stupid and illiterate white man will disdain and triumph over this worthy individual. It is disgusting to enter the house of a white man and be stared at full face in inquisitive ignorance ..." [25]**

**John Ridge**

Cherokee leader in Georgia, 1802-39
and son of Chief Major Rush

## Hey, Oklahoma is Just Like Florida and Georgia. Come On, You'll Like It There.

U.S. President Andrew Jackson's policy towards the indigenous people of America was to keep 'em moving. The Indians were occupying land coveted by the Europeans. It was desired in part because gold had been discovered in Georgia. In Jackson's first annual address to Congress in 1829, he laid out his plan to relocate Indians from the eastern United States to west of the Mississippi. His Indian policy continued throughout his administration and in his sixth annual message he said,

> **"My original convictions upon this subject have been confirmed by the course of events for several years, and experience is every day adding to their strength. That those tribes can not exist surrounded by our settlements and in continual contact with our citizens is certain. They have neither the intelligence, the industry, the moral habits, nor the desire of improvement which are essential to any favorable change in their condition. Established in the midst of another and a superior race, and without appreciating the causes of their inferiority or seeking to control them, they must necessarily yield to the force of circumstances and ere long disappear."** [26]
>
> **Andrew Jackson**
> U.S. President, 1829-37
> annual address to Congress, 1834

Congress passed the Indian Removal Act in 1830. It was opposed by the famous Tennessee congressman and frontiersman, Davy Crockett, and many other European Americans. This federal law called for removal of all eastern tribes to west of the Mississippi River. It was supposed to be a voluntary exchange of land. It wasn't. The Native Americans were not keen on leaving land they had occupied for thousands of years.

Most agree that moving people forcibly off their ancestral lands is heartless and uncaring. The Cherokees certainly did not agree with Jackson's assessment. To fight Jackson, they formed the Cherokee Nation and fought the government in the courts. They were led by the first and only elected chief of the Cherokee Nation, John Ross, who was one-eighth Cherokee.

In a Sept. 28, 1836 letter to the U.S. Senate and House of Representatives, Ross attacked the Indian Removal Act:

> **"By the stipulations of this instrument we are despoiled of our private possessions, the indefensible property of individuals. We are stripped of every attribute of freedom and eligibility for legal self-defense. Our property may be plundered before our eyes, violence may be committed on our persons; even our lives may be taken away, and there is none to regard our complaint. We are denaturalized, we are disenfranchised. We are deprived of leadership in the human family! We have neither land nor home, nor resting place that can be called our own. ... We are overwhelmed! Our hearts are sickened, our utterance is paralyzed, when we sifted on the condition in which we are placed by**

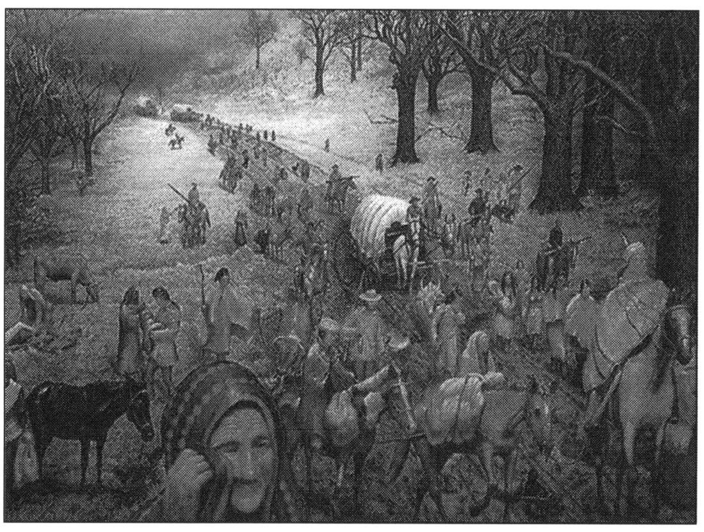

*The last of the Cherokee suffered forced removal in the infamous 1838 Trail of Tears march to the Indian Territory (present-day Oklahoma). Over a fourth of the Cherokee died on the forced march. And when they got there, the indigenous Plains Indians resented the newcomers.*

**the audacious practices of unprincipled men who have managed their strategies with so much dexterity as to impose on the Government of the United States, in the face of our earnest, solemn and reiterated protestations."** [27]

**John Ross** (1790-1866)
Principal Chief of the Cherokee Nation, 1828–1866.

While there was savagery toward the indigenous peoples of the Americas in the colonial period, it pales in comparison to the Native Americans' fate in the 19th century. This sordid chapter of American history includes the Trail of Tears, a forced journey of relocation for Native Americans of Florida, Georgia and the South to Oklahoma, Indian Territory. It continued 35 years later with the genocide of the founders of America in the slaughter of the Northern Plains tribes.

In the former instance, Southern tribes were forced to relocate to Oklahoma Indian Territory. As they sadly made the forced journey, thousands died en route. All the Eastern tribes eventually were relocated west of the Mississippi, but certainly not in accord with the government's pledge that relocation would be "on a strictly voluntary basis" (this policy was not written into the act).

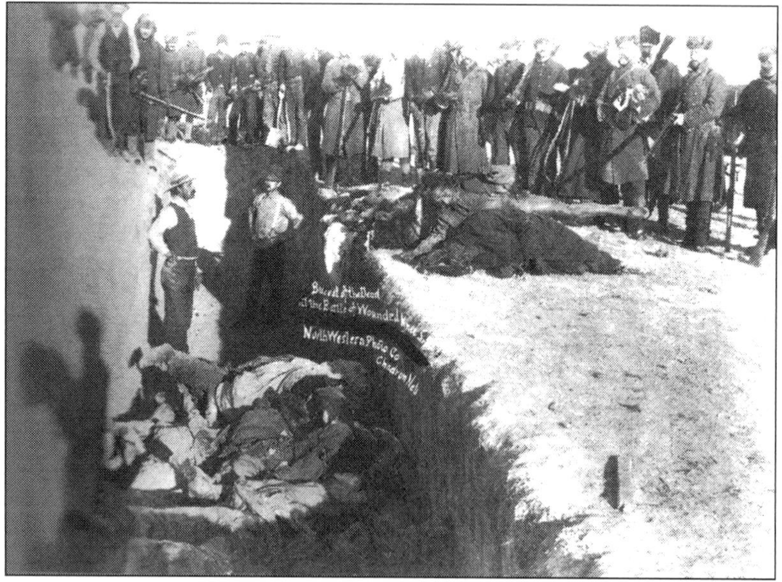


*Europeans famously massacred Native Americans at Sand Creek and Wounded Knee, but it was European germs that nearly wiped out the native population, killing almost 95%.*

Nearly all relocation was carried out under duress. Many relocation marches were accompanied by military escort of U.S. soldiers. Some tribes left only after their numbers were so decimated by broken treaties, fraudulent land deals and wars with American forces that there were no other options but to capitulate to leaving their ancient lands. [28]

## It Only Gets Worse and More Overt

Gold discovered in California in 1849 prompted development of overland routes from the East to the West Coast. This had a catastrophic effect on the native peoples of the Great Plains. The Oregon Trail disrupted the immense buffalo herds that were the keystone to the culture of the Plains Indians. Immigrants encroached on native lands and native life.

The United States' erection of forts and breaking of treaties provided more violence to the indigenous population and their way of life. [29] There were bloody Plains Wars between 1850 and 1880. The U.S. military acted cruelly and duplicitously. To subdue the historical inhabitants of the plains, the U.S. cavalry destroyed the Native Americans' possessions and exterminated the buffalo upon which they depended.

The 1864 massacre of Dull Knife's band of friendly Cheyenne at Sand Creek, Colorado is symbolic of the United States' *defacto* genocide policy. The Sand Creek Massacre was an attack on a sleepy Cheyenne village. Dull Knife's group had been directed to Sand Creek after first coming to Fort Lyon as part of a peace deal. The cavalry slaughtered as many of the Native Americans at Sand Creek as they could run down. [30]

The Native Americans, who weren't killed, were targeted for assimilation.

> "Policy-makers viewed reservations as temporary halfway houses on the road to assimilation. By the late 19th century, they were dismayed that many native people persisted in their customs and beliefs. Easterners hoping to assimilate Indians and westerners hoping to acquire reservation lands

coalesced in 1887 to pass the Dawes Severalty Act. Each individual Indian would receive between 40 and 160 acres of land, to be held in trust by the government for twenty-five years while native owners learned how to manage real estate. Homesteaders could buy any land left over. Policy-makers believed that private property would transform Indians' collective values; their cultural traditions would soon follow. The Dawes Act disregarded treaty terms nationwide, except in the arid Southwest. Although some enterprising Indians favored allotment, the vast majority opposed it, but to no avail. In *Worcester v. Georgia* (1832), the Supreme Court had confirmed the absolute plenary power of the United States over native tribes." [31]

## Custer Died For Your Sins

Vincent Deloria, Jr., the son of an Indian Episcopal clergyman, wrote *Custer Died for Your Sins* in 1969. In a November 28, 2005 opinion piece, Mary Annette Pember characterized this book as a scathing review of Indian and American relations. His *New York Times'* obituary of Nov. 13, 2005 mentions how Deloria had called the 1876 Battle of Little Big Horn – where Sioux and Cheyenne warriors defeated Gen. George Custer and his troops – a *"sensitivity training session."* [32]
Pember wrote:

> "Like his father, Mr. Deloria was a seminarian, as well as trained in law school. His deep appreciation and understanding of the power of spirituality was evident in his book *God Is Red*. It offers a look at native cosmology and describes the sophistication of Indian spirituality. It also questions the dominance of modern Christianity in American culture." [33]

In the ramp up to Custer's last stand, Custer and his troops were hunting the Lakota, Cheyenne and other tribes that were allegedly "on the war path." The Indians were "upset" because the U.S. government had unilaterally abrogated the 1868 Ft. Laramie Treaty. The treaty granted the indigenous peoples rights in perpetuity to certain lands. Now the United

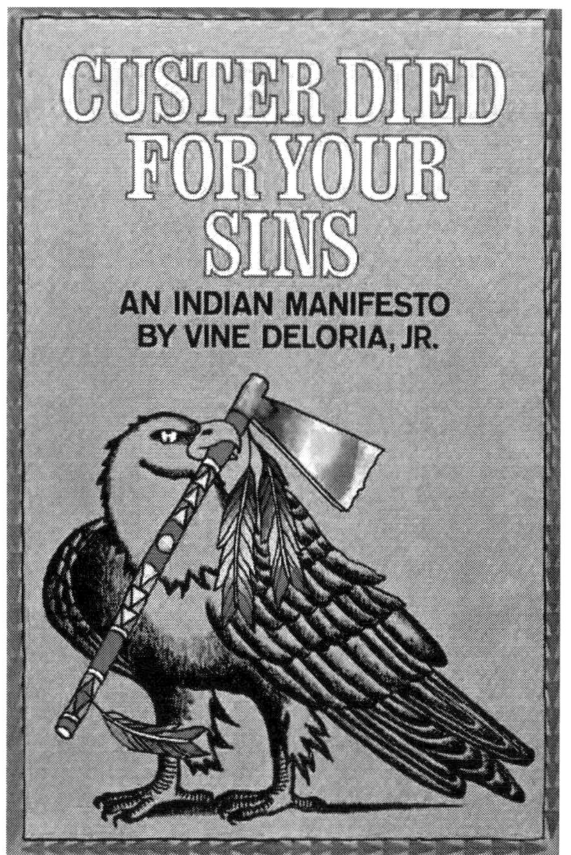


*A modern bumper sticker facetiously echoes Deloria's book title,* Custer Died for Your Sins. *In a way, Custer did. America certainly has a lot to atone for in its treatment of the original discoverers and inhabitants of "America".*

States wanted to move the Indians off their lands yet again. Why? Gold had been discovered in "them thar hills." Unfortunately it was the Black Hills, sacred to the Lakota. It was a part of the Lakota's land, per the sacred word of the federal government of the United States.

Sitting Bull, a spiritual leader of the Hunkpapa band, fought to preserve the Lakota way of life. According to both oral and written history, Sitting Bull refused to sell any part of the sacred land and move to the reservation. He objected to the reduction of the Native American lands and fought to preserve the way of life of the Native Americans.

**"I am ready to fight. My people are killed, my horses stolen; I am satisfied to fight."** [34]

**Cheyenne Chief Two Moon**
before the Battle of the Little Big Horn

The U.S. government, through the brutal actions of the Army, the numbing bureaucracy of the Bureau of Indian Affairs (BIA), the separating of children from their families, and the employment of reservation schools, systematically tried to destroy this naturalistic culture built up over millennia by the indigenous peoples of America.

In the summer of 1876, Sitting Bull had a famous dream of a great victory over the U.S. cavalry soldiers. This dream became reality at the Battle of the Little Big Horn June 25, 1876. The Lakota Nation with their allies the Cheyenne and Arapahoe defeated the 7th Cavalry under General George A. Custer, whose orders had been to bring the Sioux bands in and place them on the reservation lands.

But this was a last hurrah. Soon the buffalo were gone and the nomadic life no more. The tribes were on reservations and their children in BIA schools where they were not taught their native language or religion. Contemporary author Scott Momaday puts it this way:

> "On December 15, 1890, the great Hunkpapa leader Sitting Bull, who had opposed Custer at the Little Bighorn and who had toured for a time with Buffalo Bill and the Wild West show, was killed on the Standing Rock reservation. In a dream he had foreseen his death at the hands of his own people. This was a scant two weeks before the Wounded Knee Massacre. Killing nearly 300 of the original 350 men, women and children in the camp." [35]

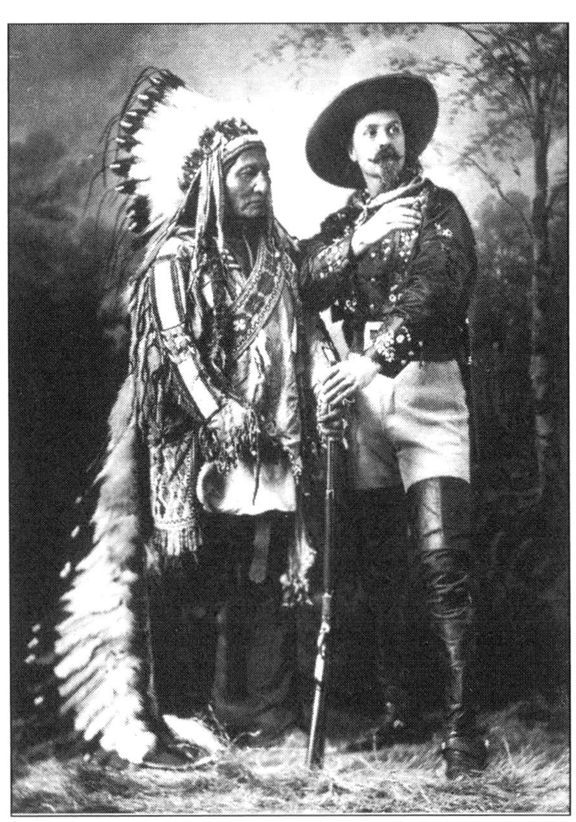

*Sitting Bull was a great Indian leader. He dreamed of the victory at the Little Big Horn before it happened. He toured with Buffalo Bill (pictured) and later had a dream foretelling the circumstances of his own death.*

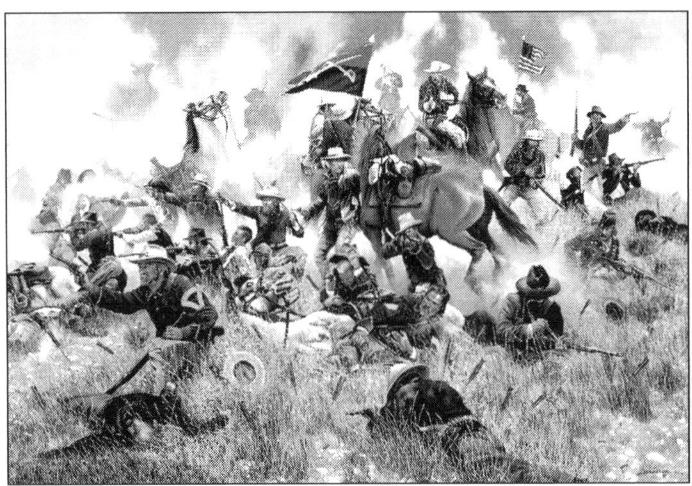

*Custer's assignment was to forcibly move the Indians off land that previously had been granted to them. In so doing, the U.S. government was violating the Fort Laramie Treaty of 1851. Custer and his men were defeated at the Battle of the Little Bighorn.*

"Sitting Bull is reported to have said, 'I am the last Indian.' In some sense he was right. During his lifetime the world of the Plains Indians had changed forever. The old roving life of the buffalo hunters was over. A terrible disintegration and

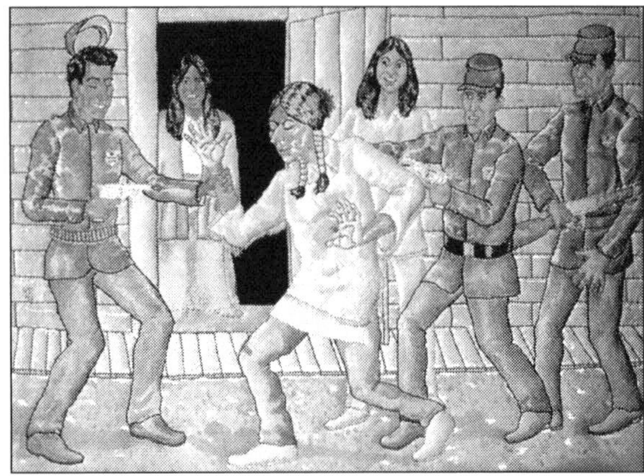

*In a misunderstanding, Sitting Bull was arrested and killed by his own tribe, an event he foretold.*

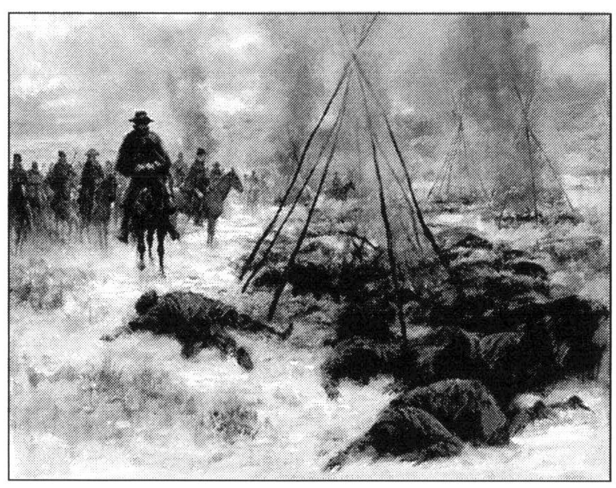

*The Indians camped at Wounded Knee were mostly old men, women and children. They did make efforts to defend themselves and 25 of the 492 soldiers and scouts that attacked them were killed. "What Wounded Knee has come to symbolize is a clash of cultures and a failed government-Indian policy; its effects still felt even today."*[36]

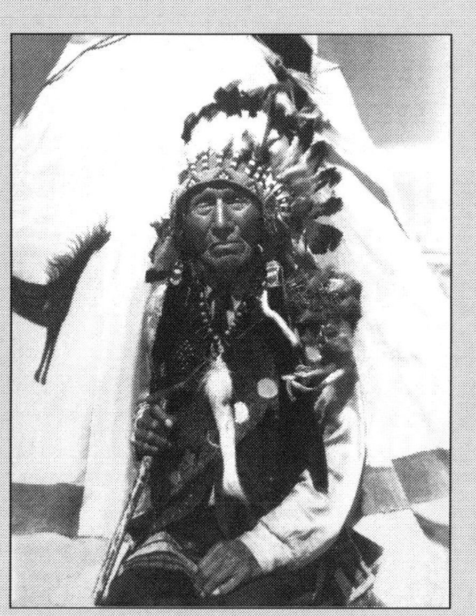

*"I did not know then how much was ended. When I look back now from the high hill of my old age, I can still see the butchered women and children lying heaped and scattered all along the crooked gulch as plain as when I saw them with eyes still young. And I can see that something else died there in the bloody mud, and was buried in the blizzard. A people's dream died there. It was a beautiful dream..."* [37]

**Black Elk,** 1863-1950
a famous medicine man of the
Oglala Lakota Sioux

### Don't Pay Any Attention to the Man Behind the Curtain

A December 17, 2006 op-ed piece by Tim Giago castigates the Wounded Knee atrocity. As a young boy, Glago lived in Wounded Knee where there is a mass grave that the Lakotas still come to pray at. Glago writes,

"Two ironies still haunt me. Six days after the bloody massacre, the editor of the *Aberdeen* (S.D.) *Saturday Pioneer* wrote in his editorial: 'The *Pioneer* has before declared that our only safety depends upon the total extermination of the Indians. Having wronged them for centuries, we had better, in order to protect our civilizations, follow it up by one more wrong and wipe these untamed and untamable creatures from the face of the earth.'

"The author of that editorial was L. Frank Baum, who later went on to write that famous children's book, *The Wonderful Wizard of Oz*. In calling for genocide against my grandmother and the rest of the Lakota people, he placed the final punctuation upon a day that will forever live in infamy amongst the Lakota." [38]

demoralization had set in with the indigenous culture – or what remained of it. If the death of Sitting Bull marked the end of an age, Wounded Knee marked the end of a culture." [39]

## Native Americans Use the Peyote Ritual to Preserve Their Culture

Peyote had long been a part of the life of the indigenous people of the American Southwest and Northern Mexico. It is known as the spirit plant. The plant gave flight to the mind and was an integral part of the Native American spiritual life for well over a thousand years. It was in the 1890s in Oklahoma that Indians not native to the southwestern United States were taught of the peyote ritual. [40] This was largely a product of the

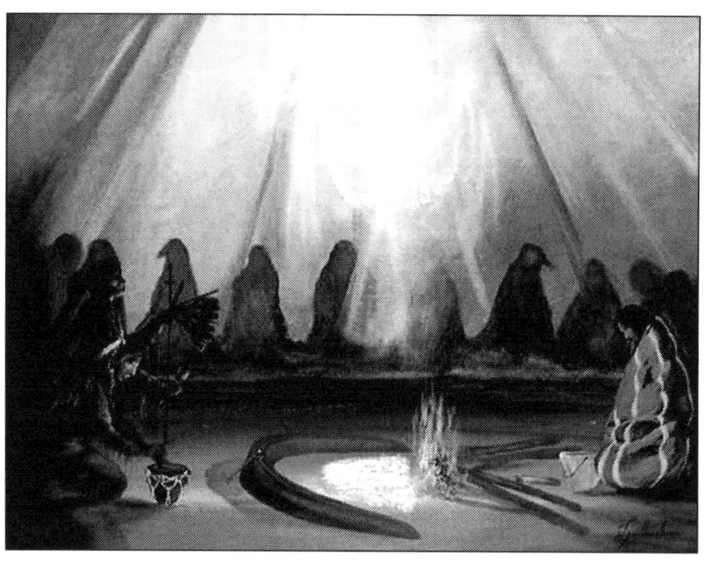

*Peyote ceremonies often took place in crowded teepees. The combination of a fire for warmth, a lot of participants, and a spiritual chanting contributed to hallucinations fueled by decreased oxygen and the consumption of peyote.*

Ghost Dance movement, an effort by Native Americans to preserve their culture and fight assimilation. The Lipan Apache had developed rituals for use of peyote in the 18th and early 19th century. They taught them to Comanche, Kiowa and Plains Apache. [41]

The Native American Church was created at the end of the 19th century to help preserve some of the last vestiges of Native American culture. This effort was necessary because of the slaughter, death by disease and systematic dismantling of the Indian way of life by European Americans over the previous 400 years. The culture of indigenous Americans had been all but wiped out by the Europeans. Two of the leaders of this movement were Quanah Parker, the last chief of the Quahadi Comanche, and John Wilson, a Caddo Indian. [42]

The Native American Church Christianized the spiritual use of peyote. Quanah Parker is generally credited with popularizing peyote use amongst Native Americans not native to the Southwest. The Native American Church combined aspects of Christianity with the many centuries-old spiritual beliefs of the indigenous Americas. It combined communal chanting, meditation and prayer. [43] The peyote ritual was incorporated as part of that cultural preservation effort.

The anthropologist James Mooney (1861-1921) was a student of the ghost dance and peyote religion. He was sympathetic to the role that these rituals played in Native American experience. He called together the leaders of this religious movement in 1918 and wrote the charter that formalized the Church.

It was only in the 1990s, that the U.S. Congress, in response to the U.S. Supreme Court's ruling in *Oregon v. Smith* (494 U.S. 872, 1990), made it crystal clear that freedom of religion also applied to those who predated the arrival of Europeans and used peyote as a spiritual vehicle.

The religious insensitivity to the discoverers of America was politically addressed at a September 1990 gathering of Indian religious leaders in Washington D.C. They implored the U.S. Congress to respect the protection of religious freedom embodied in the First Amendment to the Constitution. Winnebego Indian leader and author Reuben Snake presented an eloquent statement in support of religious freedom entitled *Native American Worship with Peyote is not Drug Abuse:*

> "The free exercise of religion was among the many features of that great Native American government (note: the Five Nations of the Iroquois Confederacy) and the freedom of religion is one which many of us take for granted today.
>
> On September 15, 1620, English subjects sailed from Plymouth, England, to seek refuge from religious persecution. The story of the Puritan pilgrims landing at Plymouth Rock in Massachusetts to achieve religious freedom is one of the best known stories in American history.
>
> It is tragic to say however, that we are now in a situation in the United States of America where

we can no longer take such a fundamental right, the free exercise of religion, for granted.

As venerable as the heritage of religious liberty has been in America, religious liberty is now in jeopardy for all minority religions." [44]

**Reuben Snake,** 1937-93
Winnebego Indian leader, 1937-1993
and co-author with Huston Smith of
*One Nation Under God: The Triumph of the Native American Church* (1996)

Snake pointed out that the court decision, which had thrown out long-standing precedents, had declared that the government no longer had shown that laws that burden and restrict religious liberty must be justified by a compelling government interest. This proposition opposing the court's decision was joined by the Baptists, the Methodists, Jewish groups, dozens of other religious groups and over 50 of America's most distinguished constitutional law professors who all sought a rehearing of the court's decision.

Mr. Snake went on to point the finger at the real culprit, which is drug-abuse hysteria:

> **"This trampling of Native American religious liberty is intolerable. Our people have been using the holy medicine, peyote, for thousands upon thousands of years.**
>
> **For the last twenty years, the American people have been suffering an epidemic of abuse of refined chemical drugs like cocaine, heroin, amphetamines, PCP, and so forth. American cities are crawling with violence and crime. This is a terrible tragedy, and this kind of drug abuse is also a problem for some Indian youth.**
>
> **But there is no peyote drug abuse problem. I defy the justices of the Supreme Court to find newspaper reports of drive-by shootings in**

## Truth in Humor

*Europeans and Americans felt (and most still feel) that their Eurocentric culture was and is superior to the culture of Native Americans. This piece of 20th-century humor gives pause for some thought on that assumption.*

### Where Did the White Man Go Wrong?

An old Indian chief sat in his hut on the reservation, smoking a ceremonial pipe, and eyeing two U.S. government officials sent to interview him. "Chief Two Eagles," asked one official, "you have observed the white man for 90 years. You've seen his wars and his material wealth. You've seen his progress, and the damage he's done." The Chief nodded in agreement. The official continued, "Considering all these events, in your opinion, where did the white man go wrong?"

The chief stared at the government officials for over a minute and then calmly replied:

> "When white man found the land, Indians were running it. No taxes, no debt, plenty buffalo, plenty beaver, women did all the work, medicine man free, Indian man spent all day hunting and fishing, and all night having sex."

Then the Chief leaned back and smiled.

> "White man dumb enough to think he could improve system like that." [45]

*Not withstanding the sexist sentiment of the joke and pejorative speech pattern attributed to the Native American, it suggests that it is possible that cultures other than Western European cultures have as good or better ways of dealing with all humans encounter in life and with achieving some tranquility in dealing with nature and our essential being. This, of course, includes the use of a variety of entheogens specific to various religious, cultures and regions.*

**connection with the holy medicine. I challenge anyone concerned about the problem of drug abuse to find examples of dope peddlers selling the holy medicine in America's school yards and play grounds. The idea is preposterous. We don't have a peyote abuse problem in this nation.**

**Yet the widespread fear, bordering on panic, about the tragedy of drug abuse has clouded the minds of the justices. In the name of the war on drugs, our guarantee of free exercise of religion has been violated. In the name of the war on drugs, the religious freedom of every American has been placed in jeopardy."** [46]

Fortunately, in 1994 America got back a little closer to what the founding fathers intended by the Constitution's First Amendment's freedom of religion clause. A 1994 bill guaranteeing religious freedom for Native Americans passed the U.S. House of Representatives on August 8, 1994 and passed the U.S. Senate on September 26, 1994. On October 6, 1994, President William Jefferson Clinton signed the American Indian Religious Freedom Act Amendments of 1994 into public law. This Act protects the traditional use of peyote by Indians for religious purposes throughout the United States.

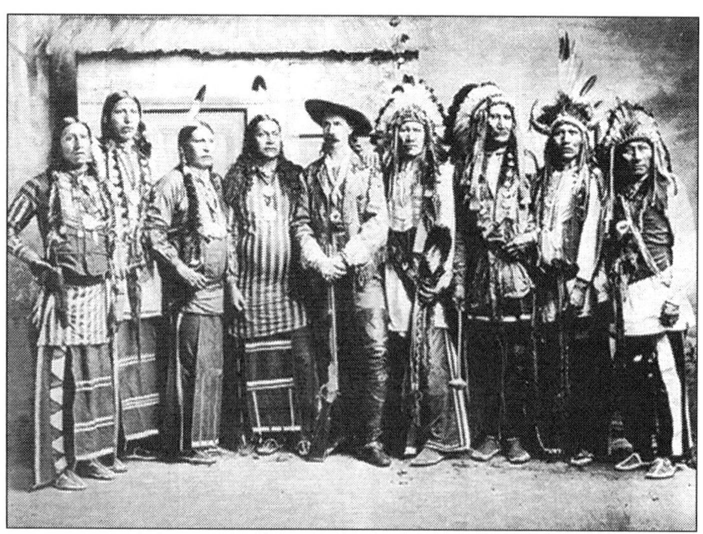

*In the late 19th and early 20th century, Native Americans became a literal side show act. Pictured is a group of Indian chiefs with Buffalo Bill. How ironic and fitting since Buffalo Bill participated in killing the buffalo and making the Plains Indians' way of life impossible to continue.*

Native Americans have a unique perspective on the hypocrisy of American rhetoric about freedom, independence and liberty:

> "All men were made by the same great spirit chief. They are all brothers. The earth is the mother of all people and all people should have equal rights upon it. You might as well expect the rivers to run backward as that any man who was born a free man should be contented when penned up and denied liberty to go where he pleases. Hear me, my chiefs! My heart is sick and tired. From where the sun now stands, I will fight no more forever." [47]

**Chief Joseph,** 1840-1904
the leader of the Wal-lam-wat-kain (Wallowa) band of Nez Perce Indians of Oregon

Chief Joseph identifies yet another reason for the failure of the prohibition of a plant. Laws can't fight human nature to be free. He concludes as illogical, the proposition that a free man will accept imprisonment. The freedom he speaks of is one of both thought and of action.

## Post-Civil War — Its Depression and Fear of "Them"

After the American Civil War (1861-65), there was a poorly-conceived and even more poorly implemented effort to integrate Negroes into American society known as Reconstruction. To Southerners, it seemed as though the North was forcing them to accept Negroes as equals. While 400 years of history cannot be erased in a few years, it's clear that Reconstruction did not provide much help to the freed slaves in either the medium or the long run. Reconstruction was a failure.

A review of Nicholas Lemann's 2006 book, *Redemption: The Last Battle of the Civil War,* is instructive:

> "Reconstruction is popularly recalled as a failed experiment in handing the reins of political power to freed slaves in the states of the former Confederacy after the South's surrender at Appomattox. The defeat of that experiment, idealized as

## Thomas' "Daddy Rice" as Jim Crow.

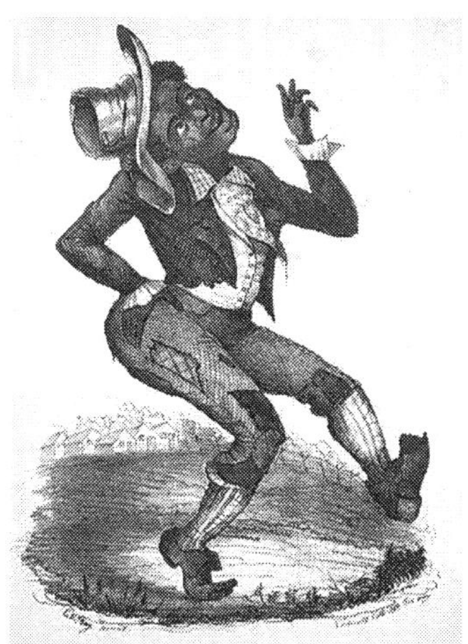

The term Jim Crow is traced back to 1828 or 1829 to a minstrel character created by a struggling white actor, Thomas Dartmouth "Daddy" Rice. Rice was one of the first to perform in Black Face (burnt cork rubbed on the face with lips outlined). He sang songs and did a foolish dance for the amusement of white people and became a popular vaudeville entertainer of the time. His Jim Crow character was an exaggerated, belittling, demeaning Negro stereotype. It soon became a popular staple of his act and somewhat of a nationwide sensation. [48] He sang and danced to the following ditty:

> First on de heel tap,
> Den on the toe
> Every time I wheel about
> I jump Jim Crow.
> Wheel about and turn about
> En do j's so.
> And every time I wheel about,
> I jump Jim Crow.
> - *From 1823 sheet music*

By the 1850s, the term Jim Crow was synonymous with other pejorative terms for Negroes. By 1875, Jim Crow was a term used to describe discriminatory laws aimed at Blacks, the so-called "Black Codes." [49] Jim Crow was a name given to a "complex system of racial laws and customs in the South that enabled white social, legal and political dominations of Blacks. Blacks were segregated, deprived of their right to vote, and subjected to verbal abuse, discrimination, and violence without redress in the courts or support by the white community." [50]

> courageous whites facing down black hordes, is enshrined in Southern memory as the time of "redemption."

Lemann uses the term redemption with intentional irony. The review continues,

> "His book offers a very contrary view, showing the initial experiment with black suffrage as a promising venture in democracy that was overthrown through a systematic and unconscionable campaign of terror that swept much of Louisiana, Alabama, South Carolina and especially Mississippi in the decade after the end of the Civil War." [51]

The economic Panic of 1873 triggered a post-Civil War depression that brought widespread unemployment. Not only was there a fear by white Southerners of losing jobs to recent immigrants from the north willing to work hard for low wages but also now having to compete for jobs with the recently freed former Negro slaves. This Panic of 1873 heralded the end to Reconstruction; it lasted less than a decade.

Reconstruction had been badly bungled. It set up Negroes (as they were politely known in that epoch) as a permanent underclass that exists to this day. Reconstruction set the stage for 100 years of overt Jim Crow and the covert and overt racism that followed. Many contemporary observers of American society, including former U.S. President Jimmy Carter, who explicitly pointed this out in the fall of 2009, that racism in America continues to the present, not withstanding the election of Barack Obama as president.

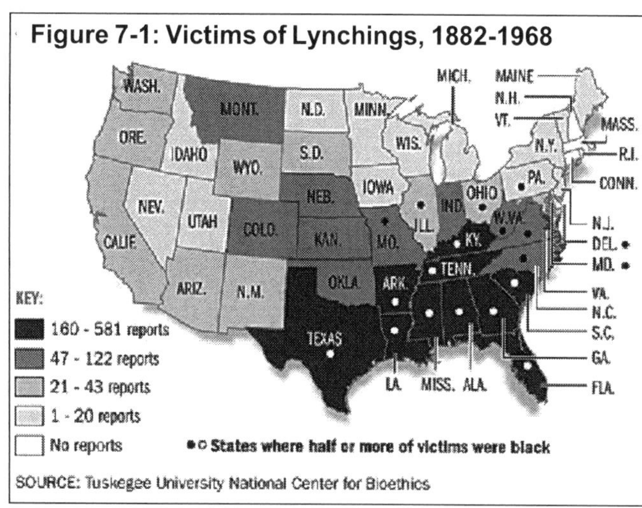


*The map shows the number and location of lynchings from 1882 to 1968.*

Post-Reconstruction was a violent, open season on Negroes. Between 1884 and 1900, there are 3,500 documented lynchings of Blacks, but the real number is surely higher. The reasons — such as they were — are appalling by any standard: being accused of looking at a white woman twice, stepping on a white man's shadow, and not going immediately to the back of a trolley. [52]

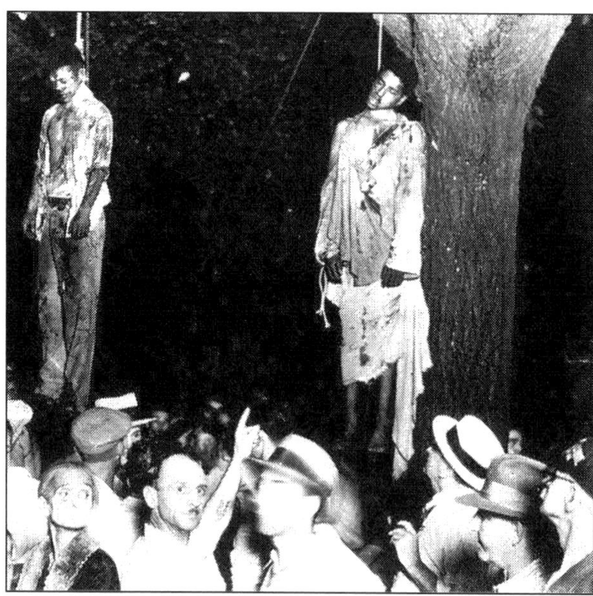

*The lynching of Thomas Shipp and Abram Smith took place in Marion, Indiana on August 7, 1930. This photograph was the inspiration for a poem by Abel Meeropol, called "Strange Fruit", which was immortalized in the song of the same name by Billie Holiday released in 1939.*

Statistics for the period from 1882 to 1951 document the racist application of lynching in that time period. Eighty-eight percent of victims were black, and ten percent were white. Fifty-nine percent of the lynchings occurred in the Southern states of Kentucky, North Carolina, South Carolina, Tennessee, Arkansas, Louisiana, Mississippi, Alabama, Georgia, and Florida.

Lynching was an aggressive, extreme effort at social intimidation and control. The underlying motivation was to keep Negroes "in their place," to prevent freedmen from voting and bearing arms, and to effectively use extra legal means for enforcement of the Black Codes. These court codes of social control had been invalidated by the Fourteenth and Fifteenth Amendments. Lynching was a tool to turn back the social changes forced on the South by the post-Civil War federal occupation during Reconstruction.

For years, States' rights was a rallying cry of conservatives, most particularly in the South. The Ninth and Tenth Amendments, which reserve to the people and the states all rights and powers not explicitly given to the federal government, were often used in the old Confederacy to support racially discriminatory laws. However, from 1914 through 1942, States' rights took one hit after another, via infringement from federal laws and liberal rulings of the U.S. Supreme Court. More and more power reserved to the several states by the Constitution was transferred to the federal government. This has included not only civil rights legislation but also federalizing drug laws.

With the Controlled Substances Act of 1970 and the Supreme Court's ruling in *Gonzalez v. Raich* (545 U.S. 1, 2005), the federal bureaucracy has been able to ignore the Ninth and Tenth Amendments by making various drugs (those in Schedule I) illegal. As Justice Sandra Day O'Connor pointed out in her dissent in that case, this successful federal effort to gain additional power not explicitly granted by the Constitution, impinged on States' rights.

The 1925 Supreme Court decision in *Linder v. United States* (268 U.S. 5) affirmed that the right to regulate the practice of medicine is reserved to the states. This decision has never been overturned. Somehow, the fact that the Constitution leaves the regulation of medicine to the States has been ignored by the federal government. Some have even speculated that the drug laws have been used to accomplish the same ends as the discriminatory laws prohibited by the 1965 civil rights legislation.

The U.S. Congress has to date neglected to outlaw lynching. It's not that Congress hasn't been given the opportunity: over 200 anti-lynching acts were introduced in the first half of the 20th century. And there certainly has been ample reason to condemn these lawless acts, which flaunt the democratically elected, republican form of government. From 1880 to 1960, more than 4,700 people are documented as being killed by lynching. These lynchings occurred in 46 states. Victims included Italians, Jews, Asians, Latinos and Blacks.

To give Congress its due, on June 13, 2005 the U.S. Senate did formally apologize for never having outlawed lynching. [53] Talk about the proverbial a day late and a dollar short!

During much of the post-Civil War period, radical racism was institutionalized in both the North and South. This radicalism stood on three legs:

(1) **Disenfranchisement:** Preventing Negroes from voting through illegal (lynching, beating) or legal (intimidation, poll taxes, literacy tests) means.

(2) **Segregation** (aka Jim Crow Laws): Laws were passed in the South to segregate Black & White people in all public accommodations, such as schools, hotels, trains and streetcars, restaurants and even cemeteries. These separate facilities were there to serve as a constant reminder by the White power structure to Blacks that they were unequal and inferior to Whites. Segregation was more subtle in the North, but still quite effective.

(3) **Economically:** When the South began to industrialize, Whites worked to exclude African Americans from these better paying jobs and forced Blacks into low-wage, rural and domestic work. The success of this enforced economic subordination helped generate permanent underemployment for a century or more. [54]

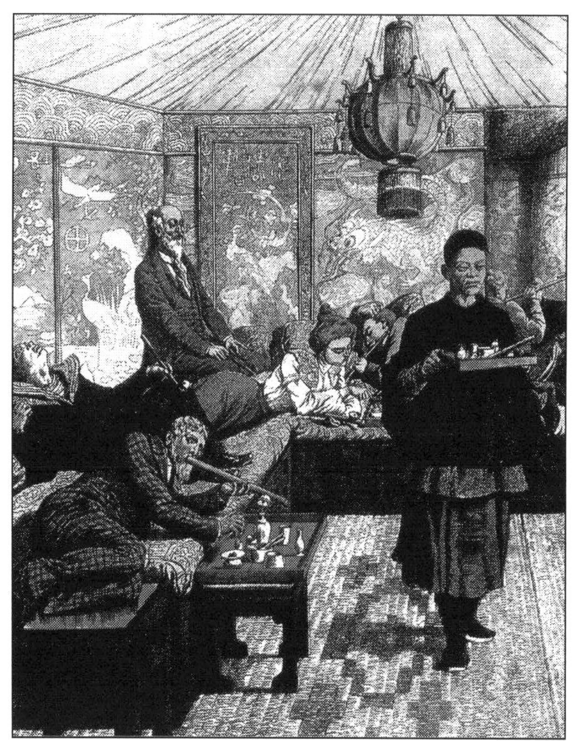

*The Anglo press tended to demonize opium dens and see them as a place to take advantage of innocent White, Protestant women. In most cases they were much more benign, similar to a men's club with opium substituted for alcohol.*

In the post reconstruction 1890s, cocaine was labeled as the cause of so-called "drug-crazed Negroes" resorting to violence against Whites. State drug laws passed in the South during this period gave racists another tool to marginalize Negroes.

## Opium is good, but not when the Chinese smoke It

After the Civil War, it was a new world. The slaves were free, the immigrants kept coming and the impact of the Industrial Revolution was obvious. Change was in the air and in 1873 the United States had a severe recession. All of this required a scapegoat and the scapegoat is *them* – the immigrants and the Negroes. Make no mistake, racism and xenophobia played a central role leading to American's present day drug laws.

Initially, the Chinese were more or less welcomed to the United States because they provided much needed manpower for the Gold Rush and building the intercontinental railway. Equally important, they worked hard and cheap. Then the Civil War came and went, followed in the early 1870s by a post-Civil War depression and jobs became scarce. This fostered a deepening xenophobia, in part because the Chinese worked hard and cheap.

The racist term "Yellow Peril" wasn't widely used until 1895 when newspaper magnet William Randolph Hearst, son of silver baron George Hearst, started publishing the insult in his two-dozen papers. But that sentiment had been abroad in the European mind for centuries. The West had long feared Asians. This fear had its roots as far back as the 13th century with Genghis Khan's invasion of Europe.

According to author Gina Marchetti, "the yellow peril combines racist terror of alien cultures, sexual anxieties, and the belief that the West will be overpowered and enveloped by the irresistible, dark, occult forces of the East. [55] These fears were magnified as a result of the 1900 Boxer Rebellion in China "against Christianity, killing Western missionaries as well as the Chinese Christian converts." Thus, the concept of the yellow peril seen as "a sea of Godless heathens who would turn on their Western 'protectors' to torture and kill them" was born in the United States. [56]

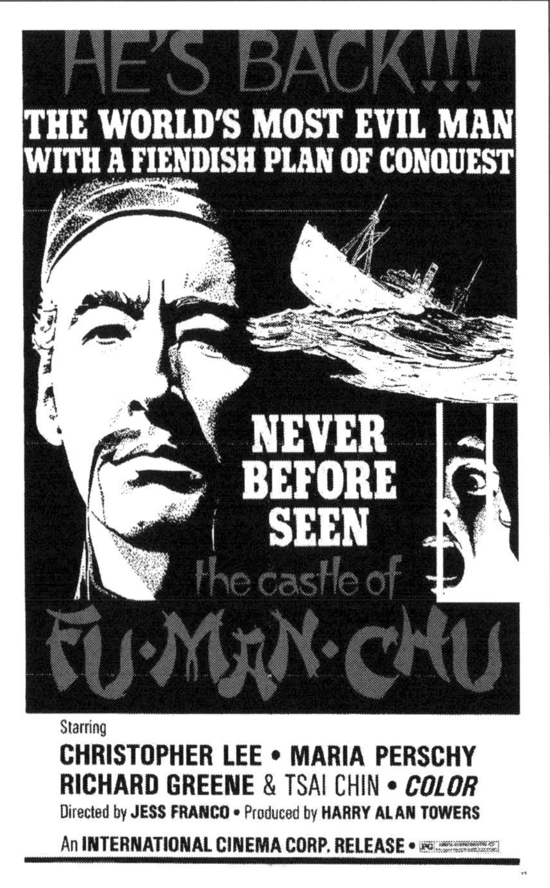


*Xenophobia. Popular literature and movies frequently port rayed Chinese as the bad guy.*

Chinese opium parlors, so-called opium dens, where Chinese retreated to relax, were used to demonize the Chinese. It was alleged that the Chinese used these supposed dens of iniquity to lure and seduce innocent White, Protestant women. In the late 1800s, lurid dime novels and magazines, such as the Police Gazette, depicted opium dens as evil, demonic places into which innocent White Protestant women were enticed only to be violated by the "heathen Chinese". In 1875 San Francisco instituted the first drug prohibition law. This law was against smoking opium and aimed squarely at the Chinese. In 1876, Virginia City, Nevada followed suit. In 1881, the federal government prohibited the importation of smoking opium.

Yet the irony of the first opium prohibition laws is that they were not directed at decreasing opiate use in patent medicine. These laws were clearly aimed at the Chinese, since these early laws only prohibited the smoking of opium. Women comprised 75% of excessive opiate users in the last quarter of the 19th century. This was as a consequence of using opiate containing nostrums such as Lydia Pinkham's Vegetable Compound for the treatment of unmentionable ills.

> "The country's first drug ban explicitly targeted the opium of 'the heathen Chinee.' Cocaine was first banned in the south to prevent an uprising of hopped-up 'cocainized' Negroes." [57]
>
> **Dan Baum & Roger Donald**
> co-authors, *Smoke and Mirrors: The War on Drugs and the Politics of Failure*, 1996

## Rum, Romanism & Rebellion

Over-exuberant nativism was used to help defeat the 1884 Republican presidential candidate, James G. Blaine. An obscure New York Republican preacher called the Democrats the party of "Rum, Romanism and Rebellion." [58] This referred to the Democrats' alleged anti-temperance attitudes, the party's popularity with Catholic immigrants, and placing the blame for the Civil War on the Democrats.

The Democrats trumpeted and exploited this remark to arouse their Irish immigrant base in New York City, galvanizing them to go to the polls in greater numbers than expected. This provided just enough additional Democratic votes so that Blaine lost New York State by 1,047 votes and lost the election to Grover Cleveland by the margin of New York State's electoral votes. [59]

Nevertheless, the American pattern of nativistic demonization and discrimination against non-Protestants and particularly non-Anglos continued to develop. By the 1880s, major elements of nativist thought – fear of foreign influence, anti-radicalism, and racism – were well established in the public mind. Fear and scapegoating, two cornerstones of American drug policy, are driven by this line of thought. To this day, the arguments of 19th-century nativists, "that the quality of immigrants had deteriorated," are being replayed.

There was no shortage of scholarly xenophobic treatises to support federal and state legislation discriminating against the Chinese. In 1881, Frederick Wines published one such report, *The Defective, Dependent and Delinquent Classes of the Population of the U.S.* Soon thereafter, the U.S. Congress passed the Chinese Exclusionary Act of 1882, excluding new Chinese immigrants from the United States. This was cheered by organized labor, which ascribed declining wages and economic woes to the, by now, despised Chinese workers. The Chinese then composed all of 0.002 percent of the nation's population. [60]

Organized labor was concerned about competition from the hard-working Chinese. At the end of the 19th and beginning of the 20th century, Samuel Gompers, the long-time president of the American Federation of Labor (AFL), carried on a decades-long vilification of the Chinese. This included Gompers' testimony before Congress as to why opium should be criminalized: "Opium gives the Chinese immigrant workers an unfair advantage in the labor market." [61]

In 1902, Gompers co-authored a booklet arguing that the racial differences between American whites and Asiatics would never be overcome. "The superior Whites," he said, "had to eradicate the Asian by law or force if necessary." Gompers believed "it was natural for the yellow man to lie, cheat and murder…." [62]

In his booklet *Some Reasons for Chinese Exclusion: Meat Versus Rice; American Manhood Against Asiatic Coolieism? Which Shall Survive?,* Gompers wrote:

> "What other crimes were committed in those dark fetid places when those innocent victims of the Chinaman's viles [sic] were under the influence of the drug, are almost too horrible to imagine. There are hundreds, aye, thousands, of our American girls and boys who have acquired this deathly habit and are doomed hopelessly doomed, beyond the shadow of redemption." [63]

## Change, Fear, Scapegoating

According to the University of Wisconsin historian Fredrick Jackson Turner, the most important change of the 1890s affecting the unique American psyche was the closing of the frontier. Turner first presented his thesis in an essay, *The Significance of the Frontier in American History* in 1893. [64] In it, he contended that an important dynamic in shaping the American psyche and character was meeting the challenges of the frontier for 400 years.

Ever since the 16th century after Columbus' 1492 trip triggered settlement of the Americas by Europeans, the United States had had a wild frontier. For four centuries, America there was a wilderness out there to explore and conquer. Now the frontier was gone. All the old clichés of Western movies were going, going, gone – the range was fenced, an increasing percentage of U.S. residents led the urban life.

Heather Cox Richardson has reworked Turner's thesis. Richardson argues that the dynamic that helped redefine America during Reconstruction was the romantic image Americans had of the West, rather than the real frontier and actual experience of living on the frontier. It was in an idealized view

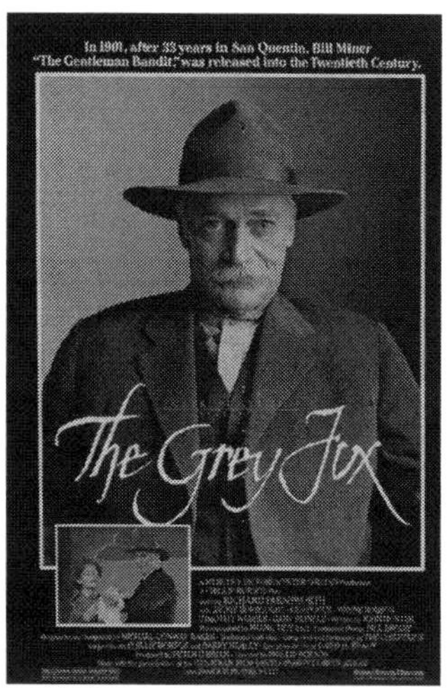


*The excellent 1982 movie* The Grey Fox *captured the spirit of the closing of the frontier. It was a fictional portrayal of a rather charming stage coach robber, who goes to jail for thirty-three years in the late 1860s. Upon getting out in 1901, he is amazed by the changes he finds – automobiles, movies, and very few stage coaches. He finds his skills are somewhat transferable and switches to robbing trains.*

of the West that Americans preserved an antebellum perception of themselves as a country of rugged individualists.

Richardson concludes that out of this mythology grew the modern middle-class opposition to what they perceived as the undeserving poor and the grasping rich. "The powerful new American identity permitted many individuals to succeed far beyond what they might have achieved elsewhere," Richardson writes, "but that exceptional openness depended on class, gender and racial bias." [65]

To this day, historians argue over the relative importance of Turner's "closing of the frontier" thesis in shaping American values versus the impact of other core American institutions such as slavery. There is no argument that he was correct about the change in American life; the rise of cities and the industrial revolution were having more influence on America than the previous top trio of influences: agriculture, discovery and adventure. Change was in the air and scapegoats were needed.

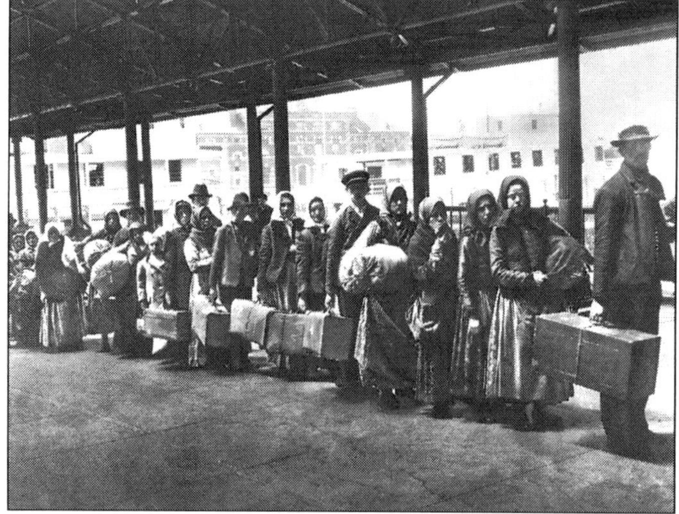

*Immigrants from eastern Europe arriving at the Ellis Island immigration inspection center in 1892. Twelve million immigrants passed through the center from 1892 to its closing in 1954.*

The 1890s were a time of serious economic depression and general unease about the future of the country. It was also the midpoint of the influx of over 35 million immigrants coming to the United States from a myriad of countries. The immigrants' origins had shifted from largely northern and western Europe to southern and eastern Europe. This shift of place of origin and often religion disturbed many immigrants who had arrived previously because the new immigrants were *them* not *us*. Both the numbers of immigrants and their differences from the majority of upper middle and upper class Americans brought an increase of anti-immigrant sentiment.

Another ten million immigrants arrived in the first decade of the 20th century, many of them from southern and eastern Europe. At the time, the total U.S. population was 92 million, so the so-called hordes of recently arriving immigrants had a dramatic impact, literally changing the face of America. Old-stock New Englanders saw "their" cities populated with more and more immigrants whom they perceived as ignorant and alien. The newcomers had different attitudes toward drugs than the bulk of the U.S. population of the time, particularly alcohol, which they were happy to party with. Some of these newcomers had experiences with the more exotic opium, hashish and pungent spices.

This changing face of the American people generated fear and concern amongst those who saw themselves as "native-born" Americans. Eugenicists felt that America's racial and biological composition – and therefore the country's future – were at risk; labor unionists blamed the immigrant for bringing down wages; the elites said that immigrants of lower-class and culturally alien backgrounds would destroy American institutions and culture. [66] As these concerns increased, ways were looked at to reinforce the American way: intimidation, lynchings, economic discrimination, and even drug laws.

The demonization of someone is an important tool of social control. It somehow allows one people to do unspeakable things to others. The conquistadores argued over whether the Indians had

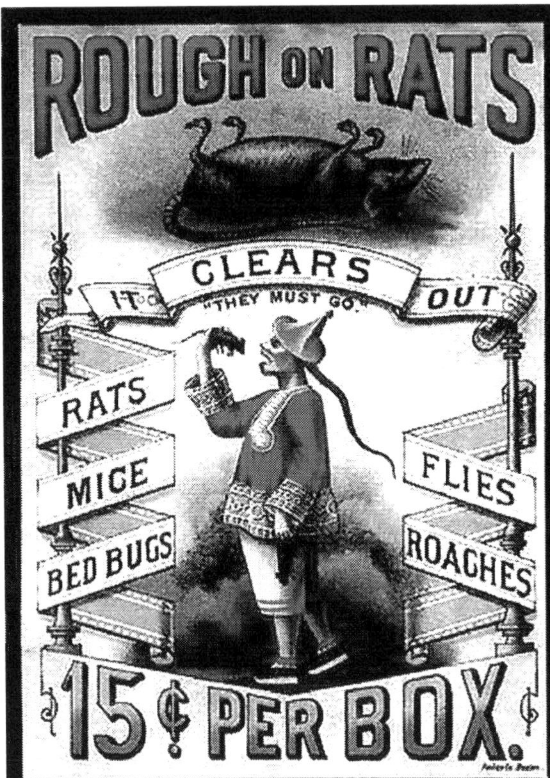


*Like many other discriminated against minorities (Italians, Jews, Moslems, Irish, Gypsies -- the list goes on and on), the Chinese were vilified as sub-human.*

souls. By the late 17th century, the non-Christian Negroes were seen as fundamentally different from Anglos. The Chinese were called vile and worse. This technique was used in the 1930s by the Germans who characterized Jews as vermin, rats, sub-human.

These depictions fit the strategy of the dominant forces in society -- the people that control the levers of power -- to demonize, dehumanize, marginalize and discriminate against the less powerful. It is an element of social, cultural, political and economic control. Sadly, little has changed over time. Demonization of one's opponent is done all the time in politics and in war. After the war, these same people are no longer demons. This is true today. Saddam Hussein was an ally of the United States when he was at war with Iran and America supported him. Ah, but circumstances changed; he was demonized, sanctions applied against his country, Iraq was eventually invaded and Saddam overthrown and hung.

Speaking in the mid-1990s, former U.S. Attorney General Ramsey Clark under President Johnson, pointed out that the U.S. sanction policies against Iraq, which at that time had been in place for fifteen years, were responsible for the deaths of over half a million innocent Iraqi women and children. He pointed out that we had demonized Saddam Hussein and by extension the Iraqi people. His point was that when you demonize people, almost any harm can be justified against them. [67]

## Medicine and Pharmacy

In the 1800s, the disciplines of medicine and pharmacy were still largely unorganized in the United States and loosely regulated, if at all. What early regulation there had been, all but disappeared during the populism of the Andrew Jackson administration. Jackson's government made no effort at regulating medicine nationally. This was a reaction against giving a monopoly to the educated (i.e., physicians), which was seen as contrary to American democracy. In addition, the Tenth Amendment, which reserves to the states all authority not explicitly granted to the federal government, limits the federal government's role in direct regulation of the practice of medicine. In the mid-1800s, most states followed the federal government's lead and repealed existing medical dispensing laws. [68]

## American Medical Association

The American Medical Association (AMA) was founded in 1847 but allopathic medicine was competing with homeopathy, naturopathy, chiropractic manipulation and just plain quacks. Medical schools, such as they were, were unregulated and could be found over garages or behind butcher shops, as well as at prestigious universities and hospitals.

Dr. David F. Musto put it this way in his book *The History of Legislative Control Over Opium, Cocaine and Their Derivatives* (1987):

> "The status of legislative control of dangerous drugs during the nineteenth century may be summed up as follows: The United States had no practical control over the health professions, no representative national health organizations to aid the government in drafting regulations, and no controls on the labeling, composition, or advertising of compounds that might contain opiates or

cocaine. The United States not only proclaimed a free marketplace, it practiced this philosophy with regard to narcotics in a manner unrestrained at every level of preparation and consumption." [69]

It took awhile for things to get sorted out. It wasn't until the early 1900s, when the influence of the journalistic muckrakers was felt, that American medicine began to clean up its act and started to transform itself into what we might recognize as the beginnings of modern medicine. In 1905, the AMA Council on Medical Education began to accredit medical schools. Soon graduation from an AMA-accredited school became a requirement to practice medicine in most states. Diploma mills, the medical schools behind garages and over butcher shops, began to disappear.

Shortly thereafter, the Carnegie Foundation funded a study to assess the low quality of American medical training. It was done for the AMA by Abraham Flexner. Work on the report began in 1907 and was completed in 1910. The Flexner Report was a milestone event in American medicine. It triggered major reform in U.S. medical education and established allopathic medicine at the top of the medical hierarchy.

But the effect of elevating allopathic medicine over its competitors – osteopathy, naturopathy and homeopathy had its professional political overtones. The Flexner Report was the beginning of the end of America's strong reliance on herbal medicine. While it did marginalize quackery, in the process it lowered the respect for phytochemicals (medicines from herbs & plants). Many medical professionals that supported traditional herbal medicine were marginalized by the Report -- some quite justifiably; others were just collateral damage.

The beginning of the 20th century was a time when allopathic medicine had lots of competition from osteopathic medicine, homeopathy, naturopathy, physiomedicolism, and electric medicine. Schools that taught these brands of medicine plus poor quality allopathic schools, particularly those not aligned with major universities, fell into rapid decline. By 1920, the number of U.S. medical schools was down to 86 from over 160 in 1900. [70] By decreasing the pool of available slots, medical schools once again became largely a male-only bastion.

Flexner's staff had included Dr. Morris Fishbein, who later became a long-time editor of the Journal of the American Medical Association and was a force in the AMA until well into the 1960s. In 1942, Fishbein said that cannabis was the best available treatment for migraine headaches. [71]

The drug policy story from the turn of the 19th century to the 1990s is a familiar one. It is chronicled in several excellent books by David F. Musto, Edward M. Brecher, and Dan Baum – respectively, *The American Disease* (1999), *Licit and Illicit Drugs* (1972), and *Smoke and Mirrors* (1997). Nevertheless, the less familiar, more distant foundations of contemporary drug policy needs to be connected with the more familiar story of American drug policies that evolved during the late 19th century and beyond into the 21st century.

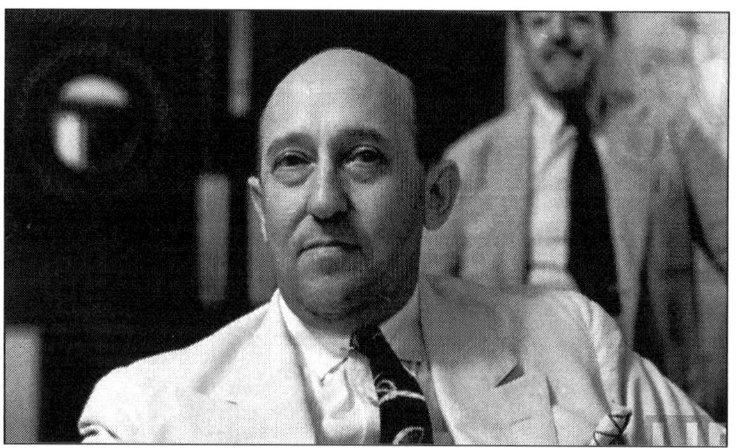

*Morris Fishbein, MD (1889-1976) was the editor of the* Journal of the American Medical Association *from 1924 to 1950. Fishbein was a staffmember in preparing the Flexner Report. He was a crusader against pseudo-medicines but a supporter of the medicinal use of marijuana.*

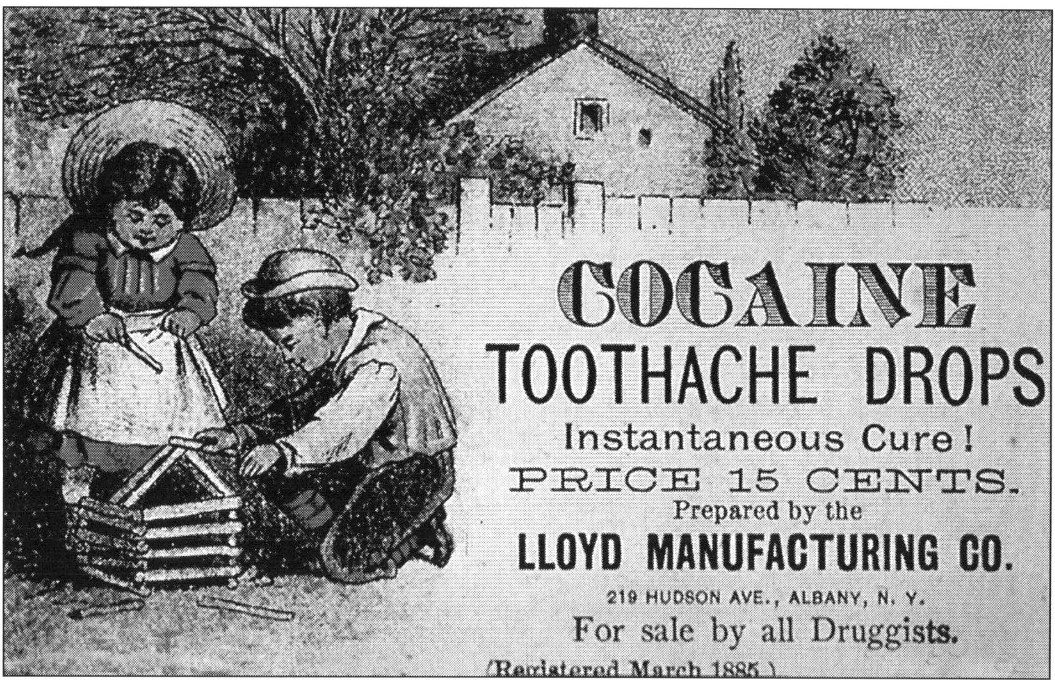


*Cocaine, opium and cannabis were the essential ingredients of many popular, so-called "patent medicines" until the United States enacted the Pure Food & Drug Act in 1906.*

# CHAPTER VIII
# 1880-1919:
# The Pure Food & Drug Act

## Patent Medicines

Patent medicines have been around since the early days of the Republic. Several factors led to the marketplace success of these medicants. Sales of these products was fueled by the desire to promote American goods over imported medicines and to create a market for herbs produced by local American farmers. Patent legislation passed by Congress in 1793 allowed people to patent their product. This included medicines.

Then as now, the ad men were important. The dramatic increase in the number of U.S. newspapers in the 19th century provided an ideal opportunity to pitch a patent medicine to the masses. Newspapers increased from 200 in the early 19th century to over 4,000 by the time of Abraham Lincoln and to 5,091 by 1870.[1] Newspapers provided the principle means and the primary medium for the successful advertising of patent medicines. They were filled with ads for these products. Another "modern" innovation used to promote patent medicines was signs on the sides of barns. Other forms of advertising for patent medicine included billboards, flyers, magazine ads and traveling medicine shows.

From before the founding of the Republic until 1914, Americans were free to buy any drug that they wanted. There was no such thing as an illegal drug in the United States until the early 20th century. Opiate-containing patent

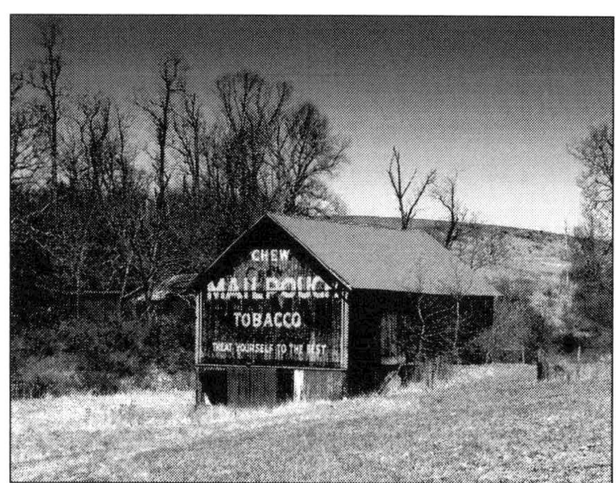


*Here is a little piece of Americana. Even before the automobile, advertisements were painted on the side of barns.*

medicines were everywhere. Patent medicines containing alcohol, opium, cocaine, cannabis and the like were available at every general store, grocery store, drug store, and even the corner saloon. No prescription was required.

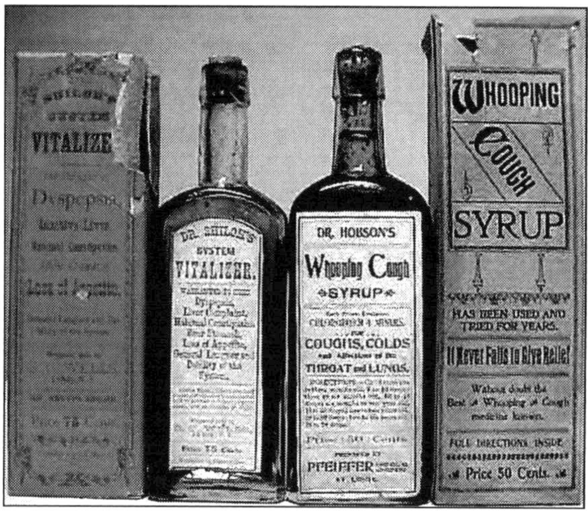


*Patent medicines were extremely popular in the 1800s. And why not? They contained alcohol, opium, cocaine, cannabis and other effective therapeutic agents. Some preparations were ineffective; others contained useless or harmful ingredients. Generally the concoctions with the most alcohol were the most popular.*

A mid-1880s Iowa survey found 3,000 stores in Iowa alone that sold opium. These outlets were serving a population of less than two million or one retail opium outlet for every 600 men, women and child in Iowa. This did not count access through the numerous physicians who dispensed it. Oh, and opium medication was available by mail, sort of like the poorly regulated Internet prescription business of today. [2] There was little if any criminal activity associated with even the inappropriate or excessive use of patent medicine containing opiates.

No doubt, easy access to opiates caused some medical problems. These warranted a medical solution, not the criminalization of these products that abounds today, which have fostered the destructive and expensive criminal justice-industrial complex.

In 1852 the American Pharmaceutical Association (APA) was founded. Like the American Medical Association (AMA), the APA wanted more respect and authority for their members. The APA 1856 constitution listed as one of their goals: "To as much as possible restrict the dispensing and sale of medicines to regularly educated druggists and apothecaries." [3] The federal Harrison Narcotics Tax Act of 1914, which required a prescription to legally possess heroin or cocaine, came along six decades later and was consistent with this goal.

In 1860, Oliver Wendell Holmes Sr. (1809-1894), an eminent physician of the Civil War era speaking to the Massachusetts Medical Society, criticized the nostrums used by many physicians, saying that if "the *medica materia*, as now used, could be sunk to the bottom of the sea, it would be all the better for mankind – and all the worse for the fishes." [4] Notwithstanding his dubious view of the 19th-century pharmacopoeia, Holmes was an opium fan. He said that it was a natural substance "which the Creator Himself seems to prescribe..." [5] In this, Holmes was in step with his colleagues.

## God's Own Medicine

Throughout much of the 19th century, the medical profession saw opium as a virtual panacea. In prescriptions of the day, physicians often abbreviated opium as: G.O.M. (God's Own Medicine). And why not! Most illnesses were little understood in the 19th century and physicians had few effective treatments. Doctors mainly treated symptoms, rather than the causes, of disease. Opium relieved many symptoms: diarrhea, teething pain, cough, and, most importantly, pain. Tuberculosis – aka TB or consumption – was rampant until well into the 20th century, and GOM is a great antitussive (cough suppressant). Opium was the most effective drug in the early American doctor's little black bag.

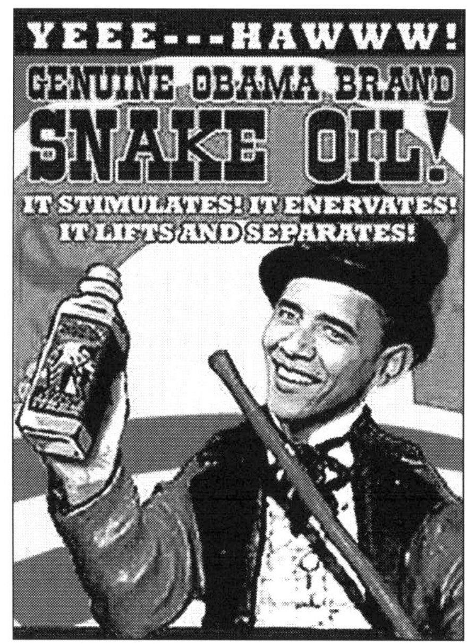


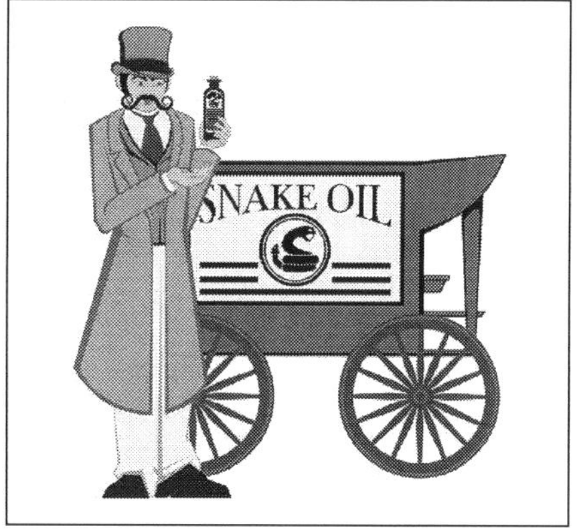


*The term "Snake Oil Salesman" is applied to anyone trying to pass off a bogus solution as the real deal. Political opponents have accused both Presidents Obama and George W. Bush of being snake oil salesmen.*

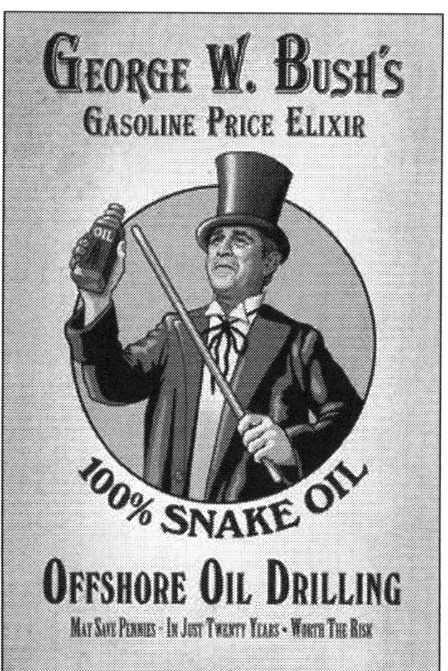


Opium has a long history as a medicine going back thousands of years. Its medicinal value was well-recognized in England. In 1680, English physician Thomas Syndenham (1625-80) praised God for opium. "Among the remedies which it has pleased the Almighty God to give to man to relieve his sufferings, none is so universal and efficacious as opium." [6] American physicians from the colonial period to the 1920s agreed with Syndenham's assessment.

Opiates (opium, morphine and, later, heroin) were ubiquitous in America. The opiates were one of the few effective ingredients in patent medicine in the so-called "Golden Age of Quackery" (roughly 1875-1910). Among many patent medicines that contained opium or morphine were the ever popular Ayer's Cherry Pectoral, Mrs. Winslow's Soothing Syrup, Darby's Carminative, Godfrey's Cordial, McMunn's Elixir of Opium, and Dover's Powder. They were advertised for teething syrups for young children, soothing syrups for diarrhea and dysentery, treatment of consumption, or for women's unmentionable ills. They were often effective for what they treated. [7]

The vast majority of opium habitués were middle-class, middle-aged white women. [8] A 1880 survey done in Michigan and Chicago, revealed that among habitual opiate users, women outnumbered men 3:1. Similar studies revealed the average age of the user was somewhere between 39 to 50. This was likely because opiates were often recommended or prescribed for menstrual cramps and menopause symptoms.

Women consumed various nostrums for, as the Lydia Pinkham's label read, "the treatment of women's unmentionable ills." The laudanum (a mixture of opium in alcohol)-filled Lydia Pinkham's Vegetable Compound was very popular. Lydia Pinkham's not only treated PMS, menopausal symptoms and arthritis, but it provided women with a socially acceptable source of alcohol in these Temperance-toned times.

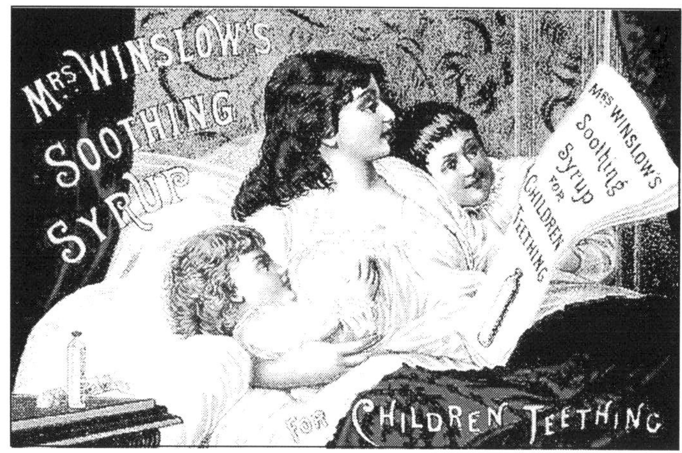


*This was just one of many opium-containing nostrums that were effective treatment for gum pain in teething infants. Like all opiate-containing patent medicine of the time, it was widely available in pharmacies and grocery stores without a prescription.*

The peak of opiate dependence in the United States occurred near the turn of the 19th to the 20th century. The number of habitual opiate users (so-called "addicts") was estimated at close to 250,000 in a population of 76 million.[9] Yet, despite the relative prevalence of this so-called addiction, the prevailing attitude at the time was that "drug addiction" was a health problem, best treated by physicians and pharmacists.

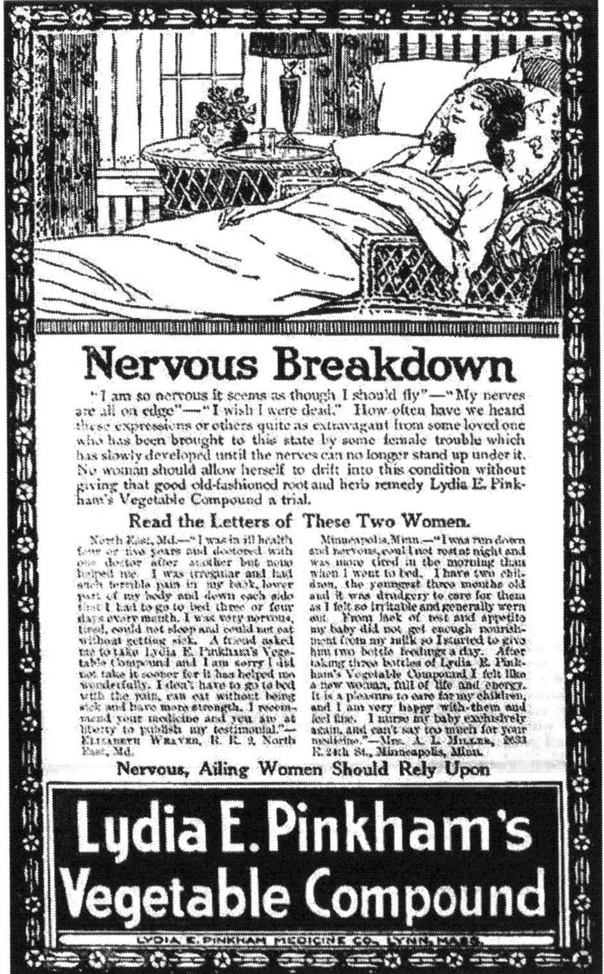


*Lydia appears to have more than a bit of the feminist in her. She asked her customers to write her for advice. She empowered her customers by providing information. She began heavy promotion of her nostrum in 1876. Her son added her picture to the product. Viola – modern advertising was born and Lydia Pinkham's became the most popular patent medicine of the day.* [10]

There was little or no crime associated with the rampant use of these narcotic substances. Maybe that's because the primary "victims" of opium use and abuse did not come from today's stereotyped, murderous, back-alley type characters. Again and again, studies published between 1871 and 1922 paint a striking portrait of the typical habitual opiate user (aka "addict") in the late 19th and early 20th century: a middle-aged, rural, middle- or upper-class white woman.[11] However, politicians and

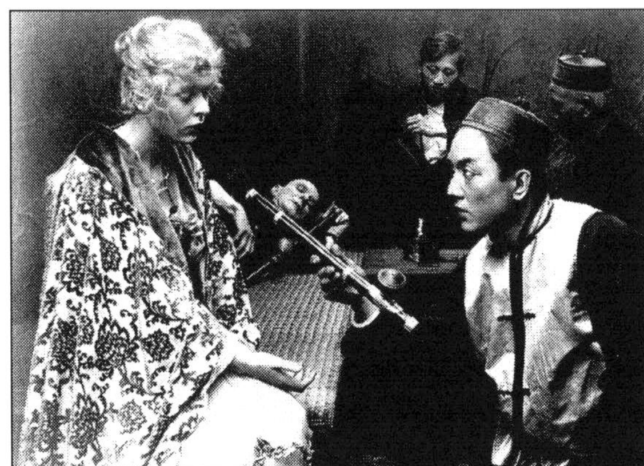

*This is a movie still from the WWI era. With this kind of material in the public media, is it any mystery why the American public was changing their mind about opiates?*

the media focused on the smoking of opium by the Chinese. Had their contribution to turn-of-the-century U.S. opiate use and abuse not been exploited, would there be a contemporary need to be examining the issue of a dysfunctional drug policy that undermines the principles and promise of this country?

## Cannabis

Cannabis had been re-introduced into Western medicine in 1839 by Dr. W.B. O'Shaugnessy. Cannabis had come to his attention while living in India for several years, where it was a commonly used medicine. He did animal and human research on cannabis while in India. When he returned to England, he gave a talk in 1839 regarding the medicinal value of cannabis in London. In 1841, O'Shaughnessy wrote *On the Preparation of the Indian Hemp or Ganja.*[12]

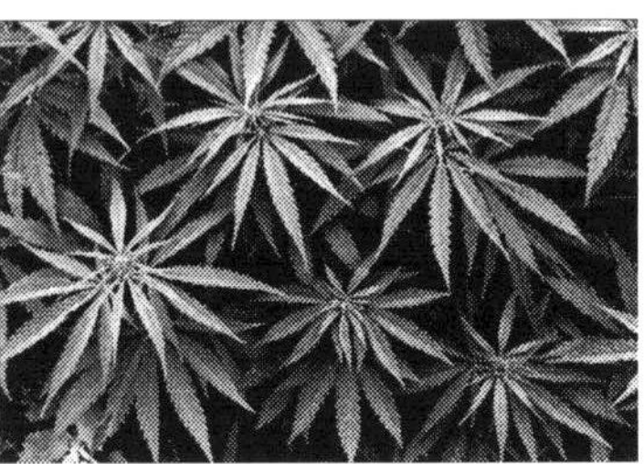

O'Shaughnessy was not just somebody who happened on the medicinal use of cannabis. By the time he demonstrated the medicinal value of cannabis to Western practitioners, he was already a well-respected physician. In 1831, he had found a treatment for cholera. On December 29, 1831 O'Shaughnessy's letter to *The Lancet* (the most prestigious British medical journal) on treatment of cholera was published. It has been characterized as "one of the shortest and yet most significant letters ever sent to the journal."[13] He showed that "the copious diarrhea of cholera leads to dehydration, electrolytic depletion, acidosis and nitrogen retention," and that "treatment must depend on intravenous replacement of the deficient salt and water."[14,15]

Cannabis was in the United States Pharmacopoeia from 1854 to 1941. From 1842 until the 1890s, *Cannabis indica*, also called Indian Hemp Extractum or *Extractum cannabis indicae*, was one of the three items (after alcohol and opium) most used in patent and prescription drugs. Cannabis remained the number three most popular medicine until 1901 when it was replaced by aspirin.[16] It was contained in preparations produced by many leading pharmaceutical companies including: Squibb, Merck, Parke Davis, and Eli Lilly.[17] Queen Victoria's personal physician, Sir J. Russell Reynolds, prescribed cannabis for relief of her menstrual cramps. He wrote in the very first issue of *Lancet* that "When pure and administered carefully, [cannabis] is one of the most valuable medicines we possess."

The doses of cannabis found in 19th-century patent medicine were pretty impressive. Using the 1983 U.S. government numbers as a yardstick, a one-day dose found in these patent medicines used by infants, children, youth, adults, women in childbirth, and senior citizens were often equal to what a current moderate-to-heavy American marijuana user probably consumes in a month or two. And as the AMA testified in 1937, cannabis created NO problems the AMA was aware of![18]

## 1894 India Hemp Commission

In the late 1800s, the British were concerned about the centuries-old tradition of using bhang, charas, and ganga (various ways of consuming cannabis) in India. Should a law be passed controlling its use or just leave things as is? In rather typical British fashion, an exhaustive study was done. Over 1300 British officers, including over 400 doctors, were interviewed. In 1895, the Indian Hemp Drug Commission published a seven-volume report containing over 3,400 pages. The commission concluded that cannabis has some medical uses, no addictive properties, and a number of positive emotional and social benefits.[19,20]

> **"In regard to the physical effects, the Commission has come to the conclusion that the moderate use of hemp drugs is practically attended by no evil results at all. Speaking generally, the Commission are of opinion that the moderate use of hemp drugs appears to cause no appreciable physical injury of any kind."**

The Commission's report concluded:

> **"There is no evidence of any weight regarding the mental and moral injuries from the moderate use of these drugs. ...Moderation does not lead to excess in hemp any more than it does in alcohol. Regular, moderate use of ganja or bhang produces the same effects as moderate and regular doses of whiskey."**[21]
>
> Report of the Indian Hemp Drugs Commission, 1894-95

Note: The commission's proposal to tax bhang was never put into effect. It may have been because one of the Indian commissioners cautioned that Moslem law and Hindu custom forbid "taxing anything that gives pleasure to the poor."[22] The Indian Hemp Drug Commission concluded that cannabis "has no addictive properties, some medical uses, and a number of positive emotional and social benefits."

However, the Europeans of the 19th century continued to be easy prey for exotic drug stories. One story that still makes the rounds is that the resin from the cannabis plant was collected by people running naked through the cannabis plantation fields, save for a rubber apron. As the story goes, the apron would get caked with the sticky cannabis resin. It would then be scraped off and made into cakes of hashish. A colorful story, but according to Martin Booth, not a word of it is true.[23]

## Cocaine

The chewing of coca leaves has been around for centuries in South America. German chemist Frederich Gaedcke isolated cocaine from the coca leaves in 1855. Soon, cocaine was being used commercially. By the 1870s, cocaine was found not only in patent medicines, but also in candy and drink. It was acceptable in polite society.

## Figure 8-1: Cannabis Time Line: 2737 BC – 2010 AD

| Date | Country | Event |
|---|---|---|
| 2737 BC | China | Listed in Shen Nung's pharmacopoeia (oldest written copy c. 100 BC) |
| 2000 BC | Egypt | Made as a drink in ancient Thebes |
| 1000 BC | India | Used as an herbal medicine |
| 500 BC | Persia | A principle sacrament of the Zoroastrians |
| 450 BC | Scythia | Inhaled as an intoxicating incense |
| 200 BC | Israel | Used as a medicine by the Essenes |
| 700 AD | Middle East | Brought divine revelation to Sufi priests |
| 1200 | Europe | Banned as a medicine by the Spanish Inquisition |
| 1480s | Italy | Criminalized by Pope Innocent VIII |
| 1802 | France | Napoleon's soldiers return from Egypt with cannabis |
| 1835 | France | Club des Hashichines established. |
| 1839 | India | Dr. William O'Shaunessy introduces medicinal cannabis to England |
| 1895 | Britain | The Indian Hemp Drug Commission Report |
| 1896 | Canada/U.S./Britain: | Sir William Osler praises cannabis for treating migraines |
| 1914 | U.S. | Cannabis successfully excluded from Harrison Narcotics Tax Act |
| 1931 | Panama Canal Zone | Siler Article |
| 1937 | U.S. | AMA testifies against Marijuana Tax Act |
| 1937 | U.S. | Harry Anslinger testifies marijuana causes aggression |
| 1942 | U.S. | Dr. Morris Fishbein, editor of *JAMA*, says cannabis best treatment for migraines |
| 1943 | U.S. | *Military Surgeon* publishes "The Marijuana Bugaboo" editorial |
| 1944 | U.S. | New York Academy of Medicine |
| 1948 | U.S. | Anslinger testifies cannabis makes users passive |
| 1949 | U.S. | First modern study on the medicinal benefits of cannabis (for epilepsy) |
| 1953 | U.S. | *Military Medicine* publishes "The Marijuana Bugaboo Revisited" |
| 1968 | Britain | Wootton Commission Report |
| 1969 | U.S. | U.S. Supreme Court finds Marijuana Tax Act unconstitutional |
| 1970 | U.S. | Controlled Substances Act passed |
| 1971 | U.S. | Nixon Marijuana Commission Report |
| 1978 | U.S. | Compassionate IND program starts |
| 1982 | U.S. | First Institute of Medicine (IOM) Report |
| 1991 | U.S. | Compassionate IND program ends |
| 1996 | U.S. | California & Arizona legalize medicinal cannabis |
| 1997 | Britain | Report of House of Lords Science & Technology Committee |
| 1999 | Britain | GW Pharmaceuticals begins research on tincture of cannabis |
| 1999 | U.S. | Calif. state legislature allocates $9 million for research on smoked cannabis' medical utility |
| 2000 | U.S. | California Marijuana Research Center opens at UCSD School of Medicine |
| 2005 | Canada | Sativex approved for sale by Health Canada |
| 2007 | U.S. | DEA ALJ rules for Dr. Lyle Craker for marijuana grow license |
| 2009 | U.S. | AG Holder suspends federal raids on legal dispensaries |
| 2010 | U.S. | UCSD School of Medicine releases 10-year CMRC report |
| 2010 | Britain | Sativex approved in Britain |
| 2012 | U.S. | Colorado and Washington legalize cannabis |

SOURCE: Montgomery, Neil M. "A Short History of Cannabis." [24]

Soon after Reconstruction ended in the early 1890s, the demonization of cocaine use by Negroes kicked in. This seems a bit odd considering that just a few years earlier, some plantation owners had encouraged cocaine use among slaves to increase their productivity.

In the Post-Reconstruction era, there was concern that Negroes didn't know their place and that they were too aggressive. According to drug policy historian Dr. David F. Musto, the fear was that access to cocaine might make Negroes "oblivious of their prescribed bounds and attack white society." [25]

Cocaine was blamed for some of this aggression. In the 1890s, some southern police chiefs even said that, due to Negroes being on cocaine, they were impervious to their bullets. These lawmen felt duty-bound to go from .32 to .38 caliber guns to be able to bring down these "drug-crazed" Negroes. [26]

Cocaine was linked to discrimination against Jews as well as Negroes. Why the Jews? They were the ones allegedly selling the cocaine to Negroes.

But cocaine had been very well-accepted in white society. The fictional Sherlock Holmes was a cocaine user as was his real-life creator, the physician Sir Arthur Conan Doyle.

THE SENATORS HAD HEARD THAT COCAINE TRANSFORMED BLACK MEN INTO POWERFUL "ZOMBIES" WHO NOT ONLY IGNORED AUTHORITY BUT WERE PHYSICALLY UNSTOPPABLE.
BLAM! BLAM! BLAM!

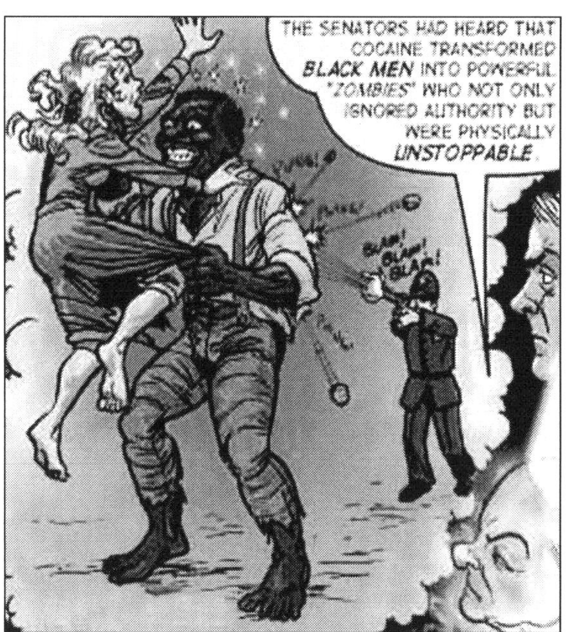

*A cartoon depicting the fanciful nightmare of southern white law enforcement officials, but which was often sworn to.*

The pioneer psychiatrist Sigmund Freud had done research with the therapeutic use of cocaine from 1884-1887. He recommended cocaine for treatment of alcohol and morphine abuse among other psychological conditions. He himself used cocaine for about 25 years. He wrote:

> "...exhilaration and lasting euphoria, which in no way differs from the normal euphoria of the healthy person ... You perceive an increase of self-control and possess more vitality and capacity for work ... In other words, you are simply normal, and it is soon hard to believe you are under the influence of any drug ... Long intensive physical work is performed without any fatigue ... This result is enjoyed without any of the unpleasant after-effects that follow exhilaration brought about by alcohol ... Absolutely no craving for the further use of cocaine appears after the first, or even after repeated taking of the drug ..." [27]
>
> **Sigmund Freud**, 1856-1939
> the founding father of psychoanalysis
> *Uber Coca (*1884)

Note: Freud died in 1939 of cancer of the mouth and oral pharynx caused by decades of inveterate cigar smoking.

Cocaine remained in accepted use in high society well into the 1920s. For example, here's a verse from a Cole Porter tune, *I Get a Kick Out of You,* from a 1934 Broadway play:

> *"Some get a kick from cocaine*
> *I'm sure that if*
> *I took even one sniff*
> *That would bore me terrifically, too*
> *Yet, I get a kick out of you."*

Some later, sanitized versions of the song revised this lyric by substituting "*Some like the perfume from Spain*" for "cocaine."

## Candy is Dandy...

Starting in 1860, a hashish candy bar was manufactured by the Ganja Wallach Hasheesh Candy Company of New York. It was a very popular maple sugar-hashish candy marketed for over 35 years in the widely distributed Sears & Roebuck catalog. An advertisement for it read: "The Arabian Gunje of Enchantment Confectionized – a most pleasurable and harmless stimulant. Cures nervousness, weakness, melancholy, etc." [28] Around the turn of the century, a candy bar containing cocaine and chocolate was advertised for "a sweet tooth or a toothache." [29]

## . . . But Liquor is Quicker

Vin Mariani (a wine from the Bordeaux region of France containing cocaine extract) was patented in 1863 by Mariani and Company. It was the most prominent cocaine product in the world. The exported variety of Vin Mariani contained 7.2 mg. of cocaine/ounce. Written testimonials were an important component of patent medicine ads and Vin Mariani was no exception. Mariani claimed Ulysses S. Grant drank their product daily and that Queen Victoria was a fan of Vin Mariani. [30] Vin Mariani was not only endorsed by the famous actress, Sarah Behrnhart, and the American inventor, Thomas Edison, but by Pope Leo XIII and Pope Pius X. But, hey, Vin Mariani was ecumenical in their ads because Vin Mariani was also endorsed by the Grand Rabbi of France. [31]

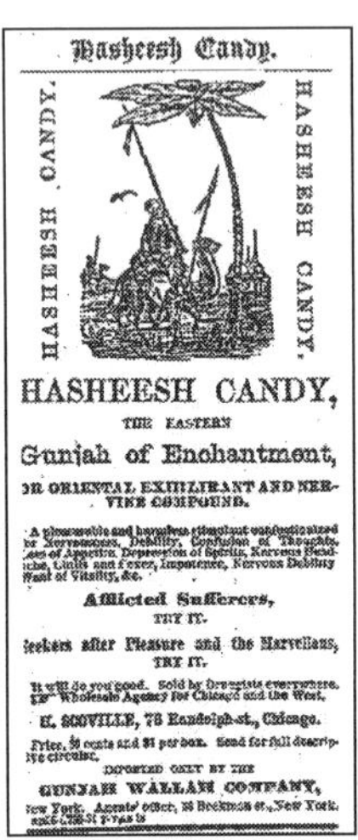


*Candy was a popular vehicle for consumption of drugs and not just sugar and chocolate. Here is an all-purpose candy, a food, a snack and a medicine (all rolled into one).*

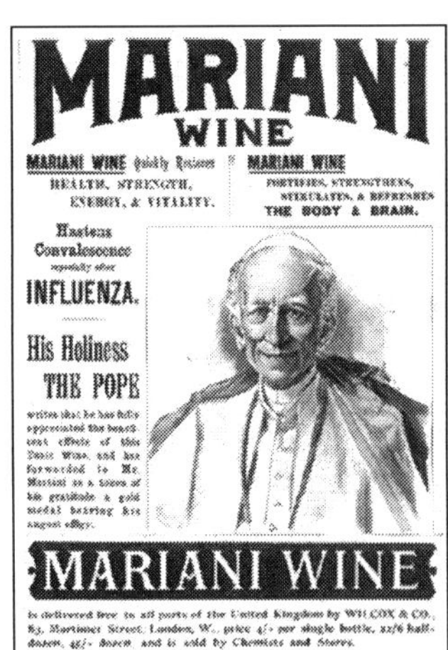


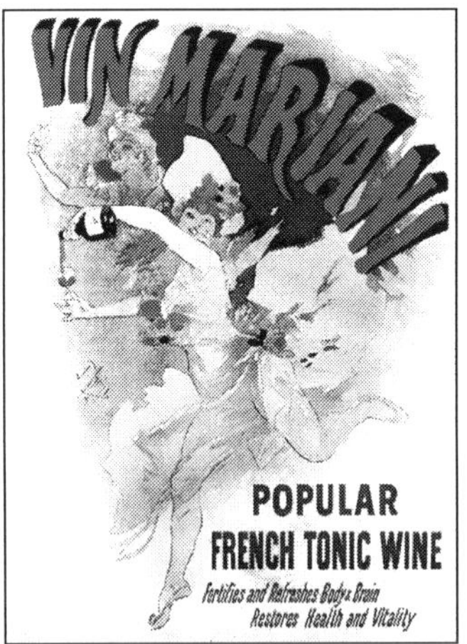


*A popular coca enhanced beverage endorsed by Pope Pious X, the 19th-century actress Sarah Bernhardt and the Grand Rabbi of France. It also claimed to be imbibed by American President Ulysses S. Grant and Queen Victoria of England.*

## Things Go Better with Coke

The most famous cocaine patent-medicine product, of course, was a secret mix of coca-leaf extract, sugar, alcohol and an extract of the caffeine-rich kola nut. It was developed by Atlanta physician, pharmacist, and former Confederate Army officer, Dr. John Stith Pemberton (1831-1888) and originally called Pemberton's French Wine Coca. It contained three parts coca leaves to one part kola nuts. [32] Pemberton's original formula was based on Vin Mariani and contained wine. [33]

## Even Coca-Cola Got in the Act

J.S. Pemberton, an Atlanta physician and pharmacist, invented Coca-Cola as a patent medicine available in drug stores. An 1885 article in the *Atlanta Journal* reported that Pemberton's French Wine Coca was composed of an extract from the Peruvian Coca leaf, the purest wine, and the Kola nut. Pemberton said, "It is the most excellent of all tonics, assisting digestion, imparting energy to the organs of respiration, and strengthening the muscular and nervous systems." [34]

In 1886, Atlanta briefly embraced prohibition of alcohol, so Pemberton took the wine out of his elixir and added sugar syrup as the sweetener. Voila! Coca-Cola was invented. The label proudly proclaimed it to be "the ideal temperance drink." Coca-Cola was soon marketed as "a remarkable therapeutic beverage," [35] the perfect beverage for a "turbulent, inventive, noisy, neurotic new America," good for "any nerve trouble, mental and physical exhaustion" and "a valuable brain tonic and cure for all nervous afflictions. [36]

Advertisements at the time declared the drink to be "one of the most delightful, cheering, and invigorating of fountain drinks." When Coca-Cola was the real thing, it may have had a little more kick than today and indeed been a bit invigorating. According to Cecil Adams in his Straight Dope column, southerners referred to Coca-Cola as "a shot in the arm." No doubt the cola was cheery and invigorating, because in 1886, a bottle of Coca-Cola contained alcohol as well as the equivalent of a contemporary line of cocaine. [37]

In 1903, the *New York Tribune* published an article linking cocaine with black crime and calling for legal

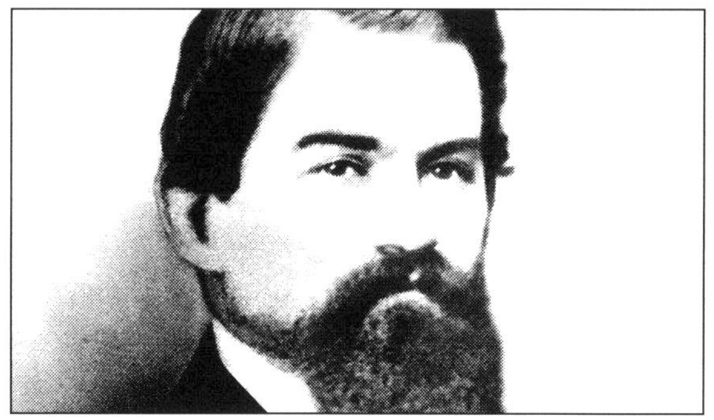

*J.S. Pemberton, an Atlanta physician, pharmacist and former Confederate Army officer, invented Coca-Cola. It was another patent medicine available in drug stores. It was sold as something to give you an energy boost. Since it contained both cocaine and caffeine, there was truth in that advertising.*

action against Coca-Cola. According to author David F. Musto, 1903 was the year the Coca-Cola Company ceased to use coca-leaf extract in its manufacturing process.[38] Other authorities cite 1902 and 1906, so the exact date cocaine was removed from Coke's formula remains a little fuzzy and the Coca Cola folks are purposely vague on the cocaine history of their product.

Coke switched from fresh to *spent* or de-cocainized coca leaves (i.e., what's left over after the cocaine has been removed) and replaced the cocaine in Coke's formula with caffeine.[39] Coke was no longer advertised as a cure for what ails you but was touted as a refreshing beverage, even though it was no longer "The Real Thing."

Today, Coca Cola allegedly contains only de-cocainized cocaine. The Coca Cola Company has conveniently forgotten their cocaine roots. The Coca-Cola museum in Atlanta does not mention the Coca-Cola elixir's connection to cocaine derived from the coca plant. Curiously, when two dried Coca Cola samples were sent to a drug testing lab in the late 1970s, they both tested positive for cocaine.[40] Who knew.

Low-potency coca products were widely available in the late 1800s and had been for at least a generation. These products were endorsed by the likes of Thomas Edison, U.S. Presidents McKinley and Roosevelt and the aforementioned Popes. All these coca-containing products were promoted as health drinks.[41] There is no evidence of widespread abuse or problems with these cocaine products.

Coca products such as tea and other beverages continue to be sold to this day in South America with no apparent health problems. There they are promoted for weight control and as a digestion aid.[42] Tourists visiting Machu Picchu, the 15th-century Inca ruins, are given a cocaine tea to help combat the lack of oxygen associated with the nearly 8,000-foot elevation.

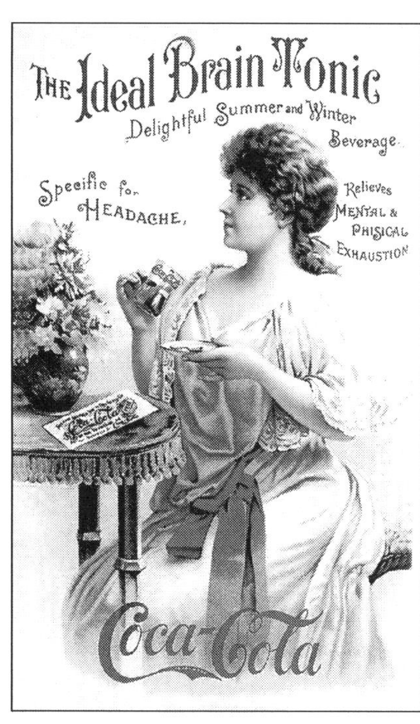


*As early as the 1890s, Coca-Cola was very popular. It contained cocaine. No one seemed to much mind until it was tied to the Reconstruction Era canard that cocaine caused Negroes to be aggressive and to lust for and attack innocent white Protestant women.*

The famed sharpshooter, Annie Oakley, was libeled by newspapers who incorrectly reported that she, not a stripper whose stage name was Annie Oakley, had been accused of theft and cocaine use. To clear her name, Oakley filed a suit against the Hearst newspapers, and other papers from St. Louis to Charleston. After six years of litigation, she prevailed and was awarded $27,600 from Hearst's Chicago paper. She won 54 or 55 other suits and the awards totaled at least $250,000 and maybe as much as $800,000. After legal expenses, she probably lost money but she was vindicated. Few people have the funds to pay for that kind of legal fight.[43] Good for Annie Oakley. Sadly, this Hearst-style smear is still rather widely used in reporting divorces, drug consumption, global warming, presidential politics and the like.

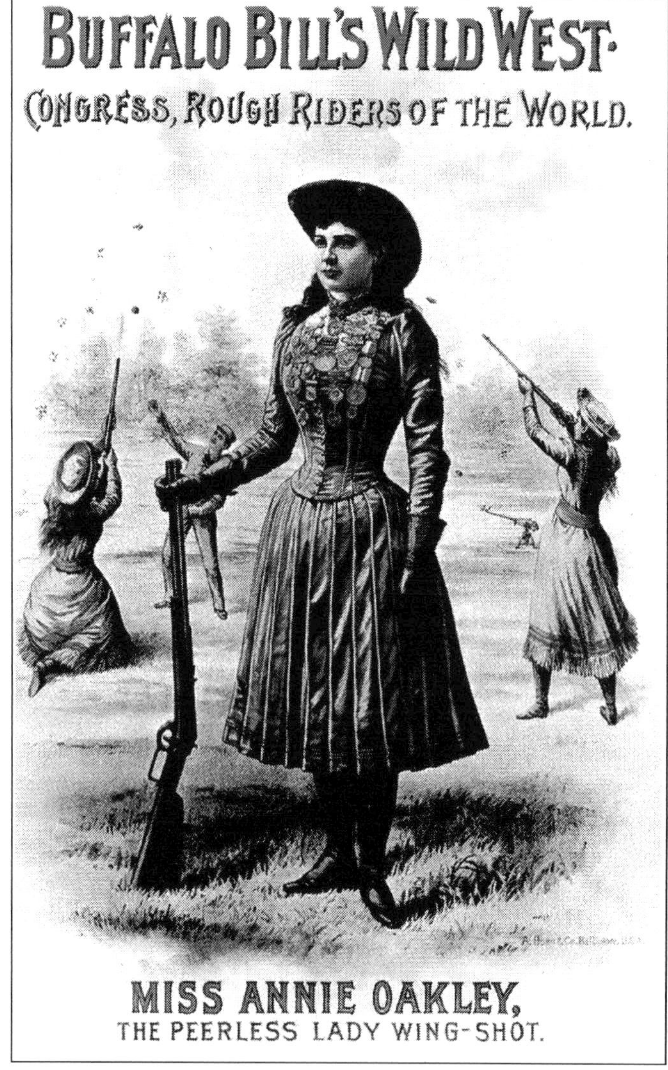


*William Randolph Hearst was unscrupulous in his zeal to sell papers. In 1903, Hearst papers smeared the great female sharpshooter, Annie Oakley. Numerous other papers picked up on Hearst's libel and reported that Oakley stood accused of theft and cocaine use. A woman burlesque performer named Maude Fontenella had been impersonating Annie Oakley for years. It was not the real Annie Oakley but the impersonator who had been so charged.*

## The Muckrakers

Turn-of-the-century muckraker-journalists wrote several exposés on American life that had a dramatic impact on the American public and which contributed to demand for the Pure Food & Drug Act. Americans demanded improved safety of food and drugs.

In 1905, Upton Sinclair published *The Jungle*, which exposed the filth and general unhealthy conditions in the meat-packing industry. The meat-packing industry revealed by Upton Sinclair makes today's *e-coli* deaths at fast-food joints look insignificant.

Patent medicines came in for their fair share of criticism, too. In 1905, *Colliers*, a popular magazine of the day, ran the "Great American Fraud" series by Samuel Hopkins Adams. Adams' article "exposed" patent medicines as a combination of snake oil, opium, herbs and cocaine – most heavily laced with alcohol. While some had real medicinal value, many were worthless and some even harmful. [44]

The patent medicine business lasts to this day but the combination of growing prohibition sentiment (most popular patent medicine contained plenty of alcohol) and the success of muckrakers and reformers in painting the patent medicine industry as a fraud and a health menace, coupled with the Pure Food and Drug Act of 1906, markedly decreased the sales of patent medicine.

The question in the early part of the 20th century was what to do about this patent medicine issue? Not everyone was a prohibitionist or into transferring powers that had historically been in the purview of state governments to the federal government. States'

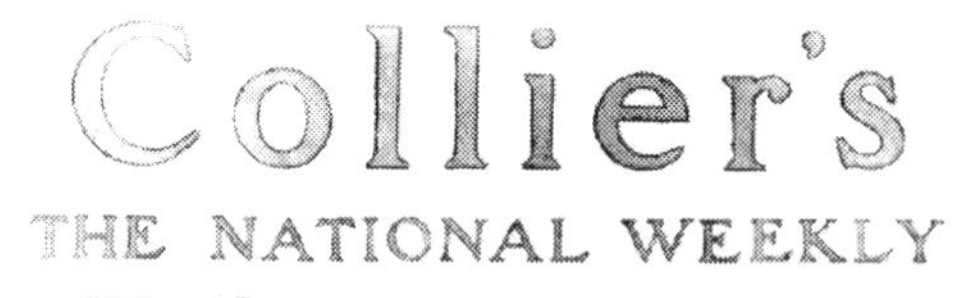


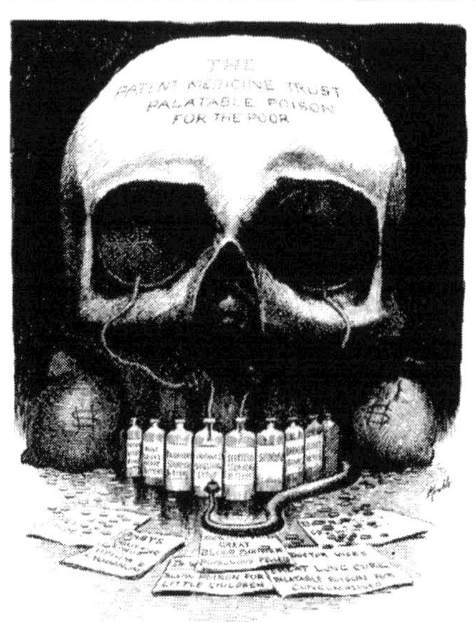


*Samuel Hopkins Adams's series, the "Great American Fraud", appeared in the popular monthly magazine,* Colliers, *in October, November and December 1905. This graphic graced the cover of Colliers trumpeting the health menace that Progressives perceived in patent medicine.*

rights and Prohibition, then as now, were both contentious issues in the early 20th century. There was little concern about what today is called "drug abuse." There was little or no violence or crime associated with use of what today might be lumped as drugs of abuse.

## Mark Twain on Self-Reliance

Mark Twain gave a speech in 1905 that was a blow for American freedom and individualism. He took *laissez-faire,* rugged-individualist approach by espousing people taking personal responsibility in drug use or nonuse. Today, the speech would most certainly not be politically correct. But it was consistent with the philosophy of the day of opposition to excessive government involvement in the lives of middle- and upper-class Americans. He defended his use of tobacco and suggested that he reached his ripe old age, not in spite of smoking, but in part because of it.

But true to the spirit of self-reliance, he did not urge others to follow his example. He said that each individual was the best judge of what was good for their health. Not bad advice, even today. The Pure Food and Drug Act of 1906 required that patent medicines carry a list of their ingredients. This was helpful in providing consumers more information so people could make better informed decisions on what they ingested. In his speech, Twain said:

> **"I have achieved my seventy years in the usual way: by sticking strictly to a scheme of life which would kill anybody else. It sounds like an exaggeration, but that is really the common rule for attaining old age. When we examine the program of any of these garrulous old people we always find that the habits which have preserved them would have decayed us ... I will offer here as a sound maxim ... That we can't reach old age by another man's road."**
>
> **"I have made it a rule never to smoke more than one cigar at a time. I have no other restriction as regards smoking. I do not know just when I began to smoke, I only know that it was in my father's lifetime and that I was discreet. He passed from this life early in 1847, when I was a shade past eleven; ever since then I have smoked publicly. As an example to others, and not that I care for moderation myself, it has always been my [practice] never to smoke when asleep and never to refrain when awake. It is a good [practice]. I mean, for me, but some of you know quite well that it wouldn't answer for everybody that's trying to get to be seventy.**
>
> **"I smoke in bed until I have to go to sleep; I wake up in the night, sometimes once, sometimes twice, sometimes three times, and I never waste any of these opportunities to smoke ... I will grant, here, that I have stopped smoking now and then, for a few months at a time, but it was not on principle, it was .. . to pulverize those critics who said I was a slave to my habit and couldn't break my bonds ... To-day it's all of sixty years that I began to smoke the limit."** [45]

In a 1998 article, "Mark Twain: An American Approach to Drugs; a View From Canada", Bruce

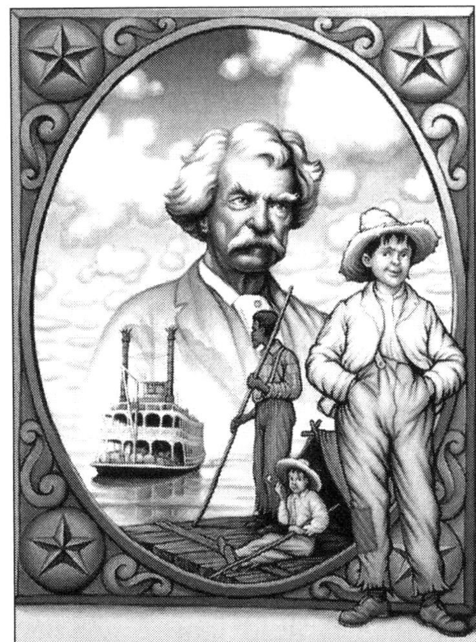

*Mark Twain skewered the conventional wisdom regarding drug use and abuse. He saw drug consumption as a personal choice and not a broader cultural or legal decision.*

K. Alexander states that "in Twain's complex analysis, the judgment about using drugs would be achieved by a kind of dynamic tension between people's understandings of their own needs and the sentiments of their families and their close society. He appeared to draw a sharp distinction between the normal human impulse to press for temperate use of drugs among one's close relatives and the 'temperance' doctrine that meant to impose abstinence on the world."[46] Alexander continues, "Should sociologists not be exploring the possibility that local forms of social control might be helpful in dealing with drug problems even though national and international drug 'wars' have clearly failed?"

---

**"There are three kinds of lies: lies, damned lies and statistics."**

**Mark Twain**

"Chapters from My Autobiography" in the *North American Review*, 1906

---

## Were the Progressives Really Progressive?

The prevailing political philosophy of the first quarter of the 20th century was dubbed Progressivism. Progressivism reflected the value system of upper middle-class America. These values included Calvinist Protestantism, Scientific Materialism and no-holds-barred Capitalism. The thought was that if certain vices interfered with work, this was not a good thing. The era embraced a robust pro-business ideology that helped create pressure for anti-vice laws. This philosophy was translated into many actions, some good (Pure Food& Drug Act, anti-trust laws) but some not so good (e.g., the Harrison Narcotic Act of 1914, Prohibition,1920-33, and anti-immigrant laws).[47]

The muckrakers' reporting stirred up enough interest and concern about the safety of patent medicine that regulating this industry became part of the Progressives reform package. Such regulation was consistent with the thinking of many prohibitionists that drugs other than alcohol should be targeted for strict control or exclusion from the marketplace. Soon the attention of reform-minded progressives included drug policy in their agenda. Mix this energy for reform with the peaking Temperance concerns, add hysterical anti-immigrant attitudes tied to opiates,

### Pure Food & Drug Act

The Pure Food and Drug Act of 1906 was passed in part because of the enormous popularity and resultant misuse of patent medicines. It had the reasonable purpose of stopping misbranded, adulterated or fraudulent products. It called for labeling medicines with their ingredients. Intoxicants in these products (e.g., alcohol, opium, cocaine, cannabis) had to be noted on the label. It left things up to the marketplace and was enormously successful at decreasing the sale and use of over-the-counter concoctions. The Pure Food and Drug Act is considered the most effective piece of drug legislation ever passed. If the United States had stopped there, it probably would have avoided the problems created by criminalization of various substances.

This law called for little more than listing a patent medicine's ingredients on the label. To date this simple labeling act has been the most effective law in decreasing substance use and abuse ever passed in U.S. history. Its effect was to immediately and dramatically lower the use of patent medicines. Within a few short years, several of the most popular patent medicines, many containing 30-50% alcohol, were no longer commercially viable and were off the market.

**The Pure Food and Drug Act of 1906 actually did four things:**

1. It created the Food and Drug Administration in Washington.

2. The Act REQUIRED that certain drugs could only be sold on prescription.

3. The Pure Food and Drug Act required that any drug that can be potentially habit-forming say so on its label. "Warning – May be habit forming" and it needed to note intoxicating ingredients.

4. It required that all drugs have the ingredients on the label.[48]

cocaine and alcohol, and voila!, the recipe for all the required political support necessary for the passage of the Pure Food and Drug Act. Its goal was positive enough – to stop misbranded, adulterated and fraudulent products.

## Harrison Narcotics Tax Act of 1914

The Harrison Narcotic Tax Act of 1914 was the first federal law criminalizing the non-medical use of a drug. The road to the 1914 Harrison Narcotics Tax Act was a long and winding one. The recipe for this unprecedented increase in federal authority at the expense of States' rights evolved over the 300 years of the West's opium trade with China, the 100 years of the Temperance Movement, post-Reconstruction racism, imperialistic gains made from the Spanish-American War, and a giant helping of xenophobia.

### The Yellow Peril

Nineteenth-century Protestant missionaries to China depicted the Chinese as deep within the powerful embrace of Satan, most definitely including the demon opium. In an effort to encourage the faithful back home to give money to save these heathens, the missionaries described the Chinese as engaging in pagan orgies of idolatry occurring with diabolical frenzy. The terms "vile", "polluted" and "diabolical" were used to describe the Chinese. Chinese men were regularly accused of defiling young girls and using "pictures, songs and aphrodisiacs" to lure them through "The Gates of Hell" to perform abominable acts. [49]

In the 1890s, internationalists with imperialist goals, most prominently Theodore Roosevelt, were eager to fight the Spanish over Cuba and Puerto Rico. The drums of war were fiercely beaten to an anti-Hispanic beat by the Hearst newspaper chain. When the Spanish-American War was over (April 25, 1898-August 12, 1898), the Philippines were part of the spoils of war for the United States. This meant that the United States had to evaluate what policy to apply to some of the Chinese minority living in the Philippines. It is argued that the Spanish-American War heralded America's entry into international imperialism. Others assert that the United States played a significant imperialist role much earlier. Regardless, the Spanish-American War definitely made the United States a player in setting international drug policy.

The demonic picture of the dope-fiend began to solidify at the turn of the 19th to the 20th century. The "fiend" wasn't the nice lady drinking her Lydia Pinkham's Vegetable Compound containing laudanum. No. The opium fiend was characterized as Chinese, smoking opium and luring vulnerable young women into their "hellish" opium dens. The fictional fiend, defined by the conventional wisdom of the time, grew out of hysteria of Americans regarding Asians, particularly the Chinese, the "Yellow Peril." Asians were seen as threatening, and not like "us". Who knew what they did while under the spell of opium? The answer, of course, is pretty much the same as the ladies sipping Lydia Pinkham's opium-laced tonic.

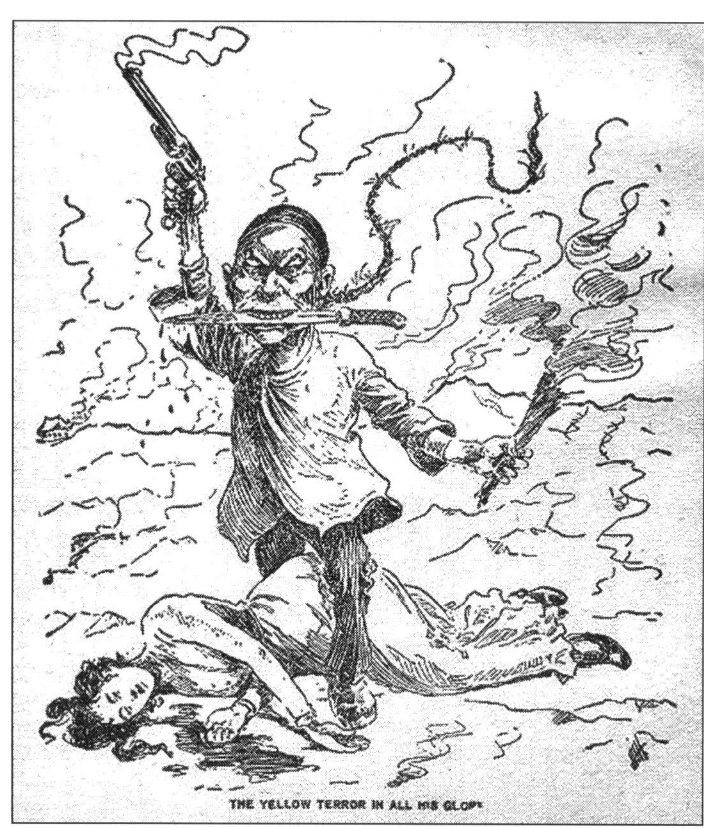


*Large numbers of Chinese began immigrating into the United States in the late 1840s to work the gold mines of California and to build the trans-continental railroad and rampant xenophobia soon followed. It was reflected in books, movies and posters such as the above editorial cartoon.*

A sign of the xenophobic times and a foreshadowing of what lay ahead, was a U.S. Senate resolution introduced in 1901 by Senator Henry Cabot Lodge. It was passed into law and forbade the sale of opium and alcohol by American traders "to aboriginal tribes and uncivilized races." Just to make sure all the "inferior" races were covered, these provisions were later extended to include "uncivilized elements in America itself and in its territories, such as Indians, Alaskans, and inhabitants of Hawaii, railroad workers, and immigrants at ports of entry." [50]

After the Spanish-American War, consistent with both the Temperance mood of those times and the Yellow Peril concerns, it was considered a moral imperative to devise a policy to control the opium smoking by the Chinese population in the Philippines. Initially, William Howard Taft, the governor of the Philippines and both a future U.S. President and Chief Justice of the Supreme Court, proposed following the tried-and-true formula of taxation. He would follow the existing Spanish policy of providing opium for the Chinese and taxing it, and using these taxes to fund their education. [51]

America's early 20th-century opium policy was driven by religious sanctimony and personal ambition. Taft's taxation idea was objected to by Christian missionaries, so President Teddy Roosevelt (1901-09) rejected that approach. In 1905, Congress approved a policy that opium could only be used for medicinal purposes. Under Taft's authority, the devising of an opiate policy for the Philippines quickly fell into the hands of two turn-of-the-century drug warriors, Episcopal Bishop Charles Brent and the politically ambitious Dr. Hamilton Wright, married to the niece of the soon to be president, William Howard Taft.

Bishop Brent and his ilk were well-meaning enough. In their effort to combat the perceived "evil" of the Chinese recreational use of opium, they created a problem where previously none had existed. By finally succeeding in making opium illegal for non-medical use, they created a great money-maker for the trio of bedfellows; organized crime, corrupt police and politicians.

Making opiates illegal resulted from Protestant religious leaders being convinced they were dealing with "evil". "They had the best of Christian intentions and missionary zeal. They took it upon themselves to judge what was right and wrong for people they didn't know and didn't understand, and then demanded that the law be used to enforce their judgment." [52]

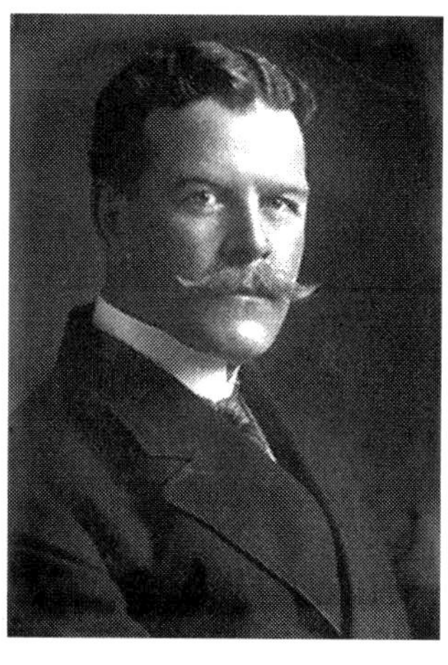

*Dr. Hamilton Wright was one of the first drug warriors. He was married to U.S. President William Howard Taft's niece and had unrealized higher political aspirations. He did succeed in getting the Harrison Narcotics Tax Act passed and the agreements for the Hague Conference included in the Treaty of Versailles following WWI. Wright and Brent helped switch the conversation from alcohol to other drugs.*

Again, this approach created more problems than it solved.

## International Conferences

Over the next decade, Bishop Brent and Dr. Wright spearheaded a series of international opium conferences promoted by the United States. These conferences set in motion the repressive international policy on opiates that is still with us. First was the Philippine Conference of 1902, which outlawed opium for the Chinese in the Philippines. This was followed by the First International Opium Commission (aka the Shanghai Conference) of 1909, which was chaired by none other than Bishop Charles Henry Brent.

The 1909 conference set the groundwork for the 1911-12 Hague Convention. The attendees included Great Britain, Austria, Hungary, France, Portugal, the Netherlands, Italy, Russia, Japan, Iran (Persia), Thailand (Siam), and the United States, culminating in the so-called World War on Opium Traffic. Their efforts were unleashed after WWI by being incorporated into the Treaty of Versailles.

These American-organized drug control conferences were well-attended by European nations. The Europeans were not that focused on the moral issue of opium control. They were much more interested in making amends for their lengthy role in promoting the opium trade in China in order to gain the Chinese as a trading partner. In 1911, a new China had emerged because Sun Yat Sun's quarter-century efforts were successful in overthrowing the Manchu dynasty.

The new Chinese government viewed opium as a major symbol of Western imperialism's corrupting influence on Eastern culture. The tattered relationship of Great Britain and the rest of Europe with China went back over 200 years. Two mid-19th-century opium wars had left more than a little lingering hostility in China toward the West. The memory was still fresh that British military power had forced China to accept importation of opium and rescind the opiate prohibition in China.

For the United States, this was a lesser motivation as Americans did not see themselves as complicit in 19th-century European imperialism in China. Still, then as now, China represented an attractive market. In 1906, China had once again cracked down on opium consumption and in particular smoking opium. Their leaders wanted to modernize China to help repel Western encroachment. They also were angered at the treatment of Chinese in America. So there was a chance for America to curry favor and get its "fair share" of trade with China. [53]

According to Dr. David F. Musto, the distinguished American medical historian, "most nations who sent representatives to these early 1900s opium conclaves were just mildly interested in the subject and were unwilling to exert much effort for the non-medical prohibition proposed by the United States. Britain was a foot-dragger due to their desire to protect the opium trade from India. *It was impossible to get general agreement that the use of opium for non-medical purposes was evil and immoral.*" [emphasis added] [54]

The rest of the world found a way of defusing the American negotiators, or so they thought. At The Hague, the Europeans figured they had stymied Wright and Brent by requiring that all European nations sign on to their drug control pact before it could become operative. The agreements reached at The Hague were just a symbolic statement to the Europeans. They figured there would never be the necessary unanimity among European nations to get the approval required for international application of these proclamations.

Sadly, the Europeans under-estimated the sanctimony and moral fervor of the early 20th-century American "Drug Warriors". Agreements developed at the Hague later became part of the treaty ending WWI, the Treaty of the Versailles. The Treaty was signed by the United States, Britain and all of Europe. The treaty had internationally criminalized what heretofore had been a medical problem of, at most, a middling concern. [55]

## Southern Support

The international agreements reached at the Hague Convention in 1912 begat the Harrison Narcotics Tax Act of 1914. The Harrison Narcotic Tax Act was a prohibition of cocaine and opiates in the guise of a Tax. Cocaine got included because of its supposed association with Negro violence. This allegation was helpful in garnering Southern Congressional support for the new law.

Democrats had won control of the House in the 1912 elections after two decades of Republican control. So support of the prohibition of drugs from southern legislators was now more important. However, southerners were resistant to the weakening of States' rights. Weakening the rights of states could interfere with local and state laws in the South, which enforced racial segregation and disenfranchised African-American voters.

But it turns out that exploiting racism against Negroes was good politics. It was about the only thing that would motivate southern U.S. Senators to vote for giving more power to the federal government at the expense of the states.

In the years and months immediately preceding the passage of the Harrison Narcotics Tax Act, racist allegations implicating both opium and cocaine became wilder. An increasing number of stories spoke of "cocaine-crazed Negroes" in the South running amuck; thus linking cocaine to what was described as aggressive Negro behavior. A February 11, 1914 story in the *New York Times,* alleged that for "most of the attacks upon white women of the South are the direct result of the 'cocaine-crazed' Negro brain." [56]

Musto notes that, "The identification of cocaine use with African Americans soon elaborated a link between cocaine and supposed African-American criminality, illustrating the tendency to find in drug use a simple explanation for complex social problems." [57]

In that *Times* article warning of the new Southern menace of Negro cocaine "fiends", Dr. Edward

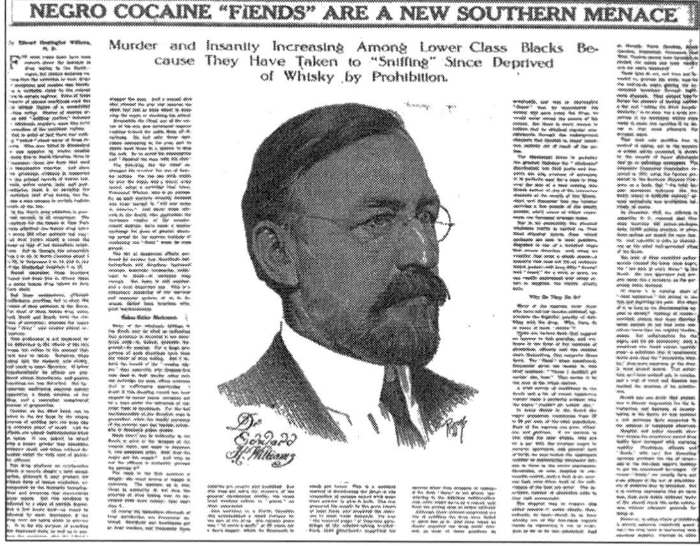
NEGRO COCAINE "FIENDS" ARE A NEW SOUTHERN MENACE

Murder and Insanity Increasing Among Lower Class Blacks Because They Have Taken to "Sniffing" Since Deprived of Whisky by Prohibition.

*Articles like this in the New York times were part of propaganda to gain the votes of Southern Congressmen for the 1914 Harrison Narcotics Tax Act. It played on bigotry and racist fears to overcome the South's strongly held support for States' rights. The Harrison Narcotics Tax Act undercut States' rights. Due to racist concerns, many southern representatives voted for the law even though it expanded federal authority at the expense of States.*

H. Williams warned of Negro marksmanship and it supported the myth of the cocaine-powered super Negro. Dr. Williams wrote, "But I believe the record of the 'cocaine nigger' near Asheville, who dropped five men dead in their tracks, using only one cartridge for each, offers evidence that is sufficiently convincing." [58]

Tales such as these made it clear to Southern politicians that in order to eliminate this terrible danger, they should suspend their support of states rights and surrender state power, which was guaranteed by the Ninth and Tenth Amendments, to the federal government and vote for the Harrison Narcotics Tax Act.

Now President Taft had made cocaine Public Enemy No. 1 by presenting a U.S. State Department report to Congress that raised hysterical race-related concerns. The report said:

> "The illicit sale of cocaine ... and the habitual use of it temporarily raises the power of a criminal to the point where in resisting arrest there is no hesitation to murder. It is most appalling in its effects than any other habit forming drug used in the United States."

The report had more helpful ammo for the prohibitionists' efforts to win over southern Congressmen. The report stated, "it has been authoritatively stated that cocaine is often the direct incentive to the crime of rape by negroes of the South and other heathens of the County." [59]

## Cannabis Excluded

Some prohibitionists wanted, but failed to include cannabis in that Act. A few voices berated those who minimized the dangers of cannabis. Charles B. Fauns, a well-known director of a drug and alcohol hospital in New York City was one. Fauns told a congressional hearing, "To my mind it is inexcusable for a man to say that there is no habit from the use of that drug. There is no drug in the pharmacopoeia today, and of all the drugs on earth I would certainly put that on the list...." [60]

Dr. William J. Schieffelin concurred with Fauns. He, too, called for the inclusion of cannabis in the proposed law. He implicated yet another minority. He testified that he had heard that it was smoked by New York City's Syrian colony and therefore it should be outlawed. [61]

So while some effort was made to include cannabis in the Harrison Act, this was never really seriously

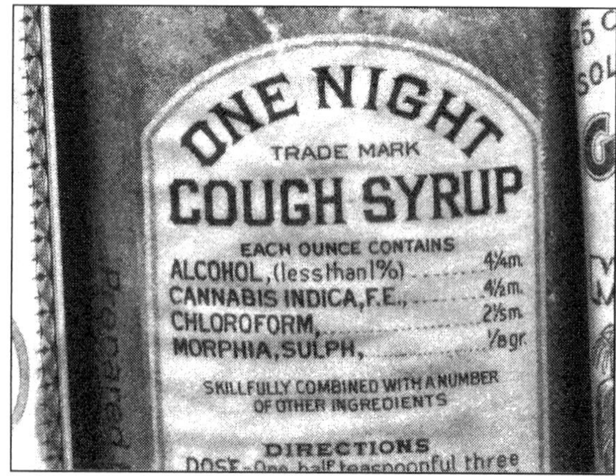


*Many patent medicines contained cannabis. These medicines were produced by well-known pharmaceutical companies such as Eli Lilly, Squibb, Merck, Parke Davis and Smith Brothers. At the end of the 19th century to the beginning of 20th, cannabis was the third most common ingredient in patent medicine.*

considered by Congress. Lobbying by pharmaceutical companies plus the lack of physician support for the idea, saw to that. Charles A. West, chairman of the National Wholesale Druggists' Association, and Albert Platt, representing New York pharmaceutical firm Lehn and Fink, spoke against the proposal. Cannabis was not included in the subsequent debate over national restrictions on narcotic drugs. [62]

## Soldier's Disease – A Useful Myth

Just as pressure to pass the Harrison Act was building, out of almost nowhere, 50 years after the end of the Civil War, the tale of "Soldier's Disease" materialized. So-called "Soldier's Disease" is supposed to be what opiate habituation was called in the late 19th century, allegedly because so many Civil War vets were habituated. This story appears to be a fabrication sewn of whole cloth. The first mention of "Soldier's Disease" in the literature is 1913. Little evidence has been found by historians to support this very late breaking news. [63]

Jerry Mandel and other historians think the influence of the Civil War on opiate abuse was vastly exaggerated and that "the soldier's disease" is a fable concocted well after the fact – 1913 to be exact – to justify the passage of this repressive drug law.

The Soldier's Disease myth is defined by Webster as "...an ill-founded belief held uncritically especially by an interested group" and exemplifies many of the basic themes of the drug warriors and support for drug prohibition. (1) Addiction is easy to acquire, (2) hard to kick and (3) is a publicly noticed, i.e., a *social*, problem." Like so much else surrounding the justification for our drug policy, Soldier's Disease is just another myth. [64]

"Soldiers Disease" is an example of how leaders create justification for laws out of phantom or at best very dubious "facts". It's clear this "Soldier's Disease" is a fictitious phenomenon. And it took another 50 years after its invention — almost a century after Appomattox — before this myth became part of drug experts' conventional wisdom. Unfortunately, this story has become a staple in most books written about drug abuse after 1960. [65]

Several historians writing about opiate abuse in the Civil War and the post-Civil War period point out

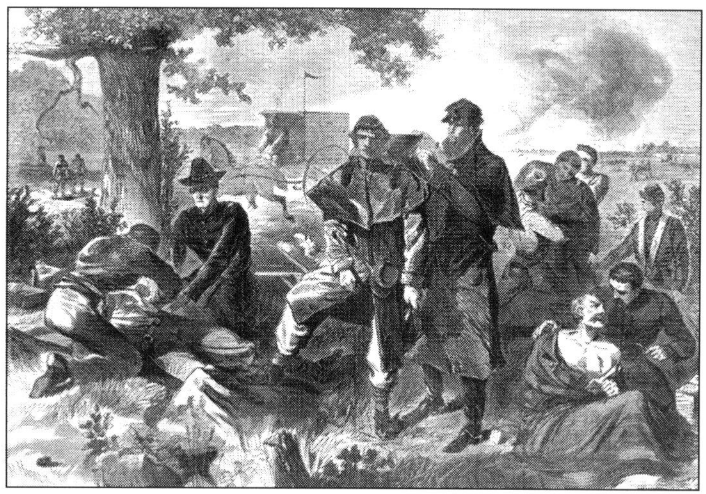

*So-called "Soldier's Disease" seems at best to be revisionist history and at worst an out-right lie. While many articles written after 1913 speak of Soldier's Disease being caused by soldiers getting hooked on morphine during and immediately after the Civil War, there is little in the literature between 1865 and 1913, almost 50 years, which confirms that allegation.*

that opiate abuse was neither closely associated with nor dispropor-tionately contri-buted to by Civil War veterans. Mandel, Mark A. Quinones and numerous others note that after the Civil War, women opiate abusers outnumbered men by 3 to 1. This is particularly surprising, knowing what is known today about posttraumatic stress disorder. There was not a high incidence of "addiction or drug use while in the service" among soldiers. [66]

Careful reviews of the contemporary post-Civil War medical literature have found little evidence pointing to the Civil War as the catalyst triggering drug addiction in America. Quite the contrary, patent medicines were already on the scene and being widely consumed long before the start of that war. [67,68,69,70]

Quinones points to the fact that there was a higher rate of addiction among southern women than men and that many Civil War veterans developed drug problems that had no record of addiction during their tour of duty. According to Quinones:

> "From a careful review of the existing literature, there is insufficient evidence to credit the Civil War as the catalyst for the onset of drug addiction in America. On the contrary, it is clear that while the Civil War may have contributed to the problem,

> drugs were already on the scene and being consumed at alarming rates long before the start of the war." [71]

Jerry Mandel documents in *The Mythical Roots of U.S. Drug Policy: Soldier's Disease and Addiction in the Civil War* (1989).

> "Even though so-called Soldier's Disease is almost certainly fictitious, it is a widely told tale in the litany of drug mythology. There was not, as first characterized in 1913, widespread addiction following massive administration of opiates during the Civil War. It represents one of the earliest and most often repeated example of a drug problem before the Narcotics laws." [72]

He and other historians think the influence of the Civil War on opiate abuse was vastly exaggerated and that "the soldier's disease" is a fable concocted well after the fact – 1913 to be exact – to justify repressive drug laws. Mandel states that there is:

> " . . . an almost total lack of contemporaneous historical mention of this condition during and after the Civil War. If this had been a real and large problem, as purported 50 and 100 years later, surely it would have been prominently mentioned at the time this alleged opiate epidemic occurred.
>
> Not one case of addiction was reported in medical records or the literature of the time. There were under ten references to addiction made in the Nineteenth Century whose cause ascribed was the Civil War; and no pejorative nickname for addicted veterans, like Soldier's Disease, appeared in the literature until 1913." [73]

## The Link Between Crime and Drugs?

A lot is heard today about drugs causing crime. Following the Civil War, there was minimal association between crime and addictions. [74]

According to Quinone, the best and only explanation that can be offered for this lack of a crime/drug association was that there was no need to resort to crime to gain access to opiates. Opiates were readily available at the corner store – drug, grocery or general – plus the occasional saloon. This is because there was no federal law controlling access to opiates until the 1914 Harrison Narcotics Tax Act.

The Harrison Act did not immediately make opiate use or acquisition illegal, but this state of affairs soon changed. The manner of the Act's implementation and court decision soon effectively criminalized the use of nonprescription opiates and even prescription opiates for habitual users. The law was tightened up by at least two Supreme Court decisions. In 1919, *Webb v. the United States* (249 U.S. 96) outlawed doctors treating habitual narcotic users with opiates, [79] and by 1924 federal law enforcement had closed the heroin maintenance clinics. [75]

Joseph McNamara, former chief of police in Kansas City, Missouri and San Jose, California and research fellow at the Hoover Institution, a conservative think tank, points out that it was NOT the police that lobbied for the Harrison Act. "It was the Protestant missionary societies in China, the Woman's Christian Temperance Union, and other such organizations that viewed the taking of psychoactive substances as sinful. These groups gradually got their religious tenets enacted into penal statutes under which the "sinners" go to jail." [76]

McNamara puts his finger on the difficulty in logically evaluating the success or failure of our current drug policy. McNamara says that it's "the conviction that the use of certain drugs is immoral" that chills the ability to scrutinize drug policy rationally and to debate the effects of the drug war. McNamara notes that when Ethan Nadelmann, director of the drug-policy reform organization, The Drug Policy Alliance, stated that it was illogical for the most hazardous drugs, alcohol and nicotine, to be legal while less dangerous drugs were illegal, he was roundly denounced.

McNamara wrote, "A leading conservative supporter of the drug war contended that while alcohol and nicotine addiction was unhealthy and could even cost lives, addiction to illegal drugs could result in the loss of one's soul. No empirical proof was given." McNamara finds that this morality-laden reasoning is why "today's ineffective and counter-productive drug laws have withstood logical analysis."[77]

Another reason is the prison-industrial complex. Where do the billions of dollars that are thrown at this medical problem go? Does it go to reforming the health care system or paying for medical care? No, it goes to pay sheriffs' police, prosecutors, judges, and prison guards — the entire bureaucratic, drug-enforcement operation. In addition, it's not cheap to build and run a prison.

Current drug laws have created a client class that supports current drug policy — not because it is good policy but because it is a jobs program.

## Going After the Physicians

With a few judicial and bureaucratic decisions and a little legislative tweaking, not only did the Harrison Narcotic Tax Act effectively criminalize opiate habituation, but also it put doctors in the Federal Bureau of Narcotics' (FBN) crosshairs.

In 1922, the U.S. Supreme Court held 6-3 that doctors could not treat habitual opiate users with opiates (*United States v. Behrman*, 258 U.S. 280). Between 1920 and 1938, almost 38,000 doctors were arrested for providing opiates to habitual opiate users and 3,000 served penitentiary sentences.[78] By outlawing opiates, the United States had created a whole new class of criminals.

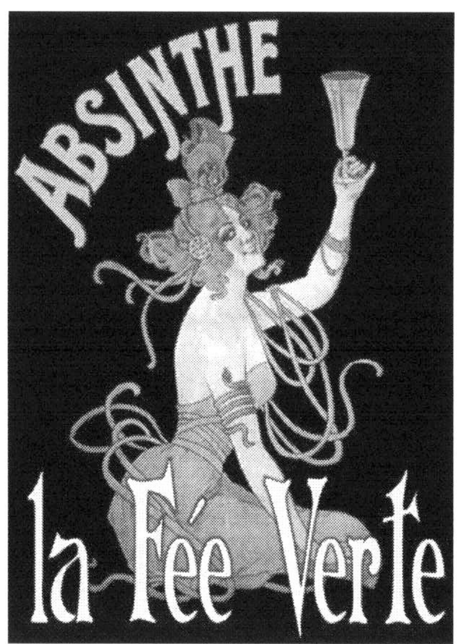


*Absinthe, a supposedly psychoactive alcohol known as "The Green Fairy", was made illegal in Europe at the end of the 19th century, which was a precursor to the banning of all alcohol in the United States in 1920.*

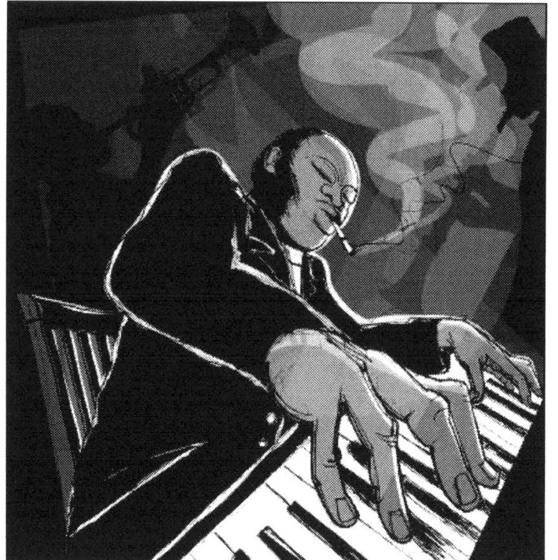

*Jazz, that uniquely American musical invention, is thought to have morphed out of "ragtime", which had originated in the bordellos of New Orleans in the early 20th century. It is well documented that marijuana was an important catalyst among the early practitioners of both genres.*

# CHAPTER IX
# 1910-19: Prelude to Prohibition

## Obtaining Heroin, Cocaine, Cannabis and Alcohol Becomes Difficult

The Harrison Act did not immediately make opiate use or acquisition illegal, but this state of affairs soon changed. The manner of the Act's implementation and court decisions soon effectively criminalized the use of non-prescription opiates and even prescription opiates for habitual users. The law was tightened up by at least two Supreme Court decisions. In 1919, *Webb v. the United States* outlawed doctors treating habitual narcotic users with opiates, [1] and by 1924, federal law enforcement had closed the heroin maintenance clinics. [2]

### Send the Sinners to Jail

Joseph McNamara, former chief of police in both Kansas City, Missouri and San Jose, California and a research fellow at the Hoover Institution, a conservative think tank, points out that it was NOT the police that lobbied for the Harrison Act. "It was the Protestant missionary societies in China, the Woman's Christian Temperance Union, and other such organizations that viewed the taking of psychoactive substances as sinful. These groups gradually got their religious tenets enacted into penal statutes under which the 'sinners' go to jail." [3]

McNamara puts his finger on the difficulty in logically evaluating the success or failure of our current drug policy. McNamara says that it's "the conviction that the use of certain drugs is immoral" that "chills" the ability to scrutinize drug policy rationally and to debate the effects of the drug war. McNamara notes that when Ethan Nadelmann, director of the drug policy reform organization, The Drug Policy Alliance, stated that it was illogical for the most hazardous drugs, alcohol and nicotine, to be legal while less dangerous drugs were illegal, he was roundly denounced.

McNamara wrote, "A leading conservative supporter of the drug war contended that while alcohol and nicotine addiction was unhealthy and could even cost lives, addiction to illegal drugs could result in the loss of one's soul. No empirical proof was given." McNamara finds that this morality laden reasoning is why "today's ineffective and counter-productive drug laws have withstood logical analysis." [4]

Another reason is the prison industrial complex. Where does the billions of dollars we are throwing at this medical problem go? Does it go to reforming our health care system or paying for medical care? No, it goes to pay sheriffs, police, prosecutors, judges, prison guards, and the entire bureaucratic drug enforcement operation. In addition, it's not cheap to build and run a prison. Our current drug laws have created a client class that supports current drug policy not because it is good policy but because it gives them a job and pays the bills.

## Heroin Maintenance: Whoever Heard of Such a Thing?

From 1919 to 1923, heroin maintenance clinics were in vogue in the United States. Most worked quite well treating opiate habituates and keeping crime down. The first morphine maintenance clinic was opened in Jacksonville, Florida. After the *Webb v. United States* decision, at least 44 communities established morphine maintenance clinics. [5] Heroin maintenance clinics in Los Angeles, New Haven, Connecticut, Jacksonville, Florida and Shreveport, Louisiana were all effective or very effective.

Apparently this was of no matter to the Narcotic Division of the Internal Revenue Service. [6] The New York Clinic, which was not well-run, with too many patients and not enough controls, was held up by the IRS as a negative model (perhaps to support an already established policy belief). This clinic's experience was used to justify a nationwide closing of all the heroin maintenance clinics. This step occurred even though the New York City heroin maintenance clinic was closed after only 11 months of operation. [7]

Later a thorough study was done of the Shreveport Clinic. [8] This included talking with the 85-year-old former director of the Shreveport Clinic, Dr. Willis Butler. During its operation, crime dropped in Shreveport. The police did not find any meaningful diversion of heroin from these clinics onto the streets of Shreveport.

But in 1923, the very effective Shreveport Heroin Maintenance Clinic and others across the country were closed. [9] After the clinic's closure, crime and illicit opiate sales in Shreveport markedly increased. [10] In a late '60s radio interview with Dr. Butler, the aging former medical director of the Shreveport Clinic continued to articulately and cogently express his support for the treatment provided there. [11]

Heroin was manufactured largely outside the United States. In 1926, the noose tightened and heroin importation was banned. The last such clinic was in Knoxville and closed in 1925. [12]

With a few judicial and bureaucratic decisions and a little legislative tweaking, not only did the Harrison Narcotic Tax Act effectively criminalize opiate habituation, it also put doctors in the Federal Bureau of Narcotics' crosshairs. Between 1920 and 1938, almost 25,000 doctors were arraigned for treating opiate abusers and 3,000 served penitentiary sentences. [13] By outlawing opiates, the United States had created a whole new class of criminals.

## Equal Opporunity Demonization: "Hindoos" and Hash

Blacks and Mexicans are not the only peoples "demonized" in conjunction with their use of cannabis. One of the first discriminated against groups over this substance were the Sikhs. The Sikhs are a religious sect from India. This discrimination resulted in the first anti-cannabis law in the United States. As Dale Gehringer, Ph.D., pointed out in his article "The Forgotten Origins of Cannabis Prohibition in California" (1999), hashish was placed into the California poison law in 1913. [14] The law was directed at Sikhs living in and around Fresno who used hashish. They worked too hard, looked diff e rent, ate different food, "smelled funny" and who knows, maybe they coveted American women. This California law came about as a result of the work of Santa Barbara pharmacist, Henry Finger, member of the California Board of Pharmacy and part of the delegation to the First International Opium Conference held at The Hague in 1911.

According to Gehringer's account,[15] Finger wanted to include cannabis prohibition with the opium ban. Finger made it clear that his request came out of concern about the "Hindoos." Finger wrote Dr. Hamilton Wright, the lead conference delegate, urging him to have the Conference take up the cannabis issue because of the "Hindoos":

> Within the last year, we in California have been getting a large influx of 'Hindoos' and they have in turn started quite a demand for cannabis indica; they are a very undesirable lot and the habit is growing in California very fast … the fear is now that they are initiating our whites into this habit … We were not aware of the extent of this vice at the time our legislature was in session and did not have our laws amended to cover this matter, and now have no legislative session for two years (January, 1913). This matter has been brought to my attention a great number of time(s) in the last two months … it seems to be a real question that now confronts us: can we do anything in the Hague that might assist in curbing this matter?"[16]

And indeed at The Hague Conference, Finger rose expressing his concern about the "Hindoos" (as he erroneously labeled the Sikhs, who, of course, are not followers of Hinduism) and their use of hashish. Finger pleaded his case that cannabis should be included amongst the drugs to be subjected to worldwide censorship. His expressed concern over the "large influx of "Hindoos" into San Francisco, who Finger alleged, were introducing "whites into their habit."[17]

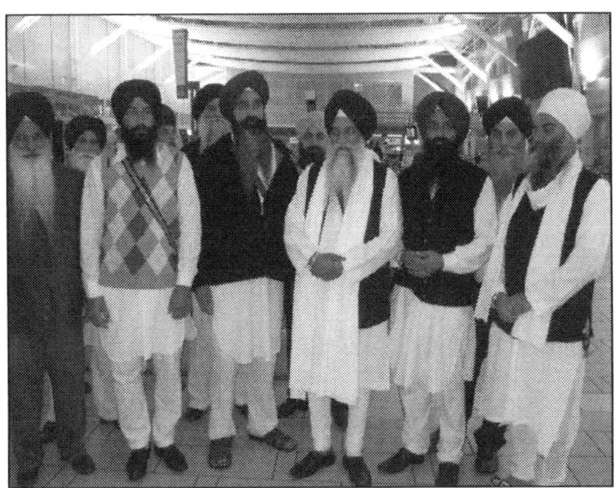

*Oddly enough, one of the initial groups demonized for using cannabis was the Sihks in the first decade of the 20th century. They used hashish, but their real sin appears to be that they were competing for jobs with Americans that came before them.*

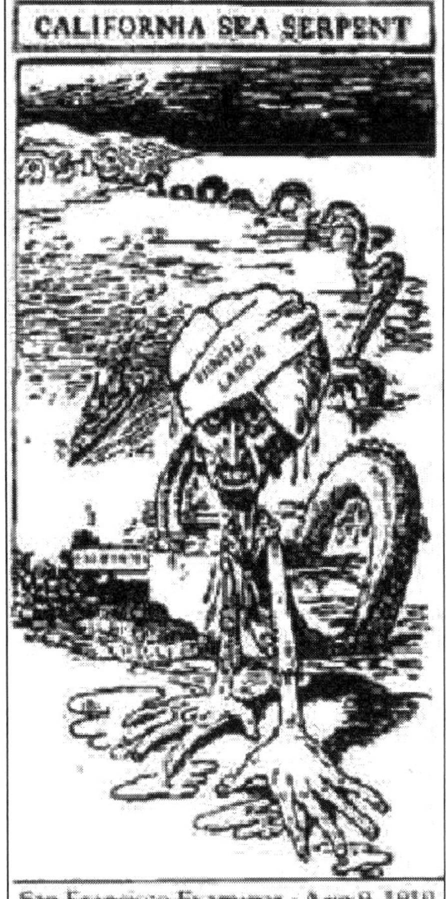


*The Sikhs are not ordinarily thought of as being a discriminated against minority. However, in 1909 they were, as this cartoon in a 1910* San Francisco Examiner *demonstrates. The bigotry directed toward the Sikhs led to the first law in the United States against cannabis. In this case it was included as a poison in California poison law.*

These concerns about the influx of "Hindoos" arose after several boatloads of Sikh immigrants from India's Punjabi region arrived in San Francisco in 1910. These so-called "Hindoos" became a popular target of anti-immigrant sentiment. Asian exclusionists protested that the "Hindoos" were even more unfit for American civilization than the Chinese. Their influx was quickly blocked by immigration authorities, leaving little more than 2,000 in the state, mostly in agricultural areas of California's Central Valley. The Sikhs were widely denounced for their supposedly outlandish customs, dirty clothes, strange food, suspect morals, but especially their propensity to work for low wages.

## Cannabis & India

Cannabis has a long history in India, the geographical base of the Sikhs. Cannabis not only is included in the oldest known *Materia Medica*, which was written circa 1100-1700 BC, but was also con-sidered holy by many Hindu sects. Shiva, the Supreme god of many Hindu sects, is said to have brought hemp a "sacred grass" down from the heavens. Shiva is known as "the Lord of Bhang" in India. This king of India gods is said to have given marijuana to the populace so they might attain elevated states of consciousness. Siddhartha is said to have eaten nothing but hemp seeds for six years while discovery his truth and becoming the Buddha.

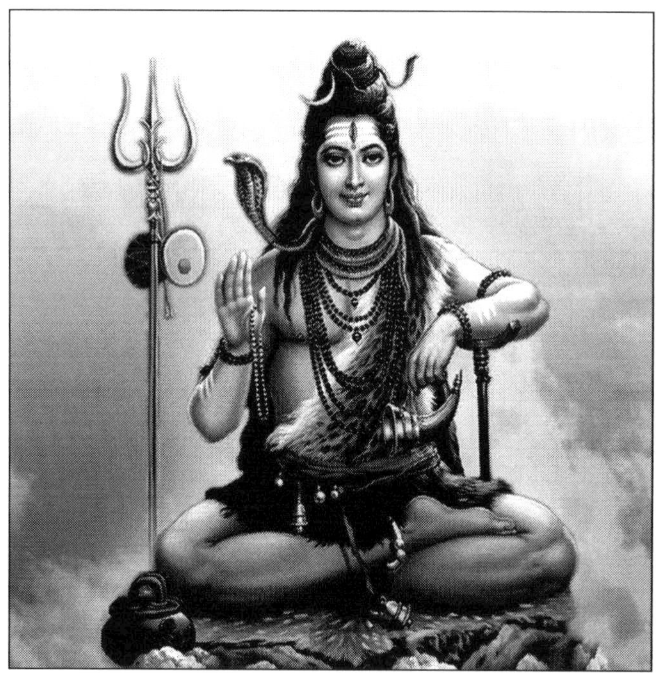

*Shiva is the Hindu God. He is said to have brought hemp "the sacred grow" down from the heavens. The Buddha is said to have eaten nothing but cannabis for seven years.*

Three grades of cannabis product are recognized in India. Bhang tended to be used by the less financially well off, whereas Charas being more expensive, was usually used by the more economically advantaged. To this day, cannabis is used in India particularly by the lower classes.

Bhang is the dried cannabis leaves, seeds and stems which is usually eaten or drunk in the form of a beverage or a confection. "The simplest bhang beverage consists of a drink made by pounding cannabis leaves with a little black pepper and sugar, and diluting with water to the desired strength."

The middle and well-to-do classes make various kinds of special (bhang) beverages by adding almonds, sugar, iced milk, and/or curds, or other flavor enhancers."[18]

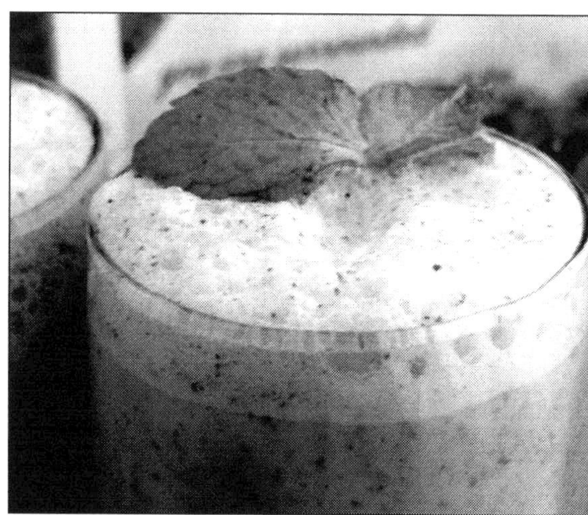

*Bhang is a tea made from cannabis plus several spices and a little milk. It's been used in India for thousands of years.*

Ganja includes some of the plant resin as well as the leaves and flowering tops. Charas is cannabis resin in pure or almost pure form, known in the West as Hash.

In 1957, the United Nations issued a report on the consumption of cannabis in India:

> **"Bhang is the Joy-giver, the Sky-filler, the Heavenly-Guide, the Poor Man's Heaven, the Soother of Grief . . . No god or man is as good as the religious drinker of bhang . . . The supporting power of bhang has brought many a Hindu family safe through the miseries of famine. To forbid or even seriously restrict the use of so gracious an herb as the hemp would cause wide spread suffering and annoyance and to large bands of worshipped ascetics, deep-seated anger. It would rob the people of solace on discomfort, of a cure in sickness, of a guardian whose gracious protection saves them from the attacks of evil influences . . .**
>
> ". . . for the vast majority of consumers, the Commission considers that the evidence shows the moderate use of ganja or charas not to be appreciably harmful . . ."[19]

United Nations Bulletin on Narcotics, 1957

## The Anti-Cannabis Movement

While the 1913 California law regarding poisons included hashish, Utah's anti-marijuana law of 1915 is usually credited with being the first state to outlaw cannabis. [20] This came about as a result of three concerns: competition from cheap Mexican labor, the return of a group of traditional polygamous Mormons from a Mormon colony in Mexico (this included Mitt Romney's grandfather), and the Mormon Church's antipathy towards intoxicants.

This whole matter became a particular issue for the Mormons as a result of the Mormon Church admitting they had made a mistake with endorsing polygamy; outlawing it in 1910. Not too surprisingly, a number of traditional Mormons left Utah. Some went to northwest Mexico with the hope of establishing a Mormon enclave with traditional Mormon values. They also looked forward to prostilytizing and converting the local Indians and Mexicans to Mormonism. They had little luck converting the Mexicans and after a few years, suffering from home sickness, many returned to Utah. They took with them a little gift from the Indians: marijuana. [21]

The Mormon Church is opposed to the use of euphoriants of any kind. So, in August of 1915, the Church, meeting in synod in Salt Lake City, decreed the use of marijuana contrary to the Mormon religion. Then, in October of 1915, the Mormon dominated state legislature met and enacted this religiously motivated prohibition as a criminal law. [22] Utah was joined by many states west of the Mississippi: Wyoming (1915), Texas (1919), Iowa (1923), Nevada (1923), Oregon (1923), Washington (1923), Arkansas (1923), and Nebraska (1927). There were also several states east of the Mississippi (e.g., Massachusetts, Maine, Indiana and Vermont) that had banned marijuana (but not cannabis); some as early as 1915. [23]

## Cannabis Becomes Marijuana

Cannabis has been many things from the most important agricultural crop in the world to a vilified drug. "To the agriculturalist, cannabis is a fiber crop; to the physician, it is an enigma; to the user, a euphoriant; to the police, a menace; to the trafficker, a source of profitable danger; to the convict or parolee and his family, a source of sorrow." [24] Use of cannabis in the Americas for other than hemp production may have existed as early as the 16th or 17th century. It is reported that slaves taken from Africa to work on sugar plantations in Brazil in the 16th century brought cannabis with them. They were allowed to plant it between the rows of cane. They would allegedly smoke it between harvests. [25] Over the centuries, the use of cannabis made its way up South America across Central America to Mexico. By the mid-19th century, its use in Mexico, particularly amongst the poor, was popular. While written of in popular media, it was rarely discussed in upper-class media. [26]

Exactly where the term marijuana itself came from is open to debate. Some say it came from the Mexican word for "Mary Jane". Others point to the Portuguese word for intoxication, "marihuango" [27] or the Mexican "mariguana", which also means intoxication. [28]

## The Mexican Revolution

Political upheaval in Mexico was the primary reason marijuana entered the United States over its southern border.

Following their 16th-century invasion and takeover of what became Mexico, the Spanish introduced an agricultural structure adapted from their feudal heritage. Called the *hacienda* system, it made virtual slaves of the workers, the peons. Peons were not allowed to own land. They worked the land for the owners much like medieval serfs. By the end of the 19th century, in an agricultural country of 10,000,000 people, only 500,000 owned more than one acre. [29]

The the excessive concentration of wealth and the suppression of civil liberties during the years of the Porfirio Diaz dictatorship (1876-1910), known as the *Porfiriato*, [30] polarized Mexican society and eventually led to bitter and destructive factional wars, which began in 1910 and lasted a decade. Collectively known as the Mexican Revolution, these wars came about due to the unequal distribution of land in Mexico and the despotic rule of Diaz.

Francisco "Pancho" Villa was one of the heroes of the Mexican Revolution. He was born a peon. At age 15, he became an outlaw when he fled for his life after killing a landowner who had raped his sister. Over time, he developed a veritable army and he and his followers developed a political agenda. His

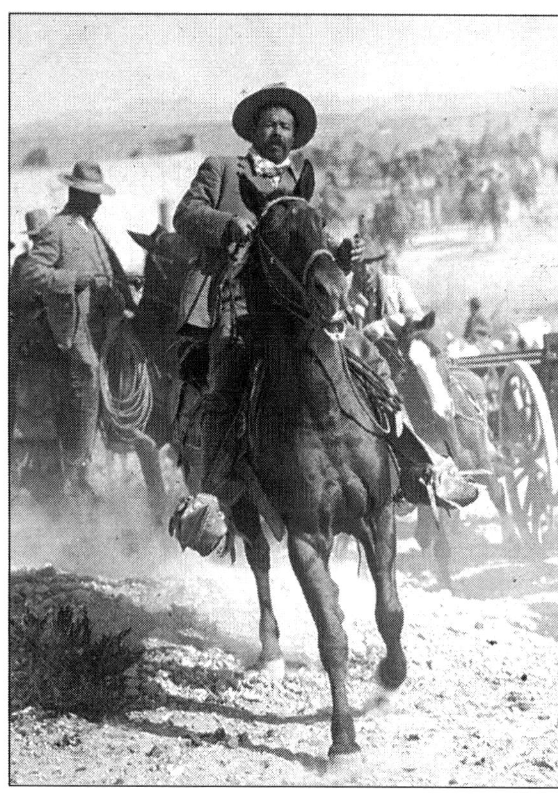

*The 1910-20 Mexican Revolution was lead in the north by Pancho Villa and his army (pictured). It generated an influx of hard-working, cheap laborers to the American West. While a boon to large ranchers, they made it making a living more difficult for small farmers. A major U. S. recession in 1913 helped fuel anti-Mexican sentiment and was followed by several U.S. states passing laws against marijuana.*

supporters wanted land reform and opposed exploitation by large land owners.

Another recruiting technique was that Villa and his men would ride into a town, attack the jail and release the prisoners from captivity. Being mostly peons, many of them would join his army. [31] He became a sort of Robin Hood in the eyes of the peon class, stealing from the rich and giving at least some of what he stole to the poor. [32] He soon assembled an army that fought both for Villa and the Revolution.

In 1913, Villa seized 1,250 square miles of the Mexican State of Sonora that William Randolph Hearst had bought for pennies an acre. [33] This land seizure probably didn't make Hearst feel particularly kindly toward Mexicans. Hearst, who is often characterized as a racist, had already shown a strong anti-Hispanic bias as evidenced by his papers' role in slanting the news about Spanish "atrocities" in Cuba to whip up enthusiasm for the Spanish-American War of 1898. [34] For the next several decades, Hearst was only too happy to have his newspapers portray marijuana as making Mexicans lazy and vicious, causing Negro men to be sexually promiscuous and leading these "hophead" black men to rape white women. [35]

Villa's followers were drawn from the poor and enjoyed marijuana. Their unofficial anthem and marching song was *La Cucaracha*. The original lyrics speak of a marijuana-smoking cockroach (hence the origin of "roach" as slang for a marijuana cigarette):

> *"La cucaracha ya no puede caminar,*
> *porque no tiene marihuana por fumar"*

This translates (roughly) as – "The cockroach can't walk anymore, because he doesn't have any marihuana to smoke." [36]

The revolution in Mexico continued after Diaz was deposed. It spilled over the border and General Pershing's army clashed with Poncho Villa. General Pershing and his men chased Villa around the Southwest. They marched to the tune, "that reflected America's attitude toward all Mexicans." [37]

> *"It's a long way to capture Villa.*
> *It's a long way to go;*
> *It's a long way across the border;*
> *Where the dirty greasers grow".*
> Sung to the tune of *It's a Long Way to Tipperary.* [38]

## The Invasion of Marijuana

The revolution in Mexico drove tens of thousands of Mexicans north into the United States looking for safety and work. While Mexico had a long historical presence from Texas to California in what is now the United States, marijuana was not much in evidence prior to this time. This is possibly because cannabis was used mostly by poor Mexicans, and the upper and middle-classes looked down on it. A greater proportion of the Mexicans that fled to the United States during and after these turbulent times were poor Mexican workers. They brought not only the word "marijuana" with them, a term heretofore practically unheard of in the United States, but their recreational and medicinal use of the herb as well.

At first jobs in agriculture and industry were plentiful and Mexicans were willing to work cheaply. However, the numbers of Mexican immigrants in the Southwest increased and jobs became scarce during the 1913-14 recession. Problems kicked up. Small farmers and ranchers resented the big ranchers that hired large numbers of Mexican laborers to work cheaply. Cheap Mexican labor gave the large ranchers further economic advantage.

During this time, a number of Southwestern states passed economically and racially motivated anti-marijuana laws. Because cannabis was widely used among Mexican workers, enforcing these anti-marijuana laws was a way to force the cheap Mexican labor back across the border. Because most Mexicans were Catholic, this made it even more tempting to pass such laws. Able states that "Protestant America considered Catholicism a religion of dark superstition and ignorance." [39]

As Mexican laborers in the West migrated farther north in increasing numbers, some of the laborers they met in the Mississippi Valley, largely Black field and factory workers, became familiar with marijuana.

As early as 1915, Hispanics were routinely vilified regarding the effects of cannabis. These were not only competitors for scarce jobs during a recession, but were Catholic and spoke Spanish. Thus they became grist for the drug "demonization" propaganda machine. It was widely reported in magazines and the press that marijuana drove Mexicans to rape white women or to go into a murderous rage. [40]

## Marijuana Also Entered the United States via New Orleans

Marijuana entered U.S. culture through both the Far West and the port of New Orleans. Hashish may have preceded the smoking of the less potent cannabis to the United States. The Centennial Exposition of 1876 in Philadelphia featured the Turkish Hashish Exposition Pavilion. A vistor could lounge at the Turkish Pavilion, use a little Turkish hashish and relax from walking the fair. It must have been a popular attraction, judging by the fact that by the 1880s every major city in the United States had hashish smoking parlors. New York alone had over 500. [41]

Smoking marijuana for recreation may have been introduced into the port of New Orleans as early as the late 1890s. Other sources suggest that 1909 was the date cannabis was first smoked in New Orleans. Whatever the date, it was likely introduced there from the Caribbean. It's known that Hindu indentured servants were brought from India to Jamaica by the British in the 1870s, to organize the cultivation of sugar cane and hemp fields. They very likely brought cannabis with them from India, smoked the flowering tops of cannabis and taught the African field workers in Jamaica about the female hemp plant's flowers. Herer states that by 1886, Black and Mexican sailors manning Caribbean sailing vessels picked up the use of cannabis and its use soon spread throughout the region. [42] Whether cannabis was used in the United States by Black slaves prior to this era is debatable.

## Jazz

Cannabis and the earliest days of jazz music are closely linked. Marijuana was popular in Storyville, New Orleans' red-light district. Storyville derived its nickname from city councilman Story, who, in 1897, introduced a law to limit prostitution to one section of town. As a consequence, this part of town carried his name. Entertainment in the bordellos of Storyville was often provided by marijuana-smoking pianists who played "ragtime". With the addition of other instruments, primarily horns, ragtime morphed into jazz in the first decade of the 20th century.

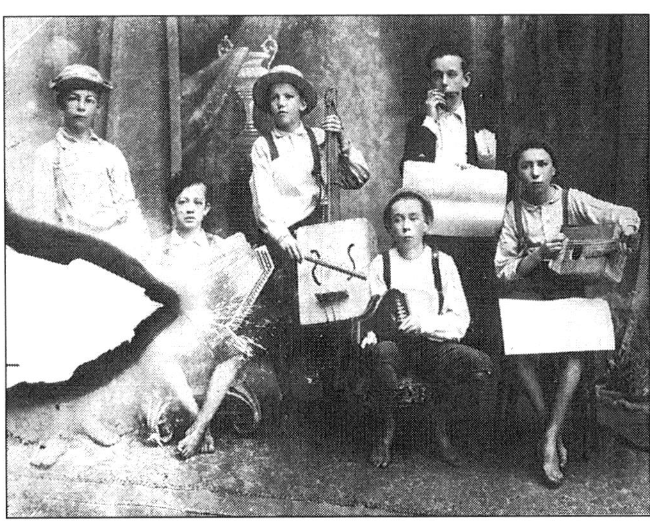

*This partially restored 1897 photograph is purportedly of the "Razzy Dazzy Spasm Band", a group of street urchins many credit with being the first "jazz" band.*

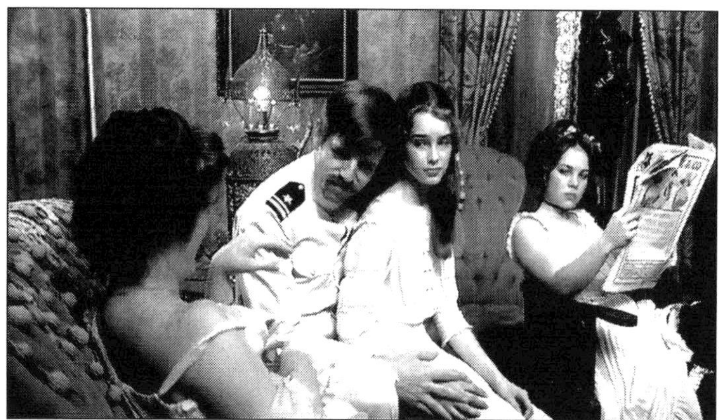

*The popular story is that jazz started in the brothels of the Storyville section of New Orleans in the early 20th century. This is a scene from a 1978 movie about a Storyville brothel.*

New Orleans was a city that took its music and dancing seriously. Storyville was the largest employer of Black musicians outside of Broadway. [43] However, ragtime and jazz were not just played in bordellos but all through the New Orleans underworld. While pianists were predominant in the bordellos, jazz bands played for social clubs, fraternities, funerals, picnics, fairs, civic celebrations, parades, and the like. [44]

Many sources credit a group of street urchins, who billed themselves as the "Razzy Dazzy Spasm Band", with being the true father of jazz. They may deserve the credit for being the first jazz band but the music was incubated and grew in the Storyville houses of ill-repute.

Ernest Abel put it this way: "It was in these bordellos, where music provided the background and not the primary focus of attention, that marihuana became an integral part of the jazz era. Unlike booze, which dulled and incapacitated, marihuana enabled musicians whose job required them to play long into the night to forget their exhaustion. Moreover, the drug seemed to make their music sound more imaginative and unique, at least to those who played and listened while under its sensual influence." [45]

Many of America's blues and jazz icons emerged from this colorful cross-cultural pollination. Harry Anslinger, the racist, first director of the Federal Bureau of Narcotics, derogatorily characterized jazz, this uniquely American creation, as a "cross-cultural contamination."

Whites in New Orleans were concerned that these gage-smoking (gage was a slang term in the Negro community for marijuana) Black musicians were spreading a very "popular new voodoo music that forced even decent white women to tap their feet. They believed that this alien music was ultimately aimed at throwing off the yoke of the whites. That music was jazz!" [46] Southern officials became alarmed because marijuana-smoking "darkie jazz musicians" were beginning to "think that they are as good as whites." By 1917, the White establishment had shuttered Storyville.

During the war years (1914-1920), Black musicians and jazz moved up the Mississippi, and as it did, many cities along the Mississippi passed laws against marijuana.

## You are Not Going to Believe This about Black Face

In many locales the Jim Crow segregation laws prohibited Black entertainers from performing in white clubs. But it turns out these Black performers were very talented, and brought in customers. In a very strange twist, some White club owners "cleverly" circumvented the racist law of the day by requiring Black performers to wear "black face". In order for a Black entertainer to be paid to perform in a White club, he/she had to be willing to pretend to be a white person pre tending to be Black. [47,48] A bizarre charade indeed. When Blacks objected to this insanity, why they were accused by Whites of being "no-good marijuana-smoking niggers." [49]

Vaudeville helped perpetuate pejorative stereotypes of all kinds; such as rural Whites as a "rube" and Jews as a "Heeb". The Black faced performers

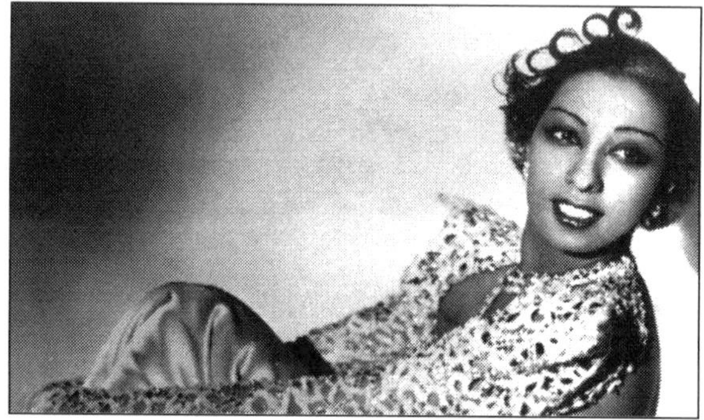

*Josephine Baker was a U.S. expatriate entertainer who wowed them in Paris. She became even more famous by adopting 12 children of different ethnicities.*

were used to portray the stereotype of the "shiftless nigger" as well as Jim Crow. The concept was so absurd that in vaudeville on occasion, some Negroes used black make-up not to be in black face but in order to look black enough. [50] Even the great Josephine Baker performed in black face. [51] Baker led an incredible life. Baker was a Black American who found great success as a singer, dancer and entertainer in France.

Her singing, dancing and comedy were only a small part of her achievements. During World War II, she helped the Red Cross and the French Resistance. After the war, she started adopting children, eventually twelve in all of diverse ethnic and national backgrounds. This was her "Rainbow Tribe." She lived with them in her chateau at Les Milandes. Because of being overly optimistic about her finances, she lost the chateau (she and her children were rescued by, among others, Princess Grace of Monaco).

When Baker toured the United States, she forced theater owners to desegregate when she performed. She did not always prevail. Her life exposed some of the absurd and disgusting aspects of racism. The Stork Club, a tony New York nightclub of the time, did not admit Blacks. But in a famous incident in 1951, Baker "arranged an admission, only to be ignored by the waiters." Walter Winchell, a well-known celebrity gossip columnist, was present. Baker called upon him to report the incident. Instead of issuing a humane, sympathetic assessment, he attacked her on his radio program and wrote to long-time FBI Director J. Edgar Hoover requesting an FBI investigation of Baker's political activities. Hoover obliged. [52]

## The Blues

The Blues are the musical foundation of jazz. Since the Middle Ages, "The word 'blues' has been associated with the idea of melancholia or depression. " [53] The American writer, Washington Irving is credited with coining the term 'the blues' as it is now defined, in 1807. [54]

What eventually became the blues was a merging of the different types of songs sung by slaves. These include the field "holler", spirituals and prison work songs. Some of these songs were filled with lyrics describing their heartache, extreme suffering and privation. [55]

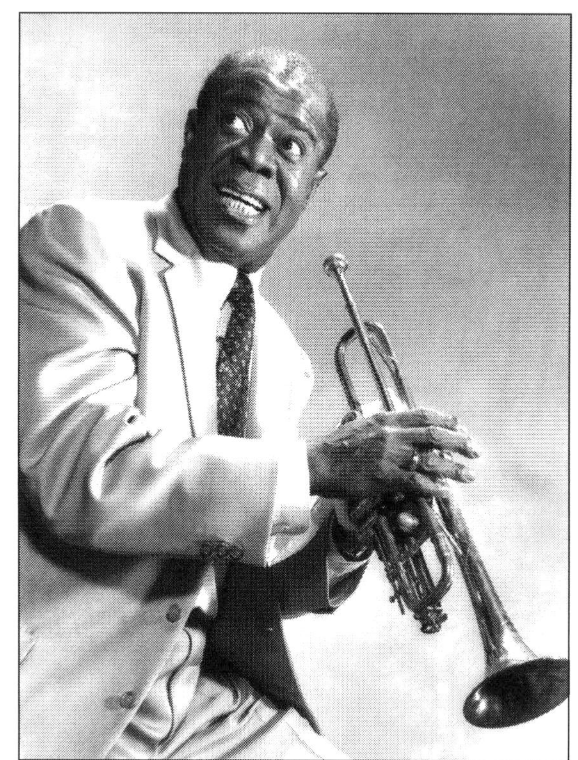

*The great jazz trumpeter, singer and entertainer Louis Armstrong (1900-71) was born in New Orleans. From the age of 25 on, he was a daily marijuana user. He said, "It makes you feel good, man. It relaxes you, makes you forget all about the bad things that happen to a Negro. It makes you feel wanted and when you're with another tea smoker it makes you feel a special sense of kinship."* [56]

The field "holler" was used by slaves as they worked in the pre-Civil War South. The field "holler" was not sung. It was yelled to the beat of the work being done. The field "holler", the spiritual, and the blues, are "notable among all human works of art for their profound despair ... They gave voice to the mood of alienation and anomie that prevailed in the construction camps of the South." [57]

The Southern prisons were another source for the Black music tradition. Prison work songs, songs of death row and murder, prostitutes, the warden, the hot sun, and a hundred other privations were fodder for the blues. [58] Many bluesmen found their songs among the prison road crews and work gangs, and many Blacks became familiar with the same songs. [59]

## Absinthe: Prohibition Practice?

Prohibition was a long time in coming. While the United States adopted the most rigid prohibition stance, it was not by any means an aberration in the world. Almost a decade before the 18th Amendment and the Volsted Act created Prohibition, we had what could be seen as a trial run for alcohol prohibition with the advent of absinthe prohibition in both Europe and the United States.

## Save the Poets from the "Green Fairy"

Absinthe, an alcoholic beverage named after its most exotic ingredient, artemsia absinthe, is usually 70-80% alcohol (140-160 proof). Absinthe was popular amongst bohemian types. Starting in the 1870s, efforts were made to cast absinthe as a demonic drink. It was finally prohibited a decade or so before Prohibition. The prohibition of absinthe in Europe and the United States contributed to the momentum for the later prohibition of alcohol.

The absinthe story illustrates that economic power, social privilege and discrimination influencing drug laws has not been confined to the United States.

Absinthe, known as "La Fee Verte" or "The Green Fairy", has been around since ancient times. Hippocrates recommended absinthe soaked in wine for jaundice and rheumatism. Artemisia absinthium (aka as wormwood) is a bitter herb. It was used for centuries as a vermifuge and digestive aid. It wasn't until 1797 that Henri-Louis Pernod opened his first Absinthe distilleries. He produced absinthe in Switzerland and in France. Its popularity in France increased in the 1840s after French soldiers, fighting in Algiers, drank absinthe to prevent malaria and other ills.

Absinthe, sometimes called "the LSD of the last half of the 19th century", is a bitter, emerald green, high-alcohol liqueur. It contains several herbs including anise (often partially substituted with star anise), Florence fennel, hyssop, Melissa, and wormwood (artemesia absinthe). Various recipes also include angelica root, sweet flag, dittany leaves, coriander, veronica, juniper, nutmeg, and miscellaneous mountain herbs. [60]

Most importantly for absinthe, it contains wormwood oil's active ingredient, Alpha-Thujon. It comes from the flowers and leaves of the medicinal plant *Artemisia absinthium*, also called wormwood. Alpha thujone is also found in the

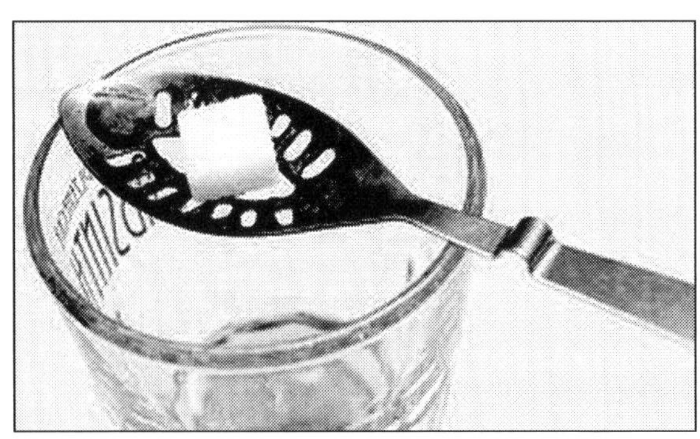

*Ceremony is an important part of both religion and drug taking. The absinthe serving ceremony involves both a special spoon with perforations and a special glass that the spoon fits over. The glass holds the absinthe liquid. A sugar cube is placed on the spoon above it. Water is dribbled (up to four parts water to one part absinthe) over the sugar, which slowly melts into the absinthe liquid below, causing a dreamy, milky appearance in the liquid.*

essential oils of the culinary herbs sage, tansy, and tarragon. Vermouth, Chartreuse and Benedictine all have small amounts of thujone in them. Vermouth made using wormwood flowers gets its name from the German "wermuth" ("wormwood").

Absinthe's alcohol content is extremely high – supposedly ranging from 45%-85% (90-170 proof) — although there is no historical evidence that any commercial vintage of absinthe was higher than 74 percent. The "buzz" is described as different from that derived from a "normal" alcoholic beverage. The absinthe drinker feels clearer and less impaired. The active ingredient, thujone, is excitatory on the brain and in small quantities has antidepressant effects.

Absinthe became popular in France in the last quarter of the 19th century. Its popularity was aided by a decades-long phylloxera blight in the French vineyards that made wine not only expensive, but scarce. In those days, wine was drunk instead of or mixed with water, as water was loaded with enough bacteria to make people sick. Dr. John Snow was just getting around to stopping a cholera epidemic in England by taking the handle off the town pump in 1862. So either wine or absinthe were often mixed with water to "purify" the water.

## Bohemian Favorite

Absinthe is said to have aphrodisiac and hallucinogenic properties. For years it was enthusiastically consumed by various thinkers, poets, writers, composers and more. During the late 1800s, the "Green Fairy" was being consumed with such glee by the Parisians that the cocktail hour "Happy Hour" was called "L'Heure Verte" (The Green Hour).

Absinthe was the muse for many artistic efforts. Oscar Wilde, Pablo Picasso, Arthur Rimbaud, Paul Verlaine, and Charles Baudelaire were all among the hedonistic, bohemian in-crowd that favored absinthe. [61] Henri de Toulouse-Lautrec, DeMoset, Edgar Degas, Emile Zola, Paul Gaugin, Victor Hebert, and Édouard Manet were all famous absinthe drinkers.

In 1859, Manet painted the *Absinthe Drinker*. He presumably had met Baudelaire over a glass of absinthe. In 1876, Degas painted his famous *Absinthe*, but it was so rudely received that he put it into storage until 1992. Picasso painted two famous pieces – the *Absinthe Drinker*, and *Woman Drinking Absinthe*. Ernest Hemingway's semi-auto-biographical character Jake observed in *The Sun Also Rises* that "absinthe made everything seem better."

But absinthe was not restricted to Europe. In the 1870s, it came to the United States. First to New Orleans, then to the bohemian/artist set in New York, Chicago and San Francisco. It attracted literary fans such as Walt Whitman, O. Henry and the aforementioned Hemingway. [62] (In modern days, actor Johnny Depp, rapper Eminem and rocker Marilyn Manson are said to enjoy the taste of absinthe.)

In its heyday, absinthe was often deliberately chosen as a prop by second- and third-rate wannabes aping the habits of these well-known nonconformists and successful artists. By indulging in absinthe, they tried to look the part of the cutting-edge artist.

With this sort of pedigree, absinthe was bound to attract the attention of the American prohibitionists. As a result, absinthe was a symbol as well as an intoxicant.

## Is There Such a Thing as Absinthism?

A condition called "absinthism" was described emerging alongside descriptions of alcoholism. Absinthism was said to be associated with gastrointestinal problems, acute auditory and visual hallucinations, epilepsy, brain damage, and increased risk of psychiatric illness and suicide. But the web page *Absinth.bz* states that absinth "does not make you hallucinate or kill your entire family." [63] Today, whether any of these symptoms are related to drinking good quality absinthe in moderate quantities is an open question.

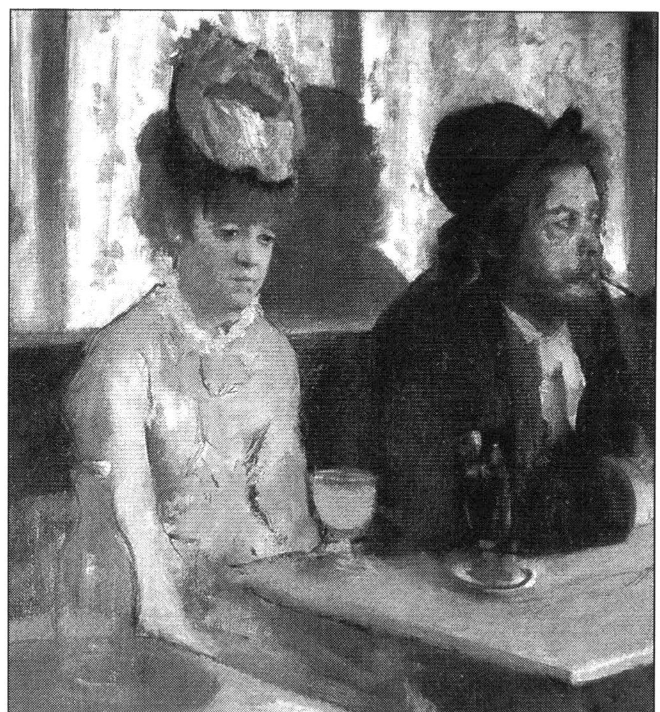

*"The Absinthe Drinker" is an 1876 painting by Edgar Degas (1834-1917). The lady appears to have drunk too much absinthe or the absinthe she drank contained too much wormwood.*

## Be Careful of the Thujone

Undistilled wormwood essential oil contains a substance called thujone, which in extremely high doses is an epileptiform and can cause renal failure. Thujone is often fingered as the major toxic and hallucinogenic ingredient in absinthe but this is very much in dispute. The supposed ill effects of the drink were blamed on that substance in 19th century so-called "studies."

More recent studies have shown that very little of the thujone present in wormwood essential oil actually makes it into a properly distilled bottle of absinthe. While thujone has some apparent psychoactivity, the principle basis for intoxication from absinthe comes from it being 75% alcohol. B. Max, in the "This and That" column in Trends in the Pharmacological Sciences, "The literature on the pharmacology of thujone is, to put it bluntly, second rate, and conclusions as to its effects have been extrapolated far beyond the experimental base." [64]

In some second rate absinthe knock-offs, the thujone content was at least seven or eight times but possibly 40 times what is allowed in today's absinthe drinks; 350 ppm in old absinthe compared to eight to nine ppm today. [65] The livers of 19th-century absinthe drinkers could easily have experienced concentrations of thujone of 20-200 umol/l. This might have presented a problem for drinkers, particularly those with a compromised liver or hematopoetic function.

In 1878, over seven million liters of absinthe were imported into the puritanical United States! But a combination of forces led to the outlawing of absinthe. Some have even likened the exaggeration of the adverse effects of absinthe to the hysteria directed at LSD in the 1960s. Here was another drug favored by the creative, the eccentric and the social critics. Mathew John Bagott cites the bigger underlying issue of change, "In retrospect absinth seems to have become the focus of fears about the changes that came with industrialization." [66]

## Prohibition of Absinthe

Heavy drinking in France became a concern in the 1850s. Absinthe was the most popular liquor in France and it was 70-80% alcohol. Wine was considered a healthful drink, so absinthe became the target for prohibitionists in France. But even more importantly, absinthe was also tied to the Bohemian lifestyle and the wine growers were much better connected politically than the absinthe distillers. [67]

The prohibition of absinthe really took off in 1905. In 1905, Jean Lanfray, a Swiss peasant of French stock, having drunk two glasses of absinthe, shot his pregnant wife and two children and attempted to kill himself. He failed, and was found the next morning collapsed across their dead bodies. He had murdered his entire family.

The man had been drinking brandy, beer and other alcoholic beverages all during the fatal day. The public focused on just one detail – the two glasses of absinthe he had drunk beforehand. Absinthe was pinned with the responsibility. People were in no doubt. It must have been the absinthe that did it.

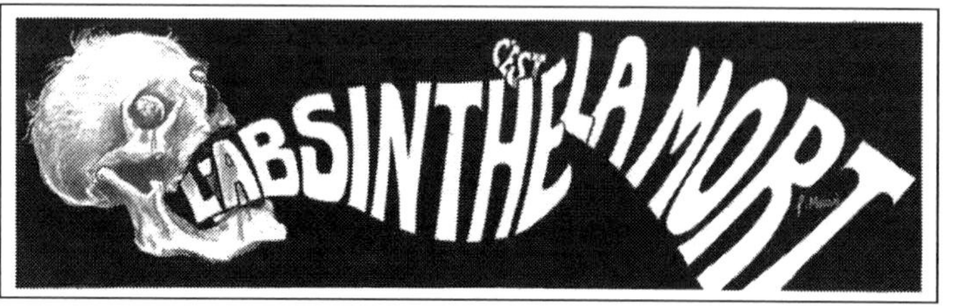


His well-publicized trial was called "The Absinthe Murders". Forgotten in the media circus was that Lanfray had a history as an extremely heavy drinker; an "alcoholic" is what he'd be called today. He habitually drank up to five liters of wine a day. Forgotten also, was that on the day of the murders, while he had indeed consumed the two absinthes before going to work – hours before the tragedy - he had also downed a crème de menthe, a couple glasses of wine to help his lunch go down, another glass of wine before leaving work, a cup of coffee with brandy in it and an aperitif on getting home, and then another coffee with marc in it. [68] In a few weeks, a petition demanding that absinthe be banned in Switzerland was signed by over 82,000 local people.

Outlawing absinthe and not wine, fit well with the relative political power of absinthe producers versus the vinticulturalists. Some of the major absinthe producers were financially powerful, but they lacked political influence in the French Chamber of Deputies where large hereditary landowners – often grape-growers – were disproportionately well represented. Worse, the owners of the biggest producer, Pernod Fils, were of Jewish origin (Arthur and Edmond Vielle-Picard, who purchased an interest in the company in 1894, were half-Jewish). Only a year earlier, the Dreyfus Affair had exposed the high level of anti-Semitism in France. The wine makers effectively targeted absinthe as a social menace. [69]

The prohibition of the high-alcohol-content absinthe offered the Prohibitionists a little practice. Absinthe was banned in Belgium in 1905. In 1908, it was officially outlawed in Switzerland. On July 25, 1912, the U.S. Department of Agriculture issued Food Inspection, banning absinthe in America. [70]

The French held out until 1915. In fact, in 1910, the French made 36 million liters of Absinthe for domestic consumption. [71] That is equal to the amount of French Champagne imported to the United States during the year 1986.

With modern science and 20/20 hindsight, the concern about absinthe appears to be based more on innuendo than facts.

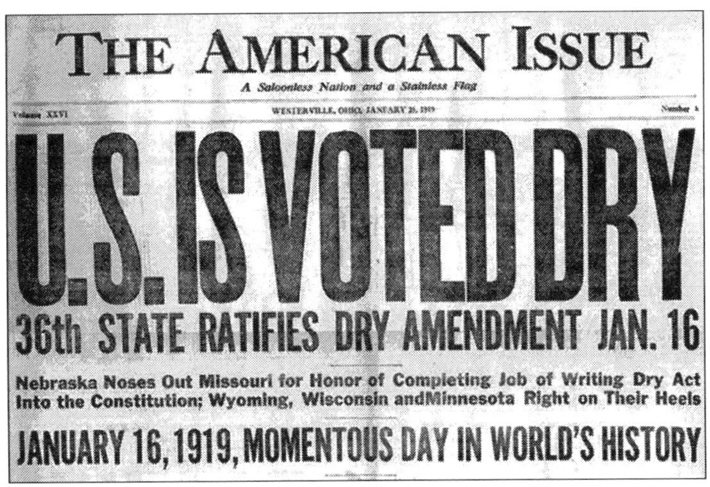

THE AMERICAN ISSUE

*A Saloonless Nation and a Stainless Flag*

Volume XXVI — WESTERVILLE, OHIO, JANUARY 25, 1919 — Number

# U.S. IS VOTED DRY

## 36th STATE RATIFIES DRY AMENDMENT JAN. 16

**Nebraska Noses Out Missouri for Honor of Completing Job of Writing Dry Act Into the Constitution; Wyoming, Wisconsin andMinnesota Right on Their Heels**

## JANUARY 16, 1919, MOMENTOUS DAY IN WORLD'S HISTORY

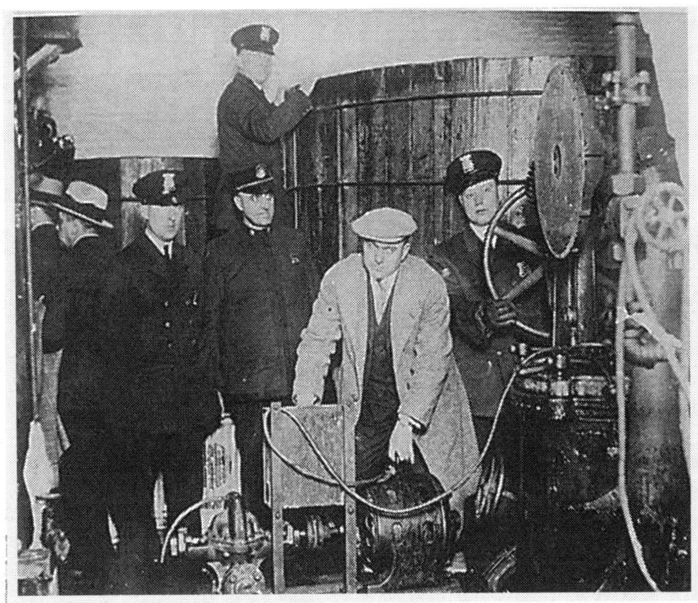

# CHAPTER X
# The Roaring Twenties and Prohibition

## Prohibition: A Moral Issue?

Prohibitionists believed users of drugs were "out of control", as if possessed by a demon. Prohibitionists saw recreational use of a "bad drug" as impossible. The Prohibitionists' goals of family integrity, decreasing both poverty and domestic violence were laudable.[1] But it turned out that Prohibition was the wrong vehicle to accomplish these ends. Prohibition was done in, not only by the "Law of Unintended Negative Consequences", but also by some very predictable negative consequences.

The real difficulties associated with Prohibition were compounded by the unstated but very transparent goal of Prohibition, which was to marginalize and punish "them," the users of the prohibited drug(s): the immigrants, the greenhorns, the nonbelievers, the infidels, the competitors for "our" jobs and "our" women.

Alcohol prohibition is a classic case of the cure being worse than the disease. It had two fundamental premises: 1) alcohol use was the primary causes of society's problems including sexual promiscuity, violence, family dissolution, labor and racial unrest, insanity, illness, child abuse, atheism, addiction, and might lead to the imminent downfall of

## Richard P. Hobson

Richard P. Hobson (1870-1937), was a naval officer who came back a hero from the Spanish-American War and later became a congressman from Alabama. He is the very embodiment of early 20th-century demagoguery. In the 1920s, after serving in Congress for several terms, he founded the International Narcotics Education Association. His concern was the alleged adverse affect of drug-using immigrants on society. Hobson framed what he perceived as an American drug problem as being a threat from immoral minority cultures within the United States and hostile nations outside the United States. So what else is new?

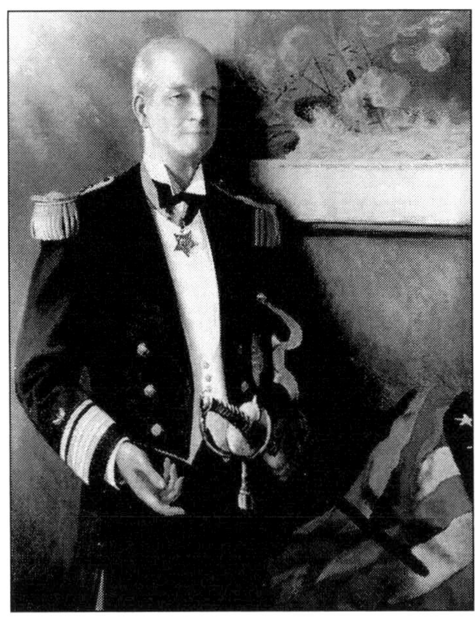

*Richard P. Hobson received a Medal of Honor as a U.S. Navel Officer in the Spanish-American War. Later elected to Congress, he was a favorite speaker for the Ku Klux Klan, who made the "Tea Baggers" of 2010 look like "pikers".*

### Save the Race

Hobson spoke out with propaganda of the worst kind in favor of the type of drug policies we have today – discrimination of "them" based on "demonization" of "them" and their drugs, combined with Draconian penalties. He believed that to save "the race" (Yes, I know, scientifically there is no such thing as race.) just about all inebriants needed to be eliminated from use.

He said, *"In America we are making the last stand of the great white race, and substantially of the human race. If this destroyer cannot be conquered in young America, it cannot in any of the old and more degenerate nations. If America fails, the world will be undone and the human race will be doomed to go down from degeneracy into degeneracy till the Almighty, in wrath, wipes the accused thing out!"* [2]

### Disinformation and Fear

Hobson, like his contemporary, Dr. Hamilton Wright, was a moralist with no compunction about spreading disinformation. For instance, even though official estimates were that there were roughly 100,000 opiate abusers in the 1920s, Hobson alleged there were millions. He said that heroin makes the user into "a desperado of the most vicious type" and that "one ounce of heroin can turn 2,000 people into addicts." [3]

He used fear, which he evoked with his colorful language, to motivate people. Hobson described heroin users as "the living dead". This metaphor conjures up the idea of retribution for a moral perversion and plants fear of the possible physical deterioration of the young body. He called drugs a "contagion"' and said drug users were "lepers among our people." This colorful language suggested substance abuse was as incurable as leprosy was at the time. He suggested drug "addiction" was "spreading like a moral and physical scourge." [4]

He gave a "clarion call" for all God-fearing people to step up to the plate and take on what he characterized as a great threat to the white race. *"We need to preach the gospel of narcotic abstinence from the pulpit, to flash it on the screen, to enact it on the stage, to proclaim it from the public platform, to depict it in the press, and, above all, to teach it in our schools. All constructive social agencies will help in fighting this peril – in setting up in the minds of all the same abhorrence that is felt for a venomous snake…"* [5]

civilization itself, and, 2) universal abstinence would greatly reduce these problems and was achievable through certain temperance remedies. [6]

## Language Frames the Issue

Language used to frame issues is often telling. The language of temperance and prohibition was moralistic and accusatory. Religion was very much a part of the Temperance story. Famed preacher and former baseball player Billy Sunday, who is referenced in that old standard *Chicago* ("Chicago, Chicago, the town that Billy Sunday could not shut down") and a fairly typical temperance leader said that "This [prohibition] is Christ's work … a holy war, and every true soldier of the Cross will be in it." [7] He mobilized the masses with his rhetoric by preaching that alcohol was:

> **...the great anaconda, which wraps its coils around home altars to cripple them, to make room for Bacchus. The vampire which fans sanity to sleep while it sucks away the lifeblood. The vulture, which preys upon the vials [sic] of the nations. It defies God, despises Jesus Christ, sins against the Holy Ghost, which is sinning against light and knowledge. Above all it murders inhumanely.** [8]

The tone and issues raised by alcohol prohibitionist Mary Hunt is typical of promoters of Prohibition. She wrote of her concern regarding "the enormous increase of immigrant population flooding us from the old world, men and women who have brought to our shores and into our politics old world habits and ideas (favorable to alcohol)" and her writing was replete with references to this "undesirable immigration" and "these immigrant hordes." [9]

The largely anti-foreign, anti-Catholic, anti-Black, anti-Irish, anti-German, anti-Semitic, and anti-urban nature of the Temperance movement has been extensively documented. In 1911, U.S. Rep. Richard Hobson of Alabama, who had strong Ku Klux Klan (KKK) support, introduced legislation that eventually became the 18th Amendment. [10] It should be no surprise that once Prohibition arrived, it was the Ku Klux Klan (KKK), that was the epitome of prohibitionist believers and the KKK strongly supported the strict enforcement of Prohibition. [11]

Hobson was popular with the Nativists and the KKK. He was the Anti-Saloon League's most popular and highest paid spokesperson. His bigoted assumptions and twisted, illogical arguments continue to be part and parcel of today's drug laws.

This is a sample of Hobson's thinking from a speech on Feb. 2, 1911 introducing legislation that eventually became the 18th Amendment, Prohibition:

> 'If a peaceable red man is subjected to the regular use of alcoholic beverage, he will speedily be put back to the plane of the savage. The Government long since recognized this and absolutely prohibits the introduction of alcoholic beverage into an Indian reservation. If a negro takes up a regular use of alcoholic beverage, in a short time he will degenerate to the level of the cannibal. No matter how high the stage of evolution, the result is the same.
>
> "In our great cities like New York, Chicago, and Philadelphia the ravages upon the average character have been so great, so many degenerates have already been produced, that the degenerate and corruptible vote not only holds the balance of power between the two great political parties and can dictate to both, but actually holds a majority of the votes, so that honest and efficient self-government as a permanent condition is now impossible. Immigrants coming in vast numbers from abroad remained chiefly in the cities. As young as our Nation is, the deadly work of alcohol has already blighted liberty in our greatest cities." [12]

And finally, the long Temperance/Prohibition crusade had become a juggernaut that could not be stopped. The last votes necessary to put the legislation over the top in Congress were generated by WWI anti-German sentiment. At the time,

German-Americans owned the vast majority of American breweries, and had for several decades. Politicians said that the grain that beer was brewed with could be better used feeding the troops. [13] The Anti- Saloon League called Milwaukee brewers "the worst of all our German enemies" and dubbed their beer "Kaiser brew." [14] So in 1917, the last few votes necessary for the 18th Amendment to the U.S. Constitution to pass the Senate were obtained.

The effects of marginalizing people of German extraction during WWI still lingered at least two generations later. Noted American humorist Garrison Keillor, creator, host and star of *A Prairie Home Companion* radio show and later a movie, was explaining how he developed his observational style of writing.

For a few years in the 1960s, Keiler was living in a small rural town near St. Cloud, Minnesota named Stearns. Here a preponderance of the inhabitants were of German heritage. As an outsider, someone who wasn't from Stearns, Keillor states that he wasn't able to have a real conversation with anyone in the town. He writes, "I didn't have long hair or a beard, didn't dress oddly or do wild things, and it troubled me. I felt like a criminal." So he would sit at the end of the bar in the town's informal gathering place and observe.

Keillor continued:

HUN RULE ASSOCIATION
WE MAKE PEOPLE POOR
WE CAUSE POVERTY AND CRIME
WE ARE AGAINST PROGRESS
WE ROB WOMEN AND CHILDREN
WE FILL PENITENTIARIES AND ASYLUMS
WE WASTE GRAIN
WASTE
RUIN
BOOZE
BOOZE
BOOZE

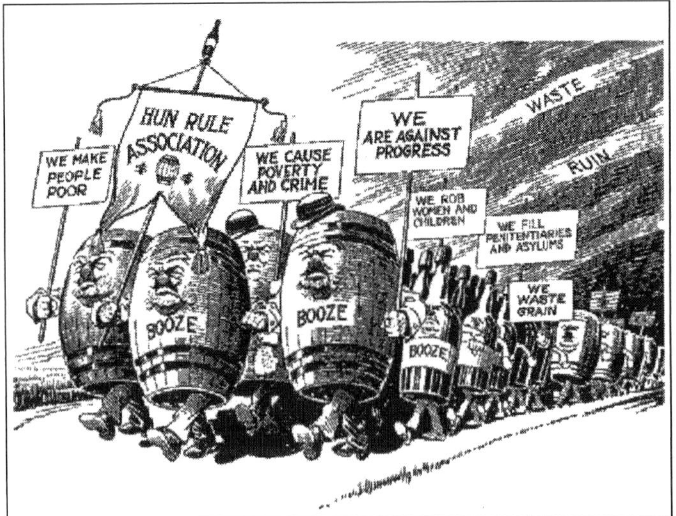

*Racism and discrimination have been a key ingredient to national drug policies. With Prohibition it was anti-German, anti-Irish and anti-immigrant propaganda.*

"This fear of outsiders was explained to me years later by a Stearns exile who said that the German population was so traumatized, first by the anti-Teutonic fevers of World War I that forbade the use of their language in schools, then by Prohibition that made outlaws of decent upstanding beer drinkers, that they never could trust auslanders again. A strange face is, to them, a cruel face. My German neighbors were a closed community, and I wasn't in it and had no part of it. Proximity does not bestow membership." [15]

## Prohibition Passes

In December 1917, after only 13 hours of debate, what was soon to become the 18th Amendment, overwhelmingly passed the U.S. Senate. [16] Shortly thereafter, the House passed the amendment after all of one day's debate. Approval by the states also occurred at warp speed. By January 1919, the requisite three-quarters of the states had made the 18th Amendment part of the Constitution. With the passage of the Volsted Act in 1920, the law was implemented.

## Demon Rum is Defeated?

From 1920 until 1933, except for medical purposes, the manufacture, sale and consumption of liquor was prohibited in America. Thus was born the Mafia. Alcohol prohibition provided the existing Italian and Jewish underworld the financial muscle to expand their criminal enterprise. This is parallel to today's Bloods & Crips fueling their criminal engine with funds made trafficking in today's illicit drugs.

Only 13 months after the 1917 Congressional vote, America had instituted what was inarguably our worst Constitutional Amendment. When alcohol Prohibition was approved, the Prohibitionists were jubilant and extremely optimistic about America's moral future. The 18th Amendment was going to purify America. Authors Aaron and Musto note that because prohibition supporters truly believed that alcohol was responsible for most crime, some towns even sold their jails. [17] They were in for a rude disappointment.

## Be Careful What You Wish For; You Just Might Get It.

Many Prohibition supporters assumed that prohibition would not be a strict, complete and absolute prohibition and that they would still have access to alcohol. These less radical supporters thought that this federal prohibition would look like some state prohibition laws which really were temperance acts and NOT prohibition. The moderate drinkers did not anticipate that prohibition would apply to them. They thought it was to control the "others", not "them".

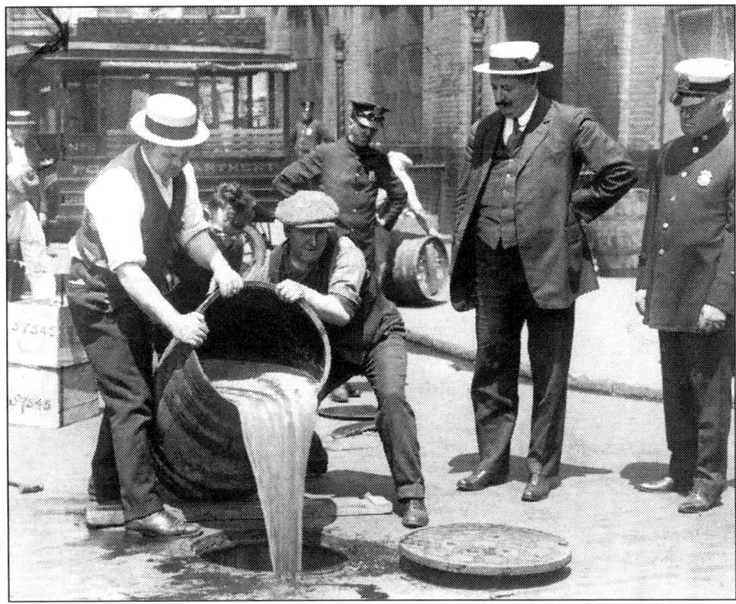

*A typical picture of "revenuers" at work destroying alcohol. It was illegal to make or sell alcohol but legal to possess it.*

## But Things Were Not "Jake"

Alcohol, however, remained available during Prohibition, particularly for the wealthy and the risk-takers. People still got drunk, still became alcoholics, still suffered delirium tremens. Drunken drivers remained a frequent menace on the highways ... The courts, jails, hospitals, and mental hospitals were still filled with drunks. [18]

---

**"Good intentions will always be pleaded for every assumption of authority. It is hardly too strong to say that the Constitution was made to guard the people against the dangers of good intentions. There are men in all ages who mean to govern well, but they mean to govern. They promise to be good masters, but they mean to be masters."** [19]

**Daniel Webster**

American statesman and senator from Massachusetts during the period leading up to the Civil War.

---

Some people drank booze smuggled in from Canada, others drank quality home brewed and distilled beverages. Many however drank "rotgut". It might be ethyl alcohol or it might not and it could be adulterated. Some folks foolishly drank methyl alcohol (rubbing alcohol) because ethyl alcohol either wasn't available or cost too much. This led to blindness and death.

"Ginger jake", a slang name for Jamaican Ginger – an alcohol extract of ginger — was an adulterant found in many bootleg beverages. It turned out that the ginger taste was pretty strong and was often itself adulterated, substituting ingredients such as molasses, glycerin, and castor oil for most of the oleoresin of ginger. This reduced the strong unpleasant ginger taste.

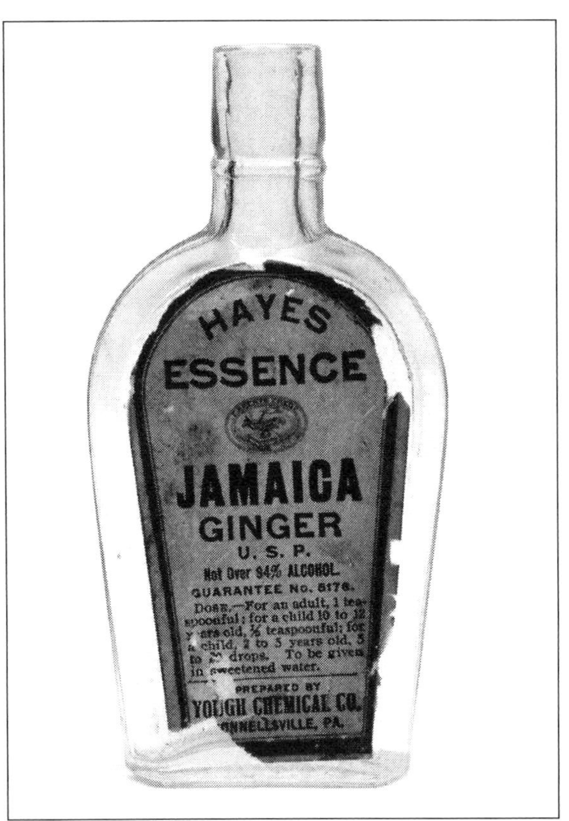


*Jamaican Ginger (Jake) couldn't kill you but some of the adulterants used to hide the ginger taste could.*

Using the wrong adulterant led to an epidemic of paralysis and death in 1930. [20] Sadly, that ginger jake was adulterated with creosol. So everything was not "jake." "Quality control" is one of the first casualties of substituting responsible government regulation with drug prohibition.

The disreputable saloon was replaced by the even less savory "speakeasy". Alcohol consumption soon switched from low-alcohol content wines and beers to distilled liquor. The consumer got more alcohol in a smaller volume, so it was less hazardous to manufacture, transport, and sell than beer or wine. Hard liquor soon became the preferred drink in speakeasies and at private parties. Respectable young women, who rarely got drunk in public before 1920, could now be seen staggering out of speakeasies, usually with their male escorts, and reeling down the streets. There were legal closing hours for saloons; the speakeasies or nightclubs, which were illegal, stayed open all hours of the day and night. [21]

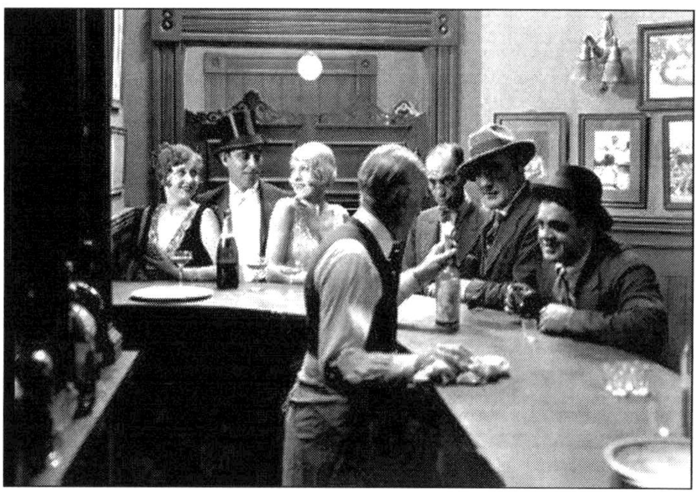

*When alcohol is taxed and regulated, saloons must serve real liquor and during specificied hours. When liquor is outlawed, there is no closing time and consumers may not get real booze.*

## Money, Money, Money: the Root of All Evil

Alcohol prohibition spawned a huge "black market" for the smuggling and sale of illegal alcohol. After all, alcohol was then, and still is, the world's most popular drug. Bootlegging was profitable and dangerous. As a prohibited item, ethyl alcohol sold at extremely high prices. There was stiff competition for this business among more than a few unsavory characters.

A lot of booze came in from off-shore in speed boats. Much of it came across the Great Lakes from Canada. One well-known speedboat bootlegger with a reputation for smuggling high quality alcoholic beverages was Bill McCoy – the original "real McCoy." [22] "Whoopee, this hooch is the real McCoy."

During Prohibition, criminals fought with each other over the territory where each bootlegger could sell illegal alcohol. This clash over territory is common with prohibited drugs. It is one of the factors accounting for the present-day high murder rate in the United States, as well as the virtual slaughter going on in Mexico, as modern day "cartels" fight over the money to be made from transporting and selling prohibited substances. The murder rate in the United States, for example, is three- to four-times that of the more drug policy permissive Netherlands. [23] It seems clear that, if more illicit drugs were taxed and regulated, we could put an end to wanton killing of innocent victims in Mexico and other places.

If America made illicit drugs legal tomorrow, it would cut off an enormous source of financial resources for gangs. These monetary resources not only support the buying of high-powered guns, but the profit to be made from prohibited drugs and protecting the source of those funds is one of the principle reasons these weapons are purchased and used. On this score, little has changed since the Prohibition of alcohol.

Illicit drugs provide the CIA with substantial off-the-books revenue. This money has funded revolution in Columbia and created unrest in Afghanistan. Making some substances illicit, and, therefore, a valuable commodity, has caused at least as much societal destabilization in the contemporary world as Prohibition did in the United States during the Roaring Twenties. While terrorism will not disappear by instituting a change in international drug policy, terrorists would have to find another source of easy, ready cash.

Disrespect and open defiance of the law were widespread during Prohibition. A week after the 18th Amendment became law, one could legally purchase small portable stills throughout the country. Also, Aaron & Musto described grape juice sold as

**Figure 10.1: U.S. Alcohol Consumption, 1910-29**

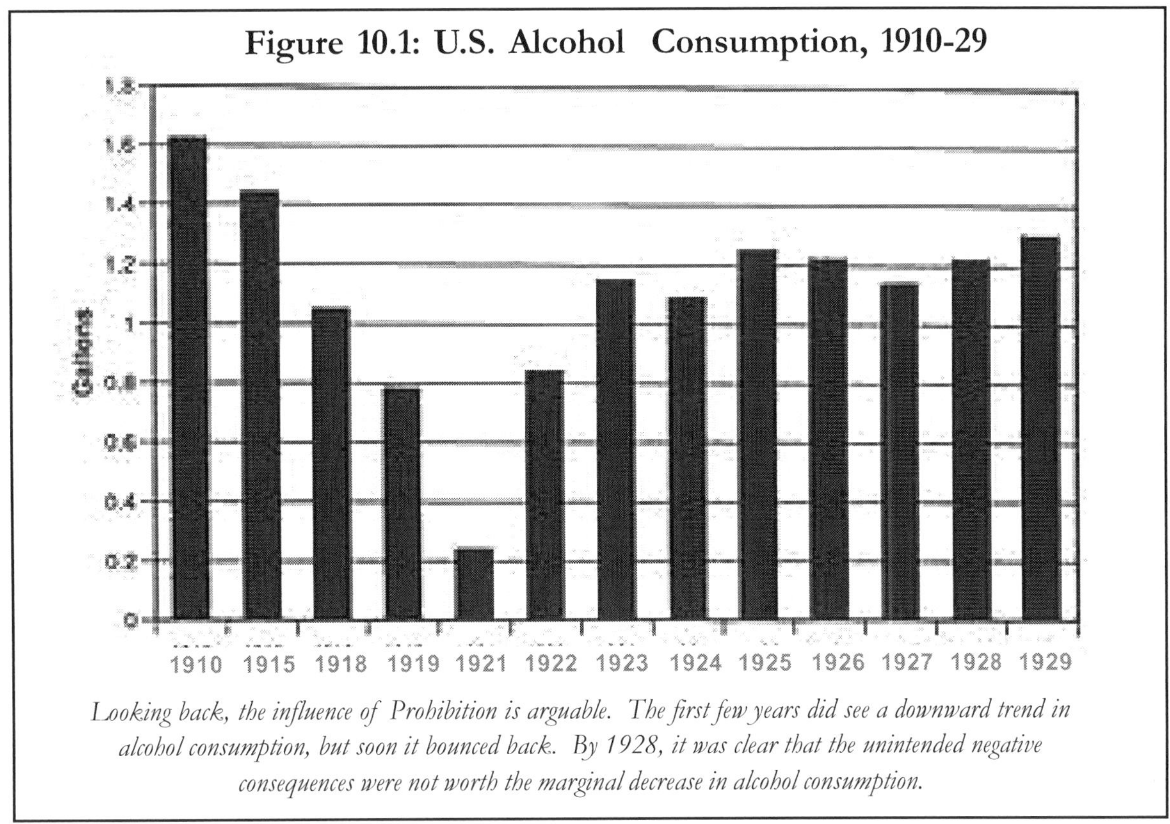


*Looking back, the influence of Prohibition is arguable. The first few years did see a downward trend in alcohol consumption, but soon it bounced back. By 1928, it was clear that the unintended negative consequences were not worth the marginal decrease in alcohol consumption.*

blocks of Rhine wine or bricks of port. These blocks/bricks carried the following warning: "After dissolving the brick in a gallon of water, do not place the liquid in a jug away in the cupboard for twenty days," because if you did, it would turn into wine. [24] Okay, you've been warned.

The mayor of New York City sent instrucitons on winemaking to his constituents. [25] Wort, or beer that had been halted in manufacturing process before the yeast was added, was readily available on the open market. The purchaser added yeast, let the wort ferment, and then filtered it. Since wort was sold before it contained alcohol, it was legal. It was sold openly throughout the entire country. [26] It's clear that Prohibition undermined respect for the rule of law. Contemporary drug prohibition has led to a similar disrespect for the law.

Songs of the day glorified bootlegging as a game the whole family could play. Here's one such ditty: [27]

> Mother makes brandy from cherries;
> Pop distills whisky and gin;
> Sister sells wine from the grapes on our
>     vine
> Good grief, how the money rolls in!

## The Roaring Twenties

After the implementation of alcohol Prohibition in 1920, coffee sales soared. For the first two or three years after Prohibition started, total alcohol use declined. [28] This decline, however, was just a continuation of a downward trend that had started several years earlier. See Figure 10.1 above. Nevertheless, the use of distilled liquors rose every year after alcohol Prohibition went into effect.

The use of alcohol went on pretty much unabated. The rich had easy access to liquor smuggled in from Canada and frequented speakeasies. Immigrants living in the cities viewed drinking as normal and refused to give up alcohol. A large percentage of normal, everyday "regular" citizens saw nothing wrong with drinking. The young saw drinking "bathtub gin" as excitement, a kick, "23 skidoo." The "speakeasies" were exciting and fun.

An openly displayed hip flask, filled with "bootleg" whiskey was a symbol of the era. Every community of any size had their "speakeasies" in which both imported and homemade alcohol could be purchased. Prohibition jump-started the Jazz Age. Keeping saloons and the drinking public supplied with liquor provided work and livelihood for tens of thousands of rumrunners, bootleggers, and beer barons. Due to Prohibition, they now all worked outside the law. [29]

## Cultures Clashing

It's arguable that America has never fully recovered from the enormous technological and societal changes that occurred between 1863 and 1933. The social changes wrought by freeing the slaves, the closing of the frontier, becoming an international power with which to be reckoned, discovery of great oil reserves, cross-country train travel, the telegraph, the telephone, electric lights, the automobile, the radio, the phonograph, and movies arguably had a more dramatic impact and effected greater cultural change than prominent post-WW II inventions: TV (which was actually invented in 1927 by Philo Farnsworth), the computer, the Internet and the cell phone.

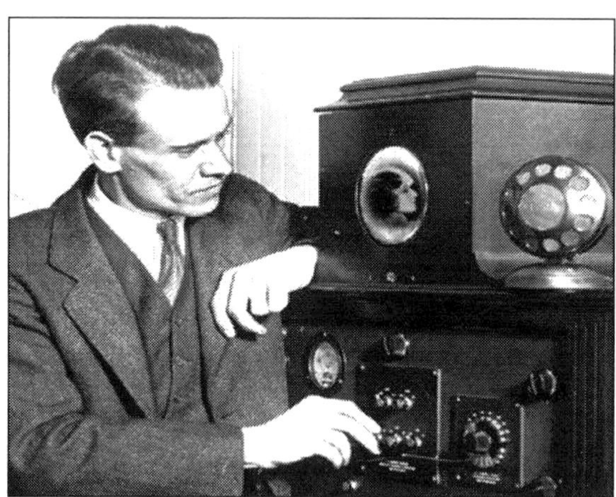

*Television was invented in 1927 by Philo Farnsworth. Here is Farnsworth with one of his early TV devices.*

From the 1860s to the 1930s, America moved from a largely rural society that stayed close to home and used few modern devices, to a very mobile, urban society with conveniences previously people had only barely imagined.

Victorian values dominated mainstream American life in the late 19th century. The Victorian value system prioritized restraint. This clashed with the dramatic cultural changes that were afoot. In the 20th century, industrialization and urbanization has widened the gap between cultural forces of the Victorian, rural, agrarian status quo and those that favored modernism or change powered by the Industrial Revolution, modern inventions and a more urban-oriented national psyche.

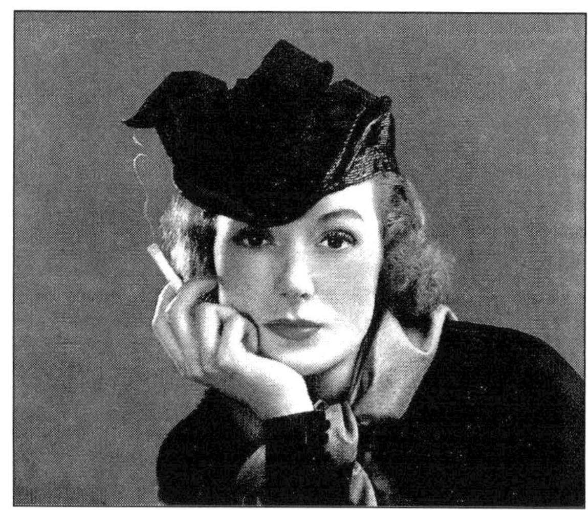

*The 1920s brought in the modern era. This decade contained the first crop of adults born in the 20th century. The combination of increased worldliness from fighting in WWI, the movies, the automobile and rebelling against Prohibition led to more smoking and drinking among women.*

There is no question that the Roaring Twenties were a milestone in this changing scene of American culture. Movies and automobile ownership became widely accessible and the three million troops (out of a national population of about 100 million) that come back from the First World War in Europe were a much more worldly lot than when they left for foreign shores. A popular song of the day spoke volumes: *How Ya Gonna Keep 'em down on the Farm after they've seen Paree?* Modern conveniences and greater worldliness heralded great changes in the average person's life.

The Roaring Twenties were a time of "bathtub gin", women smoking, bobbed hair, short skirts, loosening morals and jazz. The war was over and the post-war recession was in the rear-view-mirror. It was an era in which illegal liquor was widely available and when anyone could wink at the law and enjoy the thrill of conspiracy just by having a cocktail at "speakeasies", which were just around nearly every corner.

But those who had worked for generations for Prohibition were still in the picture. These sober, God-fearing Protestant folks were not happy with what they saw. The vision of flappers in short skirts, in the rumble seat with boys in raccoon coats, sipping on a hip flask of gin, on their way to a "speakeasy" to further flaunt the law, caused many a Prohibitionist to become almost apoplectic.

In many ways, deep cultural clashes have been a hallmark of America. The United States has an amazing resiliency, as it has endured almost a continuous round of culture clashes. These values conflicts date back to European vs. Native Americans, Tories vs. Patriots, slave owners vs. abolitionists, North vs. South, immigrants vs. Know Nothings, etc. The list goes on and on to Hippies vs. straights and Red vs. Blue states.

Unfortunately, these clashes have often led to efforts of one side to overpower the other. Drug policy is frequently a tool in these conflicts. Current U.S. drug laws exist, in part, as a backlash against the cultural, moral and ethical changes that came decades ago as America turned away from Victorian morality. "Hey, if we can't outlaw alcohol, how about expanding to heroin and cocaine and beyond?"

After over a half-century struggle, fueled by further technological and demographic change, these rural, Victorian values have given way to the relatively more relaxed morals of the late 20th century. America's draconian drug laws linger as a vestige of that bygone era.

Change breeds uncertainty and fear. Change, ancient or modern, seems to beg for scapegoats.

## *Birth of a Nation* Inspired a Rebirth of the Klan

Racism did not fade away after the end of slavery or the end of Reconstruction. The KKK did get much smaller in the first decade of the 20th century but sadly, D.W. Griffith's 1915 movie, *The Birth of a Nation*, heralded the second coming of the Klan. The movie is considered by many to be the first "great" American film.

*The Birth of a Nation* was historical fiction, loosely based on a novel, *The Clansman*, which glorified the South. The movie portrayed events around the Civil War from a Confederate point of view, with sympathetic assumptions about Southern society. The film contained all of the popular ethnic stereotypes from the 19th century. The KKK was

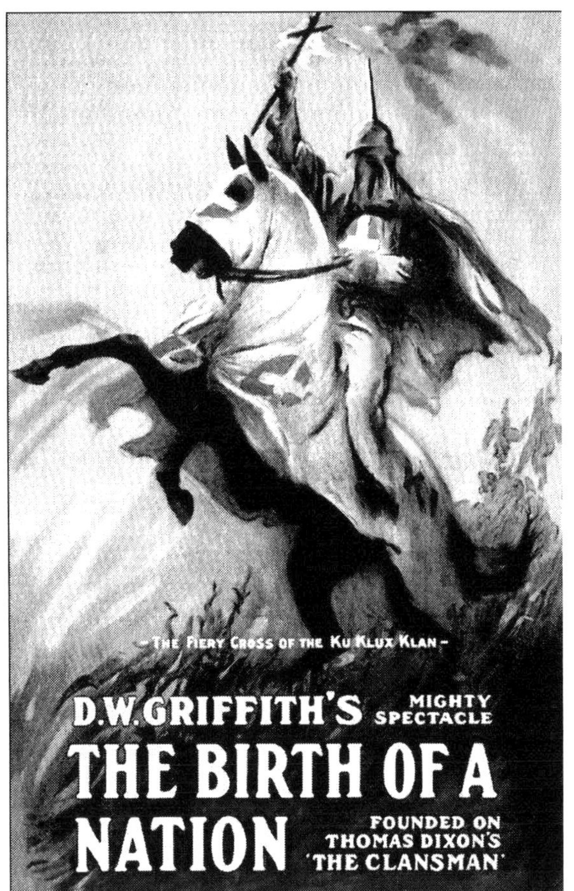


*By the early 20th century, the KKK had just about died out. The 1915 film* Birth of a Nation *by D.W. Griffin based on the pro-Clan novel* The Clansman *glamorized the Ku Klux Klan and justified their terrorist acts. The movie heralded in a revitalization of the clan.*

portrayed in a sympathetic light. They were shown as defending chaste Southern ladies from marauding and raping Black freemen. They were portrayed as saviors of the South from Black domination. The film is considered the first feature film and it was well received.

According to writer Everett Carter, the film popularized a series of irrational assumptions, which Carter referred to as "the plantation illusion."[30] This illusion is the myth that:

> (1) The antebellum (pre-war) South "was a golden age of agrarian feudal joy: wealthy autocratic landowners and happy obedient slaves".
> (2) There was perfect harmony between "colors" as long as the hierarchy was kept; and
> (3) That the "Negro" were happy to be faithful servants.

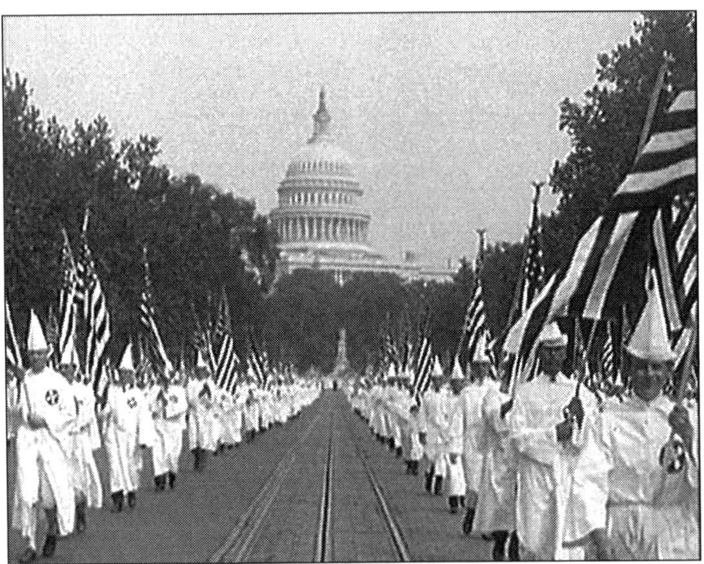

*In the early 1920s, the Ku Klux Klan gained exercise considerable political power and mobilized 50,000 Klansmen for this 1925 march on Washington, D.C.*

(4) The freed union "Negro" would be renegades wrecking terror on the South.
(5) The "mulatto" was the curse of the South because of the mixing of "Negro" bestiality with white intelligence.
(6) The "Negro "was somehow less than human.
(7) The North was seen as a "cold", harsh, industrial society."
(8) The movie exploited the Southern culture sexual fears of Negroes (rape, miscegenation, brutality)." [31]

In a 2004 article entitled "Art vs. Propaganda: *The Birth of a Nation* Viewed Today," Donato Totaro writes that these postulates "serve as a template for the film's central emotional and narrative dynamics, and, ideologically." He states that "the real concerns for Dixon and Griffith were sexual in nature and stem from a stringent Christian, Puritan, and Southern-Victorian morality and sensibility." [32]

*Birth of a Nation* was lauded by the sons and daughters of the South. They had felt put upon by Reconstruction and here was vindication via these new-fangled movies. Mrs. S.E.F. Rose, historian of the Mississippi Chapter of the United Daughters of the Confederacy, wrote a 1916 article in *Confederate Veteran*, stating "…the laws of the land had been diverted from their original purposes and trampled underfoot by ignorant and vicious negroes and adventurers who were unable properly to interpret the laws and unfit to enforce them…" [33]

This resurgent racism provided motivation for additional tightening of the Harrison Narcotics Tax Act of 1914 even beyond the Supreme Court's ruling in *United States v. Behrman*, 258 U.S. 280 (1922) limited physicians' ability to treat substance abuse. Congress then passed the Uniform Narcotic Act of 1924, which spelled the end of heroin maintenance clinics. At the state level, there was a rash of drug laws passed in the 1920s. Starting in the mid-1920s, there was a resurgence at the local level of overtly racist news articles when covering the use of recreational drugs.

## A Frenzy of Fear of Them

In the aftermath of World War I, anti-immigration forces got more grist for their demonization mill. Fear of foreign agitators (especially Communists), reached enear pidemic proportions. This frenzy of fear culminated in 1919 and the early 1920s with the Red Scare that swept the United States.

By the early 1920s, the now revived KKK was going strong. In a nation of slightly over 100 million, the Klan attracted at least five million members and possibly more. They had added anti-Semitism, anti-foreignism, and anti-immigrant to their traditional agenda of anti-Catholicism and hatred of "Negroes".

There was a symbiotic relationship between Prohibition and the poisonous tone of bigotry of the 1920s. The '20s were a wretched excess of drinking, wealth accumulation, partying, discrimination and fear. From the Sacco–Venzetti murder trial to the rise of the KKK, from the Scopes monkey trial to the "demonization" of jazz musicians and marijuana, from the Mafia to the restructured immigration laws of 1921 and 1924 – the excesses of the '20s and of alcohol Prohibition have been written about and explored *ad nauseum*.

Fear is a great motivator in humans. Fear has been used to justify not only repressive drug laws, but for many other atrocities and unsavory aspects of American history. These other matters will not be examined closely here. In the 1920s and '30s, fear ran high; first in the fear of the flood of new immigrants and then in the fear that the U.S.

economic system would never recover from what became known as the Great Depression followed by fear of the war in Europe.

The KKK and similar groups exploited fear of the "other" and the racist, anti-Catholic, anti-Semitic and xenophobic tendencies in Americans. They used phrases like "America for Americans". In the 1920s, the Ku Klux Klan had upwards of five million members, some estimate as many as 10 million, across the country. Only a kidnap, rape and murder of a young woman by a prominent Klan member, who was a strong candidate for governor of Indiana helped trim the KKK's sails.

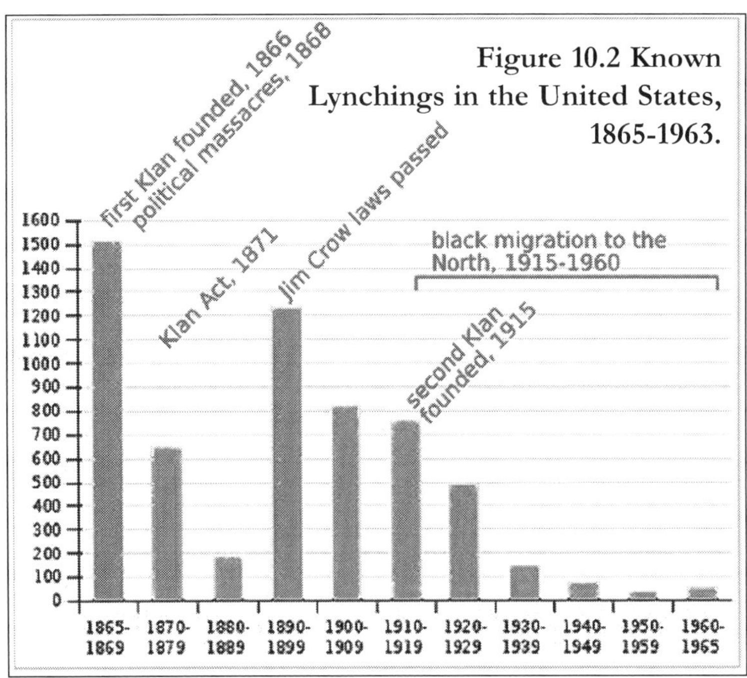

**Figure 10.2 Known Lynchings in the United States, 1865-1963.**

*A graph of known lynchings in the United States, 1865-1963. The real number was certainly higher.*

## The Demise of Rosewood, Florida

There are far too many examples of racism and violence throughout the history of this country. The destruction of Rosewood, Florida in January of 1923 by a mob of whites is one of the most egregious examples in America's unsavory history of bigotry. Rosewood's inhabitants were massacred and the town burned to the ground. Rosewood was a rarity, a town where the mostly Black population owned most of the land and businesses and was more prosperous than Whites in the neighboring shanty town of Sumner. [34]

Not surprisingly the spark that set off the Rosewood horror was when a White housewife in the nearby and poorer town was beaten by her White lover. Rather than face her husband with the truth, she cried in the street that a strange Black man did it. Her lie mutates and word spreads that she was beaten "and" raped. An armed mob soon congeals, looking for a suspect and looking toward their Black neighbors in Rosewood. The mob was soon out of control, killing and burning indiscriminately, destroying the town. in 1997, this was made into a movie, *Rosewood*, by John Singleton.

## Lynchings

Lynching, of course, was a popular form of violent intimidation, especially in the first half-century following the Civil War. The toll of lynchings tapered off in the 1930s and '40s. By the early 1940s, with the rise of Black political power in the northern cities, the advent of the Second World War and the early stages of the civil rights movement, lynchings became rarer but not rare enough. Cultural and racial violence went largely unpunished and continued in America for another 50 years, only to be supplanted by slightly subtler forms of social and economic control which continue to this day.

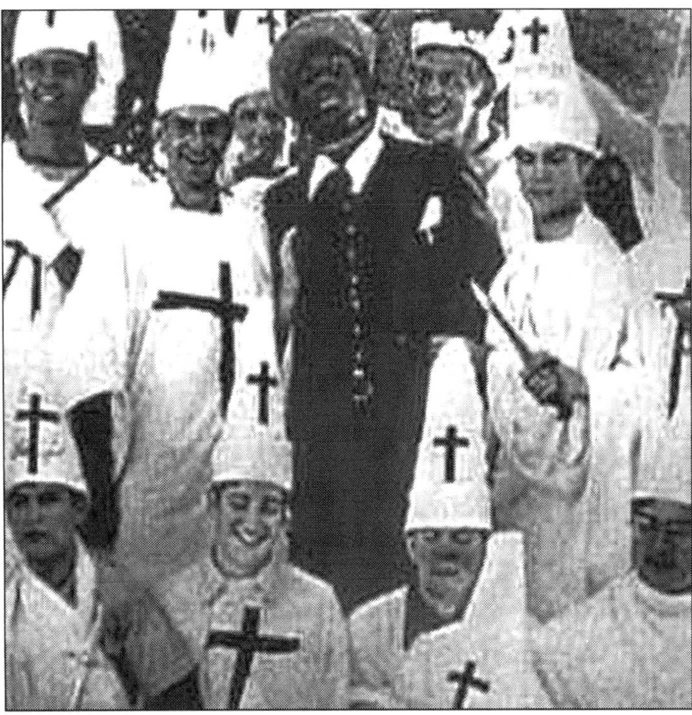

*Here is a staged mock lynching in the 1920s or '30s attributed to a fraternity at Virginia Military Institute. There were thousands of real lynchings and the KKK was implicated in many of them.*

Nowadays lynching is more often used figuratively as a label for social vilification. A modern example was during the Senate confirmation hearing for now U.S. Supreme Court Justice Clarence Thomas. Thomas referred to the allegations of sexual harassment by a Black co-worker during his 1991 U.S. Senate confirmation hearing as a "high-tech lynching."

## The Wobblies (IWW) & Joe Hill

The 1920s was a dangerous time for organized labor. Much as today, the economy was firmly controlled by big business and efforts to crush organization of labor were common and frequently hostile. The "Wobblies", or the International Workers of the World (IWW), are a case in point. At its peak in 1923, the IWW organization claimed some 100,000 dues-paying members.

The most bloody assault on the "Wobblies" in the United States occurred on November 5, 1916 at Everett, Washington. Sheriff Donald McRae led a band of deputized businessmen against the "Wobblies". The Sheriff and his men attacked the steamer Verona, killing at least five union members (six more were never accounted for and probably were lost in Puget Sound.)

The IWW, which still exists with about 2,000 members, believes all workers should be united within a single union as a class and that the wage system should be abolished. Their philosophy was a threat to the moneyed class. The IWW's goal was to promote worker solidarity in the revolutionary struggle to overthrow the employing class. Politicians and the press saw the IWW as a threat to the "free market system". The IWW's efforts generated opposition from the government, company management and their agents. These groups, functioned as vigilantes, violently fought the IWW.

The 1914 trial of Joe Hill, who was accused of murder, demonstrated the strong anti-labor bias in the United States at that time. Hill was a Swedish immigrant who became involved with the "Wobblies" in 1910. He was a songwriter, folk singer, union organizer, and itinerant worker. He traveled widely, organizing workers under the IWW banner, writing political songs and satirical poems, and making speeches. He coined the phrase "pie in the sky", which appeared in his song *The Preacher and the Slave* (a parody of the hymn *In the Sweet Bye and Bye*).

There had been a murder of a butcher in Salt Lake City by two masked gunmen. One had been shot. That evening Hill was treated for a gunshot wound. He contended he had been shot by a jealous husband. He refused to identify the adulterous wife out of chivalry and the sure knowledge that her reputation in the community would be tarnished and likely destroyed.

### Joe Hill Martyred

There was only circumstantial evidence but Hill was found guilty and sentenced to death. The case became a cause celeb. President Woodrow Wilson, Helen Keller, and people in Sweden and unions around the world all became involved in a bid for clemency. Critics charged that the trial and conviction were unfair. Hill was executed by the state of Utah on November 19, 1915.

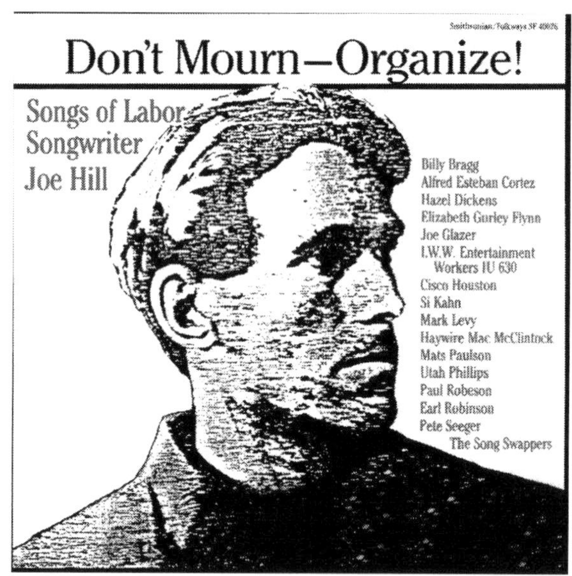


*In the first half of the 20th century, there had been clashes between big business and organized labor that were often brutal. Joe Hill, a song writer and union organizer was arrested, tried and convicted of murder on very slim evidence. The case was a cause* celebre. *He was killed by firing squad and became a martyr for union organizing.*

Hill became more famous in death than in life. His last word when he was executed by firing squad was "Fire!" Just prior to his execution, he had written to Bill Haywood, an IWW leader, saying "Goodbye Bill. I die like a true blue rebel. Don't waste any time in mourning. Organize ... Could you arrange to have my body hauled to the state line to be buried? I don't want to be found dead in Utah."[35]

His will, eventually set to music by Ethel Raim, read:

> ***My will is easy to decide***
> ***For there is nothing to divide***
> ***My kid don't need to fuss and moan***
> ***Moss does not cling to a rolling stone.***
> ***My body? – Oh. – If I could choose***
> ***I would to ashes it reduce***
> ***And let the merry breezes blow***
> ***My dust to where some flowers grow***
> ***Perhaps some fading flower then***
> ***Would come to life and bloom again***
> ***This is my Last and final Will***
> ***Good Luck to All of you.***
>
> **Joe Hill**
> Union organizer, 1879-1915

## The Red Scare

The "Red Scare" is another example of inordinate fear leading to excessive, inappropriate and ultimately un-American or at least unconstitutional activity. Attorney General A. Mitchell Palmer helped create the infamous "Red Scare" that started in 1919. He tied America's fear of Communism and immigrants together. He charged that labor unions and the Socialist and Communist parties were infiltrated with radicals who sought to overturn America's social, political, and economic institutions.

Attorney General Palmer's raids during the "Red Scare" of 1919 and 1920 were largely aimed at Italian immigrant families. As a result, many aliens were illegally detained or arrested, and some were deported with little or no basis.[36] The Palmer raids began in 1919 when Palmer and his agents started "seizing suspected anarchists and Communists and held them for deportation with no regard for due process of law."[37]

J. Edgar Hoover, later the long-time FBI director, was one of those responsible for implementing the Communist round-up of the early 1920s. Not surprisingly, his role was to develop extensive files, dossiers to identify alleged anarchist and communist enemies of the state. The Palmer raids violated the rights of thousands of American citizens and legal aliens with illegal search and seizure, wrongful arrests and even deportations.[38]

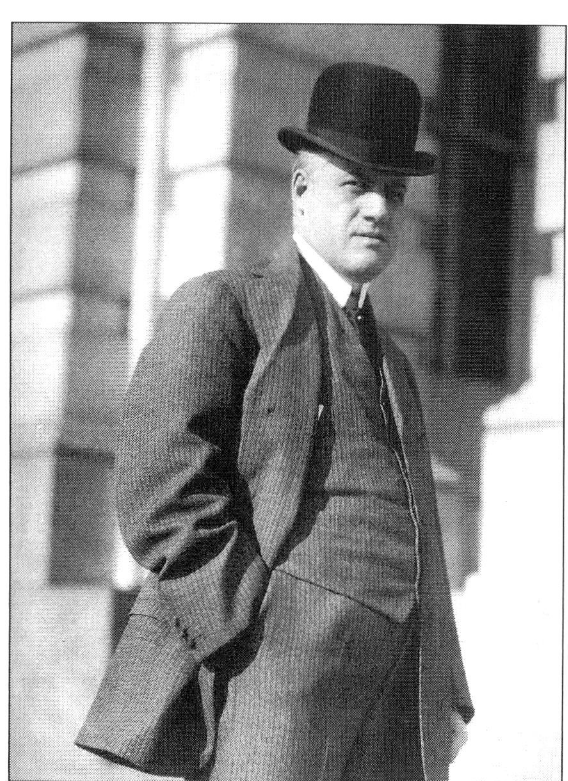

*Mitchell Palmer helped create the "Red Scare" that started in 1919. J. Edgar Hoover got his start under Palmer in keeping extensive files on alleged Communists.*

The violation of basic American Constitutional rights even for what conventional wisdom might mark as a good cause, like marginalizing the demonized and presumed bad guys, is bad for America. Ignoring American rights and freedoms undermines those very principles which have made America unique. The atmosphere of the 1920s was ripe for whipping up fear about them and their drugs; drug policy being just another tool to control those who we fear.

## DARE: Let's Do Something That Feels Good But Doesn't Work

Today's drug warriors use fear-based rhetoric to justify current governmental tactics. Present drug policies not only don't work but are counter-productive. Since 1998, the ONDCP has spent two billion dollars on public service announcements that not only do not work, but according to some studies, are counterproductive. DARE, the so-called Drug Abuse Research and Education Program, where police officers not teachers or doctors, discuss substance use and abuse, has also been shown to be a dreadful waste of money and to have NO impact on youth substance abuse.

DARE, a continuing attempt at drug-abuse prevention, is a particularly sad waste of money. It uses police officers, most of whom are not trained teachers, to address the issue of substance abuse. While there may be a feel good quality to have Officer Bill in the school room, the program is not effective. Professors Rosenbaum and Hanson of the University of Illinois at Chicago, in a 1998 study found that DARE has no impact on the long-term rate of drug use by children who go through it. This is the same result found in all major research into DARE's effectiveness. Despite the lack of evidence for its effectiveness, in 1996 it was administered in 70% of the nation's school districts, reaching 25 million students.

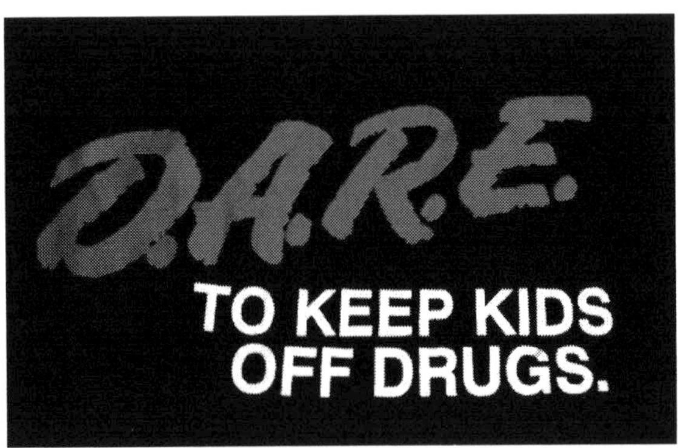


*This is the logo for the Drug Abuse Research and Education Program (DARE), a program begun in the 1980s in an effort to prevent school children from using controlled drugs. Although a series of independent studies over 1992-2009 found the program to be "ineffective' or doing more harm than good, it is still being carried out in many localities with public and private funding.* [39] *A November 2001 report by the Institute of Industrial Relations found that over $1 billion per year was being spent on DARE programs nationwide.*

---

That year 44 foreign countries also used it. The costs for this program include not just wasted taxpayer money but also the lost education time. Educators could be using that time to teach about pharmacology, physiology, childhood development, and most importantly parenting. The funds could be used to provide counseling services for children, who come from a dysfunctional home environment, and their parents.

## Controlling Immigration: Beware of "Them"

Average Americans in the 1920s worried about the effect on the economy of increased post-war immigration. The labor movement worried about the newly arrived immigrants' willingness to work for substandard wages, depressing the wages of all laborers. They called for immigration restriction.

There was concern that post-WWI immigration would increase because decreased immigration during the war had created a pent-up demand to immigrate to the United States. It was feared that soon, millions of refugees would flock to the United States and destroy the prosperity of the Roaring Twenties.

Congress was happy to respond to the public pressure, passing the National Origins Act in 1924. This law incorporated prevailing prejudices. It set immigration quotas that pointedly discriminated against Southern and Eastern Europeans. The law permitted 65,721 immigrants from Great Britain annually, but only 5,802 from Italy and 2,712 from the Soviet Union; and, no surprise, Asians were almost completely excluded. [40]

The United States has a long pattern of deliberately leaving the country's "back door" open to Mexican workers, then moving to expel them and their families years later. This has been a recurrent feature of immigration policy since the 1890s.

Arguments similar to the present day over the role of non-documented Mexican workers have been around for at least 100 years. For instance, a Texas cotton lobbyist told Congress in 1920 not to worry; the tens of thousands of Mexicans laboring in their fields were not a threat to national security. Congressmen in the 1920s faced a political problem in extending the guest workers program that had let the workers in. The cotton lobbyists suggested a wink and smile policy solution. "If you gentlemen have any objections to admitting the Mexicans by law," he said, "take the river guard away and let us alone, and we will get them all right." [41]

"Things are not the same today, but the basic dynamics do not change," said Mr. Zolberg, a professor of political science at the New School in

New York City. "Wanting immigrants because they're a good source of cheap labor and human capital on the one hand, and then posing the identity question: But will they become Americans? Where is the boundary of American identity going to be?" [42]

---

> **"The Busines of Government is Business"**
> **Calvin Coolidge**
> President of the United States, 1925-1929

---

To this day, immigration policy remains a hot button issue. Immigration is one of those complex issues with no easy answers.

Eric Schlosser, in his 2003 book, *Reefer Madness*, discusses the exploitation of legal and illegal immigrants in strengthening the strawberry industry in Guadalupe, California. In this example, even settled and legal immigrants that became growers and that take most of the risk , it's the Anglos that sell the crops who make most of the money.

## The Black Italians

It may seem strange today, but during the 1920s "racism" was a significant cause of animosity towards Italians in America. Italians' skin coloring was generally darker than the so-called "old stock" Americans. They were subject to much of the same discrimination faced by Blacks, Hispanics and Asians. [43]

Italian immigrants also suffered from anti-Catholic hostility. Julia Byrne, in her 2000 article, "Roman Catholics and the American Mainstream in the Twentieth Century", noted: "Anti-Catholic prejudice was alive and even rejuvenated in some quarters in the twentieth century. Protestant 'fundamentalists' and other new Christian denominations revived anti-Catholicism as part of an insistence on 'original' pre-Rome Christianity." [44]

Members of the Temperance movement and supporters of Prohibition were strongly against immigrants, because they linked them to excessive drinking. Immigrants were very good targets for the Temperance cause, because they could be portrayed as different. Americans fear of "them" was used to promote Prohibition. [45]

Protestants promoted an association between Italians, Catholics and immorality. The basis in part, was due to different interpretations of sin. Unlike most Calvinist branches of Christianity, Roman Catholicism does not see gambling as a sin. Traditionally, Catholicism teaches that, like alcohol, gambling can be acceptable in moderation. They are not acceptable when immoderate or when addictive. Nevertheless, the Protestants of the 1920s were quick to assail Catholics, particularly those of Italian origin, for excessive drinking, gambling, untold perversion and violence.

This anti-Italian sentiment was not new to America. Towards the end of the 19th century, Italian Catholics were characterized as being "apelike", just as the Irish were earlier and the Negroes -- both earlier and later. Italians were said to be an inferior and degraded "race" that lived immoral lives revolving around liquor.

In fact, the rate of alcoholism amongst Italians was no higher than the American average and that is the case today. But facts did not stop Nativisists from scorning Italian immigrants as "dangerous, contemptible, inferior, and disloyal – the off-scourings of the world." [46,47] These hostile, negative stereotypical portrayals are often used as a part of the argument for oppressive drug laws and chipping away at the U.S. Constitution.

## The Anarchists, the "Commies", the Immigrants; Let's Take it Out on Sacco and Vanzetti

When Sacco and Vanzetti, Italian immigrants and anarchists, were arrested in 1920 for a 1919 robbery and murder, the United States was in the midst of its first "Red Scare" and the round-up of the "Commies".

Severe poverty in the post-war years caused many American workers to be dissatisfied with the status quo. Big business and government were concerned that workers might follow the example of the Russian Bolshevik Revolution. The U.S. government was doing everything in its power to portray communism and anarchism as "un-American", and to frighten workers away from "Red" propaganda.

Sacco and Vanzetti were tried and found guilty. They spent the next six years in prison as appeal after

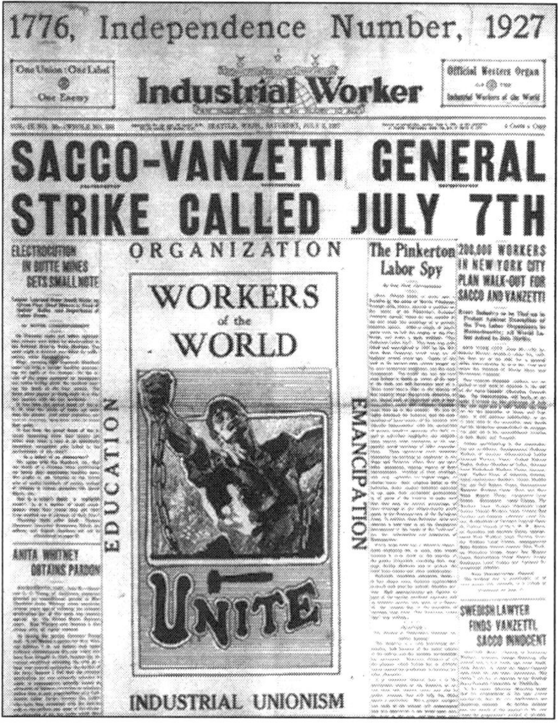
1776, Independence Number, 1927

**Industrial Worker**

# SACCO-VANZETTI GENERAL STRIKE CALLED JULY 7TH

ORGANIZATION

WORKERS of the WORLD

EDUCATION

EMANCIPATION

UNITE

INDUSTRIAL UNIONISM

The Pinkerton Labor Spy

200,000 WORKERS IN NEW YORK CITY PLAN WALK-OUT FOR SACCO AND VANZETTI

ANITA WHITNEY OBTAINS PARDON

SWEDISH LAWYER FINDS VANZETTI, SACCO INNOCENT

*Anti-Italian bias raised the real possibility that Sacco and Vanzetti were railroaded for a high-profile robbery-murder. They were unpopular Italian anarchists. Their two trials went on for seven years before they were eventually executed in 1927. At the very least, anti-Italian sentiment of the day made their trial anything but fair. The argument goes on to this day if one or both were guilty or innocent. According to two books by Francis Russell, modern tests on the evidence indicate Sacco was guilty and Vanzetti may have been innocent.* [48]

appeal was turned down. Finally, on August 23, 1927, they were executed. Judge Webster Thayer said of Vanzetti:

> "This man, although he may not have actually committed the crime attributed to him, is nevertheless morally culpable, because he is the enemy of our existing institutions."

The foreman of the jury, a retired policeman, said in response to a friend of his who ventured the opinion that Sacco and Vanzetti might be innocent, "Damn them. They ought to hang anyway." Having sentenced the two men to death, the judge boasted to a friend, "Did you see what I did to those anarchist bastards the other day?" [49]

While there is no agreement to this day as to their guilt or innocence, there was no doubt that Sacco and Vanzetti were on trial for their political beliefs. Further, the verdict was seen as the state delivering an object lesson to the U.S. working class – steer clear of anarchist thought or face the consequences. [50]

The Sacco and Vanzetti trial was built on a solid foundation of anti-Italian, anti-immigrant sentiment. Their trial was a figurative lynching, but literal lynching was a common practice in the late 19th and early 20th century. In most years in that time period, the United States had 50-100 lynchings. Negroes were far and away the most likely to be lynched. However, Italian-American immigrants were the second most commonly acounted for lynched groups. In fact, the largest mass lynching in U.S. history was of Italian-Americans. On March 14, 1891, eleven Italian-Americans were lynched in New Orleans by a mob after a jury failed to convict them of the murder of a New Orleans police chief. The eleven were falsely accused of being associated with the Mafia. The point is, of course, that irrational policy, hysteria and discrimination are a potent mix for ill and can be visited upon Black and white, poor and middle class alike.

## "Speakeasies": Hooch & Bribes – My, How the Money Rolls In

Prohibition did provide gainful employment for recent immigrants (most prominently, in our cultural memory, Jewish and Italian gangsters). It created an opportunity for Blacks and Whites to mingle in "speakeasies" where Black jazz musicians often entertained. At Harlem's famed Cotton Club, the best Negro entertainers performed before strictly all White audiences. Prohibition helped promote tobacco smoking, particularly amongst women, and gave a big boost to jazz.

Prohibition saw the illegal night clubs, dives and "clip joints" quickly replacing the previously legal, but now shuttered, friendly neighborhood saloon. As songwriter Hoagy Carmichael (writer of *Stardust*, the song that was, for decades, recorded by more artists than any other) put it, the 1920s came in "with a bang of bad booze, flappers with bare legs, jangled morals and wild weekends."

Higher class, illicit booze establishments may have been a bit pricey but you usually got what you were paying for; real alcohol and "whoopee". "Clip-

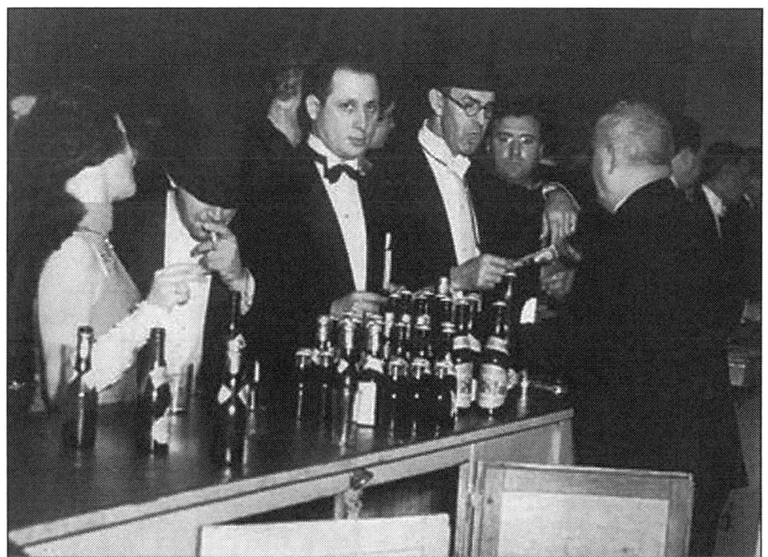

*The "speakeasy" was the illicit drinking spot that replaced the saloon. It was seen as hip. Jazz provided by Black or mixed "race" musicians, often provided the entertainment. Women openly drank and smoked.*

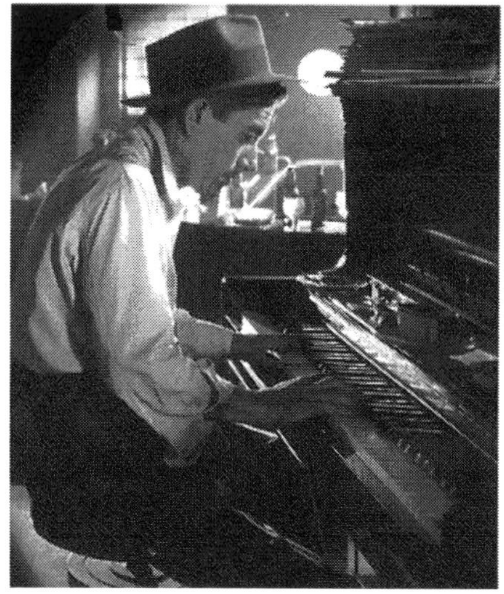

*Hoagy Carmichael, piano player and songwriter, was a popular performer in the 1920s. He wrote* Stardust, *which, until* Yesterday *by the Beatles, had been recorded by more artists than any other song.*

joints" and dives on the other hand, promised a good time but the reality was usually an exorbitant bill, frequently poor quality liquor and sometimes a beating. [51]

Combating this self-inflicted crime wave required the good citizens of the 1920s to form large police forces. Being a police officer was a pretty good job during Prohibition and the Depression. It delivered a relatively decent salary, respect, partial immunity to the law, and the opportunity to take bribes. However:

> "Seldom has any law anywhere led to greater hypocrisy or been more widely flouted. People not only continued to drink, but in greater numbers than ever. Before Prohibition, New York had 15,000 legal saloons; by the end of Prohibition it had over 30,000 illegal ones. Detroit had no fewer than 20,000 speakeasies, as illegal drinking estab-lishments became rather curiously known … Hardly anyone took the law seriously. In 1930 a journalist testified to the House Judiciary Committee that he had attended a lively party at a Detroit roadhouse where he had seen the Governor of Michigan, the chief of police of Detroit and four circuit judges, drinking lavishly.." [52]
>
> **Bill Bryson**
>
> American scholar and writer, as cited by Keith Evans in *The Longest War* (2000)

Most contemporary historians and economists generally agree that the evidence from what U.S. President Herbert Hoover called the "noble experiment" affirms sound economic theory. Economic theory predicts that the prohibition of any mutually beneficial exchange is doomed to fail. [53] Prohibition was a boon for public officials, particularly law enforcement, many of whom were on the take. Many factors brought Prohibition to an end. A compelling force was concern about corruption in law enforcement and politics.

Today's drug prohibition has as much, or more, negative consequences as alcohol prohibition. The list of prohibition-related problems is almost endless. Not only does the list of negative consequences of today's drug policies include corruption of police and public officials through bribery, but even worse, prohibition has corrupted the process. Whether it's disproportionately targeting the poor and minorities, undermining the First, Fourth, Fifth, Ninth and Tenth Amendments to the Constitution, diverting government funding from medicine and education to the criminal justice system and more: the harm to this country from modern-day drug prohibition is extensive and very troubling.

## Campaign to Repeal Prohibition

In the late 1920s and early 1930s, Prohibition's opponents made exactly the same argument for repeal as the proponents had made earlier. They

## "Texas" Guinan, 1884-1933
### Icon of the Roaring Twenties: "Hello Suckers"

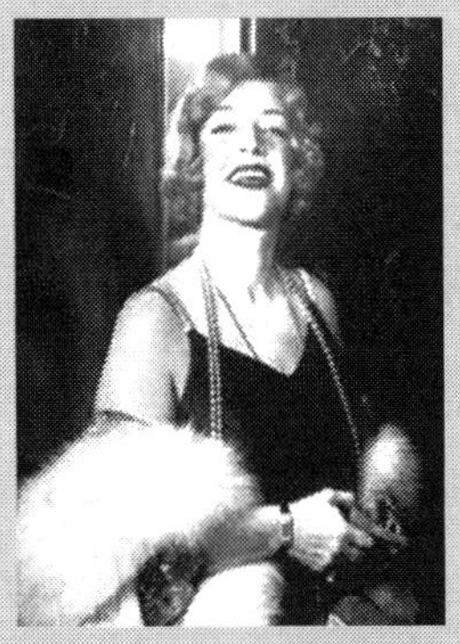

"Texas" Guinan was an icon of the speakeasy era. Even though she died in 1933, comedians on TV were still making references to her well into the 1970s. Guinan was famous or at least notorious during prohibition. Like many today, she took advantage of Prohibition to satisfy the needs of those who desired the prohibited item. She owned and ran one of the 32,000 speakeasies in New York. [54]

"Texas" Guinan was born in Waco, Texas, there she went to parochial school and sang in the church choir. The lure of Broadway, as the cliché goes, took her to New York where she had success as a singer. Her big break came in that important new cultural force making even rural Americans more worldly, the movies. Her initial film was a Western, *The Wildcat* (1917). *The Wildcat* made her America's first movie cowgirl and the pistol-packing, horseback riding Queen of the West. She added to her notoriety by going to France and entertained the troops during World War I.

"Texas" Guinan was a bigger than life singer, movie star and speak easy proprietor. She was famous for greeting her clients with, "Hello suckers."

Guinan took full advantage of the entrepreneurial opportunities offered by Prohibition. She opened a "speakeasy" called "The 300 Club". It was staffed by pretty hostesses and chorus girls, "40, count 'em 40" beautiful fan dancers. Their principal role was to get customers' minds off how much their drinks were costing.

She was arrested several times for selling illegal booze. She always claimed that any liquor in her place had been brought in by the customers and certainly had not been sold by her establishment. Who knows, maybe she was just selling expensive set-ups (e.g., glasses, mix, stirrers and the "groceries", e.g., cherries, olives, celery, etc., that decorate drinks).

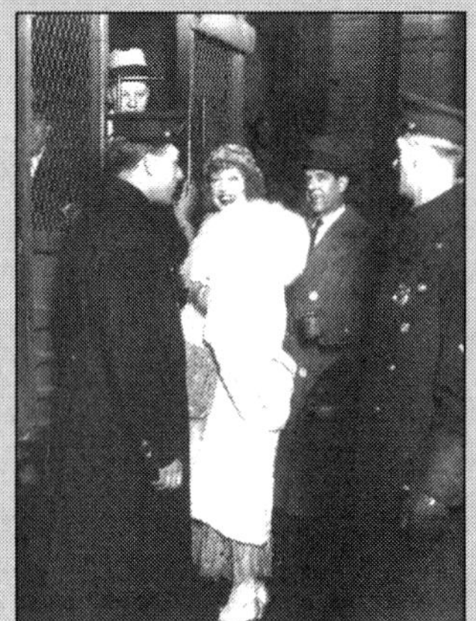

*Here is Ms. Guinan being arrested in 1927, which didn't seem to hurt her business.*

She was also accused of providing lewd entertainment. After one raid, police displayed a six by three inch square of material that they alleged was the entire costume of a dancer. The combination of the skimpy costume, dancing too suggestively and too close to the customers, were deemed way too over the top. 'Texas' replied innocently enough that the club was so crowded that there was no option but for the poor girl to dance very close to the patrons.

In 1929, Guinan starred in two sound pictures. In both *Queen of the Night Clubs* and *Broadway Through a Keyhole,* she played a speakeasy proprietress, a slightly fictionalized versions of herself. She has been portrayed in a number of movies, including *Splendor in the Grass* (1961). The production numbers in *All That Jazz* and in the musical *Chicago*, paid homage to her.

"Texas" Guinan was a colorful character who contributed many popular phrases to the language. She coined the term "butter and egg men" referring to her wealthy clientele. She noted that "a man could get hurt falling off a bar stool." After the floor show, she always encouraged her patrons to "give the little ladies a great big hand". She was "Your Mistress of Ceremonies", Texas Guinan. [55, 56]

promised repeal would provide jobs, stimulate the economy, increase tax revenue, and reduce the "lawlessness" stimulated by and characteristic of the illegal liquor industry. In the late '20s, the Association Against the Prohibition Amendment (AAPA) took over the campaign for repeal. Headed by Pierre du Pont and other powerful corporate leaders, the AAPA gathered increasing numbers of wealthy and prominent supporters.

The Wickersham Commission, a federal commission formed to study the effects of Prohibition, issued its report in 1928. This was the beginning of the end. While it was purported that its finding, supported Prohibition, the evidence it had collected confirmed the charges of the AAPA that Prohibition didn't work. [57] The general sense that the commission's report contradicted the notion that Prohibition was working was captured by Franklin P. Adams' verse in his "Conning Tower" column in the *New York World*:

Prohibition is an awful flop.
We like it.
It can't stop what it's meant to stop.
We like it.
It's left a trail of graft and slime,
It don't prohibit worth a dime,
It's filled our land with vice and crime.
Nevertheless, we're for it. [58]

In view of the numerous U.S. federal government scandals coming to light recently (e.g., in 2007 alone: abuse of the Patriot Act, political firings in the Department of Justice, waste in Iraq, NSA spying, etc.), Thomas Jefferson is prophetic. Jefferson was adamant that the government should not have power over the most personal areas of our lives, especially the foods eaten and the medicines taken.

If the government can control what goes in our body, where do they stop? Eggs, meat, sugar are all potentially unhealthy. Should they be made illegal so there is no legal sugar, eggs, or meat? This is a slippery slope. When does the public get off?

Today, it's accepted that there must be some proof that a drug is actually safe and useful. It's a question of science.

**"If people let government decide which foods they eat and medicines they take, their bodies will soon be in as sorry a state as are the souls of those who live under tyranny."** [59]

**attributed to Thomas Jefferson**

## The "Great Experiment" Ended with a Thud

In 1933, the Great Experiment was over and most everyone celebrated.

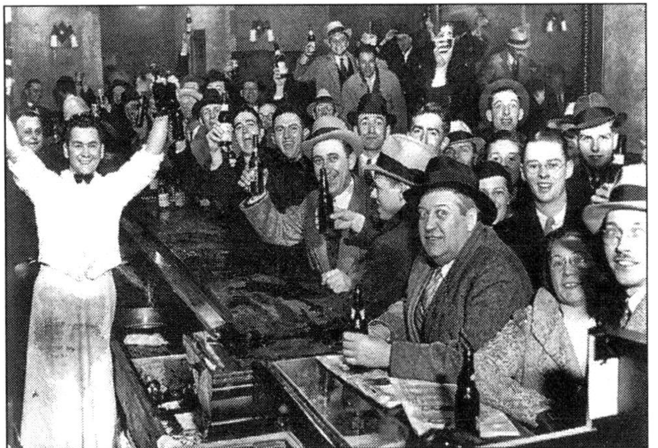

*Celebrating the end of "the Great Experiment".*

The engines that drove the repeal of the Eighteenth Amendment weren't so much a desire to return to legalized alcohol as much as the recognition that Prohibition was costly to enforce, led to corruption of public officials, provided organized crime with money to move into legal business, and fostered a disdain for the law.

But Prohibition left a residue that is with America yet. Unfortunately, one lesson apparently not fully absorbed so far, is the law of unintended negative consequences. Alcohol prohibition had plenty. And the negative consequences of today's "War on U.S. Citizens and the Constitution", also known as the "War on Drugs", are just as bad or worse than what was left from alcohol prohibition.

### Women and Cigarettes

Smoking amongst women went up dramatically as a result of Prohibition. Women were drinking in public. Smoking was chic. By 1947 (there is about a 20-year lag time in commencing a smoking habit

## Figure 10.3: Lung Cancer Rates for Men, Women, 1975-2007.

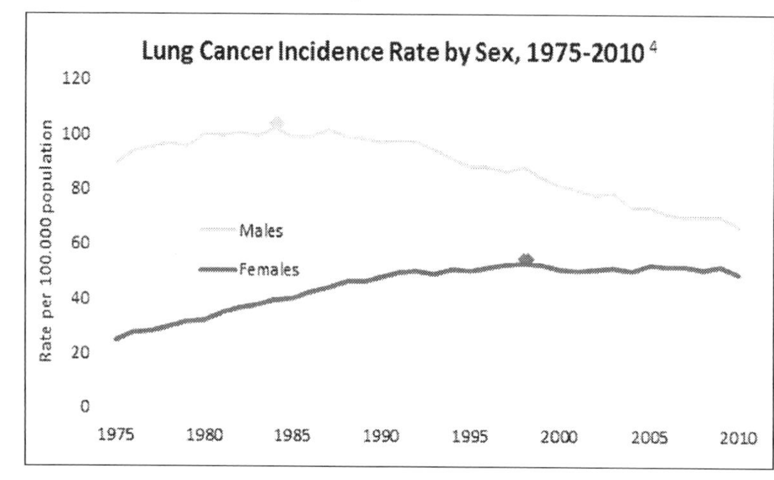


*The rate of women smoking went up in the 1920s and 1930s. This chart demonstrates that the rate of lung cancer in women increased. This increase became apparent starting in the late 1940s. It takes about 10 years of heavy tobacco smoking to significant increase lung cancer risk and 20 years to manifest.*
*SOURCE: National Cancer Center.*

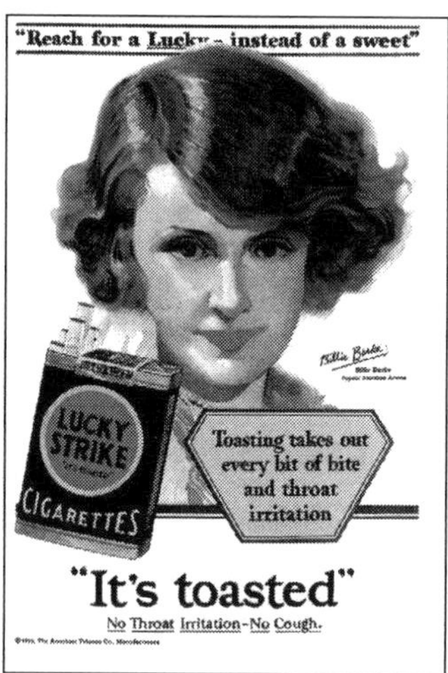


*Prior to Prohibition, smoking by women was reserved for the ultra-wealthy, hookers, and derelicts. With the advent of Prohibition and the Roaring Twenties, smoking by women became socially acceptable. Film celebrities such as Billy Burke began endorsing specific brands of cigarettes.*

> ***"The prestige of government has undoubtedly been lowered considerably by Prohibition. Nothing is more destructive of respect for the government and the law of the land than laws which cannot be enforced. It is an open secret that the dangerous increase of crime in the country is closely connected with this."***
>
> **Albert Einstein**
>
> "My First Impression of the Country," 1921

and its effect on lung cancer statistics), women's lung cancer rates were starting to catch up to men.

### Organized Crime

Not only did Prohibition fail to cut crime, improve family life and make the United States a more Christian nation, it lead to wholesale lawbreaking. Prohibition made organized crime an American institution making criminals tens of millions-of-dollars a year in 1920-dollars. The American government had unwittingly provided criminals the police power that enabled the thugs to takeover the alcohol business. To this day, in many areas the Mob still controls liquor and cigarette sales, gambling and more. [60]

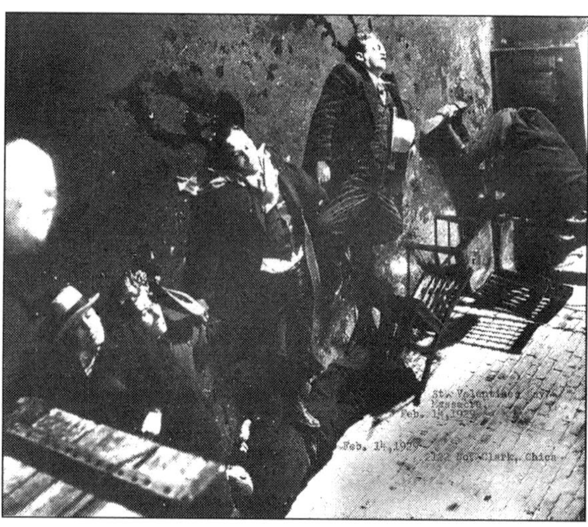

*Just as with modern prohibition, there was money to be made in the illicit alcohol trade during Prohibition. This led to turf wars. One of the most notorious involved Al Capone on the St. Valentine's Day Massacre.*

## Cannabis

By outlawing alcohol, Prohibition hastened the popularity of cannabis for recreational uses. So an unintended consequence of Prohibition was a dramatic increase in the recreational use of marijuana. Prohibition took cannabis use from something heretofore confined to a relatively small group of jazz musicians, Mexican field hands, and Jamaican sailors, and expanded its use not only amongst minorities, but "speakeasy" patrons and the Great Gatsbys of the Roaring Twenties. Cannabis was widely available in both the "speakeasies" and so-called tea houses or tea pads of the 1920s.

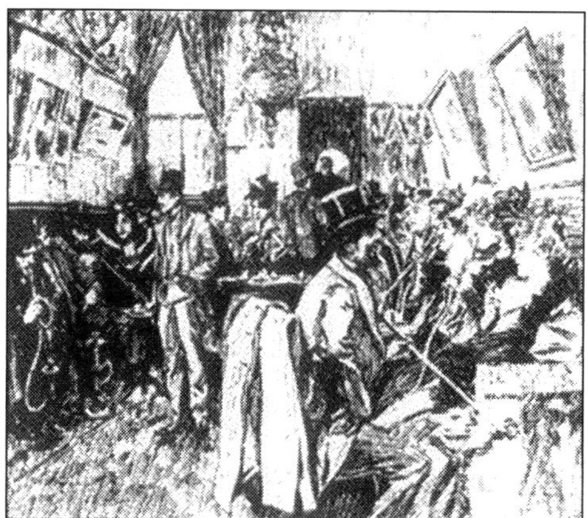

*A scene from a newly opened Turkish smoking parlor in New York City.* New York Herald, *April 28, 1895.*

---

Tea pads had started up in New York City circa 1880. By the end of the 1880s, most major American cities had hashish parlors. They were originally a spin-off of Turkish Hashish smoking parlors that were a feature in many of the World Fairs and international expositions that were held around the world from 1860-1920, such as the 1876 Philadelphia Centennial Exposition. [61]

In the early 1920s, there were over 500 such establishments in New York City alone. [62] Members of the upper class often visited these tea pads. These were places where a person could come and buy some "muggles," some "reefer," a little "mary jane", whatever you called it. A person

### Why Prohibition Failed

**by Paul Campos, Ph.D.**

*Rocky Mountain News*, July 4, 2006

"The standard story of why Prohibition failed or was a bad idea was because it couldn't 'work', fails to explain what was wrong with the attempt to make America an alcohol-free nation in the first place. It's said the attempt to make America dry was doomed to failure because our legal system lacked the resources to stamp out alcohol use, at least at an acceptable price.

"The problem with this story is it assumes that, if it were possible to eliminate alcohol use in America at an 'acceptable' cost, then this would be a desirable thing. And that is a seriously wrongheaded belief.

***"The truth about alcohol is that, for all the damage it does, its net effect on society is strongly positive. Alcoholic beverages bring both simple and sophisticated pleasures to the 75 percent of American adults who drink them at least occasionally. While it's true that 10% of people who consume alcohol create problems for themselves and their families, for the rest it serves an important role to escape from reality."***

Andrew Weil, M.D. in *The Natural Mind* (1972) makes the case that experiencing altered states of reality is necessary for mental health. Norman Taylor in *Narcotics, Nature's Dangerous Gift* (1966), argues that life is short, sad and brutal. In his view we need to have altered states to be able to live a mentally healthy life side by side with the sure knowledge that we and our loved ones will all die. Psychology professors, have noted that drinking signifies a time-out ritual, a time-out from the stresses and pressure of the rest of our reality.

Campos continues: "Alcohol encourages conviviality, making otherwise tedious social events palatable, and pleasant occasions even more enjoyable. Alcohol enhances meals, relationships, sporting events, and many other aspects of life. Human beings have recognized this for thousands of years. (For example, the ancient Greek dramas, which remain among the greatest artistic achievements of our civilization, were composed specifically for an annual festival to honor the god of wine.)

"In other words, to make America a completely sober nation, even if it were possible, would be a terrible thing."

*Paul Campos is a professor law at the University of Colorado.*

could smoke it there on a pad or take it home if they wanted.

After Prohibition, the United States was left with nothing to show for "the great experiment" but a decade of political turmoil, increased incidence of women smoking, women more willing to drink and smoke in public, promotion of recreational use of cannabis, and a lot of unemployed police officers.

However, many of the unemployed cops soon had law enforcement jobs again, thanks to the maneuvering of *über* bureaucrat Harry Anslinger, the first director of the Federal Bureau of Narcotics and Dangerous Drugs.

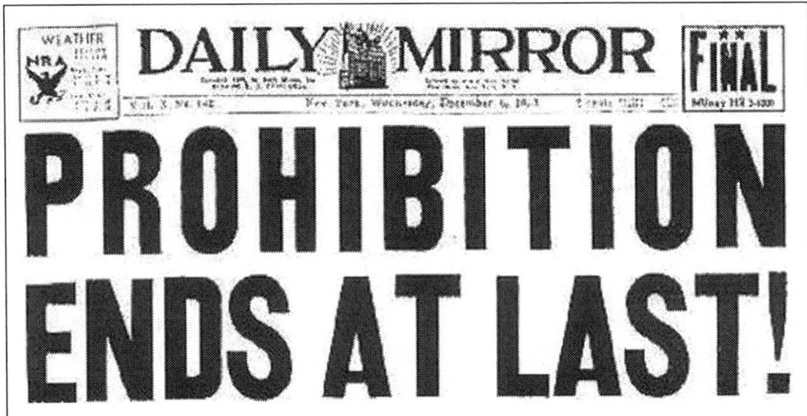

WEATHER

NRA

DAILY MIRROR

FINAL

PROHIBITION ENDS AT LAST!

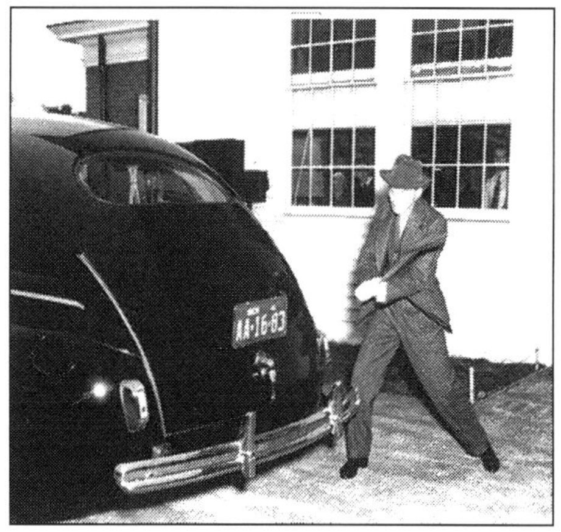


*Here is Henry Ford in 1939, hitting a hemp-powered experimental car with a sledgehammer, demonstrating that the hemp-infused acrylic body was fifteen times stronger than steel. No dent was left on the car.*

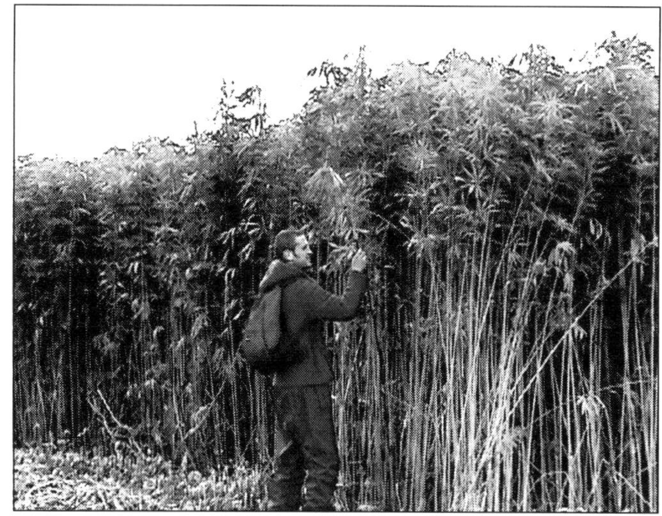

*Potential competition from less expensive hemp products motivated Dupont and other petrochemical interests to pursue the Marijuana Tax Act of 1937. Above is a modern hemp field.*

# CHAPTER XI
# 1915-1937: Marijuana Tax Act

## Was It Really Anslinger?

Harry J. Anslinger was appointed director of the U.S. Treasury Department's Federal Bureau of Narcotics (FBN) in 1930. Conventional wisdom credits him with engineering the passage of the Marijuana Tax Act of 1937. He was allegedly motivated by his racist loathing and a desire to increase his bureaucratic power. This is all true, but the back story follows a much more complicated and torturous road. The story of the potential economic impact that using modern harvesting machinery would have on elevating the competitiveness and value of hemp is compelling. Let's follow the money.

## A Remarkable Invention

The saga started in 1915 with the culmination of George Schlichten's 18-year, £400,000 (the British pound equivalent is over 20 million in 2013 dollars) effort to invent a revolutionary labor-saving hemp decorticator. His hemp decorticator harvesting machine removed the fiber from the pulp much more efficiently and less expensively than existing methods. This device eliminated the retting process, thus cutting down dramatically on the labor costs of hemp production. Had Schlichten's decorticator been put into mass production, hemp would once again be competitive for a wide variety of purposes, e.g., synthetic fabrics, paper, ethanol, biomass and building materials. In addition, hemp could be used to produce oils for paint and diesel fuel as valuable byproducts

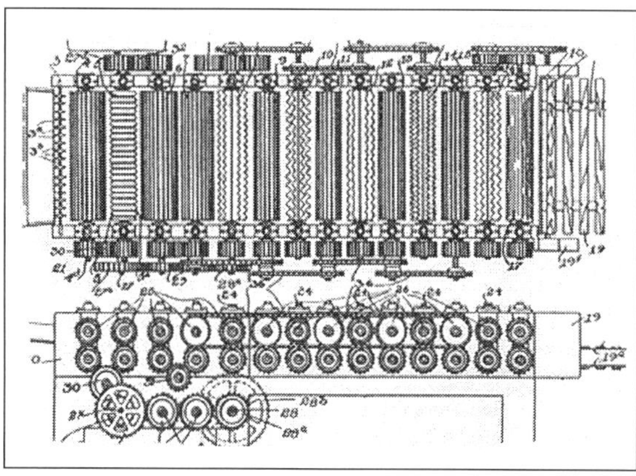

*The Hemp Decorticator: George Schlichten poured in 400,000 British punds and spent 18 years developing his hemp decorticator. He got his patent for his decorticator from the U.S. Patent Office on July 1, 1915.* [1] *Most of what is known about Schlichten comes from 24 letters he wrote in promoting his invention, which are owned by Edward W. Scripps in the Alden Library at Ohio University.*

of the plant. If this were to happen, there would be many potential industrial losers.

Starting in 1916 and even more so in the years immediately leading up the passage of the Marijuana Tax Act, hemp appeared poised to make a commercial comeback. In 1916, the U.S. Department of Agriculture (USDA) issued "Bulletin No. 404: Hemp Hurds as Paper-Making Material." The Bulletin, written by USDA scientists Dewey Lyster and Jason Merrill and printed on hemp paper, outlined exciting new hemp pulp technology. It touted the contemporary agrarian possibilities for hemp.[2]

The bulletin highlighted increased production capacity and superior quality as among the advantages of using hemp hurds for pulp. Lyster wrote in Bulletin No. 404, "Every tract of 10,000 acres which is devoted to hemp raising year by year is equivalent to a sustained pulp production capacity of 40,500 acres of average wood-pulp lands." Hence, an acre of hemp produces four times as much pulp as an acre of trees.[3,4,5,6] Schlichten had thoroughly studied many kinds of plants used for paper and he found hemp was the best. He said, "The hemp hurd is a practical success and will make Bulletin 404 come true."[7]

As WWI wore on, wood pulp became scarce. The price of wood pulp and therefore paper increased considerably over pre-war levels. Hemp paper was looking like a candidate for competition for wood pulp derived paper. At 1917 levels of hemp production, Schlichten anticipated making 50,000 tons of paper and selling it at a profit for $25/ton. This was way less than half the price of newsprint at the time, which was $80/ton. The threat to wood pump produced paper was obvious. Every acre of hemp produced four to five times as much paper as an acre of wood. Plus the hemp crop was renewable annually whereas it takes years to reproduce a comparable tree. The hemp decorticator promised to eliminate much of the need for wood-pulp paper, thus threatening to drastically reduce the value of the vast timberlands still owned by William Randolph Hearst and others in the paper business.

Schlichten got his patent for his decorticator from the U.S. Patent Office 1915[8] and by 1917 was putting the finishing touches on his brilliant invention. His decorticator could strip the fiber from nearly any plant creating both fiber and the pulp it left behind. By eliminating the retting stage of hemp fiber preparation (which loosened the fiber from the stalk, then combed out and softened the hemp fiber)[9] he decreased the labor required to prepare hemp for industrial use. Schlichten reasoned his machine would revolutionize the hemp-paper and hemp-fiber industry, just as Whitney's cotton gin had done for the cotton industry.

## Support Appears, Disappears

The process caught the eye of Harry Timken, one of the leading machinists of the day and president of the Timken Roller Bearing Company. In February 1917, Schlichten and Timkin met to discuss the decorticator. Timken, a wealthy industrialist, believed Schlichten's revolutionary machine would improve conditions for mankind. Timken had a ranch east of San Diego. He invited Schlichten to grow 100 acres of hemp on his ranch to test the economic viability and functionality of his decorticator.

In the spring of 1917, Timkin met with E.W. Scripps, a turn-of-the-century newspaper baron, to discuss

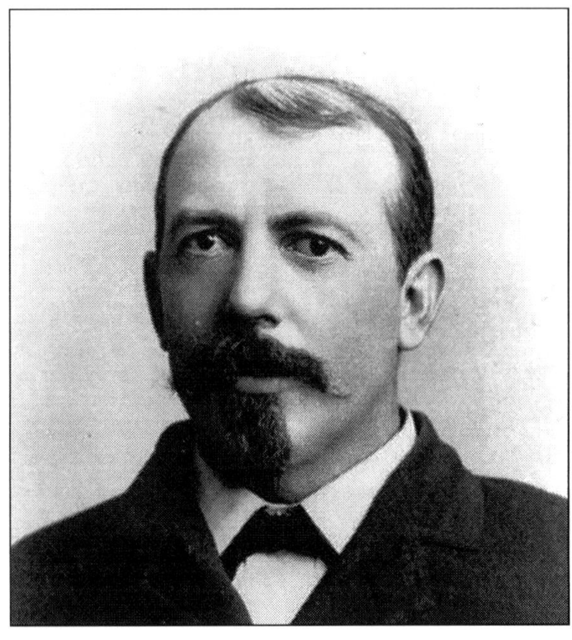

*E.W. Scripps: In the spring of 1917, Scripps, the owner of the newspaper chain bearing his name, and his business partner, Milton McRae, were interested in using hemp paper for newspapers. On the verge of making a major investment in George Schlichten's hemp decorticator, they inexplicably changed their minds.*

Schlichten's decorticator. Scripps, then 63, owned the largest chain of newspapers in the United States. His chain sold over 28 million copies per day so it required huge amounts of paper. The price of newsprint was rapidly increasing, giving Scripps an interest in the commercial viability of hemp paper.

Schlichten reportedly told Milton Alexander McRae, a Scripps business partner:

> "Don't forget, Mr. McRae, that the time will be seen when wood cannot be used for paper any more. It will be too expensive or forbidden. We have got to look for something that can be produced annually. Every acre that I produce in hemp or in cotton stock hurds will preserve five acres of forest." [10]

There were additional meetings with Timken. McRae wrote to Scripps that the decorticator was "a great invention, which will not only render great service to his country but will be very profitable finically to him." [11] On August 3, 1917, a three-hour meeting was held between Timken, Scripps, McCrae and Edward Chase, Scripps's right hand man. Transcribed by a stenographer, this excerpt typifies the initial enthusiastism of this group:

> "On August 28, Chase sent a thorough report on his investigations into hemp for paper to Scripps and McRae. This central document confirms the viability of the project Chase witnessed the decorticator at work, extolling it as "a wonderful, yet simple, invention." . . . . "The advantages of using hemp hurds are enumerated, including making pulp from an annual, to "preserve the forests, the streams and the soil." Hemp could be made into paper at a lower cost than wood pulp, Chase concluded, while using no sulphide and less soda, resin and clay than wood required. Chase noted that the Schlichten process was an advancement over that reported in Bulletin #404. He confirmed the $25 per ton price – less than half the 1917 market price for newsprint. A paper mill in San Diego was proposed. With this, Chase figured hemp could supply all Scripps Pacific Coast newspapers, with leftover pulp for side business." [12]

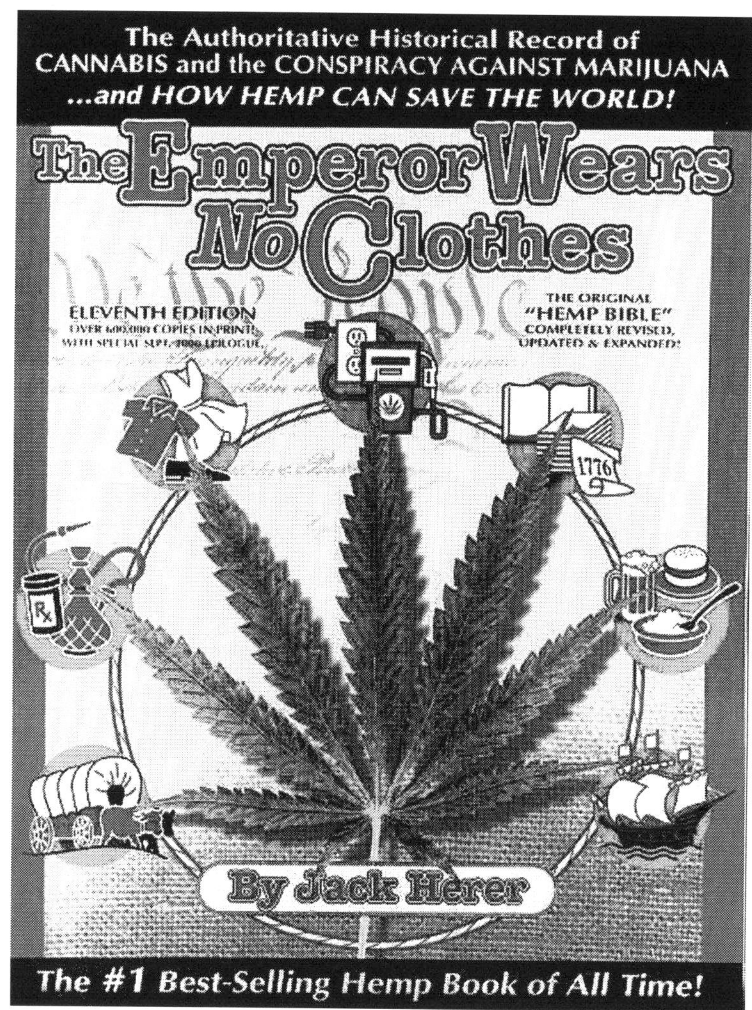


*The cover of the 11th edition of the late Jack Herer's book,* The Emperor Wears No Clothes *(originally published in 1985), quickly and dramatically illustrates the multiple economic possibilities of hemp.*

However, a short time later, and for no known reason, Chase and McRae changed their minds. [13] The correspondence with Timken became more general; less enthusiastic. Soon Chase and McRae convinced Timken beyond a reasonable doubt that hemp was not economical for newspapers. McRae then instructed Chase to drop the matter and promised Scripps he'd work on it later, but nothing else happened. Why did Scripps change his mind?

Who knows, maybe he just didn't have the courage or the need to go to a cheaper, better paper.

Without a backer, Schlichten and his machinery fell into oblivion. Schlichten sank from view and is not again mentioned in hemp literature. He died in 1924 in Solano, California.[14] But in the mid-30s, after his patent expired, interest in his decorticator again surfaced as a result of articles in *Popular Mechanics* and *Mechanical Engineering*, which pointed out the many potential applications of hemp. The economic viability of hemp was again getting some attention.

## Hemp: The Fuel of the Future?

Hemp was a very real potential threat to oil as a fuel for cars. No less than Henry Ford (1863-1947) was one of hemp's early champions as fuel for his automobiles. Ford never intended cars to use gasoline. His first Model-T was built to run on hemp-based fuel. When Ford designed the Model T, he expected that ethanol, made from renewable biological materials, would fuel the automobile.[15] Rudolf Diesel, inventor of the diesel engine, designed his engine to run on vegetable and seed oils, like hemp. In Paris at the 1898 Exposition Fair, Diesel's engine actually ran on peanut oil.[16, 17]

In 1925, Henry Ford told a *New York Times* reporter that ethyl alcohol was "the fuel of the future". This

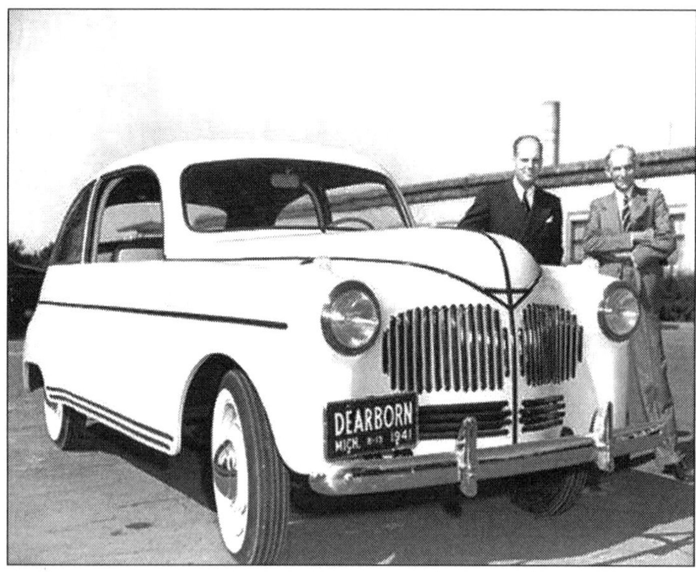


*In the 1930s Henry Ford (right) developed a car made out of vegetable matter (including hemp acrylic resin for the cars' skin and hemp fabric and insulation for the door panels) that ran on hemp oil diesel. His Model T was originally designed to run on biofuel.*

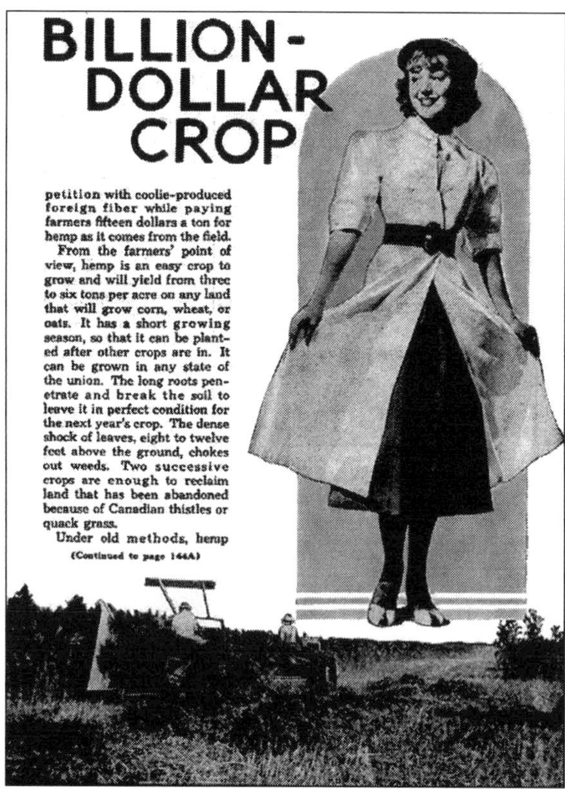

BILLION-DOLLAR CROP

petition with coolie-produced foreign fiber while paying farmers fifteen dollars a ton for hemp as it comes from the field.

From the farmers' point of view, hemp is an easy crop to grow and will yield from three to six tons per acre on any land that will grow corn, wheat, or oats. It has a short growing season, so that it can be planted after other crops are in. It can be grown in any state of the union. The long roots penetrate and break the soil to leave it in perfect condition for the next year's crop. The dense shock of leaves, eight to twelve feet above the ground, chokes out weeds. Two successive crops are enough to reclaim land that has been abandoned because of Canadian thistles or quack grass.

Under old methods, hemp

(Continued to page 144A)

*This is the famous 1938 Popular Mechanics cover and article touting hemp as the "new billion-dollar crop." This exemplifies du Pont's concern that hemp would pose strong competition to his chemical industry unless he took action.*

was an opinion widely shared within the automotive industry. "The fuel of the future is going to come from fruit like that sumach out by the road, or from apples, weeds, sawdust – almost anything," he said. "There is fuel in every bit of vegetable matter that can be fermented."[18]

> **"There's enough alcohol in one year's yield of an acre of potatoes to drive the machinery necessary to cultivate the fields for one hundred years."**[20]
>
> **Henry Ford**
>
> American industrialist, 1863-1947

In the 1930s, Ford and other companies were promising to make many of the products then being made from petroleum hydrocarbons from cannabis. Ford recognized the utility of the hemp plant. In the late 1930s, he constructed a car of resin-stiffened hemp fiber, which ran on ethanol made from hemp. According to a 1941 *Popular Mechanics* article, the hemp acrylic body was 10 times stronger than steel. [19] It was composed of 70% cellulose, which was made from straw, hemp or sisal, and 30% resin. [20]

During the 1920s, diesel engines were altered so they ran on lower-viscosity fossil fuels and not on biomass-derived fuel as Diesel had intended. [21] The petroleum industry, which was run by ruthless wealthy oil tycoons, used vicious business tactics to eliminate competition. The world is still suffering the consequences of their success.

Gasoline emerged as the dominant fuel in the early 20th century because of the ease of operation of gasoline engines with the materials then available for engine construction, a growing supply of cheap petroleum from oil field discoveries, and intense lobbying by petroleum companies for the federal government to maintain steep alcohol taxes.

Oil in those days was a major American product. The oil companies had great political clout. A noteworthy propaganda claim by petrol supporters was that any U.S. government's plans to support ethanol "robbed taxpayers to make farmers rich". In part due to the petroleum industry crushing of their fuel competitors, today the United States is making the Saudis, Kuwaitis and Iranians rich, instead of American farmers.

Hemp and other seed oils are still an enticing alternative to petroleum. Hemp grows easily in the wild in every state in America; so shortages are unlikely. And hemp, unlike oil (they just aren't making dinosaurs anymore), is renewable. Growing, harvesting, and processing hemp has much less adverse environmental impact than procuring, processing and delivering oil. Hemp fuel is biodegradable; so hemp oil spills would become fertilizer, not eco-catastrophes. [22]

In the mid-1930s, when Schlichten's patent ran out, several other inventors came out with similar, even better, very effective decorticators. Presumably, they were building on the original design of Schlichten's decorticator, but except for their use in the Hemp for Victory campaign in WWII, it was to no avail in saving the hemp (and cannabis) industry. [23] For at least the next seventy-five years the Marijuana Tax Act did in the hemp industry in the United States.

## The Build Up to the Marijuana Tax Act of 1937

There is strong circumstantial evidence that commerce had an important role in generating the Marijuana Tax Act of 1937. While the legislation, which prohibited the consumption of cannabis, was driven by business interests, it was promoted by prejudice-fueled rhetoric. "The cannabis laws were clearly aimed at demonizing and controlling minorities and other undesirables." [24]

## Hot Women, Cool Jazz, Racism, Sensational Headlines, and Lies

When Storyville, the bordello section of New Orleans and the cradle of jazz, was closed down in 1917, the jazz musicians started going north and west. During WWI, southern Blacks came up the Mississippi River to Memphis, Kansas City, St. Louis and Chicago, bringing jazz and marijuana with them. Many of these river cities soon passed laws against marijuana.

Shortly after the closing of Storyville, the Big Easy's moral crusaders focused their zeal on marijuana. In 1920, Dr. Oscar Dowling, president of the Louisiana State Board of Health, got energized about drug policy when he heard of a musician convicted of forging a doctor's signature on a marijuana prescription. He warned Louisiana's governor, John M. Parker, that marijuana is "a powerful narcotic, causing exhilaration, intoxication, delirious hallucinations, and its subsequent action, drowsiness and stupor…" and urged that something to be done about the threat to the city. [25]

In 1926, New Orleans newspapers started a racist, anti-marijuana campaign. They wrote that Cuban and South American sailors were smuggling large amounts of marijuana into New Orleans, which lead to widespread use even among children. [26] The *New Orleans Morning Tribune* ran a series highlighting marijuana as being responsible for mayhem and murder, principally by Mexicans.

The headlines were hardly the model of restraint. They blared alarms like, "School Children Found in Grip of Marijuana Habit by Investigators," "Workmen of City Lured by Muggles," and "Welfare Workers are powerless to Cope with Sinister Traffic." [27]

There were several "reefer" jazz songs in the 1930s: Louis Armstrong's "Muggles" (slang term for cannabis); Cab Calloway's "That Funny Reefer Man"; Fats Waller's "Viper's Drag"; others, by lesser-known artists, include "Viper's Moan", "Texas Tea Party", "Smokin' Reefers", "Mary Jane", and the "Mary Jane Polka". Even Benny Goodman got into the act with "Sweet Marihuana Brown". There was a 1932 Broadway show, "Smokin' Reefer", starring Clifton Webb (later Mr. Belvedere in the popular 1940's *Mr. Belvedere* movies). Lyrics included "the stuff that dreams are made of" and "the thing that white folks are afraid of"). [28]

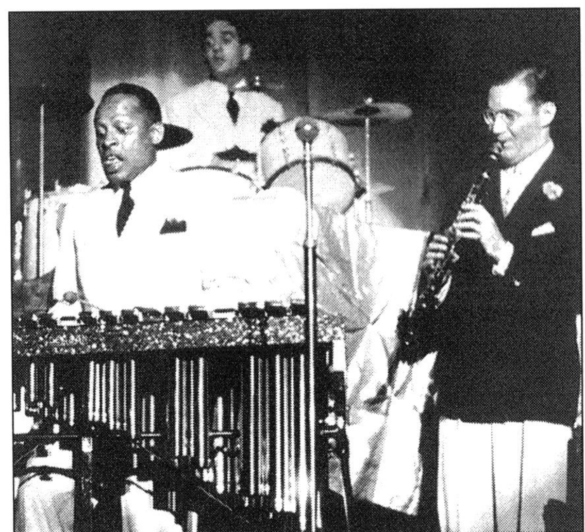

*Integrated jazz groups such as the Benny Goodman Trio infuriated racists.*

## A Simmering Caldron

American society of the 1920s and 1930s was a simmering caldron, cooking up a foul stew of demonization and discrimination. The Ku Klux Klan had millions of members across the segregated South and north into Indiana, Michigan, Missouri and southern Illinois. The Great Depression of the 1930s raised havoc with the economy. Many whites were afraid of losing their jobs to Blacks, Hispanics or immigrants, who they believed would or did work for less money.

The racist motive behind these anti-marijuana laws was obvious. Santa Barbara, Calif. pharmacist Henry Finger had fingered San Francisco's and Fresno's Hindoos and their hashish usage. And leaders of the East Coast wine and liquor distributor, W.H. Schieffelin & Co., were worried about New York City's Syrians and spoke out against their hashish habits. But it was Blacks, Jazz and the Mexican connection that seemed to push the button for marijuana control. [29]

Once the Great Depression hit, which lasted throughout the 1930s, jobs became scarce. Mexicans became doubly demonized, particularly in the southwest. Mexican immigrant field workers were real competition on the job market. This job concern fanned anti-Mexican feelings among Anglos and generated anti-immigrant societies such as the "American Coalition" and "Key Men of America." These groups were viciously anti-Mexican immigrant. The working men in the form of the American Federation of Labor lobbied against the presence of Mexican laborers. They wanted to strictly enforce immigration barriers. [Gee, this all sounds pretty contemporary.] It also mimics concerns raised in the recession of two decades earlier.

Politicians, most of who were trying to please the white working class, claimed that Mexicans were responsible for crime waves. Many were eager to marginalize the Mexican laborers, who had helped provide the energy for the economic boom of the 1920s. They wanted these Mexican laborers to leave the country, now that the Depression had set in. Indeed, a 1931 immigration law allowed the United States to forcibly remove tens of thousands of Mexican immigrants.

A 1932 article in the *Journal of Criminal Law and Criminology* was frequently referenced by other publications. It said that those under the influence of cannabis had great strength and endurance. Worse yet in the public's view, it increased sexual libido. This of course is what led to all those alleged rapes by Negroes. It also tossed in the hysterical — but totally erroneous and undocumented — information that marijuana caused irreparable brain damage and ultimately led to death. [30]

## Cannabis Becomes "Marijuana"

Throughout the period, the Hearst newspapers were regularly demonizing cannabis as "marihuana" or marijuana. William Randolph Hearst, son of obscenely wealthy Comstock Load silver baron, George Hearst, was owner and publisher of a chain of sensationalist newspapers. Reporting on Spain's actions in Cuba in 1895, Hearst and his papers exhibited strong anti-Spanish bias. In the run up to the Spanish-American War (1905), Hearst's newspapers in an effort to encourage U.S. war with Spain exaggerated the poor treatment and abuse the Cubans received at the hands of the Spainish.

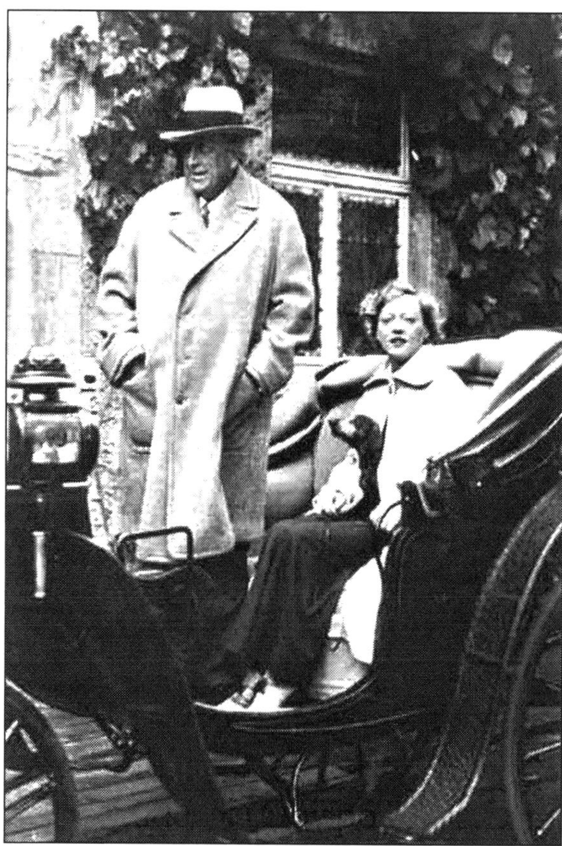

*William Randolph Hearst was the son of George Hearst, the immensely wealthy silver baron. Hearst owned a large newspaper chain and his papers are credited with fanning the flames that led to the Spanish-American War. In 1919, he began building the ostentatious Hearst Castle on 250,000 acres of California's central coast originally purchased by his father in 1865. During the 1920s and '30s, W.R. lavishly entertained celebrities and politicians at the castle with his mistress, actress Marion Davies.*

When immigration from Mexico to the United States increased after the start of the Mexican Revolution (1910), Hearst's papers' coverage of the phenomenon was based on sensationalism, exaggeration and distortion known as "yellow" journalism (named after the first comic strip character, "The Yellow Kid," which had started in a Hearst paper). Hearst-papers lambasted Mexican immigrants for laziness and contributing to crime. Rather counter-intuitively, the Hearst papers also raised concerns about Mexican immigrants unfairly competing for American jobs, and most significantly introduced "marijuana" into the American lexicon and tied in to their negative portrayal of Mexicans. Hearst papers repeatedly painted a picture of Mexicans as lazy, pot-smoking and criminally inclined.

In the ramp up to the 1914 Harrison Act, Hearst took a similarly racist approach towards reporting about Negroes and Chinese. He referred to the Chinese as "the Yellow Peril". Hearst's newspapers claimed that the majority of incidents in which Negroes were said to have raped white women, could be traced directly to cocaine. Then in the mid-1920s, after 10 years of claiming "cocaine-crazed Negroes" were raping white women, the Hearst line morphed into "marijuana-crazed Negroes" raping white women. [31]

What Hearst's motives were for the sensational hysterical stories on cannabis appearing in his newspapers are speculative. They range from nothing more than a desire to sell more newspapers, to fear of competition from hemp paper to anger at Pancho Villa, who had appropriated over 1,000,000 acres of his land in northern Mexico during the Mexican Revolution, or just the same old anti-Hispanic racist bias already exhibited by Hearst. Whatever his reasons, his papers printed many lurid, cannabis horror stories, many written by Harry Anslinger, that were Anslinger later called "the gore files". Anslinger introduced these newspaper articles at the Congressional hearings regarding the Marijuana Tax Act as "evidence" of the evils of marijuana. Upon closer historical examination, few if any of these tales proved to be true. [32]

Being an effective propagandist, Hearst did not use the term "cannabis" in discussing this issue. Cannabis was a word very familiar to most Americans. Cannabis and hemp were found in many commercial products – rope, paper, bird seed, paint, and medicine. Since the word "cannabis" was not foreign sounding nor fear-evoking to the ear of 1937 Americans, some other name, a more fear-invoking word was needed. It turned out the word was "marihuana" or marijuana, a slang term for cannabis used by far less than 3% of the 1930's American population.

Marijuana and cannabis were not presented to Americans as equal and identical because this would

**Lurid headlines and article titles**
from W.R. Hearst's newspapers
mostly from 1935

"Marihuana makes fiends of boys in thirty days – Hashish goads users to bloodlust."

"Murders due to Killer Drug Marijuana Sweeping United States."

"Murder Weed Found Up and Down Coast – Deadly Marijuana Dope Plant Ready for Harvest..."

"By the tons it is coming into this country – the deadly, dreadful poison that racks and tears not only the body, but the very heart and soul of every human being who once becomes a slave to it in any of its cruel and devastating forms ... Marihuana is a short cut to the insane asylum. Smoke marihuana cigarettes for a month and what was you're your brain will be nothing but a storehouse of horrid specters. Hasheesh makes a murderer who kills for the love of killing out of the mildest mannered man who ever laughed at the idea that any habit could ever get him ..."

"Users of marihuana become STIMULATED as they inhale the drug and are LIKELY TO DO ANYTHING. Most crimes of violence in this section, especially in country districts are laid to users of that drug."

"Was it marijuana, the new Mexican drug, that nerved the murderous arm of Clara Phillips when she hammered out her victim's life in Los Angeles? ... THREE-FOURTHS OF THE CRIMES of violence in this country today are committed by DOPE SLAVES – that is a matter of cold record."

"Marihuana influenced negroes to look at white people in the eye, step on white men's shadows, and look at a white woman twice." [33,34]

have connected marijuana to the well-known ingredient of the numerous familiar and easily obtainable popular patent medicines. Cannabis was a popular ingredient in patent medicines. Familiar cannabis-containing potions were produced by such well-known companies as Eli Lilly, Squibb, Merck and Smith Bros. These medicines had been available for nearly a century apparently harmed no one and provided others with relief. In the late 1800s, cannabis was the third most commonly used medicine in the United States after opium and alcohol. [35] It's hard to demonize what people have seen for decades with their own eyes to be essentially harmless and with practical value.

## Harry Anslinger

The Federal Bureau of Narcotics and Dangerous Drug (FBNDD, aka just the FBN) was formed in 1930, shortly before Prohibition came to an ignominious end. The FBN was responsible for enforcing federal drug laws against heroin, opium, and cocaine. Harry J. Anslinger, an agent in the federal Prohibition bureaucracy, was appointed the FBN's first director.

Anslinger had married Andrew Mellon's niece. Mellon was a wealthy financier and, not so coincidentally, the du Pont family's banker. Mellon was also secretary of the U.S. Treasury. It was in this capacity that he appointed his niece's husband, Anslinger, to be the first director of the FBN. This was a post that Anslinger held until President John F. Kennedy accepted his resignation in 1962. [36] Some reports say JFK fired him in 1961 but then re-hired him for a few months.

In 1933, Anslinger launched a national propaganda campaign, speaking across the country and writing many commentaries in newspapers and magazines – with assistance from the Hearst syndicate – against what he called the evils of "marihuana" or marijuana. Anslinger asserted a bogus relationship between marijuana (but not cannabis) with murder, mayhem, Mexicans, Negroes, jazz and sex. This became his mantra. This racist PR assault culminated in the enactment of the Marijuana Tax Act of 1937.

The U.N.'s Single Convention Treaty of 1961 required all signatory countries to adopt and maintain domestic legislation and penal measure against cannabis and other drugs. Although Anslinger wasn't an official U.S. delegate to the convention at the time (he was appointed by JFK in 1962), he was heavily involved with drafting and lobbying for the Single Convention's section on marijuana. This was Anslinger's last hurrah as FBN chief, and he believed it would make it impossible for the U.S. government to relax its marijuana policies.[37] However, Anslinger later turned against ratification of the treaty because it permitted the continued use of cannabis for "medical and scientific purposes."[38]

Anslinger worked hard to associate the word "marijuana" (that foreign, Mexican word) with depraved behavior and heinous acts. He was a great publicist. These alleged drug-crazed acts were trumpeted in lurid magazine articles he authored, including "Youth Gone Loco" and "Sex Crazing Drug Menace". His most well-known article was probably "Marijuana, Assassin of Youth", which appeared in the *America Magazine* in 1937. In it Anslinger wrote, "No one knows when he places a marijuana cigarette to his lips, whether he will become a joyous reveler in a musical heaven, a mad insensate, a calm philosopher or a crazed killer."[39]

Anslinger claimed that marijuana "can arouse in blacks and Hispanics a state of menacing fury or homicidal attack. During this period, addicts have perpetrated some of the most bizarre and fantastic offenses and sex crimes known to police annals."[40]

Even doctors open to the possibility that marijuana could lead to uncontrolled madness were disappointed when they attempted to confirm this allegation for themselves. Ernest L. Abel describes a 1922 site visit to a Texas jail by an American prison physician, Dr. M. V. Ball, one of America's few authorities on marihuana. He made this trip representing the American Medical Association to get a firsthand look at the alleged dangers of marihuana. The warden gave an inmate a marihuana cigarette to smoke so that Ball could see for himself

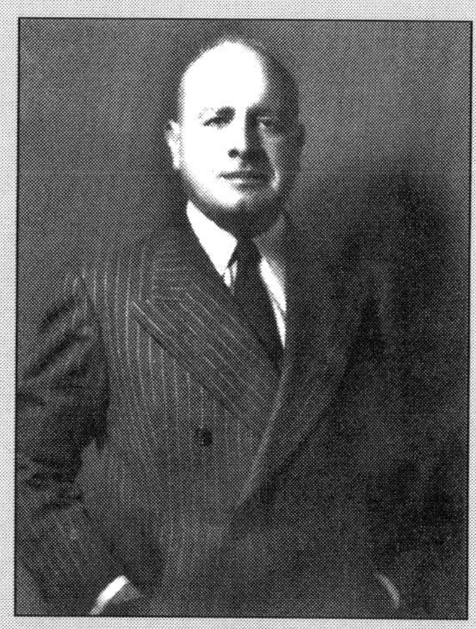

*In 1929, Harry Anslinger became head of the Federal Bureau of Narcotics. He often used Hearst's newspapers as a platform for his drug-demonization propaganda – putting the spotlight on cannabis. Anslinger made a bogus connection between "marijuana" (he didn't use the word "cannabis") and murder, mayhem, Mexicans, Negroes, jazz and sex. This became his mantra. This racist assault culminated in the 1937 Marijuana Tax Act.*

After retiring, Anslinger allegedly once mused that the FBN was a place where young men were given a license to steal and rape.[41] He was very ambitious and took advantage of the career opportunity offered by this new government agency, the FBN. In that capacity, he was able to define both the problem and the solution. As someone born in the Victorian era and as his public utterances demonstrate, he was a racist to boot Cannabis which he called marijuana was an ideal vehicle upon which to build his bureaucratic fiefdom. Anslinger used the themes of racism and violence to draw national attention to what heretofore (the consumption of cannabis) had not only been a non-problem, but had been an accepted medicine for over three-quarters of a century.

Anslinger frequented parent's and teacher's meetings, giving scary speeches about the dangers of marijuana. He worked hard at getting uniform drug laws passed in all states and in the federal Congress.

what it did to a man. To the surprise of the American prison physician and the jailer, who assured him three wiffs would drive fellows so wild that they become exceptionally difficulty to subdue, the smoker remained calm and unperturbed. [42]

## All that Jazz

Once in office, Anslinger denounced jazz as wild, untamed and primitive. He grew increasingly anxious over the popularity of dark-skinned musicians with lighter-skinned women. His racist brain reasoned that "there had to be some sort of magic chemical cocktail which some of the greatest musicians of all time were using to attract otherwise sane women of skin lighter than theirs." [43] Anslinger insisted this satanic music and the use of marijuana caused white women to seek sexual relations with Negroes.

Anslinger shared conservative public concern that the jazz scene in the 1920s and '30s led white and Black musicians to work and socialize together. Worse yet, Anslinger warned the white middle-class that Blacks and whites were dancing together in *tea houses*. Marijuana, he claimed, fueled the jazz scene.

> **"There are 100,000 total marijuana smokers in the U.S., and most are Negroes, Mexicans, Filipinos and entertainers. Their Satanic music, jazz and swing, result from marijuana usage. This marijuana causes white women to seek sexual relations with Negroes, entertainers and any others."**
>
> **Harry J. Anslinger**
> testimony to Congress, 1937
> in support of the Marijuana Tax Act

Added to Anslinger's personal dislike of jazz music was his disdain for the musicians, Black and white alike, who made it. He hated jazz musicians and what they stood for in his mind. He spent years tracking and keeping a file on many prominent jazz musicians. He threw in a few actors, singers and comedians for good measure. He spied on such greats of the time as Louis Armstrong, Count Basie, Milton Berle, Les Brown, Cab Calloway, Jimmy Dorsey, Duke Ellington, Dizzy Gillespie, Jackie Gleason, Benny Goodman, Lionel Hampton, Andre Kostelanetz, Kate Smith, and the NBC Orchestra. Anslinger dreamed of arresting them all in one huge, cross-country sweep. [44]

In 1947, Anslinger sent out the following letter to his agents:

> Dear Agent,
>
> Please prepare all cases in your jurisdiction involving musicians in violation of the marijuana laws. We will have a great national round-up arrest of all such persons on a single day. I will let you know what day. [45]
>
> Harry J. Anslinger, FBN

This plan was squelched in 1948 by his boss, Assistant Secretary of the Treasury Edward H. Foley, in a memo that read: "Mr. Foley Disapproves". [46, 47]

After doing research for the 1998, over-the-top satirical musical, *Reefer Madness: The Musical*, co-author

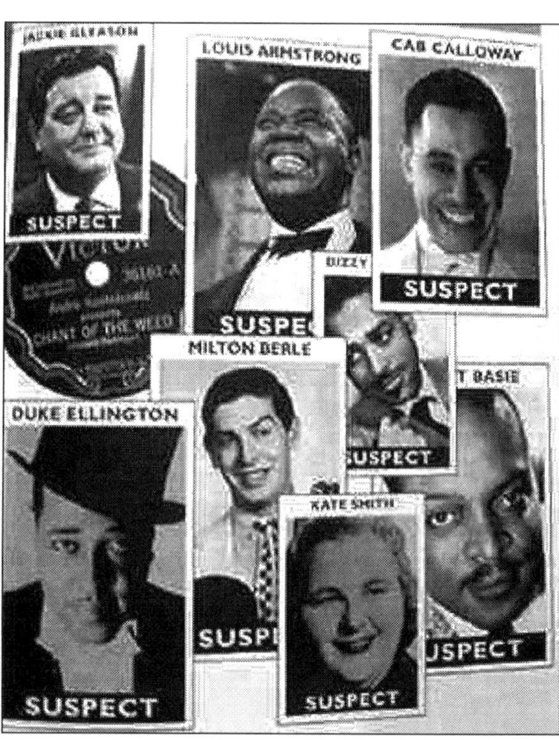


*Anslinger was on a crusade, which included targeting many jazz stars, as well as the occasional comedian and singer. This is a sampling of these targets as identified in Jack Herer's 1985 book,* The Emperor Wears No Clothes.

Some of

**Anslinger's Memorable Quotes**

regarding marijuana:

"Reefer makes darkies think they're as good as white men."

"...the primary reason to outlaw marijuana is its effect on the degenerate races."

"I believe in some cases one marijuana cigarette might develop a homicidal mania, probably to kill his brother ... All experts agree that the continued use of marijuana leads to insanity."

"Marijuana is an addictive drug which produces in its users insanity, criminality, and death."

"Marihuana leads to pacifism and communist brainwashing."

"You smoke a joint and you're likely to kill your brother."

"Marijuana is the most violence-causing drug in the history of mankind." [48]

Kevin Murphy characterized Harry J. Anslinger as someone who was "kind of an insane pit bull, a crazy racist." Murphy said "Hearst's papers would print wild stories – about this kid in Florida that hacked up his entire family with a pickax because he was high on marijuana – and Anslinger would cut out those articles and go before the Congress." [49] In the referenced Florida murder case, the perpetrator had a long, well-documented history of mental illness. Murphy thought the murders were the result of the killer's insanity and unrelated to any marijuana use, real or imagined.

## Congressional Hearings on the Marijuana Tax Act of 1937

Shortly after the U.S. Supreme Court found the 1934 National Firearms Act constitutional, Herman Oliphant, top attorney in the Department of Commerce, moved rapidly to introduce the Marijuana Tax Act to the U.S. House of Representatives. House committees such as Agriculture and Commerce could have heard the proposed act and held hearings, but it went to Ways and Means, a committee that could send it to the floor directly. Thus, the Act moved swiftly through Congress with a low profile. [50] It may be just a coincidence but the House vote was in August, a hot, unpleasant month in Washington, particularly in a time of little air conditioning. Anyone that could, usually left town.

At the hearings, Anslinger testified that cannabis was a dangerous drug that was corrupting the minds of America's youth. He said, "Marijuana is the most violence causing drug in the history of mankind." [51] Anslinger painted marijuana as an evil scourge and assigned responsibility for much of America's crimes to marijuana. Evidence, such as it was, was a fist full of clippings straight out of William Randolph Hearst's national newspapers!

---

**"History has shown Anslinger to be nothing less than a madman who craved public attention and went to great lengths to create mostly lies and distortions about what he termed the *Assassin of Youth* (the title of a book he wrote)."** [52]
(Author's note: This was actually a magazine article, although later the title of a movie.)

**Randall G. Shelden**
*Las Vegas Mercury*, 2002

---

## AMA's Opposition at the Hearings

In 1937, the American Medical Association (AMA) testified in the committee hearings in opposition to the Marijuana Tax Act. They saw no need or basis for it. There were 28 patent medicines with cannabis on the market in 1937 and no problems with cannabis were known to the AMA. [53] Their spokesperson and lobbyist, Dr. William Woodward, stated flat out that "The AMA knows of no evidence that marijuana is a dangerous drug." [54] The AMA's testimony is convincing evidence that anti-marijuana legislation was not introduced and passed due to health concerns.

Dr. Woodward was no neophyte to Congressional proceedings and hearings. He had previously been health commissioner for Washington D.C. and Boston. He had participated in drafting both the Harrison Narcotics Tax Act of 1914 and the Uniform Narcotics Code in 1926. For over 40 years, he had been testifying before Congress on a range of topics, many related to drug policy. [55]

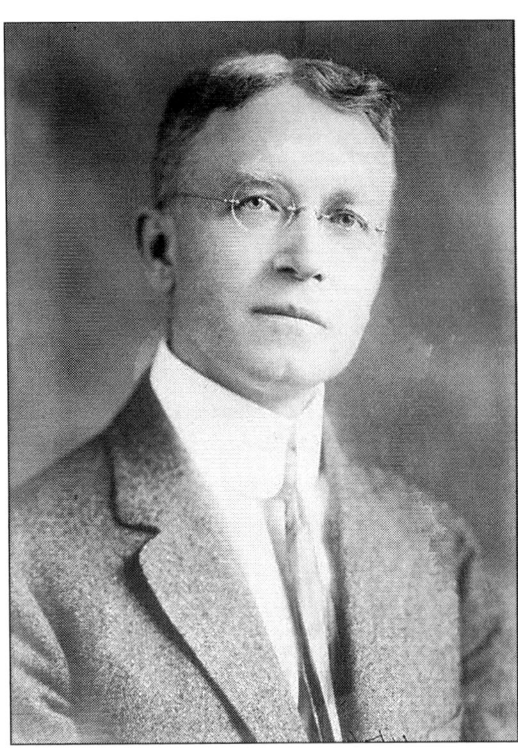

*William C. Woodward not only was a lawyer, doctor and the AMA's chief lobbyist, but he was also past president of the American Public Health Association (1914).* [84] *He had been the health commissioner of Washington, D.C. from 1893 to 1913 and later was the health commissioner of Boston. He provided the AMA's input on drug policy during Congressional hearings on the Harrison Narcotics Tax Act of 1914 and the Marijuana Tax Act of 1937.*

In his testimony, Dr. Woodward questioned the factual basis of the hearings. He claimed that the entire fabric of federal testimony was woven out of tabloid sensationalism. He alleged that Anslinger "facts" were simply a bunch of newspaper clippings. Woodward testified that there was no hard data to support the need for the law.

Woodward pointed out that Anslinger obtained no data from any government agency, bureau or department to support his outrageous allegations. [56] In preparing his testimony, Woodward had contacted the Bureau of Prisons, the Children's Bureau, the Office of Education, and the Division of Mental Health of the U.S. Public Health Service. None of them had any information to support Anslinger's wild charges. (It should be noted that latter research into Anslinger's testimony/allegations confirmed the accuracy of Dr. Woodward's testimony.)

He also slammed Anslinger for distorting earlier AMA statements that had nothing to do with marijuana to make them appear to be an AMA endorsement of Anslinger's view. Dr. Woodward made it clear that the AMA was opposed to the legislation.

Woodward was adamant that even if Congress passed the Act into law, they should not call it the Marijuana Tax Act, since no one knew what drug they were talking about. He argued for the use of the word "*cannabis*." The AMA lost on that issue, too.

The National Oil Seed Institute also testified against the Tax Act. The organization represented the high-quality machine lubrication producers and paint manufacturers. The Institute's general counsel, Ralph Loziers, vigorously described the adverse impact of outlawing hempseed oil. He testified:

> "If the Committee pleases, the hemp seed, or the seed of the cannabis sativa, is used in all the Oriental nations and also in a part of Russia as food. It is grown in their fields and used as oatmeal. Millions of people every day are using hempseed in the Orient as food. They have been doing that for many generations, especially in periods of famine ... The point I make is this – that this bill is too all inclusive. This bill is a world encircling measure. This bill brings the activities – the crushing of this great industry under the supervision of a bureau – which may mean its suppression. Last year, there was imported into the U.S. 62,813,000 pounds of hempseed. In 1935 there was imported 116 million pounds..." [57]

Matt Rens of the Rens Hemp Company seemed to catch on to DuPont's surreptitious scheming. In his testimony at the 1937 House Committee hearings, Rens prophetically said: "Such a tax would put all small producers out of the business of growing hemp, and the proportion of small producers is considerable ... The real purpose of this bill is not to raise money, is it." [58]

## The Real Deal?

Woodward's testimony provides support for those who see this as a law directed not at cannabis but at hemp. Woodward testified, that over the two-year preparation period ostensibly for a taxation bill, no one in Congress or the executive branch had informed the AMA (1) that this legislation was being discussed (2) that it was about cannabis (the scientific name of the plant in question), (3) nor asked for their input in drafting it.

> **"We cannot understand yet, Mr. Chairman why this bill should have been prepared in secret for two years without any intimation, even to the profession, that it was being prepared."** [59]
>
> **William C. Woodward, M.D.**
> American Medical Association
> representative in the Congressional hearings

Was this not an oblique reference to the two-year, behind-the-scenes lobbying of Herman Oliphant, chief counsel of the U.S. Treasury Department (1934-39), by Lammot du Pont and other commercial-industrial interests?

## Further Chicanery

Rather amazingly, when the Marijuana Tax Act bill came to a vote on the floor of the House of Representatives, only one pertinent question was asked from the floor: "Did anyone consult with the AMA and get their opinion?"

Representative Fred Vinson of Kentucky, answering for the Ways and Means Committee, replied, "Yes, we have." He stated that the committee had heard from "a Dr. Wharton." Vinson not only mistakenly identified Woodward as Wharton, he also completely turned Woodward's testimony upside down, replying that "the AMA are in complete agreement!" [60]

Because the Congress was overwhelmingly Democratic, and the AMA of the 1930s had strong Republican leanings, this memorable piece of faulty memory wasn't even necessary.

Vinson went on to become the chief justice of the U.S. Supreme Court (1946-53) and not a particularly

**The AMA's Dr. William Woodward looked for government data about the evils of cannabis and found none.**

"We are told that the use of marijuana causes crime. Yet no one has been produced from the Bureau of Prisons to show the number of prisoners who have been found addicted to the marijuana habit. An informal inquiry (by Woodward) shows that the Bureau of Prisons has no evidence on that point." [61]

He testified that he made "inquiry of the Office of Education, and they should know something of the prevalence of the habit among the school children of the country, if there is a prevalent habit – indicates that they have had no occasion to investigate and know nothing of it."

He continued that "in the Treasury Department itself, the Public Heath Service, with its Division of Mental Hygiene. The Division of Mental Hygiene was, in the first place, the Division of Narcotics. It was converted into the Division of Mental Hygiene, I think, about 1930. That particular Bureau has control at the present time of the narcotics farms that were created about 1929 or 1930 and came into operation a few years later. No one has been summoned from that Bureau to give evidence on that point. Informal inquiry by me indicates that they have had no record of any marijuana or cannabis addicts who have ever been committed to those farms."

"The bureau of Public Health Service has also a division of pharmacology. If you desire evidence as to the pharmacology of Cannabis, that obviously is the place where you can get direct and primary evidence, rather than the indirect hearsay evidence." [62]

*(Note: All Woodward quotes are from the official records of the Marijuana Tax Act hearings before the U.S. House of Representatives Ways and Means Committee in 1937, as taken from the hearing transcript printed in the Summer 2006 issue of* O'Shaughnessy's.)

memorable one. Court historians that mention this Kentucky Democrat, label him as an incompetent jurist and a Southern political hack reluctant to tamper with segregation. [63]

The bill passed, was signed into law on August 2, 1937, and became effective in December 1937. Federal and state police forces were created to enforce the law. This was a great success for those in corporate America who had put profits before ethics and a boon to the federal bureaucracy and the police profession.

## Why the stealth?

Clearly some saw hemp as a crop to be reckoned with. The February 1938 issue of *Popular Mechanics* hailed cannabis as the "New Billion-Dollar Crop," while a concurrent issue of *Mechanical Engineering* deemed hemp "The Most Profitable and Desirable Crop That Can Be Grown." A 1938 article in Popular Mechanics, "Billion Dollar Crop", (printed four months after the enactment of The Marihuana Tax Act) proclaimed that the hemp industry had a rosy future. [64]

The 1938 *Popular Mechanics* article stated:

> "Thousands of tons of hemp hurds are used every year by one large powder company for the manufacture of dynamite and TNT. The natural materials in hemp make it an economical source of pulp for any grade of paper manufactured, and the high percentage of alpha cellulose promises an unlimited supply of raw material for the thousands of cellulose products our chemists have developed." [65]

## Follow the Money

The questions are: why was hemp included in this law and was cannabis made illegal under false pretense? Was the Marijuana Tax Act just a way to boost petrochemical interests at the expense of agriculture interests?

Jack Herer, in *The Emperor Wears No Clothes* (1985 edition), and many other authorities have suggested that commerce played a major, secretive role in the passage of the Marijuana Tax Act. They believe the Act was engineered by DuPont Co., other oil/petrochemical interests, and Hearst to prevent competition from hemp.

The fate of Schlichter's decorticator suggests that this concern about competition from hemp had been present among industrialists since shortly after the 1916 USDA monograph touting the renewed commercial viability of hemp. The AMA's testimony against the Act lends considerable credence to Herer's claim that wealth, not health, was the motivation for this far-reaching piece of legislation.

Based on the research done for his musical "Reefer Madness", co-author Kevin Murphy also concluded that Hearst and DuPont were seeking to protect their investments (paper production and petrochemicals/synthetic fibers, respectively). Murphy's research led him to conclude that they joined with Andrew Mellon, DuPont's banker, to quash the competitor, hemp.

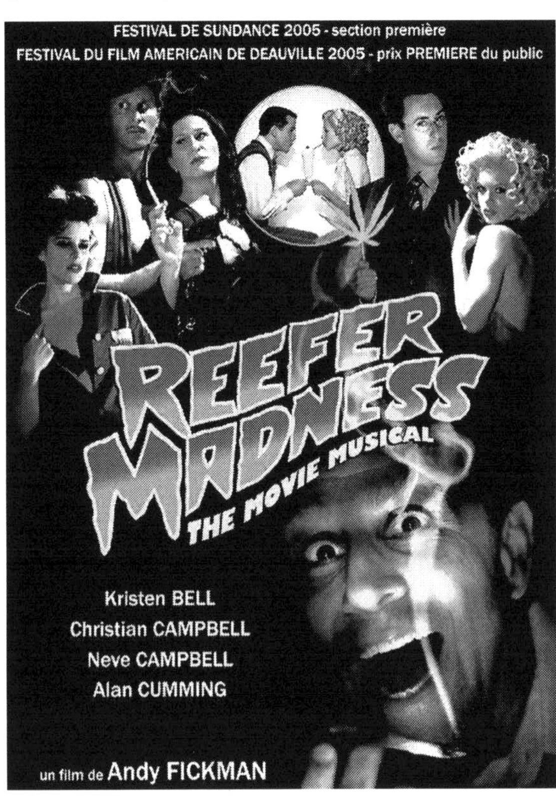


*The 1936 propaganda movie* Reefer Madness *is the ultimate kitsch. It was such an icon of misinformation that its own words were self-parody. In the first decade of the 21st century,* Reefer Madness: The Movie Musical *played to enthusiastic audiences throughout the United States that laughed at the preposterous allegations made in the original movie.*

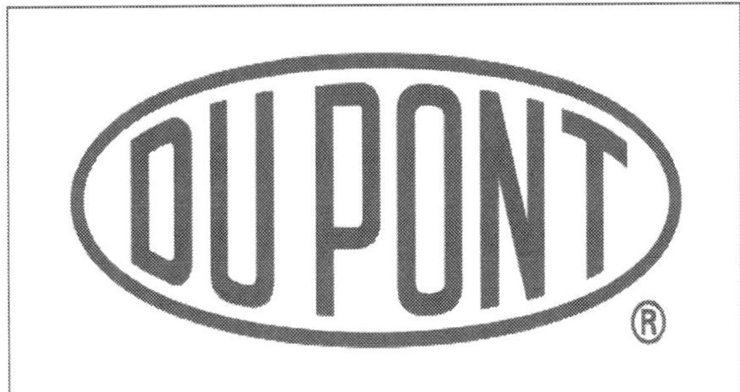


There's no question but that DuPont, Hearst and petrochemical interests had a lot to lose if they had to compete with hemp on a level playing field. Paper made from hemp cost about half as much as paper made from trees, uses 75% less chemicals, and substantially decreases biodegradation. Hemp is an annual crop; it's renewable, unlike a forest, which takes 20-30 years to grow.

Both Hearst and DuPont were heavily invested in wood-processing for paper and stood to lose a lot of their investments if paper were to be made from hemp. Hearst owned tens of thousands of acres of pine forest for pulp production. Oil, paper and fabric made from petrochemicals were all important profit centers for DuPont. In 1937, DuPont had developed the sulfate and sulfite processes for manufacture of pulp paper. DuPont also supplied Hearst with these essential chemicals, which would no longer be needed in the same quantity if paper were made from hemp

Du Pont's stake in the oil business is traced to the company's development and patenting in the 1920s and '30s of fuel additives such as tetraethyl lead. Plus, the du Pont family was heavily invested in the automobile manufacturer; General Motors Co. DuPont also had several new synthetic products such as nylon, cellophane, and other plastics. In the 1930s, they purchased the rights to produce rayon from I.M. Farben of Germany. [66] The DuPont Company was expecting that these synthetic, petrochemical-based products would be one of its main sources of income in the years ahead. [67]

At the same time, some of DuPont's competitor companies were developing synthetic products from renewable biological resources — especially hemp. Cannabis was seen as a threat because of its magnificent fiber durability, which would compete against DuPont's nylon and other synthetic fibers. Hemp's inner hurd could more safely and efficiently be used in the manufacture of paper and simple plastics. Fuel from hemp didn't need the tetraethyl lead additive that was a standard gasoline additive until the late 1970s, when its airborne pollution was discovered to be dangerous to humans.

One can imagine that there was a lot of celebrating in the du Pont and Hearst castles when the Marijuana Tax Act came into law.

## The Impact of the Act

The tax was not large but it was a nuisance. At the time, reliance on medicinal cannabis by physicians was in decline, in part due to lack of standardization of the cannabis-containing products and in part because plant based medicines were seen as old fashioned. Although the Marijuana Tax Act only made the non-medical and untaxed use of the drug illegal, many manufacturers elected not to register and pay the tax. They just stopped using cannabis in their patent medicine formula.

Even though cannabis was removed in 1941 from the United States Pharmacopoeia (USP), a semi-official compendium of commonly used pharmaceuticals, that didn't stop the long-time editor of *JAMA*, Dr. Morris Fishbein, from declaring in 1942 that cannabis was still the most effective treatment for migraine headaches. [68] Nor did it deter the New York Academy of Medicine from recommending in 1944, as part of the La Guardia Crime Commission Report, that the recreational use of cannabis should be legalized.

Dr. Tod Mikuriya, a former National Institute of Mental Health official in the late 1960s and modern medical cannabis pioneer, noted that the Federal Bureau of Narcotics was enormously successful at arresting a lot of people. He said:

> **"This law and the companion state laws have seen the incarceration of hundreds of thousands of Americans, adding up to more than 14 million wasted years in jails and prisons. Some young men have been sexually molested and gotten AIDS. This was all for the sake of poisonous, polluting industries, prison guard unions, and to reinforce some**

**white politicians' policies of racial hatred."** [69, 70, 71, 72, 73]

## Cannabis Is Medicine

Dr. Woodward's testimony in the Congressional hearing was consistent with the years of experience the AMA and American physicians had had with medicinal cannabis. Cannabis had been in the United States Pharmacopoeia since 1854. [74] At the time of the hearings in 1937, there were still at least 28 cannabis-containing medicines on the U.S. market. [75] This was only a little over 20 years after the widely acknowledged father of modern medicine, Sir William Osler, in his *Textbook of Internal Medicine*, called cannabis the best treatment for migraines. [76]

Not all government officials agreed with Anslinger's apocalyptic view of cannabis. In 1937, Assistant U.S. Surgeon General Walter Treadway was minimizing cannabis harms. He told Congress that "Marihuana is habit-forming ... in the same sense as ... sugar or coffee." [77] This was only four years after J.F. Siler, et al, published their findings that the Army need take no action to control cannabis use among the military in Panama. [78]

Dr. Woodward was a seer when it came to realizing the incredible future medicinal possibilities for cannabis. His 1937 congressional testimony included this prescient remark: "To say, however, as has been proposed here, that the use of the drug should be prevented by a prohibitive tax, loses sight of the fact that future investigation may show that there are substantial medical uses." [79]

Today, many try to stifle or marginalize discussion about cannabis by use of a pejorative vocabulary. Cannabis is often referred to as marijuana or worse, demeaned as pot, weed, dope, or devil weed. People who use cannabis are called "dopers", and people that provide it to their friends are called "drug dealers." People that use cannabis for medicinal purposes aren't "sick", or if they are, they are referred to as "dupes" or tools of the supporters of marijuana legalization.

America needs a productive discussion on drug policy. In order to have such a conversation, the use of neutral, less inflammatory terminology is needed. This discussion should be based on science, common sense, the Constitution, and not hysterical rhetoric.

## The Food, Drug, and Cosmetic Act of 1938

In 1938, the S.E. Massengill Co. introduced a new sulfa drug, Elixir Sulfanolamide. Unfortunately for the users, it contained a chemical similar to anti-freeze and over 100 people died. This triggered the Congress to pass a law requiring that drug safety be proven before a new drug was put on the market. The Federal Food, Drug, and Cosmetic Act of 1938 required the testing all new drugs for safety to gain the approval of the U.S. Food and Drug Administration (FDA). The 1938 Act remains the cornerstone of federal drug regulation.

A major, possibly unintended, result of the law was that it institutionalized the concept that single-chemical compounds were superior to plants. The law was clearly directed at manufactured pharmaceuticals, not naturally occurring plants and herbs grown for personal, not commercial use. However, it soon became conventional wisdom that single chemicals acted with more specificity and presumably better than the multiplicity of chemicals found in plants.

Soon after the 1938 Act was implemented, the FDA began to identify not only drugs that were unsafe to be marketed at all, but other drugs, such as the sulfas, which they found were not safe to be used directly by patients and must be prescribed by a physician.

The law exempted all drugs then on the market (so-called "old" drugs), which included cannabis, at least until cannabis came out of the United States Pharmacopeial Convention in 1942. The FDA soon categorized cannabis — this drug with a 100-year history of medical use in the United States and over 5,000 years of medical use by humankind — as a "new" drug.

### Drug, Herb, Vitamin, Food – Who Defines?

From 1938 to this day, there is a debate between the FDA, pharmaceutical industry, vitamin and herbal medicine purveyors, and health practitioners of various stripes over what constitutes a prescription, an over-the-counter drug, a homeopathic prescription, or a dietary supplement. Much of the ground rules for this debate were laid down in the Durham-Humphrey Amendment of 1951. The bill requires any drug that is habit-forming or potentially harmful to be dispensed under the supervision of a health practitioner as a prescription drug and must carry the statement, "Caution: Federal law prohibits dispensing without prescription." [80]

The question today is: How long is the FDA's reach? Should it include vitamins? When the FDA tried to include vitamins within their purview in the late twentieth century, Congress told them their reach exceeded their grasp. Well, what about plants and herbs or animals like the psychedelic frog?

In *From Chocolate to Morphine: Everything You Need to Know About Mind Altering Drugs* (1983), Dr. Andrew Weil and Winifred Rosen used two pages to explain that the same substances in different times, places and dosages have been variously accepted as a food, spice, ethnogeny, erotic stimulant, poison, tool of the devil and/or mind expander. Who decides? Are the food preservatives, dyes, and genetically altered plants, food or something else? The vocabulary regarding drug policy has become a "Brave New World" with "1984" double speak language. Herbs are labeled drugs, but drugs that have side effects as long as one's arm aren't dangerous. The word 'medicine' has been bastardized.

Many Americans of diverse cultural backgrounds prefer herbal medicines to prescription medicine or pills found on drug store aisles. Studies show that fully 60% of a modern physician's patients use alternative and complementary medicine and at least 40% of them neglect to share this information with their doctors. This use of herbal medicines should not be a big surprise, although many of these plant products have been used for hundreds, even thousands of years.

Some natural remedies work, at least a little; others don't work at all or have only marginal benefit. Echinacea appears to provide little or no relief for colds, glucosamine and chondroitin have been shown to provide mild relief of joint pain. Earlier studies showed that Saw Palmetto might reduce the size of the prostate in men with benign prostate hypertrophy, however, recent studies demonstrate it's no better than a placebo. The use of Rue for digestive problems or heart palpation is unproven and has safety issues. Some Latinos use Par D'Arco for arthritis and asthma. This herb can cause severe nausea, vomiting and diarrhea. And a few herbs can even be very dangerous (e.g., ephedra comfry) if used in the wrong dosage. [81]

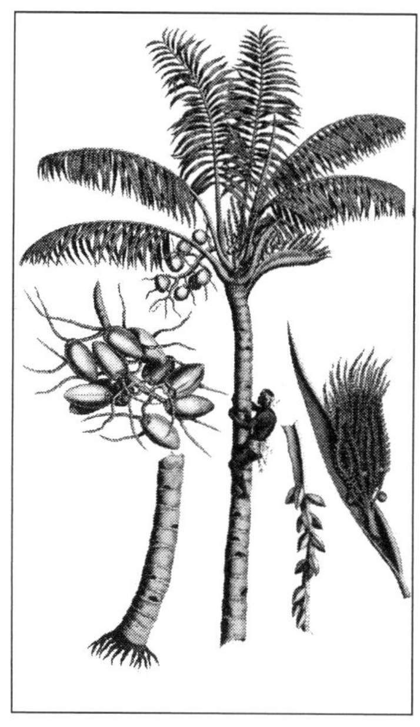

*Mayo Clinic researchers have patented an extract of the atun tree, which is native to Ambon, an island in Indonesia. This is part of a renewed effort to mine the forest for potential pharmaceuticals.*

Plants still provide us with therapeutic agents. Contemporary scientists are examining ancient herbal remedies and studying contemporary shamans in remote areas to see what can be learned for modern medicine. The focus is on which plants and herbs could be potential sources for modern medicines. A decade ago, scientists stumbled on an extract from the yew tree as a treatment for certain cancers. More recently, Eric J. Buenz, a graduate student at the Mayo Clinic, decided to research remedies recorded by the 17th-century Dutch naturalist, Georg Eberhard Rumpf, to see if they were effective.

Buenz wondered whether these 17th-century recipes could help modern day scientists find new and better drugs. Buenz and his colleagues looked into the utility of an extract from the atun tree mentioned in Rumpf's book. The claim was it could cure diarrhea. They stated that "our findings show that potential drugs can be identified by searching historical herbal texts." And the Mayo Clinic scientists have obtained a patent on the medicinal properties of the atun tree nut, in hopes someone might develop it into a drug. [82]

So which, if any, of these traditional herbal remedies should the government protect people against and how should it be accomplished? If the government is allowed to protect citizens against their presumed foolishness or bad judgment, is too dear a price being paid in the loss of American individualism, freedom and liberty?

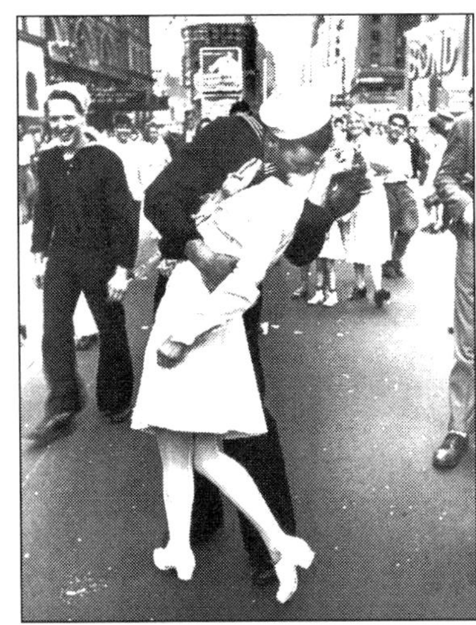

*A sailor kissing a complete stranger in Times Square on the day World War Two ended.*

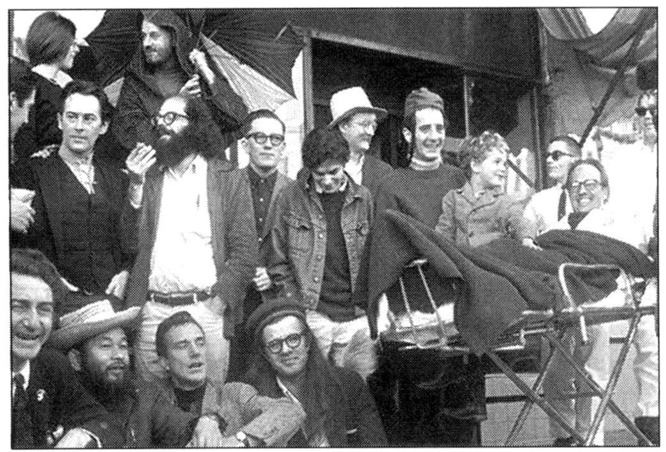

*The so-called "Beat Generation" emerged in the late 1940s. They dressed funny, wrote books and poetry, embraced homosexuality, and smoked marijuana. They were remarkably -- even iontentionally -- unconventional.*

# CHAPTER XII
# 1939-1959: WW II, Post-War Changes & The Beats

## The Germans Are Knocking

The last years of the 1930s were tumultuous. In the grand scheme of things, herbs and the role of the U.S. Food and Drug Administration paled in comparison to the more significant forces impacting people's lives. The depression was still happening and Europe was preparing for war.

As the United States approached WW II, Negroes were still very much oppressed. Nevertheless Negroes, as African Americans were then known, were getting a little more respect because of the emergence of integrated jazz groups. Jazz helped humanize African-Americans to the rest of Americans. But sports also played a big role in this uphill battle for respect. It started before the war with Jesse Owens' four gold-medal performance at the 1936 Olympics in Berlin. This was followed by Joe Louis defeating the German Max Schmeling for the heavyweight championship in 1938. It was helped along by great Negro soprano Marian Anderson singing at the Lincoln Memorial in 1939. This had been arranged by Eleanor Roosevelt, the wife of the very popular president, Franklin D. Roosevelt, after Ms. Anderson was blocked from singing at the capitol's Constitution Hall by the Daughters of the American Revolution.

## War and the Seeds of Change

World War II was a great world challenge to liberty, freedom and democracy. That conflict involved millions of troops. By comparison, with the U.S. commitment of 16,000,000 troops, the Iraq War (2002-2012) looks more like a neighbor-hood dispute.

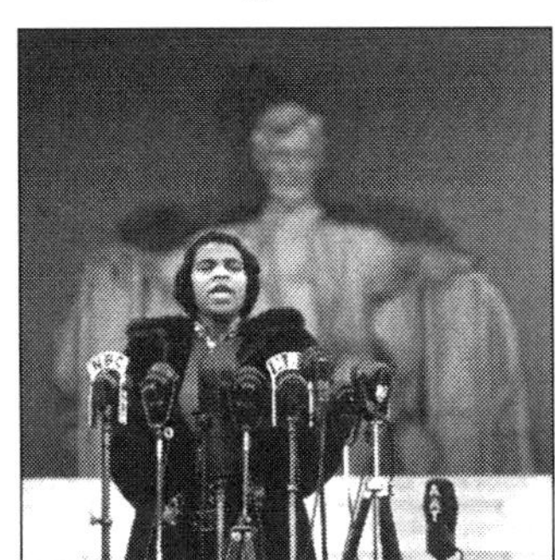

*African-American opera singer Marian Anderson singing in front of the Lincoln Memorial to an integrated audience of 75,000 in 1939 in a concert arranged by First Lady Eleanor Roosevelt.*

When it came to drugs to enhance the troops' energy, the combatants pulled out all the stops. During World War II, Army physicians on all sides (American, British, Japanese, and German) issued amphetamines to their armed forces for alleviation of battle fatigue. [1] It was also used for awhile by American and British long-range bomber pilots.

A combination of barbiturates and amphetamines was popular with American troops during WWII. It was called a "speedball". Getting up from sleep, a person got almost immediately energized with the stimulant (amphetamines), and came down with the hypnotic sedative (barbiturates). "Methamphetamine use was so widespread that Japanese citizens were given the drug to increase wartime productivity. After the war, massive stockpiles of amphetamine were marketed to the Japanese people to increase vitality and energy." [2]

Some soldiers stationed in Korea and Japan during the early 1950s mixed heroin with amphetamine and injected the combination. This was also referred to as a "speedball". [3] A later variation of the more traditional speedball, was heroin and cocaine. This practice didn't stop with WW II and the Korean War. A former Blackwater operative advised this author that amphetamines were readily available in Vietnam. [4]

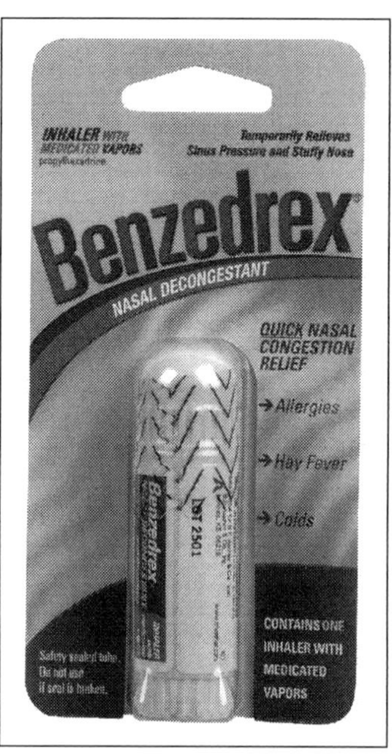


*Benzedrine inhalers contained amphetamine and were available over the counter. It was a popular recreational drug from the 1930s to the early '60s.*

Following WW II, and until well into the 1960s, physicians in the United States routinely prescribed amphetamines for treatment of depression, weight loss and narcolepsy.

### "Who put the Benzedrine in Mrs. Murphy's Ovaltine?"

Popular culture sometimes incorporates a little drug humor into entertainment. This was as true in the 1940s as it is today. Harry "The Hipster" Gibson (1915-91) was an entertainer who made jazz-influenced novelty records. He was a master pianist with a style that was a mixture of ragtime, blues, boogie, traditional jazz and a little bop influence. He wrote the song, "Who Put the Benzedrine in Mrs. Murphy's Ovaltine?", [5] with such lyrics as "she never wants to go to sleep, she says that everything is solid all reet". Lyrics like that were not appreciated in the 1940s and for awhile he was blacklisted by the music industry. Harry made a bit of a comeback in the 1970s when his lyrics were more appreciated.

## We Need Hemp to Go To War.

But the war wasn't funny. The Germans were a brutal bunch, with world domination on their minds. They presented a real threat to the existing order. In 1942, the Japanese cut off America's ability to import India hemp from the Philippines, which posed a significant problem for the war effort. Each WWII-era U.S. battleship required 34,000 feet of rope, preferably made from hemp. Hemp rope was used for towing vessels and for rigging. Hemp was also used for light duty fire hoses, webbing on parachutes and shoe laces. [6]

Something had to be done. So the United States set aside its anti-hemp stance and encouraged farmers to "Grow Hemp for Victory." Prohibiting drugs had been for maintaining power, not losing it.

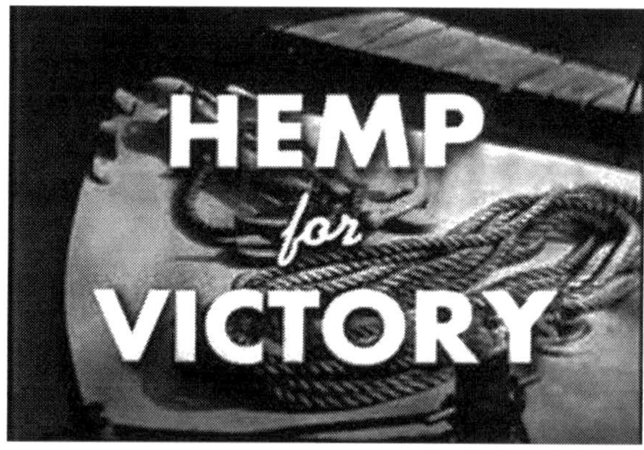


*After the onerous Marijuana Tax Act of 1937 was passed, almost all hemp used in the United States was imported. Because the World War II naval war prevented such importations, the government was forced to institute a "Hemp for Victory" program because hemp was needed in the war effort. It called for planting 300,000 acres of hemp and building 71 processing plants.* [7]

In 1942 and 1943, American farmers were shown a movie, *Hemp for Victory*, on hemp production. It was produced by the U.S. Department of Agriculture (USDA). This pro-hemp propaganda film exhorted farmers to grow hemp. It reminded farmers how to grow hemp. Growing hemp was deemed so important to the war effort that, if a farmer participated in the Hemp for Victory Campaign, both he and his sons were exempt from serving in WWII. [8]

The call to patriotism and the draft exemption were effective in dramatically increasing the acres planted in hemp in America in the early 1940s. A blurb in the August 4, 1943 *Chicago Tribune*, which was headlined "Hemp Acreage is Quadrupled in Wisconsin", noted that the 1943 hemp crop was 31,000 acres; over four times the acreage of 1942. The total acreage in hemp production for all of the United States was estimated to be 226,000 acres. [9, 10]

Dialogue in USDA's movie exhorting farmers to grow hemp stated:

> "For thousands of years, even then, this plant had been grown for cordage and cloth in China and elsewhere in the Far East. For centuries until about 1850, all the ships that sailed the western seas were rigged with hemp rope and sails. For the sailor, no less than the hangman, hemp was indispensable ... Now with Philippine and East Indian sources of hemp in the hands of the Japanese ... American hemp must meet the needs of our Army and Navy as well as our industries... The Navy's rapidly dwindling reserves. When that is gone, American hemp will go on duty again; hemp for mooring ships; hemp for tow lines; hemp for tackle and gear; hemp for countless naval uses both on ship and shore as in the days when Old Ironsides sailed the seas victorious with her hemp shrouds and hempen sails. Hemp for victory!"

The war effort saw thousands of acres of hemp planted in Iowa, Minnesota, and Wisconsin. These farmers produced 63,000 tons of hemp. [11] The Defense Plant Corporation actually built 42 hemp-processing plants throughout the Midwest. [12]

## Going, Going, Gone

> "First they came for the Communists, and I didn't speak up, because I wasn't a Communist. Then they came for the Jews, and I didn't speak up, because I wasn't a Jew. They came for the trade unionists and I was silent. Then they came for the Catholics, and I didn't speak up, because I was a Protestant. Then they came for me, and by that time there was no one left to speak up for me."

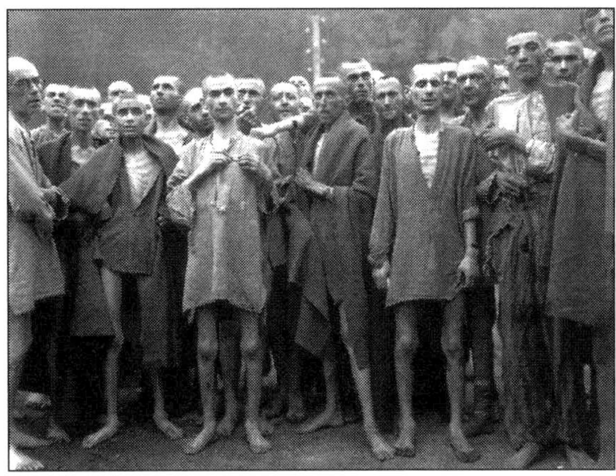

*Starving prisoners in Mauthausen concentration camp were liberated on May 5, 1945.*

These are the words of German Lutheran Reverend Martin Niemoller in 1944, speaking of the Nazis. He was arrested and placed in detainment. He survived the war and lived into the 1960s.

The words of Reverend Niemoller should stand as a warning to everyone. Incursions to the freedoms and liberties of others, will likely lead to incursions to the freedoms and liberties of everyone. Individuals must defend against such incursions or everyone may lose them for themselves.

Misinformation and demonization has taken Americans down a road of criminalization of substance use and abuse. In the process, precious Constitutional rights and liberties have been trimmed and dissipated. Drug abuse has become a modern boogeyman. This fear is clouding American's perception of the wisdom of the national's Founding Fathers. For example, trials in federal court do not permit the introduction of a medical marijuana defense. Does this sound like the idealized American justice system?

A scientific, medical, and educational drug-abuse treatment and prevention approach is much more likely to be effective and consistent with historic

American values than turning the Constitution inside out and giving the federal government unprecedented power. Some of these alternatives will be explored in latter chapters.

## West Coast Xenophobia

Side by side with handing out speed to the troops and the call to raise "Hemp for Victory", the WWII years in America saw the relentless demonization of recreational drugs and ethnic minorities. In addition to the heroin- and marijuana-using jazz musicians, the marijuana-using Mexican zoot suiters came under fire. But other xenophobic forces were at work, too.

### Internment of Japanese

In WWII, the allies (U.S. and Canadian, Australian and European forces) fought the Axis forces (Germany, Italy and Japan). On the West coast, America put 112,000-120,000 Japanese-Americans in concentration … er internment camps (some called them relocation or detention camps – but what's in a name?) and confiscated their property. This xenophobia was greater than any demonization of Germans that took place. No such internment camps were set up for German Americans. Maybe they looked too much like "us."

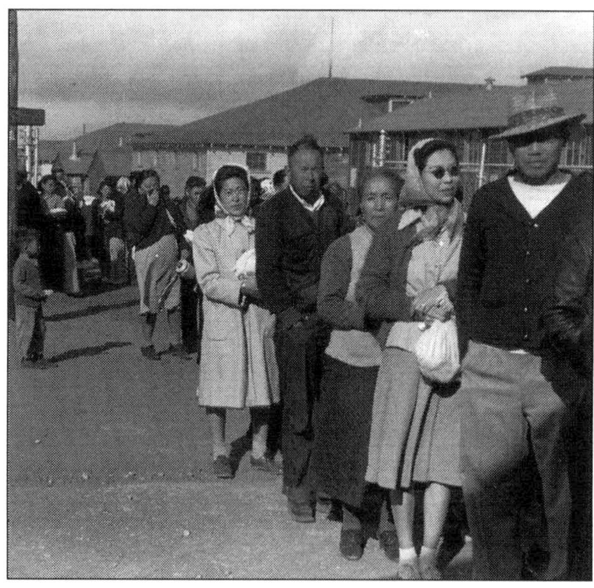

*Internment camps for Japanese-Americans are another example of America's xenophobia. Here, American citizens of Japanese descent are being herded into a "War Relocation Authority Center" in Manzanar, Calif. during WW II. Yes, America was at war, but somehow the mass internment of German-Americans never happened*

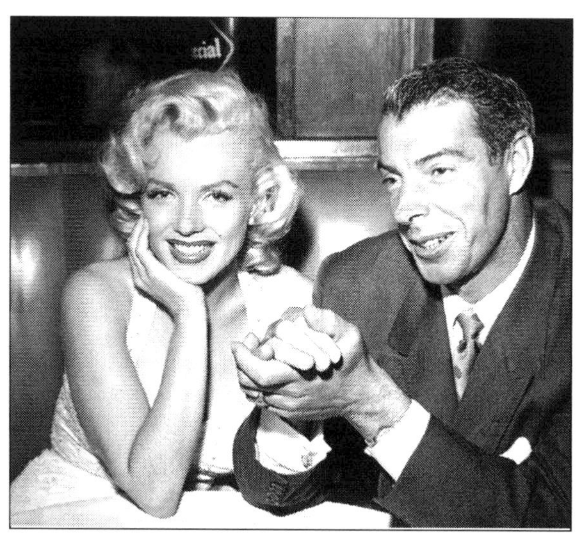

*For 13 years (1939-1951), Joe DiMaggio was the centerfielder for the New York Yankees. He has the major league record for longest hitting streak (56 consecutive games) and was once married to movie star and iconic sex symbol, Marilyn Monroe. DiMaggio was immortalized in the line in Simon & Garfunkel's song,* Mrs. Robinson: *"Where have you gone Joe DiMaggio?".*

Italians were also interred and harassed during WWII, suggesting that the anti-Italian sentiment from the 1920s was still present. During WWII, some 250 non-citizen Italian-Americans were put in internment camps on American soil. [13] Literally thousands of un-naturalized Italians were placed under surveillance and as many as 10,000 were forced to move away from the ocean and/or military facilities or had their property seized by the government.

Anti-Italian prejudice even extended to the family of the great New York Yankees center fielder, Joe DiMaggio. DiMaggio's father, a fisherman, lived in San Francisco. He was prevented from fishing in San Francisco Bay and forced to move inland. One official stated that if it had not been for Joe DiMaggio's status as a baseball player, DiMaggio's father would most likely had been sent to an internment camp. [14]

The U.S. Congress has since recognized the un-American nature of these acts, apologized, and in the very late 20th century, granted $20,000 apiece to the dwindling number of WW II Japanese internment camp survivors. The Italians are still waiting for their reparations.

## Mexican Zoot Suiters

When the controversy on interning the Japanese-Americans lulled, the Los Angeles tabloids began trumpeting a Mexican "crime wave". Propaganda attacks were directed at well-dressed Mexicans in their "zoot suits" with the "reet pleats". It was argued that the zoot suits favored by West Coast Mexican-Americans required too much fabric material. These zoot suits were actually briefly banned during the war because the yards of fabric needed to make them, it was argued, could otherwise be used for military uniforms. And these Mexicans smoked marijuana and were alleged to be engaged in a "wave" of crimes.

## The Sleepy Lagoon Murders

Demagoguery was clearly demonstrated by the shameful handling of the Sleepy Lagoon murders in Los Angeles. In this legal fiasco, the rights of 24 Mexican teenagers were violated and nine of them were railroaded into prisons for second degree murder. After serving 17 months, the so-called 38th-Street Gang members (so dubbed by the local tabloids) were released from prison but the point had been made and the damage to their lives done. The entire sad miscarriage of justice is documented and immortalized in the Broadway musical *Zoot Suit*

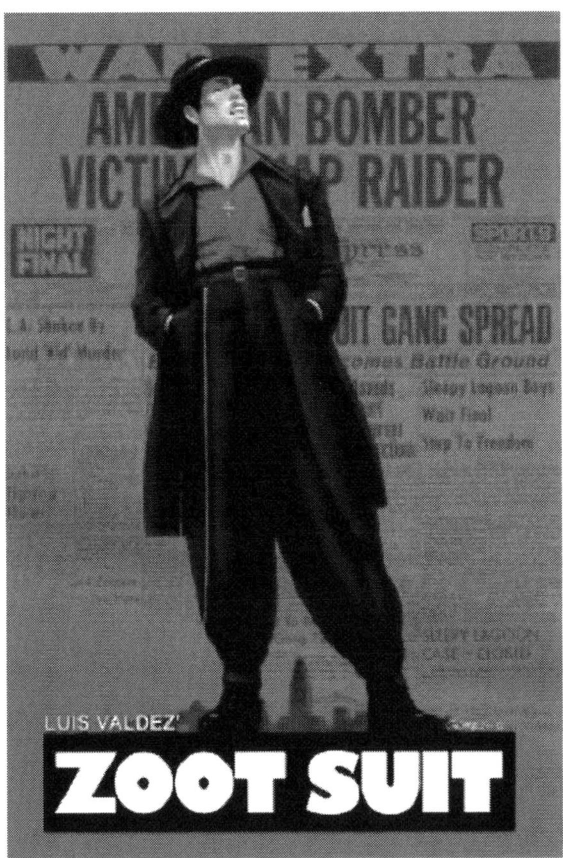


### A Crime Wave?

If there was a Mexican "Crime Wave" in Los Angeles in the Spring and Summer of 1942, the Los Angeles County Sheriff's Department was on top of the situation. They appointed E. Duran Ayres to head their Foreign Relations Bureau. Ayres produced a report on the matter that was presented to the grand jury. While he was accurate in identifying active discrimination against the Mexican "element", his grand jury testimony poured fuel on the fire of discrimination. Ayres stated that:

"Mexican-Americans are essentially Indians and therefore Orientals or Asians. Throughout history, the Orientals have shown less regard for human life than have the Europeans. Further, Mexican-Americans had inherited their 'naturally violent' tendencies from the 'bloodthirsty Aztecs' of Mexico who were said to have practiced human sacrifice centuries ago."

At one point in his report Ayres even compared the Anglo to a domesticated house cat and the Mexican to a "wild cat," suggesting that the Mexican would forever retain his wild and violent tendencies no matter how much education or training he might receive. [15]

Then came the incident at the Sleepy Lagoon.

Following a ruckus, apparently involving two Hispanic gangs at a dance, the body of Jose Diaz was found unconscious near a small pond, which was dubbed "The Sleepy Lagoon" by a reporter. Diaz later died. The autopsy revealed that Mr. Diaz was drunk at the time of his death. Whether Diaz's death was even a murder, rather than an accident, was and is still in dispute. Death was the result of blunt head trauma that was consistent with being hit by a car, a medical examiner said. Nevertheless, Henry Leyvas and 24 members of the 38th-Street Gang were arrested and charged with the murder of Mr. Diaz.

and Luis Valdez' 1981 movie of the same title, which starred James Edward Olmos. [16]

## The Zoot Suit Riots

The hysteria surrounding this trial was an excuse for increased hostility toward the Mexican-American community in Los Angeles, culminating in the Zoot Suit Riots.

The riots were triggered by a June 3, 1943 fight between eleven sailors on shore leave and a group of Mexican pachucos (a sub-culture of Hispanics in the southwestern United States at the time that wore zoot suits). The sailors alleged that they had been attacked. In response, over 200 uniformed sailors chartered twenty [17] cabs and went into East Los Angeles, the Mexican-American community in L.A.

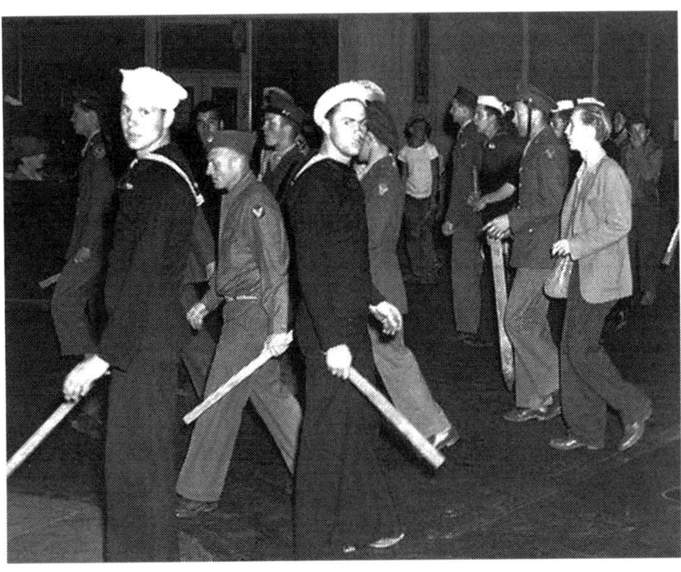

*A 1943 fight between eleven sailors on shore leave and a group of Mexican that wore "zoot suits" resulted in a riot involving hundreds of combatants. Although a later study recommended all parties involved be punished, no sailors were arrested and only Hispanics went to jail.*

These marijuana-using zoot suiters were considered fair game. Many a zoot suiter was beaten by mobs composed largely of servicemen and stripped of their zoot suits, on the spot. No sailors were arrested by the police or the sheriff. The servicemen were portrayed in the local press as heroes who were fighting the tide of the Mexican "Crime Wave" that the press had trumpeted.

Eleanor Roosevelt, wife of U.S. President Franklin D. Roosevelt, wrote in her June 16, 1943 newspaper column, "The question goes deeper than just suits. It is a racial protest. I have been worried for a long time about the Mexican racial situation. It is a problem with roots going a long way back, and we do not always face these problems as we should."

The June 18th issue of the *Los Angeles Times* slammed the first lady with an all-too-typical headline of that era: "Mrs. Roosevelt Blindly Stirs Race Discord." Governor Earl Warren (later chief justice of the U.S. Supreme Court during the Court's landmark 1950's desegregation cases) convened a committee to investigate the riots. This committee recommended punishment for all involved in the riots, servicemen and civilians alike. It should come as no surprise that charges were only filed against the Mexican-American victims; no punishment was ever meted out to the sailors. [18]

Current treatment of Mexican immigrants in the United States, both legal and illegal, is tainted with thinking similar to that which allowed and excused the Zoot Suit riots and the accompanying miscarriage of justice. Current drug laws come down disproportionately hard on Mexicans, Blacks and the poor.

In contemplating the rhetoric about the zoot suiters being unpatriotic, it's of note that Hispanics have won more Medals of Honor than any other non-white ethnic group. [19]

## LaGuardia Crime Commission

Even during the war there was an occasional note of sanity. The 1944 report on marijuana prepared for the LaGuardia Crime Commission by the New York Academy of Medicine recommended legalizing marijuana. And in 1943, Col. J.M. Phalen, editor of the semi-official military medical journal, *Military Surgeon,* wrote an editorial entitled "The Marijuana Bugaboo" that concluded, "the smoking of the leaves, flowers, and seeds of Cannabis sativa is no more harmful than the smoking of tobacco. It is hoped that no witch hunt will be instituted in the military service over a problem that does not exist." [20]

## Winds of Change

Yes, there were race riots in Detroit and the military that fought WWII was segregated. But many Black

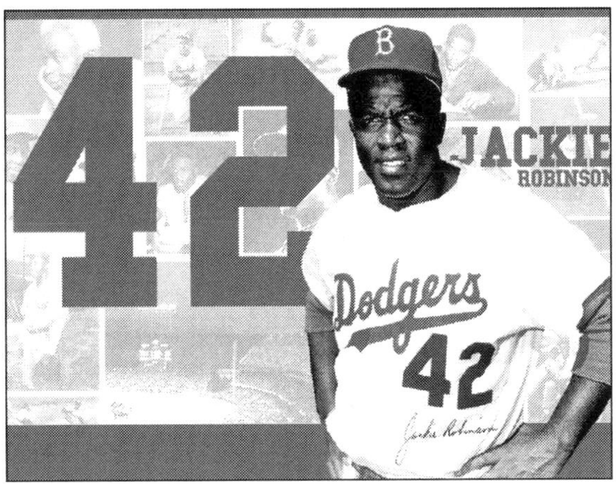


*Baseball was segregated until Jackie Robinson broke the color barrier shortly after the end of World War II. Branch Rickey, the general manager of the Brooklyn Dodgers, thought it was about time. For the next decade, Brooklyn was a strong pennant contender in part because of the skills provided by several African Americans, including Roy Campanella and Don Newcombe.*

soldiers served during WW II and there were also the heroics of the all-Negro Tuskegee Airmen. Change was in the air. Hard on the heels of the war, U.S. President Harry S Truman integrated the military and in 1947, Major League Baseball was integrated by Jackie Robinson and the Brooklyn Dodgers under the leadership of General Manager Branch Rickey.

With the end of the Second World War, the domestic demonization machine revved into high gear, in part fueled by these winds of change. But now it cast a wider net beyond race, religion, social class and national origin; the drug demonization complex spread its lengthening tentacles beyond music and went to thought.

In 1948 U.S. congressional hearings, U.S. Federal Bureau of Narcotics chief Harry J. Anslinger reversed what had been his testimony leading up to the Marijuana Tax Act of 1937. Previously, Anslinger had flatly denied any connection between cannabis and opiates and that marijuana use did not lead to other drug use. However, he now let loose the much discredited "gateway" theory. Also, he now opined that marijuana did not make a person violent, as he had previously trumpeted; it made a user passive. Anslinger asserted that the "Commies" were pushing cannabis on American youth because it made them passive dupes and easy prey for

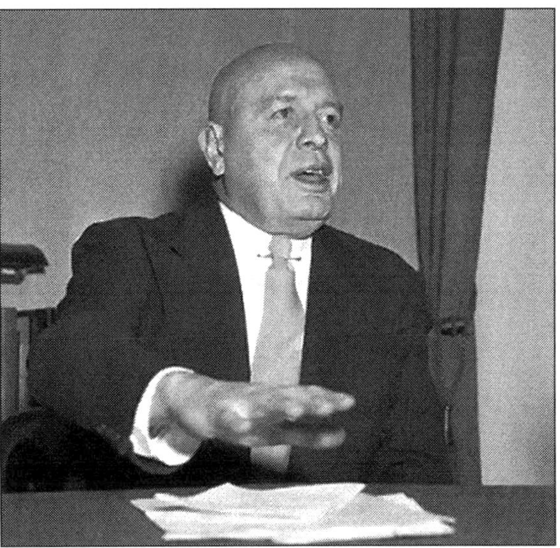

*As part of his relentless war on marijuana, U.S. Federal Bureau of Narcotics chief Harry J. Anslinger's testimony before Congress was not always consistent.*

Communism. And that it weakened the American will to fight. [21]

It's not that Americans weren't warned about straying from Constitutional protections. In 1949, Ludwig von Mises, a leading free-market economist and social philosopher of the era, delivered a stern warning against straying from our constitutional protections. By taking prohibitionist thought to its logical extension, von Mises put forth a strong Libertarian, slippery-slope argument and a chilling vision of the future.

> "Opium and morphine are certainly dangerous, habit-forming drugs. But once the principle is admitted that it is the duty of government to protect the individual against his own foolishness, no serious objections can be advanced against further encroachments. A good case could be made out in favor of the prohibition of alcohol and nicotine. And why limit the government's benevolent providence to the protection of the individual's body only? Is not the harm a man can inflict on his mind and soul even more disastrous than any bodily evils? Why not prevent him from reading bad books and seeing bad plays, from looking at bad paintings and statues and from hearing bad music?

The mischief done by bad ideologies, surely, is much more pernicious, both for the individual and for the whole society, than that done by narcotic drugs." [22]

**Ludwig von Mises**
*Human Action: A Treatise on Economics,* 1949

## The Beats

The *ennui* of the post-World War II era begat "the Beats" or beatniks. In part this movement was a reaction to the turmoil of the preceding thirty years, the depression and two world wars. The Beats were an anti-establishment movement of people disenchanted with the status quo, wanting to break away from society's racist, materialistic, capitalistic, war-generating values. Some believe that poet Allen Ginsberg could be considered the father of this movement. He and other Beat writers such as Jack Kerouac and Gary Snyder used the written word to express their dissatisfaction and frustration with what they saw as wrong with the world.

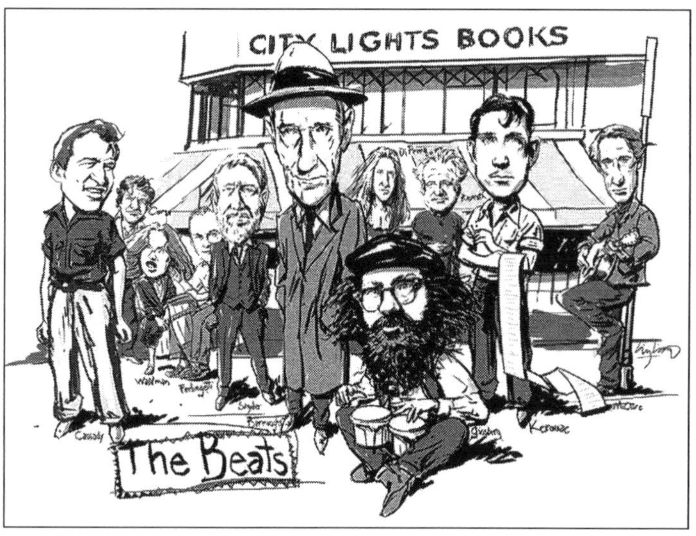


*The Beats included (left to right) Neal Cassady, Gregory Corso, Anne Waldman, Lawrence Ferlingetti on the drum, Gary Snyder, William S. Burroughs (tall, center), Diane DiPrima, Allen Ginsberg, Kenneth Rexroth, Jack Kerouak, and Michael McClure with guitar.*

In the late 1940s, "The word 'beat' was primarily used by jazz musicians and hustlers as a slang term meaning down and out, or poor and exhausted." Kerouac, author of *On the Road* went on to twist the meaning of the term "beat" to serve his own purposes, explaining that it meant "beatitude, not beat up. You feel this. You feel it in a beat, in jazz, real cool jazz." [23]

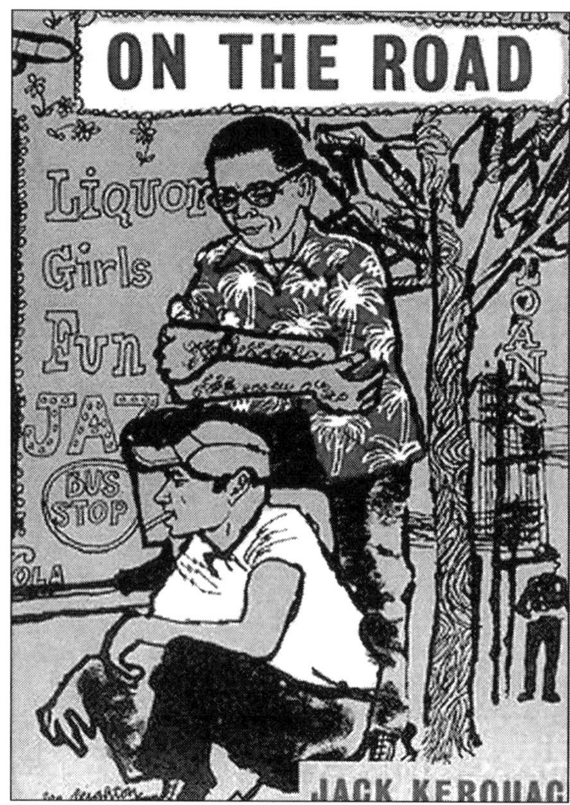


*Jack Kerouac's* On the Road *was finished in 1951 but not published until 1957. It was based on the travels of Kerouac and his friends across America in the years after WW II. The book is considered to be more-or-less a mirror of the emerging genre that came to be called the "Beat Generation." At its heart was jazz, poetry and drug use. Above is the cover of the book printed in England in the late 1950s. The graphic is by Len Deighton, a commercial artist at the time but later a popular novelist (*The IPCRESS File, *1962).*

Kerouac was into the "bop" scene. He interacted with many jazz musicians, including Zoot Sims, Miles Davis, Al Cohn and Bruce Moore. Jack Chambers wrote in *Milestones: The Music and the Times of Miles Davis* (1998) that Kerouac even got booked into the Village Vanguard nightclub to "play" regular sets, reading poetry with jazz accompaniment. And that "on his better nights, he dispensed with the poetry and took up scat singing, including a faithful rendering of a Miles Davis solo that ... was entirely accurate and something more than a simple imitation." [24]

Beat poet Allen Ginsberg said that "Howl" was all "Lester Leaps In," (Lester Young was a noted jazz woodwind player who is credited with popularizing the word "Cool"). Kerouac's *On the Road* was said to be partially inspired by Dexter Gordon's and

Wardell Gray's *The Hunt.* This passage from *On the Road* documents that connection: "Dean Moriarty (Neal Cassady) stands bowed before the big photograph listening to a wild bop record … *The Hunt*, with Dexter Gordon and Wardell Gray blowing their tops before a screaming audience that gave the record fantastic frenzied volume" demonstrates the importance of jazz to the Beats.[25] While the beats were much indebted to jazz, jazz got along just fine without the Beats.

The Beats used many of the same recreational drugs as the jazz musicians they admired. Many Beats used heroin, morphine and Benzedrine. This use was both an homage to the jazz musicians who used them, and also carried the hope that the drugs would do for them what they supposedly did for jazz greats like Charlie Parker. All of this sounds like absinthe all over again.

The influence of these drugs can be seen in the literature and biographies of beat icons William S. Burroughs, Jack Kerouac and Allen Ginsberg. Kerouac's book *On the Road* was written on a three-day-long, Benzedrine-fueled binge.

William S. Burroughs is best known for writing about his dependency on heroin. He used his heroin use and abuse as an inspiration for *Junkie* (1953), *Naked Lunch* (1959), and other books. *Junkie* was published in Britain under the pseudonym William S. Lee. It was just one of the genre of pulp-fiction drug literature popular at the time. The front cover tells it all: a man and woman hover over a syringe and, on the back cover, a woman raising her skirt to inject heroin into her thigh.

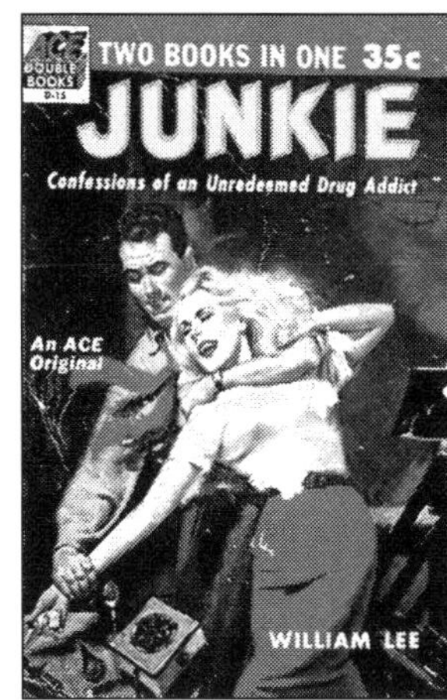


By the Fifties, the Beat movement had grown and spread. Coffee houses and jazz clubs as Beat enclaves were in all major cities and most college towns. Here were places where one could listen to music, hear poetry readings, and meet and share unconventional thoughts. From these places emerged the stereotype of the so-called "beatniks". They were usually depicted in turtleneck sweater, dark sport jacket, occasionally wearing a beret, sometimes dressed in shabby dark clothes, sporting a beard (usually a goatee), wearing sunglasses at all hours and using "drugs" while confronting conventional thinking. But the challenge to the Establishment was that the beatniks refused to conform to middle-class conventions.[26]

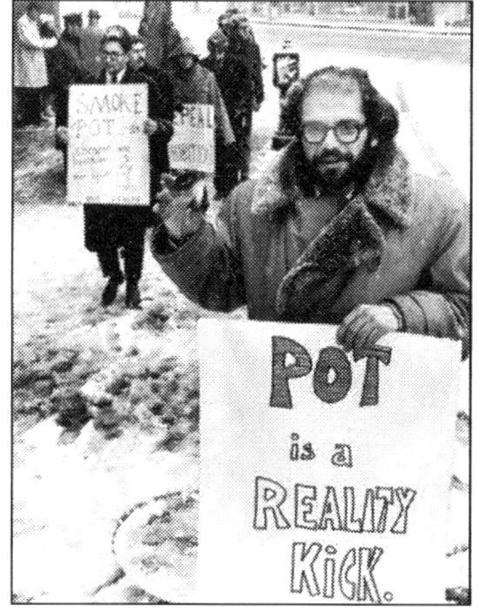


*Beat poet Allen Ginsberg smoked marijuana often and was a public advocate for its widespread use.*

The beatniks' social criticism and non-mainstream ideas were marginalized by critics focusing on prominent Beats' flagrant use of marijuana and heroin. The Beats were into ideas, and questioning comfortable materialism. They raged against the reserve, conformity and racism of the 1950s. These insurgent artists embraced the old shamanistic chemicals and newer pharmaceuticals as catalysts for creative expression.

"I saw the best minds of my generation destroyed by madness, starving hysterical naked,

dragging themselves through the negro streets at dawn looking for an angry fix,

Angel-headed hipsters burning for the ancient heavenly connection
to the starry dynamo in the machinery of night . . ."

**Allen Ginsberg**
from his poem *Howl*, 1955

Allen Ginsberg's howl of poetic protest and Jack Kerouac's exuberant be-bop yarns linked marijuana to the small but growing movement of nonconformity. During the next decade fueled by the civil rights movement and the anti-war movement, these Beatnik roots grew into a mass rebellion. The Beats use of drugs to rebel, to think and write unconventional, nonconformist ideas, helped create the youth culture that peaked during the latter stages of the Vietnam War.

## The Doors of Perception

Aldous Huxley's book, *The Doors of Perception* (1954) and his essay *Heaven and Hell* (1956) helped popularize contemporary mid-twentieth century use of hallucinogens for philosophical and spiritual reasons. (The band, The Doors, is named after Huxley's book.) His book contains an account of one day's experience with mescaline. He describes it thusly:

> "Most takers of mescaline experience only the heavenly part of schizophrenia. The drug brings hell and purgatory only to those who have had a recent case of jaundice, or who suffer form periodical depressions or a chronic anxiety ... But the reasonably healthy person knows in advance that mescaline is completely innocuous, that its effects will pass off after eight or ten hours, leaving no hangover and consequently no craving for a renewal of the dose."

He describes walking down the street and seeing a large pale blue automobile was standing at the curb. He writes at the sight of it,

> "I was suddenly overcome by enormous merriment. What complacency, what an absurd self-satisfaction beamed from those bulging surfaces of glossiest enamel! Man had created the thing in his own image – or rather in the image of his favorite character of fiction. . . I laughed till the tears ran down my cheeks."

After eating a meal Huxley and his friends got into the car and went for a drive. He recalled that:

> "The effects of the mescaline were already on the decline: but the flowers in the gardens still trembled on the brink of being supernatural, the pepper trees and carobs along the side streets still manifestly belonged to some sacred grove ... And then abruptly, we were at an intersection waiting to cross Sunset Boulevard. Before us the cars were rolling by in a steady stream – thousands of them, all bright and shiny like an advertiser's dream and each more ludicrous than the last. Once again I was convulsed with laughter ....
>
> An hour later we were back at home, and I had returned to that reassuring but profoundly unsatisfactory state known as "being in one's right mind." [27]

## Drug Hysteria Continued Unabated

Despite these cultural influences, the hysteria justifying American drug policy ramped up in the1950s. In 1951, the U.S. Congress passed The Boggs Act. The Boggs Act named cannabis as a narcotic for the first time and dictated a four-fold increase in the penalties associated with any and all narcotic violations. It also established uniform penalties for the Marijuana Tax Act and the Narcotics Drug Import and Export Act, both passed a few years previously. The Narcotics Control Act of 1956 soon followed, which introduced substantial mandatory minimum sentences for drug offenses.

The Beat generation took root during the placid, prosperous years of former General Dwight David "Ike" Eisenhower's presidency (1953-61), when the domestic issue that provoked greatest anxiety among intellectuals was conformity. Eisenhower's campaign slogan was "I Like Ike." Ike was a calming, reassuring influence on the country. His goal was to bring so-called "normalcy" back to the United States, with normalcy being broadly defined as all of Norman Rockwell's paintings laid end-to-end with economic policies endorsed by the chamber of commerce.

Still, there were some sweeping changes to America during his years in office 1953-61). Ike helped bring an end to the Korean War. He launched the interstate highway system, a project that helped end the era of small town America. It fashioned the demise of locally owned main street stores in favor of national chains in malls.

Eisenhower helped implement Truman's integrating of the military. He lowered racist government rhetoric and was of the opposition party to the more openly segregationist Southern Democrats. In 1954, two years into his first Administration, the monumental *Brown vs. Board of Education* Supreme

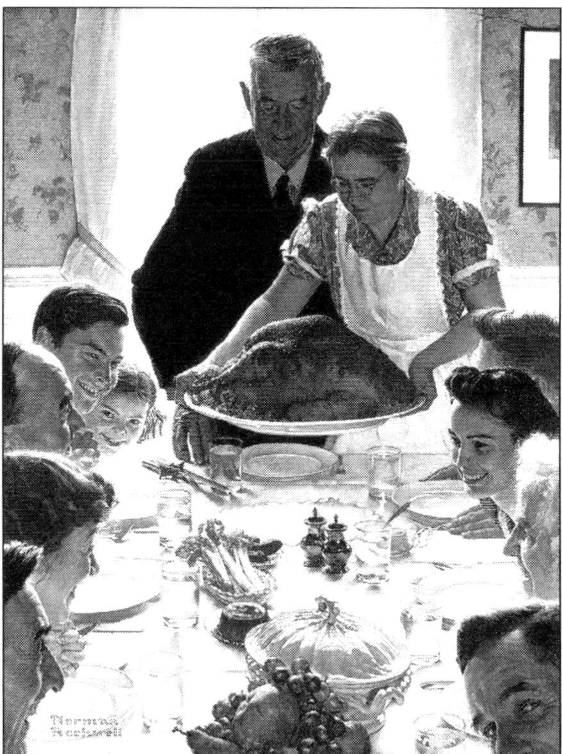

*Artist Norman Rockwell's career spanned mid-20th-century America. He painted idealized pictures of American life, which frequently graced the cover of the popular* Saturday Evening Post *magazine.*

Court decision (347 U.S. 483) eliminated "separate-but-equal" education policies throughout America. Ike sent federal troops to the South to enforce access to schools for Blacks.

However, in the view of Max Boot, senior fellow at the Council on Foreign Relations, Ike was way too cautious. "There was much to like about Ike. He ended the Korean War and avoided potential conflicts with China and the Soviet Union. He built interstate highways and balanced the budget." Boot points out that Ike "was no profile in courage when he refused to stand up to the demagogic Joseph McCarthy or to do much to enforce the Supreme Court's *Brown v. Board of Education* school integration decision.

It was left, Boot thought, to the U.S. Senate "to end McCarthy's reign of terror, and to President Lyndon B. Johnson to desegregate schools."

Boot concludes that "in the final analysis, Eisenhower was a status quo president who ratified the successful policies of his gifted predecessors – the New Deal and containment. Maybe that's what the nation needed in the 1950s." [28]

When Eisenhower left office, he famously warned America of the "military-industrial complex": the pernicious, disproportionate influence on public policy of munitions makers and those who prosper from war. This warning, unfortunately, has gone largely unheeded, as seen with Halliburton's billions in cost over-runs on no-bid contracts in the early years of the war in Iraq (2002-12). Because its former CEO was then the U.S. vice president, Richard Bruce "Dick" Cheney, these obvious transgressions were simply winked at.

Eisenhower's phrase has been modified to refer to the prison-industrial-complex to apply to the effects of drug war policies. The groups who profit from drug prohibition include but are not limited to criminal enterprises, prison guards, prison builders, law enforcement, and toxicology (urine & blood) labs.

By any rational definition, authentic substance abuse is a mental health issue. It should be approached with the same wide range of therapeutic options as other mental health problems. The current primitive "treatment" system (as opposed to real therapy) of halfway houses and so-called clean-and-sober living houses are often run by certificated felons. The reliance on moderately trained people with similar pathology issues represents an over-reliance on one modality, often to the exclusion of other more effective approaches.

## Looking Ahead

The 1950s were relatively calm, often characterized as a decade of conformity. The very sanity, prosperity and boredom of the Eisenhower era helped pave the way for the social turbulence of the 1960s. It provided lessons in idealism for the baby boomers and they translated the idealism of post-war America into action in the 1960s and '70s. The great numbers of baby boomers relative to the rest of the population gave youth a unique population clout. U.S. prosperity in the 1940s, '50s, and '60s, provided a financial cushion that afforded the economic freedom for the young to act on their idealism.

## Robert Mitchum and The Big Dope Bust of 1948

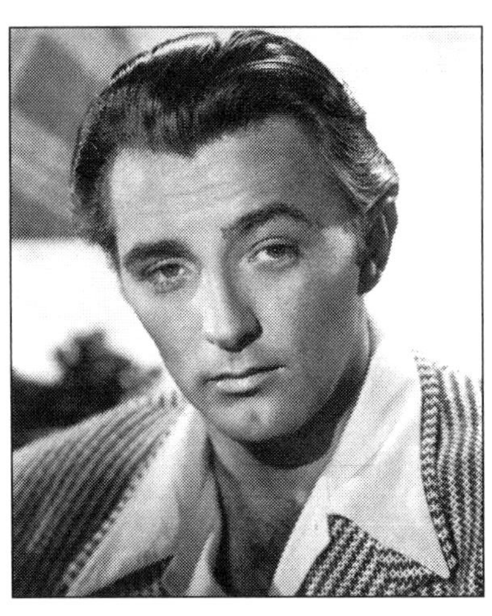

In 1948, Robert Mitchum was a rising young movie star with an Oscar nomination behind him. In that year, he was arrested for possession of marijuana in a sting by the Los Angeles cops.[29] This occurred in a raid on starlet Lila Leeds' house in Laurel Canyon where Mitchum was partying with dancer Vicki Evans, bartender-turned-real-estate-agent Robin Ford, Ms. Leeds and possibly another starlet.

One story has it that as soon as Mitchum stepped into the house, the unmistakable smell of marijuana filled his nostrils. A moment later, one of the girls handed him a joint. Shortly, L.A. detectives Barr and MacKinnon entered with guns drawn, showing her their badges. In the front room, Mitchum, Leeds and Ford were all holding marijuana cigarettes. Mitchum's cigarette pack held fifteen more joints.

It is purported that one of the other guests allegedly snuck out a bedroom window. The story goes that she almost didn't make it through the window due to the size of her back side. That actor was Marilyn Monroe. (This author got this version from discussion with a Mitchum family friend and former babysitter of Mitchum's grandchildren).[30]

It was no secret that Mitchum used marijuana. From the presence of photographers and press outside at the time of the arrest, this big celebrity "dope" bust was clearly a set up.

It was 1948 and Mitchum had been caught with marijuana. Plus he was a married man, caught partying with two young women. Shortly after the arrest, Mitchum allegedly said, "I'm ruined."

On the steps of the Los Angeles County Jail, Mitchum told the reporters and photographers waiting there, "Yes, boys, I was smoking a marijuana cigarette when they came in."[31] After posing for photographs, he speculated that his wife Dorothy would probably leave him. When the booking officer asked his occupation, Mitchum replied, "Former actor."

Attorney Jerry Giesler, who had successfully defended other prominent people in legal trouble, was retained by RKO Pictures to defend Mitchum. Both Howard Hughes' RKO and David O. Selznick's Vanguard Studios, who shared Mitchum's contract, asked the public to withhold judgment on their star. Selznick infuriated Mitchum by describing him as "a very sick man in need of medical treatment instead of a lawbreaker."

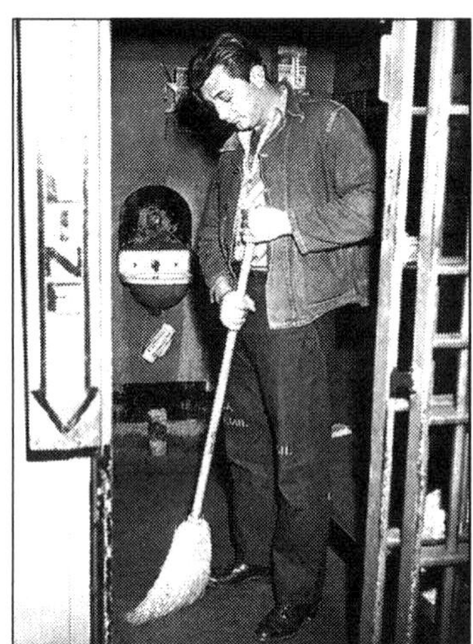

*This photo of Mitchum mopping the floor in prison blues appeared in* Life *magazine.*[32]

In this instance the studios needed to protect one of their stars. After all, the industry had around $5 million in 1947 dollars invested in Mitchum's three unreleased films: *Rachel and the Stranger* with Loretta Young, *Blood on the Moon* with Barbara Bel Geddes, and at Republic Studios, *The Red Pony* with Myrna Loy.

The following day, Louelle O. Parsons, the Hearst news-paper chain's syndicated motion picture gossip columnist, called the charge "shocking" and claimed Mitchum was "in a state of mental collapse." She quoted Selznick saying he believed Mitchum should enter a sanitarium at once "to undergo treatment for his shattered nerves." Later in the story, she reflected that, "None of the executives at RKO or Selznick studios is willing to believe that Mitchum is a real addict. They say he never gave any signs of being doped, and that he turned in some very fine performances."

Mitchum's career seemed over as the media had a circus. Headlines blared that he was "In the Grip of Demon Drugs" – a dancing slave to commie-controlled "Indian hemp."

## The Defense

As it turned out, Mitchum's lawyers, Jerry Giesler and Norman R. Tyre, did a very good job. They soon issued a statement: "There are a number of unexplained facts and peculiar circumstances surrounding the raid made yesterday in which Mitchum was involved."

Mitchum pleaded no contest. The judge sentenced both Mitchum and Leeds to a year in the county jail but suspended the sentence, placing them on probation for two years with 60 days in jail.

Mitchum served most of his time at an honor farm in Castaic. Several times, Mitchum found marijuana in his cell, apparently hidden by fellow prisoners to set him up for a snitch so they could be rewarded. Each time, he reported the find to guards. His sentence was completed without incident and on March 30 he was released.

## Observations on Jail

"I've been happy in jail," he told the waiting throng of press. The farm, he said, was "just like a weekend in Palm Springs … only you meet a better class of people."

Mitchum then told press he was going back to work as soon as he could. "I've got to. I'm broke."[34] He concluded with, "And now, if you'll excuse me, I'm heading for home."

## The Fall Out

Attorney Jerry Geisler continued working the case, trying to prove a frame-up. In early 1951, after it was exposed as a set-up, the Los Angeles Court overturned Mitchum's conviction. The court said, "After an exhaustive investigation of the evidence and testimony presented at the trial, the court orders that the verdict of guilty be sent aside and that a plea of not guilty be entered and that the information or complaint be dismissed."

Jane Greer, who appeared in Mitchum's next film, *The Big Steal*, reported that while filming in Mexico, locals were constantly trying to give him joints. The same happened to him in the states. Howard Hughes hired Kemp Niver, a former LAPD officer, to keep Mitchum out of trouble, and Niver took care of such incidents.

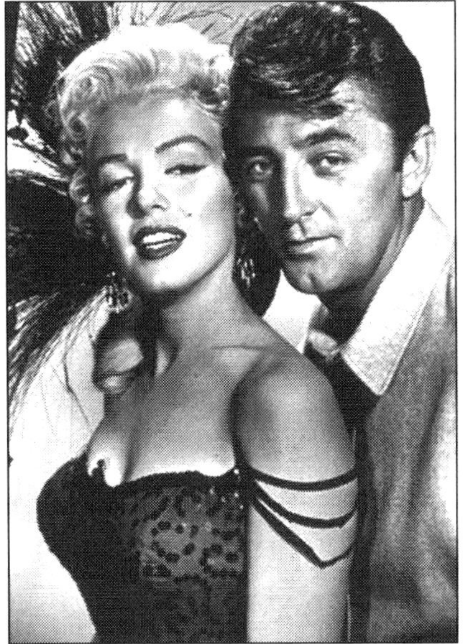

*One of Mitchum's most memorable movie roles was* River of No Return *(1954) in which he co-stared — perhaps ironically — with Marilyn Monroe.*

What is interesting is what happened next. While many times breaking drug laws in those days spelled disaster for the famous, in Mitchum's case it merely burnished his screen image as a tough guy. After being released from jail, his career continued with such films as *Cape Fear, Night of the Hunger, Ryan's Daughter* and in TV's, *The Winds of War.*

As to Miss Leeds, ironically she went on to star in a B movie with a strong anti-marijuana theme. It was titled *Wild Weed* (the original title: other titles included: *The Devil's Weed, Marijuana: The Devil's Weed*), and, the most unwieldy, *The Story of Lila Leeds and Her Expose of the Marijuana Racket.* It was also shown under the title *She Shoulda Said No.* Not so coincidentally, the film was written by Arthur Hoerl and the cinematographer was Jack Greenhalgh; both had worked on the 1936 movie, *Reefer Madness.*

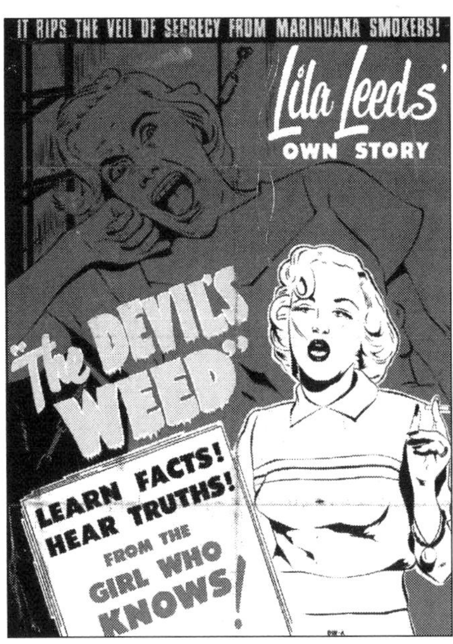


Robert Mitchum (1917-97) appeared in over 125 movies. "The Big Dope Bust of 1948" turned out to be barely a blip in his long career.

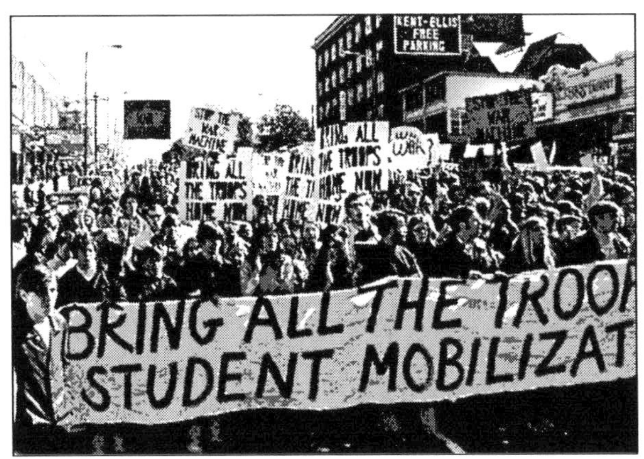


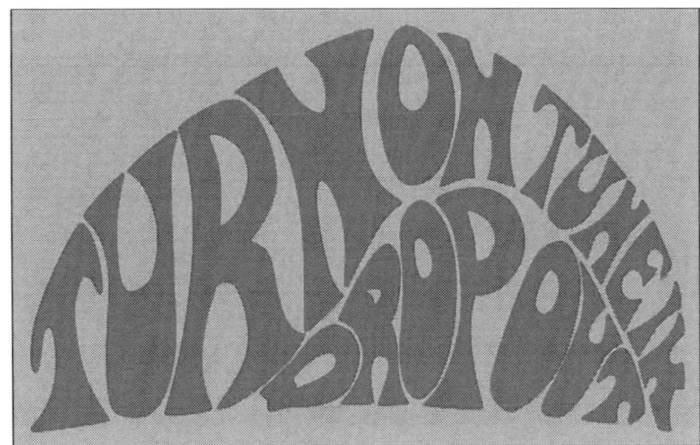


# CHAPTER XIII
## The Sixties: A Culture War Bubbles to the Surface

In the years following World War II, Americans were happy to have peace and prosperity. They were busy working and gaining the material goods that had been beyond their grasp in the 1930s and '40s. But their children had not known depression or war, only prosperity. The 1960s saw a re-emergence of sharp distinctions among generations on race, sex, drugs, war, religion and lifestyle.

In the late Fifties and early '60s, the greater acceptance of Negroes and recognition of their human worth, combined with the burgeoning economy, gave energy and motivation to the descendants of American slaves. Less and less willing to be second-class citizens, they began staging non-violent sit-ins and marches, which drew many northern middle-class supporters. The Civil Rights Movement was born.

The strides made by African-Americans or Blacks sparked additional civil rights movements among migrant workers, women, Mexican-Americans or Chicanos and Native Americans.

### The Scent of Dramatic Change

Antibiotics had lessened the real danger ofsexually transmitted diseases ( STDs). Paired with new birth control technologies, a sexual revolution was ignited. The need in WWII for more women in the workforce had provided a glimpse of what financial freedom could mean for women and had fanned the embers of feminism. Women had struggled for equal rights since the founding of the Republic but in 1963, when Betty Freidan published *The Feminine Mystic*, the Feminist Movement appeared to burst forth in full bloom.

But the glue that held all of these social movements together was the war in Viet Nam. Here the United States had an unpopular land war in Asia: a war that drafted 18-year-olds to fight and die for an uncertain cause in a far away land. In 1954, President Eisenhower approached the U.S. Senate Majority Leader Lyndon Johnson about bailing out the French forces that were pinned down at Dien Bien Phu. Johnson declined, and the French were defeated. However, the United States supplied clandestine aid to the "government" in South Vietnam under Eisenhower, which was greatly expanded under President John. F. Kennedy. Later, as president, Lyndon Johnson built up U.S. forces to 500,000 troops in Vietnam.

After 1964, the war became increasingly unpopular. The Anti-War Movement had been around since at least 1959. At first it was just a dribble, then a creek, then a river, and after the 1968 Tet offensive, it became a torrent of protest, so much so that Johnson declined to run for re-election that fall.

For a brief time, these seemingly disparate groups, representing a broad swath of America, came together to form an effective multi-dimensional force for change. But soon they were perceived by the establishment and portrayed by the media as using drugs to feed these desires for change. The mainstream media propagandized that marijuana, psychedelics and other recreational drugs were dangerous and could destroy one's brain or one's child or that users would lose their soul and go to hell. A reeling estab-lishment chose to make many of these drugs illegal or to stiffen existing penalties.

### Strom and His Daughter

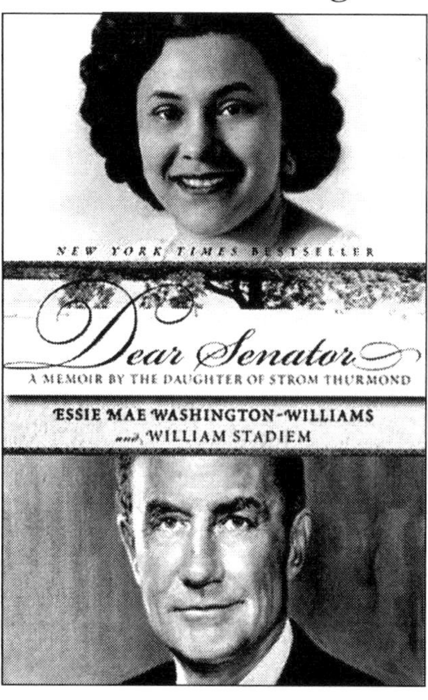


*An ironic footnote to U.S. Senator Stom Thurmond's racist legacy is that, shortly after his death, his African-American daughter publicly came forward. She was the product of a sexual liaison between a young Thurmond and his family's Negro maid in the early 1920s. It was apparently an open secret in his home state of South Carolina that Thurmond, one of the most racist U.S. senators of the last half of the 20th century, had fathered a Negro daughter. Senator Thurmond saw his daughter from time to time during his lifetime and provided some financial assistance to her in college.*

## Civil Rights

The America of the 1940s was awash with Jim Crow laws, saw regular lynching of Negroes, and found grinding poverty within a large part of the Negro community. By the 1960s, the anger, indignation and moral outrage over the plight of Negroes had been smoldering in the United States for hundreds of years. After all, Americans had even fought a civil war over slavery and race. This oppressive dis-crimination was downright un-American to an increasing number of citizens of America. In the mid-1960s, this sentiment was finally reflected in U.S. Congressional action with the passage of landmark civil rights

**Many historians say that the very slow fuse for the explosion of interest in the 1960s had been lit in 1948, when Hubert H. Humphrey . . . gave a dramatic speech at the 1948 Democratic Party Convention. . . . urging the Democrats to embrace civil rights.**

legislation during the administration of President Johnson.

Many historians say that the very slow fuse for the explosion of greater interest in support of civil rights in the 1960s had been lit in 1948, when Hubert H. Humphrey — then mayor of Minneapolis and later a Minnesota U.S. Senator and vice president under Johnson — gave a dramatic speech at the 1948 Democratic Party Convention.

Humphrey's speech publicly recognized the plight of African-Americans, deploring their oppression and urging the Democrats to embrace civil rights. Southern Democrats temporarily bolted the party and formed the segregationist "Dixiecrat" party. They ran racist South Carolina Governor Strom Thurmond for president. He carried five states.

Notwithstanding the recent monumental achievement for America with the 2008 election of Barack Obama, the echo of the Dixicrats' racism still lingers today, decades later. In 2002, U.S. Senator Trent Lott (R-Miss.), then Senate Majority Leader, gave a controversial toast at Senator Thurmond's 100th birthday celebration. He remarked, "When Strom Thurmond ran for president, [my state] voted for him. We're proud of it. And if the rest of the country had followed our lead, we wouldn't have had all these problems over all these years, either."[1] Shortly thereafter, Lott was replaced as Senate Majority Leader by Bill Frisk of Tennessee.

**Thurmond's 1948 run for the presidency as a third-party Dixiecrat, was almost 25 years before U.S. President Richard Nixon initiated his successful southern strategy to lure "conservative" Southern Democrats to permanently join the Republican fold.**

## Change Is in the Air

Still, Humphrey's high-profile oration gave Negroes hope that change could really happen, and that it would be they who would change things. However, it wasn't until the early 1960s, nearly 100 years after the end of the Civil War, that what became known as the "Civil Rights Movement" seemed to burst onto the scene, at least to the unobservant. Its leaders were largely African-Americans, with white support from the likes of aging socialists, liberals and moderates, religious leaders, and idealistic baby-boomers. Anger at this country for not living up to its purported ideals of equality helped fuel the Civil Rights Movement.

The 1960s were the nativists' worst nightmare. Finally there was a moment in history that displayed outrage over America's treatment of Blacks, Browns, and other minorities, including women. With President Kennedy, the United States had a sophisticated, northern Catholic as president, one who was willing to publicly call for equality. A culture of protest demanding the promised American values of equality, freedom and democracy was growing.

As the 1960s progressed, social activism and community organizing expanded in an attempt to redress many injustices. Federal programs like the Office of Economic Opportunity (OEO), Peace Corps and Volunteers in Service to America (VISTA) provided opportunities to fight poverty both here and abroad. Activists supported Black, Brown, and Red power. They staged sit-ins, protests, and demonstrations.

This idealism and social activism found common ground in the anti-war movement. The anti-war fervor was the glue that held these rather disparate movements together. The Establishment media tried to marginalize this opposition to the war by focusing on so-called "hippies" and their drug use and libertine sexual behavior. But this was a broadly based anti-war movement consisting of both the young and the old and both the rich and the poor, that cut across the full spectrum of the American populace.

Hippies, however defined, have long since faded from the scene. Yet the specter of this fun-loving,

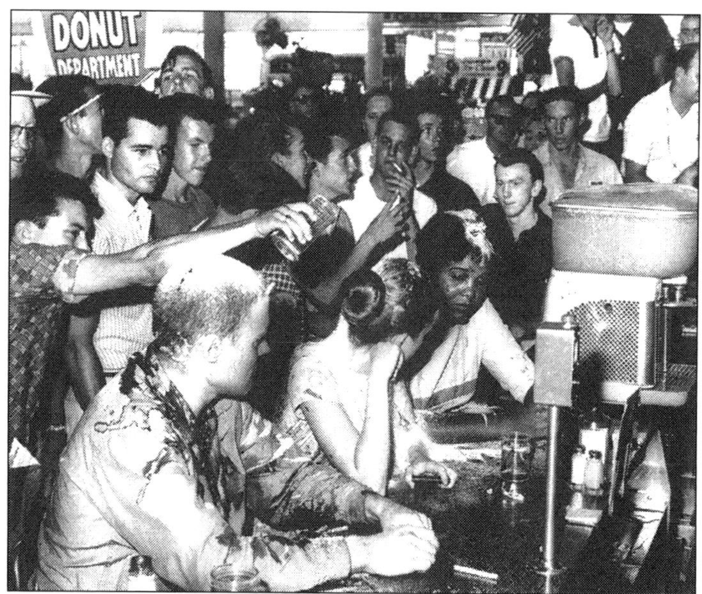

*Blacks and whites sat-in together at this Woolworth's lunch counter in the Deep South, which often led to violence against the demonstrators.*

iconoclastic, pro-peace, pro-choice, drug-using, hedonistic youth culture is still invoked as a reason to maintain our draconian drug laws. [2] With the election of Barack Obama in 2008, and his pledge not to support Drug Enforcement Agency (DEA) raids on cannabis dispensaries, the United States has begun to see some hope that American drug policy can become more functional, relevant, therapeutic and cost effective.

The experience of drug policy reform in Switzerland, Portugal, Uruguay, the Czech Republic, and the Netherlands has demonstrated that increasing emphasis on treatment and harm reduction is an effective approach to those with substance-abuse related problems. [3]

## Pop Culture

The '60s and '70s popular culture of the baby boomers, to one degree or another, supported these various movements for change, which were challenging the status quo. Alternative newspapers and progressive radio flourished in the 1960s and '70s. This support for the so-called "counter-culture" was reflected in the music of the times.

### Music

The music of that era had its roots in the folk music of musicians coming out of the depression and included such folk troubadours as Pete Seeger and Woody Guthrie and folk groups like the Weavers.

It relied heavily on the work and influences of Black blues musicians like Robert Johnson, Ma Rainy, Booker Washington, Blind Lemon Jefferson, Charley Patton, McKinley Morganfield, Muddy Waters, Sam "Lightnin'" Hopkins, John Lee Hooker, Bessie Smith and Billie Holiday. [4]

Joan Baez, Bob Dylan, Buffy St. Marie, Judy Collins, Joni Mitchell, Phil Ochs, humorist Tom Peyton, Woody's son Arlo Guthrie, Peter, Paul & Mary, and many other folk singers brought folk music into the youth culture of the '60s. Their songs had protest themes against government oppression and war. They took the words of the beat generation to a new level. [5,6,7,8] These ideas were shared by their fellow post-WWII baby boomers and were widely disseminated through records, concerts, demonstrations and alternative media.

Bob Dylan was one of the most prominent entertainer/activists of the '60s and '70s. His message provided part of the soundtrack of those turbulent years. He penned many anthems of the youth culture, including *A Hard Rain is Goin' To Fall*, *The Times They Are a' Changin'* and *Blowin' in the Wind* (the melody was based on the old Negro spiritual *No Mor' Auction Block*).

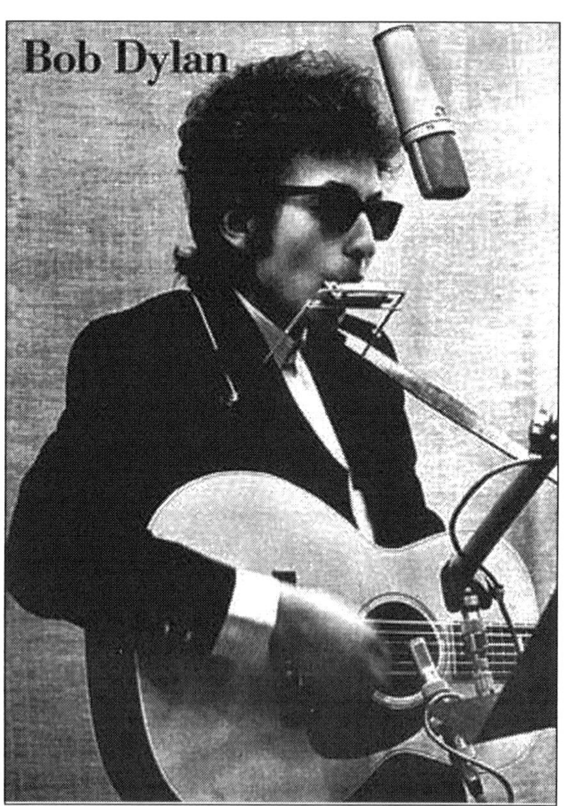


*Bob Dylan (born Robert Zimmerman) grew up in Bemidji, Minnesota, a city on the Iron Range. Early in his career, he performed in Dinky Town near the University of Minnesota. Dylan is often referred to as "the troubadour of the '60s."*

Music festivals like the Newport Jazz Festival in Rhode Island, The Monterey Jazz Festival in California, and the Sky River Rock Festival and Lighter Than Air Fair in Washington state drew large crowds of like-minded thinkers, disillusioned with the insanity of racism, sexism, and classism in U.S. society and united by their opposition to the Vietnam War and the draft. Here, the audience could not only enjoy the music, smoke marijuana, and maybe even drop some LSD, but could also share common ideas and goals. These festivals grew in size and number. Many areas banned the festivals because they were afraid of what might happen with all those "sex-crazed, dirty, dope-smoking, LSD-dropping hippies" in one place.

### Woodstock

Like most everything else about the counter culture, there are at least two interpretations of what this gathering of 500,000 to 600,000 people for this event billed as a music festival meant. The 1969 Woodstock event featured lots of music, rain, mud, nudity and drugs. It was remarkable for its peacefulness. Woodstock is often noted as being a marker of the end of the 1960s. This is perhaps true, but consider that concerns about the environment, clean energy, sustainability, sexual equality, human righteousness, and diversity are issues that are still on the political agenda of all developed nations.

Differing perceptions of the 1960s and '70s are similar to the Indian parable of the six blind men who, upon feeling different parts of an elephant (i.e. tusk, ear, tail), came to vastly different conclusions as to what kind of animal this was. Yet each, of course, believes that their version of the truth was accurate. So, too, was it true with hippies and Woodstock. In 1994, Elliot Tiber of *The Times Herald-Record* wrote, "True believers still call Woodstock the capstone of an era devoted to human advancement. Cynics say it was a fitting, ridiculous end to an era of naiveté. Then there are those who say it was just a hell of a party." [9]

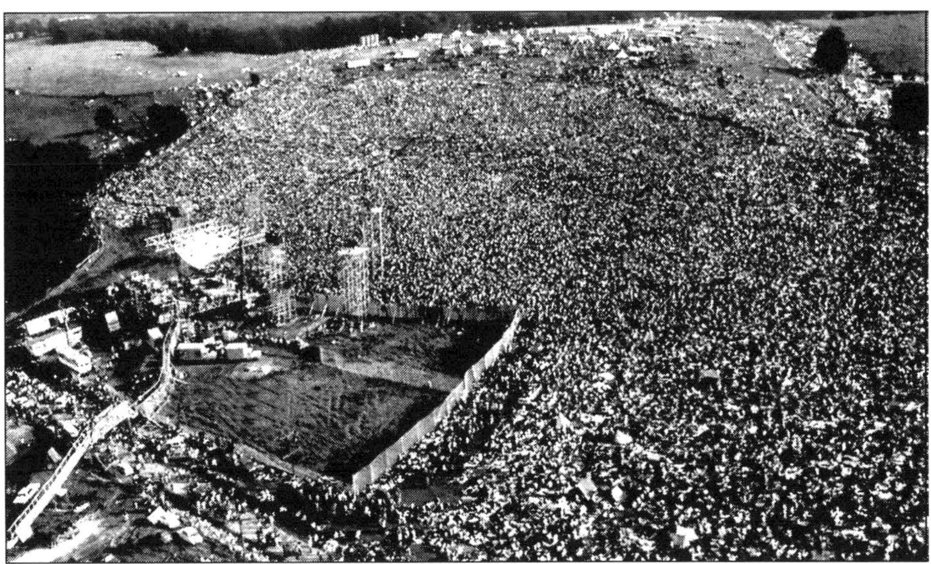

*Woodstock: This 1969, three-day rock festival on Max Yasgur's farm, about 40 miles outside of Woodstock, New York, has become iconic. Hundreds of thousands came to celebrate the anti-war, pro-hedonistic, pro-spiritual lifestyle.*

WOODSTOCK
MUSIC & ART FAIR
presents
AN
AQUARIAN
EXPOSITION
in
WHITE LAKE, N.Y.
WITH
AUGUST
15, 16, 17.
3 DAYS
of PEACE
& MUSIC

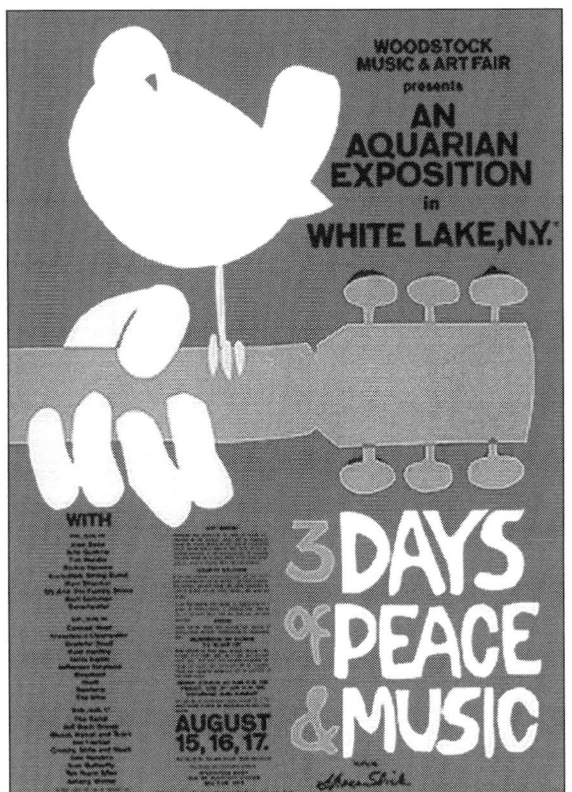

*The poster for what became known as "The Woodstock Festival", August 15, 16 and 17, 1969.*

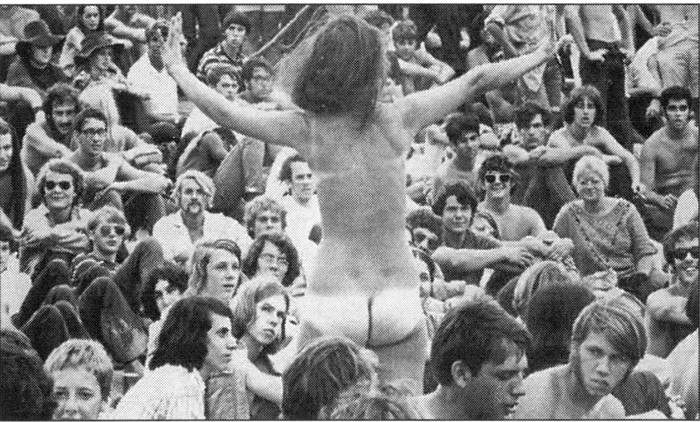

*In addition to the music, the Woodstock Festival was most noted for widespread nudity.*

The Woodstock Music and Art Fair was held at Max Yasgur's 600-acre dairy farm in the rural town of Bethel, New York, from August 15 to August 18, 1969. Bethel (Sullivan County) is 43 miles southwest of the village of Woodstock, New York, in adjoining Ulster County. Some say the festival typified the "hippie era" counterculture of the late 1960s and early 1970s. Woodstock is widely regarded as one of the greatest moments in popular music history and was listed in *Rolling Stone* magazine's "50 Moments That Changed the History of Rock and Roll." [10] The music was performed by some of the best-known musical acts of the day.

The musicians who performed at Woodstock included: Country Joe McDonald singing *Feel Like I'm Fixing to Die Rag*, Janis Joplin singing *Kosmic Blues*, and *Piece of my Heart* (in one of her two encores); the Grateful Dead singing *Mama Tried*; Creedence Clearwater Revival performing *Proud Mary* (among others); and Sly & the Family Stone singing *I Want to Take You Higher*. The Who also performed a 25-song set that included *Tommy*, while Jimi Hendrix performed his famous rendition of *The National Anthem*. Many other artists performed, including John Sebastian, Santana, and Canned Heat. The music reflected a new worldview. Charles Reich,

## Change Can Cause Anxiety Amongst the Guardians of the Status Quo

There were scary changes going on out there in the Sixties. People were getting in hot tubs naked in their backyards with members of the opposite sex. Water beds were replacing innerspring mattresses. Youth preferred marijuana over alcohol as their favored intoxicant. What happened here? To this day, there is still a clash of cultural values between the activists of the 1960s and '70s and those who pushed back against this desire for change.

The 2008 national election had two important issues – the economy and the war in Iraq. Nevertheless, the campaign of the Republican candidate, John McCain, did its best to exploit the culture clash. They tried to introduce the craziness of the 1960s into the debate by focusing on one of Democrat Barack Obama's supporters, Bill Ayers, a retired professor at the University of Illinois. Ayers had been active in the Vietnam anti-war activities and had ties to some of the movement's most radical elements. Since Obama was born in 1961, it was a bit absurd to implicate him in the '60s anti-war action. Obama pointed out that he was eight-years-old at the time of Ayers' radical efforts to end the Vietnam War.

The Obama camp played to the changing demographics and values in our society. The divide on wedge issues of gay marriage, abortion, homosexuality, global warming and drugs was supposedly reflected by the Red and Blue states. The historic election of Barak Obama was not without its subtle and not-so-subtle plays on the existing racism in the United States. This occurred both in the primaries perpetrated by Hillary Clinton and in the general election by Republican 527 groups (527 refers to the section of campaign law defining a group that is independent of the candidate).

It is generally conceded that President Obama inherited a mess from his predecessor, George W. Bush. This ugly stew, cooked over eight years, included two wars (one a war of choice), a deep recession, loss of respect from our allies, corruption by Halliburton and others in the war effort, an economy on the edge of an abyss, and the usual jails full of drug law offenders. Nevertheless, resistance to Obama's efforts to invoke the changes necessary to address these serious problems prevails. He's been strongly opposed by a right-wing movement called the "Tea Party". This movement has been accused of having racist overtones.

One of the silliest allegations is that Obama was born not in Honolulu – as his official Hawaii-issued birth certificate says and is documented by his contemporaneous birth announcement in the Honolulu newspaper – but, instead, in Kenya. At least two patently bogus alleged Kenyan birth certificates were offered as proof of this allegation. One might surmise that this strange logic is influenced by racism.

author of *The Greening of America* (1971), attributed this altered worldview in part to marijuana.

Woodstock was seen by the younger generation as a unique happening that generated "positive energy" and "good karma." This energy is one of the reasons Woodstock is remembered in music and song. The event was special. Joni Mitchell's song *Woodstock* commemorated the event and became a major hit for Crosby, Stills, Nash & Young. They were just some of the bands who created a whole new genre combining love with revolution.[11,12]

### Books/Novels

In the post-WWII era, serious writers tackled important themes: the horror of war, the meaning of life, and the need to be kind. The economic ravages of the depression and the horror of WWII spawned a generation of writers who attacked the social conventions that had created such misery. These writers included Hunter Thompson, Joseph Heller, J.D. Salinger, Philip Roth and Kurt Vonnegut.

---

**"The firebombing of Dresden, was a work of art. It was a tower of smoke and flame to commemorate the rage and heartbreak of so many who had had their lives warped or ruined by the indescribable greed and vanity and cruelty of Germany."**[13]

**Kurt Vonnegut**
*Fates Worse than Death*
(1991)

---

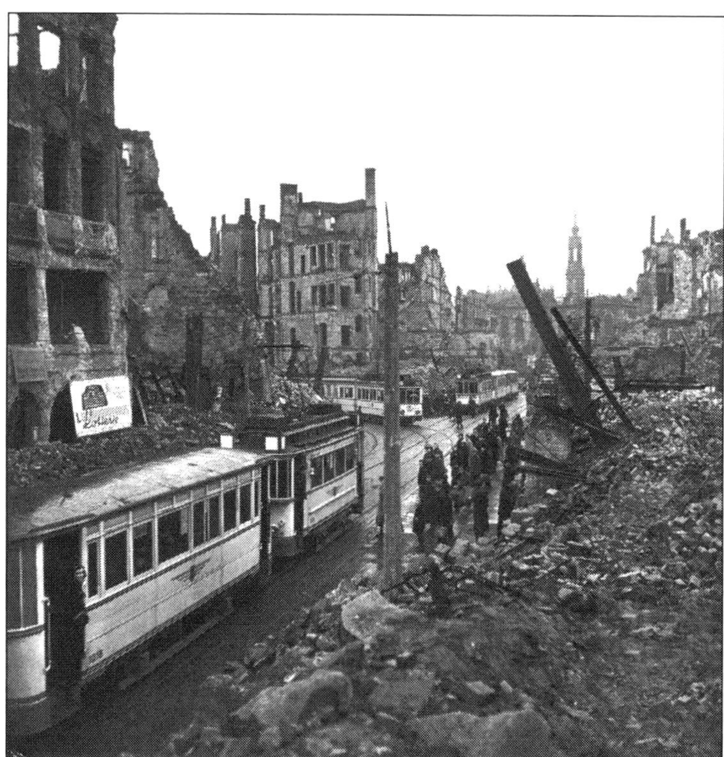

*Dresden, a city in Germany, was not a high-priority strategic WWII target. It was primarily destroyed to show that the United States and its allies could do it.*

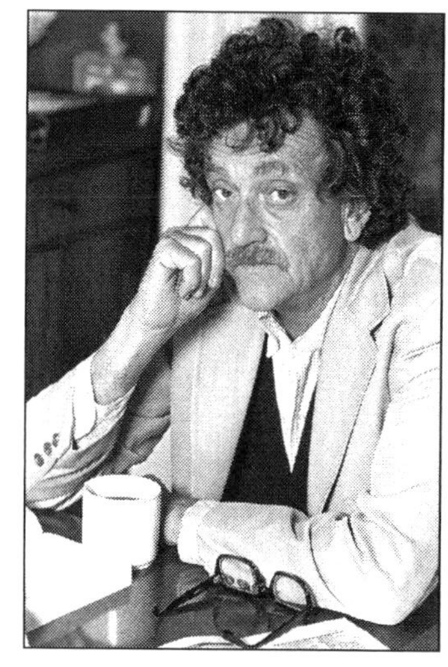

*Kurt Vonnegut was a popular writer of the 1960s and '70s. He fought in WWII and was captured by the Germans. He was in Dresden the night the Allies firebombed it to the ground. He later condemned it as senseless and useless and ironically noted that "only one person on earth clearly benefited, and I am that person." He was referring to his popular novel* Slaughterhouse Five, *which was based on his experience in Dresden.*

**"The corpses, most of them in ordinary cellars, were so numerous and represented such a health hazard, that they were cremated on huge funeral pyres, or by flamethrowers whose nozzles were thrust into the cellars, without being counted or identified."**

**Kurt Vonnegut**

*Fates Worse than Death (1991)*

Vonnegut had fought in WWII. He had been a prisoner of war in Dresden and was there when the British and Americans firebombed Dresden to rubble.

Dresden was horrific. Thousands of civilians were killed in the raids; most were burned to death or asphyxiated. Vonnegut's experience in Dresden did not improve his view of war. He had been assigned by the Germans to make vitamin supplements. The work detail saved his life because he was working with other prisoners in an underground meat locker when the warplanes started carpet-bombing the city, creating a firestorm above him. Afterward, he and his fellow prisoners were assigned to remove the dead.

His experience in Dresden was the basis of *Slaught-erhouse Five: or The Children's Crusade.* The book was pub-lished in 1969 against the backdrop of the war in Vietnam, racial un-rest and cultural and social upheaval. The novel, wrote the critic Jerome Klinkowitz, "so perfectly caught America's transformative mood that its story and structure became best-selling metaphors for the new age." [14]

In an undated speech reprinted in his "auto-biographical collage," *Fates Worse Than Death*, Vonnegut said:

> "The firebombing of Dresden was an emotional event without a trace of military importance. The Germans purposely kept the city free of major war industries and arsenals [...] so that it might be a safe haven for the wounded and refugees. There were no air-raid shelters to speak of and few antiaircraft guns. It was a famous world art treasure, like Paris or Vienna or Prague, and about as sinister as a wedding cake. I will say again what I have often said in print and in speeches, that not one Allied soldier was able to advance as much as an inch because

of the fire-bombing of Dresden. Not one prisoner of the Nazis got out of prison a micro-second earlier. Only one person on earth clearly benefited, and I am that person. I got about five dollars for each corpse, counting my fee tonight."[15]

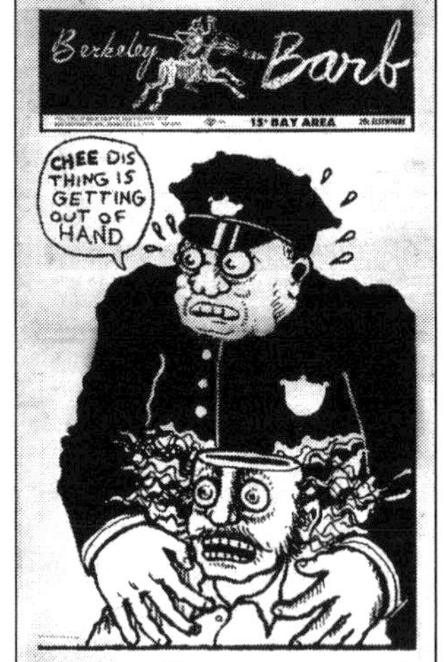


## Alternative Media

The youth, anti-war activists, free speech supporters, recreational drug users and civil-rights advocates of the 1960s felt a collective need for alternative media. An alternative media was required to question and attack religion for its hypocrisy, question the wisdom of the Vietnam War, and to talk about sex and drugs in an adult fashion. The mainstream media both shied away from these issues and seemed to squelch criticism of the status quo.

The so-called underground press, weekly newspapers put out by people in their late teens or early 20s, enraged many in the establishment. This was not only due to their opposition to the Vietnam War and their psychedelic illustrations but also their literary, visual and lifestyle endorsement of sex, drugs and rock 'n' roll. One such newspaper was the Berkeley Barb (left), which served the San Francisco Bay area.

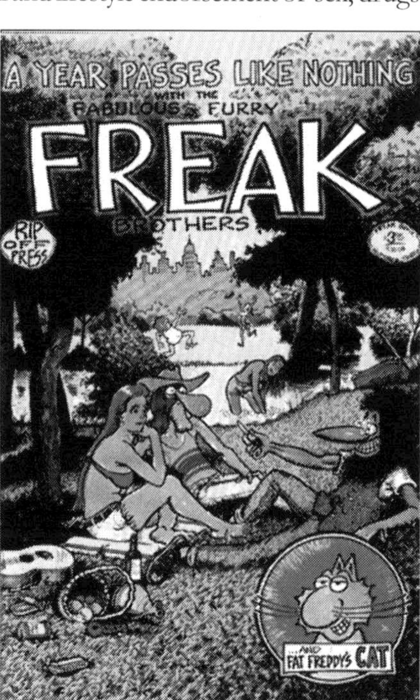


*Gilbert Shelton's <u>Fabulous Furry Freak Brothers</u> were famous for the line: "Dope will get you through times of no money better than money will get you through times of no dope."*[16]

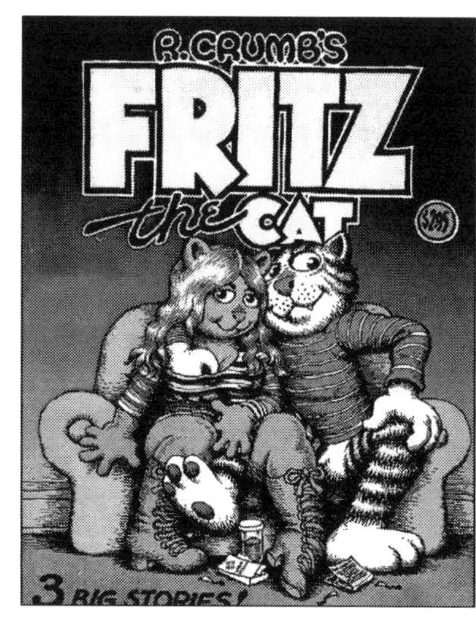


*The 1960's social criticism was captured in the counter-culture comic books satires of society, which were a parody of the wholesomeness of Disney comics.*

Underground comics were another thorn in the side of the mainstream. These often self-published comic books were usually socially relevant or satirical in nature and were meant for young adult and adult audiences. <u>ZAP Comix, Fritz the Cat, Wonder Wart Hog</u>, and artists Gilbert Shelton and R. Crumb were just part of the panoply of creative critics found in underground comics.

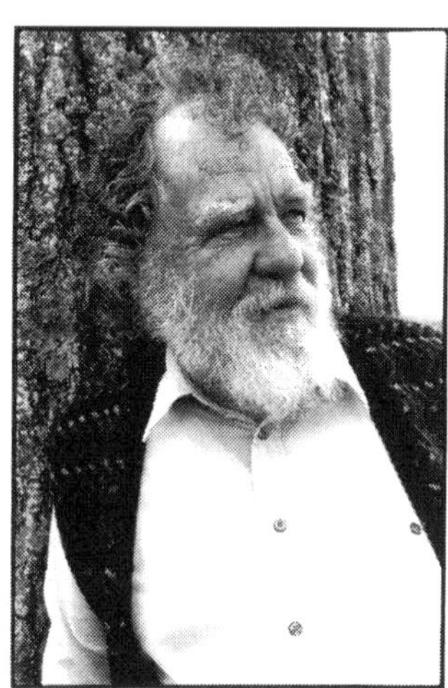

*Charles "Charley" Plymell was a bridge between The Beats and the hippies. 2011 photo.*

Charles "Charley" Plymell was a bridge between the beats and the hippies. Plymell was a "Beat" writer and poet from Kansas. He performed peyote rituals in the 1950s in Kansas City and was part of KC's jazz and benzedrine scene. Before moving to San Francisco in the 1960s, he was involved with the Beats in New York. In 1968, he shared a house in San Francisco on Gough Street with beat poet Allen Ginsberg and Neal Cassady (Jack Kerouac's buddy from *On the Road*). Here, the Beats met the Hippies. Ginsberg said that Plymell was the first to play Bob Dylan for him at a friend's house in Bolinas, then a small-town "hippy" enclave near Point Reyes, California, 50 miles up the coast from San Francisco.

Plymell was a Zelig or Forrest Gump-like character who blended into the background with prominent Beat and counter-culture characters. Besides spending a lot of time with Ginsberg and Cassady, he was also influential on underground comix artists such as R. Crumb and S. Clay Wilson. Plymell printed the first issue of Zap Comix in 1968 under the name Apex Novelties on his printing press in San Francisco.[17] He was a contemporary of influential '60s writers David Amram, Richard Brautigan and William S. Burroughs.

## A New Kind of Comedy

The '60s also ushered in a new breed of comedians. Unlike your grandfather's comics in baggy pants or women's dresses, these entertainers were satirists and social critics. They included Bob Newhart, Shelley Berman, Mort Sahl and the late Lenny Bruce. The fate of comedian and social critic Lenny Bruce is recognized today as an example of the lengths to which the establishment would go to silence a critic.

Bruce was a magnet for cops and criticism. He was arrested for obscenity and possession of narcotics nine times between 1961 and 1964. In April 1964, Lenny Bruce was busted for obscenity for his performance at a small coffee house called the Café Au Go Go in Greenwich Village, New York. Poet Allen Ginsberg became a leader of the *avant garde* in defending Bruce and the arts. He circulated a pre-trial petition containing 100 signatures, including those of Reinhold Niebuhr, Lionel Trilling, James Baldwin and Richard Burton and Elizabeth Taylor (at that time Mr. & Mrs. Burton).[18]

The trial became a cultural battlefield where articulate, intellectual witnesses took turns trying to *put away* the impassive judges. Bruce had expert witnesses from journalism, publishing houses, universities and the clergy testifying on his behalf. The defense witnesses asserted that Bruce was a brilliant social satirist. Five rebuttal witnesses, comparably credentialed, testified for the prosecution.

On the one hand, Bruce was compared to such noteworthy, influential, and frequently controversial

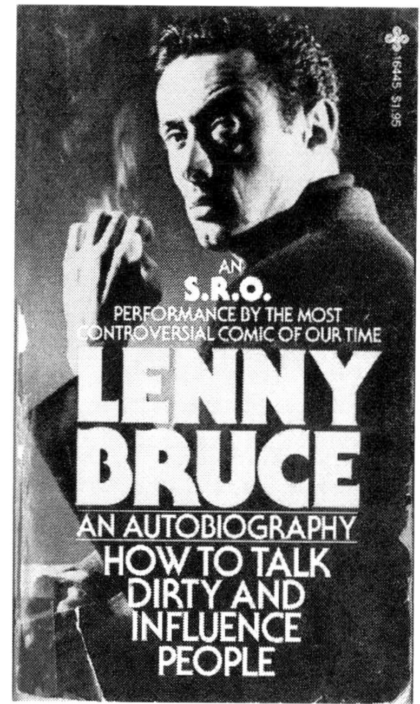


*Lenny Bruce became an icon of critical, anti-establish-ment, iconoclastic stand-up comedy. His criticism of the status quo, in particular the Catholic Church, and his use of heroin led to his many legal problems.*

writers as Francois Rabelais, Jonathan Swift, Mark Twain, James Joyce, and Henry Miller. His dirty words were a tool for social criticism. His critics, on the other hand, saw him as spewing filth, sneering at decent society, and demeaning religion.[19] Basically, there were two different views of the same picture.

A *Newsweek* article in 1964 describing Bruce's trial wrote,

> "Bruce hits his audience where they live – or think they do – in their religion, their sex lives, their politics, their prejudices and prevarications. And he does this by using many of the same shock techniques of language and behavior that modern writers, artists, and even musicians are using to cut through the crust of custom and apathy. He has become a hero to thousands of young people who want to laugh, but at something more important than Crosby's money or Hope's golf score."[20]

*Note: Singer Bing Crosby and comedian Bob Hope often appeared in musical comedies together.*

On December 23, 2003, New York Governor George Pataki issued Bruce a post-humus pardon

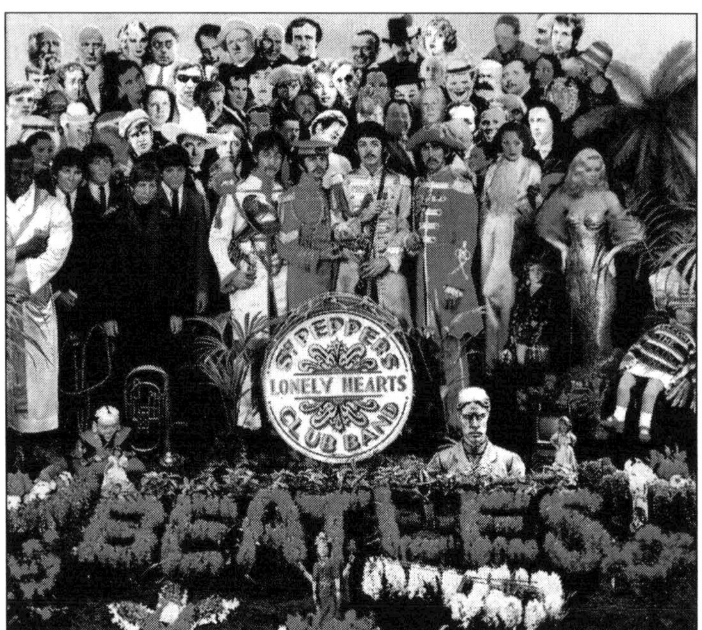


*At the height of the Beatles' popularity, John Lennon declared that the Beatles were more popular than Jesus Christ. This drew the ire of some fundamentalists who took this as a swipe at Jesus. However, Lennon was merely reporting the facts, as he saw them, of the Beatles' enormous popularity. His comment was more lamenting the phenomenon, not saying that it was the way things should be or crowing about the fact.*

from his conviction at the urging of a group concerned about the denial of free speech in the case.[21]

## Drugs & Music:

The Beatles musical foursome (John Lennon, Paul McCartney, George Harrison and Ringo Starr) had a strong impact on the culture of the 1960s. They were an integral part of the movement for greater freedom, sexual liberation, exploration of the spiritual side of drugs, and support of the Vietnam anti-war movement. Like Elvis before them, the Beatles' music was built on a base of Black rock 'n' roll. They soon expanded into contemporary themes and incorporated instruments new to Western European music, like the sitar from India. Their socially relevant, innovative music dominated the top-ten lists for the last half of the decade.

According to most accounts, The Beatles were turned on to marijuana at the Hotel Delmonico in New York in 1964 when they first met Bob Dylan. "An unusually gregarious Dylan was delighted by the Beatles' curiosity and readiness to experiment," Bob Spitz writes in *The Beatles: The Biography*. "They got right into the groove, which relaxed the recalcitrant bard, who lit joint after joint, fanning the fateful flame." The chapter ends, "[it was] *party time*. And nothing would ever be the same again."[22]

## Psychedelics

Psychedelics were part and parcel of the Civil Rights Movement, feminism, and anti-war activism of the 1960s and '70s. There was Ken Kesey and the Hog Farm's madcap, cross-country bus trip, the Summer of Love, Woodstock – and Dr. Timothy Leary with his message of "turn on, tune in, drop out." What a threat to the established order he was! A pied piper of the young, Leary pointed out in a *Playboy* interview that he saw LSD (lysergic acid diethylamide) as a spiritual sacrament, a way to open one's mind to the possibilities of life and a means to get in touch with one's eternal essence. This sounds like an echo of dangerous naturalistic religions.

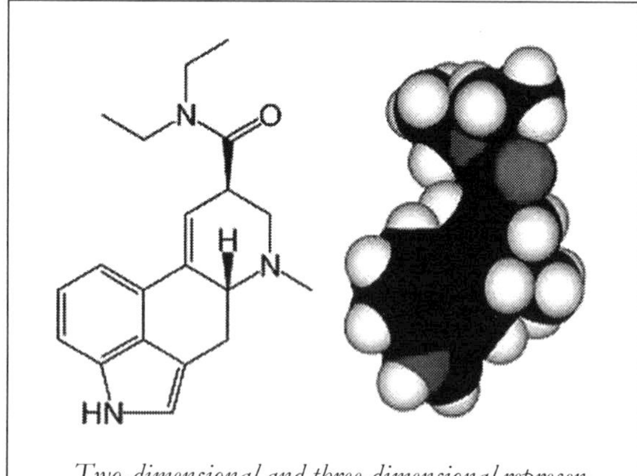


*Two-dimensional and three-dimensional representations of lysergic acid diethylamide (LSD).*

LSD had been synthesized in 1938 by Dr. Albert Hofmann working with W.A. Stoll at Sandoz Laboratories in Switzerland. He was working with the compound because Sandoz had successfully marketed ergot derivatives for treating migraine headaches and for obstetrical use.

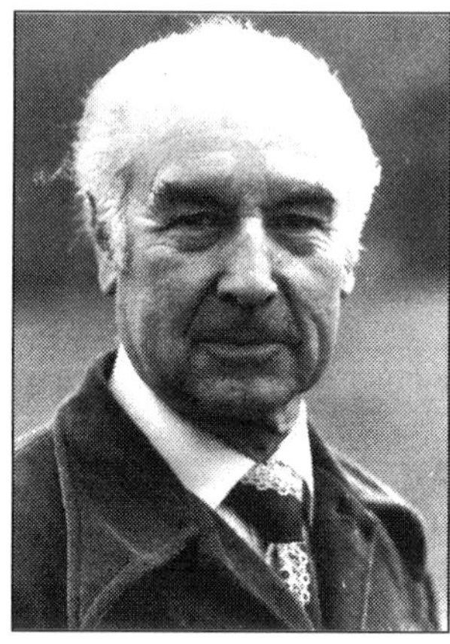

*Dr. Albert Hofmann, who invented LSD in Switzerland in 1938.*

The initial testing on animals was uneventful. But in 1943, Hoffman got some LSD on his fingers and accidentally ingested it. He experienced what he termed "a peculiar state similar to darkness characterized by exaggerated imagination." [24] The next week he took what he presumed was a small dose and kept notes. The rest is history.

---

"The characteristic property of hallucinogens, to suspend the boundaries between the experiencing self and the outer world in an ecstatic, emotional experience, makes it possible with their help, and after suitable internal and external preparation ... to evoke a mystical experience according to plan, so to speak. . . . I see the true importance of LSD in the possibility of providing material aid to meditation aimed at the mystical experience of a deeper, comprehensive reality. Such a use accords entirely with the essence and working character of LSD as a sacred drug." [24]

**Dr. Albert Hofmann**
the inventor of LSD,
who died in 2008 at the age of 102

---

## Get On the Bus

Ken Kesey, author of *Sometimes A Great Notion* (1964) and *One Flew Over the Cuckoo's Nest* (1962), an allegory of our world gone mad, is another iconic figure of the 1960s. He was born in La Junta, Colorado and raised in Oregon where he was a top high-school wrestler.

Kesey and the Merry Pranksters had a psychedelically painted, 1939 International Harvester bus they named "Further". In 1964, they went on a bus trip around the United States to spread the word for love, peace and psychedelics and against

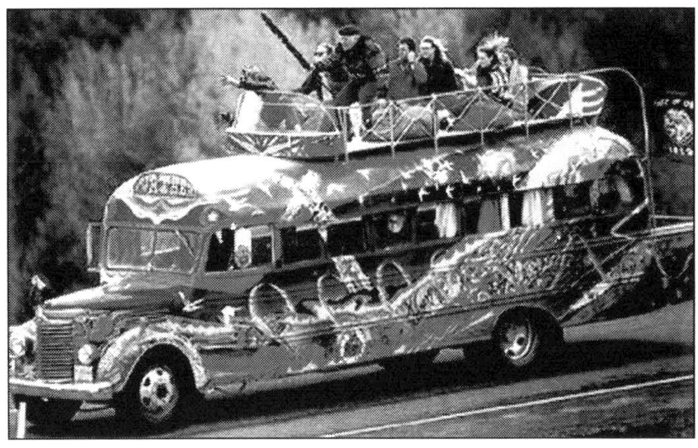

*This is Ken Kesey's famous psychedelically painted, 1939 International Harvester bus. Persons considered to be "on the bus", meant they were a member of the counterculture, and if someone was considered "off the bus", meant they were straight, a member of the establishment.*

consumerism. Further, the bus, was the source for the counter-culture slogan of the '60s, "You're either on the bus or off the bus." The meaning was clear: Riders on the bus supported love and peace and opposed war and consumerism, and endorsed a spirituality that incorporated altered states of consciousness. Kesey amd this bus trip were later immortalized in Tom Wolfe's book, *Electric Kool-Aid Acid Test* (1968).

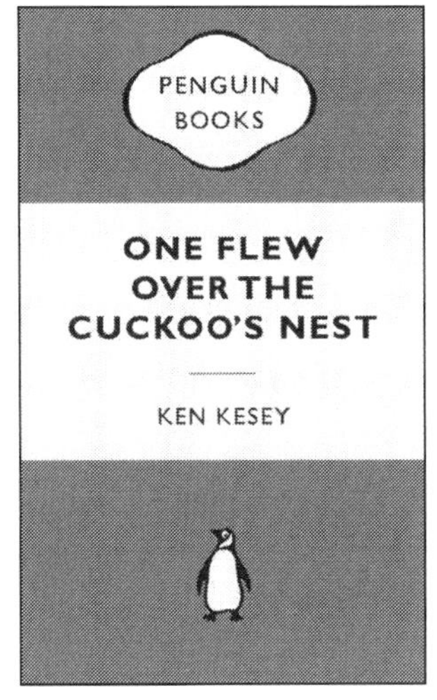


*Kesey's novel,* One Flew Over the Cuckoo's Nest *(1962), was a metaphor for wrong-headed bureaucratic action.*

## The Human Be-in

The psychedelic '60s, as they are characterized today (as opposed to the Civil Rights struggle that captured the idealism of many young Americans in the early 1960s), is said to have began with the first "Human Be-in" celebrated January 14, 1967 in San Francisco's Golden Gate Park. This was the unofficial kick-off to the so-called "Summer of Love." The Human Be-in was part rock concert, part literary event, part protest and all mass consciousness-raising.

**"My advice to people today is as follows: If you take the game of life seriously, if you take your nervous system seriously, if you take your sense organs seriously, if you take the energy process seriously, you must turn on, tune in, and drop out."** [25]

**Timothy Leary (1920-1996)**

1960's counterculture icon, American writer, psychologist, psychedelic drug researcher.

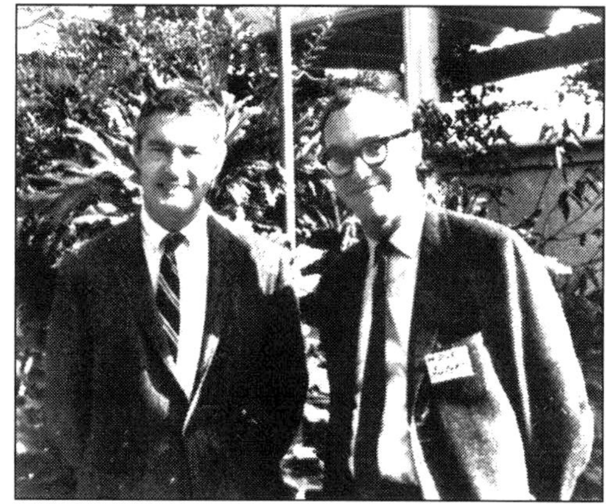

*Timothy Leary (left) and Richard Alpert in their Harvard days.*

Leary carried on many scholarly studies with psychedelics. Several were published in professional peer-reviewed, scientific journals. In one such study he stated that 70% of his subjects found that taking psilocybin in a relaxed, comfortable home environment with oriental rugs and sitar music was a positive experience. Many said it was a spiritually moving experience. Seven percent found it unpleasant. [26]

The Human Be-in was billed at the time as a Gathering of the Tribes in an effort to unite different factions of the counterculture movement. Headliners included LSD-advocate Dr. Timothy Leary, Beat poets Allen Ginsberg and Gary Snyder, comedian Dick Gregory, bands The Grateful Dead and Jefferson Airplane. [27] It was attended by over 30,000 people. The Be-in was a creation of the San Francisco counter-culture and part of the Summer of Love; a creation of the media.

THE HUMAN BE-IN
A GATHERING OF THE TRIBES
Timothy Leary
Richard Alpert
Dick Gregory
Allen Ginsberg
Jerry Rubin
MANY OTHERS
SATURDAY
JAN. 14th
1967
FREE
ALL OF SAN FRANCISCO'S ROCK BANDS
INCLUDING
SANTANA
AND
THE STEVE MILLER BAND
GOLDEN GATE PARK
SAN FRANCISCO
BRING
FLOWERS
INCENSE
FEATHERS
CANDLES
BANNERS
FLAGS
BRING
FAMILIES
ANIMALS
CYMBALS
DRUMS
CHIMES
FLUTES

*A poster for the Be-in.*

These events in celebration of life and change were common-place in the late 1960s and the '70s. Some say that the first big Be-in was held not in January 1967 but in October of 1966, on the occasion of the California law against LSD going into effect the day before.

Tom Wolfe described the scene as "thousands of heads piled in, in high costume, ringing bells, chanting, dancing ecstatically, blowing their minds one way and another and making their favorite satiric gesture to the cops, handing them flowers, burying the bastids in tender fruity petals of love. ... the thing was fantastic, a freaking mindblower, thousands of high-loving heads out there messing up the minds of the cops and everybody else in a fiesta of love and euphoria." [28]

## Turn On, Tune In, Drop Out

In the late 1950s, Ph.D. doctors Timothy Leary and Richard Alpert (now known as Baba Ram Dass) were instructors at Harvard University's Center for Personality Research.

In the fall of 1960, Leary and Alpert did university-approved research with psilocybin obtained from Sandoz. They ran an experiment on prisoners at the Massachusetts Correctional Institute to see if taking the hallucinogen psilocybin lowered recidivism. Promising initial results showed that prisoners who had taken a psilocybin trip prior to their release were less likely to violate their parole than those who had not. [29] Leary may have thought it was because "You are never the same after you've had that one flash glimpse down the cellular time tunnel." [30]

Leary and Alperts' mystique grew. Soon, they went from being Harvard faculty to being new-age gurus. They were proponents of the alleged "mind expansion" and altered perceptions caused by LSD. LSD contributed to a subculture embraced by many in the baby boomer generation. The 1960s changed music, lifestyles, attitudes toward marriage, and the substances used for recreation and enjoyment. Psychedelics (psychoactive drugs) such as dimethyltryptamine (DMT), methylene-dioxymethamphetamine (MDMA or Ecstacy), mescaline, psilocybin mushrooms, and LSD became an important part of the counterculture scene.

Counterculture advocates considered LSD a particularly potent psychotropic drug. LSD causes an altered state of consciousness and has a significant impact on perception of reality. LSD, with its ability to allow users to see things from a different perspective, was a major contributor to the counter-culture. The psychedelic experience led to a clearer recognition that reality can be relative; our view of reality is shaped by our culture, our experience, and our preconceived notions. With psychedelics, people realized there was more than one reality. LSD helped change the content of everything from university courses to cookbooks – even including many popularly held beliefs.

Alpert and Leary set up an institute (or "retreat center") in a fifty-five room mansion in Millbrook, New York, to promote the benefits of psychoactive substances. The site was owned by Mellon heir Billy Hitchcock (this is more than a bit ironic if one recalls that many people finger Andrew Mellon, Treasury Secretary under President Herbert Hoover and banker to Lammot DuPont, for the Marijuana Tax Act of 1937).

Leary was portrayed as a pied piper of the young, extolling psychedelia and LSD. It wasn't long before the mansion retreat was raided. The local cops were led by G. Gordon Liddy (Liddy eventually went to prison for his role in burglarizing the Democratic National Headquarters at Watergate as part of Nixon's 1972 reelection campaign). Leary himself later went to prison for possessing approximately a fingernail's worth of marijuana. Richard Alpert went to India and became the guru Baba Ram Dass, the very symbol of the seeker. [31]

Ken Kesey writes rather poignantly of Leary's successful prison break from the minimum security prison in San Luis Obispo, California:

> "So imagine: you're a middle-aged psychologist, an alum from West Point and a discredited prof from Harvard, serving five-to-ten years for a fall you took for your daughter at the Texas border when you relieved her of the two stupid joints she had stashed in her panties. Now you're up a power pole on top of a state prison, one eye on your wristwatch while the other contemplates the naked cable that will carry you to freedom, one way or another." Kesey reports that Leary described it as "the longest three minutes of my life." [32]

Kesey continued:

> "Now imagine being spirited out of the country and whisked to Algiers where you are taken in by fellow fugitives Eldridge and Kathleen Cleaver and the Black Panthers who intend to indoctrinate yo pampered ass! Heavy trip or what? Hemmed in by Black Panthers on one side and whitebread weather prognosticates on the other while unscrupulous Algerian cops prowl the street outside the compound eyes like hungry jackals. Might as well have stayed in San Luis Obispo." [33]

## LSD

Adam Smith, author of *Powers of Mind* (1978), points out that between 1943 and 1963, the U.S. Food and Drug Administration labeled LSD an "investigational new drug." The drug was largely used to help facilitate psychotherapy. So for over 20 years, the therapeutic use of Dr. Hofmann's chemical to treat peoples' minds brought no talk of revolution. LSD was used with little note by the media. [34]

LSD's use to aid therapy was lauded by all manner of psychological thought, including Freudians, Jungians and Rankians. Dr. Stanislav Grof, a Czechozlovakian-born Toronto psychiatrist, had popularized LSD's therapeutic use in psychiatry. Dr. Grof believed that LSD sped up the psychotherapeutic process.

LSD was described as hastening therapeutic progress by removing or lowering our defense

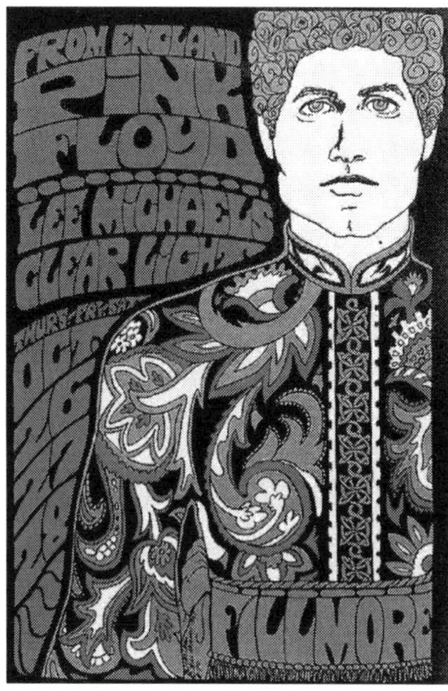


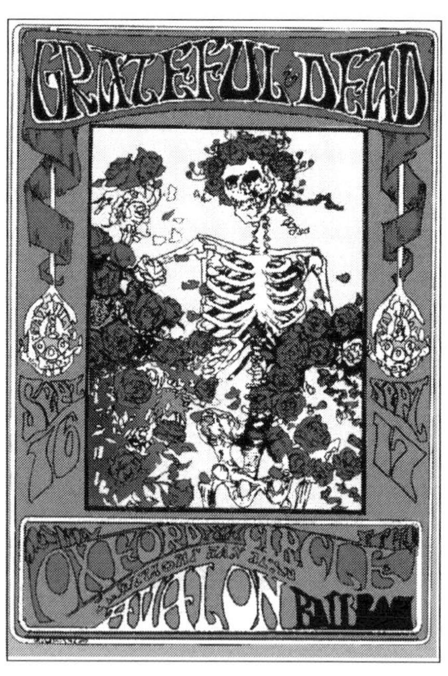


*A new art form was created, heavily influenced by the psychedelic experience, and used primarily to advertise events featuring music heavily influenced by the psychedelic experience.*

mechanism. Defense mechanisms are psychological devices such as rationalizing and projection which help protect us from too closely scrutinizing the distance between our idealized self and our self as we actually exist. For some such a revel-ation was exciting, a veritable road map on where they had to go to be a better person. For others, it was crushing and depressing to see the gap between where they were in reality as a person and how far they needed to go to attain their idealized self.

*Owsley Stanley (left), with Jerry Garcia of The Grateful Dead band, is said to have made the finest LSD available.*

Owsley (August Owsley Stanley III, sound man for The Grateful Dead band) is remembered for making the finest LSD where "everybody's trip was beautiful. [...] Orange Sunshine, a combination of lysergic acid and ergotamine tartrate, was reportedly Owsley's best product." [35] According to *The Beatles: A Biography* (2005), John Lennon made a deal to purchase a lifetime supply of LSD from Owsley. [36]

## Set, Setting & Previous Experiences

Most scientists agree that set, setting and previous experiences have a significant impact on the psychotropic drug experience. Knowing what to expect and look for helped fulfill many trippers' expectations.

In 1967, Sociology Professor Howard Becker of Northwestern University, author of *The Outsiders* (1963), wrote an article predicting that a subculture would develop around the use of LSD and that this would cause a marked decrease in so-called "bad acid trips." He felt that more sophisticated consumers would label possible LSD side effects, like excessive hallucinations, as temporary drug effects rather than permanent insanity. He also prognosticated that repeat users of LSD would become more aware of the nature and extent of LSD's side effects.

Becker reasoned that as people in this subculture became more adept at handling these adverse effects of LSD ("bad trips"), they would be less likely to panic if they did have a bad trip. As such, people using LSD for the first time were more likely to identify any adverse effects of LSD as drug effects rather than interpret these feelings of depersonalization and changes in perception as some kind of permanent mental change. The novice LSD user having a so-called "bad trip" in the company of more experienced "heads" would be less likely to panic. He or she would gain confidence from being in the hands of members of the subculture who knew what to expect.[37]

Becker was on to something. Both set and setting can have an influence in mitigating undesired effects of some drugs, as well as enhancing desired effects.[38] In fact, the incidence of so-called bad trips dropped off dramatically over the next few years.

Author Tom Wolfe put it this way:

> Leary and Alpert preached "set and setting." Everything in taking LSD, in having a fruitful-freakout-free LSD experience, depended on set and setting. You should take it in some serene and attractive setting, a house or apartment decorated with objects of the honest sort, Turkoman tapestries, Greek goatskin rugs, Cost Plus blue jugs, soft light--not Japanese paper globe light, however, but untasselated Chinese textile shades--in short, an Uptown Bohemian country retreat of the $60,000-a-year sort, ideally ... The "set" was the set of your mind. You should prepare for the experience by meditating upon the state of your being and deciding what you hope to discover and achieve on this voyage into the self. You should also have a guide who has taken LSD himself and is familiar with the various stages of the experience and whom you know and trust.[39]
>
> **Tom Wolfe**
> *The Electric Kool Aid Acid Test* (1968)

## Backlash

Things changed once LSD came into the limelight; LSD and other psychedelics soon became a full-blown divisive social issue, joining many other such issues. Steven S. Smith, a political scientist at Washington University in St. Louis, enumerated many of the contentious issues. He said, "Then came free speech, birth control pills, long hair, brotherly love, Flower Children, predators of the Flower Children, cops, narcotics, speed, laws, judges, politicians, campaigning, busts, riots, Vietnam, war resisters, the Mafia, Richard Nixon, Woodstock, confrontation."[40]

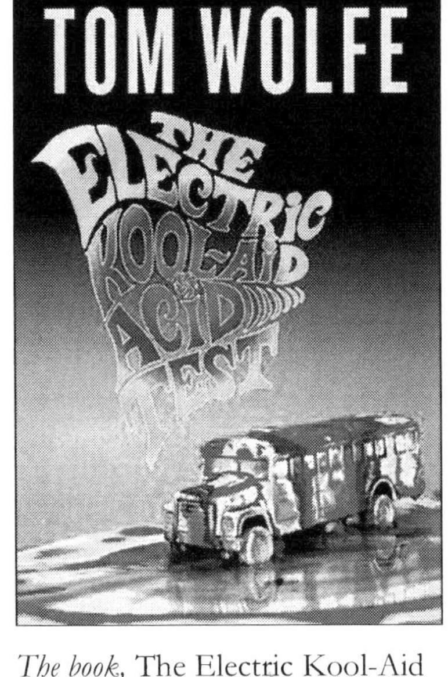


*The book,* The Electric Kool-Aid Acid Test *(1968), made journalist Tom Wolfe famous. It chronicled Ken Kesey and others and supported cultural change. It is considered a major book on the psychedelic '60s.*

The tabloids found all kinds of fiction that they promoted as fact. "LSD addicts stare at sun and become blind" was a tabloid headline in the late 1960s. It was generated by a hoax fabricated by a misguided Pennsylvania state official who wanted to scare kids away from LSD.

One tabloid ran a picture of "thalidomide babies" (children disfigured from prenatal exposure to the sedative thalidomide) that was wrongly captioned, "these were caused by LSD." Others told stories about chromosome breaks in lab experiments with LSD. The counter-culture questioned these inflammatory reports, however, asking what made LSD-induced breaks front-page news, when the same breaks were also known to occur from caffeine and aspirin yet went unreported. Could it be because the producers of coffee, tea and aspirin were major advertisers in the media?[41]

There were unflattering counterculture critiques of government, religion and the military. All of which were seen as serious threats from an establishment perspective. A full-scale counterattack ensued. This establishment effort included anti-youth, anti-liberal, anti-drug, racist, and sexist propaganda. There were agent provocateurs and many killings of Black Panther members. Others on the fringe caught up by the hostility of the time were involved in the assassinations of President Kennedy, his brother Bobby (a leading presidential candidate) and Civil Rights leader and Nobel Peace Prize winner Dr. Martin Luther King, Jr.; and the "demonization" and arrest of Leary, who was sent to federal prison for possession of less than a gram of marijuana.

Somewhat ironically, it was in the 1969 Timothy Leary case that the U.S. Supreme Court found the 1937 Marijuana Tax Act to be unconstitutional. They reasoned that it was an unconstitutional "Catch-22". If a person paid the tax, he/she could be arrested, but if the person didn't pay it, they could also be arrested.

The ruling was based on conflict between federal and State law. By registering under the Marijuana Tax Act and the Boggs amendment, one would be breaking Texas state law. This rendered the acts unconstitutional. This ruling and the hostility of two dueling Americas laid the groundwork for the passage of the Controlled Substances Act in 1970.

## The War on Poverty

After President Kennedy's assassination, President Johnson used the national moral outrage, his legislative skills as former majority leader of the U.S. Senate, and his forceful personality to push landmark civil rights legislation through Congress. These laws made it more difficult to discriminate against people on the basis of race and ethnicity.

Equally important, Johnson launched a War on Poverty in America. It spawned the Office of Economic Opportunity (OEO), an omnibus federal effort that attempted to attack the root causes of poverty, such as poor education, poor housing, crime, and limited job skills. The idea was that through federal funding of a broad array of programs, such as Head Start, subsidized job programs, job-skills training, and affordable childcare, as well as encouraging companies to expand into ghettos, the federal government could help lift people out of poverty.

### The Model Cities Program

The Model Cities Program was the centerpiece of Johnson's War on Poverty. The original idea was to pick one city in America and focus all available federal resources on that city to create a model of what could be done with such federal cooperation. Detroit was to be that model city.

The Model Cities idea was so appealing to federal legislators that soon it was suggested that there should be three cities, then 25. Eventually 225 cities got Model Cities planning grants. Many of these cities launched projects that still exist to this day. Sadly, the whole idea became so watered down by the expansion to 225 cities that there never was a one model city.

## The Vietnam War

The Vietnam War starkly revealed the fault lines in American society. The tension was simmering just below the surface. Societal differences existed regarding the war on poverty. Many did not like the idea that the government would actually spend real money to help the poor, particularly Blacks and Hispanics. As the Vietnam War wore on and Johnson lost political power, the War on Poverty drifted away.

Soon, the War on Poverty was replaced by the beginnings of the "War on Drugs". This new war made matters worse for the very people who the War on Poverty was designed to help. While the OEO and the War on Poverty are part of history, the War on Drugs is still with us. This is a war we have lost. It is a war that has cost billions, been ineffective, lost respect for the rule of law, undermined the Constitution and hasn't worked.

### War Resistance Grows

As the 1960s went on with no end to the Vietnam War in sight and with more young men being conscripted, maimed, and killed, the anti-war movement gained more and more popular support. The major turning point was the Tet Offensive by the North Vietnamese in February 1968 that produced major American losses.

Suddenly an increasing share of the American public began to believe it had been lied to about the Vietnam War. Secretary of Defense Robert McNamara's 1964 statements that there was "light at the end of the tunnel" and the "war will be over" by December 1965 were viewed as absurd. More Americans were becoming keenly aware not only that the number of young Americans drafted and killed was well into the thousands, but also that the Vietnam War was unwinnable. The light at the end of the tunnel looked more and more like an oncoming train.

Vietnam became a nightmare, both for our troops overseas and for America itself. The official reasons for our presence were even less clear than the justification for the 2003 U.S. invasion of Iraq and the war that followed. In Vietnam, as in Iraq, the motive could have been oil. The Spratley Islands off the Vietnam coast have large oil reserves; today, the Philippines and Vietnam are still contending for control of these islands and the oil reserves there.

The Cold War also contributed to the war in Vietnam. The Vietnam intervention was justified as a way to prevent the spread of communism. The United States allegedly feared a Chinese takeover of Vietnam could a result in domino effect, which would place all of Southeast Asia under Communist control. This interpretation ignored the 1,500 years of Vietnamese hatred for the Chinese. This animus was for good reason: the Chinese had invaded Vietnam at least four times through the years). The United States focused instead on suspicion of the motives and goals of the Chinese Communists.

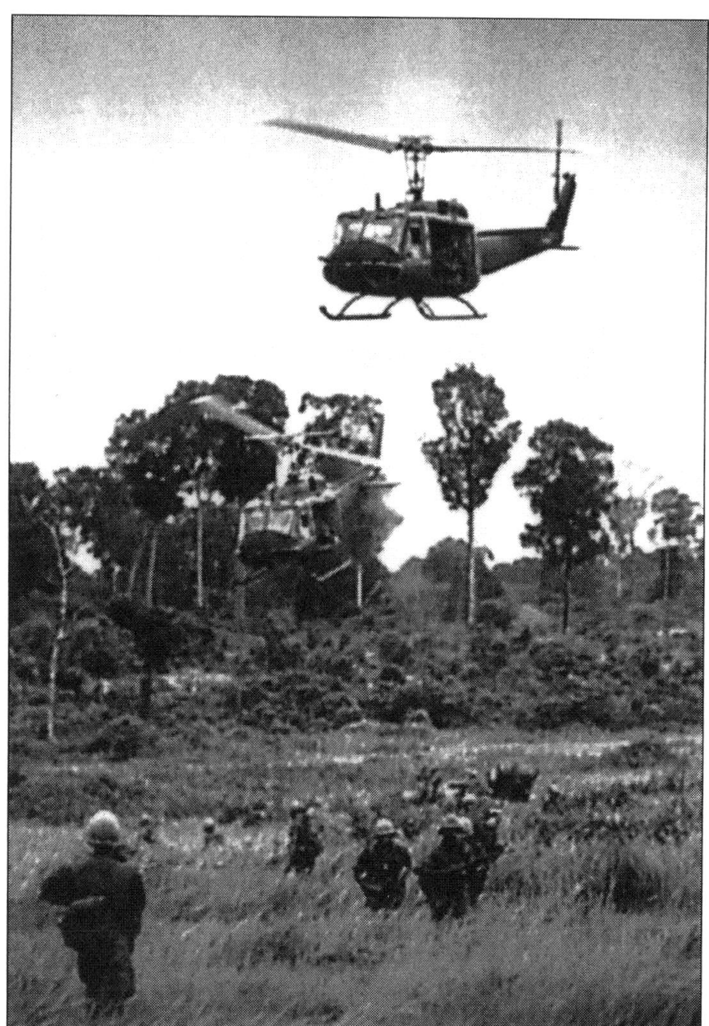

*Helicopters were an iconic symbol of the Vietnam conflict. Images of helicopters and the sound of the whirling wings figure prominently in many Vietnam War films, such as* Apocalypse Now.

## Marijuana

Because of the growing familiarity at home with marijuana and its wide availability throughout Vietnam (and likely in an effort to deal with the anxiety, depression, and Post-Traumatic Stress Disorder associated with war), many soldiers stationed in Southeast Asia began using it. It is estimated that nearly 74 percent of America's soldiers stationed in Vietnam experimented with cannabis at one time or another during their tour of duty there.[42] Later research and experience has shown cannabis to be helpful in dealing with painful memories and treating PTSD.[43]

The Vietnam War experience generated many soldiers returning to the United States with PTSD. Military men and women in Vietnam used marijuana to help them cope with the trials and tribulations of war. They were fighting a war where Vietnamese friends and enemies looked alike and children were willing to blow you up. These soldiers brought their appreciation for the relief that cannabis provided home with them. Cannabis was helpful in treating their PTSD.

As the war escalated, more and more young people were being drafted to go to Vietnam. More and more draftees were dying there. Back at home, innocent, unarmed college students protesting the war died in confrontations with the National Guard at Kent State and Jackson State universities.

Peace and an end to the war became a common goal amongst the young. The ranks of the so-called hippies and mainstream anti-war activists swelled. The establishment feared this large shift in cultural values and fought back with vigor and violence. Laws were passed aimed at criminalizing and punishing anti-establishment behavior, demonstrations, drug use, non-marital sex and anti-war activities.

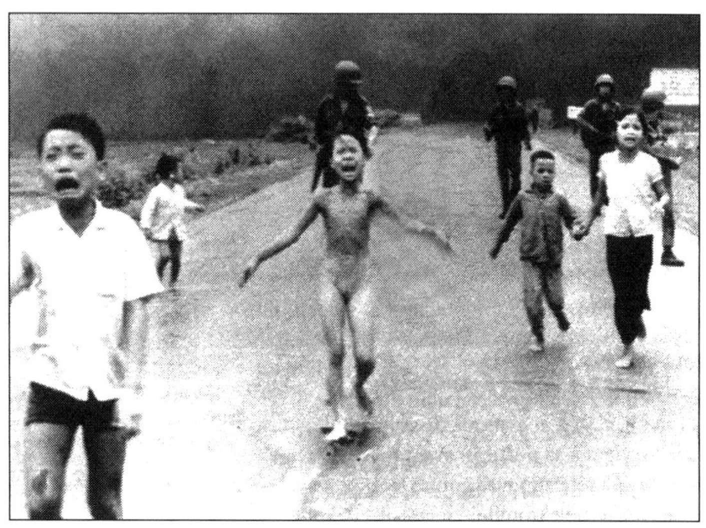

*The Vietnam War was well-covered by the media. This was the first war on television. Powerful still photos, such as above, exposed people sitting in the comfort of their own homes to the horror of war.*

Lieutenant Colonel James "Bo" Gritz was the most decorated Green Beret commander of the Vietnam War Era. At one point, U.S. General William Westmoreland pointed to Bo Gritz as the "American Soldier" for his exemplary courage in combat in Vietnam. But as the war progressed, Gritz became disillusioned.

Gritz made compelling allegations regarding the CIA and their contract airline, Air America, claiming that they were deeply involved in the transport and sale of heroin from the Golden Triangle, one of Asia's major opium-productive areas. The money from the CIA's alleged sale of drugs went to finance "off-the-books" operations (author's note: such support for as our allies in the rural mountains, the Hmong "independence fighters"), and enriched the bank accounts of some American CIA officials and high-ranking Vietnamese officers.[44]

**Official government estimates found that 30-40 percent of U.S. servicemen and women in Vietnam had used heroin, most intra-nasally (snorting). Fortunately, upon return home, all but one or two percent ceased their use of heroin.** [45]

Gritz made an effort to reform the military. In a February 1, 1988 letter to then U.S. Vice President George H.W. Bush, Gritz wrote:

**Gritz's Unanswered Plea**

"What I want to tell you very quickly is something that I feel is more heinous than the Bataan death march. Certainly it is of more concern to you as Americans than the Watergate. What I'm talking about is something we found out in Burma (May 1987). We found it out from a man named Khun Sa. He is the recognized overlord of heroin in the world. Last year (1986) he sent 900 tons of opiates and heroin into the free world. This year it will be 1200 tons. On video tape he said to us something that was most astounding: that U.S. government officials have been and are now his biggest customers and have been for the last twenty years. ... We've been embracing organized crime. Now you've all looked and heard about Ollie North, about the Contras, about nobody knowing anything. [...]

"The thing that I was most concerned about was [General Khun Sa's] offer to stop the flow of opium and heroin into the free world. Then [National Security Council staffer Tom Harvey] said, 'Bo, there's no one here that supports that.'

"And I said 'What? Vice-president Bush has been appointed by President Reagan as the number one policeman to control drug entry into the United States. How can you say there's no interest and no support when we bring back a video tape with a direct interview with a man who puts 900 tons of opium and heroin across into the free world every year and is willing to stop it?' And he said, 'Bo, what can I tell you? All I can tell you is there is no interest in doing that here.'"[46]

**James "Bo" Gritz**
1987 Speech
American Liberty Lunch Club

"January 20, 1988, I talked before your Breakfast Club in Houston, Texas. A distinguished group of approximately 125 associates of yours, including the Chief Justice of the Texas Supreme Court, expressed assurance that you are a righteous man. Almost all of them raised their hand when I asked how many of them know you personally. If you are a man with good intent, I pray you will do more than respond to this letter. I ask that you seriously look into the possibility that political appointees close to you are guilty of bypassing our Constitutional process, and for purposes of promoting illegal covert operations, conspired in the trafficking of narcotics and arms.

Please answer why a respected American Citizen like Mister H. Ross Perot can bring you a pile of evidence of wrongdoing by Armitage and others, and you, according to *TIME* magazine (May 4, page 18), not only offer him no support, but have your Secretary of Defense, Frank Carlucci tell Mr. Perot to "stop pursuing Mr. Armitage." Why Sir, will you not look into affidavits gathered by The Christic Institute (Washington, D.C.), which testify that Armitage not only trafficked in heroin, but did so under the guise of an officer charged with bringing home our POWs. If the charges are true, Armitage, who is still responsible for POW recovery as your Assistant Secretary of Defense ISA, has every reason not to want these heroes returned to us alive. Clearly, follow-on investigations would illuminate the collective cries of Armitage and others."[47]

These revelations seemed to have little impact on U.S. policy.

## The Political Scene

In 1968, opposition to the war coalesced around the presidential candidacy of former St. Thomas College professor and a veteran U.S. Senator from Minnesota, Eugene McCarthy. McCarthy entered the New Hampshire primary as an anti-war candidate and a decided underdog. Because he was scholarly and cerebral rather than a charismatic speaker, and not well-known nationally, establishment liberals initially dubbed his campaign as quixotic. But opposition to the war was reaching a cres-cendo and McCarthy's campaign caught fire with youth and those disgusted with the protracted, deadly, apparently aimless war. McCarthy garnered

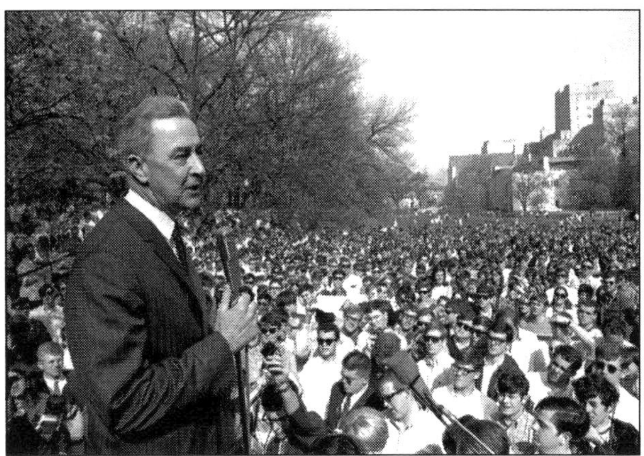

*U.S. Senator Eugene McCarthy (D-Minn.) was an erudite, former professor at a small Catholic liberal arts college in Minnesota. His entry into the 1968 Democratic primary galvanized the anti-war movement. Youth flocked to his campaign and got "Clean for Gene" (e.g., shaved their beards and mustaches and legs and armpits and exchanged their tie-died duds for more conservative appeal).*

**"This perception brought on a political crisis. President Lyndon B. Johnson was driven from the 1968 presidential race in that election year by antiwar activists, led by Minnesota Senator Eugene McCarthy and later Bobby Kennedy – whose assassination after the California primary in June brought chaos and deceit in its wake, a tumultuous, rigged Democratic convention and a bloody police riot in the streets of Chicago.**
**... this coincided with a perilous turning point in the Racial Crisis in America. The non-violent insurgence of the Civil Rights movement to overturn segregation ended in calamity, with the murder of Martin Luther King on April 4, 1968, touching off catastrophic urban riots across the country."** [48]

**Robert Potter**
Professor of Drama, UC Santa Barbara
Speech at the Dedication of the Isla Vista, Calif. Monument to those who peacfully protested the War in Vietnam. June 10, 2003

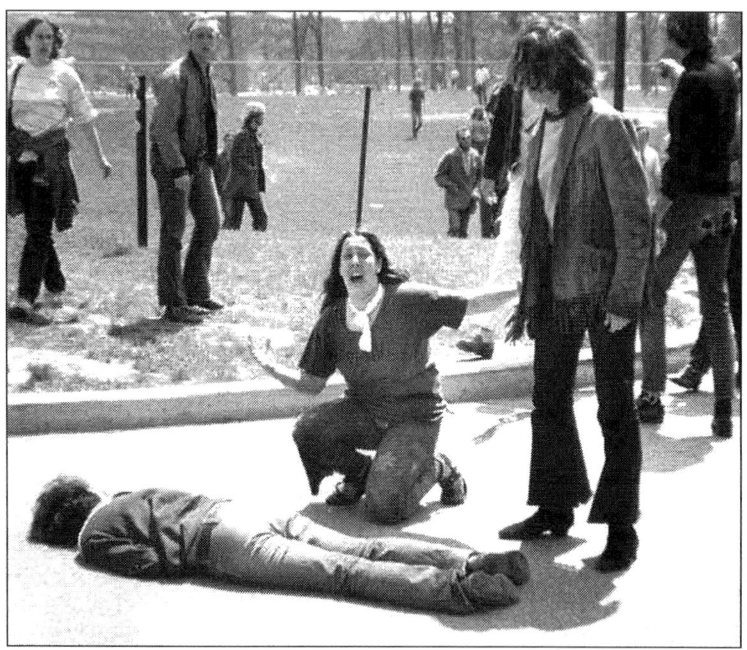

*An iconic photograph of a young woman shocked and stunned mourning over the body of one of four students shot dead by National Guardsmen at Kent State Uniersity on May 4, 1970. The students were unarmed and at least a hundred yards away from the soldiers.*

42 percent of the vote in the 1968 New Hampshire Democratic primary against the incumbent, President Lyndon Johnson. Just two weeks later, Johnson dropped out of the race.

U.S. Senator Barbara Boxer (D-Calif.) was a volunteer in McCarthy's 1968 campaign and co-founded an anti-Vietnam War group called the "Marin Alternative". In a 2005 press statement, she said: "During the Vietnam War, Senator Eugene McCarthy had the courage to stand up and be a voice for peace. He will always be remembered for that." [49] Political scientist Steven S. Smith of Washington University in St. Louis said that McCarthy "remains the most important national symbol of the peace movement and the view that the U.S. reverts to the use of force too quickly. No one has symbolized that in American politics like McCarthy has." [50]

Much of the youth drug use and unconventional dress was also a part of the anti-war protesters' lifestyle. Although many of the so-called hippies were interested in the states of mind that drugs produced – insights, images, spiritual hallucinations, and all the other mental disjunctions that were part of the mystery of the self – other recreational drug consumers were in the drug scene more for the excitement and fun of the drugs alone.

"You have offered us dreams and then urged us to abandon them. You have made us idealists and then told us to go slowly. We do not understand why you have been so offended. But as the repression continues, as the pressure increases, as the stakes become higher, and the risks greater; we can do nothing but resist more strongly. It would be unthinkable to abandon principle because we were threatened or to compromise ideals because we were repressed." [51]

**Meldon Levine**
1968 valedictory speech,
Harvard Law School

Still, others on the fringes of the movement with no political issues at all, saw beyond fun in drug use and sought power and money in illicit drugs. The term "hippie," therefore, means different things to different people. It is still used today both as a compliment and a pejorative.

## Free and Community Clinics

Beyond bringing on the Civil Rights and anti-war movements, the 1960s heralded the channeling of youthful idealism into bettering society. This included efforts to build alternative institutions such as food co-ops, drug treatment programs, legal collectives, and free and community clinics.

President Kennedy tapped into the youthful idealism of the '60s with the Peace Corps in which all Americans, but mostly young adults, were trained and sent abroad for 18 months to help villagers throughout the Third World to improve farming methods and water purification systems.

This valuing of positive change and helping others was also reflected in many domestic efforts to use skills to make this a better world. At home, there was a proliferation of recycling, environmental activism, volunteering in low-income communities, and alternative ways of delivering services.

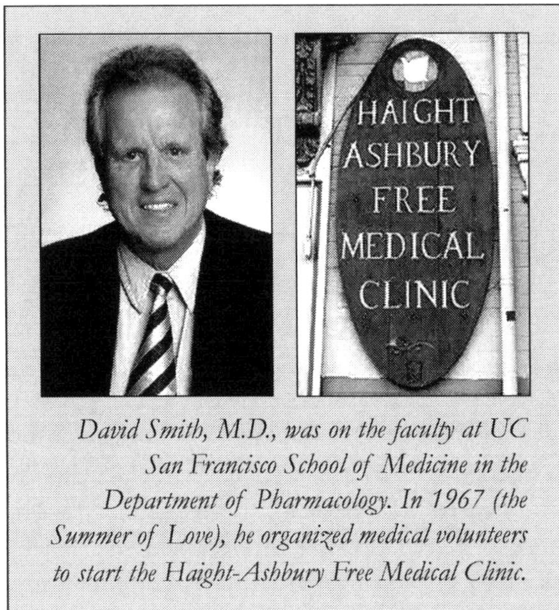


*David Smith, M.D., was on the faculty at UC San Francisco School of Medicine in the Department of Pharmacology. In 1967 (the Summer of Love), he organized medical volunteers to start the Haight-Ashbury Free Medical Clinic.*

David Smith, M.D., a faculty member at the University of California, San Francisco Medical School, started the free-clinic movement in San Francisco in the Haight-Ashbury neighborhood. The first free clinic was opened in 1967 (in either Los Angeles or San Francisco, depending on what constitutes being first), and the undisputed third was in Seattle. The free clinic movement later morphed into the community clinic movement. Many of these clinics survive to this day.

The free clinics, which began in the 1960s and early '70s, were medical facilities that often had a core paid staff but relied heavily on volunteer personnel. These clinics provided a wide range of primary medical care. The care involved conventional physical medicine, often with added components of counseling, social work, massage, acupuncture and drug-abuse treatment. Preventive medicine and health education were also often incorporated in the care. There was an effort to demystify and humanize the care. Relating to the patient as a fellow human being was considered important. The care was provided with sensitivity to cultural and ethnic differences and without eligibility requirements or financial or geographic barriers.

The word "free" meant much more than just little or no charge per patient visit; "free" meant no red tape and care provided in a non-judgmental climate. "Free" also meant a psychological tie between the clinic staff and its patients. This was part of the effort to change the country's culture by moving away from elitism and having a greater role for communication and compassion. Most free clinics were financially unsustainable, but many evolved into community clinics and joined with clinics that were originally funded by the federal government through the United States Public Health Service (USPHS) and the OEO. They have subsequently become a part of America's social safety net.

## Idealism in Flower

The workers in free clinics used social activism in medicine to help change the U.S. health-care system. They wanted to eliminate barriers to care and were proponents of not just treating the illness, but rather treating the whole person. The medical-social activism of the '60s and '70s was part of the process to make American institutions conform to the changing times and values.

A 1970s study by Dr. Charles Lewis of UCLA revealed young activist physicians to be high achievers from well-educated, affluent families; as undergraduates, 50% of them were liberal arts graduates and two-thirds were active participants in the Civil Rights movement. At the time, some in the medical establishment saw these upstarts as radicals.

These budding young professionals were looking for a vehicle to express their social concern, much as their contemporaries had in the Peace Corps in the early to mid-sixties. Doctors, nurses, medical and nursing students, college students, secretaries and just plain folks desired a vehicle to demonstrate their concern for people. For them, free clinics provided an opportunity to break away from institutional barriers and to deliver quality health care to those who needed it but, because of financial, social and/or cultural barriers, had limited access to such care.

These so-called "radical" doctors were not radical in the violent sense of blowing up hospitals or bombing clinics. No, they tore down outdated ideas as to how health care should be delivered and what a doctor's obligations are. They created new ways to treat patients and help people remain healthy. They incorporated alternative and complementary medicine into their practices; used a more humanistic, comprehensive approach; incorporated physician extenders; and focused on prevention, health education and community outreach.

As a consequence, free clinics developed and evolved over time to meet some of America's unfulfilled community needs. These needs were due to inadequate distribution of physicians, poor transportation, financial barriers, language barriers, and hostile attitudes of staff at existing facilities. Many doctors and nurses accustomed to more genteel times were put off by the casual drug use and sexual freedom of young adults of the 1960s and '70s. This generated not only hostility toward the patients they were treating, but in some cases led to poor medicine.

As Dr. David Smith put it, "establishment community medical providers select their clientele, putting up subtle barriers to those who are not acceptable for either ethnic, political or social reasons." When the Open Door Clinic in Seattle opened, the founders — including the author — stated that it was "in response to an unmet community need concerning drugs, their use and abuse, problems of drug users, and lack of accurate information concerning drugs." The free and community clinic clientele were frequently people who felt that they could not trust establishment institutions to deal with their health problems, because the "straight" people did not understand them.

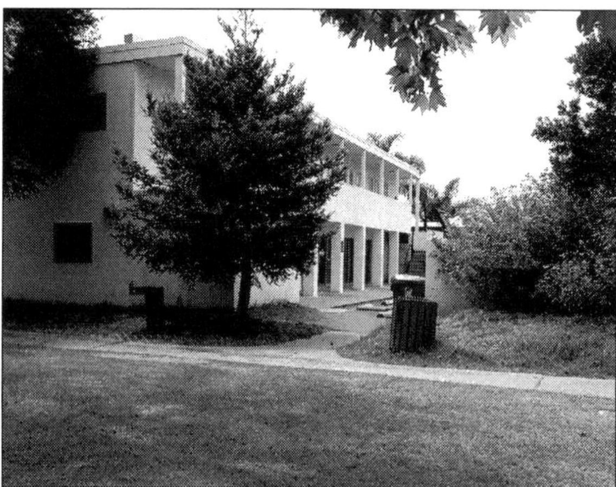

*The Isla Vista Medical Clinic in 2010. It was founded in 1970 with the aid of UC Santa Barbara, the Bank of America, local construction unions, the Isla Vista Community Council, UCSB Associated Students and literally hundreds of local citizens. It harnessed youthful idealism to address access to health care.*

## Isla Vista Open Door Clinic

In 1970, the author was intimately involved in starting the Isla Vista Open Door Clinic (now the Isla Vista Neighborhood Clinic). Isla Vista, California is a half-square mile of densely packed apartments, beach cottages and businesses inhabited mainly by students from neighboring University of California, Santa Barbara (UCSB) and the local city college.

In the 1970s, there was a chasm between Isla Vista and the Santa Barbara community. This resulted not only because of the view of Santa Barbarans that much of the population of Isla Vista supported a counterculture lifestyle, but also because of the student community's largely anti-war stance. The then more-conservative denizens of Santa Barbara (snidely referred to by Isla Vistans as Santa Barbarians) held a much more war-supportive position. This feeling of disdain directed at the youthful residents of Isla Vista was only heightened by the riots of 1970, which culminated in the burning of the Isla Vista branch of the Bank of America.

The Chairman of the Board of the Bank of America, Louis Lundberg, wrote a brief pamphlet entitled "The Lessons of Isla Vista." In this pamphlet, he explained his understanding of the frustration of the youth and the change that was taking place. He got it. If everyone understood the '60s as Lundberg did, everyone would be better off.

Many citizens of the youthful enclave felt alienated from mainstream medicine, and many physicians felt apathy toward the residents of Isla Vista. The Isla Vista community felt the necessity of having a medical clinic in town that would meet the special needs of the community. That meant the ability to handle patients who had been tear gassed, hit with tear-gas canisters, or run over by the police. It meant providing family planning and treatment for sexually transmitted diseases (STDs) in a professional, nonjudgmental manner. It meant having the knowledge and ability to treat bad trips and substance abuse problems. It meant providing

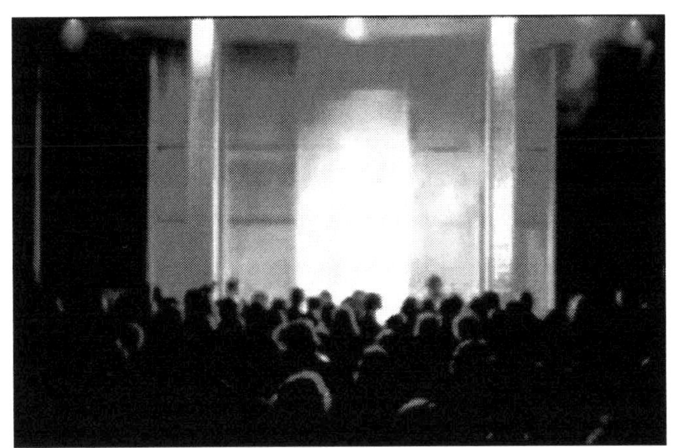

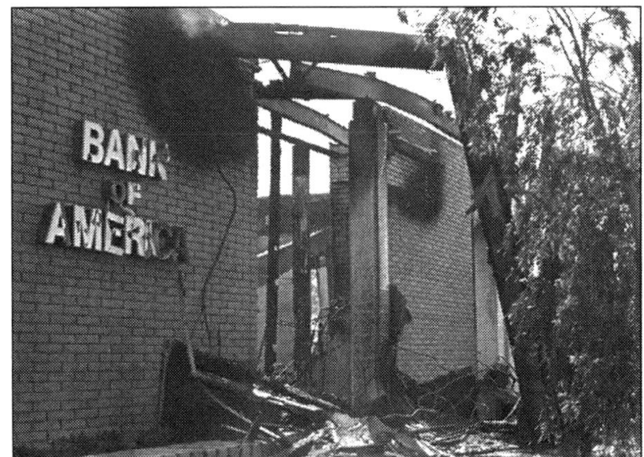


*Late on the evening of Feb. 25, 1970, hundreds of students and townies broke into the Isla Vista, Calif. branch of the Bank of America and started a fire that razed the building. Above left: the height of the inferno. Above right: the bank building the next morning. The police repression that followed over the next few months sparked a community development movement; one of the first embodiements of this wave of civic spirit was the establishment of the Isla Vista Open Door Clinic in September 1970.*

quality primary care. A medical facility was needed where all in the community would feel comfortable, and which would be accessible and acceptable – a place able to relate to the culture of the youth. This position was supported by the Santa Barbara County Health Department, UCSB administration, almost all the residents of the community, and later by the Bank of America itself.

"The struggle for just the bare necessities dominated men's lives through most of history. Then, all of a sudden, just within one lifetime, have come all of the technological breakthroughs that change all that. It was not surprising that we should all get swept up in the excitement of producing . . . . Now we wake up to realize that in the process of "conquering" nature, we were in fact destroying it. . .

There are many other issues than Vietnam. Having once been aroused by the war, having felt trapped into it by their elders, and impotent and frustrated in all their attempts to make themselves heard, these young people have begun to question everything their elders were doing; and to question everything about the society their elders created.

We have two choices as to which way we can go . . . . One course will bring bloodshed, destruction and ultimate crushing of . . . the human spirit; the other course can bring peace and with it, a hope for the rekindling of the American Dream.

The hour is late; there isn't much time. But the choice is still ours."

**Louis B. Lundburg**
Chairman, Bank of America
"The Lessons of Isla Vista" (1970)

People from the community and sympathetic health care professionals – people who felt an unmet need – worked to develop and provide the reality for that need with the Isla Vista Open Door Clinic. The facility served not only students and the young, but also the young families and later Hmong and Hispanic residents from Isla Vista and the surrounding towns of Goleta and Santa Barbara. It still exists to this day.

## Drug Abuse and Treatment

In their article "Addiction Medicine and the Free Clinic Movement," Dr. David Smith and Richard Seymour addressed the issue of discrimination in medicine, writing:

> "No area is more filled with myth and stereotype than the racial and ethnic variable in substance abuse. In recent surveys, it turns out that African-American men are less likely to drink heavily than Caucasian men. African-American men had a slightly higher incidence of alcohol and

> other drug disorders than did Caucasian men, but the differences were not significant. Racial stereotypes not only dominate in the media, but also in public policy. Seventy-five percent of the United States' prison population is African-American or non-white, and a majority of those are in prison because of substance-abuse disorders. There are currently more people in prison in the United States than in any other industrialized nation in the world. Yet we hear from the conservative elements in Congress that the answer [to drug use and abuse] is more prisons." [52]

Smith and Seymour went on to make the case for the cost effectiveness of drug abuse treatment, noting that "If people have a substance abuse problem they should see a health care professional, not go to jail. In general, addiction treatment is cost effective both from a medical and social standpoint." They pointed to a study by Dr. Andrew Mecca, Substance Abuse Coordinator done for the State of California, which showed "that every dollar invested in addiction treatment and prevention will save seven dollars in social and criminal justice costs." [53]

Things have changed. The American Society of Addiction Medicine (ASAM), a national organization of drug abuse treatment specialists, has a delegate in the American Medical Association's House of Delegates. ASAM clearly grew out of the free-clinic movement. Drug-abuse treatment long ago moved into the medical mainstream. In fact, it has become big business. Some from the free-clinic movement believe that drug-abuse treatment has grown far away from its well-intentioned roots and been turned into a cash cow for health-care corporations. Others think it is used as a subtle form of punishment, much like the old Soviet Union sending political dissidents to psychiatric hospitals.

Be that as it may, many innovative medical practices championed by the free-clinic movement have gained general acceptance. The free clinic's credo that "health care is a right, not a privilege" has become a mantra for health policy reform. These innovations have had a profound influence on health care delivery systems throughout the world. The United States has seen the growth not only of medically based in-patient and out-patient substance-abuse treatment, but also of such developments as hospital-based drop-in clinics, urgent care centers, and patient outreach, health education and early intervention programs. Free and community clinics, together with those originally founded by the USPHS and OEO, form the core of modern community health centers. The present day "Public Healthcare Safety Net" includes these old USPHS and OEO outpatient clinics, plus those originally funded through Rural Health funds or county health departments. [54]

## Is Escaping Reality Good For You?

Authors Norman Taylor, Ph.D., Andrew Weil, M.D., Thomas Szasz, Ph.D., Alexander Shulgin, Ph.D. and many other ethnogen-botanists recognize a human need for altered states and escape from reality as being essential to our mental health. They see use of psychoactive drugs as one way of dealing with the pain and ambiguities of life. Humans are keenly aware that they and all their loved ones will be on this worldly sphere for only a short time. We do not know if the universe has been here forever or was created from nothing – neither concept fits human logic. We must take our purpose – our meaning – on faith.

Throughout history, humankind has searched for exotic places, philosophies, religions, foods, herbs and drugs as relief to make the troubles of life more bearable and possibly understandable. This search for a greater understanding has included the use of plants like cannabis, datura, amanita, mescaline, opium, and the easily produced plant-based intoxicant, alcohol, not to mention manufactured pharmaceuticals.

## New Prescription Drugs

The first synthetic chemical compounds for medicinal use were developed at the end of the nineteenth century. Just a few of these manufactured psychoactive drugs include benzedrine in the late 1920s, barbiturates in the 1930s, benzodiazepines in the 1960s, Prozac™, Paxil™ and Zoloft™ in the 1990s and Effexor™, Lexapro™ and Cymbalta™ in the 21st century.

Pharmaceutical companies annually easily generate hundreds of millions of dollars in tranquilizer or

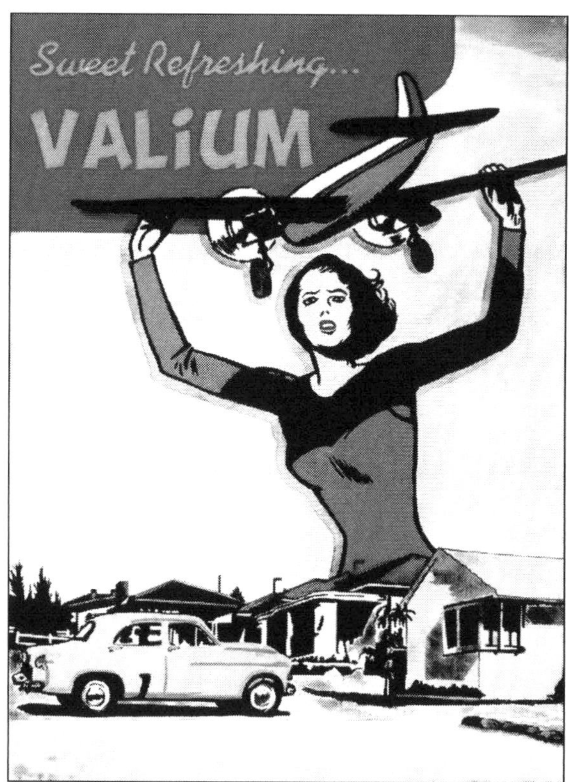


*Valium™ is an immensely financially successful tranquilizer. It has been criticized for numbing its users to the vicissitudes of life. Further, it has been shown to have significant lengthy withdrawal symptoms for a small percentage of its users.* [55]

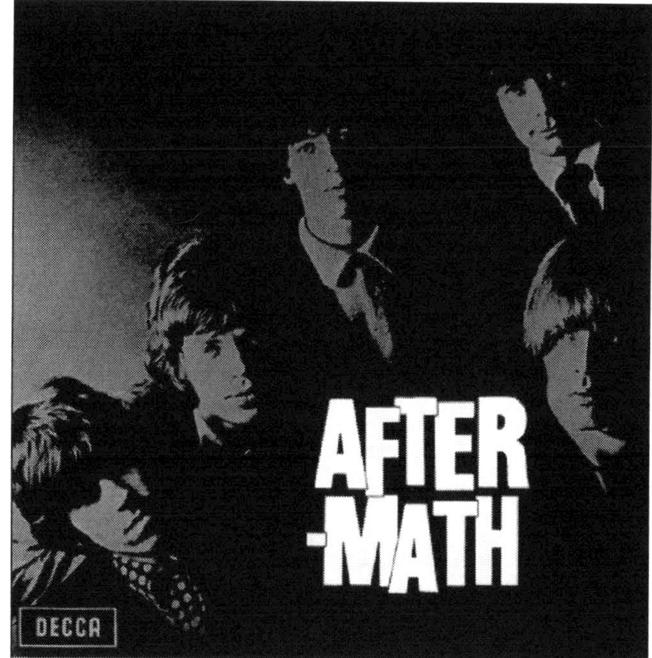


*The popular band The Rolling Stones immortalized the popularity of Valium™ amongst the suburban housewife set in their song "Mother's Little Helper", which appeared as the opening track of their 1966 album* Aftermath *and subsequently on their first compilation album,* Hot Rocks: 1964-71.

mood-elevating sales. Not surprisingly, scientists continue to search for the perfect tranquilizer. The discovery of Librium™ (chlordiazopoxide) was a giant step toward achieving this ideal; it was a drug created to help people deal with the stress-induced anxieties of life. The combination of psychological benefits and the drug's potential to make the pharmaceutical company a lot of money made Librium highly attractive.

Librium was the first in a long line of psychotropic drugs called benzodiazepines. It was followed in 1963 by its more effective cousin, Valium™ (diazapam), and dozens of analogs. These substances "quickly became the most widely prescribed mood-altering drugs in history. . . . Librium and Valium . . . were and continue to be extremely commercially successful drugs." [56]

As both medical professionals and laypeople alike know, stress reduction can also be accomplished with non-prescription herbs and teas, alcohol, meditation, yoga, stretching, walks and deep breathing. But for many, the use of prescription medicine can also be helpful.

## A Little Lobbying Never Hurt

In 1970, Valium and Librium were scheduled to be listed as "potentially addictive" under the Controlled Substances Act. Joseph Califano – a well-known, well-placed capital insider and later Secretary of the Department of Health and Human Services under President Jimmy Carter – lobbied on behalf of their manufacturer, Hoffman-LaRoche, to keep the substances excluded from this designation.

Califano convinced his old friend, Speaker of the U.S. House of Representatives, Carl Albert (D-Oklahoma), not to list these two prescription drugs in that category and to instead create a fifth schedule. According to a biography on Califano, this decision was worth billions to Califano's pharmaceutical client. Califano received a $500,000 bonus on top of his regular billings. His partner, Paul Porter (who was more in touch with such matters), thought Califano should have asked for a million. [57]

By the 1970s, Valium was the most highly prescribed pharmaceutical in the world. It was so widely used by suburban housewives that it became known as "Mother's Little Helpers." Yet in 1981, Valium™ was succeeded by an even more commercially effective benzodiazepine, Xanax™ (generic name alprazolam), which became another blockbuster product.

---

**The main problem with benzodiazepines is they can be habituating when taken over time: "Although [benzodiazepines] are safe and effective for short-term relief of anxiety and other symptoms, extended use of the compounds results in increasing tolerance and strong physical dependence."** [58]

---

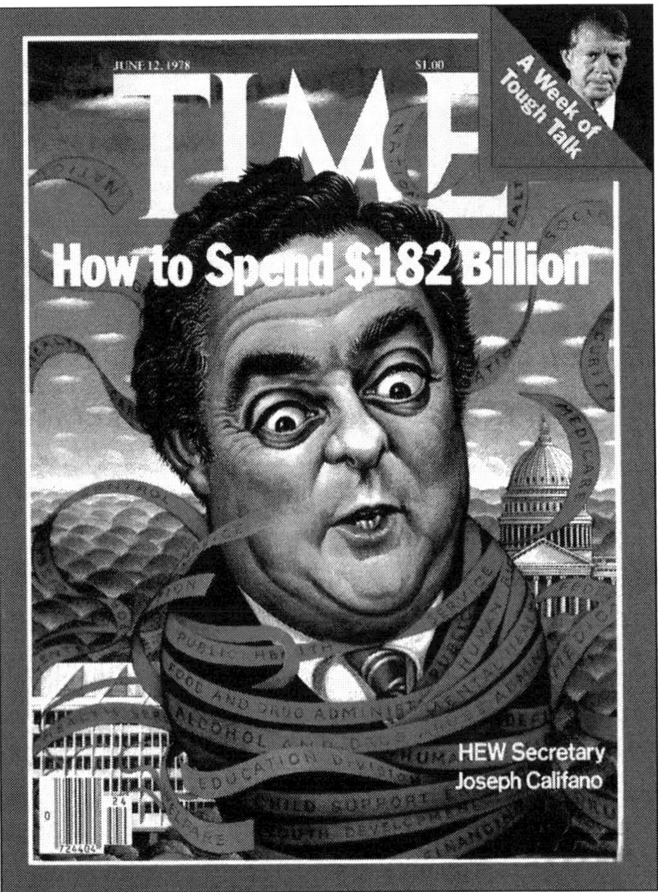


*Joseph Califano had a reputation as a drug warrior but he was not above being a paid lobbyist for drug companies. His work for Hoffman-LaRoche, manufacturer of Librium™ and Valium™, helped to make sure that Librium and Valium were not listed in the Controlled Substances Act as "potentially addictive."*

Some of the great early successes of Librium and its analogs began to be tarnished with the emergence of some problems related to benzodiazepine use. The drugs quickly entered the recreational drug scene and were frequently used in concordance with other abused substances. Studies estimate that 90% of alcohol and illicit drug abusers also abuse benzodiazepines.[59] Still, as with many drugs with abuse potential, when taken as prescribed they are very helpful in combating anxiety.

## Steele Hill Conference

Concerns were raised about Valium in the early 1970s. In 1972, Hoffman-LaRoche, the manufacturer of Valium, sponsored a retreat in Steele Hill, New Hampshire for 40 of the top U.S. drug-abuse treatment experts to discuss drug policy (of which the author was included). The principle suggestion was that Hoffman-LaRoche sponsor a series of conferences to provide education on the appropriate use of Valium to medically influential doctors throughout the country. This proposed series of seminars would have encouraged the discussion of problems associated with the long-term prescription of benzodiazepines.

The main problem with benzodiazepines is they can be habituating when taken over time: "Although [benzodiazepines] are safe and effective for short-term relief of anxiety and other symptoms, extended use of the compounds results in increasing tolerance and strong physical dependence."[60] Soon doctors discovered that when benzodiazepines were discontinued, patients could sometimes suffer potentially dangerous withdrawal symptoms, including "convulsions, tremors, abdominal and muscle cramps, vomiting, and sweating. So many people became habituated to these drugs that the problem appeared in novels, movies, jokes, and, eventually, congressional hearings."[61]

Currently, scores of benzodiazepines in a variety of strengths are on the market. They are prescribed for anxiety, stress, sleep and related conditions. One variation known as Rohypnol™ is considered to be about ten times more potent than Valium as a central nervous system depressant. Rohypnol is known as "the date-rape drug" because of its frequent use in committing said crime. Though it is not sold or manufactured in the United States, it is still smuggled into the country for illicit use.

## Cultural Bias and Business Interests vs. Science

The 1960s turned out to be just another chapter in the long history of drug policy being influenced much more by demons, discrimination, cultural bias and business interests than by science. This relatively recent history is fresh in the minds of many people alive today. Perhaps it is yet possible that we can base our public policy regarding drugs on reason, common sense, and facts.

This is reminiscent of a joke by a comedian, the late Richard Pryor, who, when caught by his wife 'flagrante delecto' said, "Who are you going to believe? Me or your lying eyes?"

Who are you going to believe? Thousands of years of human experience with psychoactive plants, tens of millions of consumers, and thousands of research studies, or bloviating politicians?

Writers like Vonnegut, Kesey and Philip Roth captured the spirit of the times. They took the ennui, sacrifice and loss generated by the economic depression of the 1930s and the death of millions in World War II, including 16 million in the Holocaust, and suggested that we could channel our outrage into creating a better world. Their work, and the contribution of so many influential writers and artists of the 1960s, pointed to a more spiritual, meaningful world, a world where happiness, self-fulfillment, and world brotherhood were the goals of everyday life. They inspired many people to imagine that these values, not greed and the acquisition of earthly goods, while plundering the earth's treasures, would be the goals of the post-World War II generation.

While many people did experience a change of political consciousness by getting on Ken Kesey's bus, most children of the '60s are left with singer/songwriter Jackson Browne's haunting question:

> "I want to know what became of the changes
> we waited for LOVE to bring?" [62]

## Rodney Dangerfield's Lifelong Romance with Marijuana

*Excerpts from a talk by Joan Dangerfield, the comedian's widow, at the "Fourth Patients Out of Time Clinical Conference On Cannabis Therapeutics" held in Santa Barbara, Calif. April 7, 2006. Reprinted in* O'Shaughnessy's, *Summer 2006.*

"If Rodney were here today he would say something brilliant. He would probably open with a marijuana joke. He'd say, 'I tell ya, that marijuana really has an effect on you. The other day I smoked a half a joint and I got so hungry, I ate the other half.'

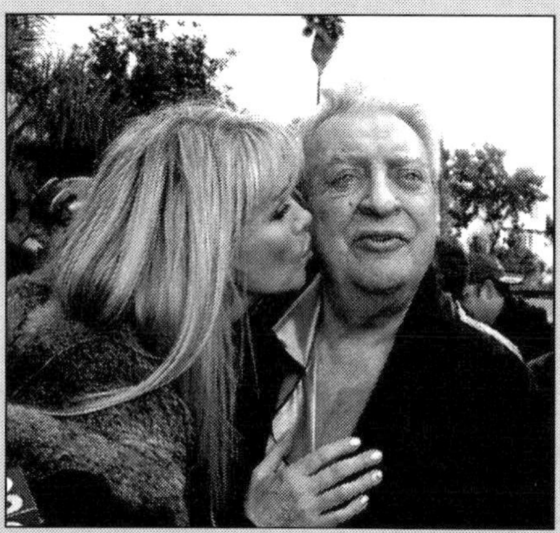

*Mr. & Mrs. Rodney Dangerfield*

Rodney first lit up back in 1942 when he was 21. He was hanging out with a comic named Bobby Byron and his friend Joe E. Ross – some of you might remember Joe E. Ross from *Car 54*. They went to the Belvedere Hotel in New York where Bobby lived.

Although he was supposed to be enjoying himself with friends, Rodney was characteristically agitated and anxiety ridden. It's how he felt every day of his life to that point. But when Rodney got high, he couldn't believe it.

For the first time in his life, he left relaxed and peaceful, and had a sense of well-being. That night, marijuana became a new friend that would be in Rodney's life for the next 62 years.

I met Rodney in 1983, and after a 10-year courtship, Rodney and I enjoyed 11 years of marriage. I must admit that when I became a part of Rodney's life, I did not approve of his marijuana use. My Mormon background hadn't given me experience with any illegal substances and I was always afraid Rodney would get arrested.

Rodney was concerned about my feelings and agreed to look for legal alternatives. We consulted the best experts we could find in search of legal anti-anxiety and pain medications and even tried Marinol™. But nothing worked for him the way real marijuana did.

I was sure that Rodney would be arrested. So I looked for, and found, Dr. David Bearman in Santa Barbara. Dr. Bearman examined Rodney and obtained records from Rodney's other doctors for review. In addition to his anxiety and depression, at the time Rodney's medical conditions included constant pain from the congenital fusion of his spine, an inoperable dislocated shoulder, a rotator-cuff tear, arthritis and ADD/ADHD.

Rodney showed the approval letter to everyone and carried miniature versions in his pockets. Ever the worried wife, I included a copy of the letter in the memory box of his casket in case the feds were waiting for him at the Pearly Gates.

After all those years of pot smoking, his memory and his joke-writing ability did not suffer and his lungs were okay. He was as sharp as ever. Even moments after brain surgery Rodney didn't miss a beat. Rodney's doctor came to his bedside after he was taken off the respirator. He said, 'Rodney, are you coughing up much?' And Rodney said, 'Last week, five-hundred for a hooker.'"

# Acknowledgements

Where does one start in thanking all those who have helped in one way or another to write this book? Some have been very close to me, helped me be the person I have become and provided necessary emotional support. Others have been essential in the actual production of the book. Still others are some of the historic figures who provided the necessary intellectual and philosophical foundation to move our knowledge of the mind and its physiology forward.

There are those who helped you down the path: my parents, who provided a supportive environment and urged me to go into medicine; my father, a pharmacist, who helped me understand the science behind how medicines work .my late brother with his humor and idealism; and my professors at the University of Washington School of Medicine, who provided encouragement, including Drs. Ron Pion, John Hampson, Thomas Holmes and James Dilley.

I appreciate what I learned from people in the free and community clinic movement - Mimi Sheridan, M.A., Kim Judson, Ph.D., Libby Kelly, Jack Delay, Kord Roosen-Runge, and Drs. Charles Huffine, David Smith and Russ Nichols.

The camaraderie, support, and suggestions of my colleagues in the Society of Cannabis Clinicians and the American Academy of Cannabinoid Medicine - Drs. Jeff Hergenrather, Greg Carter and Frank Lucido. Special thanks to Drs. Arnie Leff and Chris Fichtner, and to the late Jim Marshall for reading and commenting on the book.

Probably the most important source of knowledge was the patients I've seen throughout my career. Those who I saw for treatment of substance abuse, pain management and medicinal cannabis, helped stimulate my curiosity and appreciate therapeutic agents from the patient's point of view.

My book required many editors: They include Carmen Lodise, Amy Ford, Laura Reed, and Katherine Brown. Carmen was essential in making the book coherent. Thanks to Sonya Vega for getting the footnotes in order. Many thanks go to Donna Ryczek of Goleta Typing, who deciphered my handwriting and typed the manuscript. Great thanks to my layout men Carmen Lodise and Terrell Dunn and thanks to my publisher, Cathy Feldman, who put some much needed order and publishing professionalism into the project.

It should go without saying that this book would not exist without those who laid the scientific foundation and those who had the courage to challenge conventional thinking. The list is long but it is important to mention a few of the visionaries that contributed to the storehouse of knowledge regarding drugs, the brain, and human happiness: Shen Neng, Discordes, Dr. W.B. O'Shaughnessy, Sir William Osler, M.D., William C. Woodward, M.D., Morris Fishbein, MD, George Schlichten, Colonel James Thalen, MD, Tom Ungerleider, M.D., Norman Taylor, Ph.D., Andrew Weil, M.D.,

Tod Mikuriya, M.D., the first modern cannabis researchers, Ramsey and Davis and two grand pioneers of medicinal cannabis Lester Grinspoon, M.D. and Raphael Mechoulam,PhD.

Finally, a special thanks to Doug Daniels, Ph.D., who trusted me to teach a course in the Black Studies Department at the University of California, Santa Barbara. And particular appreciation goes to my wife Lily and my children Samantha and Benji for their ongoing love, support and patience.

# Notes

## Chapter I: Introduction to a Witch Hunt


1. Manski, Charles F., John V. Pepper and Carol V. Petrie. I*nforming America's Policy in Illegal Drugs: What We Don't Know Keeps Hurting Us.* National Research Council National Academy of Science, 2001.
2. "Collateral Damage." *Economist,* July 26, 2001.
3. McCaffrey, Barry. *Frontline Drug Wars*, 2000.
4. "U.S. President Declares War Against Drug Abuse." *People's Daily*, May 11, 2001.
5. Hardaway, Robert. "U.S. Stuck in a Quagmire." *Denver Post*, March 14, 2004.
6. Elders, Jocelyn. "All Use is Medical." *Hemptopia.*
7. Elders, Jocelyn. "Policy Project Elder." *Marijuana Policy Project.*
8. Stephan, James J. "Bureau of Justice Statistics Special Report State Prison Expenditures." *U.S. Department of Justice*, June 2004.
9. Mann, Horace. In *Report of the Superintendent of Public Instruction of the Commonwealth of Pennsylvania.* 1881.
10. Nadelmann, Ethan. "Think Again: Drugs." *Foreign Policy*, August 15, 2007.
11. Torsrud, Phillip. *America Unraveled: 2008-2012 The Political, Cultural and Economic Collapse.* iUniverse, 2012.
12. Derrida, Jacques. *Drug Prohibition and the 'Assassin of Youth'.* McGraw-Hill, 1993.
13. Bush, Lawrence. "Drugs and Jewish Spirituality." *Tikkun,* 14, no. 3 (1999.: 39-40.
14. Connolly, Kathleen, Lea McDermid, Vincent Schiraldi, and Dan Macallair. "From Classrooms to Cell Blocks: How Prison Building Affects Higher Education and African American Enrollment." *Center on Juvenile and Criminal Justice*, 1996.
15. Jackson, Richard and Benjamin Franklin. *An Historical Review of the Constitution and Government of Pennsylvania.* London: R. Griffiths, 1759.
16. Wikeke, Bill. "It's Not News that Our Kids Do Good." *Wisconsin State Journal*, July 16, 2007.
17. Nadelmann, op. cit.
18. Connolly, et. al., op. cit.
19. Bearman, David. "Medical Marijuana: Why this Issue is More Important to Health Care than Just Cannabis." *APHA 133rd Annual Meeting*, 2005
20. Norris, Mikki, Virginia Resner, and Chris Conrad. *Shattered Lives: Portraits from America's Drug War.* Creative Xpressions, 1998.
21. Derrida, op. cit.
22. "Albert Einstein." *BrainyQuote.com*, 2014. http://www.brainyquote.com/quotes/quotes/a/alberteins133991.html
23. Bearman, David, Karen Claydon, Jennifer Kincheloe, and Carmen Lodise. "Breaking the Cycle of Dependency: Dual Diagnosis and AFDC Families." *J Psychoactive Drugs,* 29, no. 4 (1997.: 359-367.
24. Chasnoff, Ira J. "Cocaine-Pregnancy and the Neonate." *Women's Health*, 15, no. 3 (1989.: 23-35.
25. Hurt, Hallam. "Slow Development in Crack Babies May be Caused by Condition of Urban Poverty, Says New Study." *Washington Post*, September 16, 1997.
26. Ibid.
27. Schuckit, Marc A. *Educating Yourself about Alcohol and Drugs: A People's Primer.* Peseus Publishing, 1995.
28. Piomelli, Daniele. "Activation of Endocannabinoid Signaling System Instriatum Precedent." *6th Internet World Congress for Biomedical Science*, 2000.
29. Alger, Bradley E. "Endocannabinoids and Their Implications for Epilepsy." *Epilepsy Currents*, 4, no. 5 (2004.: 169-173.
30. Piomelli, op. cit.
31. Norton, Amy. "Chemical Boosts Marijuana-Like Substance in the Brain." *Reuters Health*, May 3, 2000.
32. Enoch, Mary-Anne, Marc A. Schuckit, Bankole A. Johnson and David Goldman. "Genetics of Alcoholism Using Intermediate Phenotypes." *Alcoholism: Clinical and Experimental Research*, 27, no. 2 (2003.: 169-176.
33. Tomandl, Dan. "Cato Institute data." *Heartland Journal.*
34. Enoch, et. al., op. cit.
35. Hardaway, op. cit.
36. "Linder v. United States - 268 U.S. 5." *Circuit of Appeals, Ninth Circuit*, 1925.

37. Brookhiser, Richard. What Would the Founding Fathers Do? American Heritage, 2006.
38. "Gonzales v. Raich - 545 U.S. 1." *Circuit of Appeals, Ninth Circuit*, 2005.
39. Ibid.
40. Barth, Alan. *The Rights of Free Men*. Knopf, 1984.
41. *The Barbary Treaties 1786-1816: Treaty of Peace and Friendship, Signed at Tripoli November 4, 1796*. Washington: Government Printing Office, 1931.
42. Wills, Gary. *Head and Heart: American Christianities*. Penguin Press, 2007.
43. Gordon, Robert S. and Stewart Sholto-Douglas. *The Bushman Myth: The Making of the Nambian Underclass*. Westview Press, 2000.
44. *The Adams-Jefferson Letters: The Complete Correspondence*. University of North Carolina Press, 1987.
45. "Audio & Transcripts." *Nixontapes.org*, 2007.
46. Nadelmann, op. cit.
47. Torsrud, op. cit.
48. Derrida, op. cit.

## Chapter II: Ceremonial Drug Use: Religion, Shamans and Soma

1. Allen, Woody. In *Goodreads*. https://www.goodreads.com/quotes/82215-because-it-s-much-more-pleasant-to-be-obsessed-over-how.
2. Woody, op. cit.
3. Boyer, Paul and Stephen Nissenbaum. *Salem Possessed: The Social Origins of Witchcraft*. Harvard University Press, 1976.
4. Ibid.
5. Emboden, William A. *Ritual Use of Cannabis Sativa L.: A Historical-Ethnographic Survey*. Waveland Press, Inc., 1972.
6. Merlin, Mark D. *Man and Marijuana: Some Aspects of Their Ancient Relationship*. Fairleigh Dickinson University Press, 1972.
7. Knight, Margaret. *Humanist Anthology*. Prometheus Books, 1995.
8. Boyer and Nissenbaum, op. cit.
9. Ibid.
10. Robertson, John M. *A Short History of Christianity*. Kessinger Publishing, LLC, 2004.
11. Tobin, Paul. "The Rejection of Pascal's Wager: A Skeptic's Guide to Christianity." http://www.rejectionofpascalswager.net/.
12. Bierer, Donald E., Thomas J. Carlson, and Steven R. King. "Shaman Pharmaceuticals: Integrating Indigenous Knowledge, Tropical Medicinal Plants, Medicine, Modern Science, and Reciprocity into a Novel Drug Discovery Approach." *Shaman Pharmaceuticals, Inc.*, 2006.
13. Boyer and Nissenbum, op. cit.
14. Farnsworth, Norman R. "Screening Plants for New Medicines." *Biodiversity*. Washington D.C.: National Academy Press, 1988.
15. Farnsworth, Norman R., Olayiwola Akerele, Audrey S. Bingel, Djaja D. Soejarto, and Zhengang Guo. "Medicinal Plants in Therapy." *Perspectives in Biology and Medicine*, 1989.
16. Leary, Timothy. *The Politics of Ecstasy*. Ronin Publishing, 1998.
17. "Exploring Greek, Roman, and Celtic Myth and Art." http://www.loggia.com/myth/myth.html.
18. Redfern, Lore. *Cannabis and the Legacy of Soma*. 2000.
19. Merlin, op. cit.
20. Knight, op. cit.
21. Wasson, Gordon R. *Soma: Divine Mushroom of Immortality*. Harcourt Brace Javanovich, 1972.
22. Oberlies, Thomas. "Die Religion des Rgveda. Erster Teil: Das religiose System des Rgveda." *De Nobili Research Library*, no. 26, 1998.
23. Gall, Timothy L. Worldmark *Encyclopedia of Cultures and Daily Life: Koriaks*. Michigan: Gale Research Inc., 1998.
24. Carroll, Lewis. *Alice's Adventures in Wonderland*. Public Domain Books, 1997.
25. Highfield, Roger. "Santa: The Hallucinogenic Connection." *The Physics of Christmas: From the Aerodynamics of Reindeer to the Thermodynamics of Turkey*. Back Bay Books, 1999.
26. Robertson, op. cit.

27. Rudgley, op. cit.
28. Wasson, op. cit.
29. Rudgley, Richard. *The Encyclopedia of Psychoactive Substances.* St. Martin's Griffin, 2000.
30. Oberlies, op. cit.
31. Merlin, op. cit.
32. Knight, op. cit.
33. Schultes, Richard E., Albert Hofmann, and Christian Ratsch. *Plants of the Gods: Their Sacred, Healing, and Hallucinogenic Powers.* Healing Arts Press, 2001.
34. Craveri, Marcello and Charles L. Markmann. *The Life of Jesus.* Ecco Press, 1989.
35. Erowid, Nono Canasta, and K Trout. "A Brief Summary of the Relationship Between Peyote Use and the Ghost Dance." *The Vaults of Erowid*, May 2002, https://www.erowid.org/plants/peyote/peyote_history1.shtml.
36. Rudgley, op. cit..
37. Ibid.
38. Robertson, op. cit.
39. Lindsey, Hal and Carole C. Carlson. *The Late Great Planet Earth.* Zondervan, 1970.
40. Madeleine, Fredric. *The Drug Controversy and the Rise of Antichrist.* Candlestick Publishing, 1988.
41. Girard, Rene. *The Scapegoat.* John Hopkins University Press, 1989.
42. Nanda, Serena and Richard L. Warms. *Cultural Anthropology.* 9th ed. Wadsworth Publishing, 2006.
43. Harris, Sam. "The Straight Path: A Conversation with Ronald A. Howard." *Samharris.org*, April 20, 2013, http://www.samharris.org/blog/item/the-path-of-honesty.

## Chapter III: Christianity, Entheogens & Holidays

1. Berger, Pamela, *The Goddess Obscured: Transformation of the Grain Protectress from Goddess to Saint.* Boston: Beacon Press (1985).
2. Anderson, Jeff. "Christianity and the Mystery Religions." *Columbus School of Law and School of Canon Law.* 1999. http://faculty.cua.edu/pennington/churchhistory220/lectureone/Christianity_mystery_rel.htm.
3. Ibid.
4. Tobin, Paul. "The Rejection of Pascal's Wager: A Skeptic's Guide to Christianity." 2000. http://www.rejectionofpascalswager.net/.
5. Knight, Margaret. *Honest to Man: Christian Ethics Re-Examined.* Prometheus Books, 1974.
6. Robertson, John M. *A Short History of Christianity.* Kessinger Publishing, LLC, 2004.
7. Tobin, op. cit.
8. Knight, Margaret. *Humanist Anthology.* Prometheus Books, 1995.
9. Robertson, op. cit.
10. Lecky, William E. H. *History of European Morals: From Augustus to Charlemagne.* London: Longmans, Green, and Co., 1890.
11. Knight, Humanist Anthology, op. cit.
12. Craveri, Marcello and Charles L. Markmann. *The Life of Jesus.* Ecco Press, 1989.
13. Becker, Benjamin M. and David L. Gibberman. "Earl Johnson." In *On Trial! Law, Lawyers, and the Legal Profession.* Philosophical Library, 1987.
14. Knight, *Honest to Man: Christian Ethics Re-Examined*, op. cit.
15. Gibbon, Edward. *The Decline and Fall of the Roman Empire.* Wildside Press, 2004.
16. Jefferson, Thomas. *Thomas Jefferson to Horatio G. Spafford, March 17, 1814.* Letter. From The Thomas Jefferson Memorial Association, *The Writings of Thomas Jefferson.*
17. Ibid.
18. Adler, Mortimer J. *The Annals of America: Great Issues in American Life.* Encyclopaedia Britannica, 1968.
19. Wills, Garry. *What Jesus Meant.* Penguin Books, 2007.
20. Riedlinger, Thomas J. "Wasson's Alternative Candidates for Soma." *Journal of Psychoactive Drugs*, 25, no. 2 (1993.: 149-156.
21. Ibid.
22. Russell, Dan. *Shamanism and the Drug Propaganda: The Birth of Patriarchy and the Drug War.* Kalyx, 1998.
23. Allegro, John M. *The Sacred Mushroom and the Cross.* Gnostic Media Research and Publishing, 2009.

24. "The Forbidden Fruit: The History of Substance Control as it Relates to Religious Persecution and Discrimination during the Medieval and American Colonial Periods." http://etheogen.netfirms.com/articles/substance.
25. Yehoshua, Hayyim B. "Refuting Missionaries." 1998, http://mama.indstate.edu/users/nizrael/jesusrefutation.html
26. Fussell, Joseph H. *The Significance of Easter.* Theosophical University Press, 1999.
27. Price, Robert. *Christ a Fiction. Infidels*, 1997.
28. Dawkins, Richard. *The Selfish Gene.* Oxford University Press, 1990.
29. Edelen, William. "A Heartfelt Thank You to Santa Barbara." *Santa Barbara News Press*, December 4, 2005.
30. Ibid.
31. Adler, op. cit.
32. "The Origins of Christmas." www.allaboutjesuschrist.org/origin_of_christmas.
33. Day, Lorraine. "Christmas: Is it 'Christian' or Pagan?" 2006, http://www.goodnewsaboutgod.com/studies/holidays2.htm.
34. Martindale, Cyril C. "Christmas." In *The Catholic Encyclopedia.* New York: Robert Appleton Company, 1908.
35. Ibid.
36. Day, op. cit.
37. Arthur, James. *Mushrooms and Mankind: The Impact of Mushrooms on Human Consciousness and Religion.* The Book Tree, 2003.
38. Hislop, Alexander. *The Two Babylons or the Papal Worship.* New Jersey: Loizeaux Brothers, 1959.
39. "Ontario Consultants on Religious Tolerance." Religious Tolerance, http://www.religioustolerance.org/purpose.htm.
40. Arthur, op. cit.
41. Larsen, Dana. "The Psychedelic Secrets of Santa Claus." *Cannabis Culture*, December 18, 2003, http://www.cannabisculture.com/articles/3136.html.
42. Riedlinger, op. cit.
43. Wasson, Gordon R. Soma: *Divine Mushroom of Immortality.* Harcourt Brace Javanovich, 1972.
44. Larsen, op. cit.
45. "Occult Holidays and how America has Copied Many of Them." *Written Testimony*, November 25, 2004.
46. Larsen, op. cit.
47. Ibid.
48. Larsen, op. cit.
49. Furst, Peter T. "Visionary Plants and Ecstatic Shamanism." *Expedition Magazine.* http://www.penn.museum/sites/expedition/visionary-plants-and-ecstatic-shamanism/.
50. Arthur, op. cit.
51. "Occult Holidays and how America has Copied Many of Them," op. cit.
52. Ibid.
53. Ibid.
54. Clark, Cindy D. *Flights of Fancy, Leaps of Faith: Children's Myths in Contemporary America.* University of Chicago Press, 1998.
55. Irving, Washington. *Knickerbocker's History of New York.* Chicago: W.B. Conkey Company, 1809.
56. Irving, Washington. **Tour of the Prairies**. John W. Lovell Company, 1832.
57. Cooke, Mordecai C. *A Plain and Easy Account of British Fungi.* W.H. Allen & Company, 1876.
58. Highfield, Roger. *The Physics of Christmas: From the Aerodynamics of Reindeer to the Thermodynamics of Turkey.* Back Bay Books, 1999.
59. Davies, Norman. *Europe: A History.* Harper Collins, 1998.
60. Dawkins, op. cit.
61. Thomas, Stephen. "Who Does 'The Night Before Christmas' Belong to?" Lecture. *Duchess County Historical Society*, November 10, 1977.
62. Reverend Damuzi. "Easter: Sex and Drugs Celebration!" *Cannabis Culture*, May 10, 2004, http://www.cannabisculture.com/articles/3352.html.
63. Boemler, Larry. "Asherah and Easter." *Biblical Archaeology Review*, 18 (1993..
64. Ibid.
65. Boemler, op. cit.

66. Reverend Damuzi, op. cit.
67. Ratsch, Christian. *Marijuana Medicine.* Healing Arts Press, 2001.
68. Reverend Damuzi. "Witch Hunts and the War on Weed." *Cannabis Culture*, June 20, 2002, http://www.cannabisculture.com/content/witch-hunts-and-war-weed.
69. Ratsch, Christian. *Marijuana Medicine.* Healing Arts Press, 2001.
70. Beach, Edward A. "The Eleusinian Mysteries." Ball State University, http://www.bsu.edu/classes/magrath/305s01/demeter/eleusis.html.
71. Arthur, op. cit.
72. Beach, op. cit.
73. Ibid.
74. Ruck, Carl A. P. *Sacred Mushrooms: Secrets of Eleusis.* Ronin Publishing, 2006.
75. Ibid.
76. Ott, Jonathan. *Pharmacotheon.* Natural Products Company, 1996.
77. Keller, Mara Lynn. "The Eleusinian Mysteries of Demeter and Persephone: Fertility, Sexuality and Rebirth." *Journal of Feminist Studies in Religion*, 4, no. 1 (1988.: 26-39.
78. Ibid.
79. Arthur, op. cit.
80. Keller, op. cit.
81. Ott, op. cit.
82. Aggrawal, Anil. "The Story of Opium." In *Narcotic Drugs.* India: National Book Trust, 1995.
83. NicBhride, Feorag. "Bollocks and Broomsticks or, Which way is Witch?" *Prattle*, http://www.prattle.net/samhuinn02/bollocks.html.
84. Peterson, Cathy. "Witchcraft Herbal Lore and Flying Ointments." *Lady of the Earth*, 1998. http://ladyoftheearth.com/herbs/lore-flying.txt
85. McKenna, Terence. *Food of the Gods.* Bantam, 1993.
86. NicBhride, op. cit.
87. Lewis, Walter H. and Memory P. F. Elvin-Lewis. *Medical Botany: Plants Affecting Man's Health.* Wiley, 1982.
88. Johnston, Sarah I. *Ancient Religions.* Massachusetts: The Belknap Press of Harvard University Press, 2007.
89. Czolowski, Stan. "Witch's Garden." *Cannabis Culture*, November 1, 1999, http://www.cannabisculture.com/articles/78.html.
90. NicBhride, op. cit.
91. Peterson, op. cit.
92. Harner, Michael. "The Role of Hallucinogenic Plants in European Witchcraft." In *Hallucinogens and Shamanism.* New York: Oxford University Press, 1973.
93. Ibid.
94. Le Franc, Martin and Don A. Fischer. *Edition and Study of Martin LeFranc's 'Le Champion Des Dames.* University Microfilms, 1982.

## Chapter IV: 1300-1700: Bring on the Witches

1. Smitha, Frank E. "An Empire Falls: Assyria Weakens and is Overrun." FSmitha.com. http://www.fsmitha.com/h1/ch08.htm
2. "Zoroastrianism, Judaism AND Christianity." Pyracantha.com www.pyracuntha.com/z/2JC3.html
3. Kak, Subhash. "Vedic Elements in the Ancient Iranian Religion of Zarathushtra." *Vedic Religion in Ancient Iran*, p.47.
4. Shahriar Sharari. "Influence of Zoroastrianism on Other Religions," http://www.zarathushtra.com/z/article/influenc.htm
5. Taylor, Gordon Rattray. *Sex in History.* Vanguard Press, 1954.
6. Seligmann, Kurt. *The History of Magic and the Occult. Pantheon*, 1948.
7. Ibid.
8. William, Calvin H. *A Brain for All Seasons: Human Evolution and Abrupt Climate Change*, University of Chicago Press, 2003.
9. Ibid.
10. Mandia, Scott A. "Little Ice Age in Europe - Influence of Dramatic Climate Shifts in European Civilization," http://www2.sunysuffolk.edu/mandias/lia/little_ice_age.html, p. 4-6.

11. Oster, Emily. "Witchcraft, Weather and Economic Growth in Renaissance Europe," *Journal of Economic Perspectives* (2004. p. 215-228.
12. William, op. cit.
13. Mandia, op. cit.
14. Boccaccio, Giovanni. *The Decameron.* Penguin, 2003, p. 19.
15. Lapinskas, Vincas. "A Brief History Of Ergotism: From St. Anthony's Fire and St. Vitus' Dance Until Today," *Medicinos Istorija.* 2007, p. 203
16. Ibid.
17. Mandia, op. cit.
18. McKay, John P., Bennett D. Hill, and John Buckler. *A History of Western Society.* 7th Edition. University of Illinois, Georgetown University.
19. Behringer, Wolfgang. "Climate Change and Witch-Hunting. The Impact of the Little Ice Age on Moralities." *Climatic Change.* Netherlands: Kluwer Academic Publishers, 1999.
20. Behringer, op. cit.
21. "Black Death." History.com. http://www.history.com/topics/black-death
22. Levack, Brian P. "Innocent VIII: Papal Inquisitors and Witchcraft, 1484." *The Witchcraft Sourcebook.* Routledge, 2003. p. 119.
23. Sagan, Carl. *The Demon Haunted World: Science as a Candle in the Dark.* Ballantine Books: 1997. Quoted in William H. Calvin, *A Brain for All Seasons: Human Evolution and Abrupt Climate Change*, Univ. of Chicago Press: 2002.
24. Kramer, Heinrich and James Sprenger. *Malleus Maleficarum.* Digireads.com. 2010.
25. Damuzi, Reverend. "Witch Hunts and The War on Weed." *Cannabis Culture Magazine.* http://www.cannabisculture.com/articles/2309.html.
26. Hoffer, Peter Charles. *The Devil's Disciples: The Makers of the Salem Witchcraft Trials.* Johns Hopkins University Press, 1998.
27. Montgomery, Neil M. "Pot Night - A Short History of Cannabis." www.ukcia.org/research/potnight/pn4.htm
28. Linder, Douglas. "The Witchcraft Trials in Salem: A Commentary" (2007.. Available at SSRN: http://ssrn.com/abstract=1021256 or http://dx.doi.org/10.2139/ssrn.1021256
29. Ellerbe, Ellen. *The Dark Side of Christian History.* Morningstarbooks, 1995.
30. Ibid.
31. Briggs, Robin. *Witches and Neighbors: The Social and Cultural Context of European Witchcraft.* Penguin, 1998.
32. Tobin, Paul. The Rejection of Pascal's Wager: *A Skeptic's Guide to Christianity*, UK: Author's Online Ltd.,2009. www.geocities.com/paul/ritobin/
33. Kwan, Natalie. "Woodcuts and Witches: Ulrich Molitor's De lamiis et pythonicis mulieribus, 1489-1669." *Oxford Journal: German History.*
34. Ibid.
35. Pavlac, Brian A. "List of Important Events for the Witch Hunt." 2009. http://departments.kings.edu/WOMENS_HISTORY/witch/witchlist.html
36. Tobin, op. cit.
37. Huxley, Aldous. *The Devils of London.* New York, NY: Harper & Brothers, 1952.
38. Robertson, J.M. *Pagan Christs.* University Book c. 1967 (originally 1903..
39. Linder, op. cit.
40. Ibid.
41. Everything2.com. "Salem Witch Trials" http://www.everything2.com/?node=salem+witch+trials
42. Robertson, op. cit.
43. Fagan, Brian. *The Little Ice Age: How Climate Made History 1300-1850* 2000. Basic Books, 2000.
44. Yalom, Marilyn. "Oxford Companion to the Body: witch's tit." Answers.com. http://www.answers.com/topic/witch-s-tit
45. "Supernumerary Nipple." Answers.com. http://www.answers.com/topic/supernumerary-nipple
46. Barstow, Anne L. *Witchcraze: A New History of the European Witch Hunts.* HarpeOne, 1995.
47. "Witch's Tit." Everything2.com. http://everything2.com/?node=witch%27s+tit.
48. Knowles, George. "Marks of a Witch." Controverscial.com. (http://www.controverscial.com/Marks%20of%20a%20Witch.htm.

49. Ibid.
50. "Witch's Tit." Everything2.com. op. cit.
51. Ibid.
52. "Witch Prickers - Fundamentalist Christianity at its Worst." www.patregan_.freeuk.com/witchmurders.htm
53. "Bodkin." The Llewellyn Encyclopedia. http://www.llewellyn.com/encyclopedia/term/bodkin
54. Lane, Charles. "Court Eases 'No Knock' Search Ban", *Washington Post*, 2006. p. A01.
55. Burton, John. *The U.S. Supreme Court's 'No-Knock' Decision: A Frontal Assault on democratic rights*. 2006. www.wsws.org./articles/2006/june2006/supr-j20.shtml.
56. Savage, Charlie. "McCain fights exceptions to torture ban" *Boston Globe*, 2005.
57. Tobin, op. cit.
58. "Limbaugh Rejected Newsmax.com's false claim that McCain 'admitted that torture worked on him.'" http://mediamatters.org.
59. Savage, op. cit.
60. Sagan, Carl. *Demon Haunted World: Science as a. Candle in the Dark*, Random House, 1995 - and Ballantine Books, 1997.
61. "Gendercide Watch - Case Study: The European Witch Hunts c. 1450-1750 and Witch Hunts Today." Gendercide.org. http://www.gendercide.org/case_witchhunts.html
62. Gibbons, Jenny. "Recent Development in the Study of the Great European Witch Hunts." *Pomegranate*, 1998.
63. Ibid.
64. Damuzi, op. cit.
65. Kramer, Heinrich and James Sprenger, op. cit.
66. Ibid.
67. Ibid.
68. Huxley, op. cit.
69. Norris, Mikki, Chris Conrad, and Virginia Ressner. *Shattered Lives: Portraits from America's Drug War*. Creative Xpressions, 1998.
70. Sagan, op. cit.
71. Gumbel, Andrew. "An American Travesty." *Independent UK*. 2002.
72. Greene, Judith, Kevin Pranis, and Jason Zeidenberg. "Disparity By Design: How Drug-Free Zone Laws Impact Racial Disparity - and Fail to Protect Youth." *The Drug Policy Alliance*, 2006.
73. Leung, Rebecca. "Targeted in Tula, Texas?" CBS News. 2003. http://www.cbsnews.com/stories/2003/09/26/60minutes/main575291.shtl
74. Tobin, op. cit.
75. Kramer, Heinrich and James Sprenger, op. cit.

## Chapter V: 600 BC-1776 AD: Spices, Colonialism, Genocide

1. TED Case Studies. "Arab Spice Trade and Spread of Islam: SPICE Case." http://www1.american.edu/ted/spice.htm
2. Schivelbusch, Wolfgang. "Spices or the Dawn of the Middle Ages." *Tastes of Paradise: A Social History of Spices, Stimulants, and Intoxicants*. Vintage Books.
3. TED Case Studies, op. cit.
4. Crose, Patricia. *The Meccan Trade and the Rise of Spices*. Georgias Press, 2004.
5. Turner, Jack. *Spice: The History of Temptation*. Harper Collins Publishers Ltd., 2004.
6. Laufer, Berthold. *The Diamond*. Chicago Field Museum of Natural History, 1915.
7. Meurd, Stephen, and Oxford Blackwell. *All Manners of Fodo: Eating and Taste in England and France from the Middle Ages to the Present*, 1985, as cited in Kathryn A. Edwards. *Daily Life in Medieval Europe*, c. 814-1350.
8. Fernandez-Armesto, Felipe. *Pathfinders, A Global History of Exploration*. W. W. Norton & Company, 2007.
9. Laufer, Berthold, op. cit.
10. Ibid
11. TED Case Studies, op. cit.
12. Booth, Martin. *Cannabis: A History*. Picador, 2005.
13. Polo, Marco. *The Marco Polo Travels of Marco Polo*. Signet Classics, 2004.
14. Booth, op. cit.

15. Pollan, Michael. *The Botany of Desire: A Plant's-Eye View of the World.* Random House Trade Paperbacks; 1 edition, 2002.
16. Booth, op. cit.
17. Booth, op. cit.
18. Anslinger, Harry. "Statement of H. J. Anslinger." Druglibrary.org. http://www.druglibrary.org/schaffer/hemp/taxact/anslng1.htm
19. Mandel, Jerry. "Hash, Assassins and the Love of God," *Issues in Criminology 2*, 1966.
20. Booth, op. cit.
21. Cushner, Ari. "Coming to Terms With Cannabis. A Discussive History of the 1937 Marijuana Tax Act, " San Francisco State University, 2006, p. 95.
22. Anslinger, op. cit.
23. Ibid
24. Booth, op. cit.
25. Aldrich, Michael. "History of Cannabis" in *Marijuana in Medical Practice* by M.L. Mathre, McFarland & Company, Inc., Publishers - Jefferson, North Carolina and London, 1997.
26. Abel, Ernest L. Marihuana, *The First Twelve Thousand Years*, Springer, 1980.
27. Ibid
28. Lingeman, Richard. Drugs from *A to Z: A Dictionary*, McGraw-Hill, 1974.
29. Booth, op. cit.
30. Ibid
31. Bennett, Chris. "Sikhs and Cannabis." *Cannabis Culture*, 2004. http://www.cannabisculture.com/node/21460
32. Montgomery, Neil. "A Short History of Cannabis," *Pot Night - The Book*, Channel 4 Television, 1995.
33. Bennett, Chris. "Marijuana in the Bible," Patients for Medical Cannibus.com, http://patients4medicalmarijuana.wordpress.com/marijuana-info/marijuana-in-the-bible/.
34. Frazier, Wade. "The American Empire," A Healed Planet.net, http://www.ahealedplanet.net/america.htm.
35. "A Taste of Adventure," *The Economist*, 1998, http://www.economist.com/node/179810
36. David, Elizabeth. Spices, Salts and Aromatics in the English Kitchen, Grub Street Publishing; New Ed Edition, 2000.
37. Weil, Andrew T. "Nutmeg as a Narcotic," *Economic Botany*, 1965.
38. Giles Milton. *Nathaniel's Nutmeg: Or the True and Incredible Adventures of the Spice Trader Who Changed the Course of History*, Penguin,2000.
39. Dorsey, Scott. "Effects of Nutmeg & Myristicine," Erowid. Org, http://www.erowid.org/plants/nutmeg/nutmeg_info3.shtml.
40. "A Taste of Adventure," op. cit.
41. "History of the Spice Islands: Banda-part II," Baliblog.com, http://www.baliblog.com/history/history-of-the-spice-islands-banda-part-ii.html
42. Ibid
43. Zinn, Howard. "Columbus, the Indians, and Human Progress," Ch. 1, *A People's History of the United States.*
44. Brecher, Edward. *Licit and Illicit Drugs*, Little Brown & Co., 1973, p. 209.
45. Borio, Gene. "Introduction: The Chiapas Gift or the Indians Revenge," *The Tobacco Timeline*, Tobacco.org, http://archive.tobacco.org/History/Tobacco_history.html.
46. Rudgely, Richard. *Encyclopedia of Psychoactive Substances*, St. Martin's Griffin; First Edition , 2000.
47. Seig, Louis. Tobacco, Peace Pipes and Indians. Palmer Lake, CO, Filter Press, 1999.
48. Taylor, Norman. *Narcotics Nature's Dangerous Gifts.* Dell Publishing Co., 1966.
49. Borio, op. cit.
50. Taylor, op. cit.
51. Brooks, Jerome E. *The Mighty Leaf; Tobacco Through the Centuries*, Boston, MA, A. Redman, 1953.
52. Scottchristianson.org, "The Rise of the Prisoner Trade," http://www.scottchristianson.org/liberty/order/chapter.html.
53. Fahey, Joseph J. *A Peace Reader*, Paulist Pr; Rev Sub edition, 1992.
54. Ibid
55. Coe, Michael, and Sophie Coe. *The True History of Chocolate*, Thames and Hudson; 2 edition, 2007.
56. Runcie, James. "A Brief History of Chocolate," The Guardian.com, http://www.theguardian.com/lifeandstyle/2007/apr/07/foodanddrink

57. Cardwell, Glenn. "Chocolate and Health," http://glenn.server210.com/index.html
58. Wellsphere.com, "Why Do We Crave Chocolate?," http://www.wellsphere.com/women-s-health-article/why-do-we-crave-chocolate/1153857.
59. Schifano, Fabrizio, and Guido Magni. "MDMA ('Ecstasy'. Abuse: Psychological Features and Craving for Chocolate: A Case Study," *Biology and Psychiatry* 36, 763-767.
60. Ferretti, Elena, "The surprisingly scandalous history of snack foods," Foxnews.com, http://www.foxnews.com/leisure/2013/02/26/history-snack-foods/.
61. Roxby, Philippa. "Chocolate craving comes from total sensory pleasure," BBC news.com, http://www.bbc.co.uk/news/health-23449795.
62. "The Sweet Lure of Chocolate," Exploratorium.edu, http://www.exploratorium.edu/exploring/exploring_chocolate/choc_8.html.
63. Tedlock, Dennis. *Popol Vuh: The Definitive Edition of The Mayan Book of The Dawn of Life and The Glories of Gods and Kings*. Touchstone; Rev Sub edition, 1996.
64. Bensen, Amanda. "A Brief History of Chocolate," Smithsonian.com, http://www.smithsonianmag.com/arts-culture/brief-history-of-chocolate.html.
65. Coe, op. cit.
66. Rust, Randi L. "A Brief History of Chocolate, Food of the Gods." *Athena Renew*. Athena Publications, Inc.
67. Beckett, Stephen T. "The History of Chocolate," in *The Science of Chocolate*. RSC.org, http://pubs.rsc.org/en/content/chapter/bk9780854046003-00001/978-0-85404-600-3#!divabstract.
68. Blunt, Richard. "Chocolate Food for the Gods," Backwoodshome.com, http://www.backwoodshome.com/articles/blunt56.html.
69. Pace, Samantha. "Chocolate's history as rich as its taste," Minnesota Daily.com, http://www.mndaily.com/2000/02/22/chocolates-history-rich-its-taste.
70. "History of Chocolate," Essortment.com, http://www.essortment.com/history-chocolate-41087.html.
71. Diamond, Jared M. *Guns, Germs, and Steel: The Fates of Human Societies*. W. W. Norton & Company, 1999.
72. Furst, Peter T. *Hallucogens And Culture*. Chandler & Sharp Publishers, 1976.
73. Davis, Wade. *One River*. Simon and Schuster, 1998.
74. Taylor, Norman. *Narcotics, Nature's Dangerous Gift - Escape from Reality*. Dell Laurel Edition, 1966.
75. "History of Coca," Drugs-Forum.com, http://www.drugs-forum.com/forum/showwiki.php?title=History_of_Coca.
76. Davis, op. cit.
77. "History of Coca," op. cit.
78. "The Coca Leaf: Anthropological And Social Issues With The Sacred Leaf," Druglibrary.edu. http://www.druglibrary.eu/library/books/hurtado/chapter1.htm.
79. Current, John D. MD. *Pharmacology for Anesthetists*. Pedia Press. P.22
80. Diamond, op. cit.
81. "Cocaine and Crack." Drugscope.org. http://www.drugscope.org.uk/resources/drugsearch/drugsearchpages/cocaineandcrack.
82. Allen, John W. "Mushrooms and Pioneers." The Vaults of Erowid. http://www.erowid.org/library/books_online/mushroom_pioneers/mushroom_pioneers6.shtml.
83. Stafford, Peter G. and Jeremy Bigwood. *Psychedelics Encyclopedia*, edition 3, 1992, P.104.
84. Aldrich, op. cit.
85. "Mescaline." The Vault of Erowid, http://www.erowid.org/chemicals/mescaline/mescaline.shtml.
86. Schultes, Richard Evans. *Hallucinogenic Plants: A Golden Guide*. Golden Press, 1976.
87. Edley, Keith. "Rivea corymbosa - Ololiuqui." Etheology.com. http://entheology.com/plants/turbina-corymbosa-ololiuqui/
88. Taylor, op. cit.
89. Acosta, Joseph. *Natural and Moral History of the Indies*. Duke University Press, 1590.
90. Taylor, op. cit.
91. Porter, Roy and Mikulás Teich. *Drugs and Narcotics in History*. Cambridge: Cambridge University Press, 1995
92. Schultes, Richard Evans. "Teonanacatl: The Narcotic Mushroom of the Aztecs," in *American Anthropologist*, New Series, Vol. 42, No. 3, Part 1. Blackwell Publishing.
93. Ibid
94. Porter, op. cit.

95. Wassom, R. Gordon, "Hallucinogenic Fungi of Mexico", Botanical Museum of Harvard University, 1961.
96. Ibid
97. Ibid
98. "Drug Study Participants: Hallucinogen Produces Deep Mystical Experience, Foxnews.com," http://www.foxnews.com/story/2006/07/11/drug-study-participants-hallucinogen-produces-deep-mystical-experience/.
99. Ibid
100. Wassom, op. cit.
101. Wassom. op. cit.
102. Stearns, Peter N. *The Encyclopedia of World History: Ancient, Medieval and Modern; Chronologically* Arranged. James Clarke & Co Ltd, 2002.
103. Christianson, Scott. *With Liberty For Some: 500 Years of Imprisonment in America.* Northeastern, 1998.
104. "Pre-Columbian Hispaniola - Arawak/Taino Indians," World History Archives. http://www.hartford-hwp.com/archives/43a/100.html.
105. Christianson, op. cit
106. Ibid
107. Stearns, op. cit.
108. Taylor, Alan. *American Colonies: The Settling of North America*, Vol. 1. Penguin, 2002.
109. Murrin, John M. "Beneficiaries of Catastrophe: The English Colonies in America," in *The New American History,* Eric Foner, ed., p. 10. American Historical Association, 1997.
110. Taylor, Alan, op. cit.
111. Falk, Emily. *78 Things They Didn't Teach You In School: But You Do Need To Know.* Rabbit's Foot Press, 2005.
112. Wolf, Eric R. *Europe and the People Without History.* Berkeley, University of CA Press, 1982.

## Chapter VI: 1500-1863: Mercantilism, Triangular Trade, Slavery

1. Bodin, Jean. *Six Books of the Commonwealth.* Oxford, Alden Press, 1576.
2. Sieg, Louis. *Tobacco, Peace Pipes and Indians.* Filter Pr Llc, 1971.
3. Ibid
4. Taylor, Norman. *Narcotics Nature's Dangerous Gifts.* Dell Publishing Co., 1966.
5. James, King. *A Counterblast to Tobacco, 1604.* Arber, 1869.
6. "Tobacco." High Beam Business. http://business.highbeam.com/industry-reports/agriculture/tobacco.
7. Rudgley, Richard. *Encyclopedia of Psychoactive Substances.* St. Martin's Griffin; First Edition edition, 2000.
8. Borio, Gene. "The Tobacco Timeline." Tobacco.org. http://archive.tobacco.org/History/Tobacco_History.html
9. West, Jean M. "Tobacco and Slavery: The Vile Weed." *Slavery in America, 3.* http://slaveryinamerica.org/history/hs_es_slavery_tobacco_tobacco.htm.
10. Roques, Wayne J.. "Legalization: An Idea Whose Time Will Never Come." U.S. Drug Enforcement Admin., Miami Field Division: U.S. Dept. of Justice, 1994.
11. Duke, Steven B. Interview, Friday at Four. America Online, 1994.
12. Friedman, Lauren. "This Scary Map Shows Where Pregnant Women Smoke The Most." Business Insider.com. http://www.businessinsider.com/where-pregnant-women-smoke-the-most-2013-12
13. Allen, Theodore. *The Invention of the White Race, Volume 1: Racial Oppression and Social Control. Verso*; Second Edition edition, 2012.
14. Garn, Stanley M. *Human Races*. Springfield, Illinois: Rev. 2nd printing, 1962.
15. Allen, Theodore. "Summary of the Argument of the Invention of the White Race." http://clogic.eserver.org/1-2/allen.html
16. Fredricksen, George M. *The New York Review of Books.* 1997.
17. Degler, Carl N. *Neither Black Nor White: Slavery and Race Relations in Brazil and the United States* . New York, 1971.
18. Allen, op. cit.
19. McNeill, William. *History of Western Civilization: A Handbook.* University of Chicago Press; 6th Edition, 1986.
20. Hillyer, Reiko. "Origins of Slavery and Race." Columbia American History Online. http://caho-test.cc.columbia.edu/pcp/14018.html

21. Fields, Barbara Jeanne. "Slavery, Race, and Ideology in the United States of America." *New Left Review.* http://www.newleftreview.org/?view=460
22. Ibid
23. Ibid
24. Wrights, R. Lee. "The most destructive and devastating war in American history." Liberty For All. http://www.libertyforall.net/the-most-destructive-and-devastating-war-in-american-history/.
25. Mittelberger, Gottlieb. *Gottlieb Mittelberger's Journey to Pennsylvania in the Year 1750 and Return to Germany in the Year 1754.* German Society of Pennsylvania, 1898.
26. Banks, Taunya Lovell. "Dangerous Woman: Elizabeth Key's Freedom Suit - Subjecthood and Racialized Identity in Seventeenth Century Colonial Virginia (2008.." U of Maryland Legal Studies Research Paper No. 2005-28; Akron Law Review, v. 41, 2008, p. 799-837.. Available at SSRN: http://ssrn.com/abstract=672121. or http://dx.doi.org/10.2139/ssrn.672121
27. Banks, op. cit.
28. Allen, op. cit.
29. "From Indentured Servitude to Racial Slavery." PBS.org. https://www.pbs.org/wgbh/aia/part1/1narr3.html
30. Ibid
31. Sweet, Frank W. "The Invention of the One-Drop Rule in the 1830s North - Essays on the Color Line and the One-Drop Rule." Essays on the U.S. Color Line. http://essays.backintyme.biz/item/15
32. Ibid
33. Ibid
34. Ibid
35. Ibid
36. Scaruffi, Piero. "A Brief History of Blues Music," in *History of Popular Music.* Omniware, 2007.
37. Ibid
38. "Ethiopian Coffee." Selamta.net. http://www.selamta.net/Ethiopian%20Coffee.htm.
39. Toussaint-Sama, Maguelonne. "Coffee and Politics," in A History of Food. John Wiley & Sons, 2009.
40. Heathcott, Joseph. "Coffee, Capitalism and the State." *Practical Anarchy #13.* http://news.infoshop.org/article.php?story=01/08/26/6535205
41. Scheper, S. "The Fascinating History of Coffee." How to Get Focused. http://www.howtogetfocused.com/chapters/the-fascinating-history-of-coffee
42. Heathcott, op. cit.
43. Ibid
44. Ibid
45. Ibid
46. Black, Jeremy. "Apologizing for the Past? Jeremy Black explores the Eighteenth Century Atlantic Slave Trade." The Social Affairs Unit. http://www.socialaffairsunit.org.uk/blog/archives/000996.php
47. Gibson, Kenyon. "Hemp in the British Isles." Journal of Industrial Hemp. Volume 11, Issue 2, 2006 p. 57-67.
48. Shah, Anup. "Behind Consumption and Consumerism." Global Issues. http://www.globalissues.org/issue/235/consumption-and-consumerism.
49. Black, op. cit.
50. Phillips, William, Jr. and Carla Rahn Phillips. *The Worlds of Christopher Columbus.*, Cambridge University Press, 1993. pp. 56-69.
51. Ibid
52. Weil, Andrew and Winifred Rosen. *From Chocolate to Morphine: Everything You Need to Know About Mind-Altering Drugs.* Boston: Houghton Mifflin Company, 1983.
53. *Webster's New Collegiate Dictionary. College Edition*, World Publishing Co., Inc., 1974.
54. Mintz, Sydney quoted by Richard H. Robbins, in *Global Problems and the Culture of Capitalism*, (Allyn and Bacon, 1999., p. 208.
55. Allen, Theodore. "Summary of the Argument of the Invention of the White Race." Op. cit.
56. "History of Trade." History.net. http://www.historyworld.net/wrldhis/PlainTextHistories.asp?ParagraphID=dqq
57. Schlaadt, Richard G. Wellness: *Alcohol Use and Abuse.* The Duskin Publishing Group Inc. ,1992.
58. Schwartz, Stuart B. "Tropical Babylons: Sugar and the Making of the Atlantic World, 1450-1680." EH.NET, 2004.

59. McIntyre, Charshee C.L. "The Irish Precedent: The Perfecting of the System and Enslaving of the Alien." Rootsweb. http://archiver.rootsweb.ancestry.com/th/read/Melungeon/2006-03/1142765743
60. Ibid
61. Ibid
62. Morrison, Holy S. "Homily for Maine Frontier Day." 2006. Retrieved from http://www.maineulsterscots.com/docs/FrontierDay_HM_Homily_after.pdf.
63. Fitzhugh, George. *Cannibals All! or, Slaves Without Masters.* Richmond, VA, 1857.
64. Cavanaugh, James F. "Irish Slaves in the Caribbean." Clan Caomhánach. http://www.kavanaghfamily.com/articles/2003/20030618jfc.htm.
65. Ibid
66. Ibid
67. Ibid
68. Bornstein, George. "Afro-Celtic Connections From Frederick Douglass to The Commitments." Michigan Today. http://michigantoday.umich.edu/96/Mar96/mta15m96.html.
69. Ibid
70. Cavanaugh, James. "Irish Slavery." Race and History News and Views. http://www.raceandhistory.com/cgi-bin/forum/webbbs_config.pl/noframes/read/1638.
71. Ibid.
72. Ibid
73. Ibid
74. Musto, David. "The History of Legislative Control Over Opium, Cocaine and Their Derivatives." Drug Library. http://www.druglibrary.org/schaffer/history/ophs.htm
75. King, Rufus B. "The Narcotics Bureau and the Harrison Narcotics Tax Act: Jailing the Healers and the Sick." *Yale Law Review,* 1953.
76. Swan, Neil. "California Study Finds $1 Spent on Treatment Saves Taxpayers $7." NIDA Notes, Volume 10, Number 2, 1995.
77. "The History of Tea." 2B A Snob. http://www.2basnob.com/tea-history-timeline.html.
78. Ibid
79. Everage, Laura. "Coffee's Journey Throughout the World: A Brief History." Coffee Universe. http://coffeeuniverse.com/coffees-journey-throughout-the-world-a-brief-history/.
80. "The History of Tea," op. cit.
81. Robinson, Rowan. *The Great Book of Hemp: The Complete Guide to the Environmental, Commercial, and Medicinal Uses of the World's Most Extraordinary Plant.* Rochester, VT: Park Street Press, 1995.
82. Paine, Thomas. *Common Sense: and Other Writings.* New York, NY: Modern Library, 2003.
83. Russo, Ethan and Franjo Grotenhermen. *Cannabis And Cannabinoids: Pharmacology, Toxicology, And Therapeutic Potential.* New York, London, Oxford: The Haworth Integrative Healing Press, 2002.
84. Diamond, Jared M. *Guns, Germs, and Steel: The Fates of Human Societies.* W. W. Norton & Company, 1999.
85. "General Hemp Information." Hemp Basics. http://hempbasics.com/shop/hemp-information.
86. "Industrial Hemp Facts." Rediscover Hemp. http://rediscoverhemp.com/inform/industrial-hemp-facts/.
87. Russo, op. cit.
88. Herer, Jack. "The Emperor Wears No Clothes." Think or Be Beaten. http://thinkorbebeaten.com/TOBE/www.thinkorbeeaten.com/theknoll/rr/Jack_Herer_-_The_Emperor_Wears_No_Clothes_%5BHow_Hemp_Can_Save_The_World%5D.en.pdf.
89. Robinson, Rowan. *The Great Book of Hemp: The Complete Guide to the Environmental, Commercial, and Medicinal Uses of the World's Most Extraordinary Plant.* Park Street Press, 1995.
90. Solomon, David. *The Marijuana Papers.* Panther, 1972.
91. Crawford, Bryce. "Medical Marijuana: Dixie Elixirs Sold to California Company." Colorado Springs Independent. http://www.csindy.com/IndyBlog/archives/2012/04/18/medical-marijuana-dixie-elixirs-sold-to-california-company
92. Lossing, Benson J. *Diary of Gen. George Washington.* New York: Charles B. Richardson & Co.
93. Andrews, George and Simon Vinkenoog. *The Book of Grass: An Anthology of Indian Hemp.* Penguin Books, 1972.
94. Crawford, Bryce. "Medical Marijuana: Elixirs Sold to California Company." *Colorado Springs Independent,* April 18, 2012.

95. Herer, op. cit.
96. Ibid
97. "Chronology of Cannabis Hemp. " Cannabis Campaigners' Guide. http://ccguide.org/chronol.php.
98. Green, Lee. "The Demonized Seed." *Los Angeles Times.* http://articles.latimes.com/2004/jan/18/magazine/tm-hemp03.
99. Cloud, John. "This Buds Not for You." *Time Magazine.* http://content.time.com/time/magazine/article/0,9171,201911,00.html.
100. Evans, Keith. *The longest war: The short, sad story of the long war against drugs.* The Glastonbury Archive. http://isleofavalon.co.uk/GlastonburyArchive/drugwars/ke-00.html.
101. Herer, op. cit.
102. Harriss, Joseph. "How the Louisiana Purchase Changed the World." Smithsonian.com. http://www.smithsonianmag.com/history-archaeology/westward.html.
103. McGrew, Jane Lang. "History of Alcohol Prohibition", Appendix to *The technical papers of the first report of the National Commission on Marihuana and Drug Abuse, vol. 1.* Washington, D.C.: Government Printing Office, 1972.
104. Hanson, David J. "National prohibition of alcohol in the U.S." Alcohol Problems and Solutions. http://www2.potsdam.edu/hansondj/Controversies/1091124904.html.
105. Watson, Ben. *Cider, Hard and Sweet: History, Traditions, and Making Your Own.* Countryman Pr; 1st edition, 1999.
106. Ibid
107. Skilnik, Bob. *Beer and Food in American History.* Jefferson Press, 2007.
108. Rorabaugh, W.J. *The Alcoholic Republic: An American Tradition.* New York, NY: Oxford University Press, Inc.
109. McGrew, op. cit.
110. Skilnik, op. cit
111. Isaacson, Walter. *Benjamin Franklin: An American Life.* Simon and Schuster, 2004.
112. Crowley, John E. *Review of taverns and drinking in early America.* Common Place. http://www.common-place.org/vol-04/no-01/reviews/crowley.shtml.
113. "History of Alcohol Prohibition." Schaffer Library of Drug Policy. http://www.druglibrary.org/schaffer/library/studies/nc/nc2a_2.htm
114. "George Washington." *Britannica Concise Encyclopedia.* http://www.answers.com/topic/george-washington
115. Burns, Stanley and Jason Burns. "Ether frolic: Party entertainment becomes medical revolution (a pictorial history of healing.." *Clinician Reviews,* 2002.
116. Jones, Kathleen. *A Passionate Sisterhood: Women of the Wordsworth Circle.* Palgrave Macmillan, 2000.
117. Ibid
118. Burns, op. cit.
119. Ibid
120. Ibid
121. Booth, Martin. *Opium: A History.* New York, NY: St. Martin's Press.
122. Taylor, op. cit.
123. Nephalim. "Drug Prohibition: A History (Part I Pre-Prohibition.." Daily Kos. http://www.dailykos.com/story/2005/01/22/87218/-Drug-Prohibition-A-History-Part-I-Pre-Prohibition#.
124. Millegan, K. "The Boodle Boys." http://www.ctrl.org/boodleboys/boodleboys2.html
125. Ibid
126. Newsinger, John. *The blood never dried: A people's history of the British Empire.* Bookmarks, 2006.
127. Rowntree, J. *The imperial drug trade: A restatement of the opium question in the light of recent evidence and new developments in the East.* London: Methuen & Co., 1906.
128. Blackman, S.J., *Chilling out: The cultural politics of substance consumption, youth, and drug policy.* New York, NY: Shane Blackman, 2004.
129. Ibid
130. "A Social History of America's Most Popular Drugs." http://www.pbs.org/wgbh/pages/frontline/shows/drugs/buyers/socialhistory.html
131. Magagnini, Stephen. "Chinese transformed 'Gold Mountain." *Sacramento Bee,* January 18, 1998.
132. "A Social History of America's Most Popular Drugs." op. cit.
133. Magagnini, op. cit.

## Chapter VII: 1650-1900: Booze, Temperance, & Abolition


1. Waner, Jessica. *Gin and Debauchery in the Age of Reason.* Random House Trade Paperbacks, 2003.
2. .Ibid.
3. Ibid.
4. Levine, Harry G. and Craig Reinarman. "Alcohol Prohibition: Lessons from Alcohol Policy for Drug Policy." Amsterdam: CEDRO. http://www.cedro-uva.org/lib/levine.alcohol.html
5. "Benjamin Rush and His Views on Alcoholism." Health.am. http://www.health.am/psy/more/dr-benjamin-rush-and-his-views-on-alcoholism/
6. "History of Alcohol Prohibition." Schaffer Library of Drug Policy.http://www.druglibrary.org/Schaffer/LIBRARY/studies/nc/nc2a.htm.
7. Ibid.
8. Berkhout, M. & Robinson F. *Madame Joy.* HarperCollins Publishers PTY, 2000, p. 37.
9. Blackman, Shane. *Chilling Out: The Cultural Politics of Substance Consumption, Youth and Drug Policy.* McGraw-Hill International, 2004.
10. Ibid.
11. Ibid.
12. Ibid.
13. Rorabaugh, W.J. *The Alcoholic Republic: An American Tradition.* New York, NY: Oxford University Press, 1981.
14. Kenny, Kevin. *The American Irish: A History.* Longman, 2000.
15. Wohl, Anthony S. "The Function of Racism in Victorian England." http://victorianweb.org/history/race/victor9.html.
16. Ibid
17. Lender, Mark E. *Drinking in America: A History.* New York: The Free Press, 1987.
18. Wheeler, Linda. "The New York Draft Riot of 1863." Washington Post.com. http://www.washingtonpost.com/lifestyle/style/the-new-york-draft-riots-of-1863/2013/04/26/a1aacf52-a620-11e2-a8e2-5b98cb59187f_story.html.
19. Harris, Leslie M. "The New York City Draft Riots of 1863," from *In The Shadow of Slavery - African Americans in New York City, 1626-1863.* University Of Chicago Press, 2003.
20. "Know-nothing movement. " *The Columbia Electronic Encyclopedia, 6th ed.* http://www.infoplease.com/ce6/history/A0827946.html.
21. Holt, Michael. "The Know Nothing Party." http://dig.lib.niu.edu/message/ps-knownothing.html.
22. Basler, Roy P. "Letter to Joshua Speed. Abraham Lincoln Online." http://showcase.netins.net/web/creative/lincoln/speeches/speed.htm.
23. Olmsted, Frederick L. *A Journey in the Seaboard States.* New York; London: Dix and Edwards; Sampson Low, Son & Co., 1856.
24. Ibid.
25. Pinder, Sherrow O. *The Politics of Race and Ethnicity in the United States.* Palgrave Macmillan, 2013.
26. "Andrew Jackson 2nd Annual Address to Congress (1830.." Ourdocuments.gov. http://www.ourdocuments.gov/doc.php?flash=true&doc=25&page=transcript.
27. Moulton, Gary. *The Papers of Chief John Ross: 1807-1839.* University of Oklahoma Press, 1985.
28. Jennings, P. "Text of the Indian Removal Act, 1830." The Nomadic Spirit. http://www.synaptic.bc.ca/ejournal/jackson.htm.
29. Chambers II, John Whiteclay. "Plains Indian Wars." *The Oxford Campaign to American Military History*, Oxford University Press 2000.
30. Hoig, Stan. *The Sand Creek Massacre. USA:* University of Oklahoma Press, 2013.
31. "Indian History and Culture." http://www.anb.org/main-indian.html.
32. "Obituary of Vincent Deloria, Jr." *New York Times*, Nov. 13, 2005.
33. Pember, Mary Annette. *Milwaukee Journal Sentinel*, Nov. 24. 2005, p. 25A
34. "Battle of the Little Big Horn." Digital History. http://www.digitalhistory.uh.edu/disp_textbook.cfm?smtid=3&psid=706.
35. Ward, Geoffrey. *The West: An illustrated History.* Back Bay Books, 2000.
36. "Documents Relating to the Wounded Knee Massacre." Digital History. http://www.digitalhistory.uh.edu/disp_textbook.cfm?smtID=3&psid=1101.

37. Elk, Black. *The End of the Dream.* York: Pocket Books/Bison Books, 1972., pp. 224-30.
38. Giago. op. sit.
39. Giago, Tim. "The 1890 Massacre at Wounded Knee." Indianz.com. http://www.indianz.com/News/2006/017305.asp?print=1.
40. Erowid, Canasta, N., & Trout, K. "A Brief Summary of the Relationship Between Peyote Use and the Ghost Dance." The Vaults of Erowid. http://www.erowid.org/plants/peyote/peyote_history1.shtml
41. Fowler, Loretta. *The Columbia Guide to American Indians of the Great Plains.* Columbia University Press; 1st edition, 2003.
42. Ibid
43. cFikes, Jay. "A Brief History of the Native American Church." Council on Spiritual Practice. http://csp.org/communities/docs/fikes-nac_history.html.
44. Snake, Reuben. "Native American Worship with Peyote is not Drug Abuse." Criminal Justice Policy Foundation. http://www.cjpf.org/old/drug/peyote.html.
45. Eagle, White. *The Medicine of Selves Volume 3- Life & Survivor's Guilt.* White Eagle, 2011.
46. Snake, op sit
47. Fee, Chester A. *Chief Joseph: The Biography of a Great Indian.* Wilson-Erickson, 1936.
48. Rappleye, Charles. "The Uncivil War." *Los Angeles Times.com.* http://articles.latimes.com/2006/sep/17/books/bk-rappleye17.
49. Kenrick, John. *A History of the Musical Minstrel Shows. Musicals101.* http://www.musicals101.com/minstrel.htm.
50. "Creation of the Jim Crow South." ULM.edu. http://www.ulm.edu/~ryan/206/documents/jcrow.htm.
51. Wormser, Richard. *The Rise and Fall of Jim Crow.* St. Martin's Press, 2003.
52. Herer, J. The *Emperor Wears No Clothes: Hemp and the Marijuana Conspiracy.* AH HA Publishing; 12th edition, 2010.
53. Markoe, Lauren. "Senate Votes to Apologize for Failing to Outlaw Lynching". *Knight Ridder Newspapers.* https://groups.google.com/forum/#!topic/alt.obituaries/U8JWcsp4N_g.
54. Ibid
55. Marchetti, Gina. *Romance and the "Yellow Peril".* University of Cal Press, 1994.
56. Xing, Jun. *Asian America through the Lens: History, Representations, and Identities* (Critical Perspectives on Asian Pacific Americans.. Altamira Press, 1998.
57. Baum, Dan. *Smoke and Mirrors: The War on Drugs and the Politics of Failure.* Back Bay Books, 1997.
58. Summers, Mark Wahlgren. *Rum, Romanism, and Rebellion: The Making of a President, 1884* (2000. http://www.questia.com/read/104865169/rum-romanism-rebellion-the-making-of-a-president
59. Ibid
60. Wines, Frederick H. "Report on the Defective, Dependent, and Delinquent Classes of the Population of the United States, as Returned at the Tenth Census." Washington, D.C.: *Government Printing Office*, 1888.
61. Hardaway, Robert. "U.S. Stuck in a Quagmire." *The Denver Post*, March 14, 2004.
62. Gompers, Samuel. "Some Reasons for Chinese Exclusion." *American Federation of Labor*, 1902.
63. Ibid.
64. Turner, Frederick J. "The Significance of the Frontier in American History." *American Historical Association*, 1893.
65. Richardson, Heather C. *The Reconstruction of America after the Civil War.* Yale University Press, 2008.
66. Lehtinen, V. "America Would Lose its Soul." University of Helsinki, 2002.
67. "Former US Attorney General Ramsey Clark on Why Sanctions are Genocide." Mediaroots. http://www.mediaroots.org/former-us-attorney-general-ramsey-clark-on-why-sanctions-are-genocidal/.
68. Hogan, Daniel B. "The Effectiveness of Licensing History, Evidence, and Recommendations." *Law and Human behavior, 7* (2B.. p. 119.
69. Musto, David F. "The History of Legislative Control Over Opium, Cocaine and Their Derivatives." *Schaffer Library of Drug Policy.* http://www.druglibrary.org/schaffer/history/ophs.htm.
70. Beck, Andrew H. "The Flexner Report and Standardization of American Medicine." *JAMA*, Vol. 291, No. 17, 2004.
71. Russo, Ethan B. and Franjo Grotenhermen. *The Handbook of Cannabis Therapeutics: From Bench to Bedside* (Haworth Series in Integrative Healing.. Routledge, 2006.

## Chapter VIII: 1880-1919: Pure Food & Drug Act


1. "Emergence of Advertising in America - EAA. Timeline." Duke University Libraries Digital Collections. http://library.duke.edu/digitalcollections/eaa/timeline/.
2. Brecher, Edward M. *Licit And Illicit Drugs; the Consumers Union Report on Narcotics, Stimulants, Depressants, Inhalants, Hallucinogens, And Marijuana - Including Caffeine, Nicotine And Alcohol.* Consumers Union; First Edition edition, 1972.
3. Musto, David. *The American Disease: Origins of Narcotic Control.* Oxnard University Press, 1999, pg. 258.
4. "Oliver Wendell Holmes." Medical Antiques. http://www.medicalantiques.com/civilwar/Medical_Authors_Faculty/Holmes_Oliver_Wendell_Sr..htm.
5. Holmes, Oliver W. *Medical essays: Webster's French thesaurus edition.* Icon Group International, Incorporated, 2008.
6. Goodman, Louis and Alfred Gilman. *Goodman and Gilman's The Pharmacological Basis of Therapeutics.* Macmillan Publishing Company; 6th edition, 1982.
7. Brecher, Edward M. "Nineteenth-century America - a 'dope fiend's paradise.'" Schaffer Library of Drug Policy. http://www.druglibrary.org/schaffer/library/studies/cu/cu1.html.
8. Ibid
9. Musto, David. "The History of Legislative Control over opium cocaine and their derivatives." Schaffer Library of Drug Policies. http://www.druglibrary.org/schaffer/history/ophs.htm
10. "From Quackery to Bacteriology: The Emergence of Modern Medicine in 19th Century America." Utoledo.edu. http://www.utoledo.edu/library/canaday/exhibits/quackery/quack-index.html.
11. Musto, op. cit.
12. Ibid
13. Aldrich, Michael R. " The Remarkable W.B. O' Shaughessy." *O'Shaughnessy's*, Spring 2006.
14. Ibid
15. Coakley, Davis. *Irish Masters of Medicine.* Dublin: Town House, 1992.
16. Aldrich, op. cit.
17. Herer, Jack. "The Emperor Wears No Clothes." Jack Herer.com. http://www.jackherer.com/thebook/chapter-twelve/.
18. Ibid
19. "Transcripts of House Hearings on the Marijuana Tax Act." Origin of the Hemp-Marijuana Myth. http://webstation19.8k.com/archives/37HEAR.HTM.
20. Montgomery, Neil M. "A Short History of Cannabis." Pot Night - The Book. http://www.ukcia.org/research/potnight/pn4.htm
21. Mikuriya, Tod. "Physical, Mental, and Moral Effects of Marijuana: The Indian Hemp Drugs Commission Report." Schaffer Library of Drug Policy. http://www.druglibrary.org/schaffer/library/effects.htm.
22. Ibid
23. Montgomery, Neil M. "A Short History of Cannabis." In *Pot Night.* Channel 4 Television, 1995.
24. Taylor, Norman. "The Pleasant Assassin: The Story of Marihuana," in The Marijuana Papers by Timothy Leary, et al. Bobbs-Merrill, 1996.
25. Booth, Martin. *Cannabis: A History.* Picador, 2005, p. 8-9.
26. Musto, op. cit.
27. Herer, op. cit.
28. Freud, Sigmund. *Über Coca.* EOD Network, 2012.
29. Herer, op. cit.
30. Brownless, Nick, Nick Constable, Gareth Thomas and Robert Ashton. *The Little Box of Drugs: Unbiased and Unadulterated Commentary on the Drugs Debate.* Sanctuary Publishing, 2004.
31. Gottlieb, Adam. *The Pleasures of Cocaine.* Ronin Publishing, 1999.
32. "Vintage Wine." Cocaine.org. http://cocaine.org/cocawine.htm.
33. "Is it true Coca-Cola once contained cocaine?" The Straight Dope. http://www.straightdope.com/columns/read/384/is-it-true-coca-cola-once-contained-cocaine.
34. Hamblin, James. "Why We Took Cocaine Out of Soda. " *The Atlantic.com.* http://www.theatlantic.com/health/archive/2013/01/why-we-took-cocaine-out-of-soda/272694/.
35. Ibid

36. Becker, Howard S. "History, Culture and Subjective Experience: An Exploration of the Social Bases of Drug-Induced Experiences." *Journal of Health and Society Behavior*, Vol. 8, No. 3., 1967.
37. "Is it true Coca-Cola once contained cocaine?" op. cit.
38. Hamblin, op. cit.
39. Musto, op.cit.
40. "100 years of altered states." *The Observer.* http://observer.theguardian.com/drugs/story/0,,686503,00.html.
41. "Cocaine: A Short History." Drugfreeworld. http://www.drugfreeworld.org/drugfacts/cocaine/a-short-history.html.
42. Harris, Mark. "Weed, Booze, Cocaine and Other Old School 'Medicine' Ads." Pharmacy Techs.net. http://www.pharmacytechs.net/blog/old-school-medicine-ads/.
43. Ibid
44. "Biography: Annie Oakley." PBS.org. http://www.pbs.org/wgbh/americanexperience/features/biography/oakley-annie/.
45. Adams, Samuel Hopkins. *The Great American Fraud.* Chicago : American Medical Association, 1907.
46. Bruce K. Alexander. "Mark Twain and the American Approach to Drugs: A View from Canada." *Psychnews International*, Volume 3, Issue 4 , 1998.
47. Ibid
48. Lupien, John Craig. *Unraveling an American Dilemma: The Demonization of Marijuana.* Pepperdine University, 1995.
49. Whitebread, Charles. "History of the Non Medical Use of Drugs in the United States." Schaffer Library of Drug Policy. http://www.druglibrary.org/schaffer/history/whiteb1.htm/
50. Williams, Samuel. *The Middle Kingdom.* New York: John Wiley, 1848, p. 96.
51. Sinclair, Upton. *The Jungle.* Dover Publications, 2001.
52. Musto, David F. "The history of legislative control over opium, cocaine, and their derivatives." *Schaffer Library of Drug Policy.* http://www.druglibrary.org/schaffer/History/ophs.htm.
53. Evans, Keith. *The Longest War; The Short, Sad Story Of The Long War Against Drug.* Isle ofAvalo. http://www.isleofavalon.co.uk/GlastonburyArchive/drugwars/ke-02.html.
54. Musto, op. cit.
55. Evans, op. cit.
56. Ibid
57. Williams, Edward H. "Negro Cocaine 'Fiends' Are A New Southern Menace." *New York Times*, 1914.
58. Musto, David, in *Dying to Get High Marijuana as Medicine* by Wendy Chapkis & Richard J. Webb. NYU Press, 2008.
59. Williams, op. cit.
60. Philip Bean. *Drugs and Crime.* Routledge, 2013.
61. "Marijuana - The First Twelve Thousand Years." Schaffer Library of Drug Policy. http://druglibrary.org/schaffer/hemp/history/first12000/11.htm.
62. Ibid
63. Ibid
64. Mandel, Jerry. "The Mythical Roots Of U.S. Drug Policy: Soldier's Disease And Addicts In The Civil War." Schaffer Library of Drug Policy. http://www.druglibrary.org/schaffer/history/soldis.htm.
65. Ibid
66. Ibid
67. Quinones, Mark A. "Drug Abuse During the Civil War (1861-1865)." Informa Health Care. http://informahealthcare.com/doi/abs/10.3109/10826087509028357?journalCode=sum.
68. Swatos, William H., Jr. "Opiate Addiction in the Late Nineteenth Century: A Study of the Social Problems, Using Medical Journals of the Period." *International Journal of Addictions, 7*, 1972.
69. Musto, op. cit.
70. Mandel, op. cit.
71. Quinones, op. cit.
72. Quinones, Mark as quoted in *American Civil War Pharmacy, A History of Drugs, Drug Supply and Provision and Therapeutics for the Union and Confederacy* by Michael A. Flannery. Binghamton, NY: CRC Press, 2004.
73. Mandel, op. cit.
74. Ibid

75. Quinones, op. cit.
76. Anslinger, H.J. "The Physician and Narcotics Law." *Tulane Law Review*, Vol. XX, No. 3, 1946. Schaffer Library of Drug Policy. http://www.druglibrary.org/schaffer/history/physician_and_feds.html.
77. Brecher, op. cit.
78. "The War on Drugs is Lost." Old National Review. http://old.nationalreview.com/12feb96/drug.html.
79. Wallechinsky, David and Irving Wallace. *The People's Almanac*. Doubleday, 1975.

## Chapter IX: 1910-1919: Prelude to Prohibition

1. *Webb v. United States*. Justia.com. http://supreme.justia.com/cases/federal/us/249/96/.
2. Breche, Edward. "Supplying heroin legally to addicts," in *The Consumers Union Report on Licit and Illicit Drugs. Schaffer Library of Drug Policy*. http://www.druglibrary.org/schaffer/library/studies/cu/cu13.html.
3. "National Review." Old National Review. http://old.nationalreview.com/12feb96/drug.html.
4. Ibid
5. White, William L. "History of Drug Policy, Treatment, and Recovery." http://www.williamwhitepapers.com/pr/2004Historyofdrugproblems%26policy.pdf.
6. Ibid
7. Ibid
8. "Swiss System in the US." *The Drug Policy Forum of Texas*. http://www.dpft.org/heroin.htm.
9. Sweenie, Tracie. "On Dignity, Human Rights and Misguided Critics of Methadone Treatment" Op-Ed from Brown. http://www.brown.edu/Administration/News_Bureau/Op-Eds/Lewis4.html.
10. Ibid
11. Tallaksen, Amund. "Reflections on 'Addicts Who Survived.'" Points: The Blog of the Alcohol and Drugs History Society. http://pointsadhsblog.wordpress.com/2013/04/11/reflections-on-addicts-who-survived-amund-tallaksen/.
12. "Timeline of Events in the History of Drugs." INPUD International Diaries. http://inpud.wordpress.com/timeline-of-events-in-the-history-of-drugs/.
13. Ibid
14. Gieringer, Dale. "The Origins of Cannabis Prohibition in California." *Contemporary Drug Problems*, Federal Legal Publications, New York 1999.
15. Ibid.
16. Wright, Hamilton as cited in "The Origins of California's 1913 Cannabis Law," by Gieringer, Dale. *Journal of Contemporary Drug Problems*, 1999.
17. Chopra, I. C., R. N. Chopra. "The Use of the Cannabis Drugs in India." UNODC. http://www.unodc.org/unodc/en/data-and-analysis/bulletin/bulletin_1957-01-01_1_page003.html.
18. Abel, Ernest. "Reefer Racism," in *Marihuana The First Twelve-Thousand Years*. Springer, 1980.
19. Chopra, op. cit.
20. "History of the Medical Use of Marijuana, Marihuana," in *A Signal of Misunderstanding, the Report of the US National Commission on Marihuana and Drug Abuse*, 1972.
21. Brecher, Edward. "The Consumers Union Report on Licit and Illicit Drugs." Schaffer Library of Drug Policy. http://www.druglibrary.org/schaffer/library/studies/cu/cu54.html.
22. "A Social History of America's Most Popular Drugs." PBS. http://www.pbs.org/wgbh/pages/frontline/shows/drugs/buyers/socialhistory.html.
23. "History of the Medical Use of Marijuana, Marihuana," op. cit.
24. Ibid
25. Ibid
26. "The Early State- Marijuana Laws." Schaffer Library of Drug Policy. http://www.druglibrary.org/olsen/dpf/whitebread05.html.
27. "History of Marijuana as Medicine - 2900 BC to Present." Procon.org. http://medicalmarijuana.procon.org/view.timeline.php?timelineID=000026.
28. Ibid.
29. Rosenberg, Jennifer. "Pancho Villa." About.com. http://history1900s.about.com/cs/panchovilla/p/panchovilla.htm.
30. Ibid.

31. Carter, Everett. *Cultural History Written with Lightning: The Significance of The Birth of a Nation.* Lexington,Kentucky: University of Kentucky Press, 1983.
32. Ibid
33. Catchpole, Karen. "California's Cowboy Coast." American Cowboy. http://www.americancowboy.com/travel/trips/californias-cowboy-coast.
34. Ibid
35. Ibid
36. Ibid.
37. Ibid.
38. Carter, op. cit.
39. Ibid.
40. Ibid.
41. "Reefer Madness Rears Its Ugly Head." UKCIA.org. http://www.ukcia.org/potculture/20/madness.html.
42. Herer, Jack. *The Emperor Wears No Clothes: Hemp and the Marijuana Conspiracy.* AH HA Publishing, 2010.
43. Scaruffi, Piero. "A Brief history of Blues Music," in *History of Popular Music.* Omniware, 2007.
44. Ibid.
45. Abel, op. cit.
46. Scarutti, op. cit.
47. "Blackface! Minstrel Shows." Black-Face.com. http://black-face.com/minstrel-shows.htm.
48. Kenrick, John. "A History of the Musical Minstrel Shows." Musicals 101. http://www.musicals101.com/minstrel.htm.
49. "Blackface! Minstrel Shows," op. cit.
50. Ibid
51. Jules-Rosette, Bennetta. *Josephine Baker in Art and Life: The Icon and the Image.* University of Illinois Press, 2007.
52. Ibid
53. Ojibwa. "Origins of English: Blue." Daily Kos. http://www.dailykos.com/story/2012/08/04/1116727/-Origins-of-English-Blue.
54. Baker, Robert M. "A Brief History of the Blues." The Blue Highway. http://thebluehighway.com/blues/history.html.
55. Scaruffi, op. cit.
56. Elliot, Steve. "Louis Armstrong." Toke Signals. http://tokesignals.com/cannabis-quote-of-the-day-louis-armstrong/.
57. Ibid
58. Baker, op. cit.
59. Ibid.
60. Allen, Gary. "The Green Fairy Flies High." Leite's Culinaria. http://leitesculinaria.com/37206/writings-absinthe.html.
61. "How the Absinthe Ban Came to Be." Absinthe 101. http://www.absinthe101.com/absinthe-ban.html.
62. "The history of absinthe." Absinthe Fever. http://www.absinthefever.com/absinthe/history.
63. "Absinth effects." Absinth.bz. http://www.absinth.bz/articles/absinth-effects.html.
64. Max. B. "This and that: Clots, creamers and canals." *Trends in Pharmacological Sciences.* Volume 9, Issue 4, 1988, p. 122-124.
65. "Absinthe and Its Silver-Tongued Marketers - Thujone's Role in Absinthe Sales." Mutineer Magazine. http://www.mutineermagazine.com/blog/2010/11/absinthe-and-its-silver-tongued-marketers-thujones-role-in-absinthe-sales/.
66. Baggott, Matthew. "Absinthe: Frequently Asked Questions and Some Attempted Answers." The Vaults of Erowid. http://www.erowid.org/chemicals/absinthe/absinthe_faq.shtml.
67. "Absinthe Reference." Fee Verte. http://www.feeverte.net/faq-absinthe.html.
68. Black, Annetta, Mark Casey, and Rachel. "Site of 'The Absinthe Murders.'" Atlas Obscura. http://www.atlasobscura.com/places/site-absinthe-murders.
69. "The Prohibition of Absinthe." Green Devil. http://www.greendevil.com/absinthe_legal.html.
70. Dolittle, Dunlap, Mitchell. "Food Inspection Decision 147 - The US Ban on Absinthe." The Wormwood Society. http://www.wormwoodsociety.org/index.php/history-articles/469-food-inspection-decision-147-the-us-ban-on-absinthe.

71. "Absinthe Reference." Fee Verte, op. cit.

## Chapter X: The Roaring Twenties and Prohibition

1. "Prohibition II." Newspeak Dictionary. http://www.newspeakdictionary.com/ct-prohibition.html.
2. Hobson, Richmond Pearson. *The Great Destroyer.* BiblioLife, 2009.
3. Ibid.
4. Ibid.
5. Ibid.
6. Musto, David F. "Opium, Cocaine and Marijuana in American History." *Scientific American*, 1991.
7. "Timeline of Events in the History of Drugs." Black Poppy Mag. http://blackpoppymag.wordpress.com/timeline-of-events-in-the-history-of-drugs/.
8. Hanson, David J. "National Prohibition of Alcohol in the U.S." Alcohol Problems and Solutions, http://www2.potsdam.edu/alcohol/Controversies/1091124904.html#.U3VBUfldU1M.
9. Ibid.
10. Moore, L.J. "Historical Interpretation of the 1920s Klan: The Traditional View and the Popular Revision." *Journal of Social History*, 1990.
11. Ibid.
12. Hobson, op. cit.
13. McCann, Dennis. "Anti-German Sentiment Aided Alcohol Prohibition's Approval." *Milwaukee Journal*, 1998.
14. Ibid.
15. Keillor, Garrison. *In Search of Lake Wobegon.* Studio, 2001.
16. "The Eighteenth Amendment." Alcohol Problems and Solutions. http://www2.potsdam.edu/hansondj/Controversies/The-Eighteenth-Amendment.html#.Utb2KtJdWqk.
17. Aaron, Paul and David Musto. *Temperance and Prohibition in America: A Historical Overview.* Washington, DC: National Academy Press, 1981.
18. Aaron and Musto, op. cit.
19. Webster, Daniel. "Daniel Webster quote - 'good intentions.'" Free Republic. http://www.freerepublic.com/focus/f-chat/2943047/posts.
20. Munsey, Cecil. "Paralysis In A Bottle: The `Jake Walk Story.'" Bottles and Extras, 2007.
21. "Anti-Saloon League of America Yearbook." Anti-Saloon League of America. Westerville, Ohio: *American Issue Press,* 1920, p. 8. Cited by Mulford, Harold A. *Alcohol and Alcoholism in Iowa*, 1965. Iowa City, IA: University of Iowa, 1965, p. 9.
22. Hanson, op. cit.
23. Reinarman, Craig.. *The Dutch Example Shows that Liberal Drug Laws can be Beneficial.* Greenhaven Press, 2000.
24. Aaron and Musto, op. cit.
25. Feldman, Herman. *Prohibition: Its Economic and Industrial Aspects.* New York: D. Appleton and Company, 1928.
26. "Did Alcohol Use Decrease During Alcohol Prohibition?" Schaffer Library of Drug Policy. http://druglibrary.org/prohibitionresults1.htm.
27. Singer, Allen J. *Stepping Out in Cincinnati, Queen City Entertainment, 1900-1960.* Arcadia Publishing, 2012.
28. Sinclair, Andrew. Prohibition: The Era of Excess. Little, Brown & Co., 1962.
29. Ibid.
30. Carter, Everett. *Cultural History Written with Lightning: The Significance of The Birth of a Nation.* Lexington,Kentucky: University of Kentucky Press, 1983.
31. Rose , Mrs. S. E.F. *The Ku Klux Klan or The Invisible Empire.* CreateSpace Independent Publishing Platform, 2012.
32. Totaro, Donato. "Birth of a Nation: Viewed Today." *Off Screen*, February 29, 2004.
33. Rose, op. cit.
34. D'Orso, Michael. *Like Judgment Day: The Ruin and Redemption of a Town Called Rosewood.* Grosset, 1996.
35. Zinn, Howard. A People's History of the United States: 1492 to Present. Harper Perennial Modern Classics, 2005.
36. Avrich, Paul. *Sacco and Vanzetti: The Anarchist Background.* Princeton University Press, 1991.
37. Ibid.
38. Ibid.

39. "Ineffective DARE Program Remains Popular." Alcohol Problems and Solutions, http://www2.potsdam.edu/alcohol/Controversies/20070705122620.html#.U3ZShvldU1M.
40. "National Origins Act of 1924." *Office of the Historian, Bureau of Public Affairs.*
41. Bernstein, Nina. "100 Years in the Back Door, Out the Front." *The New York Times*, 2006.
42. Ibid.
43. Bryne, Julie. "Roman Catholics and the American Mainstream in the Twentieth Century." *National Humanities Center*, 2000.
44. Ibid.
45. "National Prohibition of Alcohol in the U.S." Alcohol Problems and Solutions. http://www2.potsdam.edu/hansondj/Controversies/1091124904_6.html#.Utb7G9JdWqk.
46. Ibid.
47. Blackman, Shane. "Drug Prohibition & the Assassin of Youth," in *Chilling Out: The Cultural Politics of Substance Consumption, Youth and Drug Policy*. McGraw-Hill, 2004.
48. Avrich, op. cit.
49. Ibid.
50. Ibid.
51. "The Language of The Jazz Age - 1920s Slang." 1920s and 20s Fashion and Music.com. http://www.1920s-fashion-and-music.com/1920s-slang.html#ixzz2qVIWxd2u
52. Evans, Keith. "The Longest War." 2000.
53. Thornton, Mark. *The Economics of Prohibition*. Ludwig Von Mises Institute, 2007.
54. Popik, Barry. "Give This Little Girl a Big Hand!" Barrypopik.com.
55. Ibid.
56. Ibid.
57. Berman, Jay S. *Prophets Without Honor: The Wickersham Commission and the Development of American Law Enforcement*. Michigan State University, 1973.
58. Ibid.
59. "Weed Quotes." Marijuana Games, http://marijuanagames.org/weed-quotes/.
60. Blackman, op. cit.
61. Hanson, op. cit.
62. Ibid.
63. Ibid.
64. Abel, E. L. Marihuana: *The First Twelve Thousand Years*. Springer, 1980.
65. "Marijuana Smoking in Panama." In *The Military Surgeon*. Schaffer Library of Drug Policy, 1933.
66. Ibid.

## Chapter XI: 1915-1937: Marijuana Tax Act

1. Robinson, Rowan. *The Great Book of Hemp*. Park Street Press, 1995.
2. Lyster, Dewey and Jason Merrill. "Hemp Hurds As Paper Making Material." *Bulletin 404, U.S. Dept. of Agriculture*, 1916.
3. Ibid.
4. "Billion-Dollar Crop." *Popular Mechanics*, 1938.
5. "U.S. Agricultural Indexes." 1916 through 1982.
6. Lyster and Merrill, op. cit.
7. "Schlichten Papers." Innvista, 2013. http://www.innvista.com/health/foods/hemp/schlichten-papers/
8. Ibid.
9. Robinson, op. cit.
10. "E.W. Scripps Papers, 1868-1926." Ohio University Library, 2009. http://www.library.ohiou.edu/archives/mss/mss117.html
11. Ibid.
12. "Schlichten Papers," op. cit.
13. Ibid.
14. Ibid.
15. "Henry Ford: 1863-1947." Hempcar TransAmerica. http://www.hempcar.org/ford.shtml
16. "A History of Biofuels: A History of the Diesel Engine." *Yakayo Biofuels.*

17. Ibid.
18. "Henry Ford: 1863-1947," op. cit.
19. "Billion Dollar Crop," op. cit.
20. "Henry Ford: 1863-1947," op. cit.
21. "A History of Biofuels: A History of the Diesel Engine," op. cit.
22. Robinson, op. cit.
23. "Schlichten Papers," op. cit.
24. Herer, Jack. *The Emperor Wears No Clothes*. AH HA Publishing, 2010.
25. Musto, David F. "The History of the Marihuana Tax Act of 1937." *Archives of General Psychiatry*, 1972.
26. Ibid.
27. Ibid.
28. Webb, Clifton. *Smokin' Reefers*. Flying Colors, 1932.
29. Musto, op. cit.
30. "Marihuana." *Journal of Criminal Law and Criminology*, 1932.
31. "Harrison Narcotics Tax Act, 1914." *Drug Reform Coordination Network*.
32. McWilliams, op. cit.
33. Abel, Ernest L. *Marijuana - The First Twelve Thousand Years*. Schaffer Library of Drug Policy, 1980.
34. Ibid.
35. Robinson, op. cit.
36. McWilliams, John C. *The Protectors: Harry J. Anslinger and the Federal Bureau of Narcotics, 1930-62*. University of Delaware Print, 1990.
37. Lee, Martin A., *Smoke Signals: A Social History of Marijuana - Medical, Recreational, and Scientific*. Scribner, 2012. page 77
38. Booth, Martin, Cannabis: A History, Picador, 2003. p. 250
39. Whitebread, Charles II. *The Marijuana Conviction*. University of Virginia Press, 1974.
40. Ibid.
41. Ibid.
42. Abel, op. cit.
43. McWilliams, op. cit.
44. Herer, op. cit.
45. Guither, Pete. "Why Is Marijuana Illegal?" Drug War Rant, http://www.drugwarrant.com/articles/why-is-marijuana-illegal/.
46. Nelson, Robert A. *Hemp & Health*. Rex Research, 1999, http://www.rexresearch.com/hhusb/hmphlth.htm.
47. Herer, op. cit.
48. Abel, op. cit.
49. Sheldon, Randall G."Local View: Reefer Madness Strikes Again." *Las Vegas Mercury*, October 31, 2002. http://cannabisnews.com/news/14/thread14624.shtml.
50. Lee, Green. "The Demonized Seed." *Los Angeles Times*, January 18, 2004
51. Herer, op. cit.
52. Abel, op. cit.
53. Woodward, William. In "Taxation of Marihuana." Testimony. Committee on Ways and Means, May 4, 1937, http://www.druglibrary.org/schaffer/hemp/taxact/woodward.htm.
54. Ibid.
55. Aldrich, Michael. "History of Marijuana Tax Act." O'Shaughnessy's.
56. Woodward, op. cit.
57. Ibid.
58. Whitebread, op. cit.
59. Woodward, op. cit.
60. Ibid.
61. Ibid.
62. Ibid.
63. McWhirter, Cameon and Bill Rankin. *Atlanta Journal and Constitution*, 2003.
64. "Billion Dollar Crop," op. cit.

65. Ibid.
66. Herer, op. cit.
67. Ibid.
68. Fishbein, Morris and Queine, M. "Migraine Associated with Menstruation." *JAMA*, 1942.
69. Mikuriya, Tod H. *Marijuana Medical Papers: 1839-1972*. Symposium Publishing, 2007.
70. Sloman, Larry. *Reefer Madness: The History of Marijuana in America.* Grove Press, 1979.
71. Lindsmith, *Alfred. The Addict and the Law.* Indiana U. Press, 1965.
72. Whitebread, op. cit.
73. Woodward, op. cit.
74. Ibid.
75. Ibid.
76. Russo, Ethan, Mary Lynn Mathre, Al Bryne, Robert Velin, Paul J. Back, Juan Sanchez-Ramos, and Kristin A. Kirlin. "Chronic Cannabis Use in the Compassionate Investigational New Drug Program: An Examination of Benefits and Adverse Effects of Legal Clinical Cannabis." *Journal of Cannabis Therapeutics*, 2002, no. 2.
77. Abel, op. cit.
78. J.F. Sn. ER, Colonel, M.C. "Marijuana Smoking in Panama." *The Military Surgeon*, 1933.
79. Woodward, op. cit.
80. "What We Do." *U.S. Food and Drug Administration*, 2013.
81. "Ancient Remedies Being Tried Once Again." *Santa Barbara News Press*, 2007.
82. Buenz, Eric J. *Searching Historical Herbal Texts for Potential New Drugs.* BMJ Publishing Group, 2006.

## Chapter XII: 1939-1959: WW II, Post-War Changes and the Beatst

1. Baker, Robert. "A Brief History of the Blues." *The Blue Highway*, 1995.
2. Duncan, John. "Neurological Morbidity and the Behavioral Correlates of Methamphetamine Abuse." *University of Oklahoma*, http://www.ou.edu/cls/online/lstd4753/pdf/neurological_morbidity.pdf. Casey, Elaine. "History of Drug Use and Drug Users in the United States." *Schaffer Library of Drug Policy*, November 1978, http://www.druglibrary.org/schaffer/history/casey1.htm.
3. Lomax, Alan. *The Land Where the Blues Began.* Pantheon Books, 1993.
4. Pareles, Jon & Romanowski, Patricia. *The Rolling Stone Encyclopedia of Rock and Roll.* Rolling Stone Press, 1983.
5. Tanner, Paul & Gerow, Maurice. *A Study of Jazz* William C. Brown Publishers, 1984.
6. Tiber, Elliott. "The Times Herald Record." Woodstock Commemorative Edition, 1994.
7. Greene, Michael J. "California Hemp History." CDS Consulting, http://www.votehemp.com/PDF/Hemp_in_California_5-29-10.pdf.
8. "Hemp Acreage is Quadrupled in Wisconsin." *Chicago Tribune*, August 4, 1943.
9. Ibid.
10. Frank, Mel. *The Marijuana Grower's Guide.* Red Eye Press, 1993.
11. Nelson, Robert A. "Hemp Husbandry." Rex Research, 2000, http://www.rexresearch.com/hhusb/hh11stcr.htm.
12. "Italian American History." The Quagliata Family Genealogy Project, http://quagliatagenealogy.com/iahistory.html.
13. Peppers, John G. "Violence Against Italians in the US." Electrical Audio, July 10, 2007.
14. Alvarez, Luis. *The Power of the Zoot: Youth Culture and Resistance during World War II.* Berkeley: University of California Press, 2008.
15. Ibid.
16. Ibid.
17. "Mrs. Roosevelt Blindly Stirs Race Discord." *Los Angeles Times*, 1943.
18. Alvarez, op. cit.
19. Ibid.
20. Phalen, J. M. Col. "The Marijuana Bugaboo." *Military Surgeon*, 1943.
21. McWilliams, John C. *The Protectors: Harry J. Anslinger and the Federal Bureau of Narcotics, 1930-62.* University of Delaware Print, 1990.
22. Mises, Ludwig V. *Human Action: A Treatise on Economics.* 1949.
23. Kerouac, Jack. *On the Road.* Penguin Books, 1999.

24. Chambers, Jack. "Milestones: The Music and the Times of Miles Davis." 1998.
25. Gordon, Dexter & Gray, Wendell. *The Hunt.*
26. Baker, op. cit.
27. Huxley, Aldous. *The Doors of Perception.* 1954.
28. "Max Boot - Publications." *Council of Foreign Relations.*
29. "Robert Mitch Arrested with Two Actresses in Marijuana Raid." *St. Petersburg Time*s, September 2, 1948.
30. "Robert Mitchum's Canyon Drug Bust - 1948." L.A. Stories, http://www.seastwood.com/backup310/mitchumbust.htm.
31. Young, Paul. *L.A. Exposed: Strange Myths and Curious Legends in the City of Angels.* St. Martin's Griffin, 2002.
32. "Mitchum Images." Sprintmail.com.
33. Siegel, Dick. "The Big Dope Bust of 1948 That Sent Robert Mitchum to Jail." *National Enquirer*, April 6, 2014.
34. "Mitchum Images," op. cit.

## Chapter XIII: The Sixties: A Culture War Bubbles to the Surface

1. Hulse, Carl. "Lott's Praise for Thurmond Echoed His Words of 1980." *The New York Times*, December 11, 2002, http://www.nytimes.com/2002/12/11/us/lott-s-praise-for-thurmond-echoed-his-words-of-1980.html.
2. Elders, Joycelyn. "Myths About Medical Marujuana." *The Providence Journal.*
3. Robinson, Rowan. *The Great Book of Hemp.* Park Street Press, 1995.
4. Baker, Robert M. "A Brief History of the Blues." The Blue Highway. http://thebluehighway.com/blues/history.html.
5. George-Warren, Holly, Patricia Romanowski and Jon Pareles. *The Rolling Stone Encyclopedia of Rock & Roll.* Touchstone, 2001.
6. Tanner, Paul and Maurice Gerow. *A Study of Jazz.* William C. Brown Publishers, 1973.
7. Tiber, Elliot. "How Woodstock Happened." In *The Times Herald Record.* 1994.
8. "50 Moments That Changed the History of Rock and Roll." *Rolling Stone,* June 24, 2004, http://www.rollingstone.com/music/news/50-moments-that-changed-rock-and-roll-otis-and-jimi-burn-it-up-20040624.
9. Tiber, op. cit.
10. "50 Moments That Changed the History of Rock and Roll," op. cit.
11. Tiber, op. cit.
12. George-Warren et al., op. cit.
13. Smith, Dinitia. "Kurt Vonnegut, Novelist Who Caught the Imagination of His Age, Is Dead at 84." *The New York Times,* April 12, 2007, http://www.nytimes.com/2007/04/12/books/12vonnegut.html?pagewanted=all.
14. Vonnegut, Kurt. *Slaughterhouse-Five.* Dell Publishing, 1991.
15. Vonnegut, Kurt. *Fates Worse Than Death.* Berkley Trade, 1992.
16. Shelton, Gilbert. *The Fabulous Furry Freak Brothers Omnibus.* Knockabout Comics, 2008.
17. Estren, Mark. *A History of Underground Comics.* Ronin Publishing, 1993.
18. Goldman, Albert. "The Trial of Lenny Bruce." *The New Republic*, September 12, 1964.
19. Ibid.
20. "Bruce's Trial." *Newsweek,* July 20, 1964.
21. Kifner, John. "No Joke! 37 Years After Death Lenny Bruce Receives Pardon." *The New York Times,* December 24, 2003, http://www.nytimes.com/2003/12/24/nyregion/no-joke-37-years-after-death-lenny-bruce-receives-pardon.html.
22. Wolfe, Tom. *The Electric Kool-Aid Acid Test.* Picador Publishing, 2008.
23. Spitz, Bob. *The Beatles: The Biography.* Back Bay Books, 2006.
24. Wasson, Gordon R., Albert Hofmann, Carl A. P. Ruck, Huston Smith, and Peter Webster. *The Road to Eleusis: Unveiling the Secret of the Mysteries.* North Atlantic Books, 2008.
25. Stafford, Peter. *Psychedelics Encyclopedia.* Ronin Publishing, 1993.
26. Swift, Dusty. *A Different Drum: A Story about Coming of Age in the Sixties and Having to Choose Between Peace and War.* Bloomington: iUniverse Publishing, 2011.
27. Wolfe, op. cit.
28. Smith, Adam. *Powers of Mind.* New York: Ballantine Books, 1975.

29. Wasson, et. al., op. cit.
30. Wasson, et. al., op.  cit.
31. Adam Smith, op. cit.
32. Adam Smith, op. cit.
33. Casey, Elaine. "History of Drug Use and Drug Users in the United States." In *Facts About Drug Abuse*, 1978.
34. Adam Smith, op. cit.
35. Casey, op. cit.
36. Casey, op. cit.
37. Spitz, op. cit.
38. Adam Smith, op. cit.
39. Adam Smith, op. cit.
40. Wolfe, op. cit.
41. Wolfe, op. cit.
42. Robinson, op. cit.
43. Potter, Robert. "Bob Potter's Speech at the Ceremony Dedicating the Monument to the Worldwide Peace Movement During the Vietnam War era in Isla Vista's Perfect Park." Speech, Isla Vista, CA, June 10, 2003. http://www.islavistahistory.com/downloads/BobPotterSpeech.pdf.
44. Robinson, op. cit.
45. Gritz, Bo. "The CIA and Opium." Speech, American Liberty Lunch Club. http://www.druglibrary.org/schaffer/Misc/ciaopium.htm.
46. Gritz, op. cit.
47. Gritz, op. cit.
48. Pine, Art. "Eugene McCarthy; Candidacy Inspired Antiwar Movement." *Los Angeles Times*, December 11, 2005, http://articles.latimes.com/2005/dec/11/nation/na-mccarthy11.
49. Ibid.
50. Smith, David E. and Richard B. Seymour. "Addiction Medicine and the Free Clinic Movement." *Journal of Psychoactive Drugs* 29, no. 2 (1997.: 155-160.
51. Ibid.
52. Ibid.
53. Ibid.
54. Hanson,, David. "Librium." *Chemical & Engineering News.*
55. Ibid.
56. Califano, Joseph A. "High Society: How Substance Abuse Ravages America and What to Do About it." The *New England Journal of Medicine* 359 (2008.: 1413-1414.
57. Ibid.
58. Ibid.
59. Hanson, op. cit.
60. Ibid.
61. Browne, Jackson. "The Pretender." In *The Pretender*, 1976.
62. Califano, op. cit.

# About the Author

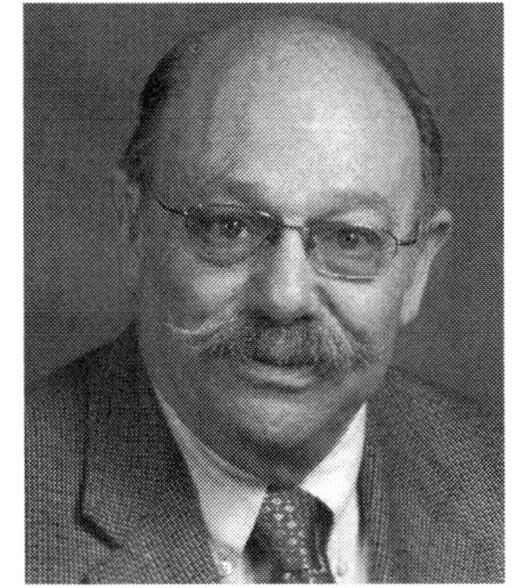

David Bearman received his M.D. from the University of Washington School of Medicine. He has served at all levels of government including the U.S. Public Health Service, Director of Health Services at San Diego State University, Health Officer and Director Sutter County Health Department and Medical Director and Director of Medical Services for the Santa Barbara Regional Health Authority (now CenCal).

Dr. Bearman has a long and illustrative career in the field of drug abuse treatment and prevention. He was prominent in the community clinic movement, having started the third Free Clinic in the country in Seattle, then directing the Haight Ashbury Drug Treatment Program, and in 1970 founding the Isla Vista Medical Clinic. He was Medical Director of Santa Barbara County Methadone Maintenance Clinic and Ventura County Opiate Detox Program, and Zona Seca, an outpatient drug treatment program..

He is a leader in the field of cannabinoid medicine and is a co-founder of the American Academy of Cannabinoid Medicine, on the board of Americans for Safe Access and the Advisory Board for Patients Out of Time. The Wall Street Journal Health Blog declared him their Doctor of the Day.
He has taught courses on the physiology and history of substance use and abuse at UCSF, UCSB, and SDSU, been a consultant to Hoffman LaRoche, NIDA and the National PTA, made numerous professional presentations and consulted widely and has been an expert witness in over 400 civil, criminal, and family court cases. Currently he is Zona Seca's Medical Consultant, maintains a private practice, as well as frequently serving as an expert witness.

Dr. Bearman developed an early interest in medicine when working in his father's pharmacy in Rice Lake, Wisconsin as a high school and college student. He graduated from the University of Wisconsin in 1963 with a degree in Psychology and in 1967 obtained his M.D. degree from the University of Washington School of Medicine. He now maintains a private practice as a specialist in pain management and cannabinoid medicine in Goleta, California where lives with his wife, Lily (a career counselor). They have two children, Samantha and Benjamin.

Made in the USA
San Bernardino, CA
29 July 2016

# SOCIAL PROBLEMS
## and the quality of life

Fifteenth Edition

**Robert H. Lauer**
*Alliant International University*

**Jeanette C. Lauer**
*Alliant International University*

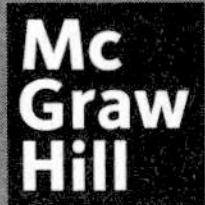

To Jon, Kathy, Julie, Donna, Jeffrey, Kate, Jeff, Nina, Krista, Benjamin, David, John Robert, Addie, and Robbie.

". . . the greatest of these is love."

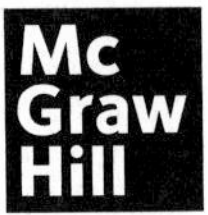


SOCIAL PROBLEMS AND THE QUALITY OF LIFE, FIFTEENTH EDITION

Published by McGraw Hill LLC, 1325 Avenue of the Americas, New York, NY 10019. 

This book is printed on acid-free paper.

1 2 3 4 5 6 7 8 9 LWI 27 26 25 24 23 22

ISBN 978-1-264-30036-5 (bound edition)
MHID 1-264-30036-0 (bound edition)
ISBN 978-1-265-78185-9 (loose-leaf edition)
MHID 1-265-78185-0 (loose-leaf edition)

Portfolio Manager: *Sarah Remington*
Product Developer: *Elisa Odoardi*
Marketing Manager: *Rasheiter Calhoun*
Content Project Managers: *Melissa M. Leick and Katie Reuter*
Buyer: *Laura Fuller*
Content Licensing Specialist: *Shawntel Schmitt*
Cover Image: *sujin Jetkasettakorn/rufous/123RF*
Compositor: *MPS Limited*



**Library of Congress Cataloging-in-Publication Data**

Names: Lauer, Robert H., author. | Lauer, Jeanette C., author.
Title: Social problems and the quality of life / Robert H. Lauer, Jeanette C. Lauer.
Description: Fifteenth edition. | New York, NY : McGraw Hill Education, [2023] | Includes bibliographical references and index.
Identifiers: LCCN 2021019786 (print) | LCCN 2021019787 (ebook) | ISBN 9781264300365 (paperback) | ISBN 9781265781859 (looseleaf) | ISBN 9781265780807 (ebook)
Subjects: LCSH: United States–Social conditions. | Quality of life–United States. | Social problems–United States.
Classification: LCC HN57 .L39 2023 (print) | LCC HN57 (ebook) | DDC 306.0973–dc23
LC record available at https://lccn.loc.gov/2021019786
LC ebook record available at https://lccn.loc.gov/2021019787



mheducation.com/highered

# brief contents

# contents

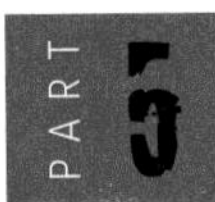

## PART 5 Global Social Problems 475

### 14 War and Terrorism 476



### 15 The Environment 512

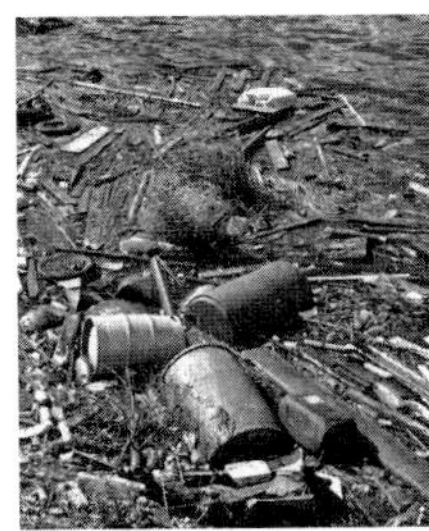

Steve Allen/Brand X Picture/ Alamy Stock Photo

# list of figures

# list of tables

# preface

People everywhere want to maximize the quality of their lives. There is widespread agreement that a high quality of life requires such things as a good education, freedom from fear of crime, good housing, meaningful work, and good health. A high quality of life, then, can only be attained if people deal with the social problems that detract from that quality. As we point out in the first chapter of this text, a social problem is, by definition, a condition or pattern of behavior that is incompatible with people's desired quality of life.

To deal with a problem, you must understand it—how it affects one's quality of life, what causes it, what tends to maintain it. Sociologists have used three theoretical perspectives to answer these questions in order to analyze and deal with social problems. We discuss the three major perspectives in Chapter 1 and show how we use elements from each to analyze individual problems and talk about how the problem can be attacked.

We do not mean to give the impression here that either understanding a problem or attacking it is a simple matter. Even experts disagree on such things. The factors that combine to cause and perpetuate any particular problem are many and complex. We have seen students feel overwhelmed as they study these factors. As one said: "I don't see how society can ever deal with some of these problems. The more I understand about what causes them, the more hopeless I feel."

It is interesting to note, therefore, that some problems are less serious than they were when this book was in its first edition. Among other things, poverty among the aged has declined, many crime rates have dropped, divorce rates have declined, the cold war and the accompanying arms race between the superpowers have come to an end, and air and water pollution levels have decreased significantly. Other problems, however, are still as serious—or even more so. For instance, addictions continue to ruin lives and traumatize families; domestic and international terrorism are of the highest concern to citizens and the government; war remains a vexing problem; white-collar crime is more widespread and more of a threat to the economy than previously recognized; health problems afflict great numbers of people, many of whom have no health insurance; racial minorities have lost some of the gains made in previous years; poverty has increased among some groups; increasing numbers of single parents mean increasing problems for children; equitable opportunities remain elusive for homosexuals; and the threats posed by such things as global warming and toxic wastes are more serious than previously thought. These advances and setbacks are all discussed in the text.

## Changes in the Fifteenth Edition

A social problem is a product of social definition. That is, something becomes a problem, and becomes a more or less serious problem, as it is so defined by the people of a society. People's definitions of problems and the problems themselves continually change.

Each new edition of a social problems text, therefore, strives to capture the current status of an ever-changing phenomenon. To achieve this goal, we have updated all materials in this edition with hundreds of new references as well as the most recent data available from the government and other sources.

There are changing concerns among the public as well as changing emphases among researchers. To reflect current interests and concerns more adequately, we have included new or expanded materials on such topics as white-collar crime, domestic terrorism, human trafficking, the "Me Too" movement, the Black Lives Matter movement, student loans, the COVID-19 pandemic, and the Flint, Michigan, drinking water crisis.

## Organization

We have divided the book into 5 parts and 15 chapters. Part 1 introduces students to social problems. Chapter 1 discusses the various tools needed, including the difference between social problems and personal problems, sociological theories and methods, and fallacious ways of thinking.

In Part 2, we look at a cluster of problems that involve behavior that deviates from social norms. Chapters 2 through 5 cover the problems of alcohol and other drugs, crime and delinquency, violence (including rape), and sexual deviance (prostitution and pornography).

Part 3 examines problems that involve social inequality. Poverty (Chapter 6) is inequality in income and wealth. Gender and sexual orientation comprise another area of inequality (Chapter 7), as women and homosexuals strive to gain equal rights. Racial and ethnic inequality (Chapter 8) include the multiple ways in which there is disparity in valued things between the various racial and ethnic groups in the nation.

Part 4 focuses on problems of social institutions. Chapters 9 through 13 cover the institutions of government and politics, work and the economy, education, family, and health care. These institutions are factors in other kinds of social problems but are also problematic in themselves.

Finally, Part 5 covers two global social problems: war and terrorism (Chapter 14) and the environment (Chapter 15). These problems pose a threat to civilization itself and cannot be understood apart from their global context.

## Learning Aids

We use a variety of learning aids to facilitate understanding of the materials:

- Chapter-opening vignettes personalize the various problems. They make each problem not just a set of facts, but a social reality that disrupts and diminishes the quality of people's lives in concrete, understandable ways.
- Chapter objectives and marginal key terms keep students on track as they work through the chapters.
- Global Comparison boxes add dimension to students' understanding of social problems by seeing how they work out in another nation or nations.

- Dealing with the problems is as important as knowing what causes them. Each chapter, therefore, contains a section, called Solutions: Public Policy and Private Action, that suggests ways to ameliorate each problem. We have found that most students are like the one quoted near the beginning of this preface—they don't simply want to know about problems; they also want to know what can be done to address those problems. We do not claim that the suggestions will eliminate the problems. But they do demonstrate that problems have solutions, and the solutions are always, to some extent, up to each individual.
- Marginal icons identify places in the text where we show how people use the fallacies of thinking discussed in Chapter 1 to draw erroneous conclusions about social problems.
- End-of-chapter summaries, key terms lists, study questions, and Internet resources and exercises provide students with ample review, study materials, and self-learning projects.

## Supplements

As a full-service publisher of quality educational products, McGraw Hill does much more than sell textbooks. The company creates and publishes an extensive array of print and digital supplements for students and instructors. This edition of *Social Problems* is accompanied by a set of comprehensive supplements.

### For the Student

- McGraw Hill Connect® provides students with an eBook, personalized study path, and assignments that help them conceptualize what they learn through application and critical thinking. Access this title at https://connect.mheducation.com.

### For the Instructor

The fifteenth edition of *Social Problems and the Quality of Life* is now available online with Connect, McGraw Hill Education's integrated assignment and assessment platform. Connect also offers SmartBook® 2.0 for the new edition, which is the first adaptive reading experience proven to improve grades and help students study more effectively. All of the title's website and ancillary content is also available through Connect, including:

- Instructor's Manual/Testbank—chapter outlines, key terms, overviews, lecture notes, discussion questions, a complete testbank, and more.
- PowerPoint Slides—complete, chapter-by-chapter slide shows featuring text, tables, and visuals.
- Create—a unique database publishing system that allows instructors to create their own custom text from material in *Social Problems* or elsewhere and deliver that text to students electronically as an e-book or in print format via the bookstore.

## Remote Proctoring & Browser-Locking Capabilities

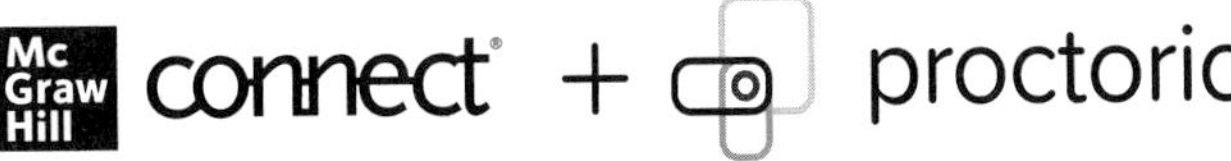


New remote proctoring and browser-locking capabilities, hosted by Proctorio within Connect, provide control of the assessment environment by enabling security options and verifying the identity of the student.

Seamlessly integrated within Connect, these services allow instructors to control students' assessment experience by restricting browser activity, recording students' activity, and verifying students are doing their own work.

Instant and detailed reporting gives instructors an at-a-glance view of potential academic integrity concerns, thereby avoiding personal bias and supporting evidence-based claims.

## Writing Assignment

Available within McGraw Hill Connect® and McGraw Hill Connect® Master, the Writing Assignment tool delivers a learning experience to help students improve their written communication skills and conceptual understanding. As an instructor you can assign, monitor, grade, and provide feedback on writing more efficiently and effectively.

## Acknowledgments

Many people are important in producing a book. The staff at McGraw Hill have been most helpful and supportive. Time and again, we are impressed with the quality of work done by the various editors with whom we worked. We appreciate each of them, and particularly Sameer Jena, who worked with us on this latest edition. We would also like to thank the academic reviewers who are listed on page xviii; their suggestions have, we believe, enhanced this book.

**Robert H. Lauer**

**Jeanette C. Lauer**

# **Students:** Get Learning that Fits You

## Effective tools for efficient studying

Connect is designed to help you be more productive with simple, flexible, intuitive tools that maximize your study time and meet your individual learning needs. Get learning that works for you with Connect.

## Study anytime, anywhere

Download the free ReadAnywhere app and access your online eBook, SmartBook 2.0, or Adaptive Learning Assignments when it's convenient, even if you're offline. And since the app automatically syncs with your Connect account, all of your work is available every time you open it. Find out more at **www.mheducation.com/readanywhere**

***"I really liked this app—it made it easy to study when you don't have your text-book in front of you."***

- Jordan Cunningham,
Eastern Washington University

Calendar: owattaphotos/Getty Images

## Everything you need in one place

Your Connect course has everything you need—whether reading on your digital eBook or completing assignments for class, Connect makes it easy to get your work done.

## Learning for everyone

McGraw Hill works directly with Accessibility Services Departments and faculty to meet the learning needs of all students. Please contact your Accessibility Services Office and ask them to email accessibility@mheducation.com, or visit **www.mheducation.com/about/accessibility** for more information.

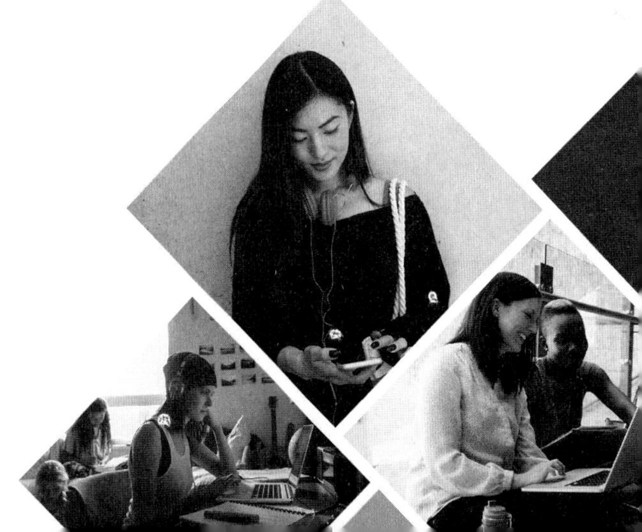

Top: Jenner Images/Getty Images, Left: Hero Images/Getty Images, Right: Hero Images/Getty Images

# reviewer acknowledgments

Cezara Crisan
*Purdue University Northwest*

F. Kurt Cylke
*SUNY Geneseo*

Lutz Kaelber
*University of Vermont*

Edward Avery-Natale
*Mercer County Community College*

Stacy Sanders
*Southeast Technical College*

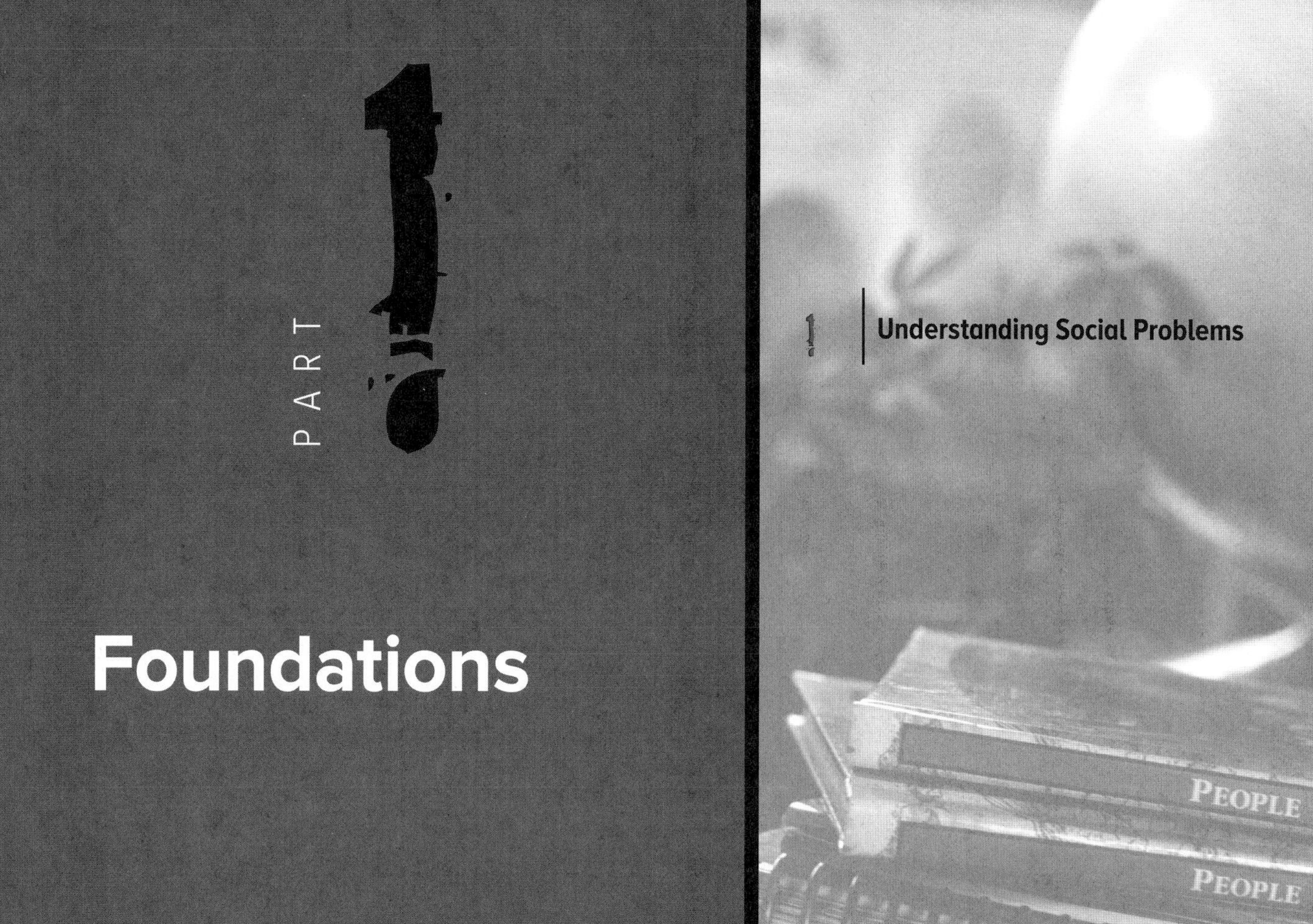

Dynamic Graphics/JupiterImages

A Chinese philosopher remarked that one should not attempt to open clams with a crowbar. In other words, any task demands the proper tools. Part 1 of this book is about the proper tools for the study of social problems. What kind of perspective should you bring to the study? What kind of information do you need, and what are the proper ways to gather it? Unless you answer such questions appropriately, you cannot answer the vexing question of how to deal with social problems. This part, then, prepares you to delve into particular problems. It shows you how to use the proper tools to open the "clams."

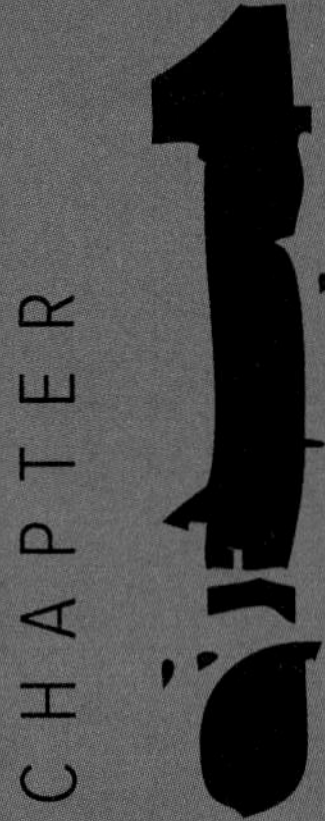

CHAPTER 1

# Understanding Social Problems

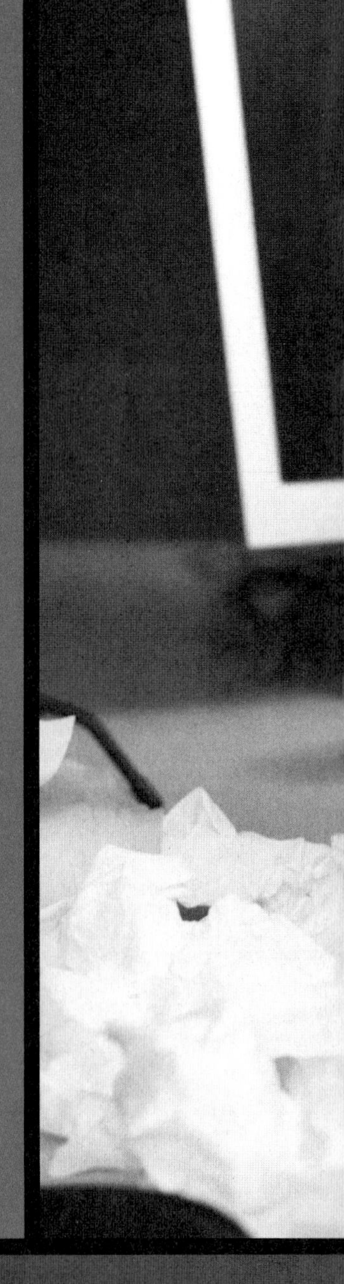

OBJECTIVES

1. Explain the difference between personal and social problems.
2. Understand the model used to explain social problems.
3. Discuss the fallacies of thinking, including how they have been used to explain social problems.
4. Explain the meaning of social research.
5. Give examples of different kinds of social research and describe how they have been used to study social problems.

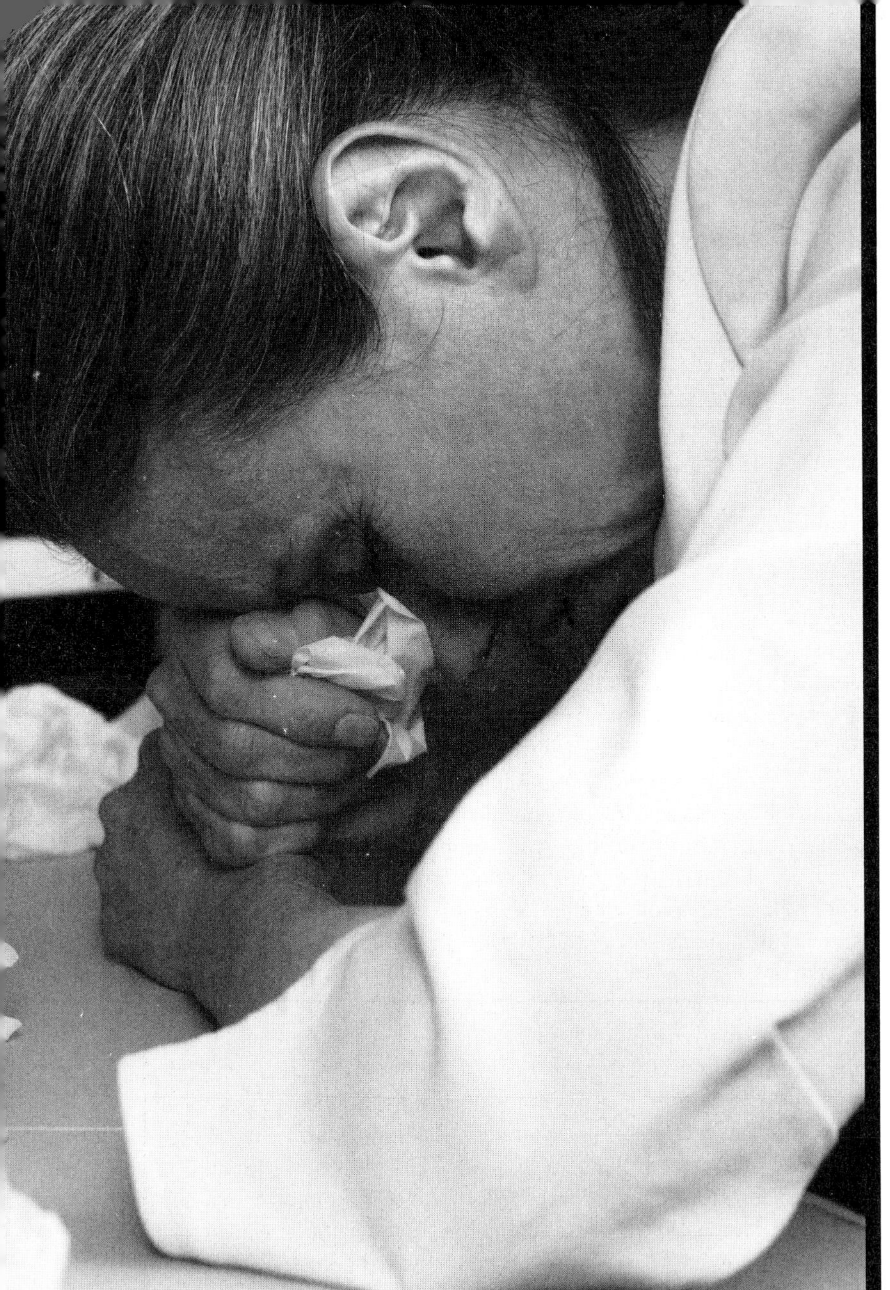

Beathan/Fuse/Getty Images

### "Why Is It My Fault?"

Marie, her husband Jim, and their two children had a good life until he lost his job. Stress built up, their marriage fell apart, and he moved to another state. Marie's life has never been the same:

*I've never gotten any financial help from Jim since we were divorced. I went to work. It was really hard, raising two kids by myself and working full-time. But we were making it. And I enjoyed working—having people tell me I was doing a good job. Then the company downsized and I was laid off. It's been awful since then.*

*For the first time in my life, I know what it's like to be poor. I know what it's like to try to get help from the government. And you know one of the worst things? It's feeling ashamed. It's feeling like for some reason it's my fault, like there's something I could have done to avoid it. Why is this my fault? I keep telling myself I shouldn't feel that way, but I can't help it.*

## Introduction

Who is at fault if you are poor? Are you responsible because you are lazy and unwilling to work or because you are a spendthrift and refuse to properly manage your finances? If so, you have a personal problem. Or are there other factors such as the state of the economy that are responsible for your situation? If so, you are caught up in a social problem. Later in this chapter we define social problems precisely. As a preliminary definition, however, think of social problems as behaviors or conditions that are caused by factors external to individuals and that detract from the quality of life.

Actually, "we are all part of some social problem" (Lopata 1984:249). In fact, we are all part of the biggest social problem of all—the race to save the planet (Brown 2000; Mezey 2020). These assertions will become increasingly clear in subsequent chapters. In addition, many individuals are wrestling with several problems at once. For example, the stress of poverty may lead to health problems, both mental and physical. If the impoverished individual is a woman or a minority, the stress may be intensified. The individual also may have to deal with unemployment or underemployment, poor performance at school by a child, and the threat of victimization by criminals. Indeed, social workers deal with families who are coping simultaneously with the majority of problems discussed in this book.

But what exactly is a social problem? How do sociologists decide what is or isn't a social problem? And once you identify something as a social problem, how do you go about analyzing it so that you can understand it? The first part of this chapter answers these questions. We begin by looking at the difference between personal problems and social problems because Americans tend to make all problems personal. That is, they believe that the problem is in some way *the fault of the individual who is struggling with it.* As you shall see, however, to say that a problem is social means that its causes, its consequences, and the way to deal with it all involve the social structure in which individuals live.

Social scientists do not arbitrarily decide which problems are social. Rather, they focus on those conditions that arise from contradictions in the society and that diminish people's quality of life. There is considerable consensus throughout the world on the kinds of things important to the quality of life, so the same kinds of problems tend to be identified in all societies.

Once a problem is identified, because large numbers of people agree that it detracts from their quality of life, we analyze and understand it by looking at the numerous social factors involved in creating and maintaining the problem. Only then can we realistically discuss ways to address the problem. The model we provide later in this chapter shows the kinds of factors that sociologists have found to be important.

Finally, we discuss two important tools of analysis for social problems—critical thinking skills and methods of research. These tools enable us to get valid information about the social factors involved in the problems—information that is crucial to making a realistic and useful analysis from which we can deduce effective ways to address the problem.

## Personal versus Social Problems

**personal problem**
a problem that can be explained in terms of the qualities of the individual

**social problem**
a condition or pattern of behavior that contradicts some other condition or pattern of behavior; is defined as incompatible with the desired quality of life; is caused, facilitated, or prolonged by social factors; involves intergroup conflict; and requires social action for resolution

We define a **personal problem** as one whose causes and solutions lie within the individual and his or her immediate environment. A **social problem,** on the other hand, is one whose causes and solutions lie outside the individual and the immediate environment. This distinction is not based on the individual's experience of suffering because a certain amount of suffering may occur in either case.

C. Wright Mills (1959:8–9) made a similar distinction, calling personal problems the "personal troubles of milieu" and social problems the "public issues of social structure." He offered many illustrations of the difference between the two. If one individual in a city is unemployed, that individual has a personal trouble. The person may have personality problems, may lack skills, or may have family difficulties that consume all of his or her energy. But if there are 100 million jobs in a society and 150 million people are available for work, this is a public issue. Even without personal problems, a third of the people will be unemployed. Such a problem cannot be resolved solely by dealing with individual personalities or motivations.

Similarly, a man and woman may have personal troubles in their marriage. They may agonize over their troubles and ultimately separate or divorce. If theirs is one of few marriages that experience such problems, you may conclude that they have personal problems and their marriage broke up because of some flaw in their personalities or in their relationship. But when the divorce rate soars and millions of families are broken up, you must look for causes and solutions beyond the personalities of individuals. The question is no longer "What is wrong with those people?" but "What has happened to the **institution** of marriage and the family in our society?"

**institution**
a collective pattern of dealing with a basic social function; typical institutions identified by sociologists are the government, economy, education, family and marriage, religion, and the media

Whether you define a problem as social or as personal is crucial. The distinction determines how you perceive the causes of the problem, the consequences of the problem, and *appropriate ways* to cope with the problem.

## The Causes of Problems

When asked why there is poverty in affluent America, a 31-year-old female bank teller said the poor themselves are to blame because most of them "are lazy and unreliable . . . and the little money they do make is spent on liquor and nonnecessities rather than for their economic advancement." This is a common approach, namely, that problems are personal. *The victim is blamed as both the source and the solution of the problem.*

Similarly, African Americans are said to have problems because they don't work to advance themselves. If you accept such an individualistic explanation, you are not likely to support government programs designed to raise the status of African Americans. National polls found that 81 percent of whites but only 45 percent of African Americans believe that the latter have as good a chance as whites to get any kind of job for which they are qualified (Polling Report 2020). When people believe that we already have equal opportunity, they will not support new laws or programs. This is well illustrated by the fact that a majority of African Americans (76 percent) but a minority of whites (48 percent) believe that the nation needs voting rights legislation to address the issue of state laws in recent years that tended to suppress the vote of minorities. Thus, the way problems are defined—as social or personal—has important consequences for identifying causes. In turn, the kind of causes identified affects the way problems are handled.

A word of caution is in order here. We are not arguing that *all* problems are social problems, nor that personal problems have no social factors, nor that social problems are free of any personal elements. There are certainly psychological and, in some cases, physiological factors at work. The point is that if you do not look beyond such factors, you will have a distorted view about the causes of problems.

## The Consequences of Problems

Viewing a problem as either personal or social leads you to identify very different consequences as well as different causes. Consider, for example, a father who can obtain only occasional work and whose family, therefore, lives in poverty. If the man defines his problem as the result of his own inadequacies, he likely will despise himself and passively accept his poverty. Consider, for example, the garbage collector who placed the blame for his lowly position entirely on himself: "Look, I know it's nobody's fault but mine that I got stuck here where I am, I mean . . . if I wasn't such a dumb— . . . no, it ain't that neither . . . if I'd applied myself, I know I got it in me to be different, can't say anyone did it to me." This man defined his problem as personal and, consequently, viewed himself as inadequate.

The *sense of inadequacy*—blaming or downgrading oneself—is not uncommon among those victimized by social problems. Some children who grow up in impoverished homes view themselves unfavorably, believing that their impoverishment is proof of their inferiority. Some women who are beaten by their husbands feel they have done something to deserve the abuse. Some people who lose their jobs during an economic crunch believe they are failures even though they had no control over what happened.

If a problem is defined as personal, *individual strategies* are employed to cope with the problem. Thus, the individual looks inward for a solution. Sometimes that solution is found in an *escape mechanism,* such as neurosis, physical illness, heavy drinking, or self-destructive behavior. At other times a solution is sought from specialists such as psychotherapists or religious advisors who help the person to change. These specialists may facilitate adjustment to the problem but not ultimately resolve it. If America's troubled families sought the help of counselors, they might learn to cope with or endure their troubles. But troubled families would continue to appear just as frequently.

Identifying something as a social problem presents it from a much different perspective and leads to far different conclusions and actions. Thus, if a man defines his poverty as the result of a declining economy, he may join in collective action such as a social movement, a rent strike group, or an organization set up to relieve the plight of the poor. Rather than blame himself for his poverty, he sees it as a *social* problem and takes action to redress it.

Or consider the problem of rape. Whether rape is defined as a social or personal problem makes a great deal of difference (Figure 1.1). Defining it as a personal problem either *blames the victim* or *castigates the offender.* Defining it as a social problem recognizes the need for *collective action* that attacks factors outside the individual.

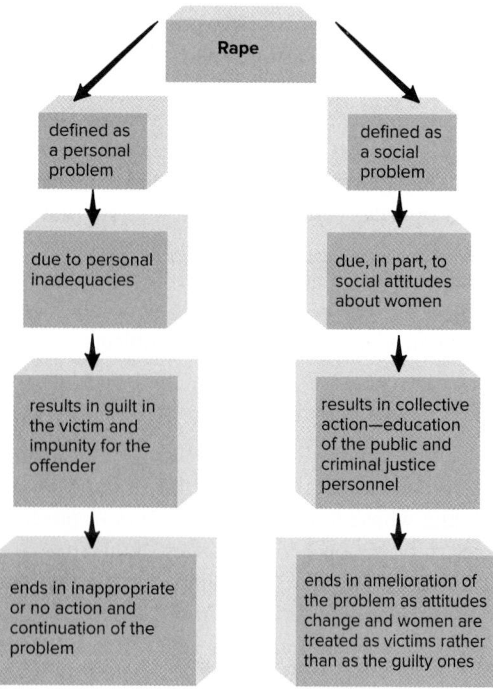


**FIGURE 1.1**
Some Possible Differences When a Problem—Rape in This Case—Is Defined as Social or Personal.

Several cases of rape (as reported in the news media) illustrate the need to consider it a social rather than a purely personal problem. A physician, 39 years old, married, and the father of two children, confessed to raping 22 women and sexually attacking at least 10 other women, one of whom was a nun. The doctor was a respected member of his community by day but an attacker of women by night. A teenage girl who decided to follow others and cool off in a park fountain on a hot July day was raped by two young men while at least three adults ignored her screams for help. Another young woman met a man at a New Year's Eve party. The man's sister, whom the young woman knew, introduced them. The man drove the two women home, dropped his sister off first, then asked if he could come up to the young woman's apartment for coffee. He was a genial, polite man, and since she had no reason to suspect him, she agreed. Once in her apartment, however, the man forced her to participate in various sex acts. When she prosecuted, she discovered that the man was on parole for a prior rape conviction. Yet people who had been at the party testified on the man's behalf, claiming that they had seen the couple talking and that the woman had been drinking. The man was acquitted. Subsequently he was brought to trial again for the alleged rape of a 13-year-old girl.

How can we account for these rapes? Were the victims at fault in these cases? Did they bring it on themselves by luring their attackers? A female student told us, "My father always said that if a woman was raped, it was her fault, that she somehow provoked the guy to do it." Or can the rapes be attributed to mentally ill or evil males? Are the rapists "sick" individuals who need therapy? Or are they evil men who ought to be castrated? You can blame the victims and say that they have personal problems–their wayward behavior. Or you can accuse the rapists of having personal problems–disturbed or evil natures. Neither will resolve the problem. Women who fight, scream, and risk their physical well-being (and even their lives) to ward off an attacker can hardly be said to be luring the man–and there was no evidence that the attackers were mentally ill.

Nor would castration solve the problem. Contrary to popular belief, castration does not prevent a man from having sexual relations. Castration has been used in a number of European countries to punish sex offenders, but of 39 offenders in West Germany who had voluntarily agreed to castration, 11 could still have sexual relations a number of years afterward, and 4 of the men had sex one to three times a week (Heim 1981).

Rape, in sum, is not a personal problem that can be solved by individual efforts. Like other social problems, rape requires collective action to attack such things as the social attitudes that legitimate exploiting women and a legal system that may treat the victim as harshly as the rapist does. Important differences, thus, result from defining a problem as social rather than personal. Unless problems like rape are defined as social, causes may not be identified nor solutions found.

## A Model for Understanding

Given that problems are social and not merely personal, how do we go about understanding them? First let's define precisely what we mean by a *social problem:* It is *a condition or pattern of behavior that (1) contradicts some other condition or pattern of behavior and is defined as incompatible with the desired quality of life; (2) is caused, facilitated, or prolonged by factors that operate at multiple levels of social life; (3) involves intergroup conflict; and (4) requires social action to be resolved.* We explain this definition in the following pages. It uses major insights of sociological theories and is the basis for the model we use in discussing each of the problems in this book.

**structural functionalism**
a sociological theory that focuses on social systems and how their interdependent parts maintain order

**conflict theory**
a theory that focuses on contradictory interests, inequalities between social groups, and the resulting conflict and change

**symbolic interactionism**
a sociological theory that focuses on the interaction between individuals, the individual's perception of situations, and the ways in which social life is constructed through interaction

**interaction**
reciprocally influenced behavior on the part of two or more people

**contradiction**
opposing phenomena within the same social system

**norm**
shared expectations about behavior

**role**
the behavior associated with a particular position in the social structure

**values**
things preferred because they are defined as having worth

**stratification system**
arrangement of society into groups that are unequal with regard to such valued resources as wealth, power, and prestige

**attitude**
a predisposition about something in one's environment

**ideology**
a set of ideas that explain or justify some aspect of social reality

## A Theory-Based Model

There are three major theoretical perspectives in sociology: **structural functionalism, conflict theory,** and **symbolic interactionism.** Each theory has distinctive emphases that are useful for understanding social phenomena. Structural functionalism focuses on social systems and the way in which their interdependent parts maintain order. Conflict theory focuses on contradictory interests of groups, inequalities in society, and the resulting conflict and change. Symbolic interactionism focuses on the **interaction** between individuals, the importance of knowing individuals' perspectives to understand their behavior, and the ways in which social life is constructed through interaction.

To illustrate these three approaches, consider the problem of crime. A structural-functional approach would point out the way that rapid change has weakened social solidarity and social institutions like the family, so that insufficient order is maintained. A conflict approach would note that the powerful groups in society define the kind of behavior that is crime (resulting in higher rates among the poor), and that much crime results from the lack of opportunities for the poor and for racial or ethnic minorities. A symbolic interactionist approach would stress the fact that people learn criminal behavior by interacting with, and accepting for themselves the perspective of, others who approve of such behavior. Figure 1.2 briefly summarizes the theories, how they are used to understand social problems, and how they can be applied to another problem—poverty.

Some sociologists use only one of the theoretical approaches to analyze social problems. We believe that all three approaches are necessary. Each of the theoretical approaches to crime is valid. Our model, therefore, incorporates emphases of each perspective (Figure 1.3). In essence, the model posits mutual influence between social structural factors, social psychological/cognitive factors, and social interaction. Social problems arise when people define **contradictions** among these various elements as incompatible with their quality of life.

Each of the three theories contributes to this model. In structural functionalism, a problem involves a system of interdependent parts, including institutions (collective means of dealing with basic social functions such as government, the family, the mass media, and the economy), **norms** (shared expectations about behavior), **roles** (behavior associated with particular positions in the social structure), and **values** (things preferred because they are defined as having worth). The parts are interrelated and exert pressure to maintain the system.

According to conflict theory, however, contradictions and inequalities exist between the parts of the system that generate conflict between groups. This is manifest in the **stratification system,** the pattern of inequality of wealth, power, and prestige that exists in all societies.

And according to symbolic interactionism, social interaction and the perspectives of individuals, including their **attitudes** (predispositions of individuals toward something) and **ideologies** (sets of ideas that explain or justify some aspect of social life), are important components of the system. Only as you understand how an individual perceives his or her social world can you understand that individual's behavior.

The pairs of arrows in the model indicate *mutual influence.* For example, social structural factors affect the way people interact. Norms and roles may lead a white person and a Black person to treat each other as equals at the factory but not in other settings. The influence can go both ways: patterns of social interaction can alter the social structural factors. In recent years, for instance, women have interacted with men in ways that have altered the female role. Similarly, African Americans have persisted in interacting with whites in ways that have changed traditional roles. An ideology of white

| | Structural Functionalism | Conflict Theory | Symbolic Interaction |
|---|---|---|---|
| Assumptions of the theory | Society is an integrated system of interdependent parts, bound together by shared values and norms. | Society is a system of diverse groups, with conflicting values and interests, vying with each other for power, wealth, and other valued resources. | Society is an arena of interacting individuals who behave in accord with their definitions of situations and who create shared meanings as they interact. |
| How the theory might explain social problems generally | Problems arise out of social disorganization, a state in which consensus about norms has broken down. | Problems are the result of dominance over, and exploitation of, some groups by others. | A situation or form of behavior becomes a problem when people define it as such. |
| How the theory might explain poverty | Political, economic, and educational institutions are not functioning adequately (often because of rapid social change), so that old arrangements are obsolete before new arrangements are in place. | The upper and middle classes oppress and exploit the poor through such things as using political and economic institutions for their own benefit and creating ideologies that blame the poor and justify their poverty. | Poverty became a social problem in the United States when people accepted the influential media's definition of it as such; people remain poor when they define their poverty as the result of their own deficiencies. |
| Illustration of the explanation | Schools train increasing numbers of students for jobs that are diminishing in number as firms adjust to the changing global economy and "outsource" many of those jobs. | Upper- and middle-class lawmakers regularly support corporate welfare (e.g., subsidies and tax breaks) but reject such welfare ideas for the poor as a guaranteed minimum annual income. | The public did not consider poverty as a social problem until the publication of Michael Harrington's influential book *The Other America* in 1962. |

**FIGURE 1.2** Theoretical Explanations of Poverty.

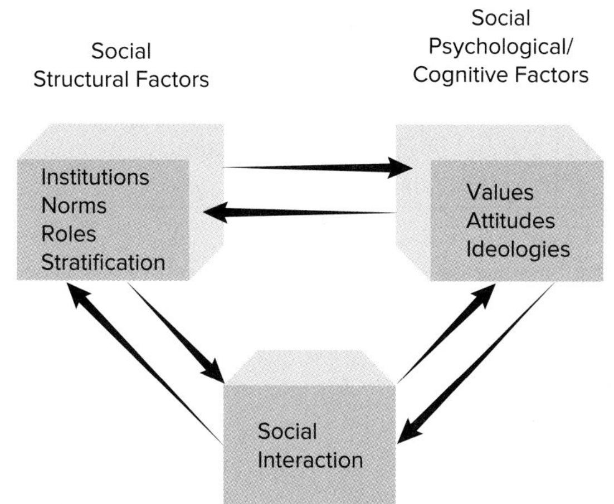


**FIGURE 1.3** A Model for the Analysis of Social Problems.

supremacy can help to create and maintain Blacks in a subservient role, but as minorities refuse to accept the role and assume instead the same kinds of roles as whites, the ideology will be rejected by increasing numbers of people.

By the very nature of social life, there are numerous *contradictions* among the elements in Figure 1.3. This means that opposing phenomena exist within the same social system. The phenomena are opposed in the sense that both cannot be true or operative. When the contradictions are defined as incompatible with the *desired quality of life,* you have a social problem. For example, the limited opportunities available in the economy are a contradiction to the ideology that all people should support themselves by working. The contradiction, as we shall see in Chapter 6, is incompatible with the desired quality of life of the poor.

By our definition, not all societal contradictions signal social problems, only those defined as detracting from the quality of life. In other words, objective data alone do not compose a problem. In accord with symbolic interactionism, only when people define a situation as problematic and persuade others to view it in the same way is there a social problem (Fine 2000). For instance, religion tends to be a unifying force, proclaiming a duty to love, make peace, and establish brotherhood. Recent terrorist acts by Islamic extremists and religious conflict in various nations contradict this peaceful role. Still, religion generally is not considered a social problem by most observers.

Whether people generally define something as detracting from their quality of life depends upon such things as how the problem is presented in the media (including the increasingly influential Internet blogs), how the problem squares with people's experiences, how readily people can understand the various facets of the problem, and how political leaders shape public opinion on issues (Hawdon 2001; Sacco 2003; Maratea 2008).

Finally, consider gender equality as another example of the usefulness of the model. Among the opposing phenomena involved in the problem are:

1. The *ideology* of equal opportunity versus the *reality* of limited opportunities for female participation in the economy.
2. The *value* of the pursuit of happiness versus the *narrowness* of the traditional female *role.*
3. The *value* of human dignity versus male-female *interaction* in which females are treated as intellectual inferiors.

Each of these oppositions has consequences that are incompatible with the desired quality of life of many women.

### Quality of Life

What is this *quality of life* that plays so prominent a role in determining whether a contradiction is defined as a social problem? Thoreau captured its meaning in his desire to avoid discovering, at the point of death, that

> I had not lived. I did not wish to live what was not life, living is so dear; nor did I wish to practise resignation, unless it was quite necessary. I wanted to live deep and suck out all the marrow of life. (Thoreau 1968:113)

The desire to "live deep," to maximize the quality of life, is reflected in a proliferation of studies in recent decades. In quality-of-life studies, cities and states are evaluated in terms of such aspects as equality of opportunity, agriculture, crime rates, technology, education, climate, the economy, cultural opportunities, and health and welfare. They are then ranked according to their overall "quality of life."

After decades of these studies, there is considerable agreement about what Americans define as important to the quality of their lives (Ferriss 2000). In essence, they evaluate their quality of life according to how well they are doing financially, physically, emotionally, socially, and culturally. Americans want well-paying and meaningful work and financial security. They want good health, access to good health care facilities, opportunity for a good education, opportunity to participate in cultural activities, and opportunity to live and work in areas with minimal crime. Americans also want respect from others, self-respect, and a sense of personal worth. Finally, they want to live without fear and with reasonable freedom from stress.

One effort to categorize and quantify quality of life in nations is the Social Progress Index (Institute for Strategy and Competitiveness 2020). The Index uses three broad categories: basic human needs (such as nutrition, medical care, and sanitation); foundations of well-being (health, environmental quality, access to basic knowledge and information); and opportunity (personal rights and freedom, tolerance, access to advanced education). In 2020, 163 nations were rated. The highest score went to Norway, the lowest to South Sudan. The United States was in 28th place, lower than Canada, Japan, South Korea, and most European countries.

When people are asked about their quality of life, they indicate a lowered quality when they lack the kinds of things in the Index. Thus, researchers have found a reduced quality of life reported because of such things as personal health problems (Alonso et al. 2004; LaGrow et al. 2011), work demands that interfere with nonworking time (Rice, Frone, and McFarlin 1992), environmental problems (Tickell 1992), and the experience of financial problems and status inequality (Coverdill, Lopez, and Petrie 2011).

Americans are not unique in their view of what constitutes a high quality of life. Studies of other nations show that people everywhere value many of the same things that Americans do (Ventegodt et al. 2005; Liu 2006; Headey, Muffels, and Wooden 2008). Quality of life, then, involves far more than income. You may be able to purchase security devices for your home, but you can't buy total peace of mind when the newspapers regularly remind you of the pervasiveness of crime. You may be able to afford the best seats in the house, but that's meaningless if your community lacks cultural opportunities. You may live in the most expensive area available, but you can't shut out the polluted air that engulfs your property.

Moreover, undesirable conditions that diminish the quality of life affect you both directly and indirectly. For example, some people are the direct victims of criminal activity: assaults, muggings, robberies, rapes, swindles, and so forth. But everyone has some *fear of criminal victimization,* even people who have never been directly victimized. This fear may put limits on where they go or what they do or how secure they feel—limits that reduce the quality of their lives.

In sum, there are numerous contradictions in society that create conditions incompatible with the desired quality of life. Everyone is affected, though some suffer far more than others. Because of the diminished quality of life, we define these contradictions and the conditions they create as *social problems.*

## Multiple Levels of Social Problems

Social problems are manifested at *multiple levels of social life.* The factors that cause, facilitate, and help to perpetuate social problems are found at the individual level (e.g., attitudes), group levels (e.g., ideologies of terrorist groups), societal levels (e.g., the government), and in some cases, global levels (e.g., globalization of the economy).

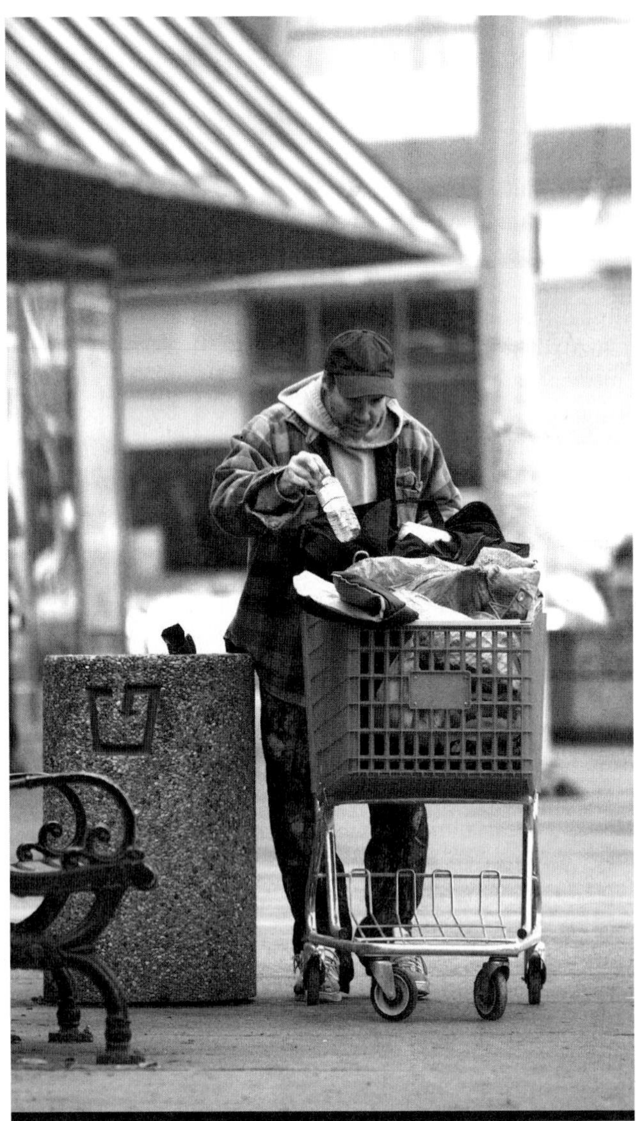

Explaining social problems requires many factors rather than a single cause.
Con Tanasiuk/Design Pics

Think, for example, about the problem of racial and ethnic relations (for brevity's sake, we shall refer to this problem by the commonly used phrase "race problem," though the "problem" is not race per se, but the relation between people of diverse racial and ethnic backgrounds). We could analyze the problem in terms of a stratification system in which racial minorities are disadvantaged, kept in inferior roles, and systematically subjected to discrimination. Such arrangements restrict interaction between the races and justify prejudice and claims that the disadvantaged group is naturally inferior.

Or we could analyze the problem in terms of attitudes of prejudice combined with a value of individualism (meaning that the government should not force people to interact with other races). Add to this an ideology that defines the oppressed race as inferior and therefore deserving of an inferior position. These values, attitudes, and ideology explain and perpetuate a structure in which the oppressed race remains in the least desirable roles, institutional positions, and socioeconomic stratum. Furthermore, interaction between the races is restricted, permitting little opportunity for reevaluation and change.

The point is, as our model indicates, *mutual influence* exists among the various factors at differing levels of social life. Prejudice restricts interaction and restricted interaction fosters prejudice. The two feed on each other. Similarly, education can be structured in such a way as to deprive minorities of adequate learning, thereby justifying an ideology of racial inferiority; but the ideology can also justify inaction in securing adequate education for minorities.

The multiple-level factors, in sum, work together to maintain the problem. Meantime, inequalities in the system lead people to act in their own behalf to bring about change; and interaction is never so confined as to prevent the development of new values, attitudes, and ideologies. Eventually, there may be changes in interaction patterns and in the social structure.

The pressure to change may arise as members of the oppressed race react to the contradiction between an ideology of the free pursuit of happiness and the realities of their situation. They may use the ideology and the contradiction to shape new attitudes and values among the oppressed and the oppressors. They may create new ideologies, such as a myth of their own superiority. They may strive to alter patterns of interaction and elements of the social structure. They may try to change the content of education, the power structure of government, and the practices and policies of the economy.

Thus, understanding and dealing with a social problem is never a simple matter. A social problem cannot be reduced to one thing, such as the race problem being due merely to prejudice or poverty's being due merely to people's failure to work. All the factors in our model enter into each problem.

## Social Action for Resolution

Social problems often give rise to *protest groups* and intergroup conflict as expressions of social action. Protest groups arise because not everyone in the society defines a particular situation the same way. For example, the contradiction between the ideals of American life and the reality of life for most African Americans is not defined by all Americans as incompatible with the quality of life. Some deny that African Americans have less access than whites to the desirable aspects of American life. In other words, they deny the existence of a contradiction.

If all Americans denied the contradiction, there would be no racial problem in this country (even though a foreign observer might see the contradiction). On the other hand, if all Americans affirmed the contradiction and demanded change, the problem might be quickly resolved. Because the contradiction is defined differently by different collectivities, intergroup conflict plays a part in resolving social problems.

We use the term *collectivity* here in reference to members of opposing groups in the conflict who agree on particular issues. The race problem, for example, is not simply a matter of white versus minority. The abortion problem is not just a case of Catholics versus Protestants. Gender inequality is not simply men versus women. Poverty is not merely rich versus poor. In each case there are members of both groups on either side of the issue.

All social problems are characterized by opposing groups with differing ideologies and contrary definitions of the contradiction. One side will argue that the contradiction is incompatible with the desired quality of their lives, while the other side will argue that there is no contradiction, that the contradiction is necessary, or that the contradiction exists but is not rooted in the social system (in other words, the victims of the contradictions are blamed for their plight). Such conflict is the context in which efforts to resolve problems take place.

In subsequent chapters we discuss the ways in which problems may be attacked by social action (both public policy and private action). There are many reasons resolution of most social problems through social action are slow and agonizing: problems are manifested at multiple levels of social reality; numerous factors are involved in causing and maintaining problems; intergroup conflict surrounds most problems; and efforts to resolve a problem may ameliorate one problem but create new problems (Fine 2006).

## The Changing Nature of Social Problems

One additional factor adds to the difficulty of resolving social problems—both the definition and the objective aspects of a particular problem change over time. Sometimes the change may be so rapid that an issue barely has time to be a problem. Until the exceptionally hot and dry summer of 1988, the public did not respond much to the warnings of scientists about global warming (Ungar 1992). That summer brought the problem to the public's attention. When the summer passed, the problem's importance waned in the public mind as other issues rose to the fore. Although virtually all scientists agree that global warming is occurring, there is still dispute in the nation as to whether it is a social problem.

Thus, problems may *rise and decline in perceived importance,* as illustrated by the problem of poverty. Views of poverty have changed over time. A 1952 edition of a social problems text omitted the two chapters on poverty that had appeared in the original 1942 edition (Reinhardt, Meadows, and Gillette 1952). The omission reflected the belief in the 1950s that poverty was largely a problem of the past. (Even the 1942 edition reflected more the opinion of sociologists than that of the public.) Gallup opinion polls about the most important problems facing the nation, taken since November 1935, show that the public did not consider poverty an important problem until 1965 (Lauer 1976). Concerns about poverty peaked in the 1960s and 1970s then tended to diminish. Only 3 percent of those surveyed mentioned poverty as a problem in a 2016 poll (Poling Report 2020). And by 2020, only 1 percent in a Gallup poll named poverty as one of the nation's most important problems.

The objective conditions of poverty also have changed over time: the amount of poverty has changed (as measured by some standard such as family income); the composition of the poor has changed (such as the relative proportions of racial, ethnic, and age groups); and the organization of antipoverty efforts has changed (such as the vigor and focus of protest groups and official attitudes and programs).

Recognizing such changes in problems is important for both understanding and action. For example, many people continue to identify poverty as essentially a problem of work—the poor are unemployed. As you will see, the problem of poverty would be little changed even if every able-bodied person in America had a job. It is true that during the depression of the 1930s a considerable number of the impoverished were unemployed. Many people who lived through that period continue to associate poverty with unemployment, failing to recognize the changed nature of the problem. Today, a large number of poor people are working but still live in poverty. Therefore, to continue associating the two concepts is to misunderstand the contemporary problem and thereby fail to take appropriate action.

As you study the various problems, you will see fluctuations in all of them. Some appear to be getting better, and some appear to be getting worse. It is important to remember that improvement does not mean that the problem is resolved (gains can be quickly lost in the ongoing struggle for justice and equality), nor does deterioration mean that the problem is hopeless (lost ground may be regained and new ground may be gained dramatically when appropriate social action is taken).

## Analyzing Social Problems

The definition of the term "social problems" that we presented earlier in this chapter shapes our approach to each problem considered in this book. First, we "get the feel" of the problem by seeing how it affects people's lives and examining how the problem involves a contradiction and is defined as incompatible with the desired quality of life. Second, we analyze the multiple-level factors involved in the problem. We do not relate every factor identified in Figure 1.3 to each problem: Research has not yet identified the components of every problem. Yet in each we see the multiple-level components that show how the problem arises and is perpetuated. Third, we consider various ways to attack the problem. Our examination is sketchy (any adequate treatment would require a book in itself), but we do discuss some kinds of both public policy and private action that can ameliorate each problem.

Before we turn to specific problems, we need to address an additional issue. Seemingly reasonable statements are made about every social problem. For example, following the series of highly publicized killings by preteens and teenagers in the 1990s, explanations ranged from the pampering of criminals by the legal system to violence in video games and movies to mental illness. How do you know which of these explanations, if any, are correct? Or to put it another way, how do you distinguish opinion from valid analysis?

**critical thinking**
the analysis and evaluation of information

First, you need to *develop critical thinking skills.* **Critical thinking** is the process of carefully attending to spoken or written information in order to evaluate its validity.

Make sure you understand the information; then evaluate it by asking such questions as whether it is logical and reasonable. One important way to evaluate information is to look for any *fallacies of thinking.* These fallacies are commonly used when people analyze social problems. You will find illustrations throughout this book on how fallacies lead to misunderstandings.

Second, you need to examine how sociologists research social problems by gathering data to test various explanations. The data may lead you to revise your explanations. Remember, the study of social problems is not an exercise in speculation; it needs explanations that are supported by evidence. Let's look, then, at fallacious ways of thinking and at methods of social research.

## Critical Thinking: Recognizing Fallacies

Nine different fallacies have been used to analyze social problems. An important aspect of critical thinking is the ability to recognize these fallacies. This ability enables you not only to assess the validity of information and arguments presented by others but also to make your own analyses with logic and clarity.

### Fallacy of Dramatic Instance

**fallacy of dramatic instance** overgeneralizing

The **fallacy of dramatic instance** refers to the tendency to *overgeneralize,* to use one, two, or three cases to support an entire argument. This mistake is common among people who discuss social problems. It may be difficult to counter because the limited number of cases often are a part of an *individual's personal experience.* For example, in discussing the racial problem in the United States, a man said to us: "Blacks in this country can make it just as much as whites. I know a Black businessman who is making a million. In fact, he has a better house and a better car than I have." We pointed out that this successful businessperson is an exception. The man dismissed the point: "If one guy can make it, they all can." The fallacy of dramatic instance mistakes a few cases for a general situation.

This fallacy is difficult to deal with because the argument is based partly on fact. There are, after all, African Americans who are millionaires. Does this mean there is no discrimination and that any Black person can attain success? To use another example, many Americans believe that welfare recipients are "ripping off" the rest of us, that we are subsidizing their unwillingness to work and supporting them at a higher standard of living than we ourselves enjoy. Is this true? Yes, in a few cases. Occasionally, newspapers report instances of individuals making fraudulent use of welfare. But does this mean that most welfare recipients are doing the same? Do people on welfare really live better than people who work for a living?

The point is, in studying social problems, you must recognize that exceptions exist. To use such cases in support of your argument is to fall into the trap of the fallacy of dramatic instance because social problems deal with general situations rather than with individual exceptions.

As this fallacy suggests, the fact that you hear about a lazy poor person or a rich African American or a corrupt politician does not mean that such cases represent the typical situation. Millions of people are involved in the problems of poverty, race, and government. *Systematic studies* are needed to determine whether the one or two cases you know about represent the norm or the exception. For instance, the fact that there are Black and Hispanic millionaires is less important than the government report showing that in 2019 the median annual household income for non-Hispanic whites was $76,057, whereas that for Hispanics was $56,113 and that for African Americans was $45,438 (Semega et al. 2020). That same year, 7.3 percent of non-Hispanic whites, 15.7 percent of Hispanics, and 18.8 percent of African Americans lived in poverty. Such figures are more pertinent to the race problem than are cases that represent exceptions to the general pattern.

We are not saying that individual examples or cases are unimportant or unusable. At various points throughout this book (including the chapter-opening vignettes) we use examples of people's experiences. These examples are not given as proof or even as evidence. Rather, we use them to *illustrate the impact of social problems on people's quality of life.* These examples may dramatize better than statistics the ways in which people's lives are adversely affected by social problems.

## Fallacy of Retrospective Determinism

**fallacy of retrospective determinism**
the argument that things could not have worked out any other way than they did

The **fallacy of retrospective determinism** is the argument that things could not have worked out any other way than the way they did. It is a *deterministic* position, but the determinism is aimed at the past rather than the future. The fallacy asserts that what happened historically *had* to happen, and it *had* to happen just the way it did. If you accept this fallacy, the present social problems are inevitable. Whether the issue is racial discrimination, poverty, war, or the well-being of the family, the fallacy of retrospective determinism makes it unavoidable.

This fallacy is unfortunate for a number of reasons. History is more than a tale of *inevitable tragedies.* History is important for understanding social problems. You cannot fully understand the tensions between America's minority groups and the white majority unless you know about the decades of exploitation and humiliation preceding

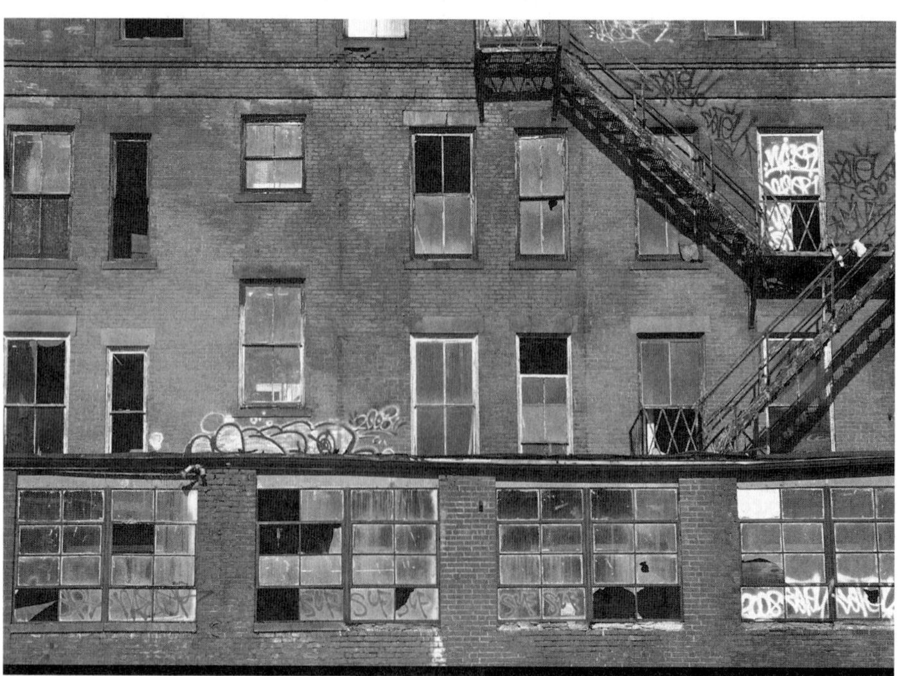

Those who are born poor are likely to remain poor. Their poverty, however, is caused by social conditions, not fate.
Denis Tangney Jr./Getty Images

the emergence of the modern civil rights movement. Your understanding will remain clouded if you regard those events as nothing more than an inevitable process. Similarly, you cannot fully understand the tension between the People's Republic of China and the West if you view it only as a battle of economic ideologies. It is vital to know that the tension is based in the pillage and humiliation to which China was subjected by the West. Yet your understanding will not be enhanced by the study of history if you regard the Western oppression of China in the 19th century as inevitable.

If you view the past in terms of determinism, you have little reason to study it and are deprived of an important source of understanding. Furthermore, the fallacy of retrospective determinism is but a small step from the stoic *acceptance of the inevitable.* That is, if things are the way they have to be, why worry about them? Assuming that the future also is determined by forces beyond your control, you are left in a position of apathy: There is little point in trying to contest the inevitable.

This fallacy is probably less common in discussions about social problems than the fallacy of dramatic instance, but it does appear in everyday discussions. For example, in responding to the question about the causes of poverty in America, a 64-year-old service station owner told us: "Go back through history, it's traditional; there's no special reason, no cause for it. We can't get away from it. It has just always been this way." A businessman expressed a similar fatalism: "I don't actually know the cause of poverty, but it's here to stay and we must learn to live with it. We have to take the good with the bad."

An individual might view social problems in deterministic terms for reasons other than intellectual conviction. Determinism can relieve you of responsibility and can legitimate a lack of concern with efforts to effect changes you do not want. Whatever the basis for affirming determinism, the outcome is the same: You may as well accept the problem and learn to live with it, because it is inevitably and inextricably with you.

## Fallacy of Misplaced Concreteness

Some people have a tendency to explain some social problems by resorting to **reification**—making what is abstract into something concrete. "Society," for example, is an abstraction. It is not like a person, an animal, or an object that can be touched. It is an idea, a way of thinking about a particular collectivity of people. Yet we often hear people assert that something is the fault of "society" or that "society" caused a certain problem. This is the **fallacy of misplaced concreteness.** In what sense can society "make" or "cause" or "do" anything? To say that society caused a problem leaves you helpless to correct the situation because you haven't the faintest notion where to begin. If, for example, society is the cause of juvenile delinquency, how do you tackle the problem? Must you change society? If so, how?

**reification**
defining what is abstract as something concrete

**fallacy of misplaced concreteness**
making something abstract into something concrete

The point is that "society" is an abstraction, a concept that refers to a group of people who interact in particular ways. To *attribute social problems to an abstraction* like "society" does not help resolve the problems. Sometimes people who attribute the cause of a particular problem to society intend to *deny individual responsibility.* To say that society causes delinquency may be a way of saying that the delinquent child is not responsible for his or her behavior.

You can recognize the social causes of problems without either attributing them to an abstraction like society or relieving the individual of responsibility for his or her behavior. For instance, you could talk about the family's role in delinquency. A family is a concrete phenomenon. Furthermore, you could say that the family itself is a victim of some kind of societal arrangement, such as government regulations that tend to perpetuate poverty, cause stress, and create disruption in many families. You could say that families can be helped by changing the government regulations that keep some of them in poverty and, thereby, facilitate delinquent behavior.

Society, in short, does not cause anything. Rather, problems are caused by that which the concept of society represents—people acting in accord with certain social arrangements and within a particular cultural system.

## Fallacy of Personal Attack

**fallacy of personal attack** argument by attacking the opponent personally rather than dealing with the issue

A tactic among debaters is to attack the opponent *personally* when they can't support their position by reason, logic, or facts. This tactic diverts attention from the issue and focuses it on personality. We call this the **fallacy of personal attack** (philosophers call it *ad hominem*). It is remarkably effective in avoiding the use of reason or the consideration of evidence in discussing a social problem. In analyzing social problems, this fallacy can be used either to attack an opponent in a debate about a problem or to *attack the people who are the victims of the problem.* Ryan (1971) called this "blaming the victim" and said it involves nearly every problem in America.

Historically, the poor have suffered from this approach. Instead of offering sympathy or being concerned for the poor, people may label the poor as disreputable and, consequently, deserving of or responsible for their plight. People who are not poor are relieved of any responsibility. In fact, government efforts to alleviate poverty are even thought to contribute to the problem by taking away any incentive of the poor to help themselves, and leading them instead to become sexually promiscuous, irresponsible, and dependent on others (Somers and Block 2005). Attitudes have been changing. Increasing numbers of Americans agree that the poor are victims of circumstances beyond their control. Still, by 2019, 42 percent of Americans polled said that "poor life chances" are the main reason for poverty, and 40 percent pinned the problem of drugs and alcohol (Ekins 2019).

The meaning and seriousness of any social problem may be sidestepped by attacking the intelligence or character of the victims or of those who call attention to the problem. Name-calling and labeling, thereby, change the social problem into a personal problem.

## Fallacy of Appeal to Prejudice

**fallacy of appeal to prejudice** argument by appealing to popular prejudices or passions

In addition to attacking the opponent, a debater may try to support an unreasonable position by using another technique: **fallacy of appeal to prejudice.** (Philosophers call it argument *ad populum.*) With this fallacy, debaters use popular prejudices or passions to convince others of the correctness of their position. When the topic is social problems, debaters use *popular slogans* or *popular myths* to sway people emotionally rather than using reasoning from systematic studies.

Some slogans or phrases persist for decades and are employed to oppose efforts to resolve social problems. "Creeping socialism" has been used to describe many government programs designed to aid the underdogs of society. The term is not used when the programs are designed to help business or industry, or when the affluent benefit from the programs. As someone remarked, "What the government does for me is progress; what it does for you is socialism."

In some cases, the slogans use general terms that reflect *traditional values.* Thus, the various advances made in civil rights legislation—voting, public accommodations, open housing—have been resisted in the name of the "rights of the individual." These slogans help to perpetuate the myth that legislation that benefits African Americans infringes on the constitutional rights of the white majority. More recently, those who continue to oppose same-sex marriage, even though it is now legal, argue that they are simply acting in *defense of marriage and the family*. They claim that same-sex marriage will further damage or even destroy the traditional family life that is the bedrock of a stable society.

Unfortunately, in the absence of other information or evidence, people tend to rely on myths to assess situations. Thus, some Americans continue to assume that rape is often the woman's fault because she has sexually provoked the man. These Americans either have seen no evidence to the contrary or have dismissed the evidence as invalid. Unfortunately, myths tend to become so deeply rooted in people's thinking that when people are confronted by new evidence, they have difficulty accepting it.

Myths are hard to break down, but if you want to understand social problems, you must abandon popular ideas and assumptions and resist popular slogans and prejudices that cloud your thinking. Instead, you must make judgments based on evidence.

## Fallacy of Circular Reasoning

The ancient Greek physician Galen praised the healing qualities of a certain clay by pointing out that all who drink the remedy recover quickly—except those whom it does not help. The latter die and are not helped by any medicine. Obviously, according to Galen, the clay fails only in incurable cases. This is an example of the **fallacy of circular reasoning:** using conclusions to support the assumptions that were necessary to draw the conclusions.

**fallacy of circular reasoning** using conclusions to support the assumptions that were necessary to make the conclusions

Circular reasoning creeps into analyses of social problems. Someone might argue that Hispanics are inherently inferior and assert that their inferiority is evident because they hold only menial jobs and do not do intellectual work. In reply, you might point out that Hispanics are not doing more intellectual work because of discriminatory hiring practices. The person might then counter that Hispanics could not be hired for such jobs anyway because they are inferior.

Similarly, you might argue that homosexuals are sex perverts because they commonly have remained secretive about their sexual preference. But, we counter, the secrecy is due to the general disapproval of homosexuality. No, you reply, homosexuality is kept secret because it is a perversion. Thus, in circular reasoning people bounce *back and forth between assumptions and conclusions.* Circular reasoning leads nowhere in the search for an understanding of social problems.

## Fallacy of Authority

Virtually everything you know is based on some authority. You know comparatively little from personal experience or personal research. The authority you necessarily rely on is someone else's experience, research, or belief. You accept notions of everything from the nature of the universe to the structure of the atom, from the state of international relationships to the doctrines of religion—all on the basis of some authority. Most people accept a war as legitimate on the authority of their political leaders. Many accept the validity of capital punishment on the authority of law enforcement officers. Some accept that use of contraceptives is morally wrong on religious authority. Most rely on the authority of the news media about the extent and severity of various problems.

The knowledge that you acquire through authority can be inaccurate and can exacerbate rather than resolve or ameliorate social problems. The **fallacy of authority** means an *illegitimate appeal to authority.* Such an appeal obtrudes into thinking about social problems in at least four ways.

**fallacy of authority** argument by an illegitimate appeal to authority

First, the *authority may be ambiguous.* Thus, appeal is made to the Bible by both those who support and those who oppose capital punishment. Supporters of capital punishment point out that the Bible, particularly the Old Testament, decreed death for certain offenses. Opponents counter that the death penalty contradicts New Testament notions of Christian love. An appeal to this kind of authority, then, is really an appeal to a particular interpretation of the authority. Because the interpretations are contradictory, people must find other bases for making judgments.

Second, the *authority may be irrelevant to the problem.* The fact that a man is a first-rate physicist does not mean he can speak with legitimate authority about race relations. Most of us are impressed by people who have significant accomplishments in some area, but their accomplishments should not overwhelm us if those people speak about a problem outside their area of expertise.

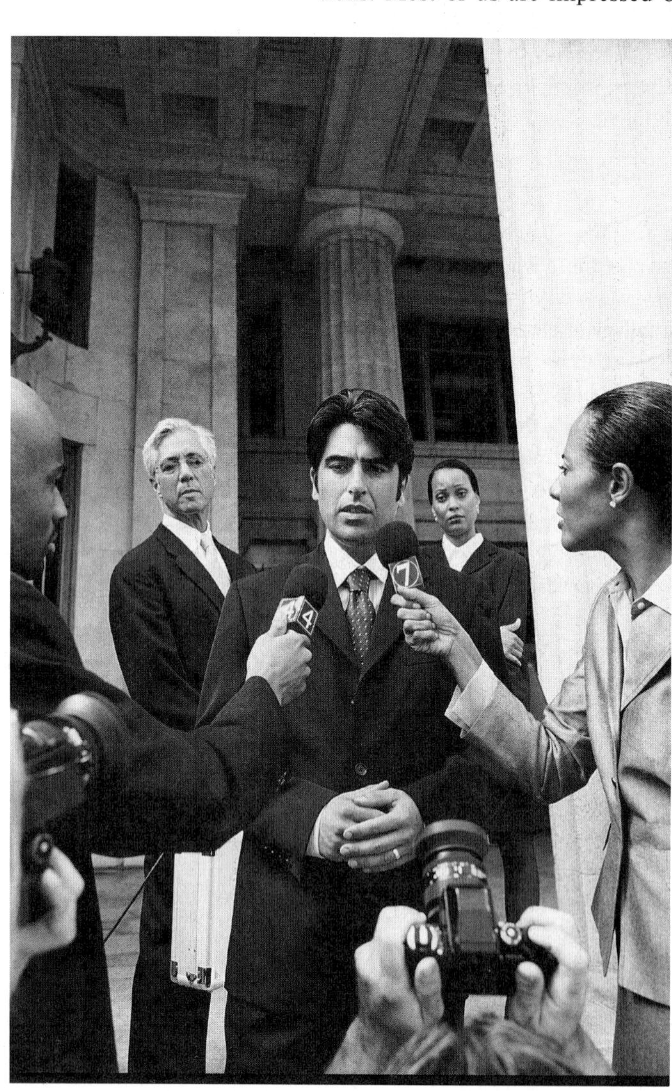

We rely on authorities for information, but authorities are not always right.

Jim Arbogast/Masterfile

Third, the *authority may be pursuing a bias* rather than studying a problem. To say that someone is pursuing a bias is not necessarily to disparage that person because pursuing it may be part of a job. For example, military officers are likely to analyze the problem of war from a military rather than a moral, political, or economic perspective. This is their job—and this is why decisions about armaments, defense, and war should not be left solely to the military. From a military point of view, one way to prevent war is to be prepared to counter an enemy attack. The nation must be militarily strong, according to this argument, so that other nations will hesitate to attack—and military strength requires the most sophisticated technology, a stockpile of weaponry, and a large, standing military force.

The shortcomings of this line of reasoning were dramatically illustrated by the incidents of September 11, 2001, when terrorists seized jetliners and crashed them into the World Trade Center towers in New York City and the Pentagon in Washington, D.C. At the time, the United States was clearly the strongest military power in the world. Nevertheless, the terrorists struck and they struck effectively. As we discuss in Chapter 14, the notion of defending against enemies must now be reexamined in light of a new face of war in the world.

Although some people pursue a bias as a normal part of their work, others pursue it because of *vested interests.* That is, the authority may deliberately or unconsciously allow biases to affect what he or she says because it is personally advantageous. The head of a corporation that builds private prisons and argues that the private sector can deal with prisoners more effectively than can the government will obviously benefit from public policy that privatizes state and federal prisons. The corporate executive who talks about federal overregulation would clearly benefit if the government withdrew from consumer protection programs. Political leaders credit their own policies when crime rates fall and point to uncontrollable circumstances when crime rates rise. Their policies may have no effect on crime rates, but they benefit if they can persuade people that their actions have lowered the rate or will do so in the future.

Finally, *the authority may simply be wrong.* This problem often occurs when one authority cites another. For example, in 2003, the Census Bureau issued a report on the foreign-born population of the United States (Schmidley 2003). The report showed the years of entry of the 32.5 million foreign-born people now living in the nation: 4.1 million came before 1970, 4.6 million came during the 1970s, 7.96 million came during the 1980s, and 15.8 million came after 1990. Suppose we wanted information about immigration patterns, and we consulted newspapers instead of the Census Bureau. We examined three respectable sources and found the following interpretations of the report. A national financial paper said that the number of immigrants continued to grow at "a blistering pace." An urban newspaper reported that immigration continued at a steady pace during "the past two years." And a national newspaper claimed that the Census Bureau report stated that the number of foreign-born coming to live in the United States has "slowed considerably"! Clearly, when one authority cites another, it is best to check out the initial authority before drawing any conclusions.

## Fallacy of Composition

That the whole is equal to the sum of its parts appears obvious. That what is true of the part is also true of the whole likewise seems to be a reasonable statement, but the former is debatable, and the latter is the **fallacy of composition.** As economists have illustrated, the notion that *what is valid for the part is also valid for the whole* is not necessarily true. Consider, for example, the relationship between work and income. If a farmer works hard and the weather is not adverse, the farmer's income may rise; but if every farmer works hard and the weather is favorable, and a bumper crop results, the total farm income may fall. The latter case is based on supply and demand, whereas the former assumes that a particular farmer outperforms other farmers.

**fallacy of composition** the assertion that what is true of the part is necessarily true of the whole

In thinking about social problems, *you cannot assume that what is true for the individual is also true for the group.* An individual may be able to resolve a problem insofar as it affects him or her, but that resolution is not available to all members of the group. For example, a man who is unemployed and living in poverty may find work that enables him to escape poverty. The work may require him to move or to work for less money than someone else, but still he is able to rise above poverty. As you will see in our discussion of poverty, however, that solution is not possible for most of the nation's poor. Thus, something may be true for a particular individual or even a few individuals and yet be inapplicable or counterproductive for the entire group of which the individuals are members.

## Fallacy of Non Sequitur

A number of the fallacies already discussed involve non sequitur, but we look at this way of thinking separately because of its importance. Literally, non sequitur means *"it does not follow."* This **fallacy of non sequitur** is commonly found when people interpret statistical data.

**fallacy of non sequitur** something that does not follow logically from what has preceded it

For example, data may show that the amount of welfare payments by state governments has increased dramatically over the past few decades. What is the meaning of such data? You might conclude that the number of people unwilling to work has

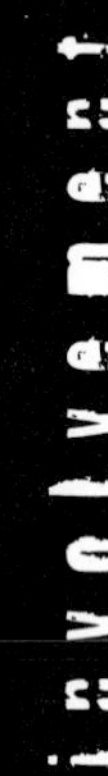

## HOW, AND HOW NOT, TO THINK

"Use it or lose it" is a common saying. We might paraphrase that and say "Use it and learn it." That is, one of the best ways to learn something is to use it and not simply to memorize it. For this involvement, therefore, we are asking you to learn the fallacies by using them.

Select any social problem in which you are interested. Show how people could use each of the fallacies to "explain" that problem. Construct nine different explanations that are one or two sentences long. Try to make your explanations sound reasonable. Test them by sharing them with someone and seeing how many you can get the other person to accept. If the entire class participates in this project, gather in small groups and have each member share his or her explanations. Group members should then try to identify the fallacy in each of the explanations. Be sure not to present the fallacies in the order in which they appear in the book.

As an alternative, use simple observation to test the accuracy of common (or your own) notions about people involved in particular social problems. For instance, visit a gay bar. Or attend a meeting of gay activists, a feminist group, Alcoholics Anonymous, or an environmental group. Ask a number of people to describe the typical member of the group you visit, and compare their responses (and your own preconceptions) with your observations.

increased and that more and more "freeloaders" are living off the public treasury, but there are other explanations. The increase may reflect adjustments due to inflation, better efforts to get welfare money to eligible recipients, or a rise in unemployment due to government action to control inflation.

Daniel Bell (1960) showed how statistics on crime can be misleading. In New York one year, reported assaults were up 200 percent, robberies were up 400 percent, and burglaries were up 1,300 percent! Those were the "facts," but what did they mean? A crime wave? Actually, the larger figures reflected a new method of crime reporting that was more effective in determining the total amount of crime. An increase in reported crime rates can mean different things, but it does not necessarily signify an actual increase in the amount of crime.

One other example involves studies of women who work. Some employers believe that women are not desirable workers because they are less committed to the job than men, as indicated by their higher turnover rate. Women do indeed have a higher rate of turnover than men. But what does this mean? Are women truly less committed to their jobs?

When you look at the situation more closely, you find that the real problem is that women tend to be concentrated in lower-level jobs. Also, women who quit a job tend to find another one quickly. Thus, women may be uncommitted to a particular low-level job but strongly committed to work. Furthermore, if you look at jobs with the same status, the turnover rate is no higher for women than men.

These illustrations are not meant to discourage you from drawing conclusions. Instead, they are reminders of the need for thorough study and the need to avoid quick conclusions, even when those conclusions seem logical on the surface. Contrary to popular opinion, *"facts" do not necessarily speak for themselves.* They must be interpreted in light of the complexities of social life and with the awareness that a number of different conclusions can usually be drawn from any set of data.

### Fallacies and Mass Media

In subsequent chapters, we discuss how mass media contribute to particular social problems. Here we want to point out how the media contribute to misunderstandings by committing or facilitating the various fallacies.

In some cases, the media may inadvertently create fallacious thinking by the way something is reported. For instance, a newspaper story about someone who is guilty of welfare fraud, which omits the fact that such fraud represents only a tiny minority of recipients, can lead readers to commit the fallacy of the dramatic instance: The story proves that those on welfare are cheats who want handouts rather than responsibility. Or a story in a religious magazine about a formerly gay man who is now married to a woman, which omits any mention of the numerous gays who have tried and failed to change their sexual orientation, can lead readers to commit the fallacy of non sequitur: If one man can do it, they all can.

Because the media represent authority in the matter of information, they are particularly prone to the fallacy of authority. That is, they might provide information that is misleading or wrong. It may be a case of bias on the part of those gathering and/or presenting the information. It may be a case of misunderstanding the original source of the information. Or it may be a case of the original source itself being wrong. For example, in 2006 a survey commissioned by the American Medical Association found a startlingly high rate of binge drinking and unprotected sex on the part of female college students while on spring break (Rosenthal 2006). The study, reported widely on TV and in newspapers, was based on a "random sample." It turned out, however, that the sample was not random. Those who participated were volunteers, and only one-fourth of them had actually been on a spring break trip. In essence, then, no conclusions about college women in general could be drawn from the survey.

We do not intend to commit the fallacy of dramatic instance ourselves by suggesting that such incidents are typical or even very common. Rather, they illustrate the need to be alert, thoughtful, and cautious about the things you read and hear about social problems.

## The Sources of Data: Social Research

The various "intellectual blind alleys" we have described create and help to perpetuate myths about social problems. *Social research* is designed to gain information about social problems so that you can have a valid understanding of them and employ realistic efforts in resolving them.

Not everything called research is scientifically valid. Therefore, you need to use critical thinking skills as well as information and arguments to evaluate research. Some so-called social research aims to shape rather than gain information. For example, we once received a letter from a U.S. congressman inquiring about our attitudes toward labor unions. Actually, the letter attempted to shape information, and the questionnaire that accompanied it was designed to enlist support for the congressman's antiunion stance. The letter began by saying, "What will happen to your state and local taxes—your family's safety—and our American way of life, if the czars of organized labor have their way in the new Congress?" It used such phrases as "henchmen," "power hungry union professionals," "rip-offs which enrich the union fat cats at your expense," and "freedom from union tyranny." The questionnaire itself requested yes-or-no responses to questions such as "Do you feel that anyone should be forced to pay a union boss for permission to earn a living?" Clearly, this inquiry resorted to *the fallacies of personal attack and appeal to prejudice.* A critical-thinking approach would treat the results as little else than an illustration of people with biases against labor unions.

If you want to gain information and discover the nature of social reality, you must use scientific social research. Scientific research is both rational and *empirical.* That is, it is logical and comes to conclusions based on evidence rather than speculation or feelings. The stages of such research typically include a clear statement of the problem or issue to be researched; formulation of *hypotheses* so that the problem or issue is in researchable form; selection of the appropriate method, including the sample; collection of the data; analysis of the data; and interpretation and report of the conclusions. A guiding principle throughout the foregoing stages is the desire to discover evidence, not to confirm preconceptions.

Many different methods are used in social research. We look at four methods that have yielded important information about social problems: survey research, statistical analysis of official records (particularly of government data), experiments, and participant observation.

## Survey Research

**survey**
a method of research in which a sample of people are interviewed or given questionnaires in order to get data on some phenomenon

**socioeconomic status**
position in the social system based on economic resources, power, education, prestige, and lifestyle

**variable**
any trait or characteristic that varies in value or magnitude

The **survey** uses interviews and/or questionnaires to gain data about some phenomenon. The people from whom the information is gathered are normally a *sample* (a small number of people selected by various methods from a larger population) of a *population* (a group that is the focus of the study). The data include everything from attitudes about various matters to information such as gender, age, and **socioeconomic status.** You can learn two important aspects of social reality from surveys. First, you can discover the *distribution of people along some dimension.* For example, you can learn the proportion of people who say they will vote Republican or Democratic in an election; the proportion of people who favor, oppose, or are neutral about capital punishment; or the proportion of people who believe that homosexuals should be allowed to marry. Second, you can discover *relationships among* **variables.** (A *variable* is any trait or characteristic that varies in value or magnitude.) For instance, you can investigate the relationship between people's positions in the stratification system (socioeconomic status) and their attitudes toward the race problem, gender inequality, or the plight of the poor.

Survey research is probably the most common method used in sociology. Let's examine one piece of such research that deals with the problem of wife rape. The example illustrates both the technique of survey research and the kind of information that survey research can yield about a social problem.

Can a man rape his wife? In our experience, students have diverse opinions. Some believe that wife rape is as serious an offense against a woman as rape by a stranger. Others believe that rape makes no sense in the context of marriage, that sex in marriage is "his right" and "her duty" (Durán, Moya, and Megias 2011), a view that is supported by a long legal tradition. The so-called marital rape exemption goes back to 17th-century England, when Chief Justice Matthew Hale declared that a husband cannot be guilty of raping his wife "for by their mutual matrimonial consent and contract the wife hath given up herself in this kind unto the husband which she cannot retract" (quoted in Russell 1982:17). This decision was based on the idea that wives are property and that sex is a wife's duty. It was the prevailing legal guideline in the United States until the 1970s. In 1977, Oregon deleted the spouse-immunity clause from the rape statute, and a man was tried (though not convicted) for wife rape the next year. Marital rape is now a crime in all 50 states, and it is estimated that 10 to 14 percent of all married women and 40 to 50 percent of battered women will experience it (Martin, Taft, and Resick 2007).

Apart from public and legal opinions, is it reasonable to speak of wife rape? Does the wife suffer the same kinds of trauma as other rape victims? In a pioneering study whose results remain valid, Diana Russell (1982) investigated the question of wife rape by surveying a random sample of 930 women in the San Francisco Bay area. ("Random" does not mean they were chosen at random, but that they were carefully selected using a method that gave every woman in the area an equal chance of being chosen.) She interviewed the 644 women who were or had been married. About 14 percent, or one in seven, told about "sexual assaults" by their husbands that could be classified as rape. The wives were raped by force, by the threat of force, and by their inability to consent to sexual intercourse because of being drugged, asleep, or somehow helpless. The forced sex included oral and anal sex as well as sexual intercourse.

Some of the women said their husbands threatened to beat them if they did not submit. Others said they were held down forcibly. In a few cases, weapons were used to intimidate them or they were beaten with fists or objects. Overall, 84 percent of the wives indicated that some kind of force was used. Pushing and pinning down were the most common kinds of force employed by the husbands, but 16 percent of the women said that their husbands hit, kicked, or slapped them, and 19 percent said they were beaten or slugged. About 1 out of 10 of the women pointed out, without being asked, that they had been injured during the attack, ranging from bruises to broken bones and concussions.

The husbands also made verbal threats and even used weapons: 13 percent of the husbands had guns and 1 percent had knives. Twenty-one percent threatened to kill their wives. These wives were obviously and understandably intimidated.

What about the argument that forced sex with one's husband cannot possibly be as traumatic as forced sex with a stranger? Russell compared the responses of her sample with those of women who had been raped by strangers; acquaintances; authority figures; and friends, dates, or lovers. In terms of the proportion of women who reported being "extremely upset" by the incident, the proportions were 65 percent of those raped by a relative other than the husband (usually a childhood rape), 61 percent of those raped by a stranger, 59 percent of those raped by a husband, 42 percent of those raped by an acquaintance, 41 percent of those raped by an authority figure, and 33 percent of those raped by a friend, date, or lover (Russell 1982). Further, the same percentage—52 percent—of women who were raped by their husbands and women who were raped by a relative other than the husband indicated "great long-term effects" on their lives, compared to 39 percent of those raped by a stranger, and smaller percentages of those involved in the other kinds of rape.

Clearly, wife rape is no less traumatic than other kinds of rape and is more traumatic than many kinds. Women who had been raped by their husbands suffered, among other effects, increased negative feelings toward their husbands and men generally; deterioration of the marriage (including divorce); changed behavior patterns (drinking more, or never remarrying if a divorce resulted); increased fear, anxiety, anger, or depression; and increased negative feelings about sex. Two of the raped women tried to commit suicide.

Russell's research has clear implications for dealing with the problem. Many states still have various forms of the marital rape exemption on their statute books. In some cases, a distinction is made between rape by a husband and rape by someone else, with the former being a less serious offense; but Russell's research shows that rape by a husband is a serious offense from the victim's point of view. Such research not only provides insight but also suggests realistic ways of resolving a problem.

### Statistical Analysis of Official Records

Suppose you want to see how *self-esteem* enters into various social problems. For instance, you might want to see whether prejudice and discrimination affect the self-esteem of minorities, whether negative attitudes about growing old affect the self-esteem

**mean**
the average

of the aged, or whether rapists or other offenders have low self-esteem. You could use a questionnaire to measure self-esteem, then compute the **mean** (average) scores of your respondents.

Let's say that the mean score of a random sample of offenders was 8.9 and the mean score of a random sample of average citizens of the same age, gender, and socioeconomic status was 10.2. The offenders have lower self-esteem. But is the difference between 8.9 and 10.2 a significant one? If not, how much difference would be required before you could say that it was significant—that is, before you could say with some confidence that the two groups differ in level of self-esteem?

**test of significance**
a statistical method for determining the probability that research findings occurred by chance

The question can be answered by using a **test of significance,** which is a technical way of determining the probability that your findings occurred by chance. That is, if the difference is not significant statistically, then you cannot say that offenders have a lower self-esteem than nonoffenders. A different set of samples might yield scores of 9.4 for both groups, or a slightly higher mean for offenders than for nonoffenders. If the difference is statistically significant, however, you can say with some confidence that offenders generally have lower self-esteem than nonoffenders.

We will not examine details of tests of significance; they require greater knowledge of statistics. Note, however, that many of the findings about social problems discussed in this book—whether gathered through survey research, experiment, or official records—have been subjected to statistical tests. This gives you confidence that the results reflect significant differences between the groups and, if the samples were adequate, that the results apply to more groups than the ones tested. Thus, you can make general statements about, say, women in America without having surveyed the majority of American women.

Some other questions can be asked about data gathered in research. For example, you might want to know how many of the offenders scored high, medium, and low in self-esteem. To get this information, you need a **frequency distribution,** which we use in subsequent chapters. The frequency distribution provides information not available in the mean.

**frequency distribution**
the organization of data to show the number of times each item occurs

As Table 1.1 shows, you can have different frequency distributions with the same number of cases and the same mean. If the scores in the table represented thousands of income dollars of women in an organization, you would draw different conclusions about the women's economic well-being in the two cases even though the means were the same.

**median**
the score below which are half of the scores and above which are the other half

Another question that can be asked is, "What is the **median** score?" The median is the score below which half the scores fall and above which the other half fall. This

**TABLE 1.1**
Frequency Distribution of Two Sets of Hypothetical Data

| | Number In: | |
|---|---|---|
| Score | Set A | Set B |
| 1 | 10 | 3 |
| 2 | 2 | 10 |
| 3 | 2 | 7 |
| 4 | 6 | 0 |
| Mean score | 2.2 | 2.2 |

**TABLE 1.2**
Frequency Distribution, Mean, and Median of Two Sets of Hypothetical Income Data

| | Number of Families | |
|---|---|---|
| Income Level | Set A | Set B |
| $ 1,000 | 2 | 1 |
| 2,000 | 1 | 2 |
| 3,000 | 1 | 1 |
| 4,000 | 1 | 0 |
| 5,000 | 2 | 1 |
| 10,000 | 0 | 2 |
| Mean | $3,000 | $4,714 |
| Median | 3,000 | 3,000 |

furnishes important information for dealing with things such as income distribution. For instance, if A and B represent two communities in Table 1.2, the mean incomes of the two are quite different. You might conclude that the people in community B are better off than those in community A. Actually, the median income is the same for both A and B, and the higher mean for B is due to the two families with very high incomes. Thus, *extreme figures* will affect the mean but not the median. When you find a big difference between the mean and the median, you know extremes are involved.

Statistical analysis is useful for several types of research. Suppose you want to see whether women are discriminated against with respect to income. You will need a frequency distribution of male and female incomes as well as mean and median income for the two groups. This information can be obtained from government census data: The analysis has already been made, and you need only interpret it. You do not need to make a test of significance because census data involve the entire population; tests of significance are used only when you want to know the probability that your findings about a sample are true for the population.

Not all official records are analyzed statistically, and not all are as complete as census data. Yet many data are available that you can use to improve your understanding of social problems. An example of the utility of the statistical analysis of official records is provided by Jacobs and Carmichael's (2002) study of the death penalty. The researchers raised the question of why the death penalty exists in some states but not others. Is it simply a matter that some people believe the penalty is an effective crime deterrent while others do not? Or are other factors at work as well?

Using various theoretical considerations, the researchers set up hypotheses about the impact of economic, political, and racial factors on the death penalty. They tested the hypotheses by using official records, including whether a state had the death penalty, the extent of economic inequality in the state, the unemployment rate, the proportion of African Americans and Hispanics, the proportion of families headed by a woman, the extent of public conservatism (measured by the ideologies of the state's elected congresspeople), and the strength of the Republican Party (measured by whether the governor was Republican and the proportion of Republicans in the state legislature).

In accord with their hypotheses, the researchers found that states with the largest Black populations, the greatest economic inequality, Republican dominance in the state legislature, and stronger conservative values were more likely to have the death penalty. In accord with our model, the researchers identified multiple social factors associated with the death penalty—institutions, stratification, values, and ideologies—and they showed that whether a state has the death penalty is not simply a matter of believing in its value as a deterrent to crime. Economic threats, racial divisions, and ideologies all enter into the matter.

## Experiments

**independent variable** the variable in an experiment that is manipulated to see how it affects changes in the dependent variable

**dependent variable** the variable in an experiment that is influenced by an independent variable

In essence, the *experimental method* involves manipulation of one or more variables, control of other variables, and measurement of the consequences in still other variables. The manipulated variables are called the **independent variables,** while those that are measured to see the ways they have been affected are called the **dependent variables.** To see whether the independent variables cause change in the dependent variables, the experimenter uses *both an experimental group and a control group.* Measurements are taken in both groups, but the control group is not exposed to the treatment (the independent variable).

Suppose you want to set up an experiment to test the hypothesis that prejudice is increased by negative interpersonal encounters with people of other races. You get a group of white volunteers, test them on their level of prejudice, and select 20 who score about the same (that is, you control for level of prejudice). You then divide them into two groups and give each group the same brief lecture by an African American. One group is treated kindly by the lecturer, while the other group is treated in an abusive manner. Following the lecture, you again test the 20 subjects for their level of prejudice.

If the 10 who hear the abusive lecturer increase their level of prejudice while the 10 who listen to the kindly lecturer show no increase, the hypothesis is clearly supported. In practice, experiments never come out this neatly. Some people who listen to the abusive speaker will not increase their level of prejudice, and some who listen to the kindly speaker will show more prejudice afterward. In other words, factors other than just the interpersonal contact are at work. The experimenter tries to control the setting and the subjects in order to minimize the effect of these other factors.

The utility of experiments is illustrated in a study of how using a cell phone while driving affects other drivers (McGarva, Ramsey, and Shear 2006). One-third or more of all drivers use cell phones while driving, and cell phone users are more likely than others to be involved in collisions. Is it possible that using cell phones increases the amount of hostility and road rage in others when users are seen driving in ways that are frustrating or hazardous? If so, then cell phone usage while driving may be a factor in the total amount of violence in our society.

How could we find out? McGarva, Ramsey, and Shear (2006) set up two experiments to observe reactions to drivers on cell phones. In the first experiment, one of the researchers drove an older car on some two-lane roads within the city limits of a Midwestern town. The car was equipped with a hidden camera that recorded drivers behind the researcher's car. When a car approached from the rear, the researcher slowed down to 10 miles per hour less than the posted speed limit. In some cases, the researcher appeared to talk on a cell phone while driving slowly (the experimental group); in other cases, the researcher drove with both hands on the wheel (the control group).

In the second experiment, when the researcher's car was at a red light and another car was waiting behind it, the researcher's car paused approximately 15 seconds after

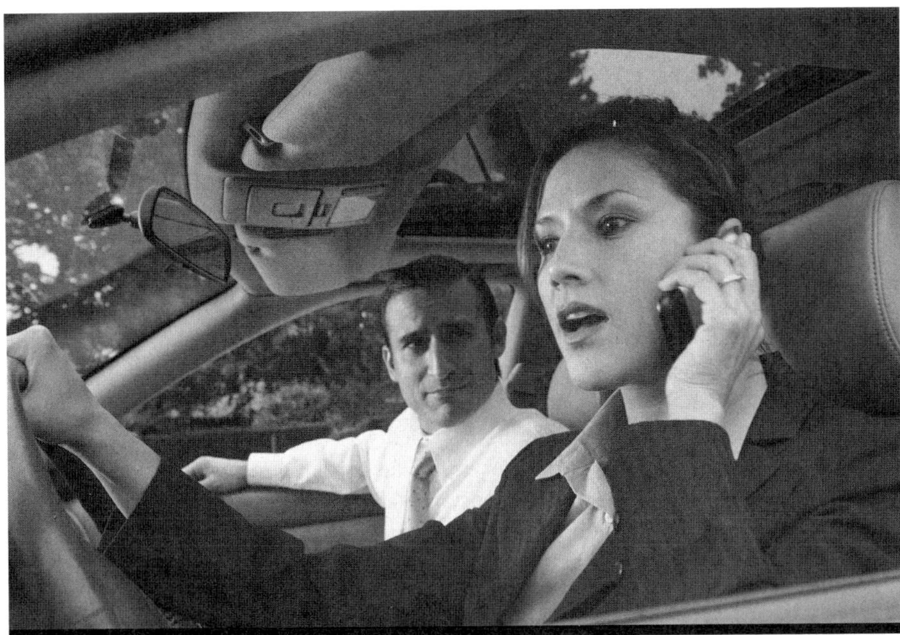

Drivers on cell phones increase the amount of roadway aggression.

David Buffington/Getty Images

the light had turned green. Again, in some cases the researcher appeared to be talking on a cell phone (the experimental group) while in other cases the researcher simply sat in the car with both hands on the wheel.

In both experiments the researchers found that when the driver appeared to be talking on a cell phone, men in other cars honked their horns more quickly and frequently than when the driver was not on a cell phone. Women in other cars tended to use their horns less, but judgments of their facial expressions concluded that they were more angry when the researcher was on a cell phone than when the researcher had both hands on the wheel.

The researchers concluded that the use of cell phones by drivers adds to the growing problem of roadway aggression. It would be useful to know whether those frustrated drivers with elevated levels of hostility act more aggressively or violently afterward. Such a question illustrates why researchers invariably point out that additional research is necessary.

## Participant Observation

**Participant observation,** the last method we consider, involves a number of elements, including interaction with subjects, participation in and observation of pertinent activities of the subjects, interviews, and use of documents and artifacts. In participant observation, the researcher directly participates in and observes the social reality being studied. The researcher is both a part of and detached from the social reality being studied.

**participant observation** a method of research in which one directly participates and observes the social reality being studied

However, there are differences in the extent to which the researcher is involved in the social reality being studied. The relative emphasis on participation versus observation, and whether the researcher reveals his or her identity to participants, are decisions that must be made (and are matters of ethical debate). For instance, if a researcher uses observation to study poverty, he or she might live in an impoverished community and pretend to be a poor person. Or the researcher might acknowledge that research is being conducted while he or she participates in community activities. The researcher might decide to participate only in selective community activities that he or she specifically wants to observe. Or the researcher could choose to be primarily an observer, watching poor children in a schoolroom behind a one-way mirror. Which will yield the best information? Which, if any, would be considered unethical? Researchers must answer such questions.

As an example of participant observation research, we looked at Gwendolyn Dordick's (2002) research into a transitional housing program for the homeless. Numerous programs exist to deal with the problem of homeless people. How effective are these programs? This question needs to be addressed in order to frame public policy and provide guidelines for private efforts to attack the problems.

Dordick pointed out that the initial emphasis on setting up emergency shelters and giving monetary assistance for housing has given way to programs that combine temporary shelter with a variety of social services. The services are designed to address the basic causes of homelessness, such as substance abuse, mental illness, and chronic unemployment. Homeless individuals or families are given temporary shelter while they take advantage of the services to deal with the cause of their homelessness. The goal is to make the homeless "housing-ready."

Dordick spent 18 months as a participant observer in On the Way, a transitional program for homeless, single, substance-abusing men. Her goals were to determine the meaning of "becoming housing-ready" and to see how effective the program was in making people housing-ready.

Dordick did not live in the home where the program was run, but she visited it nearly 100 times, spending two to six hours there each time. She joined in staff and community meetings, observed group therapeutic activities, and hung out with people in the home and in the residents' rooms. She also conducted interviews with current and past staff members and residents.

The services provided by On the Way included mental health counseling, education, job training, and training in independent living skills. Basic questions Dordick tried to answer were: How does one know when a resident is housing-ready, prepared to live on his or her own? How do the staff know when to tell a resident that he or she is ready to move on? The ability to pay rent or the eligibility for government subsidy were not among the criteria used. Rather, the staff used very subjective means such as the "quality of sobriety." A staff member found it very difficult to define precisely what he meant by quality of sobriety. He just had a sense of it from his own experience.

So how well did the program work? While Dordick was there, and during the year following her research, seven residents and two resident managers left On the Way. One secured his own apartment and another moved to a permanent subsidized housing facility. The others moved in with relatives or girlfriends. As Dordick summed it up, there was no transition to independent living for most of them. It was just a matter of substituting "one set of dependencies for another" (Dordick 2002:27).

By the use of participant observation, then, Dordick was able to evaluate the effectiveness of one program designed to help the homeless. The minimal success of this program does not mean that the homeless are hopeless. It means that we must keep searching for effective ways to help.

## Summary

You need to distinguish between personal and social problems. For the former, the causes and solutions lie within the individual and his or her immediate environment. For the latter, the causes and solutions lie outside the individual and his or her immediate environment. Defining a particular problem as personal or social is important because the definition determines the causes you identify, the consequences of the problem, and how you cope with the problem.

The model we use to analyze social problems treats them as contradictions. It emphasizes that multiple-level factors cause and help perpetuate problems. You must understand social problems in terms of the mutual influence between social structural factors, social psychological or cognitive factors, and social interaction.

In addition to attending to the multiple factors involved, two additional tools are necessary for an adequate understanding of social problems. One is to use critical thinking skills to identify fallacious ways of thinking that have been used to analyze social problems and that create and perpetuate myths about those problems. The other is to understand the methods of social research. An adequate understanding of social problems is based on research and not merely on what seems to be reasonable.

Nine different fallacies have been used to analyze social problems. The fallacy of dramatic instance refers to the tendency to overgeneralize, to use a single case or a few cases to support an entire argument. The fallacy of retrospective determinism is the argument that things could not have worked out differently. The fallacy of misplaced concreteness is the tendency to resort to reification, to make something abstract into something concrete. The fallacy of personal attack is a form of debate or argument in which an attack is made on the opponent rather than on the issues. Appeal to prejudice is the exploitation of popular prejudices or passions. Circular reasoning involves the use of conclusions supporting assumptions necessary to make those conclusions. The fallacy of authority is an illegitimate appeal to authority. The fallacy of composition is the idea that what is true of the part is also true of the whole. Finally, non sequitur is drawing the wrong conclusions from premises even though the premises themselves are valid.

Four methods of social research that are useful for understanding social problems are survey research, statistical analysis of official records, experiment, and participant observation. Survey research employs interviews and questionnaires on a sample of people in order to get data. Statistical analysis of official records may be simple (computing means, medians, and frequency distributions) or relatively complex (computing tests of significance). Experiment involves manipulation of one or more variables, control of other variables, and measurement of consequences in still other variables. Experiments frequently take place in a laboratory setting, where the researcher has a high degree of control over what happens. Finally, participant observation involves both participation and observation on the part of the researcher; the researcher is both a part of and detached from the social reality being studied.

## Key Terms

**Attitude**
**Conflict Theory**
**Contradiction**
**Critical Thinking**
**Dependent Variable**
**Fallacy of Appeal to Prejudice**
**Fallacy of Authority**
**Fallacy of Circular Reasoning**
**Fallacy of Composition**
**Fallacy of Dramatic Instance**
**Fallacy of Misplaced Concreteness**
**Fallacy of Non Sequitur**
**Fallacy of Personal Attack**
**Fallacy of Retrospective Determinism**
**Frequency Distribution**
**Ideology**
**Independent Variable**
**Institution**
**Interaction**
**Mean**
**Median**
**Norm**
**Participant Observation**
**Personal Problem**
**Reification**
**Role**
**Social Problem**
**Socioeconomic Status**
**Stratification System**
**Structural Functionalism**
**Survey**
**Symbolic Interactionism**
**Test of Significance**
**Values**
**Variables**

## Study Questions

1. Using rape or some other problem as an example, how would you distinguish between a personal and a social problem?

2. What difference does the distinction between personal and social problems make in understanding the causes and consequences of problems?
3. Define each of the concepts in the authors' model and illustrate how each can enhance understanding of social problems.
4. What is meant by "quality of life," and in what way is it a part of social problems?
5. Illustrate each of the nine fallacies of thinking by showing how each can be used to "explain" a social problem.
6. How is survey research used to study social problems?
7. In what ways are official records useful for the study of social problems?
8. How do you set up a scientific experiment to research a social problem?
9. What did participant observation teach you about a program designed to help the homeless, and how did the researcher go about being a participant observer?

## Internet Resources/ Exercises

1. Explore some of the ideas in this chapter on the following sites:

**http://www.asanet.org** The official site of the American Sociological Association. Includes press releases and other information of value to students of social problems.

**http://www.sssp1.org** Official site of the Society for the Study of Social Problems, with access to the *SSSP Newsletter.* Links to other sites relevant to social problems.

**www.davidcoon.com/soc.htm** A list of sociology sites on the Internet, including links to many sites useful in dealing with social problems.

2. The journal *Social Problems* is published by Oxford. Go to its site: **https://academic.oup.com/socpro**. Find the journal and examine the table of contents over the past year. Compare the kinds of problems dealt with in the articles with those explored in this text, with those you think are of concern to most Americans, and with those of most concern to you personally. Is the journal dealing with the issues of most concern?

3. Input the term "fallacies" into your search engine. Select a number of sites and compare their materials with those in the text. Are there other fallacies that should be included in the text? Are there fallacies that seem more appropriate than some of those described in the text for understanding social problems? In addition to those dealt with in the text, what other fallacies do you find helpful for understanding patterns of thinking?

## For Further Reading

Best, Joel. *Damned Lies and Statistics: Uncovering Numbers from the Media, Politicians, and Activists.* Berkeley: University of California Press, 2001. Discusses the various ways people use and misuse statistics as they think about and report on social problems.

Black, Beth, ed. *An A to Z of Critical Thinking.* New York: Continuum, 2012. Gives definitions and examples of more than 130 terms and concepts employed in critical thinking. Helps you to better understand the differences between such things as facts, fallacies, arguments, logic, and opinions.

Diestler, Sherry. *Becoming a Critical Thinker: A User Friendly Manual.* 4th ed. New York: Prentice-Hall, 2004. A comprehensive but accessible survey of critical thinking on controversial issues, including exercises to hone your skills.

Gilbert, Nigel, ed. *Researching Social Life.* 3rd ed. Thousand Oaks, CA: Sage, 2008. Shows how qualitative and quantitative methods can be used to research social phenomena.

Rapley, Mark. *Quality of Life Research: A Critical Introduction.* Thousand Oaks, CA: Sage, 2003. A critical introduction to the concept of quality of life and the ways in which people research it. Uses an interdisciplinary approach in its analysis.

Spiegelhalter, David. *The Art of Statistics.* New York: Pelican Books, 2019. A very readable discussion of how to understand and use statistical data.

Sribnick, Ethan G., ed. *A Legacy of Innovation: Governors and Public Policy.* Philadelphia: University of Pennsylvania Press, 2008. Explores the role of state governors vis-à-vis the federal government in addressing a number of social problems.

## References

Alonso, J., et al. 2004. "Health-related quality of life associated with chronic conditions in eight countries." *Quality of Life Research* 13:283-98.

Bell, D. 1960. *The End of Ideology.* New York: Free Press.

Brown, L. R. 2000. "Challenges of the new century." In *State of the World 2000,* ed. L. R. Brown et al., pp. 3-21. New York: W. W. Norton.

Coverdill, J. E., C. A. Lopez, and M. A. Petrie. 2011. "Race, ethnicity and the quality of life in America, 1972-2008." *Social Forces* 89:783-805.

Dordick, G. A. 2002. "Recovering from homelessness: Determining the 'quality of sobriety' in a transitional housing program." *Qualitative Sociology* 25:7-32.

Durán, M., M. Moya, and J. L. Magias. 2011. "It's his right, it's her duty: Benevolent sexism and the justification of traditional sexual roles." *Journal of Sex Research* 48:470-78.

Ekins, E. 2019. "Welfare, work, and worth national survey." Cato Institute website.

Ferriss, A. L. 2000. "The quality of life among U.S. states." *Social Indicators Research* 49 (January):1-23.

Fine, G. A. 2000. "Games and truths: Learning to construct social problems in high school debate." *Sociological Quarterly* 41 (Winter):103-23.

——. 2006. "The chaining of social problems: Solutions and unintended consequences in the age of betrayal." *Social Problems* 53:3-17.

Hawdon, J. E. 2001. "The role of presidential rhetoric in the creation of a moral panic." *Deviant Behavior* 22:419-45.

Headey, B., R. Muffels, and M. Wooden. 2008. "Money does not buy happiness: Or does it?" *Social Indicators Research* 87:65-82.

Heim, N. 1981. "Sexual behavior of castrated sex offenders." *Archives of Sexual Behavior* 10 (1):11-19.

Institute for Strategy and Competitiveness. 2020. *Social Progress Index*. Harvard Business School website.

Jacobs, D., and J. T. Carmichael. 2002. "The political sociology of the death penalty." *American Sociological Review* 67:109-31.

LaGrow, S., et al. 2011. "Determinants of the overall quality of life of older persons who have difficulty seeing." *Journal of Visual Impairment & Blindness* 105:720-30.

Lauer, R. H. 1976. "Defining social problems: Public opinion and textbook practice." *Social Problems* 24 (October):122-30.

Liu, L. 2006. "Quality of life as a social representation in China." *Social Indicators Research* 75:217-40.

Lopata, H. Z. 1984. "Social construction of social problems over time." *Social Problems* 31 (February):249-72.

Maratea, R. 2008. "The e-rise and fall of social problems: The blogosphere as a public arena." *Social Problems* 55:139-60.

Martin, E. K., C. T. Taft, and P. A. Resick. 2007. "A review of marital rape." *Aggression and Violent Behavior* 12:329-47.

McGarva, A. R., M. Ramsey, and S. A. Shear. 2006. "Effects of driver cell-phone use on driver aggression." *Journal of Social Psychology* 140:133-46.

Mezey, N. 2020. "Start spreading the news: Illuminating the effects of climate change as a social problem." *Social Problems* 67:605-15.

Mills, C. W. 1959. *The Sociological Imagination*. New York: Oxford University Press.

Polling Report. 2020. The Polling Report website.

Reinhardt, J. M., P. Meadows, and J. M. Gillette. 1952. *Social Problems and Social Policy.* New York: American Book.

Rice, R. W., M. R. Frone, and D. B. McFarlin. 1992. "Work-nonwork conflict and the perceived quality of life." *Journal of Organizational Behavior* 13 (March):155-68.

Rosenthal, J. 2006. "Precisely false vs. approximately right." *New York Times,* August 27.

Russell, D. E. H. 1982. *Rape in Marriage.* New York: Macmillan.

Ryan, W. 1971. *Blaming the Victim.* New York: Pantheon Books.

Sacco, V. F. 2003. "Black hand outrage: A constructionist analysis of an urban crime wave." *Deviant Behavior* 24:53-77.

Schmidley, D. 2003. The *Foreign-Born Population in the United States: March 2002.* Washington, DC: Government Printing Office.

Semega, J., et al. 2020. "Income and poverty in the United States: 2019." U.S. Government Publishing Office.

Somers, M. R., and F. Block. 2005. "From poverty to perversity: Ideas, markets, and institutions over 200 years of welfare debate." *American Sociological Review* 70:260–87.

Thoreau, H. D. 1968. *Walden and the Essay on Civil Disobedience.* New York: Lancer.

Tickell, C. 1992. "The quality of life: What quality? Whose life?" *Environmental Values* 1 (Spring):65–76.

Ungar, S. 1992. "The rise and (relative) decline of global warming as a social problem." *Sociological Quarterly* 33 (4):483–501.

Ventegodt, S., et al. 2005. "Global quality of life (QOL), health and ability are primarily determined by our consciousness." *Social Indicators Research* 71:87–122.

PART

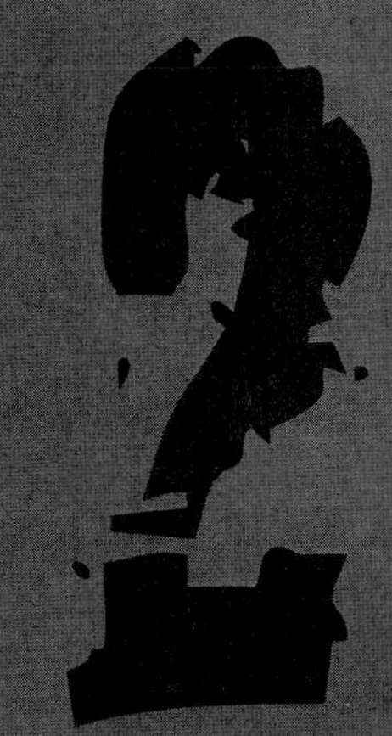

# Problems of Behavioral Deviance



Dynamic Graphics/JupiterImages

What do such actions as prostitution, drug addiction, and arson have in common? They all involve behavior that deviates from social norms. As such, most Americans view the behavior as within the individual's control and responsibility. That is, if a person engages in prostitution, uses drugs, or robs a store, it is a matter of his or her free choice. Further, because it is a choice that violates social norms, the person who engages in any kind of behavioral variance is likely to be (1) condemned and punished, (2) defined as "sick" and given therapy, or (3) both.

As you will see, the matter is not as simple as this view suggests. If, for example, you define crime as any infraction of the law—including such activities as speeding or failing to report income on tax returns—few if any Americans are innocent of crime. Like all problems discussed in this book, problems of behavioral deviance are complex issues that involve social contradictions, are defined as having adverse effects on the quality of life, and have multilevel causes.

CHAPTER

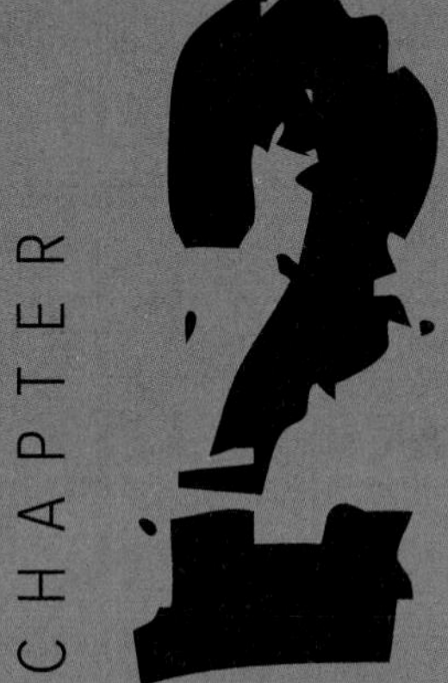

# Alcohol and Other Drugs

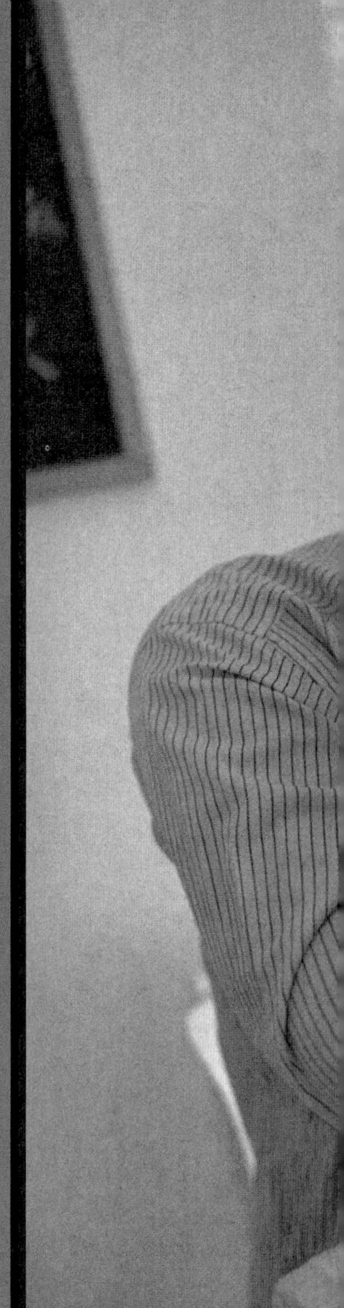

OBJECTIVES

1. Learn the types and effects of alcohol and various other drugs.
2. Identify the patterns of use in the United States.
3. Explain the personal, interpersonal, and societal consequences of the use and abuse of alcohol and other drugs.
4. Understand the varied social structural factors that facilitate and help perpetuate the problem.
5. Describe the kinds of attitudes and ideologies that underlie America's problem of alcohol and other drugs.

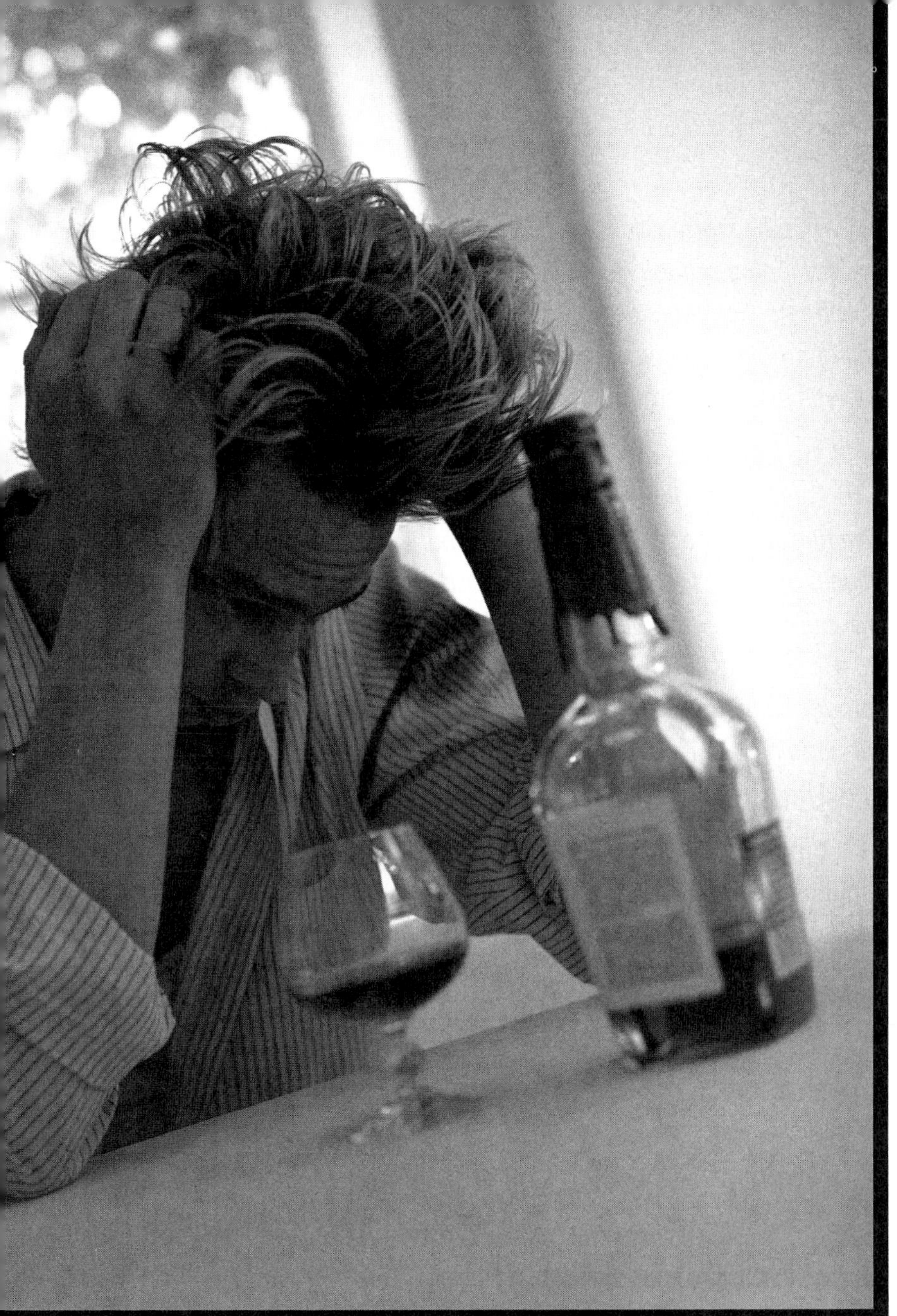
Scott T. Baxter/Getty Images

## Despair and Hope

Two voices illustrate the trauma of drug abuse. The first is a cocaine addict, a man mired in despair. The second is the parent of an alcoholic, a mother who has hope after years of despair.

- Mark, the cocaine addict, grew up in a small southern town. After two years of college, he found a good-paying job in a large city. For a while, his life seemed to be on a fast, upward track:

*But I lost it all because I got hooked on crack. I wanted to hang out with the fast people. But crack is a double-edged sword. It makes you feel great, but it tears your life apart. I was always able to meet every challenge of my life. But I can't beat this drug thing. My company paid tens of thousands of dollars to send me through two rehabilitation programs. I didn't get any better, so they fired me. I've had a heart operation, but I'm still smoking. Coke is a cruel mistress, man. She don't care who she takes from. And she doesn't give anything back.*

Mark, now homeless, is resigned to a dismal existence. In his own mind, he will never be anything other than a cocaine addict.

- Betty, the mother of an alcoholic, is also a victim of the drug problem. Her years of pain underscore the fact that it is not only the abusers who suffer destructive consequences. Her son, Curt, is sober at the present time. But Betty vividly remembers the years of abuse:

*He was only 14 when he started drinking. I don't know why. But he began avoiding us, and skipping school. He spent a lot of time alone in his room when he was at home. For years I cried for my boy. But I refused to admit that he had a drinking problem. My husband told me that Curt was getting drunk, but I insisted it was just his allergies.*

*When he was 18, he left home. You can't imagine the pain I felt. But three months later, he suddenly appeared at the kitchen door. He was dirty, hungry, and thin. I gave him some food. He stayed home, but a year later he came home drunk again and was foul-mouthed. My husband told him to go to bed, and when he sobered up he should leave our house. He did, but three months later he called. He was desperate. We got him into a short-term treatment center, then brought him home again. My husband died shortly after that. I was afraid Curt would go off on another binge, but he's stayed with me and is working now and helping support me.*

Betty is hopeful but also apprehensive about Curt's long-term prospects. Like everyone connected with a person who abuses alcohol, she can only live day by day. The grimness on her face as she tells her story powerfully expresses her uncertainty.

## Introduction

Americans have had ambivalent feelings about alcohol and other drugs throughout their history. In general, the colonists regarded alcoholic beverages as one of God's gifts to mankind. As Furnas (1965:18) noted, our forebears "clung long to the late medieval notion that alcohol deserved its splendid name, *aqua vitae*, water of life." Drunkenness was punished, but drinking was generally considered one of life's pleasures. Yet by the 19th century a growing temperance movement began urging its members to abstain from all alcoholic beverages (Furnas 1965:67).

Until the beginning of the 19th century, the use of opium and its derivatives was less offensive to Americans than smoking cigarettes or drinking. After the Civil War, however, some Americans began to warn about the dangers of **addiction.** Eventually these warnings became part of national policy, as seen in the war on drugs that began in the 1980s.

**addiction**
repeated use of a drug or alcohol to the point of periodic or chronic intoxication that is detrimental to the user or society

**abuse**
improper use of drugs or alcohol to the degree that the consequences are defined as detrimental to the user or society

This ambivalence about drugs is based partly on the distinctions among use, **abuse,** and addiction. The abuse of alcohol and other drugs, not the use, creates the problem. We define *abuse* as the *improper use of alcohol and other drugs to the degree that the consequences are defined as detrimental to the user or to society.* Addiction is a form of abuse. Addiction has been called a "brain disease" because continued abuse of a drug causes changes in brain function that drive the addict to compulsively seek and use the drug (Leshner 1998).

Not every case of abuse involves addiction. A man may not be an alcoholic, but he may get drunk and kill someone while driving his car. A woman may not be hooked on any drugs, but she may be persuaded to try LSD, have a "bad trip," and commit suicide.

Our focus in this chapter is on abuse, including addiction. We look at alcohol and other drugs, discussing their effects on users, patterns of use, effects on the quality of life, multilevel factors that create and perpetuate the problems, and ways people have attempted to cope.

## Alcohol

The use and abuse of alcohol is the nation's most serious health problem. We examine first the effects of this troublesome drug.

### Effects

All alcoholic beverages contain the same drug, ethyl alcohol or ethanol, but the proportion varies in different beverages. An individual can consume about the same amount of alcohol by drinking a pint of beer, a glass of wine, or a shot (1.5 ounces) of whiskey. What happens when that alcohol is ingested? The alcohol is burned and broken down in the body at a relatively constant rate. If an individual drinks slowly, there is little or no accumulation of alcohol in the blood; but if an individual consumes alcohol more quickly than it can be burned in the body, the *concentration of alcohol in the blood increases.*

A small amount of alcohol can result in changes in an individual's mood and behavior, and the effects become more serious as the concentration of alcohol in the blood increases (National Institute on Alcohol Abuse and Alcoholism 2019). A blood alcohol level of about 0.05 percent (one part alcohol to 2,000 parts blood) can make the individual feel a sense of release from tensions and inhibitions. This mild euphoria is the aim of many people who drink moderately. As the alcohol level increases, however, there is an increasing loss of control because alcohol acts as a depressant on brain functions. At the 0.10 percent level, the individual's motor control is affected—hands, arms, and legs become clumsy. At 0.20 percent, both the motor and the emotional functions of the brain are impaired, and the individual staggers and becomes intensely emotional. This is the level at which someone is defined as drunk.

At 0.30 percent, an individual is incapable of adequately perceiving and responding to the environment and may go into a stupor. At 0.40 or a higher percent, the individual lapses into a coma and may die.

What do these numbers mean in actual drinks? Suppose you are a 150-pound individual who drinks on an empty stomach. After drinking two bottles of beer or the equivalent (11 ounces of wine, 2 highballs, or 2 cocktails), you will feel warm and relaxed. After three bottles of beer or the equivalent, you will start experiencing more intense emotions and are likely to become talkative, noisy, or morose. Four bottles of beer or its equivalent produces clumsiness and unsteady walking and standing. At this point, you are legally drunk in most states. If you drink four bottles of beer or the equivalent on an empty stomach, it takes about eight hours for all the alcohol to leave your body.

The damaging effects of alcohol abuse are most obvious in the *alcoholic*—the individual who is addicted to alcohol. Alcoholism is defined in terms of four symptoms (National Institute on Alcohol Abuse and Alcoholism 2019): (1) a craving or compulsion to drink; (2) loss of control to limit drinking on any particular occasion; (3) physical dependence, so that withdrawal symptoms (nausea, sweating, shakiness, anxiety) are experienced if alcohol use ceases; and (4) tolerance, the need to drink increasingly greater amounts in order to get "high." Because the effects can be so deleterious and the use of alcohol is so widespread, many experts consider alcohol abuse the major drug problem in the United States today.

## Patterns of Use

**binge drinking**
having five or more drinks on the same occasion

A majority of adult Americans are drinkers. In 2019, 85.6 percent of Americans aged 18 or over reported drinking at some point in their lives, 79.5 percent reported drinking in the last year, 25.8 percent reported **binge drinking** (five or more drinks on the same occasion), and 6.3 percent reported heavy alcohol use (binge drinking on 5 or more days in the past month) (National Institute on Alcohol Abuse and Alcoholism 2019). Alcohol use varies by age, of course, but a considerable amount of drinking occurs among the young. In fact, in 2019, 4 percent of 8th-, 9 percent of 10th-, and 14 percent of 12th-grade students reported binge drinking (Forum on Child and Family Statistics 2020).

Among adults, the pervasiveness of the problem is seen in the fact that alcohol use and impairment affects 15 percent of the workforce (Frone 2006). Some drink before work and some during work. Millions work while under the influence of alcohol, and millions more work with a hangover. By their own admission, then, tens of millions of Americans have a problem with alcohol abuse.

Drinking patterns vary across different groups, though all groups are affected to some extent. American Indians probably have the highest rates of use and abuse of alcohol. Compared to the general population, they begin drinking at an earlier age, drink more frequently and in greater amounts, and have a higher alcohol-related death rate (Friese et al. 2011; Landen et al. 2014; Cole et al. 2020). Alcohol is involved in about one of every six American Indian deaths.

Among other racial/ethnic groups, whites have the highest rate of current use (56.8 percent), followed by Hispanics (43.7 percent), African Americans (41.7 percent), and Asian Americans (36.8 percent) (National Center for Health Statistics 2019).

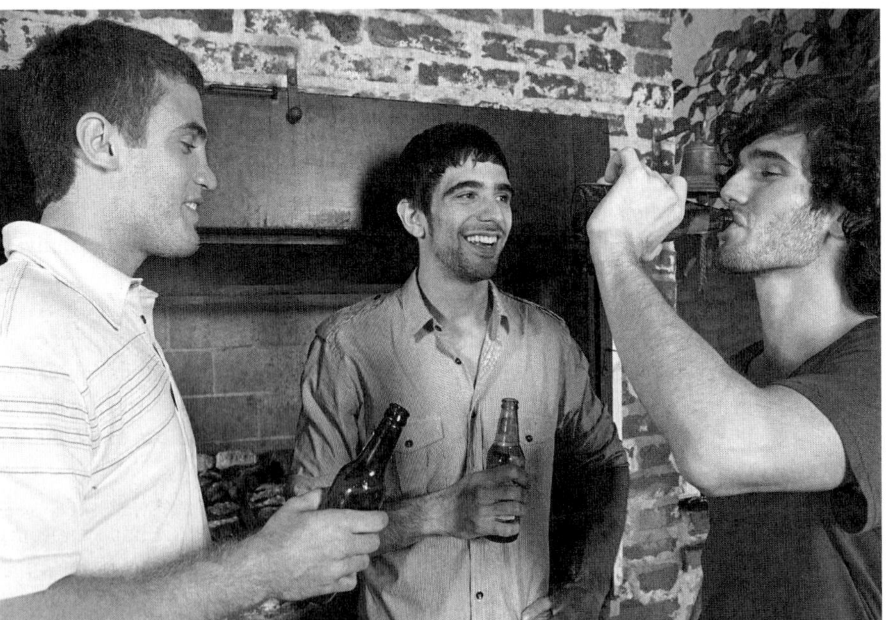

Alcohol use and abuse are more likely to take place in groups.
Image Source/Getty Images

Interestingly, the rate of drinking varies considerably among the various subgroups of Hispanics, with Mexican Americans and Puerto Ricans having much higher rates than other Hispanics and than the general population (Caetano, Ramisetty-Mikler, and Rodriguez 2008). Across all racial and ethnic groups, men drink more than women. Gender differences are decreasing, but *alcohol abuse and alcoholism are primarily male problems.*

As noted above, while alcohol abuse is more common among adults, it is a problem for younger age groups as well. A national survey reported that 15 percent of youth drank before the age of 13 (Centers for Disease Control and Prevention 2019a). A survey of college students reported that on an average day during a one-year period, 2,179 full-time college students took their first drink of alcohol (Lipari and Jean-Francois 2016). And more than a third of the students engaged in binge drinking in the past month. Binge drinkers are far more likely than others to have unprotected sex, to drive after drinking, to fall behind in school, to be aggressive, and to be involved in property damage. Interestingly, going to a four-year college is associated with higher rates of heavy drinking for whites, but with lower rates for African Americans and Hispanics (Paschall, Bersamin, and Flewelling 2005).

Alcohol abuse, then, is found in all age groups. And for the very young, it can be lethal–excessive drinking results in thousands of deaths a year among underage youth in the United States and in the fact that the earlier a child begins drinking the more likely that child is to become dependent on alcohol or other drugs and to have alcohol-related behavior problems (Roeber 2007; Hingson, Heeren, and Edwards 2008; Cheadle and Whitbeck 2011).

Thus, the skid-row image of the alcohol abuser is false. Those most likely to drink frequently and to consume higher quantities of alcohol per drinking session are young, white, male, and comparatively well-to-do (Moore et al. 2005).

## Alcohol and the Quality of Life

Alcohol, like other drugs, has some medical benefits when used in moderation. In fact, there is evidence that moderate drinkers, compared to both abstainers and heavy drinkers, have a lower rate of coronary heart disease and are less likely to have a heart attack (Mukamal and Rimm 2001). Alcohol abuse, on the other hand, is highly deleterious to the quality of life.

*Physical Health.* The physical consequences of alcohol abuse contradict the American *value of physical well-being.* As mentioned earlier, the immediate effects of intoxicating levels of alcohol include impaired motor performance. The long-range effects of abuse include more than 30 medical problems such as cirrhosis of the liver, infectious diseases, cancer, diabetes, mental health problems, cardiovascular disease, liver and pancreas disease, brain damage, gastrointestinal problems, and early death (Rehm 2011). It is estimated that alcohol abuse is responsible for 3.2 to 3.7 percent of all cancer deaths (Nelson et al. 2013). Brain damage is also common, affecting the cognitive functioning of the individual (Cairney, Clough, Jaragba, and Maruff 2007; Mukherjee, Vaidyanathan, and Vasudevan 2008). At any given time, the neuropsychological functioning of the alcoholic–as measured by such things as eye-hand coordination and spatial ability–will be equivalent to that of someone about 10 years older. In *terms of cognitive ability,* in other words, alcoholism costs the user about 10 years of life.

Heavy drinking also may result in muscle diseases and tremors. Heart functioning and the gastrointestinal and respiratory systems may be impaired by prolonged heavy drinking. Whereas moderate alcohol consumption protects the heart, heavy consumption increases the risk of strokes. The ills of the gastrointestinal system range from nausea, vomiting, and diarrhea to gastritis, ulcers, and pancreatitis. Problems of the respiratory system include lowered resistance to pneumonia and other infectious diseases. Among women, alcohol abuse can result in menstrual cycle irregularity, inability to conceive, and early onset of menopause (Gavaler 1991; Carroll, Lustyk, and Larimer 2015). Among men, alcohol can lead to sterility and erectile dysfunction (Kumsar, Kumsar, and Dilbaz 2016).

Alcohol abuse can lead to early death (Costello 2006). A study of male veterans found that the death rate among alcoholics was 2.5 times higher than that of nonalcoholics, and that alcoholics in the 35- to 44-year-old age group were 5.5 times as likely to die as were nonalcoholics of the same age (Liskow et al. 2000). Alcohol abuse is now the third leading preventable cause of death in the United States, and the problem may be increasing: from 2000 to 2018 the rate of alcohol-induced deaths increased from 10.7 per 100,000 to 15.3 per 100,000 (Spencer, Curtin, and Hedegaard 2020).

Alcohol plays a role in various kinds of physical trauma. Consider the following (Rivara et al. 1997; Greenfeld 1998; Males 2010; Fierro, Morales, and Alvarez 2011; Terry-McElrath, O'Malley, and Johnston 2014):

Alcohol use is associated with an increased risk of injury and violent death (suicide or homicide) in the home.

About 35 percent of violent victimizations involve an offender who had been drinking.

Two-thirds of the victims of intimate violence report that alcohol was a factor in the attack.

Intoxicated drivers are more prone to road rage, are involved in nearly a third of all fatal accidents, and are the sixth leading cause of death for teenagers.

Alcohol also affects the unborn children of women who drink. The most severe cases are those of *fetal alcohol syndrome* (Burd, Cotsonas-Hassler, Martsolf, and Kerbeshian 2003). The health problems of children born with fetal alcohol syndrome are head and face deformities; major organ problems that result in heart defects, ear infections, hearing loss, poor eyesight, and bad teeth; and problems with the central nervous system, leading to such problems as mental retardation, hyperactivity, stunted growth, learning disorders, epilepsy, and cerebral palsy (Streissguth 1992; Aronson and Hagberg 1998; Burd et al. 2003).

Alcohol abuse generally, and the fetal alcohol syndrome in particular, illustrate an important point–social problems have consequences at the community level as well as the individual level. In a real sense, a community can become the victim of a problem, for social problems can strain the community's resources and deprive it of the positive contributions that could otherwise be made by people caught up in the problems.

This point is dramatized in American Indian communities (Parker et al. 2010). Alcohol is a factor in about one out of every six American Indian deaths. A study of the fetal alcohol syndrome among American Indians pointed out some of the consequences, including an overload on community institutions (such as sheltered care), dramatic increases in health care costs, and problems of adoption and foster home placement (May 1991). Add to those costs the loss to the community of positive contributions that could be made by those who are abusing alcohol or those suffering from fetal alcohol syndrome. Thus, the community at large, as well as individuals, suffers.

*Psychological Health.* The *desire for psychological well-being* is contradicted by the various degrees of impairment that result from alcohol abuse. Even a small amount of alcohol can reduce the individual's sensitivity to taste, smell, and pain. Vision can be affected by large amounts of alcohol (one factor in the dangers of driving while drinking). Continued heavy use of alcohol is associated with major depression and with impaired cognitive functions such as memory and visuospatial ability (Schuckit, Smith, and

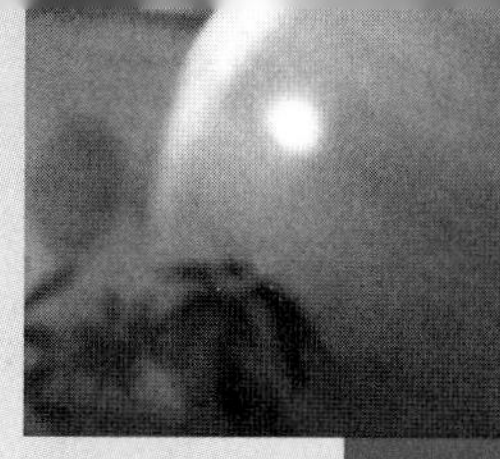

global comparison

## ALCOHOLISM IN EASTERN EUROPE

In the 10th century, a Slavic prince noted that drink was the joy of the people. "We cannot live without it," he asserted. Time appears to have borne out his observation. Slavs and other Eastern European people drink, on average, far more than Americans and have high rates of alcoholism. The problem worsened considerably after the breakup of communism began in 1989.

A World Health Organization survey found that worldwide the consumption of alcohol was about 6.13 liters per person per year aged 15 years and older. The amount for the United States was 9.44 liters. But in Eastern Europe, consumption levels ranged from a low of 12.4 liters for Bulgaria to 15.8 liters for Russia. In other words, Eastern European people drink double or more the worldwide average. Russians purchase 250 million cases of vodka a year. This is three times the amount sold in all the rest of the world and more than the total amount of hard liquor sold in the United States.

It is not surprising, then, that the average life span for Russian men is only 58. Nor that Russia has about 8 million alcoholics; the rate is more than double that of the United States.

Other Eastern European nations face similar problems with alcoholism and consequent health problems and premature death. In Poland, the annual per capita consumption of pure alcohol is around 3 gallons, a figure twice as high as the 1987 rate. In Hungary, cirrhosis of the liver is the leading cause of death of men aged 36 to 60. The number of alcoholics in Hungary doubled from 1989 to 1992.

Why do the Eastern Europeans drink so heavily? There is no simple answer. During the communist era, it was popular to blame alcoholism on the repressiveness of the regimes. But as we just noted, alcoholism increased rapidly after the breakdown of communism.

A number of factors seem to be at work. In the new market economies, alcohol is much cheaper than it was under communism. In the mid-1980s, the average Polish worker's monthly salary could buy 11 liters of vodka. By the mid-1990s, it could buy 35 liters! In the transition to capitalism, Eastern Europeans have also faced high rates of unemployment and considerable insecurity about the future, conditions that tend to breed higher rates of alcohol abuse. Finally, the Eastern Europeans have a long tradition—stretching back hundreds of years—of heavy drinking. The combination of all these factors has created the highest rates of alcoholism in the world.

SOURCES

*Chicago Tribune*, April 23, 1995; U.S. News & World Report, April 15, 1996; McKee and Shkolnikov 2001; Mackenbach et al. 2008; World Health Organization 2011.

Kalmijn 2013; Nguyen-Louie et al. 2015; Caetano, Vaeth, and Canino 2019). Such problems occur because alcohol adversely affects the brain. In the alcoholic, the adverse effects are severe (National Institute on Alcohol Abuse and Alcoholism 2019; Vanheusden et al. 2008). At least half of all alcoholics have difficulty with problem solving, abstract thinking, memory tasks, and psychomotor performance. Severe alcoholics may succumb to *alcohol amnestic disorder* (short-term memory impairments) or *dementia* (general loss of intellectual abilities, impaired memory, and possible personality change). Some alcohol abusers take the final solution to their despair: Alcohol abuse is associated with a substantial proportion of suicides (Roy 2003; Mann et al. 2006).

One popular belief is that alcohol "releases inhibitions," so that the person who drinks "loosens up" and may, for example, be more motivated toward sexual activity. Actually, heavy drinking inhibits sexual performance, and alcoholics report a deficient sex life or even impotence (Peugh and Belenko 2001). Another belief is that a drink in the evening helps the individual to relax and thereby to sleep better. Whatever the value of one drink, having several drinks before going to sleep decreases the amount of dreaming, which can impair concentration and memory and increase anxiety, irritability, and a sense of tiredness.

*Interpersonal Problems.* Alcohol abuse leads to *problems of interaction* both within and outside the family. Pregnant women who drink put their unborn children at risk even if they

## "I'D KILL BEFORE I'D DRINK"

We once attended a meeting of Alcoholics Anonymous with a friend who had been "dry" for a short time. As we drove through the countryside to the small town where the group met, the friend kept commenting on the beauty of the scenery. He was enchanted by what we thought was a fairly common view on a warm spring evening. But his years as an alcoholic had been a living hell, and in the course of rediscovering what life can be like when you are free of addiction, he was finding beauty in the commonplace. "I really think," he told us, "that if someone tried to force me to take a drink I would kill them." The thought of ever returning to alcohol terrified him.

One of the best ways to understand the impact of addiction on an individual is to talk with an ex-addict. If you do not know an ex-alcoholic, contact Alcoholics Anonymous and attend one of their open meetings. Ask one or two members if they would be willing to discuss their understanding of why they became addicted, what their life was like when they were addicted, and what finally led them to seek the help of AA.

List the adverse effects on the quality of life discussed in this chapter that apply to your informants. Based on your interviews, make a report, oral or written, of your recommendations for dealing with the problem of alcoholism.

do not drink heavily enough to induce fetal alcohol syndrome. In a small study, children aged 10–18 who were exposed prenatally to alcohol had lower levels of moral maturity and higher rates of delinquency than those not exposed (Schonfeld, Mattson, and Riley 2005).

Early use of alcohol by children is associated with an increased risk of violence in young adulthood (Green, Doherty, Zebrak, and Ensminger 2011). It is also associated with early sexual activity, with all its potential hazards, including pregnancy and disease (Phillips-Howard et al. 2010). Alcoholic husbands are more likely to have an extramarital affair and to engage in risky sexual behavior (not using condoms) than are nonalcoholic husbands (Hall, Fals-Stewart, and Fincham 2008). Marriages in which one spouse has alcohol abuse disorder are more prone to break up (Crawford 2014). Adult alcoholics have poorer relationships generally with friends, coworkers, spouses, and children (McFarlin, Fals-Stewart, Major, and Justice 2001). Alcohol is associated with aggressive behavior, which leads to ill will and conflict with others (Harford, Wechsler, and Muthen 2003; Graham, Osgood, Wells, and Stockwell 2006; Duke et al. 2011). This aggression may result in a severe form of violence against acquaintances or dates or family members (Xue, Zimmerman, and Cunningham 2009; Rothman et al. 2011). Homes in which one or both spouses abuse alcohol have higher rates of both verbal and physical abuse (Stuart, Moore, Ramsey, and Kahler 2003, 2004; Snow et al. 2006). A comparative study of alcohol and homicide in Russia and the United States concluded that 73 percent of the homicides in Russia and 57 percent of those in the United States involve the use of alcohol (Landberg and Norstrom 2011).

Even if an alcoholic does not become abusive, his or her behavior is certain to cause stress within the family. Mates and children of alcoholics tend to develop physical and psychological problems of their own (Tempier et al. 2006; Keller et al. 2011). Children tend to develop behavior disorders (Haber et al. 2010). And compared to those from nonalcoholic homes, the children of alcohol abusers are more likely to have poorer self-concepts, higher rates of drug use, and higher rates of anxiety, depression, alcoholism, and other disorders when they become adults, as well as lower rates of marriage and of marital quality when they do marry (Obot, Wagner, and Anthony 2001; Watt 2002; Osborne and Berger 2009). The intensity of the stress in an alcoholic home is illustrated by the widow who declared herself to be the happiest person alive because her husband had finally drunk himself to death and thereby set her and her children free.

*Economic Costs.* Alcohol abuse is costly to the nation. A study of underage drinking alone put the cost higher than the price of the drink (Miller, Levy, Spicer, and Taylor 2006). In one year, underage drinking resulted in 3,170 deaths and 2.6 million other harmful events, costing around $61.9 billion in medical expenses, work loss, and lost quality of life.

Overall, the cost of alcohol abuse is more than $250 billion (National Institute on Drug Abuse 2020). The costs include the expenses of the arrest, trial, and imprisonment of people who are drunk (in some cities, more than half of all arrests are for drunkenness). They include business losses: People with drinking problems are absent from work about two and a half times as often as others. Moreover, when they are on the job, they may have problems of interaction. Costs to industry are as much as $10 billion a year because of lost work time and lowered productivity of alcoholic employees. All these costs represent resources that could be channeled into activities and programs to enhance the nation's quality of life.

## Contributing Factors

The factors that contribute to the alcohol problem both maintain demand and guarantee supply. The problem is embedded in the American way of life.

*Social Structural Factors.* Being a part of a *group whose norms and behavior condone drinking* is the most powerful predictor of an individual's drinking (Simons-Morton et al. 2016; Hamilton and Dehart 2019). Males, in fact, use alcohol to bond with each other and to enhance their sense of importance and power (Liu and Kaplan 1996). Some groups establish a tradition of periodic heavy drinking. For example, about half of those people who drink and attend fraternity or sorority parties engage in heavy drinking in those settings (Harford, Wechsler, and Seibring 2002). Off-campus parties and bars are also settings in which heavy drinking takes place among college students. The hazards of such drinking go beyond any immediate effects. A national study of college and university students found that those who were drunk prior to the age of 19 were significantly more likely than others to become alcohol dependent and frequent heavy drinkers, to report that they drove after drinking, and to sustain injuries requiring medical attention after drinking (Hingson et al. 2003).

Integration into a group in which the use of alcohol is approved does not mean the individual will abuse it. Many people use alcohol without becoming addicted. A lower rate of alcoholism is correlated with the following characteristics (National Institute on Alcohol Abuse and Alcoholism 2019):

1. Children are given alcohol early in life in the context of strong family life or religious orientation.
2. Low-alcohol-content beverages–wines and beers–are most commonly used.
3. The alcoholic beverage is ordinarily consumed at meals.
4. Parents typically provide an example of moderation in drinking.
5. Drinking is not a moral question, merely one of custom.
6. Drinking is not defined as a symbol of manhood or adulthood.
7. Abstinence is as acceptable as drinking.
8. Drunkenness is not socially acceptable.
9. Alcohol is not a central element in activities (like a cocktail party).
10. There is general agreement on what is proper and what is improper in drinking.

Under such conditions, a group or an entire society could have high per capita rates of alcohol consumption and relatively low rates of alcoholism. Group norms are an important factor in alcohol use and abuse, but they need not demand abstinence to prevent abuse. Both Jews and Italians in the United States use alcohol as part of a traditional way of life, but alcoholism in those groups is extremely low. The norms of many religious groups also make abuse less likely. Thus, active participation in religion is associated with lower levels of drinking (Bjarnason et al. 2005; Jessor, Costa, Krueger, and Turbin 2006).

*Role problems* that generate emotional distress can lead to alcohol abuse (Holahan et al. 2001; Lemke, Brennan, Schutte, and Moos 2007). People trying to cope with role conflict may resort to alcohol for relief. Those under stress at school or work and those who believe that alcohol relieves stress are more likely to drink (Park, Armeli, and Tennen 2004; Crosnoe 2006). Undesirable role changes also may lead to alcohol abuse. A major loss (for example, divorce or death of a spouse) or separation can result in alcohol abuse, particularly for men. The stress resulting from financial strain, from poverty, or from unfair treatment because one is a member of a minority group can also lead to alcohol abuse (Mulia, Ye, Zemore, and Greenfield 2008; Shaw, Agahi, and Krause 2011). Whether from poverty or racial/ethnic identity or both, those who are severely disadvantaged have a two to six times greater risk of having alcohol problems.

Three kinds of *family experiences* are involved in alcohol abuse. First, abuse is more likely when the individual grows up in a family where there is a history of alcoholism or where there is poor marital quality or violence between the parents (Warner, White, and Johnson 2007; Bossarte and Swahn 2008; Hair et al. 2009). Second, alcohol abusers are more likely to come from *broken homes* (Wolfinger 1998; Bjarnason et al. 2003). Third, alcohol abuse is associated with various *problematic relationships within the family*, including dysfunctional marriages and troubled parent-child relationships (Silberg, Rutter, D'Onofrio, and Eaves 2003; Whisman, Uebelacker, and Bruce 2006; Hoffmann and Bahr 2014). Problem drinking among adolescents is associated with homes in which the parents express hostility to the adolescents or in which there is severe family conflict (Conger et al. 1991; Smith, Rivers, and Stahl 1992).

The *mass media also contribute to alcohol abuse*. Researchers who examined 601 popular movies found that 92 percent depicted drinking (Sargent et al. 2006). The researchers surveyed thousands of adolescents to determine the relationship between watching movies and drinking. There was an association between higher exposure to movie alcohol use and drinking by the adolescents. The researchers concluded that exposure to movie alcohol use is a risk factor for early-onset teen drinking. Similarly, television programs show a great deal of drinking with no negative consequences; adolescent viewers of such drinking are more likely to drink themselves (Pinkleton, Fujioka, and Austin 2000). A survey of alcohol advertising on radio showed that nearly half of the ads were placed in programs for which the local audience was disproportionately underage youth, thus adding yet another influence of the media on underage drinking (Centers for Disease Control and Prevention 2006). Additionally, a study of problem drinking among Black women found higher rates of abuse among women who lived in an area where they were exposed to outdoor alcohol advertising (Kwate and Meyer 2009). And a survey of middle-school youth reported an average of two to four ads a day on their handheld computers, putting the students at risk for earlier or more frequent drinking (Collins et al. 2016).

Finally, any social structural factors that increase stress levels are likely to increase the prevalence of alcohol abuse (Young-Wolff, Kendler, and Prescott 2012; Jones-Webb et al. 2016). In the United States, a *rapidly changing structure* has been associated with increased alcoholism. Both the high rate around 1830 and the increased consumption in the 1960s and 1970s have been associated with stresses induced by a rapidly changing society (Rorabaugh 1979). Another source of stress is a sense of *powerlessness*. You are not comfortable when you feel powerless. Yet the world situation, national problems, your work, and other organizations with which you are involved may induce a sense of powerlessness. If you feel powerless, you are more likely to drink heavily and to have a drinking problem (Seeman, Seeman, and Budros 1988).

*Social Psychological Factors.* *Attitudes* toward drinking and drunkenness tend to be different from attitudes toward use and abuse of other drugs. Although alcoholism is a major factor in death and disease, there is little public outcry. Parents who would be horrified to find their children smoking marijuana have allowed them to drink spiked punch or other alcoholic beverages at parties.

The importance of attitudes is underscored by the fact that heavy drinkers have more positive and more indulgent attitudes about the use of alcohol. They are likely to believe that their drinking is no different from that of others in the groups to which they belong and that their own drinking is not enough to be called a problem (Wild 2002). For example, a large proportion of college students overestimate the amount of drinking by their peers (Pedersen and LaBrie 2008; Lewis et al. 2011). And their misperceptions are strongly related to the amount of alcohol they consume: They drink as heavily as they believe that others are drinking. In addition, some male college students associate heavy drinking with masculinity (Wells et al. 2014). In other words, the masculine image they want for themselves is affirmed when they engage in heavy drinking.

The problem of alcoholism is further complicated by ideologies—by *the ideology that transforms it into a personal rather than a social problem, and the campus ideology that heavy drinking at parties is both acceptable and the way to maximize one's fun*. Many Americans believe that the alcoholic can recover if he or she "really wants to change"—that alcoholism is basically a problem of individual self-control. And many students believe that heavy drinking, drinking contests, and hangovers are all legitimate ways to maximize their pleasure and prove their mettle.

## Solutions: Public Policy and Private Action

Instead of asking what can be done for an alcoholic, you need to ask first what kind of alcoholic you are dealing with. Experts are attempting to sort out the special needs of the alcoholic with psychiatric problems, the chronically relapsing alcoholic, the alcoholic's family members who may be both victims of and contributors to the problem, and addicted adolescents and women. Special programs are being developed for these special needs.

Whatever the special needs may be, of course, the alcoholic is likely to need one or more of the following: *individual therapy, drug therapy, behavior therapy,* or *group therapy*. Drug therapies involve administration of either a nausea-producing agent along with an alcoholic beverage or a "deterrent agent" that causes intense headaches and nausea when alcohol is consumed. Obviously, drug therapy requires close supervision by a physician.

In group therapy, the alcoholic is in a group with other alcoholics and with a therapist as facilitator. The task of the group members is to attain insight into their individual reasons for drinking and to get control over drinking. A form of group therapy that is quite successful and does not utilize a professional therapist is Alcoholics Anonymous (AA), which was started by alcoholics. Members gather regularly in small groups to share their experiences and to sustain each other in sobriety. Each member is available to every other member at any time help is needed—when, for example, a member needs to talk to someone in order to resist the urge to drink. Those who join AA begin by admitting they are powerless over alcohol and lack control of their own lives. This admission is significant because it opposes the ideology discussed earlier (an ideology, incidentally, held by alcoholics as well as by others). New members also agree to surrender to a Higher Power (as they understand it), to make amends to those harmed by their drinking, and to help other alcoholics become sober.

Millions of alcoholics have sought help through AA, which is still one of the most effective ways to deal with alcoholism (Connors, Tonigan, and Miller 2001; McKellar, Stewart, and Humphreys 2003; Moos and Moos 2004). Of course, not everyone who comes to AA will break the habit; no form of help can claim a 100 percent success rate. The extent to which a particular form of help will succeed depends on, among other things, factors in the social background of the individual seeking help. For instance, a study of adolescent problem drinkers found that those with a background of religious participation found it easier to integrate into the AA program than did those with little or no religiosity (Kelly, Pagano, Stout, and Johnson 2011).

Two spin-offs of AA that are designed to help family members of the alcoholic are Al-Anon and Alateen. Al-Anon is for the alcoholic's spouse or significant other. It helps the person both to deal with the problems caused by the alcoholic and to see his or her own contribution to the interpersonal problems that may be a factor in the alcoholism. Members of Al-Anon learn to take care of their own needs and to stop focusing their lives around the alcoholic's problems. Alateen uses the same principles to help the teenaged children of alcoholics. Frequently, the sponsor of an Alateen group is a member of Al-Anon.

Behavior therapy is based on the principle of rewarding desired behavior in order to reinforce behavior. The reward can be quite simple, such as the pins given at Alcoholics Anonymous meetings to recognize extended periods of sobriety. Or the rewards can be more substantial, such as the vouchers or tokens given by some therapists for each week or month of sobriety; these vouchers or tokens can be exchanged for various kinds of retail goods or entertainment (gift certificates for stores, restaurants, etc.). The use of vouchers or tokens is a form of behavior contracting (also called contingency contracting or contingency management), which is more effective than methods designed to educate, confront, or shock the alcoholic (Miller and Wilbourne 2002).

A somewhat recent trend is so-called brief therapy. Rather than attending therapy sessions over an extended period of time, the alcohol abuser has only a few sessions with a therapist. At a minimum, brief therapy with alcohol abusers involves a 15-minute initial contact and at least one follow-up. A survey of research studies done of brief behavioral interventions for risky and harmful alcohol use reported that 12 months after the counseling, the clients had reduced their average number of drinks per week 13 to 34 percent more than those who did not have the therapy (Whitlock et al. 2004). During counseling, the patient receives an assessment of his or her health status, advice, help in goal setting, a motivational message, and other kinds of help.

The problem of alcoholism also has been attacked through various other programs and facilities. Among these are community care programs, which allow alcoholics to remain in their homes and communities while undergoing treatment. Other programs remove alcoholics from their environments. Throughout the nation, there are hundreds of *halfway* houses for alcoholics, places where they can function in a relatively normal way while receiving therapy. Most of these locations have Alcoholics Anonymous groups, counseling, and other services available to the alcoholics. Alcoholics who are acutely ill may have to be hospitalized for a period of time before going to a halfway house or returning to their homes.

Ultimately, to resolve the problem, the social bases of alcoholism must be attacked through public policy. As with other drugs, *enforcement as well as prevention and education programs* are needed. Research has shown that raising the minimum legal drinking age to 21, increasing alcohol taxes, and intensifying the enforcement of drinking-and-driving laws all reduce the number of alcohol problems (Hollingworth et al. 2006; Fell et al. 2016).

Prevention and education programs face difficulty because group norms and alternative means of coping with stress are involved. Nevertheless, there is evidence that educational programs can help reduce the negative effects of alcohol (Flynn and Brown 1991).

Educational programs must help people understand not only the dangers of alcohol but also ways they can deal with the pressure to drink. For instance, adolescents, who are most likely to give in to peer pressure, can resist drinking even in high-pressure situations by using a number of cognitive and behavioral techniques. These techniques include defining themselves as nondrinkers and defining drinkers in negative terms (e.g., drinkers are weak), developing strong refusal skills, finding alternative activities (such as volunteering or religious activities), and limiting direct exposure to high-risk situations (such as not going to a party at which heavy drinking will occur and may even be expected) (Weitzman and Kawachi 2000; Brown, Parks, Zimmerman, and Phillips 2001; Guo, Hawkins, Hill, and Abbott 2001; Grekin, Sher, and Krull 2007; Wallace et al. 2007).

Finally, both informal and formal measures can be taken to help those victimized by alcohol-impaired driving and to ameliorate or prevent further victimization. At an informal level, peer intervention—trying to stop a friend or acquaintance from driving drunk—has been shown to be effective in the bulk of cases (Collins and Frey 1992).

At a formal level, campaigns against alcohol-impaired drivers began in the 1980s when a California woman founded Mothers Against Drunk Drivers (MADD). She took action after her teenaged daughter was killed by a man who was not only drunk but out on bail from a hit-and-run arrest for drunken driving just two days prior to the accident. Within two years, the group had chapters in more than 20 states. Other groups formed as well—Students Against Driving Drunk (SADD) and Remove Intoxicated Drivers (RID). As a result of the work of these organizations, a number of states have taken measures to reduce the risks to citizens from alcohol-impaired drivers, including raising the drinking age, using roadside sobriety tests, and suspending licenses of offenders. In some states, a driver with a blood alcohol content of more than 0.10 automatically loses his or her license for 90 days, regardless of the outcome of the court case. As a result of these varied formal and informal measures, the proportion of fatal crashes that were alcohol-related declined from 60 percent of all fatal crashes in 1982 to 41 percent in 2006 (Maguire 2012).

*Follow-Up.* Has anyone close to you—a family member or friend—ever had a problem with alcohol? How did it affect the person's behavior and relationship with you? Describe any efforts or programs that didn't help, and any that did.

## Other Drugs

Although alcohol abuse is the major drug problem, the use and abuse of other drugs affect nearly all Americans directly or indirectly. We begin our examination of the problem by looking at the different kinds of drugs and their effects.

### Types and Effects

Seven main types of nonalcoholic drugs and some of their possible effects are summarized in Figure 2.1. We should note that these do not include all drugs, only some of

**FIGURE 2.1**
Some Commonly Abused Drugs and Their Effects

| Category and Name | Commercial and Street Names | *Intoxication Effects/* Potential Health Consequences |
|---|---|---|
| **Cannabinoids** | | *Euphoria; slowed thinking and reaction time; confusion; impaired balance and coordination/* cough, frequent respiratory infections; impaired memory and learning; increased heart rate, anxiety; panic attacks; addiction. |
| Hashish | Boom, chronic, hash, hemp, gangster | |
| Marijuana | Dope, grass, joints, pot, weed, blunt, ganja, mary jane | |
| **Depressants** | | *Reduced anxiety; feeling of well-being; lowered inhibitions; slowed pulse and breathing; lowered blood pressure; poor concentration/* fatigue; confusion; impaired coordination, memory, judgment; addiction; respiratory depression and arrest; death.<br><br>*Also, for barbiturates—sedation, drowsiness/* depression; unusual excitement; fever; irritability; slurred speech; dizziness; life-threatening withdrawal.<br><br>*For benzodiazepines—sedation, drowsiness/ dizziness.*<br><br>*For flunitrazepam*—visual and gastrointestinal disturbances; urinary retention; memory loss for the time under the drug's effects. |
| Barbiturates | Amytal, Seconal, Phenobarbital; barbs, reds, yellows, yellow jackets | |
| Benzodiazepines | Ativan, Librium, Valium, Xanax; candy, downers, tranks | |
| Flunitrazepam* | Rohypnol; Mexican valium, R2, roofies, rope | |

**FIGURE 2.1**
Continued

| Category and Name | Commercial and Street Names | *Intoxication Effects/* Potential Health Consequences |
|---|---|---|
| **Hallucinogens** | | *Altered states of perception and feeling; nausea/*persisting perception disorder (flashbacks). |
| LSD | Lysergic acid diethylamide; acid, boomers, cubes, yellow sunshines, blue heaven | *Also, for LSD and mescaline*—increased body temperature, heart rate, blood pressure; loss of appetite; sleeplessness; numbness; weakness; tremors. |
| Mescaline | Buttons, cactus, mesc, peyote | *For LSD*—persistent mental disorders. |
| Psilocybin | Magic mushroom, purple passion, shrooms | *For psilocybin*—nervousness; paranoia. |
| **Opioids and Morphine Derivatives** | | *Pain relief; euphoria; drowsiness/*constipation; confusion; sedation; respiratory depression and arrest; addiction; unconsciousness; coma; death. |
| Codeine | Empirin with Codeine, Robitussin A-C; Cody, schoolboy | |
| Heroin | Diacetylmorphine; brown sugar, dope, H, smack, skunk | *Also, for heroin—staggering gait.* |
| Morphine | Rosanol; M, miss emma, monkey | |
| Oxycodone HCl | Oxy, O.C., killer | |
| Hydrocodone bitartrate | Vicodin; vike | |
| **Stimulants** | | *Increased heart rate, blood pressure, metabolism; feelings of exhilaration, energy,* |

(*continued*)

**FIGURE 2.1**
Continued

| Category and Name | Commercial and Street Names | *Intoxication Effects/* Potential Health Consequences |
|---|---|---|
| Amphetamine | Dexedrine; bennies, black beauties, speed, uppers, crosses, hearts | *increased mental alertness*/rapid or irregular heart beat; reduced appetite; weight loss; heart failure; nervousness; insomnia. |
| Cocaine | Cocaine hydrochloride; blow, bump, C, candy, coke, crack, snow, charlie, rock | *Also, for amphetamine—rapid breathing*/tremor; loss of coordination; irritability; anxiousness; restlessness; delirium; panic; paranoia; impulsive behavior; aggressiveness; addiction; psychosis. |
| MDMA (methylenedioxy-methamphetamine) | Adam, clarity, ecstasy, Eve, lover's speed, molly, X, XTC | |
| Methamphetamine | Desoxyn; chalk, crank, crystal, glass, ice, speed | *For cocaine—increased temperature*/chest pain; respiratory failure; nausea; abdominal pain; strokes; seizures; headaches; malnutrition; panic attacks. |
| Methylphenidate | Ritalin; JIF, R-ball, skippy, the smart drug | *For MDMA—mild hallucinogenic effects; increased tactile sensitivity; empathic feelings*/impaired memory and learning; hyperthermia; cardiac toxicity; renal failure; liver toxicity. |
| Nicotine | Cigarettes, cigars, smokeless tobacco, snuff, chew | *For methamphetamine—aggression, violence, psychotic behavior*/memory loss; cardiac and neurological damage; impaired memory and learning; addiction. |
| | | *For nicotine*—adverse pregnancy outcomes; chronic lung disease; cardiovascular disease; stroke; cancer; addiction. |

FIGURE 2.1
Continued

| Category and Name | Commercial and Street Names | Intoxication Effects/ Potential Health Consequences |
|---|---|---|
| **Other Compounds** | | *For anabolic steroids—no intoxication effects/* hypertension; blood clotting and cholesterol changes; liver and kidney cancer; hostility and aggression; in males, prostate cancer, reduced sperm production, shrunken testicles, breast enlargement; in females, menstrual irregularities, development of masculine characteristics (e.g., a beard). |
| Anabolic steroids | Anadrol, Oxandrin, Equipoise; roids, juice | |
| Inhalants | Solvents (paint thinners, gasoline, glues), gases (butane, propane, aerosol propellants); laughing gas, poppers, snappers | *For inhalants—stimulation; loss of inhibition/*headache; nausea or vomiting; slurred speech; loss of motor coordination; wheezing; unconsciousness; cramps; weight loss; muscle weakness; depression; memory impairment; damage to cardiovascular and nervous systems; sudden death. |

*A rape drug, associated with sexual assaults.
SOURCE: National Institute on Drug Abuse, "Commonly Abused Drugs," NIDA website, 2006 and 2012.

those that are more commonly abused. New *designer drugs* continue to appear, some of which are performance-enhancing drugs for athletes. In addition, **psychotherapeutic drugs** have become an important source of abuse. Psychotherapeutic drugs are prescription drugs—pain relievers, tranquilizers, stimulants, and sedatives—that are used for their intoxication effects rather than for medical purposes.

**psychotherapeutic drugs** prescription drugs, including pain relievers, tranquilizers, stimulants, and sedatives, that are used for intoxication effects rather than medical purposes

For some drugs, the intoxication effects vary depending on the chemical composition, the amount taken, the method of administration, and the social situation in which the drug is administered. In other words, you need to know more than the physiological effects of a drug to understand the experience of the individual taking it.

There are no intrinsic and automatic effects of a particular drug on every individual who takes it. Rather, the *effects vary according to how they are defined* (Becker 1953). A famous experiment by Schachter and Singer (1962) found that individuals who have a physiological experience for which there is no immediate explanation (e.g., you find your heart racing but don't know why) will *label the experience* with whatever information is available. Thus, one person may label a sensation as joy, while another labels the same sensation as anger or fear.

**placebo**
any substance having no physiological effect that is given to a subject who believes it to be a drug that does have an effect

In this experiment, some students received an injection of the hormone epinephrine, and others received a **placebo.** Among the physiological effects of epinephrine are palpitation, tremor, and sometimes accelerated breathing and the feeling of being flushed. All the students were told they had received the drug in order to determine its effects on their vision. Some were given no information on any side effects, some were correctly informed of those effects, and others were misinformed about the effects. While waiting for the effects, each student was sent to a room where a student who was an accomplice of the experimenter created a situation of euphoria for some of the students and of anger for others. Students who had been injected with epinephrine and who had received either no information or misinformation about side effects "gave behavioral and self-report indications that they had been readily manipulable into the disparate feeling states of euphoria and anger" (Schachter and Singer 1962:395).

Similarly, based on 50 interviews, Becker (1953) found that *defining the effects of marijuana as pleasurable is a learning process.* First, the person must learn the technique of smoking marijuana. Then he or she must learn what the effects of the drug are and learn to associate those effects with its use. For example, if intense hunger is an effect, the user must learn to define that hunger as a sign of being high. Finally, the person must learn to define the effects as pleasurable rather than undesirable. Effects such as dizziness, thirst, and tingling of the scalp can be defined as undesirable or as symptoms of illness. Yet by interacting with others who define those effects as desirable, the user can learn to define them as desirable.

Legal drugs can harm or kill you just as effectively as illicit ones. In addition to alcohol, tobacco is one of the deadliest drugs in American society. In 1997 the Liggett Group, the maker of Chesterfield cigarettes, openly acknowledged that smoking is both addictive and deadly (Vedantam, Epstine, and Geiger 1997). Being legal does not mean that a drug is harmless. Sometimes it is difficult, however, to determine how harmful the drug is, as illustrated by the recent (2004) advent of electronic cigarettes (also called e-cigarettes).

E-cigarettes are smoked by vaporizing a liquid composed of nicotine, flavorings, and other chemicals. They are touted as a healthful alternative to regular tobacco products, a way to reduce tobacco-related deaths as smokers switch to them (Levy et al. 2016). However, it appears that smokers who use e-cigarettes do not stop smoking tobacco, and those who begin with e-cigarettes tend to move on to tobacco products (Leventhal et al. 2015; Sutfin et al. 2015). By 2018, 14.9 percent of adults had ever used an e-cigarette, and 3.1 percent were current users (Villarroel, Cha, and Vahratian 2020). Some adverse effects of using e-cigarettes are already known (Higham et al. 2016). More, including effects of second-hand inhalation, may be known in the future.

Finally, increasing attention is being paid to the *abuse of psychotherapeutic drugs.* Of course, such drugs have enormously increased our physical and mental well-being. Countless numbers of people would have been unable to function as well or at all and would have died sooner without the use of prescription drugs. Nevertheless, those drugs can be abused to one's detriment as well as used to one's enhanced health.

In some cases, the abuse is the unintended by-product of attempts at self-medication. A national survey of Americans aged 57 through 85 concluded that nearly 1 in 25 were at risk for a major drug-drug interaction with the potential for adverse health consequences (Qato et al. 2008). Another study looked at death certificates and found that the proportion of deaths due to mixing prescription with nonprescription drugs (including alcohol) increased nearly 3,200 percent over a two-decade period (Phillips, Barker, and Eguchi 2008).

More commonly, however, psychotherapeutic drugs are taken for their intoxication effects, and they rank second, after marijuana, as the drug of choice for Americans. In recent years, the concern has grown about the misuse of opioid painkillers (Percocet, Vicodin, OxyContin, and illegal heroin). A dramatic rise in the number of prescriptions and the number of nonmedical uses of the drugs led some experts to call the problem an "epidemic" (Binswanger and Gordon 2016). A survey in Maine, for example, reported that in 2014 opioids were dispensed to 22.4 percent of the residents, enough to give every person in Maine a 16-day supply (Piper et al. 2016). Nationally, in 2014 more than 28,000 Americans died from an overdose of one of the opioids.

## Patterns of Use

It is difficult to know the number of drug users in the United States. Not all users are addicts, and not all addicts are known to the authorities. There is wide variation in use, depending on such factors as the type of drug and the age, sex, race/ethnicity, and social class of the user. Alcohol is the most widely used drug, followed by tobacco and marijuana. Among Americans aged 18 years or older, 14.1 percent used tobacco in 2017 (National Center for Health Statistics 2019). This was down from 30.4 percent in 2002, part of a continuing decline in tobacco use. And marijuana usage in 2017 was 9.6 percent of those aged 12 years or older.

Illicit drug use varies by a number of demographic factors (National Center for Health Statistics 2019). The proportion of current users is higher for males (12.8 percent) than for females (9.1 percent). With regard to age groups, the proportion who are current users varies from 2.0 percent for 12- to 13-year-olds to 7.7 percent for those 35 years and older. The highest rate is the 18- to 25-year-old group—24.2 percent.

Use also varies by race/ethnicity. The proportion of users of illicit drugs in 2017, was as follows, from highest to lowest: Native Americans, 17.67 percent; African Americans, 13.1 percent; whites, 11.6 percent; Hispanics, 9.8 percent; and Asian Americans, 4.5 percent. Finally, drug use is higher in the lower than in the middle or upper social classes (Barbeau, Krieger, and Soobader 2004). In general, then, *the highest rates of drug use and abuse occur among those who are male, young, and poor.*

Table 2.1 shows the proportion of current users of various drugs by age group. These proportions are, of course, smaller than the proportion of those who have ever used the drugs. For example, compared to the proportion who are current users, the

**TABLE 2.1**
Use of Selected Drugs (percent who used in last 30 days)

| | | Age Group | | |
|---|---|---|---|---|
| Substance | Total | 12–17 Years | 18–25 Years | 26–34 Years |
| Any Illicit Drug | 11.2 | 7.9 | 24.2 | 17.4 |
| Marijuana | 9.6 | 6.5 | 22.1 | 14.8 |
| Psychotherapeutics | 2.2 | 1.5 | 4.5 | 3.7 |
| Alcohol | 51.7 | 9.9 | 56.3 | 64.2 |
| Heavy Alcohol Use | 6.1 | 0.7 | 9.6 | 8.8 |

SOURCE: National Center for Health Statistics website.

proportion who have ever tried an illicit drug is close to half the adult population (Maguire 2012).

*Trends.* Drug use rose rapidly after 1960 and peaked in 1979 (U.S. Department of Health and Human Services 1995). During the 1980s, the upward trend stopped and even reversed for most drugs. Since then, drug use has fluctuated. For example, the proportion of high school seniors who are current users of any illicit drug was 16.4 percent in 1991, reached a high of 26.2 percent in 1997, and stood at 23.7 percent in 2019 (Miech et al. 2020).

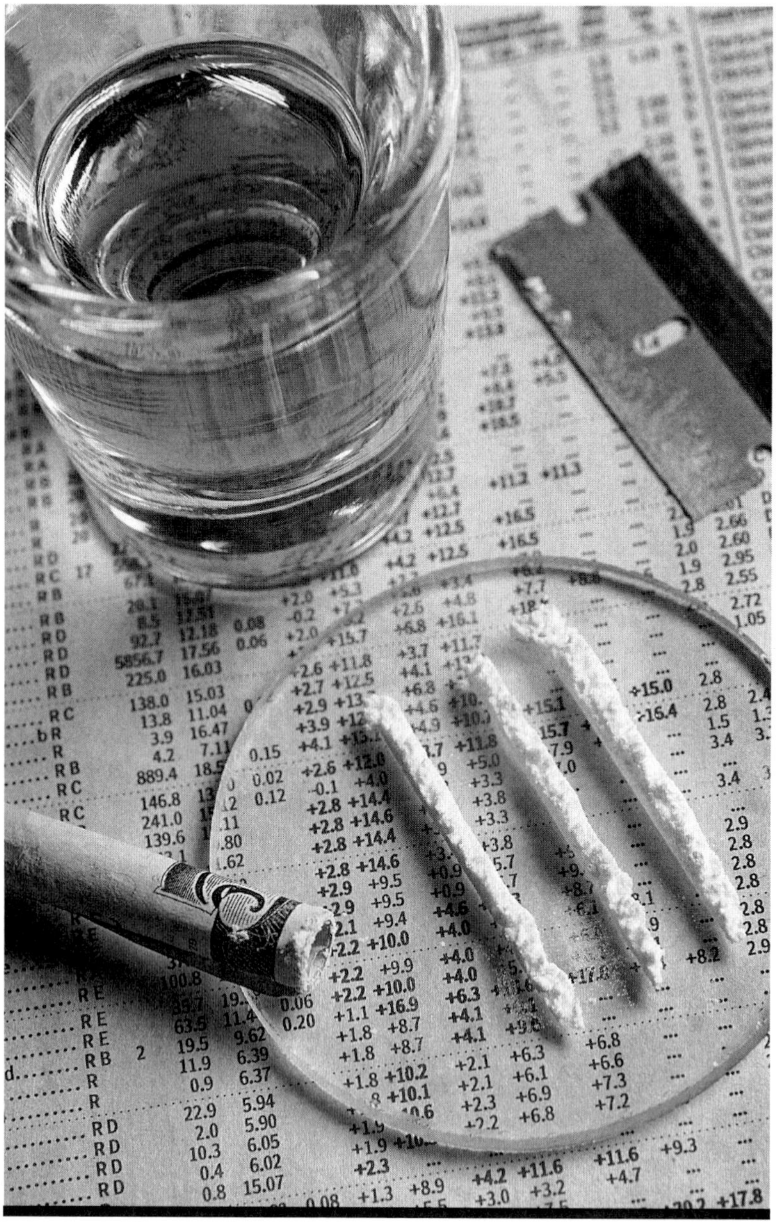

To some extent, the variation in rates of usage may reflect changing definitions of the effects. For instance, when cocaine became popular during the 1980s, one of the appealing aspects was the claim that it gave users a great "high" without undesirable physical effects. However, most people now seem to realize that cocaine and crack (an especially dangerous form of cocaine that can be smoked) may lead to both physical and mental health problems, including chronic sore throat, hoarseness, chronic coughing, shortness of breath, depression, hallucinations, psychosis, and death from overdose (Smart 1991).

*Multiple Use.* A question often raised is whether the use of one drug leads to the use of others. A number of studies have investigated the question, and in general they support the conclusion that there is a *tendency for multiple use* (Martin, Clifford, and Clapper 1992; National Center on Addiction and Substance Abuse at Columbia University 1998). Smokers are likely to drink alcohol (Costello, Dierker, Jones, and Rose 2008). Those who use alcohol and/or tobacco may move on to abuse prescription drugs or to use marijuana and then hard drugs (White et al. 2007; Sintov et al. 2009). And youth who abuse prescription drugs also have higher rates of tobacco use, heavy drinking, and the use of illicit drugs like marijuana and cocaine (National Institute on Drug Abuse 2014).

Multiple use of drugs is common.

Ingram Publishing

Nevertheless, we cannot say that the use of one drug causes the individual to experiment with another drug. To do so would be the *fallacy of non sequitur*. At this point, we can only say that whatever leads an individual to experiment with one substance may lead that individual to experiment with others.

fallacy

*Age of Initiation.* Drug use is beginning at an increasingly earlier age (Johnson and Gerstein 1998). Among those born in the 1930s, for example, only alcohol, cigarettes, and marijuana were used by more than 1 percent of people before the age of 35. For those born between 1951 and 1955, 10 drugs were used by more than 5 percent of people before the age of 35.

In both rural and urban areas, children begin experimenting with drugs as early as the third grade (McBroom 1992). Inhalants are more likely the first drugs with which children experiment (Fritz 2003). As many as 6 percent of American children have tried an inhalant by the fourth grade. Young children also experiment with smoking and drinking alcohol (Miech et al. 2019). In 2015, 7 percent of 8th graders said they had started smoking in grade 6 or earlier. And 26 percent had tried alcohol and 10.9 percent said they had been drunk one or more times. Still another survey, by The Centers for Disease Control and Prevention (2019b), found that 5.6 percent had tried marijuana before the age of 13.

In their teen years, young people have increasing exposure to, and opportunities for, drug use. Few users begin experimenting as adults. Adults who smoke, for example, typically become daily smokers before the age of 20 (Centers for Disease Control and Prevention 1995). Similarly, adults who use other kinds of drugs, including heroin, typically begin at an early age (Epstein and Groerer 1997).

## Drugs and the Quality of Life

It is clear that drug abuse is a widespread problem in America and affects both abusers and nonabusers. Residents in drug-trafficking neighborhoods are often terrorized by and fearful of dealers and users. As we discuss the effects of *abuse on the quality of life of individuals*, keep in mind how whole communities are affected.

*Physical Health.* Drug abuse contradicts the American *value of physical well-being*. A person may experiment with drugs because they seem to hold the promise of fulfillment, but the fulfillment is elusive; greater and greater quantities are consumed, and ultimately the person suffers physical and psychological deterioration.

The *physical harm resulting from the use of illegal drugs includes* (U.S. Department of Justice 1992:10):

1. Death.
2. Medical emergencies from acute reactions to drugs or toxic adulterants.
3. Exposure to HIV infection, hepatitis, and other diseases resulting from intravenous drug use.
4. Injury from accidents caused by drug-related impairment.
5. Injuries from violence while obtaining drugs in the drug distribution network.
6. Dependence or addiction.
7. Chronic physical problems.

This list is greatly abbreviated, of course. For example, consider the *multiple consequences of using a drug such as methamphetamine* (National Institute on Drug Abuse 2005). Even small amounts can result in increased wakefulness, decreased appetite, increased respiration, hyperthermia, irritability, insomnia, confusion, tremors, convulsions, anxiety, paranoia, and aggressiveness. Methamphetamine also can cause irreversible damage to blood vessels in the brain, producing strokes, irregular heartbeat, and, ultimately, cardiovascular collapse and death. The point is, drug use involves a long list of physical, psychological, and social consequences that are destructive.

Drug abuse is now the main preventable cause of illness and premature death in the United States. Each year hundreds of thousands of Americans die from smoking, alcohol abuse, and the use of illicit drugs (Hedegaard, Minino, and Warner 2020). Early death from illegal drugs is often associated with an overdose of the drug. Heroin slows the vital functions of the body, and if a sufficient amount of the drug is ingested, those vital functions will completely stop. The addict can never be sure how much of the drug constitutes an overdose, nor can he or she be sure about the purity of the drug. Also, the *addict's tolerance level can vary* from one day to another, depending on how much of the drug has been used. If the addict manages to avoid death by overdose, he or she still may die from infections carried by the needle. Thus, the user *is at risk not merely from the drug itself but from other factors associated with drug use.*

The health consequences go beyond the addict herself in the case of a pregnant woman. Cocaine and tobacco use are both associated with a significant risk of spontaneous abortion (Ness et al. 1999). Children who survive the risk and are born to addicted mothers have a significant number of perinatal medical problems, behavioral problems in early infancy, and developmental deficiencies in their cognitive and psychomotor skills (Singer et al. 2002). Children of mothers who smoked during pregnancy are also more likely to be born with heart defects (Malik et al. 2008).

*Tobacco Use Is a Global Problem.* In the United States, tobacco use causes more physiological damage than any nonalcoholic drug and is the leading cause of preventable death—mortality among smokers is two to three times as high as that among those who never smoked (Carter et al. 2015). Globally, tobacco causes about 6 million deaths each year (World Health Organization 2016). About 600,000 of those deaths are due to secondhand inhalation.

The consequences of tobacco use are well established. Among the known consequences of smoking are increased probability of lung cancer and other respiratory diseases, increased risk of heart disease, increased risk of colorectal cancer, and increased probability of complications during childbirth (LaCroix et al. 1991; Botteri et al. 2008; Kabir et al. 2008). The risks are dramatized by the fact that a 29 percent decline in smoking prevalence in Massachusetts over a 10-year period was associated with a 31 percent decline in deaths due to coronary heart disease (Kabir et al. 2008). There are, of course, people who smoke regularly and live to a "ripe old age," but using them to counter the systematic evidence is the *fallacy of dramatic instance*. What matters is not the few exceptions, but the great numbers who support the conclusions.

fallacy

Moreover, nonsmokers who are exposed to a smoking environment also may suffer. Nonsmokers who live or work in a smoking environment are more likely than those not in such an environment to develop coronary heart disease or lung cancer (U.S. Department of Health and Human Services 2006). Thus, thousands of nonsmokers die each year as a result of inhaling secondhand smoke. Pregnant women exposed to secondhand smoke have increased odds of giving birth before full term or of low birth weight for a full-term baby (Ghosh, Wilhelm, and Ritz 2013). Researchers also have found that babies are more likely to develop a respiratory tract infection and to die of sudden infant death syndrome when they are exposed to smoke (Pollack 2001; Blizzard et al. 2003). Smoking parents also increase the chances of their children developing asthma and, in later life, lung cancer (Scott 1990; Sturm, Yeatts, and Loomis 2004). As a result of such findings, smoke-free environments at work and in public places are becoming common.

Some consequences of other drugs were briefly noted in Figure 2.1. We need to examine in more detail, however, the effects of marijuana, which have been a matter of controversy.

*Marijuana.* Although the nonmedical use of marijuana is now legal in some states, controversy continues over its effects. Is it simply a way to relax? Can it enhance the quality of life? Or do the hazards of usage outweigh any benefits? Clearly there are hazards (Office of National drug Control Policy 2003b; National Academies of Sciences, Engineering, and Medicine 2017). The hazards include

1. Acute effects of marijuana intoxication:
   a. Impaired memory, thinking, speaking, and problem solving.
   b. Impaired time perception.
   c. Increased heart rate (as high as 160 beats per minute).
   d. Reddening of the eyes.
   e. Impaired psychomotor performance (resulting in automobile accidents and deaths).
2. Chronic effects:
   a. Adverse effects on the respiratory system, similar to those of cigarettes.
   b. Reduced sperm count in males.
   c. Possible adverse effects on children when the mother uses the drug, including lowered birth weight and more fetal abnormalities.
   d. Interference with the normal pattern of sex hormones, impairing their release from the brain.
   e. Mental health problems, including psychoses, anxiety, and depression.

While it is true that marijuana poses a greater threat to well-being than was once believed, it also may have more medical uses than previously thought—including treating glaucoma patients, relieving the pain of cancer patients, ameliorating the side effects of chemotherapy, and relieving the suffering of asthmatics. Undoubtedly, research on the effects of marijuana will continue.

*Psychological Health.* Americans value psychological as well as physical health. The search for "happiness," "peace of mind," or "contentment" is common. The short-range euphoria that follows drug use is misleading because the long-range effects of drug abuse contradict the *quest for psychological well-being.* In essence, drug use leads to poorer mental health, and multiple use intensifies the detrimental effects (Booth et al. 2010). For example, the high that is produced by a drug such as crack can be followed by severe depression. You need only listen to the stories of addicts or ex-addicts to realize the devastation to psychological health that results from drug abuse. You also should note that, in contrast to the common belief that people turn to drugs for relief from distress, a study of adolescents found that users did not start drugs because of preexisting psychological distress; rather, the drug use led to both physical and psychological impairments (Hansell and White 1991).

The greater the use, the more intense the problems. A study of 161 adolescents reported that increased drug use was associated with increased depression, decreased self-esteem, and a deterioration of purpose in life (Kinnier, Metha, Okey, and Keim

1994). Even smoking is associated with psychological problems. Nicotine-dependent individuals are more likely to have problems with depression, anxiety, and lower self-esteem (Croghan et al. 2006; Hu, Davies, and Kandel 2006; McCaffery et al. 2008). By midlife, heavy smoking can lead to cognitive impairment and decline (Richards, Jarvis, Thompson, and Wadsworth 2003; Nooyens, van Gelder, and Verschuren 2008). And a mother who smokes while pregnant can decrease her baby's IQ (Olds, Henderson, and Tatelbaum 1994).

Similarly, marijuana use poses serious mental health problems (Office of National Drug Control Policy 2003b). Regular use by adolescents impairs memory, attentional ability, learning, and psychomotor performance (Solowij et al. 2002). Adolescents who seek relief from depression through marijuana may actually intensify their depression (Office of National Drug Control Policy 2008; Womack et al. 2016). An English study found that marijuana users increase their chances of developing a psychotic disorder later in life by about 40 percent (Moore et al. 2007). And a study of Italian men who used only marijuana found that 83 percent were dependent on the drug, 46 percent abused it, and 29 percent of occasional users had at least one emotional disorder (Troisi, Pasini, Saracco, and Spalletta 1998).

The dangers of marijuana have increased because the drug is stronger than it used to be (Office of National Drug Control Policy 2003b). Marijuana with 2 percent tetrahydrocannabinol (THC) can result in severe psychological damage, including paranoia and psychosis. Currently, however, average levels are 6 percent THC, or three times the amount that can cause serious damage to the user.

*Interpersonal Difficulties.* In addition to a sense of physical and psychological well-being, the desired quality of life for Americans demands harmonious relationships. This value is contradicted by relationship problems that tend to result from drug abuse.

A variety of interpersonal problems are associated with drug use and abuse (U.S. Department of Justice 1992; Office of National Drug Control Policy 2003b). They include arguing with family and friends, feeling suspicious and distrustful of people, encountering troubles at school or work, and getting into trouble with the police. Drug users are three to four times more likely than nonusers to engage in criminal behavior (Bennett, Holloway, and Farrington 2006). Marijuana users experience less cohesion and harmony in their relationships and have more relationship conflict than nonusers (Brook, Pahl, and Cohen 2008). Inhalant users have higher rates of both childhood and adult antisocial behavior than nonusers, including bullying, starting fights, using weapons, and being physically cruel toward others (Howard et al. 2010). Children whose parents abuse drugs are almost three times more likely to be abused and more than four times more likely to be neglected than are children of nonabusing parents, and they are also likely to have emotional, academic, and interpersonal problems (Reid, Macchetto, and Foster 1999; Wilens et al. 2002).

Interpersonal problems may continue for addicts even after they no longer abuse drugs. The ex-addict may attempt to compensate for past failures and assume a role of leadership. The outcome may be a power struggle between the ex-addict and his or her mate. In other cases, there may be unrealistic expectations about the outcome of treatment. The mate of an ex-addict may expect immediate and dramatic changes, and when such changes do not appear, the result can be disillusionment or bitterness. Also, the ex-addict may find that long-term or permanent damage has been done to his or her relationships.

*Economic Costs.* All social problems involve certain *economic costs,* and these affect the quality of life. The more money required to deal with a social problem, the less money there is for other desired services and programs.

Determining the exact dollar cost of any social problem is difficult. The costs of the drug problem include some that can be measured and some that can only be estimated. There is, of course, a cost to the user–the expense of maintaining the habit (for some, hundreds of dollars a week or more) and the loss of earnings over their life span.

The measurable costs to the nation are staggering. Federal funding for various drug control programs was $35.6 billion for 2020. State and local expenditures and other costs cannot be easily estimated. They include (U.S. Department of Justice 1992:127):

Criminal justice expenditures on drug-related crime.

Health care costs of injuries from drug-related child abuse and accidents.

The cost of lost productivity due to absenteeism and inefficiency and errors of users at the workplace.

Loss of property values due to drug-related neighborhood crime.

Property damage from drug-related activities.

Loss of agricultural resources, which are used for cultivation of illegal drugs.

Toxins introduced into public air and water supplies by drug production.

Emotional and physical damage to users as well as their families, friends, and co-workers.

Overall, drug control programs cost the federal government hundreds of billions of dollars. And the cost continues to rise each year.

## Contributing Factors

The various contributing factors have a double-barreled effect: They maintain demand by encouraging use of drugs, and they guarantee a supply.

*Social Structural Factors.* As with alcohol, *group norms* are one of the most important factors in the problem of other drugs, creating *peer pressure* that leads individuals to drug use. For the most part, young people do not take drugs to relieve emotional distress but to be accepted by their peers–and the pressure begins in elementary school.

**Group Norms.** Group norms are important for adults as well. Being *integrated into a group in which drug use is approved* is one of the strongest factors associated with drug use at all ages (Kilmer et al. 2006; Edwards, Witkiewitz, and Vowles 2019). The "group" may be your family, your friends, or your peers at school or work. A survey of 1,802 fourth- and fifth-grade pupils found perceived family use to be the strongest influence on the children's drug use (Bush, Weinfurt, and Iannotti 1994). A study of employees who abused drugs reported that they tended to come from families with substance abuse problems and that they, in turn, associated with substance-abusing friends (Lehman, Farabee, Holcom, and Simpson 1995).

Some Americans who regard themselves as respectable citizens find it difficult to imagine following group norms when those norms are illegal. They need to realize that people all follow the norms of their groups and follow them for basically the same reasons. The respectable citizen who abides by the norm that the appearance of one's house and yard should be neat and clean derives satisfaction and a sense of acceptance from that normative behavior. Similarly, the youth who uses drugs finds certain *rewards*–including admiration, respect, and acceptance–in that usage when it is the norm of his or her group.

**Role Problems.** Role problems are a second social structural factor in the drug problem. *Role problems create stress* in the individual, who may then use drugs to deal with the problems and their consequent stress (Goeders 2003). Indeed, when you consider that the first use of a drug like tobacco is likely to be a highly unpleasant experience, it is reasonable that strong forces are at work to develop the habit. Once a youth tries a cigarette, either peer pressure or stress can lead to subsequent tries, but stress seems to lead the individual more quickly to develop the habit (Hirschman, Leventhal, and Glynn 1984). Of course, the student role is inherently stressful for most people. For some, the stress is sufficiently severe to search for relief in drugs. A study of college students found that students who experience academic strain have higher levels of depression, and some try to relieve the depression with the nonmedical use of prescription stimulants (Ford and Schroeder 2009).

What kinds of role problems create such stress? One is the socially devalued role. That is, certain roles rank low in terms of such things as social acceptance. Those in such roles may become victims of prejudice and discrimination. The role of immigrant is one such role. Thus, an investigation of adult immigrants in the Midwest found a higher rate of drug use among those who had experienced discrimination (Tran, Lee, and Burgess 2010).

**role conflict**
a person's perception that two or more of his or her roles are contradictory, or that the same role has contradictory expectations, or that the expectations of the role are unacceptable or excessive

A second stress-generating role problem is **role conflict.** Two or more roles may be contradictory—as, for example, when a woman experiences a contradiction between her role as a physician and her role as a wife because she does not have time to meet the expectations of both her patients and her husband. Contradictory expectations may impinge upon a single role, as when a physician's patients demand the right of abortion and his or her peers and friends define abortion as illegal and immoral. An individual may define the expectations of a role as somehow unacceptable or excessive, as when a physician feels overwhelmed by the multiple demands made upon his or her time and professional skills.

Physicians have been deliberately used in the examples here because of the high rate of drug addiction among doctors. The actual cause of addiction is not known, but it probably is rooted in a combination of easy access to drugs and the stresses of the role. Drug abuse is a symptom of stress, and role problems do generate stress in the individual. To the extent that particular roles are especially likely to create problems, people who occupy those roles will be particularly vulnerable to stress and perhaps to using drugs to deal with stress.

An important point here is that role conflict is a social phenomenon, not an individual phenomenon. It is not a particular doctor who is oppressed by the demands of the role; rather, all doctors must come to terms with the role of a physician in American society. The expectations attached to the role tend to create the same problems for everyone who occupies the role.

Another role problem that can generate stress and increase the likelihood of drug abuse is a *role change that is defined as undesirable.* Such a role change occurs when a spouse dies. Suddenly a person is no longer a husband or a wife—that role has been lost.

After the loss (which may be the result of separation or divorce as well as death), the individual must work through the grief process. A person copes with a significant loss by passing through a series of emotional phases. The process may take as long as two or more years. Typically, the initial phase is shock, followed by a period of numbness, or lack of intense emotion. In the next phase, the individual wavers between fantasy and reality, overcomes fantasies, and then experiences the full impact of the loss. A period of increasing adjustment follows, punctuated sporadically by episodes of painful memories. Finally, if the full grief process has been experienced, the individual accepts the loss and reaffirms his or her life. The grief process is painful, and some individuals may resort to drugs.

**Family Experiences.** Family experiences also are involved in the use and abuse of drugs. Families that are strong, healthy, and highly cohesive tend to inhibit the use and abuse of drugs (Wilens et al. 2002; Dorius, Bahr, Hoffman, and Harmon 2004). Family values and practices such as religious involvement, parental supervision, and eating dinner together are associated with less likelihood of drug abuse (National Center on Addiction and Substance Abuse at Columbia University 1998; Reboussin et al. 2019).

However, the three kinds of family experiences that contribute to the alcohol problem also are involved in the abuse of other drugs. First, as noted earlier in this chapter, drug abusers are more likely to come from homes in which other family members are abusers (Kilpatrick et al. 2000; Farmer et al. 2019).

Second, drug abusers are more likely to come from broken homes than are nonabusers. Adolescents who grow up in single-parent homes are more likely to use tobacco and illegal drugs than those who live with both parents (Flewelling and Bauman 1990). Looking at overall drug involvement (including alcohol), rates are higher among those whose homes are disrupted by divorce than those who grow up in intact homes (Wolfinger 1998).

Third, drug abuse is associated with various problematic relationships within the family. Parental conflict and *alienation between youth and their parents* can result in drug use and abuse (Fish, Maier, and Priest 2015). A study of adolescents reported that those with authoritarian fathers (which typically results in parent-child conflict) are more likely to use drugs (Bronte-Tinkew, Moore, and Carrano 2006). Heroin users also reported an unhappy parental marriage, parental coldness, and conflict with parents. In addition, they were likely to have mothers with some kind of physical or emotional illness. Thus, the use and abuse of all kinds of drugs are likely to be associated with disturbed family relationships.

Of course, the sense of rejection and alienation from parents can follow from drug use rather than precede it. Even if it is true, for instance, that a young person first uses drugs because of his or her group's norms and then becomes alienated from his or her parents, this alienation is likely to perpetuate the drug use. Thus, even if alienation is not one of the causes of initial use, it is likely to be a cause of continuing use.

**Government.** A fourth structural factor is the government, and especially the *government's definition of drug use as illegal.* For some drugs, the illegal status is the consequence of social and political processes rather than of scientific evidence. Why, for example, is tobacco legal while other drugs are not? Once a drug is declared illegal, criminal elements enter the drug traffic in order to profit from black-market dealings. In essence, illegality raises the cost of maintaining the drug habit, deeply involves criminals in the drug traffic, strains the criminal justice system, and leads the addict to undesirable behavior. Criminal involvement results from the potential for high

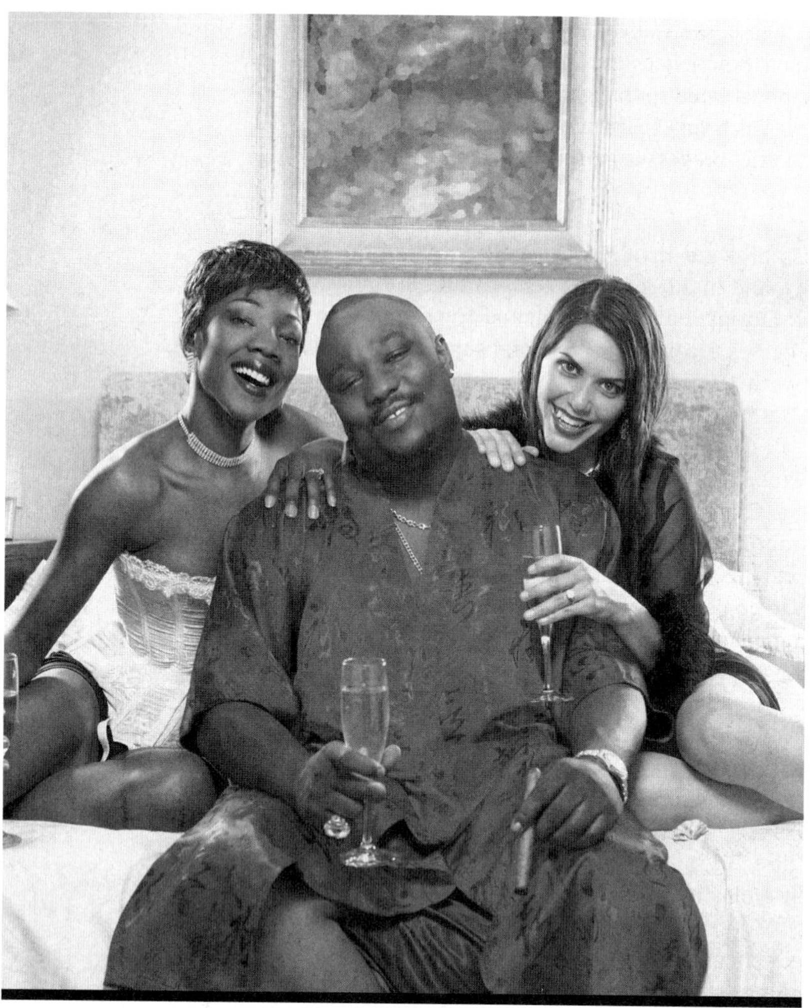

Ads portray drug users as leading happy glamorous lives.
Plush Studios/Blend Images LLC

profits. For example, the street value of heroin may be 50 times or more its wholesale cost and 10,000 times the amount paid to the farmer who supplies the opium! Similar profits are realized in the sale of other illicit drugs, which is one reason pushers risk prison to ply their trade.

**Economy.** A fifth structural factor is the *economy*. The economy supports the drug problem in at least two ways. First, many people who get involved in the distribution, sale, and/or use and abuse of drugs come from the margins of the economy. That is, they are from the more impoverished families and have little hope of achieving any kind of financial success apart from that which drugs appear to offer them. Second, the legal drugs–alcohol and tobacco–are marketed freely and openly, and the industries are so profitable that they exert enormous pressure on the government to remain a legitimate part of the economy, including pressure to allow their products to be advertised in markets that will reach young people.

**Mass Media.** The mass media can contribute to the drug problem by allowing celebrities to laughingly discuss their use of marijuana and their abuse of alcohol. Movies, TV programs, magazines, and the Internet provide outlets for those who send the message–a message likely to be particularly effective to the young–that people should not miss experiencing the use of illegal drugs and the abuse of legal drugs. Such a message turns the once-popular phrase about drug use, "just say no," on its head. The message now is "just say yes," because it's an experience you won't want to miss.

Popular movies and music can reinforce the message (Chen, Miller, Grube, and Waiters 2006). To see drug use romanticized in a movie or to hear the use of drugs celebrated in rap or song lyrics is likely to influence at least some people to emulate the behavior.

In essence, a part of the culture has become an advocate of drug usage and has thereby increased the number of people who are users and abusers. A study of adolescents who took up smoking reported that a third of the youth nominated a movie star who smoked on-screen as one of their favorites (Distefan, Pierce, and Gilpin 2004). And a study of fifth and eighth grade students found that those who saw actors and actresses smoking in movies were more likely than others to begin smoking themselves (Wills et al. 2007).

Finally, the mass media also affect usage through the advertising of legal drugs. Some studies have found that ads are more influential than peers on adolescents' decisions to start smoking (Evans et al. 1995). Research over a three-year period in California concluded that a third of all experimentation with smoking resulted from advertising (Pierce et al. 1998). Cigarette ads in the United States have declined considerably, but a study of sixth and eighth grade students in India reported that exposure to tobacco ads was significantly related to increased tobacco use (Arora, Reddy, Stigler, and Perry 2008).

**Supply.** Although the structural factors that create the *demand for drugs* are crucial, there is also a *powerful organization of supply*. Massive amounts of coca, marijuana, and opium, for example, are grown in Latin America, processed in refineries, and smuggled into the United States. Hundreds of tons of cocaine alone are produced and smuggled into the United States each year (Office of National Drug Control Policy 2003a). About three-fourths of the coca grown for processing the cocaine is from Colombia. Of all the cocaine that enters the nation, 72 percent passes through the Mexico/Central America corridor, 27 percent moves through the Caribbean, and the other 1 percent comes directly from South America. The main ports of entry are central Arizona, El Paso, Houston, Los Angeles, Miami, and Puerto Rico.

Some of the drug suppliers have their own armies and use terrorist activities to intimidate officials. In addition, smugglers exploit the massive corruption that exists at all layers of government (including law enforcement agencies) and among businesspeople (who may "launder" drug money) in the United States and Latin America.

The supply network in Latin America and elsewhere is so powerful and the potential profits are so enormous that efforts to cut off supplies have been fruitless. Cut off at one point, smugglers find alternatives. Efforts to stop the supply should not be abandoned, but many experts agree that as long as there is demand and profits are high, the suppliers will find a way to provide drugs.

*Social Psychological Factors.* People *who have positive attitudes* toward drug use are more likely to become users. Both adolescents and adults underestimate their risks from using legal or illegal drugs (Strecher, Kreuter, and Kobrin 1995; Ayanian and Cleary 1999). Abusers may not be unaware of risks, but the value to them of the psychic effects—euphoria, pleasure, and change of mood—exceeds any concern they have about risks. As reported in a study of psychotherapeutic drug abusers in Florida, the psychic effects are one of the most important motivations for using drugs (Rigg and Ibanez 2010). The two other most frequently named reasons were "to sleep" and "for anxiety/stress."

The quest for psychic effects also was noted in a study of people who had reached a physical and/or emotional crisis from their drug abuse (Table 2.2). Those who reach a crisis stage are also likely to recognize their dependence and to admit their suicidal intentions.

**TABLE 2.2**
Motivation for Drug Abuse by Age, Race, and Sex of Abuser and Selected Drugs (percent of mentions)

| | Psychic Effects | Dependence | Self-Destruction | Other |
|---|---|---|---|---|
| All mentions | 38 | 22 | 33 | 7 |
| Age | | | | |
| 15 and under | 60 | 7 | 22 | 10 |
| 16–19 | 57 | 17 | 20 | 6 |
| 20–29 | 36 | 28 | 30 | 7 |
| 30–39 | 23 | 24 | 46 | 9 |
| 40–49 | 16 | 21 | 53 | 10 |
| 50 and over | 13 | 14 | 61 | 12 |
| Race | | | | |
| White | 39 | 18 | 35 | 8 |
| Black | 33 | 35 | 24 | 7 |
| Other | 41 | 27 | 26 | 6 |
| Sex | | | | |
| Male | 46 | 29 | 19 | 6 |
| Female | 31 | 15 | 45 | 9 |

SOURCE: U.S. Department of Justice, Drug Enforcement Administration, Drug Abuse Warning Network, Phase II Report, July 1973–March 1974 (Washington, DC: Government Printing Office).

Two other motivations we should note are *boredom and curiosity*, which are likely to be factors particularly among adolescents (De Micheli and Formigoni 2002; Adams et al. 2003). Adolescents with too few demands on their time may find themselves attracted to experimenting with drugs simply to relieve the boredom. Others may have a natural curiosity that spurs them to want to know what the drug experience is like. Unfortunately, if they define that first experience as highly gratifying, they may continue to use and ultimately abuse the drug.

Motivations may change over the years. A study of adolescents who use marijuana found that things such as boredom, the psychic effects, and fitting in with peers were still factors in using drugs (Patrick et al. 2019). But by 2016 they had become less important than using the drug to cope with the stresses and challenges of daily life.

Finally, *ideology* is a factor in the drug problem. In fact, positive attitudes, group norms, and ideologies about drug use reinforce each other. Friedenberg (1972) identified the following ideology about marijuana:

1. People who are enjoying themselves without harming others have an inalienable right to privacy.
2. A drug whose effect is to turn its users inward upon their own experience, enriching their fantasy life at the expense of their sense of need to achieve or relate to others, is as moral as alcohol, which encourages a false gregariousness and increasingly pugnacious or competitive behavior.
3. Much of the solicitude of the older generation for the welfare of the young merely expresses a desire to dominate and control them for the sake of adult interests and the preservation of adult status and authority.

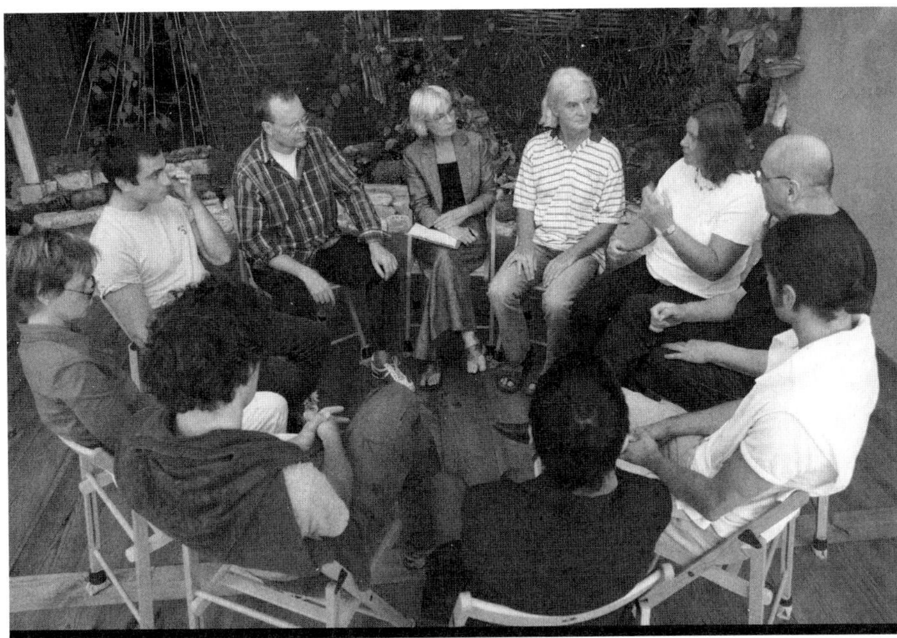

Group therapy can be effective in the treatment of some addicts.
Manchan/Getty Images

This ideology, like all ideologies, serves the purpose of explaining and validating certain behavior, thereby reinforcing the behavior.

## Solutions: Public Policy and Private Action

Is it possible to eliminate the drug problem? No society we know of has completely solved the problem. Even China, which seemed to have eradicated the problem, has experienced renewed problems of drug abuse (Lu and Wang 2008).

Still, progress can be made, and the severity of the problem can be lessened. For that to happen, programs must attack the social bases as well as treat individual addicts and also focus on *reducing demand rather than stopping the supply.* For example, as noted in this chapter, demand and use are highest in the lower social classes. Public policy that enables those in the lower strata to better their lot will also reduce the demand for illegal drugs. We are not saying that enforcement is useless but only that treatment as well as programs of education and prevention must be given at least as much, and perhaps more, attention and support. Demand for some drugs may be reduced through legislation. A study of 10 years of tobacco control in New York City found that such measures as high excise taxes and smoke-free air laws resulted in a decline of 28 percent in adult smoking and 52 percent in youth smoking (Kilgore et al. 2014). While those who quit smoking will have lingering effects on their health, they will still extend their life span by as much as 20 years (Kramarow 2020).

*Enforcement Programs.* Enforcement programs involve efforts to prevent drugs from entering the country or from being produced within the country. It also includes the capture, prosecution, and imprisonment of users, dealers, and pushers. A controversial form of enforcement is mandatory testing of employees at the workplace.

Some people feel that such testing is a violation of an individual's civil liberties. Yet federal law now requires railroads, airlines, and trucking companies to develop and administer drug-testing programs, and many other firms are setting up programs on their own. Federal law also bans smoking on all domestic airplane flights. Many states have passed laws restricting smoking in restaurants and regulating smoking in private workplaces. These regulations have reduced the risk of heart attacks and heart disease associated with breathing secondhand smoke (National Academy of Sciences 2009).

Some local-level strategies are enforcing the laws on drugs other than tobacco (Mazerolle, Kadleck, and Roehl 2004). In street enforcement programs, police watch the hot spots for drug sales and arrest both the seller and the buyer. In some cases, police will seize the assets of a buyer, such as the buyer's car. They also may use a *reverse sting.* Undercover police pose as dealers and arrest users who ask to buy drugs.

*Community policing by citizens* offers another means of enforcement (Xu, Fiedler, and Flaming 2005). In the case of drugs, citizens organize to eliminate the conditions that facilitate drug sales. Among other things, they may set up a drug hotline, lobby for new laws and jail space, and set up neighborhood cleanup projects.

*Treating Addicts.* The purpose of treating an addict is to reduce or eliminate his or her dependence on the drug. Because there is no single cause for all addictions, however, there is no single treatment that will work for everyone (Rodgers 1994). One method that has claimed some success with cocaine addicts is a form of behavioral therapy—contingency contracting (Petry and Martin 2002). In contingency contracting, the addicts make an agreement with the therapist to pay a severe penalty if urine tests reveal that they have ingested any of the drug during the week. For instance, a nurse signed a contract in which she agreed that she would write a letter to her parents confessing her drug habit and asking that they no longer give her any financial support. She would write a second letter to the state board of nursing in which she would confess her habit and turn in her license.

**detoxification**
supervised withdrawal from dependence on a drug

With heroin addicts, a first step is **detoxification,** *the elimination of dependence* through supervised withdrawal. One of the more common methods of treating heroin addiction is *methadone maintenance.* In methadone maintenance, the addict orally ingests the drug methadone, which is considered less dangerous than heroin and has a number of properties that allow the addict to lead a more normal life than is possible with heroin. Methadone may also be used in the detoxification program, but detoxification involves the elimination of all drug use–including the methadone after it helps mitigate withdrawal symptoms.

Although there is some disagreement as to whether methadone maintenance is more effective than drug-free treatment programs, it is clear that the methadone program reduces the use of heroin (Marsch 1998). Unfortunately, methadone cannot be prescribed by a physician but must be dispensed at a licensed clinic (Wren 1997). In addition, methadone is itself a drug that is abused (Belluck 2003). And even when it succeeds in enabling users to overcome their heroin addiction, it may cause them, as found in a Danish study, to feel inferior and vulnerable (Järvinen and Miller 2010).

A more recent form of treatment is *brief intervention therapy* (Rodgers 1994). In a relatively few sessions, the therapist seeks to establish a warm and supportive relationship with the addict, while giving advice, exploring various ways to deal with the addiction, and helping the addict see that he or she must take responsibility for getting free of the addiction. The therapist also instills a sense of empowerment in the addict—not only "I *have* to do this," but "I can do this."

Addiction is more than physiological, of course. Relationships are involved. Consequently, successful treatment must enable the individual to cope with the conditions that led to the addiction. For many people, this treatment involves group therapy.

One type of group therapy is *family therapy*. Because, for example, adolescent drug abuse is a symptom of family problems in many cases, family therapy may be the most effective mode of treatment (Reilly 1984). For adults, small-group therapy may be helpful. Cocaine Anonymous emerged in the 1980s (Cohen 1984). It is run by former addicts and provides group support to the addict as a means of breaking the habit.

Another variation of group therapy that may be combined with individual therapy is the *drug treatment center*. The efficacy of the centers is a matter of debate. However, one study showed that 80 percent of the treated addicts were off hard drugs after completing a program at an inpatient or an outpatient center (Biden 1990).

A form of group therapy that is effective for some people involves *religious or religious-type experiences*. A religious orientation enables many people to abstain from experimenting with drugs or to stop using drugs (Hei 2019). Adolescents who are high in religiosity are less likely to use drugs (National Survey on Drug Use and Health 2004). In a nationwide survey, the National Center on Addiction and Substance Abuse at Columbia University (1998) found that teenagers who attend services at least four times a month are less likely to use tobacco or marijuana than those attending less than once a month.

Finally, a more recent form of group therapy involves the use of peer support (Levy, Gallmeier, and Wiebel 1995). Peer support is not new, of course, but the program—"outreach-assisted peer support"—is unique in that it targets active addicts who are not in treatment and who may decide to continue drug use while in the group. Whether they opt for total abstinence or for reduced or controlled usage, addicts may join the group.

*Education and Prevention Programs.* Most of the money allocated to the drug problem goes into enforcement, but many people believe that education and prevention are as important—if not more so—because they reduce the demand. Thus, a nationally representative sample of high school seniors found that those who said they would not use marijuana in the coming year gave a number of reasons for their decision that showed they had been well educated about the effects of drugs (Terry-McElrath, O'Malley, and Johnston 2008). The most frequent reasons were the psychological and physical harm involved and the fact that they did not want to get high.

The value of prevention and education programs is also evident in the significant decline of tobacco use in cities and states that have implemented such programs, which include an increase in the tax on cigarettes, requiring smoke-free work sites, and placing antismoking ads in the mass media (Bauer et al. 2005; Frieden et al. 2005; Netemeyer, Andrews, and Burton 2005; Sung et al. 2005). Programs in schools, of course, must begin early because drugs are available even in elementary schools. In fact, the National Institute on Drug Abuse (2004) recommends that prevention programs begin in preschool. It recommends that programs from first grade through high school increase the academic and social competence of students so that they gain the skills needed to resist drug use.

Much of what young people learn, of course, occurs outside the schools. Antidrug advertising has helped make youth attitudes less favorable toward drugs and less likely to use them. Pressure can be exerted on the media to portray drug use, if at all, negatively. For example, smoking shown in movies declined from 1950 to the early 1980s, but in 2002 it was at the same level it was in 1950 (Glantz, Kacirk, and McCulloch 2004).

Parental behavior is also a factor in prevention. Miller-Day (2008) studied the ways parents express their expectations about alcohol or other drug use to their children. She found seven different strategies: let the children use their own judgment; give hints that the children shouldn't use drugs; have a "no tolerance" rule; give information about drug use; threaten punishment; reward nonuse; and ignore the issue. The only strategy to have a significant effect on usage was the "no tolerance" rule. As one subject explained it: The parents said "they would not put up with me doing it and that was that."

Finally, *decriminalization of drug use* is a possible way to attack the social bases of the problem. Although decriminalization would reduce the demand for illegal drugs, it is a controversial issue (Cussen and Block 2000; Sher 2003). Advocates claim that it would resolve many aspects of the problem. It would help safeguard our civil liberties (people would have the option to choose whether to use drugs and could choose usage with legal impunity). Drug traffic would no longer be profitable (making it useless for organized crime). The courts would not be overwhelmed with cases of drug violators. Addicts would not be required to engage in criminal activity to support their habits. The reduction of crime would improve the quality of life in the inner cities. Taxes could be lowered, or the money and other resources now spent on enforcement could be used for better purposes.

Opponents argue that decriminalization would only exacerbate the problem. People would get a wrong and destructive message, namely that drug use is OK. Cheaper, readily available drugs would increase the rate of addiction. The health costs of dealing with abusers would skyrocket. Families would be harmed when an addicted member could no longer provide monetary or emotional support. Children would be harmed when an addicted parent or parents abuse and neglect them. Children born to a mother who used drugs during pregnancy would face various and permanent physical, emotional, and social disabilities. And both the individual abuser and the society would suffer the loss of a meaningful and productive life.

Whatever stance one takes on decriminalization, therefore, should be taken with caution. There are strong arguments both for and against legalization. Recently, a number of states have legalized marijuana, and this might eventually provide data that will guide future action. We say "might" because in other nations such as Great Britain, the Netherlands, and Switzerland where some drugs have been legalized, there is disagreement about the effectiveness of the move. The issue is likely to be controversial for the foreseeable future.

*Follow-Up.* Do you favor the decriminalization of drugs as a way to ease the problem? Why or why not?

## Summary

The problem of alcohol and other drugs is one of abuse and not merely of use. Various drugs have various effects, and the effects depend on the method of administration, the amount taken, and the social situation as well as the chemical composition of the drug. Alcohol is the most widely used drug, and its effects can be extremely deleterious. Many experts consider alcohol abuse much more serious than abuse of other drugs.

Around 1980, drug use of all kinds began to decline for the first time in two decades. In the 1990s, patterns of use fluctuated. Although less than in the peak years, use and abuse are still quite high. A majority of Americans drink, and a substantial number say that drinking has been a source of trouble in their families. Millions of Americans indicate that they are current users of marijuana. Many users tend toward multiple drug use. Most alcohol abusers are young and male but not poor, whereas other drug addicts tend to be young, male, and poor.

The meaning of the drug problem for the quality of life is seen in the consequences for physical health, psychological health, interpersonal relationships, and economic costs. Abusers suffer various undesirable effects in all areas, and they inflict suffering on others. The nation as a whole also suffers great economic cost because billions of dollars per year are involved in lost services and in efforts to combat the deleterious effects of abuse.

Various structural factors contribute to the problem. An important one is group norms. Integration into a group that approves drug use is one of the most reliable predictors of use. Role problems, including being in a socially devalued role, role conflict, and undesirable role change, create stress in the individual and that stress can lead to abuse. Abusers are more likely to come from homes in which family members are abusers, from broken homes, or from homes with problematic relationships. The government's definition of many drugs as illegal has several implications: more people are classified as criminal; previously classified criminals become deeply involved in the drug traffic; the criminal justice system is strained; and users and abusers are led into various kinds of undesirable behavior. Finally, the suppliers of illegal drugs are organized effectively and take advantage of corruption, so that a supply will always be available when there is a demand and profits are high.

Among social psychological factors is the alienation of users from the larger society. Many people believe drug use produces desirable psychic effects. These positive attitudes toward drug use combine with group norms and various ideologies that develop in groups. The ideologies explain and validate drug use.

In treating the problem, efforts to help the individual abuser or reduce the supply available to users have far exceeded efforts to get at the social roots of the problem. If it is to be dealt with effectively, both approaches are needed—attacks on the social factors as well as treatment of individual abusers.

## Key Terms

**Abuse**
**Addiction**
**Binge Drinking**
**Detoxification**
**Placebo**
**Psychotherapeutic Drugs**
**Role Conflict**

## Study Questions

1. What is meant by the statement that Americans have had ambivalent feelings about alcohol and other drugs throughout their history?
2. Identify the various types of drugs and briefly note their effects on people.
3. Who are the most likely users and abusers of alcohol and other drugs?
4. How do the use and abuse of alcohol and other drugs affect physical health?
5. What are the consequences of alcohol and other drugs for psychological health?
6. How does alcohol affect interpersonal relationships?
7. Indicate the economic costs of drug use and abuse.
8. In what ways do group norms affect patterns of drug use?
9. What kind of role problems enter into drug use and abuse?
10. How do social institutions contribute to the problem?
11. What are the attitudes and ideologies that are important in understanding the drug problem?
12. Name some steps that can be taken to alleviate the problem of alcohol and other drugs.

## Internet Resources/Exercises

1. Explore some of the ideas in this chapter on the following sites:

**http://www.nida.nih.gov** The National Institute on Drug Abuse site contains news, publications, and links to other sources.

**https://www.niaa.nih.gov** The National Institute on Alcohol Abuse and Alcoholism has useful information and data on all aspects of alcohol abuse.

**http://ash.org** The Action on Smoking and Health home page provides information on nonsmokers' rights, smoking statistics and information, and help for stopping.

2. Look at Figure 2.1 in the text. Select five drugs and get detailed information on them from the National Institute on Drug Abuse site. If everyone had this information, how many people would still experiment with the drugs? Give arguments both for maintaining that nobody would be a user and for asserting that some would still be users.

3. Search the Internet for "drug use" and "tobacco." Find sites that defend people's right to be users. List the reasons, and respond to them with materials in the text.

## For Further Reading

Brandt, Allan. *The Cigarette Century: The Rise, Fall, and Deadly Persistence of the Product That Defined America*. New York: Basic Books, 2009. An account by a medical professor of how cigarettes affect us culturally, biologically, and healthwise as well as a discussion about the deception of the public by the tobacco industry.

Cheever, Susan, John Hoffman, Susan Froemke, and Sheila Nevins. *Addiction: Why Can't They Just Stop?* New York: Rodale Books, 2007. Uses personal narratives, experts, and statistical data to show the difficulty of breaking an addiction and the impact that addiction has on other people, the social order, and the economy.

Dodes, Lance M. *The Heart of Addiction: A New Approach to Understanding and Managing Alcoholism and Other Addictive Behaviors*. New York: Harper Collins, 2002. Identifies myths about addiction and discusses the common elements in addictions of all types. Includes addiction problems of particular groups and ways to get help.

Hepola, Sara. *Blackout: Remembering the Things I Drank to Forget*. New York: Grand Central Publishing, 2016. A writer shares the story of her addiction to alcohol, including the blackouts, loss of memory, sex with strangers, loss of friends, and finally the painful process of getting sober.

Jersild, Devon. *Happy Hours: Alcohol in a Woman's Life*. New York: HarperCollins, 2001. Both statistics and personal stories highlight the increasingly serious problem of women's abuse of alcohol, including the unique challenges women face as they try to overcome their addiction.

Kuhn, Cynthia, Scott Swartzwelder, and Wilkie Wilson. *Buzzed: The Straight Facts About the Most Used and Abused Drugs from Alcohol to Ecstasy*. 3rd ed. New York: Norton, 2008. Three professors from the Duke University Medical Center discuss the history, effects, and hazards of 12 kinds of drugs, then probe such topics as the role of the brain, the nature of addiction, and legal issues.

Nuff, David. *Drugs Without the Hot Air: Making Sense of Legal and Illegal Drugs*. 2nd ed. Cambridge: UIT Cambridge Ltd, 2020. An expert uses case studies to discuss what drugs are, how they work, their effects, and why people use them.

## References

Adams, J. B., et al. 2003. "Relationships between personality and preferred substance and motivations for use among adolescent substance abusers." *American Journal of Drug and Alcohol Abuse* 29:691–712.

Aronson, M., and B. Hagberg. 1998. "Neuropsychological disorders in children exposed to alcohol during pregnancy." *Alcoholism: Clinical and Experimental Research* 22 (April):321–24.

Arora, M., K. S. Reddy, M. H. Stigler, and C. L. Perry. 2008. "Associations between tobacco marketing and use among urban youth in India." *American Journal of Health Behavior* 32:283–94.

Ayanian, J. Z., and P. D. Cleary. 1999. "Perceived risks of heart disease and cancer among cigarette smokers." *Journal of the American Medical Association* 281 (April 28):1019–21.

Barbeau, E. M., N. Krieger, and M. Soobader. 2004. "Working-class matters: Socioeconomic disadvantage, race/ethnicity, gender, and smoking in NHIS 2000." *American Journal of Public Health* 94:269–78.

Bauer, J. E., et al. 2005. "Longitudinal assessment of the impact of smoke-free worksite policies on tobacco use." *American Journal of Public Health* 95:1024–29.

Becker, H. S. 1953. "Becoming a marijuana user." *American Journal of Sociology* 59 (November): 235–42.

Belluck, P. 2003. "Methadone, once the way out, suddenly grows as a killer drug." *New York Times*, February 9.

Bennett, T., K. Holloway, and D. P. Farrington. 2006. "Does neighborhood watch reduce crime?" *Journal of Experimental Criminology* 2:437–58.

Biden, J. R., Jr. 1990. "They're out there crying for help." *Los Angeles Times*, March 14.

Binswanger, I. A., and A. J. Gordon. 2016. "From risk reduction to implementation." *Substance Abuse* 37:1–3.

Bjarnason, T., et al. 2003. "Alcohol culture, family structure, and adolescent alcohol use." *Journal of Studies on Alcohol* 64:200–8.

——. 2005. "Familial and religious influences on adolescent alcohol use." *Social Forces* 84:375–90.

Blizzard, L., A. Ponsonby, T. Dwyer, A. Venn, and J. A. Cochrane. 2003. "Parental smoking and infant respiratory infection." *American Journal of Public Health* 93:482–88.

Booth, B. M., et al. 2010. "Longitudinal relationship between psychological distress and multiple substance use." *Journal of Studies on Alcohol and Drugs* 71:258–67.

Bossarte, R. M., and M. H. Swahn. 2008. "Interactions between race/ethnicity and psychosocial correlates of preteen alcohol use initiation among seventh grade students in an urban setting." *Journal of Studies on Alcohol and Drugs* 69:660–65.

Botteri, E., et al. 2008. "Smoking and colorectal cancer." *Journal of the American Medical Association* 300:2765–78.

Bronte-Tinkew, J., K. A. Moore, and J. Carrano. 2006. "The father-child relationship, parenting styles, and adolescent risk behaviors in intact families." *Journal of Family Issues* 27:850–81.

Brook, J. S., K. Pahl, and P. Cohen. 2008. "Associations between marijuana use during emerging adulthood and aspects of the significant other relationship in young adulthood." *Journal of Child and Family Studies* 17:1–12.

Brown, T. L., G. S. Parks, R. S. Zimmerman, and C. M. Phillips. 2001. "The role of religion in predicting adolescent alcohol use and problem drinking." *Journal of Studies on Alcohol* 62:696–705.

Burd, L., T. M. Cotsonas-Hassler, J. T. Martsolf, and J. Kerbeshian. 2003. "Recognition and management of fetal alcohol syndrome." *Neurotoxicology and Teratology* 25:681–88.

Bush, P. J., K. P. Weinfurt, and R. J. Iannotti. 1994. "Families versus peers: Developmental influences on drug use from grade 4-5 to grade 7-8." *Journal of Applied Developmental Psychology* 15 (July-September): 437–56.

Caetano, R., S. Ramisetty-Mikler, and L. A. Rodriguez. 2008. "The Hispanic Americans baseline alcohol survey." *Journal of Studies on Alcohol and Drugs* 69:441–48.

Caetano, R., P. A. C. Vaeth, and G. Canino. 2019. "Comorbidity of lifetime alcohol use disorder and major depressive disorder in San Juan, Puerto Rico." *Journal of Studies on Alcohol and Drugs* 80:546–51.

Cairney, S., A. Clough, M. Jaragba, and P. Maruff. 2007. "Cognitive impairment in Aboriginal people with heavy episodic patterns of alcohol use." *Addiction* 102:909–15.

Carroll, H. A., M. K. Lustyk, and M. E. Larimer. 2015. "The relationship between alcohol consumption and menstrual cycle." *Archives of Women's Mental Health* 18:773–81.

Carter, B. D., et al. 2015. "Smoking and mortality." *New England Journal of Medicine* 372:631–40.

Centers for Disease Control and Prevention. 1995. "Health-care provider advice on tobacco use to persons aged 10–22 years—United States, 1993." *Morbidity and Mortality Weekly Report*, 44 (November 10).

——. 2006. "Youth exposure to alcohol advertising on radio." *Morbidity and Mortality Weekly Report*, 44 (November 20).

——. 2019a. "Trends in the prevalence of alcohol use." CDC website.

——. 2019b. "Trends in the prevalence of marijuana, cocaine, and other illegal drug use." CDC website.

Cheadle, J. E., and L. B. Whitbeck. 2011. "Alcohol use trajectories and problem drinking over the course of adolescence." *Journal of Health and Social Behavior* 52:228–45.

Chen, M. J., B. A. Miller, J. W. Grube, and E. D. Waiters. 2006. "Music, substance use, and aggression." *Journal of Studies on Alcohol* 67:373–81.

Cohen, S. 1984. "Cocaine Anonymous." *Drug Abuse and Alcoholism Newsletter* 13 (3).

Cole, A. B., et al. 2020. "Health risk factors in American Indian and non-Hispanic white homeless adults." *American Journal of Health Behavior* 44:631–41.

Collins, M. D., and J. H. Frey. 1992. "Drunken driving and informal social control: The case of peer intervention." *Deviant Behavior* 13 (January–March):73–87.

Collins, R. L., et al. 2016. "Alcohol advertising exposure among middle school-age youth." *Journal of Studies on Alcohol and Drugs* 77: 384–92.

Conger, R. D., F. O. Lorenz, G. H. Elder Jr., J. N. Melby, R. L. Simons, and K. J. Conger. 1991. "A process model of family economic pressure and early adolescent alcohol use." *Journal of Early Adolescence* 11 (November): 430–49.

Connors, G. J., J. S. Tonigan, and W. R. Miller. 2001. "A longitudinal model of intake symptomatology, AA participation, and outcome." *Journal of Studies on Alcohol* 62:817–25.

Costello, D. M., L. C. Dierker, B. L. Jones, and J. S. Rose. 2008. "Trajectories of smoking from adolescence to early adulthood and their psychosocial risk factors." *Health Psychology* 27:811–18.

Costello, R. M. 2006. "Long-term mortality from alcoholism." *Journal of Studies on Alcohol* 67:694–99.

Crawford, J. A. 2014. "DSM-IV alcohol dependence and marital dissolution." *Journal of Studies on Alcohol and Drugs* 75:520–29.

Croghan, I. T., et al. 2006. "Is smoking related to body image satisfaction, stress, and self-esteem in young adults?" *American Journal of Health Behavior* 30:322–33.

Crosnoe, R. 2006. "The connection between academic failure and adolescent drinking in secondary school." *Sociology of Education* 79:44–60.

Cussen, M., and W. Block. 2000. "Legalize drugs now!" *American Journal of Economics and Sociology* 59:525–36.

De Micheli, D., and M. L. Formigoni. 2002. "Are reasons for the first use of drugs and family circumstances predictors of future use patterns?" *Addictive Behaviors* 27:87–100.

Distefan, J. M., J. P. Pierce, and E. A. Gilpin. 2004. "Do favorite movie stars influence adolescent smoking initiation?" *American Journal of Public Health* 94:1239–44.

Dorius, C. J., S. J. Bahr, J. P. Hoffman, and E. L. Harmon. 2004. "Parenting practices as moderators of the relationship between peers and adolescent marijuana use." *Journal of Marriage and Family* 66:163–78.

Duke, A. A., et al. 2011. "Alcohol dose and aggression." *Journal of Studies on Alcohol and Drugs* 72:34–43.

Edwards, K. A., K. Witkiewitz, and K. E. Vowles. 2019. "Demographic differences in perceived social norms of drug and alcohol use among Hispanic/Latinx and non-Hispanic white college students." *Addictive Behaviors* 98:1-7.

Epstein, J. F., and J. C. Groerer. 1997. "Heroin abuse in the United States." *OAS Working Paper.* Rockville, MD: SAMHSA.

Evans, N., A. Farkas, E. Gilpin, C. Berry, and J. P. Pierce. 1995. "Influence of tobacco marketing and exposure to smokers on adolescent susceptibility to smoking." *Journal of the National Cancer Institute* 87 (October):1538–45.

Farmer, R. P., et al. 2019. "Family aggregation of substance use disorders." *Journal of the Study of Alcohol and Drugs* 80:462–71.

Fell, J. C., et al. 2016. "Assessing the impact of twenty underage drinking laws." *Journal of Studies on Alcohol and Drugs* 71:249–60.

Fierro, I., C. Morales, and F. J. Alvarez. 2011. "Alcohol use, illicit drug use, and road rage." *Journal of Studies on Alcohol and Drugs* 72:185–93.

Fish, J. N., C. A. Meier, and J. B. Priest. 2015. "Substance abuse treatment response in a Latino sample." *Journal of Substance Abuse Treatment* 49:27–34.

Flewelling, R. L., and K. E. Bauman. 1990. "Family structure as a predictor of initial substance use and sexual intercourse in early adolescence." *Journal of Marriage and the Family* 52 (February):171–81.

Flynn, C. A., and W. E. Brown. 1991. "The effects of a mandatory alcohol education program on college student problem drinkers." *Journal of Alcohol and Drug Education* 37 (1):15–24.

Ford, J. A., and R. D. Schroeder. 2009. "Academic strain and non-medical use of prescription stimulants among college students." *Deviant Behavior* 30:26–53.

Forum on Child and Family Statistics. 2020. *America's Children in Brief: Key National Indicators of Well-Being, 2020.* Washington, DC: Government Printing Office.

Frieden, T. R., et al. 2005. "Adult tobacco use levels after intensive tobacco control measures." *American Journal of Public Health* 95:1016-23.

Friedenberg, E. Z. 1972. "The revolt against democracy." In *The Prospect of Youth,* ed. T. J. Cottle, pp. 147-56. Boston: Little, Brown.

Friese, B., et al. 2011. "Drinking behavior and sources of alcohol." *Journal of Studies on Alcohol and Drugs* 72:53-60.

Fritz, G. K. 2003. "Inhalant abuse among children and adolescents." *The Brown University Child and Adolescent Behavior Letter* 19:8.

Frone, M. R. 2006. "Prevalence and distribution of alcohol use and impairment in the workplace." *Journal of Studies on Alcohol* 67:147-56.

Furnas, J. C. 1965. *The Life and Times of the Late Demon Rum.* New York: Capricorn.

Gavaler, J. S. 1991. "Effects of alcohol on female endocrine function." *Alcohol Health and Research World* 15 (12):104-9.

Ghosh, J. K. C., M. Wilhelm, and B. Ritz. 2013. "Effects of residential Indoor air quality and household ventilation on preterm birth and term low birth weight in Los Angeles County, California." *American Journal of Public Health* 103:686-94.

Glantz, S. A., K. W. Kacirk, and C. McCulloch. 2004. "Back to the future: Smoking in the movies in 2002 compared with 1950 levels." *American Journal of Public Health* 94:261-63.

Goeders, N. E. 2003. "The impact of stress on addiction." *European Neuropsychopharmacology* 13:435-41.

Graham, K., D. W. Osgood, S. Wells, and T. Stockwell. 2006. "To what extent is intoxication associated with aggression in bars?" *Journal of Studies on Alcohol* 67:382-90.

Green, K. M., E. E. Doherty, K. A. Zebrak, and M. E. Ensminger. 2011. "Association between adolescent drinking and adult violence." *Journal of Studies on Alcohol and Drugs* 72:701-10.

Greenfeld, L. A. 1998. *Alcohol and Crime.* Washington, DC: Government Printing Office.

Grekin, E. R., K. J. Sher, and J. L. Krull. 2007. "College spring break and alcohol use." *Journal of Studies on Alcohol and Drugs* 68:681-88.

Guo, J., J. D. Hawkins, K. G. Hill, and R. D. Abbott. 2001. "Childhood and adolescent predictors of alcohol abuse and dependence in young adulthood." *Journal of Studies on Alcohol* 62:754-62.

Haber, J. R., et al. 2010. "Effect of paternal alcohol and drug dependence on offspring conduct disorder." *Journal of Studies on Alcohol and Drugs* 71:652-63.

Hair, E. C., et al. 2009. "Parent marital quality and the parent-adolescent relationship: Effects on adolescent and young adult health outcomes." *Marriage & Family Review* 45:218-48.

Hall, J. H., W. Fals-Stewart, and F. D. Fincham. 2008. "Risky sexual behavior among married alcoholic men." *Journal of Family Psychology* 22:287-92.

Hamilton, H. R., and T. Dehart. 2019. "Needs and norms." *Journal of Studies on Alcohol and Drugs* 80:340-48.

Hansell, S., and H. R. White. 1991. "Adolescent drug use, psychological distress, and physical symptoms." *Journal of Health and Social Behavior* 32 (September):288-301.

Harford, T. C., H. Wechsler, and B. O. Muthen. 2003. "Alcohol-related aggression and drinking at off-campus parties and bars." *Journal of Studies on Alcohol* 64:704-11.

Harford, T. C., H. Wechsler, and M. Seibring. 2002. "Attendance and alcohol use at parties and bars in college." *Journal of Studies on Alcohol* 63:726-33.

Hedegaard, H., A. M. Minino, and M. Warner. 2020. "Drug overdose deaths in the United States, 1999-2018." National Center for Health Statistics website.

Hei, W. M. 2019. "Dimensions of religiosity." *Journal of Studies on Alcohol and Drugs* 80:358-65.

Higham, A., et al. 2016. "Electronic cigarette exposure triggers neutrophil inflammatory responses." *Respiratory Research* 17:56.

Hingson, R. W., T. Heeren, and E. M. Edwards. 2008. "Age at drinking onset, alcohol dependence, and their relation to drug use and dependence, driving under the influence of drugs, and motor-vehicle crash involvement because of drugs." *Journal of Studies on Alcohol and Drugs* 69:192-201.

Hingson, R., T. Heeren, R. Zakoes, M. Winter, and H. Wechsler. 2003. "Age at first intoxication, heavy drinking, driving after drinking, and risk of unintentional injury among U.S. college students." *Journal of Studies on Alcohol* 64:23-31.

Hirschman, R. S., H. Leventhal, and K. Glynn. 1984. "The development of smoking behavior: Conceptualization and supportive cross-sectional survey data." *Journal of Applied Social Psychology* 14 (May-June):184-206.

Hoffmann, J. P., and S. J. Bahr. 2014. "Parenting style, religiosity, peer alcohol use, and adolescent heavy drinking." *Journal of Studies on Alcohol and Drugs* 75:222-27.

Holahan, C. J., R. H. Moos, C. K. Holahan, R. C. Cronkite, and P. K. Randall. 2001. "Drinking to cope: Emotional distress and alcohol use and abuse." *Journal of Studies on Alcohol* 62:190-98.

Hollingworth, W., et al. 2006. "Prevention of deaths from harmful drinking in the United States." *Journal of Studies on Alcohol* 67:300-8.

Howard, M. O., et al. 2010. "Inhalant use, inhalant-use disorders, and antisocial behavior." *Journal of Studies on Alcohol and Drugs* 71:201-9.

Hu, M., M. Davies, and D. B. Kandel. 2006. "Epidemiology and correlates of daily smoking and nicotine dependence among young adults in the United States." *American Journal of Public Health* 96:299-308.

Järvinen, M., and G. Miller. 2010. "Methadone maintenance as last resort." *Sociological Forum* 25:804-23.

Jessor, R., F. M. Costa, P. M. Krueger, and M. S. Turbin. 2006. "A developmental study of heavy episodic drinking among college students." *Journal of Studies on Alcohol* 67:86-94.

Johnson, R. A., and D. R. Gerstein. 1998. "Initiation of use of alcohol, cigarettes, marijuana, cocaine, and other substances in U.S. birth cohorts since 1919." *American Journal of Public Health* 88 (January):27-33.

Jones-Webb, R., et al. 2016. "Effects of economic disruptions on alcohol use and problems." *Journal of Studies on Alcohol and Drugs* 77:261-71.

Kabir, Z., G. N. Connolly, L. Clancy, H. K. Koh, and S. Capewell. 2008. "Coronary heart disease deaths and decreased smoking prevalence in Massachusetts, 1993-2003." *American Journal of Public Health* 98:1468-69.

Keller, P. S., et al. 2011. "Parent problem drinking, marital aggression, and child emotional insecurity." *Journal of Studies on Alcohol and Drugs* 72:711-22.

Kelly, J. F., M. E. Pagano, R. L. Stout, and S. M. Johnson. 2011. "Influence of religiosity on 12-step participation and treatment response among substance-dependent adolescents." *Journal of Studies on Alcohol and Drugs* 72:1000-11.

Kilgore, E. A., et al. 2014. "Making it harder to smoke and easier to quit." *American Journal of Public Health* 104:65-8.

Kilmer, J. R., et al. 2006. "Misperceptions of college student marijuana use." *Journal of Studies on Alcohol* 67:277-81.

Kilpatrick, D. G., et al. 2000. "Risk factors for adolescent substance abuse and dependence." *Journal of Consulting and Clinical Psychology* 68:19-30.

Kinnier, R. T., A. T. Metha, J. L. Okey, and J. M. Keim. 1994. "Adolescent substance abuse and psychological health." *Journal of Alcohol and Drug Education* 40 (Fall):51-56.

Kramarow, E. A. 2020. "Health of former cigarette smokers aged 65 and over." National Center for Health Statistics website.

Kumsar, N., S. Kumsar, and N. Dilbaz. 2016. "Sexual dysfunction in men diagnosed as substance use disorder." *Andrologia* 48:1229-35.

Kwate, N. O. A., and I. H. Meyer. 2009. "Association between residential exposure to outdoor alcohol advertising and problem drinking among African American women in New York City." *American Journal of Public Health* 99: 228-30.

LaCroix, A. Z., et al. 1991. "Smoking and mortality among older men and women in three communities." *New England Journal of Medicine* 324 (June 6):1619-25.

Landberg, J., and T. Norstrom. 2011. "Alcohol and homicide in Russia and the United States." *Journal of Studies on Alcohol and Drugs* 72:723-30.

Landen, M., et al. 2014. "Alcohol-attributable mortality among American Indians and Alaska Natives in the United States, 1999-2009." *American Journal of Public Health* 104:S343-49.

Lehman, W. E. K., D. J. Farabee, M. L. Holcom, and D. D. Simpson. 1995. "Prediction of substance use in the workplace: Unique contributions of personal background and work environment variables." *Journal of Drug Issues* 25 (2):253-74.

Lemke, S., P. L. Brennan, K. K. Schutte, and R. H. Moos. 2007. "Upward pressures on drinking." *Journal of Studies on Alcohol and Drugs* 68:437-45.

Leshner, A. I. 1998. "Addiction is a brain disease—and it matters." *National Institute of Justice Journal* (October):2-6.

Leventhal, A. M., et al. 2015. "Association of electronic cigarette use with initiation of combustible tobacco product smoking in early adolescence." *Journal of the American Medical Association* 314:700-7.

Levy, D. T., et al. 2016. "The application of a decision-theoretic model to estimate the public health impact of vaporized nicotine product initiation in the United States." *Nicotine and Tobacco Research*, published online.

Levy, J. A., C. P. Gallmeier, and W. W. Wiebel. 1995. "The outreach assisted peer-support model for controlling drug dependency." *Journal of Drug Issues* 25 (3):507-29.

Lewis, M. A., et al. 2011. "They drink how much and where? Normative perceptions by drinking contexts and their association to college students' alcohol consumption." *Journal of Studies on Alcohol and Drugs* 72:844-53.

Lipari, R. N., and B. Jean-Francois. 2016. *A day in the life of college students aged 18 to 22: Substance use facts.* Substance Abuse and Mental Health Services Administration. Rockville, MD.

Liskow, B. I., et al. 2000. "Mortality in male alcoholics after ten to fourteen years." *Journal of Studies on Alcohol* 61:853-61.

Lu, L., and X. Wang. 2008. "Drug addiction in China." *Journal of the New York Academy of Sciences* 1141:304-17.

Liu, X., and H. B. Kaplan. 1996. "Gender-related differences in circumstances surrounding initiation and escalation of alcohol and other substance use/abuse." *Deviant Behavior* 17 (1):71-106.

Mackenbach, J. P., et al. 2008. "Socioeconomic inequalities in health in 22 European countries." *New England Journal of Medicine* 358:2468-81.

Maguire, K. 2012. *Sourcebook of Criminal Justice Statistics.* Bureau of Justice Statistics website.

Males, M. 2010. "Traffic crash victimizations of children and teenagers by drinking drivers age 21 and older." *Journal of Studies on Alcohol and Drugs* 71:351-56.

Malik, S., et al. 2008. "Maternal smoking and congenital heart defects." *Pediatrics* 121:810-16.

Mann, R. E., R. F. Zaleman, R. G. Smart, B. R. Rush, and H. Suurvali. 2006. "Alcohol consumption, alcoholics anonymous membership, and suicide mortality rates, Ontario, 1968-1991." *Journal of Studies on Alcohol* 67:445-53.

Marsch, L. A. 1998. "The efficacy of methadone maintenance interventions in reducing illicit opiate use, HIV risk behavior and criminality." *Addiction* 93 (April):515-32.

Martin, C. S., P. R. Clifford, and R. L. Clapper. 1992. "Patterns and predictors of simultaneous and concurrent use of alcohol, tobacco, marijuana, and hallucinogens in first-year college students." *Journal of Substance Abuse* 4 (3):319-26.

May, P. A. 1991. "Fetal alcohol effects among North American Indians." *Alcohol Health and Research World* 15 (3):239-48.

Mazerolle, L., C. Kadleck, and J. Roehl. 2004. "Differential police control at drug-dealing places." *Security Journal* 17:61-69.

McBroom, J. R. 1992. "Alcohol and drug use by third, fourth, and fifth graders in a town of 20,000." *Sociology and Social Research* 76 (April):156-60.

McCaffery, J. M., G. D. Papandonatos, C. Stanton, E. E. Lloyd-Richardson, and R. Niaura. 2008. "Depressive symptoms and cigarette smoking in twins from the National Longitudinal Study of Adolescent Health." *Health Psychology* 27:207-15.

McFarlin, S. K., W. Fals-Stewart, D. A. Major, and E. M. Justice. 2001. "Alcohol use and workplace aggression." *Journal of Substance Abuse* 13:303-21.

McKee, M., and V. Shkolnikov. 2001. "Understanding the toll of premature death among men in Eastern Europe." *British Medical Journal* 323:1051-55.

McKellar, J., E. Stewart, and K. Humphreys. 2003. "Alcoholics Anonymous involvement and positive alcohol-related outcomes." *Journal of Consulting and Clinical Psychology* 71:302-8.

Miech, R. A., et al. 2020. *Monitoring the Future National Survey Results on Drug Use.* Ann Arbor: Institute for Social Research.

Miller, T. R., D. T. Levy, R. S. Spicer, and D. M. Taylor. 2006. "Societal costs of underage drinking." *Journal of Studies on Alcohol* 67:519-28.

Miller, W. R., and P. L. Wilbourne. 2002. "Mesa Grande: A methodological analysis of clinical trials of treatments for alcohol use disorders." *Addiction* 97:265-77.

Miller-Day, M. 2008. "Talking to youth about drugs: What do late adolescents say about parental strategies?" *Family Relations* 57:1-12.

Moore, A. A., et al. 2005. "Longitudinal patterns and predictors of alcohol consumption in the United States." *American Journal of Public Health* 95:458-65.

Moore, T. H. M., et al. 2007. "Cannabis use and risk of psychotic or affective mental health outcomes." *The Lancet* 370:319-28.

Moos, R. H., and B. S. Moos. 2004. "Long-term influence of duration and frequency of participation in Alcoholics Anonymous on individuals with alcohol use disorders." *Journal of Consulting and Clinical Psychology* 72:81-90.

Mukamal, K. J., and E. B. Rimm. 2001. "Alcohol's effects on the risk for coronary heart disease." *Alcohol Research and Health* 25:255-61.

Mukherjee, S., S. K. Das, K. Vaidyanathan, and D. M. Vasudevan. 2008. "Consequences of alcohol consumption on neurotransmitters." *Current Neurovascular Research* 5:266-72.

Mulia, N., Y. Ye, S. E. Zemore, and T. K. Greenfield. 2008. "Social disadvantage, stress, and alcohol use among black, Hispanic, and white Americans." *Journal of Studies on Alcohol and Drugs* 69:824-33.

National Academies of Science, Engineering, and Medicine. 2017. *The Health Effects of Cannabis and Cannabinoids*. Washington, DC: The National Academies Press.

National Academy of Sciences. 2009. "Smoking bans reduce the risk of heart attacks associated with secondhand smoke." NAS website.

National Center for Health Statistics 2019. "*Health, United States, 2018*." Hyattsville, MD: National Center for Health Statistics.

National Center on Addiction and Substance Abuse at Columbia University. 1998. *Back to School 1998: The CASA National Survey of American Attitudes on Substance Abuse*. Washington, DC: National Center on Addiction and Substance Abuse.

National Institute on Alcohol Abuse and Alcoholism. 2019. "Alcohol facts and statistics." NIAAA website.

National Institute on Drug Abuse. 2004. "Preventing drug use among children and adolescents." NIDA website.

——. 2005. "NIDA infofacts: Methamphetamine." NIDA website.

——. 2014. "Adolescents and young adults." NIDA website.

——. 2020. "Costs of substance abuse." NIDA website.

National Survey on Drug Use and Health. 2004. "Religious beliefs and substance use among youths." *The NSDUH Report,* January 30.

Nelson, D. E., et al. 2013. "Alcohol-attributable cancer deaths and years of potential life lost in the United States." *American Journal of Public Health* 103:641-8.

Ness, R. B., et al. 1999. "Cocaine and tobacco use and the risk of spontaneous abortion." *New England Journal of Medicine* 340 (February 4):333-39.

Netemeyer, R. G., J. C. Andrews, and S. Burton. 2005. "Effects of antismoking advertising-based beliefs on adult smokers' consideration of quitting." *American Journal of Public Health* 95:1062-66.

Nguyen-Louie, T. T., et al. 2015. "Effects of emerging alcohol and marijuana use behaviors on adolescents' neuropsychological functioning over four years." *Journal of Studies on Alcohol and Drugs* 76:738-48.

Nooyens, A. C. J., B. M. van Gelder, and W. M. M. Verschuren. 2008. "Smoking and cognitive decline among middle-aged men and women." *American Journal of Public Health* 98:2244-50.

Obot, I. S., F. A. Wagner, and J. C. Anthony. 2001. "Early onset and recent drug use among children of parents with alcohol problems." *Drug and Alcohol Dependence* 65:1-8.

Office of National Drug Control Policy. 2003a. *Cocaine.* Washington, DC: Government Printing Office.

——. 2003b. *What Americans Need to Know about Marijuana*. Washington, DC: Government Printing Office.

——. 2008. *Teen Marijuana Use Worsens Depression*. Washington, DC: Government Printing Office.

Olds, D. L., C. R. Henderson Jr., and R. Tatelbaum. 1994. "Prevention of intellectual impairment in children of women who smoke during pregnancy." *Pediatrics* 93 (February):228-33.

Osborne, C., and L. M. Berger. 2009. "Parental substance abuse and child well-being." *Journal of Family Issues* 30:341-70.

Park, C. L., S. Armeli, and H. Tennen. 2004. "The daily stress and coping process and alcohol use among college students." *Journal of Studies on Alcohol* 65:126-35.

Parker, T., et al. 2010. "Beyond the prison bubble." *NIJ Journal* 268:31-36.

Paschall, M. J., M. Bersamin, and R. L. Flewelling. 2005. "Racial/ethnic differences in the association between college attendance and heavy alcohol use." *Journal of Studies on Alcohol* 66:266–74.

Patrick, M. E., et al. 2019. "Reasons high school students use marijuana." *Journal of Studies on Alcohol and Drugs* 80:15–25.

Pedersen, E. R., and J. W. LaBrie. 2008. "Normative misperceptions of drinking among college students." *Journal of Studies on Alcohol and Drugs* 69:406–11.

Petry, N. M., and B. Martin. 2002. "Low-cost contingency management for treating cocaine- and opioid-abusing methadone patients." *Journal of Consulting and Clinical Psychology* 70:398–405.

Peugh, J., and S. Belenko. 2001. "Alcohol, drugs, and sexual function." *Journal of Psychoactive Drugs* 33:223–32.

Phillips, D. P., G. E. C. Barker, and M. M. Eguchi. 2008. "A steep increase in domestic fatal medication errors with use of alcohol and/or street drugs." *Archives of Internal Medicine* 168:1561–66.

Phillips-Howard, P. A., et al. 2010. "Wellbeing, alcohol use and sexual activity in young teenagers." *Substance Abuse Treatment, Prevention, and Policy* 5:27–34.

Pierce, J. P., et al. 1998. "Tobacco industry promotion of cigarettes and adolescent smoking." *Journal of the American Medical Association* 279 (February 18):511–15.

Pinkleton, B. E., Y. Fujioka, and E. W. Austin. 2000. "The role of interpretation processes and parental discussion in the media's effects on adolescents' use of alcohol." *Pediatrics* 105:343–49.

Piper, B. J., et al. 2016. "Use and misuse of opioids in Maine." *Journal of Studies on Alcohol and Drugs* 77: 556–65.

Pollack, H. A. 2001. "Sudden infant death syndrome, maternal smoking during pregnancy, and the cost-effectiveness of smoking cessation intervention." *American Journal of Public Health* 91:432–36.

Qato, D. M., et al. 2008. "Use of prescription and over-the-counter medications and dietary supplements among older adults in the United States." *Journal of the American Medical Association* 300:2867–78.

Reboussin, B. A., et al. 2019. "Social influences on drinking trajectories from adolescence to young adulthood in an urban minority sample." *Journal of Studies on Alcohol and Drugs* 80:186–95.

Rehm, J. 2011. "The risks associated with alcohol use and alcoholism." *Alcohol Research and Health* 34:135–43.

Reid, J., P. Macchetto, and S. Foster. 1999. *No Safe Haven: Children of Substance-Abusing Parents*. Washington, DC: National Center on Addiction and Substance Abuse.

Reilly, D. M. 1984. "Family therapy with adolescent drug abusers and their families: Defying gravity and achieving escape velocity." *Journal of Drug Issues* 14 (Spring):381–91.

Richards, M., M. J. Jarvis, N. Thompson, and M. E. J. Wadsworth. 2003. "Cigarette smoking and cognitive decline in midlife." *American Journal of Public Health* 93:994–98.

Rigg, K. K., and G. E. Ibanez. 2010. "Motivations for non-medical prescription drug use." *Journal of Substance Abuse Treatment* 39:236–47.

Rivara, F. P., et al. 1997. "Alcohol and illicit drug abuse and the risk of violent death in the home." *Journal of the American Medical Association* 278 (August 20):569–75.

Rodgers, J. E. 1994. "Addiction—A whole new view." *Psychology Today*, September–October, pp. 32–39.

Roeber, J., et al. 2007. "Types of alcoholic beverages usually consumed by students in 9th–12th grades—Four states, 2005." *Morbidity and Mortality Weekly Report* 56:737–40.

Rorabaugh, W. J. 1979. *The Alcoholic Republic: An American Tradition*. New York: Oxford University Press.

Rothman, E. F., et al. 2011. "Drinking style and dating violence in a sample of urban, alcohol-using youth." *Journal of Studies on Alcohol and Drugs* 72:555–66.

Roy, A. 2003. "Distal risk factors for suicidal behavior in alcoholics." *Journal of Affective Disorders* 77:267–71.

Sargent, J. D., T. A. Wills, M. Stoolmiller, J. Gibson, and F. X. Gibbons. 2006. "Alcohol use in motion pictures and its relation with early-onset teen drinking." *Journal of Studies on Alcohol* 67:54–65.

Schachter, S., and J. E. Singer. 1962. "Cognitive, social, and psychological determinants of emotional state." *Psychological Review* 69 (September):379–99.

Schonfeld, A. M., S. N. Mattson, and E. P. Riley. 2005. "Moral maturity and delinquency after prenatal alcohol exposure." *Journal of Studies on Alcohol* 66:545–54.

Schuckit, M. A., T. L. Smith, and J. Kalmijn. 2013. "Relationships among independent major depressions, alcohol use, and other substance use and related problems over 30 Years in 397 families." *Journal of Studies on Alcohol and Drugs* 74:271-79.

Scott, J. 1990. "Parents' smoking linked to children's lung cancer." *Los Angeles Times,* September 6.

Seeman, M., A. Z. Seeman, and A. Budros. 1988. "Powerlessness, work, and community: A longitudinal study of alienation and alcohol use." *Journal of Health and Social Behavior* 29 (September):185-98.

Shaw, B. A., N. Agahi, and N. Krause. 2011. "Are changes in financial strain associated with changes in alcohol use and smoking among older adults?" *Journal of Studies on Alcohol and Drugs* 72:917-25.

Sher, G. 2003. "On the decriminalization of drugs." *Criminal Justice Ethics* 22:12-15.

Silberg, J., M. Rutter, B. D'Onofrio, and L. Eaves. 2003. "Genetic and environmental risk factors in adolescent substance use." *Journal of Child Psychology and Psychiatry and Allied Disciplines* 44:664-76.

Simons-Morton, B., et al. 2016. "The effect of residence, school status, work status, and social influence of alcohol use among emerging adults." *Journal of Studies on Alcohol and Drugs* 77:121-32.

Singer, L. T., et al. 2002. "Cognitive and motor outcomes of cocaine-exposed infants." *Journal of the American Medical Association* 287:1952-60.

Sintov, N. D., et al. 2009. "Predictors of illicit substance dependence among individuals with alcohol dependence." *Journal of Studies on Alcohol and Drugs* 70:269-78.

Smart, R. G. 1991. "Crack cocaine use: A review of prevalence and adverse effects." *American Journal of Drug and Alcohol Abuse* 17 (March):13-26.

Smith, P. D., P. C. Rivers, and K. J. Stahl. 1992. "Family cohesion and conflict as predictors of drinking patterns: Beyond demographics and alcohol expectancies." *Family Dynamics of Addiction Quarterly* 2 (2):61-69.

Snow, D. L., et al. 2006. "The role of coping and problem drinking in men's abuse of female partners." *Violence and Victims* 21:267-85.

Spencer, M. R., S. C. Curtin, and H. Hedegaard. 2020. "Rates of alcohol-induced deaths among adults aged 25 and over in urban and rural areas." National Center for Health Statistics website.

Solowij, N., et al. 2002. "Cognitive functioning of long-term heavy cannabis users seeking treatment." *Journal of the American Medical Association* 287:1123-31.

Strecher, V. J., M. W. Kreuter, and S. C. Kobrin. 1995. "Do cigarette smokers have unrealistic perceptions of their heart attack, cancer, and stroke risks?" *Journal of Behavioral Medicine* 18 (February):45-54.

Streissguth, A. P. 1992. "Fetal alcohol syndrome: Early and long-term consequences." In *Problems of Drug Dependence 1991,* ed. L. Harris. Rockville, MD: National Institute on Drug Abuse.

Stuart, G. L., T. M. Moore, S. E. Ramsey, and C. W. Kahler. 2003. "Relationship aggression and substance use among women court-referred to domestic violence intervention programs." *Addictive Behaviors* 28:1603-10.

——. 2004. "Hazardous drinking and relationship violence perpetration and victimization in women arrested for domestic violence." *Journal of Studies on Alcohol* 65:46-53.

Sturm, J. J., K. Yeatts, and D. Loomis. 2004. "Effects of tobacco smoke exposure on asthma prevalence and medical care use in North Carolina middle school children." *American Journal of Public Health* 94:308-13.

Sung, H., et al. 2005. "Major state tobacco tax increase, the master settlement agreement, and cigarette consumption." *American Journal of Public Health* 95:1030-35.

Sutfin, E. L., et al. 2015. "The impact of trying electronic cigarettes on cigarette smoking by college students." *American Journal of Public Health* 105:e83-e89.

Tempier, R., et al. 2006. "Psychological distress among female spouses of male at-risk drinkers." *Alcohol* 40:41-49.

Terry-McElrath, Y. M., P. M. O'Malley, and L. D. Johnston. 2008. "Saying no to marijuana: Why American youth report quitting or abstaining." *Journal of Studies on Alcohol and Drugs* 69:796-805.

——. 2014. "Alcohol and Marijuana use patterns associated with unsafe driving among U.S. high school seniors." *Journal of Studies on Alcohol and Drugs* 75:378-89.

Tran, A. G. T. T., R. M. Lee, and D. J. Burgess. 2010. "Perceived discrimination and substance use in Hispanic/ Latino, African-born black, and Southeast Asian immigrants." *Cultural Diversity and Ethnic Minority Psychology* 16:226-36.

Troisi, A., A. Pasini, M. Saracco, and G. Spalletta. 1998. "Psychiatric symptoms in male cannabis users not using other illicit drugs." *Addiction* 93 (April):487–92.

U.S. Department of Health and Human Services. 1995. "Preliminary estimates from the 1994 national household survey on drug abuse." *Advance Report Number 10* (September).

——. 2006. *The Health Consequences of Involuntary Exposure to Tobacco Smoke*. Washington, DC: Government Printing Office.

U.S. Department of Justice. 1992. *Drugs, Crime, and the Justice System*. Washington, DC: Government Printing Office.

Vanheusden, K., et al. 2008. "Patterns of association between alcohol consumption and internalizing and externalizing problems in young adults." *Journal of Studies on Alcohol and Drugs* 69:49–57.

Vedantam, S., A. Epstine, and B. Geiger. 1997. "Tobacco firm says smoking is addictive." *San Diego Union-Tribune,* March 21.

Villarroel, M. A., A. E. Cha, and A. Vahratian. 2020. "Electronic cigarette use among U.S. adults, 2018." National Center for Health Statistics website.

Wallace, J. M., et al. 2007. "Religiosity and adolescent substance use: The role of individual and contextual influences." *Social Problems* 54:308–27.

Warner, L. A., H. R. White, and V. Johnson. 2007. "Alcohol initiation experiences and family history of alcoholism as predictors of problem-drinking trajectories." *Journal of Studies on Alcohol and Drugs* 68:56–65.

Watt, T. T. 2002. "Marital and cohabiting relationships of adult children of alcoholics." *Journal of Family Issues* 23:246–65.

Weitzman, E. R., and I. Kawachi. 2000. "Giving means receiving: The protective effect of social capital on binge drinking on college campuses." *American Journal of Public Health* 90:1936–39.

Wells, S., et al. 2014. "Linking Masculinity to Negative Drinking Consequences." *Journal of Studies on Alcohol and Drugs* 75:510–19.

Whisman, M. A., L. A. Uebelacker, and M. L. Bruce. 2006. "Longitudinal association between marital dissatisfaction and alcohol use disorders in a community sample." *Journal of Family Psychology* 20:164–67.

White, H. R., N. Jarrett, E. Y. Valencia, R. Loeber, and E. Wei. 2007. "Stages and sequences of initiation and regular substance use in a longitudinal cohort of black and white male adolescents." *Journal of Studies on Alcohol and Drugs* 68:173–81.

Whitlock, E. P., M. R. Polen, C. A. Green, T. Orleans, and J. Klein. 2004. "Behavioral counseling interventions in primary care to reduce risky/harmful alcohol use by adults." *Annals of Internal Medicine* 140:557–68.

Wild, T. C. 2002. "Personal drinking and sociocultural drinking norms." *Journal of Studies on Alcohol* 63:469–75.

Wilens, T. E., et al. 2002. "A family study of the high-risk children of opioid- and alcohol-dependent parents." *American Journal on Addictions* 11:41–51.

Wills, T. A., et al. 2007. "Movie exposure to smoking cues and adolescent smoking onset." *Health Psychology* 26:769–76.

Wolfinger, N. H. 1998. "The effects of parental divorce on adult tobacco and alcohol consumption." *Journal of Health and Social Behavior* 39 (September):254–69.

Womack, S. R., et al. 2016. "Bidirectional associations between cannabis use and depressive symptoms from adolescence through early adulthood among at-risk young men." *Journal of Studies on Alcohol and Drugs* 77: 287–97.

World Health Organization. 2011. "Action needed to reduce the health impact of harmful alcoholism." WHO website.

——. 2016. "Ambient air pollution: A global assessment of exposure and burden of disease." WHO website.

Wren, C. S. 1997. "Ex-addicts find methadone more elusive than heroin." *New York Times,* February 2.

Wright, H. I., J. S. Gavaler, and D. Van Thiel. 1991. "Effects of alcohol on the male reproductive system." *Alcohol Health and Research World* 15 (12):110–14.

Xu, Y., M. L. Fiedler, and K. H. Flaming. 2005. "Discovering the impact of community policing." *Journal of Research in Crime and Delinquency* 42:147–86.

Xue, Y., M. A. Zimmerman, and R. Cunningham. 2009. "Relationship between alcohol use and violent behavior among urban African American youths from adolescence to emerging adulthood." *American Journal of Public Health* 99:2041–48.

Young-Wolff, K. C., K. S. Kendler, and C. A. Prescott. 2012. "Interactive effects of childhood maltreatment and recent stressful life events on alcohol consumption in adulthood." *Journal of Studies on Alcohol and Drugs* 73:559–69.

CHAPTER

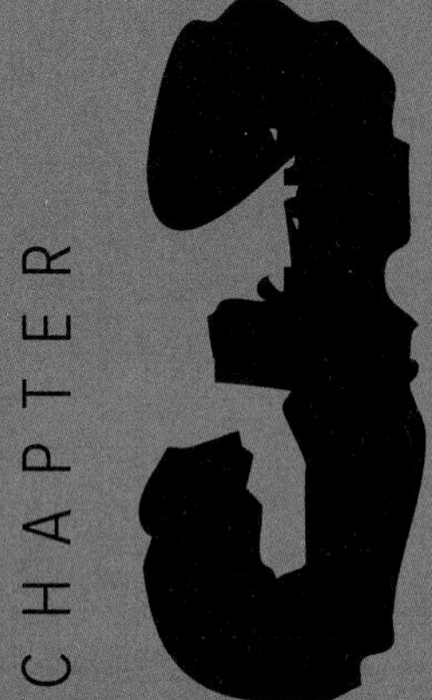

# Crime and Delinquency

## OBJECTIVES

1. Know the different kinds of crime.
2. Explain the ways in which crime data are obtained, and describe the problems inherent in official records.
3. Discuss the amount and distribution of crime in the United States.
4. Identify the varied consequences of crime in regard to the quality of American life.
5. Explain the factors that contribute to the problem of crime.
6. Discuss the varied and sometimes contradictory suggestions for reducing crime.

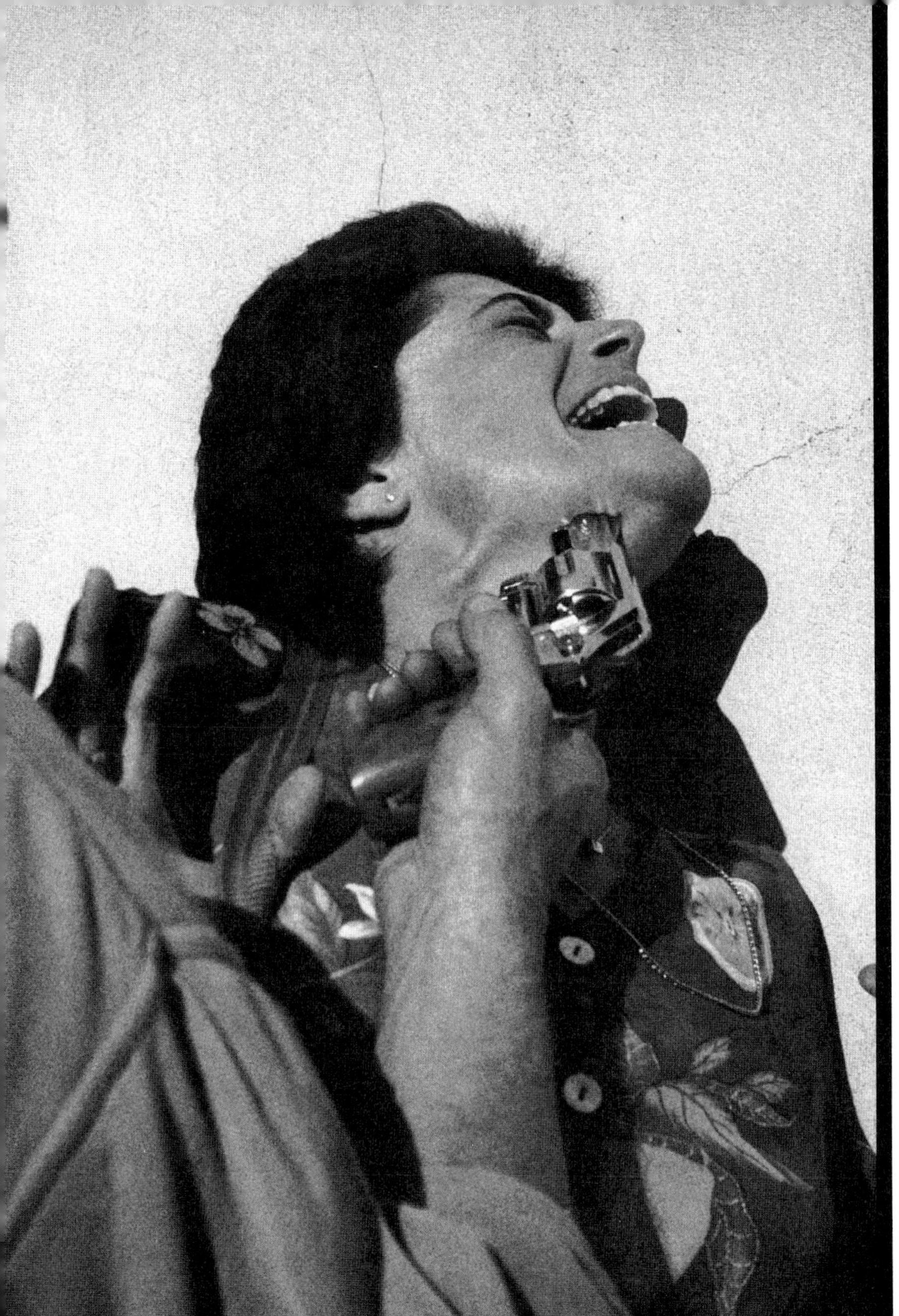

Laurent Hamels/Photoalto/PictureQuest

## A Victim Recovers

Marcia, in her 20s, is one of the few survivors of an attack by a serial killer and rapist. After her assailant was sentenced to die for the murder of five young women and the rape of two others, Marcia told her story publicly. Like others, she felt a kind of double victimization:

*I was only 22 when he appeared in my bedroom doorway, a bandanna covering his features, a knife raised high as he leaped toward my bed. A week before, he had been a visitor in my home, passing the time during the week he stayed as the houseguest of a neighbor.*

*Nothing could have prepared me for the viciousness I would experience in the following hours, reduced from a human being to an "it" in the mind and actions of this man. He dragged me around my house by the neck for several hours, forced me to do unspeakable things and twice strangled me into unconsciousness. I fully expected to die before the night passed, hoping only to die with some dignity. He is 14 inches taller than me and twice my weight. I began to fight him with my mind. It became critical that I showed no fear because when I showed fear, he fed on it. I told him excuses for his behavior. Each time he hurt me, I chastised him almost cheerfully as though I was his friend. Four and a half hours after it started, he walked away of his own accord. I had managed to convince him that he had nothing to fear from me.*

*Just as nothing could have prepared me for him, nothing prepared me for the seven years ahead, in which I would keep alive these hideous memories for the appeasement of an overburdened and overindulgent criminal defense system. I remember being disheveled and in shock in my living room and the policeman asking me how committed I was to prosecuting my assailant. I told him that I would do whatever I had to do. I could not have known that it would take seven years and three trials. I had to describe to three juries in painful detail the kind of agony he meted out to his victims. Despite my anger that the families of the victims and myself have been further victimized to this extent by a system that gave him every reasonable—and unreasonable—concession and delay over the years, I do not regret my decision to testify.*

*In the end, I can only mourn at the tragic waste he represents, not only in his victims—and I am no longer one of them—but in himself. However, I'm not so noble as to keep back some satisfaction that this random killer should find that the blood on his hands is also his own.*

## Introduction

Americans frequently get upset or angry about the problem of crime. A small child is killed, a mother is strangled by her estranged husband, or a businessman cheats people out of their retirement. Such crimes enrage people and can lead to an increased demand for law and order.

Is there reason for such concern? After all, crime rates have generally been falling since about 1990, and some have fallen dramatically (see Table 3.2). Still, there is an enormous amount of crime in the nation (Figure 3.1). For example, the murder rate was 9.4 per 100,000 in 1990, but down to 5.0 in 2019. The victimization rate for all other violent crimes fell from 31.3 per 1,000 people aged 12 and above in 1991 to 21.0 in 2019 (Morgan and Truman 2020). Property crime rates have also declined. Such figures are encouraging, but they take on a different cast when you realize that in 2019 there were still 5.8 million Americans victimized by violent crime and 12.8 million victimized by property crime (burglary and theft). Or think of it this way: It is doubtful if any American can reach adulthood without being the victim of a crime or having a family member or acquaintance who has been a victim. In short, despite the declining rates, crime remains a serious social problem.

Major crimes like murder, robbery, and theft capture people's attention and generate concern. But historian Herbert Butterfield suggested that a society can be destroyed by crimes involving "petty breaches of faith" of "very nice people" (Butterfield 1949:54). These two contrasting points of view form the theme of this chapter: Crime is a social problem that pervades American society, and it *includes both respectable and nonrespectable citizens.*

First, we look at the varieties of crime and define crime and delinquency. We then examine the extent of crime in the United States, the effects that crime and delinquency have on the quality of life, and the kinds of sociocultural factors that contribute to the problem. Finally, we discuss measures that can be taken and have been taken to resolve the problem.

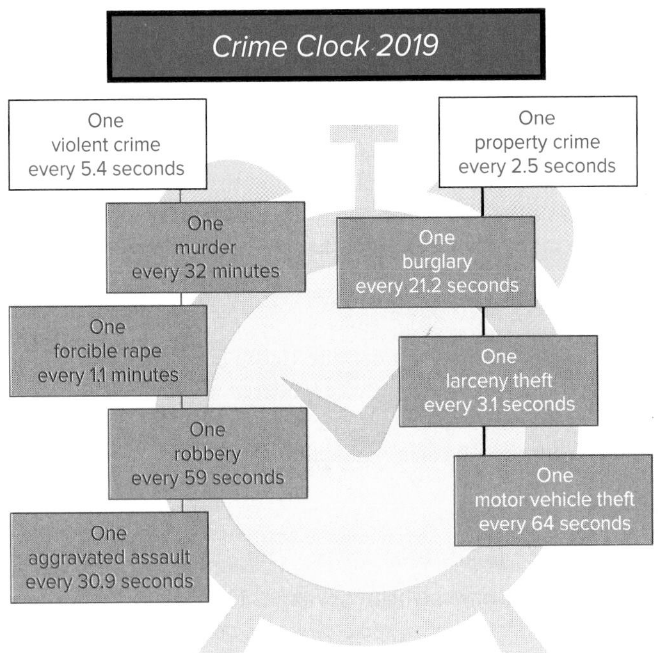


**FIGURE 3.1**
The Crime Clock Dramatizes the Extensiveness of Crime in the United States.
Source: Morgan and Truman 2020.

## The Varieties of Crime

Technically, crime is any violation of the criminal law. However, as you will see when we examine white-collar crime, this definition is inadequate. Nevertheless, we begin with a discussion of the kinds of acts embodied in the criminal law—acts that are defined as threatening to the state or to citizens whom the state is obligated to protect.

### Predatory Crime

When the word *crime* is mentioned, people generally think of **predatory crimes**—*acts that have victims who suffer loss of property or some kind of physical harm.* Property crimes are more common, but the public generally defines crimes against persons as more serious. Less than 10 percent of all crime involves acts such as murder and rape, but these violent acts are the ones that arouse the greatest public apprehension.

**predatory crimes**
acts that have victims who suffer loss of property or some kind of physical harm

A commonly used measure of *crime rates*—the *Federal Bureau of Investigation Crime Index*—covers eight major felonies, all serious violations of the criminal law, and all predatory crimes. The FBI defines them as follows (Federal Bureau of Investigation 2002): (1) *Murder and non-negligent manslaughter* are willful killing of a person. Not included are deaths by negligence, suicide, accident, and justifiable homicide. (2) *Aggravated assault,* "an unlawful attack by one person upon another for the purpose of inflicting severe bodily injury," usually involves a weapon. (3) *Forcible rape* is defined as actual or attempted sexual intercourse "through the use of force or the threat of force." (4) *Robbery* is the use of force or threat of force to take something of value from a person. (5) *Burglary*—by definition the "unlawful entry of a structure to commit a felony or theft"—does not necessarily mean force was used to gain entry. (6) *Larceny-theft* is the "unlawful taking or stealing of property or articles without the use of force, violence, or fraud." It includes shoplifting, picking pockets, purse snatching, and the like. (7) *Motor vehicle theft* includes both actual and attempted theft of any motor vehicle. (8) Finally, *arson* is any "willful or malicious burning or attempt to burn, with or without intent to defraud, a dwelling house, public building, motor vehicle or aircraft, personal property of another, etc."

Because not all predatory crimes are included in the FBI Index, the Index cannot be used as an indication of the total amount of crime in the society. Fraud, for example, is not counted, nor are many of the white-collar crimes that we discuss.

### Illegal Service Crimes

Illegal service crimes do not involve a definite victim but rather *a relationship between a criminal and his customer.* The illegal service rendered might be drugs, gambling, prostitution, or high-interest loans. Although these relationships violate the law, they are not likely to be reported because the criminal and the customer probably prefer to have the service available.

### Public Disorder Crimes

Public disorder crimes also have no definite victim. They involve behavior that *is treated as criminal only when it occurs before some audience that will be offended.* These crimes include behavior such as disorderly conduct, drunkenness, and indecent exposure. Public disorder crimes are more common than predatory or illegal service crimes, according to arrest figures.

### Crimes of Negligence

Crimes of negligence involve an *unintended victim or potential victim.* They include actions such as reckless driving and other infractions of the law by automobile drivers. The "criminal" in this case is not deemed to be deliberately trying to harm anyone. Rather, the behavior is a threat or a nuisance from which the public should be protected. Negligence crimes and public disorder crimes compose the bulk of police work in the United States.

### Cybercrime

Cybercrime is the use of the computer to engage in criminal activity. Victims include individuals, organizations, and, potentially, an entire nation (Shawn 2011). A nation can be attacked by terrorist groups that hack into government records or disrupt the financial or military system in some way. Organizations such as businesses and corporations are victimized when hackers steal information that can be used to gain a competitive advantage. One company, for example, reported a loss of years' worth of research and development valued at $1 billion. And the loss occurred almost overnight!

Organized crime is increasingly operating over computer networks (Shawn 2011). Rather than robbing banks at gunpoint, they break into the computer systems of financial institutions and steal a wealth of data that can then be sold or used for financial gain.

As for individual victims, the FBI has identified a multitude of scams and frauds (Federal Bureau of Investigation 2010). Two of these are newer versions of "phishing" (you get an e-mail that claims to be from your bank or credit card company asking you to update your information and password). The newer versions are "smishing" (which combines texting and phishing) and "vishing" (which combines voice and phishing).

The criminals set up an automated dialing system that calls people in a particular area or that uses telephone numbers stolen from banks or credit unions. Victims get a message telling them there's a problem with their account or that their ATM card needs to be reactivated. The victims also receive a telephone number or a website they must contact to address the problem. Victims are then asked for personal information that enables the criminal to steal the victim's money from bank accounts, use the victim's charge cards for purchases, create a false ATM card, and so on.

Cybercrime has become such a serious matter that the FBI and the National White Collar Crime Center established the Internet Crime Complaint Center in 2000. According to the FBI website, the center received 469,361 complaints in 2019, representing losses to victims of $3.5 billion. Two of the more common complaints involved payments for merchandise that was never delivered and identity theft (illegal use of a bank account or credit card).

## White-Collar Crime

**white-collar crime** crimes committed by respectable citizens in the course of their work

**White-collar crime** is the crime of "respectable" people. The term was coined by Edwin Sutherland (Sutherland and Cressey 1955), who said that white-collar crimes are *committed by respectable people in the course of their work.* White-collar crimes include consumer fraud, which may be the most widespread of all the crimes (Rosoff, Pontell, and Tillman 2002); environmental offenses; insider trading in stocks; securities fraud; government corruption; cybercrime; and misleading advertising.

In an effort to categorize the various kinds of white-collar crime, Edelhertz (1983) suggests four types. First are "personal," or "ad hoc," crimes. The individual in this case generally does not have a face-to-face confrontation with the victim. Cheating on federal and state income taxes is one example of such a crime.

A second type of white-collar crime involves "abuses of trust," which are crimes committed by people who have custody of someone else's wealth (e.g., embezzlement) or who have the power to make decisions (e.g., accepting a bribe to make a favorable decision).

Third are crimes that are "incidental to and in furtherance of organizational operations," though they are not part of the purpose of the organization. Violations of antitrust laws and the federal Corrupt Practices Act fit in here. Or on a smaller scale, Edelhertz says that this "most troublesome" of the four categories involves such issues as fraudulent Medicare or Medicaid claims and the false weight on purchases at the grocery store. Edelhertz calls this third category the most troublesome because the offenders do not think of themselves as criminals and generally have high status in their communities. Nevertheless, the outcome is victimization of people. Consider, for instance, the problem of deceptive advertising. The advertising agency and the corporate executives who pay for ads do not think of themselves as engaging in criminal activity. Yet millions of Americans buy products based on this deceptive advertising.

The fourth category is white-collar crime carried on as a business by full-time con artists. This category includes actions from stock swindles to street games in which people are cheated out of their money.

White-collar crime abounds at all levels: individuals, small businesses, large corporations, and governmental agencies. Examples of individuals include cyber criminals, some of whom work out of their homes to defraud companies. At the small business level, numerous cases of fraud emerged in the first decade of this century in financial schemes. For example, two men who had gained a reputation for making shrewd, profitable investments in the stock market bilked hundreds of millions of dollars

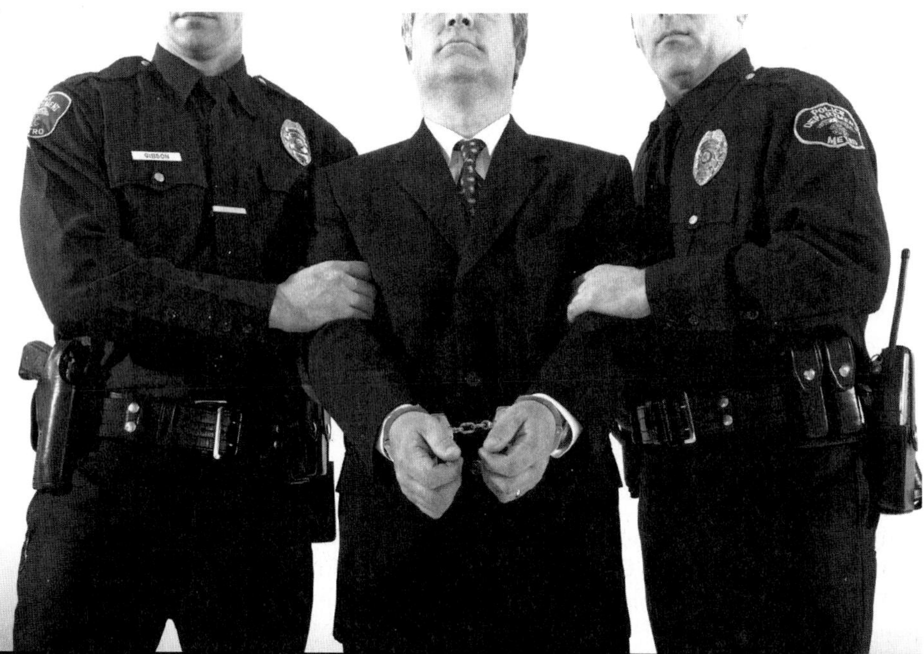
White-collar criminals are usually high-status individuals who appear to be successful and respectable.

UpperCut Images/Alamy Stock Photo

from investments made by public pension funds and universities (Kouwe 2009). The investors were unable to recover their losses because the men had spent it on a lavish lifestyle.

Large corporations also get involved in white-collar crime, including, in recent years, a brokerage firm that committed 2,000 felonies, a health care organization that paid bribes and kickbacks to doctors, a health maintenance organization that defrauded government health programs, an accounting firm that set up fraudulent shelters to help rich clients evade billions of dollars in taxes, and the Enron Corporation's "creative" accounting practices and manipulation of energy markets (McClam 2005). The Enron case illustrates how far-reaching the effects of corporate crime can be. Among other things, the actions of the Enron executives resulted in California energy costs that soared when markets were manipulated, hurting countless individuals and businesses that could not afford the higher rates; investors lost huge sums of money and many, including Enron employees, lost their life savings and retirement when the corporation collapsed; and many Enron employees lost their jobs.

Although some Enron officials received prison sentences, in many cases of corporate crime the only punishment meted out is a fine. In fact, some of the "crimes" are not defined as illegal by the law. Corporate lawyers are skilled at advising business executives on ways to avoid breaking the law while engaging in questionable practices. Sometimes their advice may be counterproductive: Perhaps the most devastating example of corporate crime was the Camp fire in 2018 (Rosenblatt 2020). It was the most destructive wildfire ever in California, causing 85 deaths, numerous injuries, and the loss of 18,804 structures. The fire raged over nearly 240 square miles. It started from a faulty transmission line. The Pacific Gas and Electric company acknowledged their responsibility because of inadequate maintenance of the power lines. The company was ordered to pay over $25 billion to victims and local government agencies.

It was because of such incidents, Sutherland argued that many practices of respectable people that are not defined by the law as crimes should be treated as crimes. He asserted, in fact, that businesspeople were more criminalistic than people of the ghettoes. A major difference is that criminal law distinguishes between the two groups, so that some acts that logically could be defined as crime are not in the criminal law. Further, some acts involving businesses and corporations are handled by government commissions rather than the criminal justice system. You can reasonably argue that when a company advertises a 6 percent interest rate on installment payments and actually collects 11.5 percent, it is committing fraud. The executives of the company will not be charged with fraud; the company will merely be ordered by the Federal Trade Commission (FTC) to stop advertising the false rate.

Even when the offense is covered by the criminal law, white-collar criminals may receive less severe punishment or escape punishment altogether. For one thing, the number of white-collar crimes prosecuted declined 28 percent in the early 2000s as concern shifted to homeland security and prosecution of illegal immigration (Marks 2006). For another thing, when fines are levied against companies, they may have their fines reduced later or the fines may go unpaid (Mendoza and Sullivan 2006). Still, the courts have sentenced a number of executives to prison terms in recent years, ranging from 1 to 150 years. Experts applaud such convictions, arguing that white-collar crime is at least as serious as, or even more serious than, the violent acts of street criminals. Street criminals tax the patience and resources of society, but white-collar criminals are like an insidious corrosion that slowly but surely destroys.

## Organized Crime

The term "organized crime" brings up images of Al Capone, machine guns, the Mafia, the Mob, La Cosa Nostra, the Syndicate, and films like *The Untouchables* and *The Godfather.* Is organized crime such a phenomenon in the United States? Are there groups that control the criminal activities of cities, regions, or even the entire nation? Criminologists themselves do not agree on the exact nature of organized crime, but there is some consensus on five characteristics of **organized crime:** the determination of a group of people to make money by any means necessary, the provision of illegal goods and services to people who want them or can be coerced into taking them, the use of political corruption to maintain and extend the activities, the persistence of the activities by the same organizations over successive generations of people, and a code of conduct for members (e.g., see Berger 1999). There is also likely to be some involvement in legitimate business, which is used to launder illegal funds or stolen merchandise. For instance, profits from drug sales may be claimed as legitimate profits of a legitimate business by manipulating its accounting records.

**organized crime**
an ongoing organization of people who provide illegal services and goods and who maintain their activities by the aid of political corruption

The activities of organized crime include gambling, prostitution, drugs, extortion, loan-sharking, and various legitimate enterprises (such as restaurants) that are used to launder money received from the illegal activities (Motivans 2003). There is, however, no single organization that controls all organized crime at the international or national level. Rather, there are numerous and diverse groups.

Although the Mafia and La Cosa Nostra are the most well-known organized crime groups, the Federal Bureau of Investigation (2009) points out that the face of organized crime has changed over time. The current concerns of the Bureau are with Russian mobsters who fled to the United States in the wake of the Soviet Union's collapse; groups from African countries like Nigeria that engage in drug trafficking and financial scams;

Chinese tongs, Japanese Boryokudan, and other Asian crime rings; and enterprises based in Eastern European nations like Hungary and Romania. These groups engage in various illegal activities, including drug trafficking, extortion, murder, kidnapping, home invasions, prostitution, illegal gambling, loan sharking, insurance/credit card fraud, stock fraud, and the theft of high-tech components. They also engage in human trafficking, particularly in bringing Chinese migrants and selling them into sex or sweatshop slavery.

Organized crime is no longer the province of any particular racial or ethnic group. Rather, it involves diverse groups who use it to gain economic and social mobility.

## Juvenile Delinquency

The concept of juvenile delinquency is a modern one. Until the late 19th century, juvenile offenders were regarded as incapable of certain crimes or were treated as adults in the criminal justice system. This concept changed in the 19th century when a group of reformers set out to redeem the nation's wayward youth (Platt 1969). These "child savers" helped establish the juvenile court system in the United States. As a result, juveniles were treated differently from adults, and certain behavior that was once ignored or handled in an informal way came under the jurisdiction of a government agency. Thus, the *concept of delinquency* was "invented" in America in the 19th century.

The nation's first *juvenile court* was established in 1899 in Illinois. All states now have juvenile court systems. The court's primary responsibility is to protect the welfare of youth, and its secondary task is to safeguard the community from youthful offenders. This orientation has given juvenile judges considerable discretion to make whatever decisions they deem necessary for the juveniles' protection and rehabilitation.

Three types of juveniles come under the court's jurisdiction. (A *juvenile* is typically defined as someone between the ages of 7 and 17.) *Youthful offenders* are those who engage in behavior for which adults can be tried in a criminal court. All predatory crimes are included here. Further, in the mid-1990s most states overhauled their laws so that more youths can be tried as adults in a criminal court and offenders are no longer protected by the confidentiality of juvenile court proceedings. The second type of juvenile handled by the juvenile court is the *status offenders,* those who violate the juvenile court code rather than the criminal code. Behavior such as truancy, running away from home, and breaking the curfew is included in this category. Finally, the court deals with *minors in need of care*–those who are neglected or abused and in need of the court's care. They do not fall into the category of delinquent, but they are the responsibility of the juvenile court.

The range of behavior defined as delinquent tends to be broad. Perhaps as many as 90 percent of all young people have engaged in behavior that would fall under the jurisdiction of juvenile court, including activities such as fighting, truancy, and running away from home. In some states, statutes define delinquency so broadly that virtually all juveniles could be categorized as delinquent. Delinquency, then, includes a much greater range of behavior than does crime.

## Juvenile Violence and Juvenile Gangs

Perhaps "delinquency" is a term that does not sufficiently capture the *severity of the problem of youth crime.* According to the FBI, youths under the age of 18 account for 9.8 percent of all violent crime and 11.1 percent of all property crime.

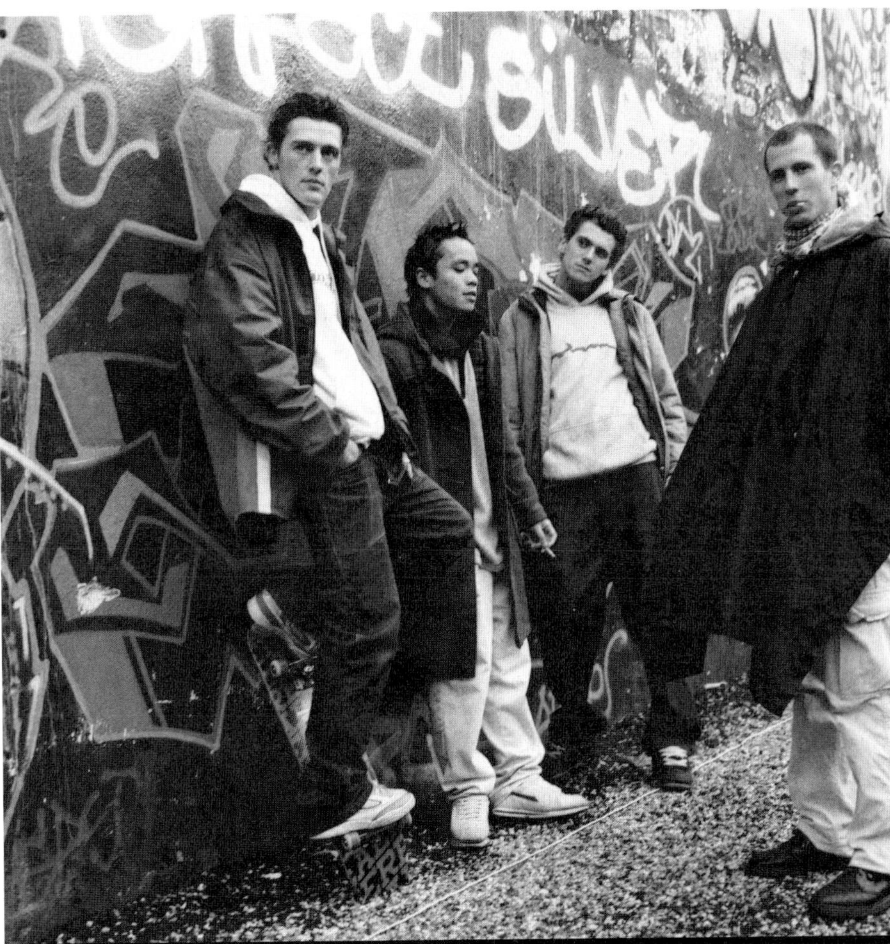

Youths join gangs for a variety of reasons, among them being the desire to gain status and escape poverty.

Patrick Sheandell O'Carroll/PhotoAlto/Getty Images

Part, but not all, of the problem of juvenile violence stems from juvenile gangs. There are about 1.4 million gang members in tens of thousands of gangs in the nation (Finelli 2019). And hundreds of thousands of youth join the gangs each year. *The proliferation of gangs, along with involvement in drugs and the ready availability of guns, has exacerbated the problem of violent crime by youths.* Gang members account for a disproportionate number of arrests for serious offenses (Thornberry, Huizinga, and Loeber 2004; Harrell 2005).

Juvenile gangs are now pervasive, appearing everywhere from large metropolitan to rural areas of the nation. The gangs exist in all 50 states. An increasing number of females are joining gangs. One study found that in high-risk, high-crime neighborhoods, 29.4 percent of girls and 32.4 percent of boys said they were members of a gang. The girls join because of such problems as family abuse and the appeal of being an integral part of a group (Miller 2001).

One reason for the increasing number of gangs is that the conditions that spawn the gangs—poverty, discrimination, and lack of legitimate opportunities—continue to exist throughout the nation. Once gangs appear in an area, they *tend to perpetuate themselves by setting models for each succeeding generation.* They also are perpetuated by a small number of members who stay in the gangs into adulthood and even parenthood.

Youths who enter gangs may be *socialized quickly into violence* (Taylor 2009). Entry into the gang itself may require the new member to be beaten by the others. Fighting among members is common and may be even more frequent than fighting with outsiders. Such violence has a number of purposes, including disciplining, demonstrating courage and toughness, establishing individual status within the group, and gaining the skills necessary to defend the gang's "turf" (Kennedy and Baron 1993).

Youths join gangs for various reasons. One of the more important is that the gang enables them to gain status (Alleyne and Wood 2010). They also, of course, gain income from the illegal activities of the gang. In impoverished areas, there are few opportunities for the young to gain either money or status, so gang membership can be very appealing.

Gangs engage in various kinds of crime, including smuggling, armed robbery, assault, auto theft, drug trafficking, extortion, fraud, identity theft, murder, and weapons trafficking. They are also involved in about 16 percent of all homicides in the nation (Egley, Howell, and Harris 2014). In many communities, gangs commit as much as 80 percent of the crime. Selling drugs is the major means for gangs to maintain their operations and the lifestyles of their members. Some gangs use such fronts as clothing stores, hair salons, and music recording and production companies to launder the money they get from selling drugs.

## The Extent of Crime and Delinquency

How widespread are crime and delinquency? The question is difficult to answer because of certain problems with official statistics. Here we examine ways to gather data, look at problems with official records, and then draw conclusions about the extent of crime and delinquency.

### Sources of Data

The three basic sources of data on crime are *official records, victimization studies,* and *self-reports.* A frequently used official record are the data published annually by the FBI. As noted previously, the FBI's Crime Index includes only eight major felonies. A great deal of crime—indeed, most crime—does not appear in this annual report. Other official sources include municipal police records and the records of juvenile courts. Because juvenile courts have no uniform system of reporting, we can only estimate the number of delinquency cases processed annually.

Victimization studies secure information from the victims of crime rather than from officials or official records. A victimization study usually involves interviews at a representative sample of homes. People in those homes are asked whether they or members of their families have been the victims of a crime or crimes during the previous year. The major source of victimization data is the National Crime Victimization Survey conducted annually by the Department of Justice.

In contrast to the *FBI data,* which are based on statistics gathered from thousands (but not all) of law enforcement authorities in America's cities and towns, the National Crime Victimization Survey includes both a greater range of crimes and crimes never *officially reported.* Because of nonreporting, the Victimization Survey data are sometimes twice as high as those of the *FBI.*

Self-reports are usually used with youths. The youths are asked whether they engaged in any of a number of different kinds of criminal activity. Various techniques are used to try to ensure honesty and accuracy, and there is evidence that self-reported crime by young people is fairly accurate.

## Problems with Official Records

If you attempt to estimate the crime rate from official records, you encounter a number of problems. First, quite a number of crimes are *undetected.* There are two ways to get an estimate of the amount of undetected crime. One is by asking people whether they have ever committed various crimes. When allowed to respond anonymously, people will often admit to a number of felonies for which they were never convicted as a criminal. The other way is to ask people whether they have been victims of the various crimes and then compare their responses with official records.

Second, *a substantial number of crimes are never reported to the police* (Carson et al. 2020). The rate of reporting varies with the type of crime (Figure 3.2), and the reasons for not reporting also vary (Table 3.1). Official figures under-report nearly every kind of crime.

A third problem with official records is that *definitions of crime change* and the *methods of reporting crime change.* Because a crime is a violation of the criminal law, any change in the law changes the amount of crime. In the early 1930s a considerable number of inmates in federal prisons were there for crimes that would not have been crimes a few years earlier. They were serving time for violating laws related to the Eighteenth Amendment to the Constitution–the amendment that established Prohibition.

Changes in the method of reporting crime can result in an apparent crime wave that may really be a "crime reporting" wave. For example, some years ago the FBI discovered that police were reporting only about half the number of property crimes that insurance companies were reporting. A new system was implemented, and during the next year there was an enormous increase in the police-reported rate of assaults, robberies, and burglaries. The rates reflected the new reporting methods but not necessarily any increase in the actual rate of crime.

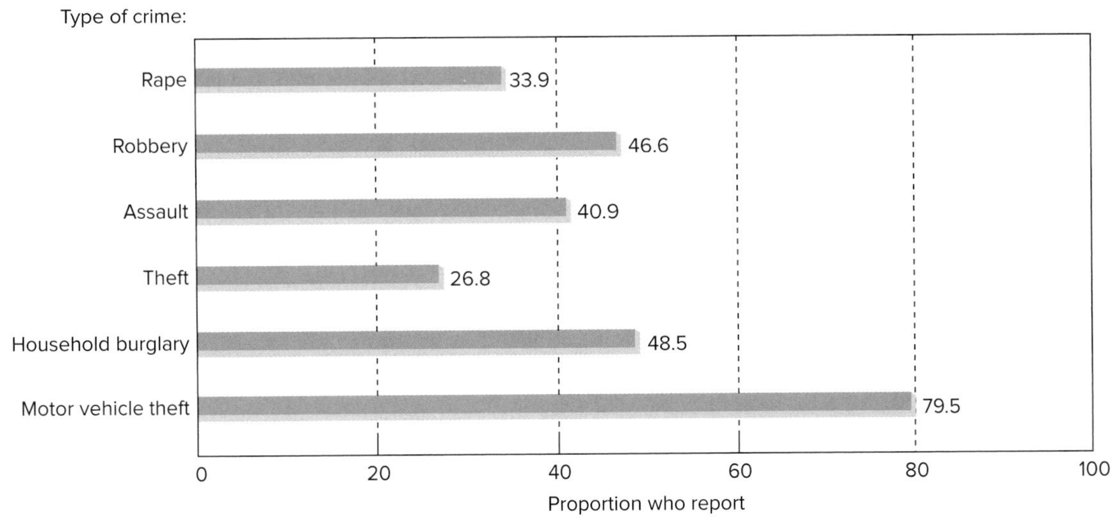


**FIGURE 3.2** Reporting Victimizations to the Police.

Source: Morgan and Truman 2020.

| Reason | All Crimes, Total | Crimes of Violence: Robbery | Crimes of Violence: Assault | Property Crimes: Burglary | Property Crimes: Auto Theft | Property Crimes: Theft |
|---|---|---|---|---|---|---|
| Reported to another official | 13.0 | 5.4 | 14.2 | 5.2 | 3.4 | 8.3 |
| Personal/private | 20.7 | 12.2 | 21.8 | 7.0 | 7.9 | 5.3 |
| Object recovered, offender unsuccessful | 17.3 | 11.2 | 18.5 | 21.4 | 16.3 | 26.7 |
| Not important enough | 6.2 | 1.9 | 7.1 | 6.2 | 0.0 | 4.4 |
| Lack of proof | 3.4 | 10.2 | 2.1 | 12.1 | 13.1 | 9.9 |
| Police wouldn't want to be bothered | 6.3 | 11.4 | 5.8 | 10.9 | 3.1 | 10.5 |
| Police ineffective or biased | 4.6 | 17.8 | 3.1 | 6.9 | 15.3 | 3.8 |
| Fear of reprisal | 7.3 | 5.8 | 7.3 | 1.0 | 1.3 | 0.5 |
| Inconvenient | 4.7 | 7.5 | 4.2 | 3.5 | 6.4 | 4.1 |
| Other reasons | 15.7 | 13.8 | 15.6 | 10.3 | 24.2 | 10.4 |

**TABLE 3.1**
Reasons for Not Reporting Crimes to the Police (in percent not reported)

SOURCE: U.S. Department of Justice 2008:110.

A fourth problem with official records involves *police procedures.* Whether some behavior is defined officially by the police as criminal depends on factors other than the behavior itself. For instance, the police may be caught in political cross-pressures when they decide whether to report offenses. If they report offenses, they may be blamed for failing to stem the rising tide of crime. If they fail to report them, they may be blamed for being unresponsive. There also may be pressure to keep reported offenses low in order to make areas more attractive to business, residents, and tourists.

A final problem with official records relates to *changing expectations* in society. At one time in U.S. history, many crimes in slum areas and sections of cities populated by minority groups were unreported. Indeed, the police were not necessarily even notified when criminal offenses occurred. In recent decades, the poor and minority groups expect and demand adequate protection. Although a great many crimes are never reported, there is evidence that more are now being reported than in the past, thus making the rate of crime appear to be increasing.

These qualifications to the reliability of official records suggest that the amount of crime in the nation is considerably greater than official records indicate. They also suggest that caution must be exercised when comparing rates across time and drawing a quick conclusion that a "crime wave" is in process. However, when official records are used in conjunction with victimization studies and other evidence, the conclusions are more reliable.

## The Amount of Crime and Delinquency

What do the data reveal about the amount of crime and delinquency in America? The amount differs depending on whether you look at FBI or victimization data. According to FBI data, rates of serious crime fluctuate over time. However, there has been a general downward trend in rates over the past few decades. Still, most rates were far higher by the end of 2019 than they were in 1960 (Table 3.2).

| Year | Violent Crime: Murder | Forcible Rape | Robbery | Aggravated Assault | Property Crime: Burglary | Larceny/ Theft | Auto Theft |
|---|---|---|---|---|---|---|---|
| Number (1,000) | | | | | | | |
| 1960 | 9.1 | 17.2 | 108 | 154 | 912 | 1,855 | 328 |
| 1970 | 16.0 | 38.0 | 350 | 335 | 2,205 | 4,226 | 928 |
| 1980 | 23.0 | 82.1 | 549 | 655 | 3,759 | 7,113 | 1,115 |
| 1990 | 23.4 | 102.6 | 639 | 1,055 | 3,074 | 7,946 | 1,636 |
| 2000 | 16.0 | 90.0 | 408 | 912 | 2,051 | 6,972 | 1,160 |
| 2019 | 16.4 | 98.2 | 268 | 821 | 1,118 | 5,086 | 722 |
| Rate (per 100,000) | | | | | | | |
| 1960 | 5.1 | 9.6 | 60 | 86 | 509 | 1,035 | 183 |
| 1970 | 7.9 | 18.7 | 172 | 165 | 1,085 | 2,079 | 457 |
| 1980 | 10.2 | 36.4 | 244 | 291 | 1,668 | 3,156 | 495 |
| 1990 | 9.4 | 41.2 | 257 | 424 | 1,236 | 3,195 | 658 |
| 2000 | 5.5 | 32.0 | 145 | 324 | 729 | 2,477 | 412 |
| 2019 | 5.0 | 29.9 | 81.6 | 250 | 340 | 1,550 | 22 |

**TABLE 3.2**
Crime and Crime Rates by Type, 1960 to 2019

SOURCE: U.S. Census Bureau 1975:153; Federal Bureau of Investigation website.

Victimization data also show fluctuating rates over time. Table 3.3 gives the rates for 2019. Overall, there were 21 violent victimizations for every 1,000 people aged 12 or older and 101 property crimes for every 1,000 households. About one out of every eight households, therefore, experienced some kind of property crime in 2019.

Obtaining information about white-collar crime is difficult. The FBI has some information on specific kinds of white-collar crime but acknowledges that it is impossible to give an accurate, overall portrait. Still, it is clear that unethical and illegal behaviors abound in business and industry. Much of the business crime, however, involves insiders,

| Type of Crime | Number (1,000s) | Rate |
|---|---|---|
| Crimes of violence | 5,813 | 21.0 |
| Rape/sexual assault | 459 | 1.7 |
| Robbery | 534 | 1.9 |
| Assault | 4,819 | 17.4 |
| Aggravated assault | 1,019 | 3.7 |
| Simple assault | 3,800 | 13.7 |
| Property crimes | 12,818 | 101.4 |
| Household burglary | 2,178 | 17.2 |
| Motor vehicle theft | 496 | 3.9 |
| Theft | 10,144 | 80.2 |

**TABLE 3.3**
Victimization Rates, Personal and Household Crimes, 2019 (per 1,000 persons aged 12 or older or per 1,000 households)

SOURCE: Morgan and Truman 2020.

including businesspeople at the higher levels of the organization. The loss caused by owners and executives is far greater than that caused by rank-and-file employees. Bank employees steal more from banks than do robbers. And businesses are offenders as well as victims, engaging in criminal activity against consumers and customers. Indictments for criminal activity and fines for serious misbehavior occur regularly among both small businesses and the nation's largest corporations.

Finally, this nation has an enormous amount of delinquency. Keep in mind, however, that delinquency by definition includes some relatively trivial kinds of behavior. Juveniles may be arrested for conduct that would not be defined as criminal on the part of an adult (e.g., violation of curfew, running away from home, and possession of an alcoholic beverage). But juveniles also are involved in serious crimes. In 2019, 7.1 percent of all arrests involved youth under 18 years of age (FBI website). Clearly, a disproportionate number of juveniles are responsible for crimes.

## The Distribution of Crime

Crime is unequally distributed in the United States. There are variations by region, by state, and by population size. For example, the murder rate for the nation as a whole in 2019 was 5.0 per 100,000 inhabitants (FBI website). The highest rate, however, was in cities with populations between 1/2 and 1 million inhabitants–12.5 per 100,000 inhabitants, or more than double the overall rate. Cities of that size also had a rate of auto theft that was more than double the rate for the nation as a whole.

Group variations also exist. In general, males, young people, racial/ethnic minorities, and the poor have higher rates of victimization than others. For example, the 2019 murder rates varied by race/ethnicity (41.6 percent of the victims were white, 53.7 percent were African American, and 17.0 percent were Hispanic) and by gender (78.3 percent were male).

## The Criminal Justice Process

To understand the problem of crime in the nation, it is important to know about the criminal justice process. What happens when you report a crime to the police? The path from the reporting to the final settlement is long and complex. Here we can only give you a sketch of the process to illustrate its complexity.

After a crime is reported and law enforcement officers verify that it has indeed been committed (a proportion of incidents reported to the police are not defined by them as crimes), a suspect must be identified and apprehended. Frequently, extensive investigation is required to properly identify the suspect. After an arrest is made, information about the suspect and the case is given to the prosecutor, who will decide whether to file formal charges with the court. If charges are not filed, the suspect is released.

A suspect who is charged is brought before a judge or magistrate without any unnecessary delay. The judge or magistrate informs the accused of the charges and decides whether there is probable cause to detain the suspect. If the offense is a minor one, a decision about guilt and penalty can be made at this point. If the offense is serious, the process continues. In many jurisdictions, the next step is a preliminary hearing, which is an effort to decide whether there is probable cause to believe that the accused committed a crime within the jurisdiction of the court. If the judge does not find probable cause, the case is dismissed. If the judge finds probable cause, or if the accused waives the preliminary hearing, the case can be turned over to a grand jury. The grand jury hears the evidence and decides whether there is enough to justify a trial. If so, the grand jury issues an *indictment,* which gives the basic facts of the offense charged against the accused.

Once the indictment is filed, the accused is scheduled for *arraignment,* at which time the accused is informed of the charges, advised of his or her rights, and asked to enter a plea to the charges. In most cases, the accused will plead guilty in order to take advantage of *plea bargaining.* Generally, plea bargaining means that the prosecution and defense agree to a lesser offense or to only one of the original charges. Plea bargaining allows the offender to get a lighter sentence, assures the prosecutor that the offender will not be totally acquitted, and saves everyone the time and expense of a court trial. If the plea is "Not guilty," or if the plea is "Guilty" but is refused by the judge (the judge may believe that the accused was coerced into the plea), the case proceeds to trial. The trial can be by jury, or the accused may request that the case be decided by a judge.

If the trial results in conviction, the defendant may appeal to a higher court. If no appeal is made, or if the appeals are rejected, the offender must submit to the sentence imposed by the judge or jury. Sometimes a sentence is handed down only after a sentencing hearing in which the defense presents mitigating circumstances to help minimize the severity of the sentence.

This process is not followed exactly in every jurisdiction, and the juvenile justice system differs in a number of important ways. Yet this explanation outlines the basic process and shows how decisions are made at a number of points in the process. Decision at each point may result in the release of the accused. The system reflects the American belief that the accused is presumed innocent until proven guilty. The result is, as Figure 3.3 shows for federal cases for one year, that half or fewer of those arrested for crimes will likely be convicted and incarcerated.

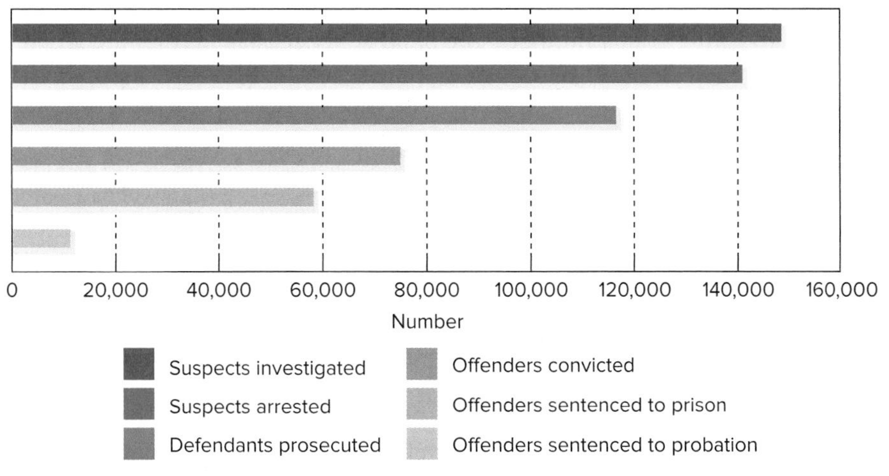


**FIGURE 3.3**
Federal Criminal Case Processing, 2004.
Source: U.S. Department of Justice 2006:1.

## Crime, Delinquency, and the Quality of Life

Widespread crime contradicts American values of freedom from fear, of well-being, and of the right to keep personal property. Crime, by definition, often involves exploitive or violent relationships and thereby contradicts both the *values and ideology* about America being a land of opportunity for all. The "land of opportunity" notion loses some of its appeal for those who fear that their success can make them victims if it attracts criminal activity. Thus, crime diminishes the quality of life by exacting high physical, psychological, and economic costs.

### Physical and Psychological Costs of Crime

Crime causes physical and psychological suffering. Although it is difficult to measure, there is evidence that this suffering is considerable. Crime affects physical and emotional health, increases fear, and fosters alienation.

**trauma**
physical or emotional injury

*Physical and Mental Health.* The victim of a crime experiences **trauma.** The victim may be temporarily or permanently injured, either physically or emotionally (Randa and Reyns 2020). A fourth of all violent crime victims, and half of rape victims, are injured (Simon, Mercy, and Perkins 2001). Emotional trauma such as anxiety, depression, shame, humiliation, or despair is also likely (Hochstetler et al. 2014). A substantial number of crime victims get mental health counseling or therapy, or join a support group every year.

White-collar crime also takes its toll on Americans' physical and mental health. Some people have lost their businesses or life savings because of fraud. Identity theft can cause severe stress because victims may be denied loans, housing, education, or job opportunities and can even be arrested for crimes they did not commit (Morton 2004). Consumers have suffered financial and health losses because of corporate practices, including the practice of not fully informing the public about potential problems with various products. To learn that you have undergone a medical procedure or taken a prescription drug that negatively affects your health is an emotionally traumatic experience.

*Fear and Its Consequences.* Widespread crime can produce pervasive fear in a society. With the falling crime rates since the early 1990s, the fear of crime also diminished. Still, a 2016 Gallup poll found that 53 percent worry a "great deal" about crime (Davis 2016). And a third or more of all Americans admit they are afraid to walk alone at night. The fear generated by crime means that everyone loses—victims, people who are afraid they might be victims, and residents and businesspeople in high-crime areas.

*Alienation.* Sutherland (1968) argued that white-collar crime has a psychological impact that cannot be measured in monetary terms alone. He pointed out that such crimes create an atmosphere of distrust in a society, lowering social morale and creating widespread social disorganization. People not only become cynical about social institutions (illustrated by the common belief that all politicians are crooked), but they also have a tendency to develop a social Darwinist approach to life. ("It's a dog-eat-dog world and you have to look out for yourself above all else.") In a sense, then, white-collar crime may be more damaging to a society than predatory crime. It indicates that the whole society is corrupt—that fraud, theft, and exploitation pervade the paneled offices of professionals as well as the littered streets of the slums. White-collar crime, thus, produces a pervasive sense of distrust and **alienation** and suggests that the society is sick.

**alienation**
a sense of estrangement from one's social environment, typically measured by one's feelings of powerlessness, normlessness, isolation, meaninglessness, and self-estrangement

### Economic Costs of Crime

A great many factors must be taken into account when we try to assess the economic losses due to crime. These factors include the personal loss of property; expense of insurance; cost of loan sharks, false advertising, and shoddy workmanship on consumer goods; work absences and lost wages resulting from physical and emotional trauma; medical cost for treating injuries; cost of maintaining security systems and other crime prevention measures; and cost of maintaining the criminal justice system. The criminal justice system alone (including local, state, and federal levels of government) costs hundreds of billions of dollars each year.

Some costs cannot even be measured. Consumers pay higher prices because of organized crime's involvement in legitimate business and because of business losses from crimes (including employee theft). Shoplifting adds to the cost of retail items. Many crimes of fraud, embezzlement, and arson-for-profit are never detected. Some crimes go unreported because the victims are afraid (blackmail or retaliation), embarrassed (con games), or involved in illegal activity (gambling).

When the costs are added, including direct losses due to personal and household crime and the cost of maintaining the criminal justice system, crime costs Americans hundreds of billions of dollars every year.

## Contributing Factors

Like crime itself, the factors that generate and sustain crime involve both respectable and nonrespectable elements of society.

### Social Structural Factors

*Age Structure of the Population.* As we noted earlier in this chapter, a disproportionate amount of crime is committed by young males. Males account for nearly three out of four of all arrests and eight out of ten arrests for violent crime (FBI website). Thus, a partial explanation for the decreasing crime rates of the 1990s and early 2000s is the decline in the number of young males (Phillips 2006).

As the age structure of the nation shifts, with smaller or larger proportions falling into the lower age categories, crime rates should vary accordingly; but we must be cautious about predictions because no single factor is involved in the amount of crime. Although the current younger generation is more violent than previous ones, the homicide rates have fallen for them also, in part because of the shrinking urban market for crack cocaine (much of the increased killing in the late 1980s and early 1990s occurred in urban crack markets) (Rosenfeld 2002).

*Hot Spots.* Cohen and Felson (1979) developed a "routine activities" approach to crime. They focused on circumstances rather than the characteristics of offenders. In particular, they emphasized the importance of *likely offenders, suitable targets,* and *a lack of capable guardians* occurring at a particular place and time. "Capable guardians" can include anything from the presence of police to alarm systems. The convergence, or lack of convergence, of these three factors, along with the socioeconomic context, explain why certain areas become "hot spots," or locales of high crime rates (Weisburd and Mazerolle 2000; He, Paez, and Liu 2017).

Van Koppen and Jansen (1999) used this approach to explain daily, weekly, and seasonal variations in robbery rates. Robbers' expectations of the amount of money available at a particular time and place constitute the suitable target, whereas the increased number of dark hours during the winter mean less adequate guardianship. Bryjak (1999) explained the drop in burglary rates in the 1990s in terms of increased guardianship of suitable targets; namely, the fact that more people are spending time in their homes because of personal computers, cable television, VCRs, and video games. This approach also helps explain fraud (Holtfreter, Reisig, and Pratt 2008), cybercrime victimization (Holt and Bossler 2009), juvenile crime (Weisburd, Groff, and Morris 2011), and using the cell phone for sexting (sending sexually explicit photos or videos) (Wolfe et al. 2016). The juvenile crime study focused on Seattle, Washington, where the researchers discovered that half of all juvenile crime occurred in less than 1 percent of street segments, concentrating in public and commercial areas where youth gathered rather than in residential areas.

Other research, covering 52 nations over a 25-year period, suggests that this approach may apply more to property crime than to personal crime (Bennett 1991). At any rate, the convergence of offenders, suitable targets, and inadequate guardianship in a lower socioeconomic setting helps explain a certain amount of crime (Hipp, Bauer, Curran, and Bollen 2004). It follows that changing any one of the factors may alter crime rates. For example, convenience stores are targets for robbery. Some local governments have passed ordinances requiring convenience stores to have at least two clerks on duty at all times. These additional clerks may reduce the amount of armed robbery by increasing the number of capable guardians.

**differential association theory**
the theory that illegal behavior is due to a preponderance of definitions favorable to such behavior

*Norms.* The **differential association theory** of crime and delinquency emphasizes the importance of *norms.* The theory states that potential or actual criminals or delinquents have their significant interactions with people whose norms violate the criminal law. Consistent with the theory, researchers have found that delinquents tend to spend more time with friends who are delinquent than with those who are nondelinquent (Haynie 2002). Delinquents who grow up in impoverished areas are also likely to live with one parent, to be unemployed, and to be school dropouts.

Thus, the lower-class delinquent may have few or no experiences with people who could motivate him or her to accept the norms of the larger society. The delinquent is drawn to a group because of the need for companionship, and the group develops norms that violate the law. Because *group membership* is more meaningful to this youth than anything else he or she has experienced, those norms are accepted and followed. Those youths, on the other hand, who have their significant interactions with people who affirm the norms of the larger society—family, religious groups, and so on—are much less likely to engage in delinquent behavior (Johnson, Jang, Larson, and De Li 2001; Pearce and Haynie 2004).

Norms are involved in white-collar crime also. Certain practices in business and industry may be justified on the basis that everyone does them, that they are necessary for continuing one's enterprise, or that they are acceptable to those in authority. News accounts have reported corporate executives justifying illegal behavior on the grounds that their competitors engaged in the behavior; so if they did not, they would lose business and profits. American businessmen have paid off influential foreigners in order to secure contracts for business, and then shrugged off the practice by pointing out that the alternative was to not do business in those foreign countries. Such practices are learned early. A study of 133 MBA students found them likely to decide to further market and produce a hypothetical drug that was about to be recalled by the Food and Drug Administration when coworkers and the board of directors agreed with that decision (Piquero, Tibbetts, and Blankenship 2006).

*The Politics of Control: The Prison.* The United States has a higher proportion of its population incarcerated than does any other Western nation. While the proportion has gone down some since 2009, 1.43 million Americans (a rate of 432 per 100,000) were in state and federal prisons in 2019 (Carson 2020). Both the number and the rate are far higher than past decades. For example, in 1990 the number was 738,894, a rate of 294. 15 per 100,000. In addition to those in prisons, there are hundreds of thousands more in jails (a jail is a locally administered institution that has authority to retain adults for 48 hours or longer; a prison is a state or federally administered facility for correction only). As a result, the incarceration rate in the United States is about seven times the rate in Europe (World Population Review 2021). The prison population is so large that one in nine government employees works in corrections, and many states spend more money each year on prisons than they do on education.

The high rate of incarceration is a political decision. There are alternative ways of dealing with criminals (see Global Comparison). Some people believe that **rehabilitation** should be the focus of the criminal justice system, whereas others believe criminals should be put into prisons for *punishment* and *isolation from society*. Still others believe that rehabilitation should be combined with the punishment of imprisonment. To address the issue, we examine what happens in the nation's prisons and jails. A basic problem is that, as Petersilia (2011) put it, "we have a corrections system that does not correct." Rehabilitation programs can be effective in reducing **recidivism** (repeated criminal activity and incarceration), but not all prisoners have access to rehabilitation programs, particularly the kind that are effective (such as high-school equivalency diploma programs, vocational training, and drug treatment). This is the case in the nation's jails, where only a fraction of the total jail population has access to any programs other than religious services (Freudenberg et al. 2005). The need for programs of support and rehabilitation is underscored by the fact that *people in jails have high rates of infectious and chronic diseases, substance abuse, mental health problems, and suicide rates that are far higher than those in prisons and in the larger society* (Freudenberg et al. 2005; Mumola 2005). On average, a prisoner stays in jail about 17 days, though some may remain for a year or more because of the shortage of prison space. The prisoner, who may be frightened, confused, or emotionally disturbed, has no one to talk with except other prisoners.

**rehabilitation**
resocializing a criminal and returning him or her to full participation in society

**recidivism**
repeated criminal activity and incarceration

Among those jails that do have rehabilitation programs, basic adult education is the most common, followed by vocational training. Only the larger jails (those with 250 or more inmates) are likely to have such programs.

Even if rehabilitation programs are available, the *nature of prison life reduces the probability that rehabilitation will occur.* In addition, the longer the time spent in prison, the more the likelihood of recidivism. For one thing, jails and prisons are seriously overcrowded (Welsh 2002). Because there are too many prisoners for the amount of space available, nearly two-thirds of prison inmates are confined to units with less than 60 square feet of space, and a third spend 10 or more hours a day in that space. Such conditions are stressful and make any efforts at rehabilitation difficult. In addition, the stress is sufficiently severe that it makes many prisoners—particularly those with a history of incarceration—more vulnerable to infectious diseases and other physical and emotional illnesses that arise out of stress (Massoglia 2008). A national survey of jails and prisons reported that about four out of ten prisoners suffer from a chronic medical condition (Wilper et al.

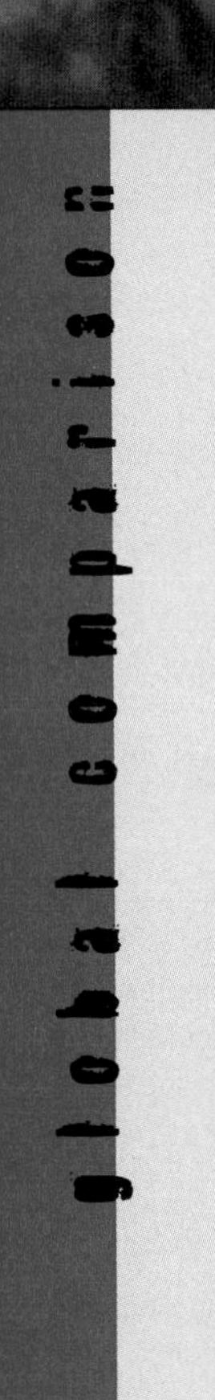


## ALTERNATIVES TO IMPRISONMENT: GERMANY AND ISRAEL

The fact that the United States has a higher proportion of its population in jails and prisons than any other country in the world does not mean that the nation also has higher crime rates or more effective policing (which would catch greater numbers of criminals). The high incarceration rate reflects the societal attitude that criminals should be removed from society and punished. Would alternatives to imprisonment be beneficial for both the criminal and society? Evidence from Germany and Israel suggest that they would.

German courts make use of suspensions, probation, fines, and community service. Judges have lifetime appointments and sole authority to sentence offenders who are 18 to 20 years old. Hard-line judges continue to use imprisonment, whereas liberal judges try to use alternatives. The alternatives are common. In one year, for example, 634,735 adults were sentenced under the criminal law. The most frequent sentence, meted out to 80 percent of the offenders, was a fine. Of those sentenced to prison, two-thirds received a suspended sentence with probation. Only 6 percent actually went to prison.

Researchers have found that those imprisoned had higher rates of recidivism than did those given alternative sanctions. Even if the imprisonment included job training, offenders had a harder time getting a job after release than did those who had an alternative sanction. A study of regions reported that the proportion of offenders increased over a period of four years by 7 percent where imprisonment was the norm, and fell by 13 percent where alternative sanctions were the norm.

In Israel, the Kibbutz Resocialization Program is an effort to put offenders into a close-knit society that will change them into respectable citizens. The offenders are placed with an adoptive family, put into a cohesive work group, and expected to become productive members of the kibbutz.

A study of 27 long-term offenders assigned to a kibbutz found that, three years after being assigned, three-fourths of them had no additional criminal activity: nine were working full-time, five served in the army, five were engaged or married, and eight remained in the kibbutz as members.

Thus, programs in both nations offer evidence that alternatives to imprisonment may be a more effective way to deal with some kinds of criminals. If the goal is to rehabilitate, alternatives may work better than imprisonment.

SOURCES: National Institute of Justice 1996; Fischer and Geiger 1996; Jehle 2005.

2009). In addition, two-thirds of those in federal and state prisons and nearly half of those in jails were on a psychiatric medication.

Far from serving as a deterrent to further crime or as a place of rehabilitation, the jail or prison at best keeps criminals away from the public for a period of time. At worst, the prison becomes a *training ground* for making criminals more competent and more committed to a life of crime. If the abnormal circumstances of the prison, including extended, close association with hardened offenders, does not ensure continued criminal behavior, the stigma of having been in prison probably will. The prison itself is a *dehumanizing institution,* and people who enter it are unlikely to escape being brutalized, hardened, and better trained in criminal behavior. The same kind of threats to well-being found in the larger society must be faced by those in prison. Homicides, sexual assault, and gang formation and violence characterize prison life (Allender and Marcell 2003; Beck and Harrison 2006). It is estimated that about 4 percent of prisoners experience sexual assault by a fellow inmate or a prison staff person that ranges from unwanted touching to rape (Beck 2013). Sexual violence also occurs in juvenile facilities, both youth-on-youth and staff-on-youth (Beck, Harrison, and Guerino 2010).

involvement

## CODDLING CRIMINALS

Many Americans believe that one way to deal with the problem of crime is to stop "coddling" criminals. Actually, it is true that some criminals are coddled. Consider, for example, the following cases from the American system of justice:

*Item:* The portfolio manager of two mutual funds cheated investors out of almost $10 million. He was sentenced to six months in prison and put on five years' probation.

*Item:* The manufacturer of drugs watered down an antidote for poisoned children with a useless substance. He was given one year's probation and a $10,000 fine.

*Item:* A judge in a state supreme court was involved in receiving and transporting $800,000 in stolen U.S. Treasury bills. He was fined $10,000 and sentenced to one year in prison.

These cases are just a few examples of the numerous white-collar crimes in which the offenders received very light punishment.

In this chapter we have stressed the seriousness of white-collar crime. How aware are the people in your area of the extent and corrosiveness of this crime? For one week, note any articles in your local newspaper that talk about crime. Assuming that the newspaper gave an accurate picture of the problem of crime in your area, how much and what kind of a crime problem exist? Do you think your paper is sensitive to the significance of white-collar crime? Make a list of various crimes, including street crimes and white-collar crimes. Ask some people in your community to rank them by seriousness, and ask them why they ranked them as they did. How do they feel about the different kinds of crime?

About 12 percent of youth in juvenile facilities report experiencing one or more incidents of sexual assault, with assaults by staff far more common than assaults by other youth. All of this takes place in a setting that almost seems designed to create degradation and humiliation (Tregea and Larmour 2009). It is not surprising, then, that self-injurious behaviors, including attempts at suicide, occur in correctional facilities (Smith and Kaminski 2011).

Normal behavior and feelings are impossible in prison. The prison is a **total institution,** a place where the totality of the individual's existence is controlled by various external forces. Offenders who enter the maximum security prison are immediately deprived of valuable things: liberty, goods and services, heterosexual relationships, autonomy, and security (from attacks of other prisoners). Moreover, they are in a place with a high proportion of disturbed individuals. Over half of those in state prisons, 45 percent of those in federal prisons, and 64 percent of those in local jails have or have had some kind of mental health problem, including serious mental illness, breakdowns, and brain damage (James and Glaze 2006; Lovell 2008). The constraints of prison life are so severe that an individual must focus on survival rather than personal development or change.

**total institution**
a place in which the totality of the individual's existence is controlled by external forces

The combination of the inmate code and the demands of the authorities virtually eliminates any possibility of individual growth or personal lifestyle. There is a popular notion that "stone walls do not a prison make" and that even in a cell the individual's mind is free to roam and explore, but only a rare individual can transcend the forces that impinge on him or her and thereby avoid the dehumanization of the prison.

The *inmate code* contributes to the **dehumanization.** The code requires that an inmate must never report infractions of rules by another inmate and must never notice anything. For example, an inmate walking down a prison corridor saw a fellow inmate lying on the floor, bleeding. He had an impulse to help the man on the floor but went to his cell instead. Other inmates who discussed the incident with the prison psychiatrist agreed with the behavior. They pointed out that if the man had called a guard, the guard would have suspected him of having struck the man on the floor or would have

**dehumanization**
the process by which an individual is deprived of the qualities or traits of a human being

intensely questioned him. Further, any other inmate who saw him call the guard would have accused him of "snitching." Had he stopped to help the fallen man, he might have been beaten by the man's attacker. Also, to personally help would suggest a homosexual relationship between the two inmates.

Finally, to survive in such an inhuman context, inmates practice and hone the same skills they used in their criminal careers. The most likely outcome of a prison sentence, then, is an improvement of criminal skills and thus the high probability of a continued criminal career and an eventual return to prison.

*The Family Background of Offenders.* Because the *family plays a significant role in the socialization of children,* much attention is focused on family background to discover why young people become delinquents. Many family factors have been associated with delinquency, but the most important is the *quality of the relationships between parents and children.*

In essence, there is less delinquency among those youths whose parents value, love, accept, and spend time with them (Brody et al. 2001; Milkie, Nomaguchi, and Denny 2015). In contrast, rates of delinquency are higher among youths in abusive, troubled, or disrupted families (Thornberry, Huizinga, and Loeber 2004; Fagan 2005; Wu et al. 2014; Shukla and Wiesner 2016). Rates of homicide are higher in cohorts of youth with a higher percentage born to unwed mothers, suggesting again the importance of the family in crime rates (O'Brien, Stockard, and Isaacson 1999).

When there are poor relationships in the family, parental moral and emotional authority is weakened. The diminished authority tends to weaken children's bonds to the social order and increases the likelihood of delinquency (Browning and Loeber 1999). Don't commit the *fallacy of retrospective determinism* here. Not all children from such families are delinquents. Family background helps you *understand* why some youths become delinquent, but it does not condone delinquency or absolve delinquents of responsibility for their behavior.

fallacy

*Adult criminals are also likely to have had troubled family relationships* (Grogan-Kaylor and Otis 2003). We are not saying that the criminal behavior began in adulthood, of course. In fact, virtually all criminal careers (other than white-collar crime) begin before the age of 18. A large number of youths who engage in serious delinquent behavior will continue their criminal activities as adults.

*Social Stratification and Crime.* Crime and delinquency are related to the social stratification system in three ways: (1) The kind of behavior considered criminal is defined by those who have power within the system. (2) Different kinds of crime tend to be committed within different strata of the system. (3) Disproportionate numbers of criminals come from different socioeconomic levels.

A good deal of the behavior of relatively powerless people is defined as criminal whereas similar behavior among more powerful people is not defined as criminal. This finding is true especially when the behavior involves monetary exploitation. A corporate executive might support the definition of employee theft as criminal but would not define false advertising and exploitation of consumers as theft or crime. A physician might deplore abuses of the welfare system, labeling them criminal fraud, but think little about prescribing expensive brand-name drugs rather than less expensive generic counterparts because, in part, his or her retirement plan rests on investments in the pharmaceutical industry. In both cases, the people who influence the defining process are the *holders or wielders of power in society,* and they *do not define their own behavior as criminal.*

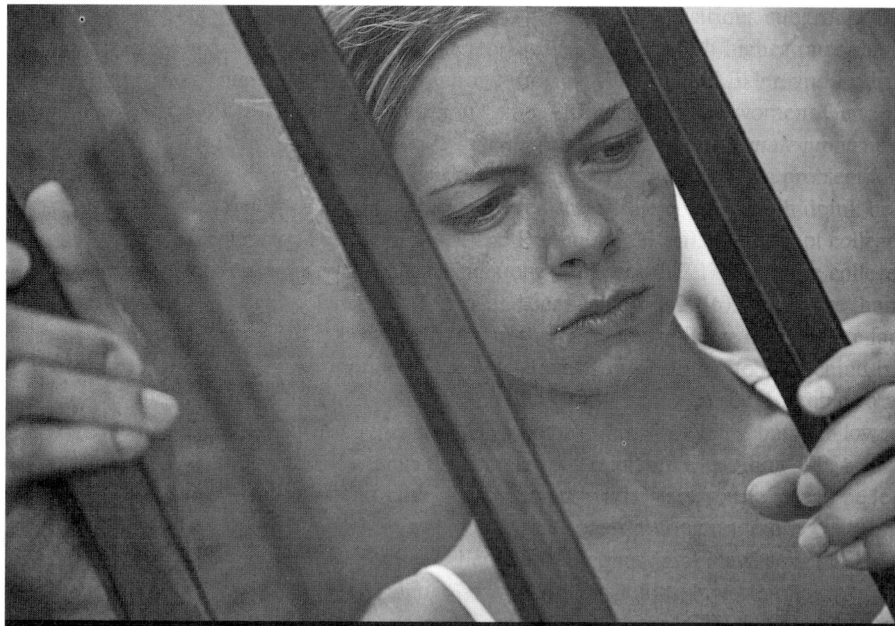

Prison life is dehumanizing.
Kristy-Anne Glubish/Design Pics

The second way in which social stratification intersects with crime and delinquency involves the kinds of crime committed. Those in the lower socioeconomic strata are more likely to be both the offenders and the victims of delinquency, property crime, and violent crime, including murder of a family member (Markowitz 2003; Diem and Pizarro 2010). In contrast, white-collar criminals are more likely to come from the middle and upper strata.

Delinquency, violence, and property crime are more characteristic of those people struggling to survive the deprivations of a seriously unequal society. Thus, there is more delinquency among those who face ongoing and severe economic problems (Agnew et al. 2008). Unable to buy their needed goods and services, deprived youth resort to various kinds of delinquent and criminal behavior. Basically, the more impoverished an area and the fewer opportunities it offers for dealing with economic deprivation, the higher the rates of crime (Lee and Ousey 2001; Weiss and Reid 2005).

The third way the stratification system is related to crime is in the disproportionate number of criminals who come from the lower socioeconomic strata (Western, Kleykamp, and Rosenfeld 2006). As suggested earlier, part of the reason is that the powerless and deprived are more likely to be defined as criminals. Several studies over the last few decades have revealed many consistencies in the characteristics of people *labeled as criminals.* Their general *powerlessness* and their location in the stratification system are clear. Criminals are more likely to (1) lack *social anchorage* in the sense of growing up in a stable family that is integrated into the community, (2) come from a lower-income family, (3) be young, (4) be male, and (5) come disproportionately from a minority group.

In sum, *the powerless are more likely to be defined as criminals throughout the criminal justice system.* They are more likely to be suspects and more likely to be arrested. In some states, judges have the option of withholding **adjudication** of guilt from people placed on probation. The judge's decision, then, determines whether *the individual will*

**adjudication**
making a judgment; settling a judicial matter

*carry the stigma of being a convicted felon.* Those people most likely to carry that stigma are the powerless–the poor and minorities. We are not saying that these people are innocent; rather, we are pointing out the unequal treatment received by those in the lower strata.

## Social Psychological Factors

Respectable people define crime as reprehensible–but how do criminals define it? In a classic and creative analysis, Katz (1988) pointed out that a part of the explanation of crime is found in the fact that criminal acts possess certain "sensual dynamics." Each kind of crime has a certain appeal, one that results in the criminal's feeling good or even exhilarated. In line with this, Lopez (2008) found a number of different reasons why adolescents commit property crimes. They included the usual reasons of stress and economic gain, but also included the "thrills" the offender experienced when successful. Katz also discussed the property crime of robbery, which typically involves considerable risk and minimal gain. What makes robbery attractive, according to Katz, is not just the money gained, but the excitement, adventure, and sense of conquest in the act. "In virtually all robberies, the offender discovers, fantasizes, or manufactures *an angle of moral superiority* over the intended victim" and makes "a fool of his victim" (Katz 1988:169, 174).

Other kinds of crimes have their own emotional rewards. The murderer may gain a sense of righteous revenge. Youths in street gangs may gain a sense of triumph over a destructive and dehumanizing environment. The point is that crime has *both emotional and material rewards for people* (Meadows and Anklin 2002). In part, motivation to continue a criminal career may lie in the emotional rewards.

Attitudes as well as emotions are important in crime. We noted earlier that the attitudes that prison conditions generate in inmates help to perpetuate crime. *Attitudes of respectable people* also contribute to the problem by providing necessary support for much officially defined crime, even though they don't view themselves as culpable or as contributors to crime. The assertion has been made that prostitution could not continue without official support. Certainly it could not continue without the support of the respectable clientele it serves or without the overt or covert support of the police.

Automobile theft is another example of crime supported by respectable people. Upwardly mobile young men in business and the professions sometimes buy stolen luxury cars for a fraction of their retail cost. They may know, or at least suspect, that they are buying a stolen car. Such crimes would have no payoff without these respectable customers. ("After all," they reason, "if I don't buy it, someone else will.")

fallacy

Attitudes of respectable people that stigmatize criminals contribute to continuation of the criminal careers (Pager 2003; Davies and Tanner 2003). Often, the very people who decry crime resist providing any help to the criminal. They get mired in the *fallacy of circular reasoning.* They believe that criminals can't be trusted in respectable jobs, then condemn criminals for not becoming respectable people. The ex-criminal who sincerely wants to become respectable becomes the victim of the process.

*Attitudes toward white-collar criminals* are ambivalent. Generally, unless the acts are flagrant and overt violations, white-collar criminals may not be prosecuted as criminals. However, white-collar criminals are not as invulnerable to the criminal justice system as they once were, in part because of a reaction to the Watergate scandal of the Nixon administration. Some white-collar criminals receive stiff penalties and sentences for their offenses. Nevertheless, their chances for leniency are far greater than are those for other criminals. In addition, white-collar criminals do not face the same kinds of hurdles when they try to reenter society following imprisonment (Kerley and Copes 2004). Unless such criminals have multiple arrests or are arrested and imprisoned before the age of 24, they are able to secure stable employment much easier than are other offenders.

Finally, in looking at the social psychology of *committed criminals or delinquents,* you find a distinctive set of attitudes, values, and other attributes. For these individuals, delinquency or crime has become a way of life. They have a *"subterranean" set of values*—hedonism, a focus on immediate gratification, and the ability to outwit and con others. They appear to be untouched by punishment, continue their deviant ways, and account for much of the crime in the nation. For them, deviance is a way of life. This finding is illustrated by studies that have examined the *self-concepts of delinquents.* Typically, the studies reveal congruence between attitudes toward the self and behavior. Low self-esteem fosters delinquent behavior, and the behavior, in turn, may raise the individual's self-esteem (Mason 2001). The delinquent behavior is a protection of the self as well as a rejection of law-abiding society.

## Solutions: Public Policy and Private Action

Our discussion of the causes of crime suggests the kinds of actions that will reduce the amount of crime. For example, whatever ameliorates economic deprivation reduces crime rates (Hannon and Defronzo 1998; Rosenfeld 2002). Intensive police patrolling of "hot spots" reduces crime rates (Rosenfeld 2002; Zimring 2011). Reducing drug use brings a decline in crime (Blumstein and Rosenfeld 1998). Youth curfew laws cut down on the number of offenders in hot spots and reduce burglary, larceny, and simple assault (McDowall, Loftin, and Wiersema 2000). Finding employment for older offenders reduces recidivism (Uggen 2000; Duwe 2015). Prevention programs that help youths by fostering a healthy family life, making communities safe, encouraging the young to stay in school, and developing skills and healthy lifestyle choices can reduce the number of youths who begin a life of crime (Coolbaugh and Hansel 2000). Stronger laws can aid the fight against white-collar crime (Goldsmith 2004). Setting up a neighborhood watch program tends to reduce the amount of crime in the area (Bennett, Holloway, and Farrington 2006). And being in a stable relationship with a law-abiding woman reduces a man's likelihood of continued criminal activity (Forrest 2014; Andersen, Andersen, and Skov 2015). Various other programs hold promise, but first we must look at the issue of punishment versus rehabilitation.

### Punishment or Rehabilitation?

Will crime be reduced by punishing or by rehabilitating criminals? Should criminals be required to reimburse their victims? Are criminals themselves victims, people who can be rehabilitated with the proper methods, or are their offenses unjustified acts that demand punishment? Can you trust a criminal to become a law-abiding citizen again? Such questions are behind the various solutions proposed for the problem of crime.

For many centuries the societal reaction to crime was simply one of punishment in order to deter others who might consider the same acts. Now more people advocate *rehabilitation instead of punishment.* In this view, the criminal has the potential to become a law-abiding citizen and should be given the opportunity to do so. Even if this view is true, some people would argue that *criminals should make restitution* to their victims, and in recent years some courts have required offenders to do so. Usually, the restitution is a cash payment large enough to offset the loss, and the payment may be reduced to fit the earning capacity of the offender. But what kind of payment can be made to compensate for emotional trauma? Sometimes services that benefit the victim directly or indirectly also may be required or substituted for the cash payment.

Experts who advocate rehabilitation face the problem of the offender's *reintegration* into the community. How can offenders be reintegrated into society? Because many offenders got in trouble because of the environment in which they lived, reintegration requires community resources such as vocational counseling and employment to restructure the offender's life. The goal is to help the offender find a legitimate role in the community.

That goal will not be easy. As Talbot (2003) notes, about 1,600 people leave state and federal prisons each day. Most come out with nothing more than a small amount of money ($20 to $200) and a one-way bus ticket. Some are drug abusers who received no treatment. Some are sex offenders who received no counseling. Some are high school dropouts who took no classes and received no training in job skills. Many are sick (HIV, tuberculosis, and hepatitis C). And only about one in eight received any kind of prerelease program to prepare them for life outside the prison.

As ex-convicts try to cope with life in the community, they may find themselves spending a good deal of their time dealing with parole officers, going to public assistance agencies, finding adequate housing, and using various community services (Halushka 2020). And the best that most of them can do for employment is to find a low-paying job that has little or no stability (Fernandes 2020).

Clearly, the task of reentry is massive. Nevertheless, rehabilitation is possible; recidivism rates can be reduced. In particular, recidivism is less likely when the offender is able to secure housing and employment and complete treatment programs (community-based programs tend to be more effective than those based in prisons) (Makarios, Steiner, and Travis 2010; Clement, Schwarzfeld, and Thompson 2011).

## Capital Punishment

Some people advocate a *get-tough* policy on crime, including the use of *capital punishment*. Many states and the District of Columbia do not allow the death penalty, even though it was reinstated as constitutional by the Supreme Court in 1976. At the end of 2018, 2,628 prisoners were being held under the sentence of death (Snell 2020). Of those prisoners, 98 percent were male, 56 percent were white, 42 percent were Black, and 15 percent were Hispanic. As with so many other aspects of American life, racial/ethnic background affects the criminal justice process.

Although a 2020 Gallup poll found that 55 percent of Americans favor the death penalty for murderers, capital punishment is controversial from both a moral and a criminal justice point of view. From a moral point of view, the question is whether the state has the right to kill someone as punishment for murder. Opponents of capital punishment view it as extreme and inhumane—an official form of the same heinous crime committed by the individual. Furthermore, they argue, keeping an individual on death row is a form of torture, as underscored by the fact that suicide and natural causes, rather than execution, are the leading cause of deaths of prisoners on death row (Locke 1996). The appeals process can take so long that some prisoners literally die of natural causes, and the process of waiting is so agonizing that many commit suicide or become mentally ill.

In addition, critics point out the danger of executing people who are innocent. Using DNA tests and discovering other evidence has led to the exoneration and release of hundreds of prisoners sentenced to death, some of whom were on death row for a decade or more (Westervelt and Cook 2008).

Religious groups take varying positions on the moral issue (Falsani 1996). Protestants and Jews are divided. The official Roman Catholic position, as defined in a 1995 encyclical by Pope John Paul II, is one of opposition. The Pope argued for nonlethal means of combating crime.

From the criminal justice point of view, is capital punishment an effective deterrent for murder? Experts disagree. Stack (1990) found a 17.5 percent drop in homicide rates in South Carolina in months with publicized executions. In contrast, Bailey (1990) and Hong and Kleck (2017) found no drop in homicide rates after publicized executions. Sorenson, Wrinkle, Brewer, and Marquart (1999) found no evidence of deterrence in Texas (the most active execution state in recent times) from 1984 through 1997. Finally, states without capital punishment tend to have lower homicide rates than states with it.

Arguments about the effectiveness of punishment versus rehabilitation go on. Advocates of punishment and isolation are correct when they contend that prisons do not rehabilitate. But rehabilitation programs can be effective. In fact, rehabilitative efforts may need to be combined with punishment. There is strong evidence that punishment is a deterrent to crime. However, the *certainty of punishment* is as important as the severity of punishment for purposes of deterrence (Matthews and Agnew 2008; Zhang, Smith, and McDowell 2009). To the extent that people are convinced that, if caught, they will be punished (rather than avoiding punishment through legal maneuvers), crime rates fall.

Thus, the criminal justice system in the United States should be revamped in two ways: First, punishment for crime must be made more certain. Second, efforts must be made, through reform of prisons or through innovative alternatives, to establish effective rehabilitation programs. Certainty of punishment will act as a deterrent for some criminals and will remove others from society, whereas more effective rehabilitation programs will effect change in others and help them live socially useful lives.

## Innovative Alternatives

Some innovative alternatives to the present system, including some that are popular with citizens and law enforcement officials, are ineffective in reducing crime. In a comprehensive study of crime prevention programs, researchers concluded that the following are among the programs that do not lower crime: gun buyback programs, drug prevention classes that focus on fear or on building self-esteem, increased arrests or raids on drug market locations, correctional boot camps using military basic training, "Scared Straight" programs in which juvenile offenders visit adult prisons, intensive supervision on parole or probation, and community mobilization against crime in high-crime poverty areas (Sherman et al. 1998).

In contrast, the researchers identified about 30 programs that show promise for dealing with crime, including community policing with meetings to set priorities, greater respect by the police for arrested offenders (may reduce repeat offending), higher numbers of police officers in cities, monitoring of gangs by community workers and law enforcement officials, mentoring programs for youths, prison-based vocational education programs for adult inmates, enterprise zones to reduce unemployment, drug treatment in jails followed by urine testing in the community, and intensive supervision and aftercare of juvenile offenders.

NEIGHBORHOOD
CRIME WATCH
We immediately report
all SUSPICIOUS PERSONS and
activities to our Police Dept.

Community programs can reduce crime.

S. Meltzer/PhotoLink/Getty Images

*Private prisons* (that is, prisons privately owned and operated under contract with a state) are an alternative that may be no better, or even worse, than the prisons operated by the government. Advocates claim that private prisons can lower costs and reduce recidivism. A recent study found no difference in the behavior of inmates with one exception—men in private prisons were a little less likely to engage in institutional violence (El Sayed, Morris, and DeShay 2020). However, an early study found that private prisons are *not* more cost-effective (Pratt and Maahs 1999). And an Oklahoma study concluded that recidivism was actually higher among those who had been in a private prison (Spivak and Sharp 2008). The failure of private prisons is underscored by the fact that in 2016 the Justice Department announced it was going to phase out the use of private prisons for federal prisoners because the private facilities are less safe and less effective at providing correctional services (Zapotosky and Harlan 2016). Other nations have experimented with private prisons also. A study of one in Scotland found that, compared to the government prisons, the private prison had lower morale and greater risks to both the inmates and the prison staff (Taylor and Cooper 2008).

### Community Action and Involvement

Crime prevention is not just a matter of official action. A number of community programs can reduce crime (Loeber and Farrington 1998; Sherman et al. 1998). Parents, neighborhood groups, and school personnel can work together to teach children values and to encourage and reward law-abiding behavior. Community-based afterschool recreational programs may help reduce local juvenile crime. In fact, community organizations are crucially important. Research shows that for every new nonprofit community organization in a city of 100,000, there will be a drop of 1.2 percent in murders, a drop of 1 percent in other violent crimes, and a drop of 0.7 percent in property crimes (Atchison 2018).

Even the physical arrangements in a community affect crime. Greener surroundings in the inner city and increased lighting reduce both the fear of crime and the amount of actual crime (Kuo and Sullivan 2001; Clarke 2008). Always having two workers in convenience stores at night lessens the likelihood of robbery, and neighborhood parks and recreational facilities can provide alternatives to gang activity.

Finally, whatever can be done to enhance cohesion in a community will deter crime. Three researchers who examined violent crime in urban neighborhoods concluded that the more that residents trust each other, share values, and are willing to intervene in the lives of children (e.g., to stop truancy and graffiti painting), the lower the rate of crime will be (Sampson, Raudenbush, and Earls 1997).

## Aid to Victims

An important public policy effort involves *aid to the victims.* Aid to victims is provided by governments to prevent a double victimization—once by the offender and again by the criminal justice system. Some problems faced by the victim of a crime include a lack of transportation to court, difficulty in retrieving stolen property from the police, threats by defendants if the victim testifies, and the amount of time consumed by the various procedures in the criminal justice system. An aid program can compensate for some of these losses incurred by the victims.

Most states now have compensation programs to help the victims of violent crime. Awards vary from small amounts to tens of thousands of dollars. Some states require the victim to show financial need, and most require that the crime be reported to police and the claim filed within a specified time period (ranging from a few days to a number of months).

The compensation programs provide for the recovery of medical expenses and lost earnings. In a number of states, money to aid victims is accumulated through penalties assessed against offenders or by expropriating the money earned by offenders resulting from their crimes (e.g., by writing a book).

*Follow-Up.* Do you think prisons should primarily punish or primarily rehabilitate inmates? Based on your answer, design the "perfect" prison to achieve your goals.

## Summary

Crime is one of the problems about which Americans are most concerned. Technically, crime is any violation of the criminal law. Therefore, the acts defined by law as crime vary over time. We classify crime into four broad types: (1) Predatory crime, which includes white-collar crime, is an act that causes a victim to suffer physical harm or loss of property. (2) Illegal service crimes involve offenses such as drugs or prostitution. (3) Public disorder crimes have no definite victim but are acts that offend the public. (4) Crimes of negligence involve an unintended victim or potential victim. Cybercrime may be either predatory or illegal service, whereas white-collar crime is primarily predatory. Organized crime involves groups of people in an ongoing organization who provide illegal goods and services and who use predatory crime and political corruption to maintain their activities. The term "juvenile delinquency" covers a broad range of behavior, frequently including fighting, truancy, and running away from home. Juvenile gangs may get involved in a range of criminal activities, from predatory crime to illegal goods and services.

Crime and delinquency are widespread, as measured by various indexes—official records, victimization studies, or self-reports. Crime is not uniformly distributed, however; the likelihood of being a victim depends on the kind of crime; where the person lives; and his or her sex, race, age, education, and income.

Crime diminishes the quality of life and exacts physical, psychological, and economic costs. Crime threatens physical and mental health. It generates fear, which restricts the activities of people. White-collar crime can lead to pervasive cynicism and alienation. Crime costs the nation billions of dollars yearly, and the costs are increasing.

Norms are an important sociocultural factor contributing to the problem of crime and delinquency because they encourage members of certain groups to engage in criminal behavior. In particular, norms that are counter to the law have developed among lower-class youths and groups of businesspeople and professionals.

The political aspects of crime control contribute to the problem, especially through the nation's prison system. Prisons make rehabilitation unlikely because they tend to dehumanize offenders, remove them further from noncriminal social control, and make them more competent in criminal activity.

The family may be a factor in crime. A disproportionate number of delinquents come from families with poor relationships between parents and children or from broken homes. Adult offenders are likely to have had troubled family backgrounds.

The stratification system also relates to crime. Monetary exploitation of others is more likely to be defined as crime among lower-class people than among middle- and upper-class people. The lower class has a greater proportion of violent crime and delinquency, whereas middle and upper classes have more white-collar crime. A lower-class individual is more likely to be defined as a criminal by the processes of the criminal justice system.

Emotionally, crime may provide a certain thrill or reward to offenders. Many attitudes tend to perpetuate crime. Crimes are facilitated by the attitudes of respectable people about their own behavior—especially their use of the services offered by criminals. Stigmatizing criminals tends to keep them in criminal careers. Minimizing the seriousness of white-collar crime also encourages it. Finally, the attitudes, values, and other social psychological characteristics of some criminals and delinquents form a consistent set that makes for a way of life. Having deviant values and attitudes and thinking of themselves as people who engage in criminal or delinquent behavior, they tend to maintain their way of life even when they are punished.

## Key Terms

**Adjudication**
**Alienation**
**Dehumanization**
**Differential Association Theory**
**Organized Crime**
**Predatory Crimes**
**Recidivism**
**Rehabilitation**
**Total Institution**
**Trauma**
**White-Collar Crime**

## Study Questions

1. Define and illustrate the various types of crime.
2. What are the problems in obtaining accurate data on the amount of crime?
3. How much crime is there in the United States, and where is a person most likely to be a victim?
4. How does crime affect physical and psychological well-being?
5. What is the cost of crime in economic terms?

6. How is the amount of crime affected by the age structure of the population?
7. What is the role of norms in criminal activity?
8. How do prisons help or worsen the problem of crime?
9. In what ways do the family and the social stratification system contribute to the problem of crime?
10. How do the attitudes of respectable people bear on the amount of crime in the nation?
11. What can be done to reduce crime?

## Internet Resources/Exercises

1. Explore some of the ideas in this chapter on the following sites:

**http://www.fbi.gov** The FBI site offers current crime news, information about the most wanted criminals, and crime data.

**http://www.usdoj.gov** The Department of Justice site gives information about all kinds of crime and crime prevention, and includes a link to the Bureau of Justice Statistics.

**http://journals.sagepub.com/home/ijo** This is the site for the International Journal of Offender Therapy and Comparative Criminology. You can read the abstracts of articles published in the journal from 1966 to the present.

2. Log on to the international journal site. Find and read the abstract of an article that focuses on a topic in criminology that interests you and that involves a country other than the United States. Search the Internet to see if additional materials on the topic are available. How do your findings compare with information in the text? What conclusions would you draw about the effectiveness of the criminal justice system in different countries?

3. Investigate how victimization rates have varied over time. The Department of Justice site has the data. Chart the data for various crimes over a period of three decades. How do the patterns of the crimes compare with each other? How do they compare with the FBI data in Table 3.2? What are some possible explanations for the patterns?

## For Further Reading

Bedau, Hugo, and Paul Cassell. *Debating the Death Penalty: Should America Have Capital Punishment?* New York: Oxford University Press, 2003. Gives the pro and con arguments for the death penalty, including the perspectives of judges, lawyers, philosophers, and a state governor who put a moratorium on the death penalty in Illinois.

Duran, Robert J. *Gang Life in Two Cities: An Insider's Journey.* New York: Columbia University Press, 2013. A Latino and former gang member, Duran shows why belonging to a gang is not primarily a way to participate in crime but a way to adapt to oppressive social environments.

Elliott, A. Larry, and Richard J. Schroth. *How Companies Lie: Why Enron Is Just the Tip of the Iceberg.* New York: Crown Business, 2002. Two corporate consultants argue that a new business culture has arisen that justifies any means used to increase profits, including those that are illegal or unethical. The notorious Enron case is but one example.

Hassine, Victor. *Life Without Parole.* 4th ed. New York: Oxford University Press, 2008. Law school graduate Victor Hassine, convicted of a capital offense in 1981 and sentenced to life in prison without parole, describes what it is like to be confined to prison amidst such things as rape, gangs, violence, and prison politics.

Ross, Jeffrey Ian, ed. *Varieties of State Crime and Its Control.* Monsey, NY: Criminal Justice Press, 2000. Case studies of government crimes in the United States and other nations, including political corruption and various kinds of violence and repression by governments against their citizens.

Roth, R. *American Homicide.* Cambridge, MA: Belknap Harvard, 2009. A history professor explores the process of America's shift from being one of the least homicidal Western nations in the mid-18th and early 19th centuries to one of the most homicidal societies in the world today.

Simpson, Sally, and Carole Gibbs, eds. *Corporate Crime.* Burlington, VT: Ashgate, 2007. A collection of classic and contemporary articles that examine every aspect of the problem of corporate crime in the United States and other nations.

Whitman, James Q. *Harsh Justice: Criminal Punishment and the Widening Gap between America and Europe.* Oxford, England: Oxford University Press, 2003. Shows the many different ways in which American justice is harsher than that of Europe, including the U.S. prison system, the number of punishable kinds of behavior, and the length of sentences.

## References


Agnew, R., S. K. Matthews, J. Bucher, A. N. Welcher, and C. Keyes. 2008. "Socioeconomic status, economic problems, and delinquency." *Youth & Society* 40:159–81.

Allender, D. M., and F. Marcell. 2003. "Career criminals, security threat groups, and prison gangs." *FBI Law Enforcement Bulletin* 72:8–12.

Alleyne, E., and J. I. Wood. 2010. "Gang involvement: Psychological and behavioral characteristics of gang members, peripheral youth, and nongang youth." *Aggressive Behavior* 36:423–36.

Andersen, S. H., L. H. Andersen, and P. E. Skov. 2015. "Effect of marriage and spousal criminality on recidivism." *Journal of Marriage and Family* 77:496–509.

Atchison, N. 2018. "Community organizations have important role in lowering crime rates." Brennan Center for Justice website.

Bailey, W. C. 1990. "Murder, capital punishment, and television: Execution publicity and homicide rates." *American Sociological Review* 55 (October):628–33.

Beck, A. 2013. "Sexual victimization in prisons and jails reported by Inmates, 2011–12." Bureau of Justice Statistics website.

Beck, A. J., and P. M. Harrison. 2006. "Sexual violence reported by correctional authorities." *Bureau of Justice Statistics Special Bulletin,* July.

Beck, A. J., P. M. Harrison, and P. Guerino. 2010. "Sexual victimization in juvenile facilities reported by youth, 2008–09." *Bureau of Justice Statistics Special Report.* BJS website.

Bennett, R. 1991. "Routine activities: A cross-national assessment of a criminological perspective." *Social Forces* 70:147–63.

Bennett, T., K. Holloway, and D. P. Farrington. 2006. "Does neighborhood watch reduce crime?" *Journal of Experimental Criminology* 2:437–58.

Berger, J. 1999. "Panel is proposed to fight corruption in trash industry." *New York Times,* March 16.

Blumstein, A., and R. Rosenfeld. 1998. "Assessing the recent ups and downs in U.S. homicide rates." *National Institute of Justice Journal* (October):9–11.

Brody, G. H., et al. 2001. "The influence of neighborhood disadvantage, collective socialization, and parenting on African American children's affiliation with deviant peers." *Child Development* 72:1231–46.

Browning, K., and R. Loeber. 1999. "Highlights of findings from the Pittsburgh youth study." *OJJDP Fact Sheet #95.* Washington, DC: Government Printing Office.

Bryjak, G. I. 1999. "Multiple reasons for lower crime rates." *San Diego Union-Tribuine,* March 28.

Butterfield, H. 1949. *Christianity and History.* London: Fontana Books.

Carson, E. A. 2020. "Prisoners in 2019." Bureau of Justice Statistics website.

Carson, K. W., et al. 2020. "Why women are not talking about it." *Violence Against Women* 26:271–95.

Clarke, R. V. 2008. "Improving street lighting to reduce crime in residential areas." *Problem-Oriented Guides for Police Response Guide No. 8.* Washington, DC: Center for Problem-Oriented Policing.

Clement, M., M. Schwarzfeld, and M. Thompson. 2011. *The National Summit on Justice Reinvestment and Public Safety.* Bureau of Justice Statistics website.

Cohen, L. E., and M. Felson. 1979. "Social change and crime rate trends." *American Sociological Review* 44 (August):588–607.

Coolbaugh, K., and C. J. Hansel. 2000. "The comprehensive strategy: Lessons learned from pilot sites." *Juvenile Justice Bulletin.* Washington, DC: Government Printing Office.

Davies, S., and J. Tanner. 2003. "The long arm of the law." *The Sociological Quarterly* 44:385–404.

Davis, A. 2016. "In U.S., concern about crime climbs to 15-year high." Gallup Poll website.

Diem, C., and J. M. Pizarro. 2010. "Social structure and family homicides." *Journal of Family Violence* 25:521–32.

Duwe, G. 2015. "The benefits of keeping idle hands busy." *Crime and Delinquency* 61:559–86.

Edelhertz, H. 1983. "White-collar and professional crime." *American Behavioral Scientist* 27 (October-November):109–28.

Egley, A., J. C. Howell, and M. Harris. 2014. "Highlights of the 2012 national youth gang survey." Office of Juvenile Justice and Delinquency Prevention website.

El Sayed, S. A., R. G. Morris, and R. A. DeShay. 2020. "Comparing the rates of misconduct between private and public prisons in Texas." *Crime and Delinquency* 66:1217–41.

Fagan, A. A. 2005. "The relationship between adolescent physical abuse and criminal offending." *Journal of Family Violence* 20:279–90.

Falsani, C. 1996. "Churches, clergy split on capital punishment." *Chicago Tribune,* May 24.

Federal Bureau of Investigation. 2002. "Crime in the United States: 2002." FBI website.

——. 2009. "Move over Mafia: The new face of organized crime." FBI website.

——. 2010. "Smishing and vishing and other cyber scams to watch out for this holiday." FBI website.

——. 2019. "Hate crime statistics." FBI website.

Fernandes, A. D. 2020. "On the job or in the joint." *Crime and Delinquency* 66:1678–1702.

Finelli, G. A. 2019. "Slash, shoot, kill." *Family Court Review* 57:243–57.

Fischer, M., and B. Geiger. 1996. "Resocializing young offenders in the kibbutz." *International Journal of Offender Therapy and Comparative Criminology* 40 (1):44–53.

Forrest, W. 2014. "Cohabitation, relationship quality, and desistance from crime." *Journal of Marriage and Family* 76:539–56.

Freudenberg, N., J. Daniels, M. Crum, T. Perkins, and B. E. Richie. 2005. "Coming home from jail." *American Journal of Public Health* 95:1725–36.

Goldsmith, M. 2004. "Resurrecting RICO: Removing immunity for white-collar crime." *Harvard Journal on Legislation* 41:281–317.

Grogan-Kaylor, A., and M. D. Otis. 2003. "Effect of childhood maltreatment on adult criminality." *Child Maltreatment* 8:129–37.

Halushka, J. M. 2020. "The runaround: Punishment, welfare, and poverty survival after prison." *Social problems* 67:233–50.

Hannon, L., and J. Defronzo. 1998. "The truly disadvantaged, public assistance, and crime." *Social Problems* 45:383–92.

Harrell, E. 2005. "Violence by gang members, 1993-2003." *Bureau of Justice Statistics Crime Data Brief,* June.

Haynie, D. L. 2002. "Friendship networks and delinquency." *Journal of Quantitative Criminology* 15:99–134.

He, L., A. Paez, and D. Liu. 2017. "Persistence of crime hot spots." *Geographical Analysis* 49:3–22.

Hipp, J. R., D. J. Bauer, P. J. Curran, and K. A. Bollen. 2004. "Crimes of opportunity or crimes of emotion? Testing two explanations of seasonal change in crime." *Social Forces* 82:1333–72.

Hochstetler, A., et al. 2014. "The criminal victimization-depression sequela." *Crime and Delinquency* 60:785–806.

Holt, T. J., and A. M. Bossler. 2009. "Examining the applicability of lifestyle-routine activities theory for cybercrime victimization." *Deviant Behavior* 30:1–25.

Holtfreter, K., M. D. Reisig, and T. C. Pratt. 2008. "Low self-control, routine activities, and fraud victimization." *Criminology* 46:189–220.

Hong, M., and G. Kleck. 2017. "The short-term deterrent effect of executions." *Crime and Delinquency* 64:939–70.

James, D. J., and L. E. Glaze. 2006. "Mental health problems of prison and jail inmates." *Bureau of Justice Statistics Special Report,* September.

Jehle, J. M. 2005. *Criminal Justice in Germany.* Berlin: Federal Ministry of Justice.

Johnson, B. R., S. J. Jang, D. B. Larson, and S. De Li. 2001. "Does adolescent religious commitment matter?" *Journal of Research in Crime and Delinquency* 38:22–44.

Katz, J. 1988. *Seductions of Crime: Moral and Sensual Attractions of Doing Evil.* New York: Basic Books.

Kennedy, L. W., and S. W. Baron. 1993. "Routine activities and a subculture of violence: A study of violence on the street." *Journal of Research in Crime and Delinquency* 30 (February):88–112.

Kerley, K. R., and H. Copes. 2004. "The effects of criminal justice contact on employment stability for white-collar and street-level offenders." *International Journal of Offender Therapy and Comparative Criminology* 48:65–84.

Kouwe, Z. 2009. "2 money managers held in new Wall St. fraud case." *New York Times,* February 26.

Kuo, F. E., and W. C. Sullivan. 2001. "Environment and crime in the inner city." *Environment and Behavior* 33:343–67.

Lee, M. R., and G. C. Ousey. 2001. "Size matters: Examining the link between small manufacturing socioeconomic deprivation and crime rates in nonmetropolitan communities." *Sociological Quarterly* 42:581–602.

Locke, M. 1996. "Suicide, natural causes: How most inmates die on death rows." *Chicago Tribune,* March 6.

Loeber, R., and D. P. Farrington. 1998. *Serious and Violent Juvenile Offenders: Risk Factors and Successful Interventions.* Newbury Park, CA: Sage.

Lopez, V. 2008. "Understanding adolescent property crime using a delinquent events perspective." *Deviant Behavior* 29:581–610.

Lovell, D. 2008. "Patterns of disturbed behavior in a supermax population." *Criminal Justice and Behavior* 35:985-1004.

Makarios, M., B. Steiner, and L. F. Travis. 2010. "Examining the predictors of recidivism among men and women released from prison in Ohio." *Criminal Justice and Behavior* 37:1377-91.

Markowitz, F. E. 2003. "Socioeconomic disadvantage and violence." *Aggression and Violent Behavior* 8:145-54.

Marks, A. 2006. "Prosecutions drop for U.S. white-collar crime." *Christian Science Monitor,* August 31.

Mason, W. A. 2001. "Self-esteem and delinquency revisited (again)." *Journal of Youth and Adolescence* 30:83-102.

Massoglia, M. 2008. "Incarceration as exposure." *Journal of Health and Social Behavior* 49:56-71.

Matthews, S. K., and R. Agnew. 2008. "Extending deterrence theory." *Journal of Research in Crime and Delinquency* 45:91-118.

McClam, E. 2005. "Role in tax scam admitted by KPMG." *San Diego Union-Tribune,* August 30.

McDowall, D., C. Loftin, and B. Wiersema. 2000. "The impact of youth curfew laws on juvenile crime rates." *Crime and Delinquency* 46 (January):76-91.

Meadows, R. J., and K. L. Anklin. 2002. "Study of the criminal motivations of sentenced jail inmates." In *Visions for Change: Crime and Justice in the Twenty-First Century,* 3rd ed., ed. R. Muraskin and A. R. Roberts, pp. 287-302. New York: Prentice-Hall.

Mendoza, M., and C. Sullivan. 2006. "Uncle Sam struggling to collect on fines." *San Diego Union-Tribune,* March 19.

Milkie, M. A., K. M. Nomaguchi, and K. E. Denny. 2015. "Does the amount of time mothers spend with children or adolescents matter?" *Journal of Marriage and Family* 77:355-72.

Miller, J. 2001. *One of the Guys: Girls, Gangs, and Gender.* New York: Oxford University Press.

Morgan, R. E., and J. L. Truman. 2020. "Criminal victimization, 2019." Bureau of Justice Statistics website.

Morton, H. 2004. "Identity thieves." *State Legislatures* 30:30-41.

Motivans, M. 2003. "Money laundering offenders, 1994-2001." *Bureau of Justice Statistics Special Report.* Washington, DC: Government Printing Office.

Mumola, C. 2005. "Suicide and homicide in state prisons and local jails." *Bureau of Justice Statistics Special Report,* August.

National Institute of Justice. 1996. "Alternative sanctions in Germany: An overview of Germany's sentencing practices." *Research Preview,* February.

O'Brien, R. M., J. Stockard, and L. Isaacson. 1999. "The enduring effects of cohort characteristics on age-specific homicide rates, 1960-1995." *American Journal of Sociology* 104 (January):1061-95.

Pager, D. 2003. "The mark of a criminal record." *American Journal of Sociology* 108:937-75.

Pearce, L. D., and D. L. Haynie. 2004. "Intergenerational religious dynamics and adolescent delinquency." *Social Forces* 82:1553-72.

Petersilia, J. 2011. "Beyond the prison bubble." *NIJ Journal,* #268, pp. 267-31.

Phillips, J. A. 2006. "The relationship between age structure and homicide rates in the United States, 1970 to 1999." *Journal of Research in Crime and Delinquency* 43:230-60.

Piquero, N. L., S. G. Tibbetts, and M. B. Blankenship. 2006. "Examining the role of differential association and techniques of neutralization in explaining corporate crime." *Deviant Behavior* 26:159-88.

Platt, A. 1969. *The Child Savers: The Invention of Delinquency.* Chicago: University of Chicago Press.

Pratt, T. C., and J. Maahs. 1999. "Are private prisons more cost-effective than public prisons?" *Crime and Delinquency* 45 (July):358-71.

Randa, R., and B. W. Reyns. 2020. "The physical and emotional toll of identity theft victimization." *Deviant Behavior* 41:1290-1304.

Rosenblatt, J. 2020. "Deadliest corporate crime in U.S. will end with 84 guilty pleas." Bloomberg News website.

Rosenfeld, R. 2002. "Crime decline in context." *Contexts* 1:25-34.

Rosoff, S. M., H. N. Pontell, and R. H. Tillman. 2002. *Profit without Honor: White-Collar Crime and the Looting of America.* 2nd ed. New York: Prentice-Hall.

Sampson, R. J., S. W. Raudenbush, and F. Earls. 1997. "Neighborhoods and violent crime: A multilevel study." *Science* 277 (August 15):918-24.

Sherman, L. W., et al. 1998. *Preventing Crime: What Works, What Doesn't, What's Promising.* Washington, DC: Government Printing Office.

Shawn, H. 2011. "Responding to the cyber threat." FBI website.

Shukla, K., and M. Wiesner. 2016. "Relations of delinquency to direct and indirect violence exposure among economically disadvantaged, ethnic-minority mid-adolescents." *Crime and Delinquency* 62:423-55.

Simon, T., J. Mercy, and C. Perkins. 2001. *Injuries from Violent Crime, 1992-98*. Washington, DC: Government Printing Office.

Smith, H. P., and R. J. Kaminski. 2011. "Self-injurious behaviors in state prisons." *Criminal Justice and Behavior* 38:26-41.

Snell, T. L. 2020. "Capital punishment, 2018." Bureau of Justice Statistics website.

Sorenson, J., R. Wrinkle, V. Brewer, and J. Marquart. 1999. "Capital punishment and deterrence: Examining the effect of executions on murder in Texas." *Crime and Delinquency* 45 (October):481-93.

Spivak, A. L., and S. F. Sharp. 2008. "Inmate recidivism as a measure of private prison performance." *Crime & Delinquency* 54:482-508.

Stack, S. 1990. "Execution publicity and homicide in South Carolina: A research note." *Sociological Quarterly* 31 (4):599-611.

Sutherland, E. H. 1968. "White collar criminality." In *Radical Perspectives on Social Problems*, ed. Frank Lindenfeld, pp. 149-60. New York: Macmillan.

Sutherland, E. H., and D. R. Cressey. 1955. *Principles of Criminology*. 5th ed. Philadelphia: J. B. Lippincott.

Talbot, M. 2003. "Catch and Release." *Atlantic Monthly*, January/February, pp. 97-100.

Taylor, P., and C. Cooper. 2008. "'It was absolute hell': Inside the private prison." *Capital & Class* 96:3-30.

Taylor, S. S. 2009. "How street gangs recruit and socialize members." *Journal of Gang Research* 17:1-27.

Thornberry, T. P., D. Huizinga, and R. Loeber. 2004. "The causes and correlates studies." *Juvenile Justice* 9:3-19.

Tregea, W., and M. Larmour. 2009. *The Prisoners' World: Portraits of Convicts Caught in the Incarceration Binge*. New York: Lexington Books.

U.S. Census Bureau. 1975. *Historical Statistics of the United States, Colonial Times to 1970*. Washington, DC: Government Printing Office.

U.S. Department of Justice. 2006. *Compendium of Federal Justice Statistics, 2004*. Washington, DC: Government Printing Office.

Uggen, C. 2000. "Work as a turning point in the life course of criminals." *American Sociological Review* 67:529-46.

Van Koppen, P. J., and R. W. J. Jansen. 1999. "The time to rob: Variations in time of number of commercial robberies." *Journal of Research in Crime and Delinquency* 36 (February):7-29.

Weisburd, D., and L. G. Mazerolle. 2000. "Crime and disorder in drug hot spots." *Police Quarterly* 3:331-49.

Weisburd, D., E. Groff, and N. Morris. 2011. "Hot spots of juvenile crime: Findings from Seattle." *Juvenile Justice Bulletin*. OJJDP website.

Weiss, H. E., and L. W. Reid. 2005. "Low-quality employment concentration and crime." *Sociological Perspectives* 48:213-32.

Welsh, W. N. 2002. "Court-ordered reform of jails." In *Visions for Change: Crime and Justice in the Twenty-first Century*, 3rd ed., ed. R. Muraskin and A. R. Roberts, pp. 390-407. New York: Prentice-Hall.

Western, B., M. Kleykamp, and J. Rosenfeld. 2006. "Did falling wages and employment increase U.S. imprisonment?" *Social Forces* 84:2291-2311.

Westervelt, S. D., and K. J. Cook. 2008. "Coping with innocence after death row." *Contexts* 7:32-37.

Wilper, A. P., et al. 2009. "The health and health care of US prisoners." *American Journal of Public Health* 99:666-72.

Wolfe, S. E., et al. 2016. "Routine cell activity and exposure to sext messages." *Crime and Delinquency* 62:614-44.

World Population Review. 2021. "Incarceration rates by country, 2021." WPR website.

Wu, E. Y., et al. 2014. "Paternal hostility and maternal hostility in European American and African American families." *Journal of Marriage and Family* 76:638-51.

Zapotosky, M., and C. Harlan. 2016. "Justice Dept. to end use of private prisons." *San Diego Union Tribune*, August 19.

Zhang, L., W. W. Smith, and W. C. McDowell. 2009. "Examining digital piracy." *Information Resources Management Journal* 22:24-44.

Zimring, F. E. 2011. "How New York beat crime." *Scientific American*, August, pp. 75-79.

CHAPTER

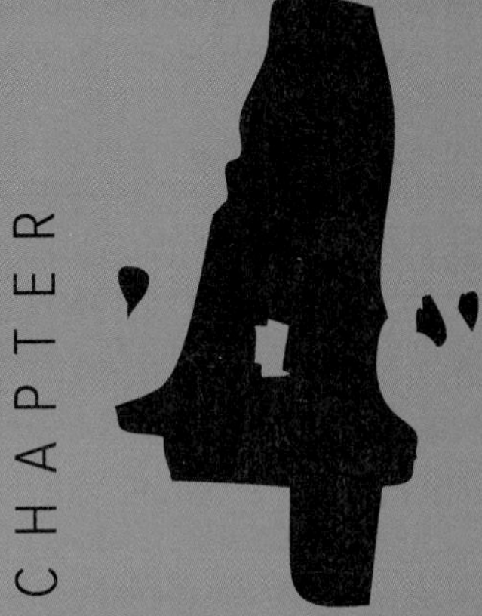

# Violence

OBJECTIVES

1 Gain a sense of the extent of violence in the United States.

2 Understand the human consequences of violent behavior.

3 Identify the factors that lead people to be violent, including societal factors that impinge on the violent individual.

4 Explain the consequences for the victim of both completed and attempted rapes.

5 Know the varied causes of rape.

6 Suggest ways to deal with violence, including rape.

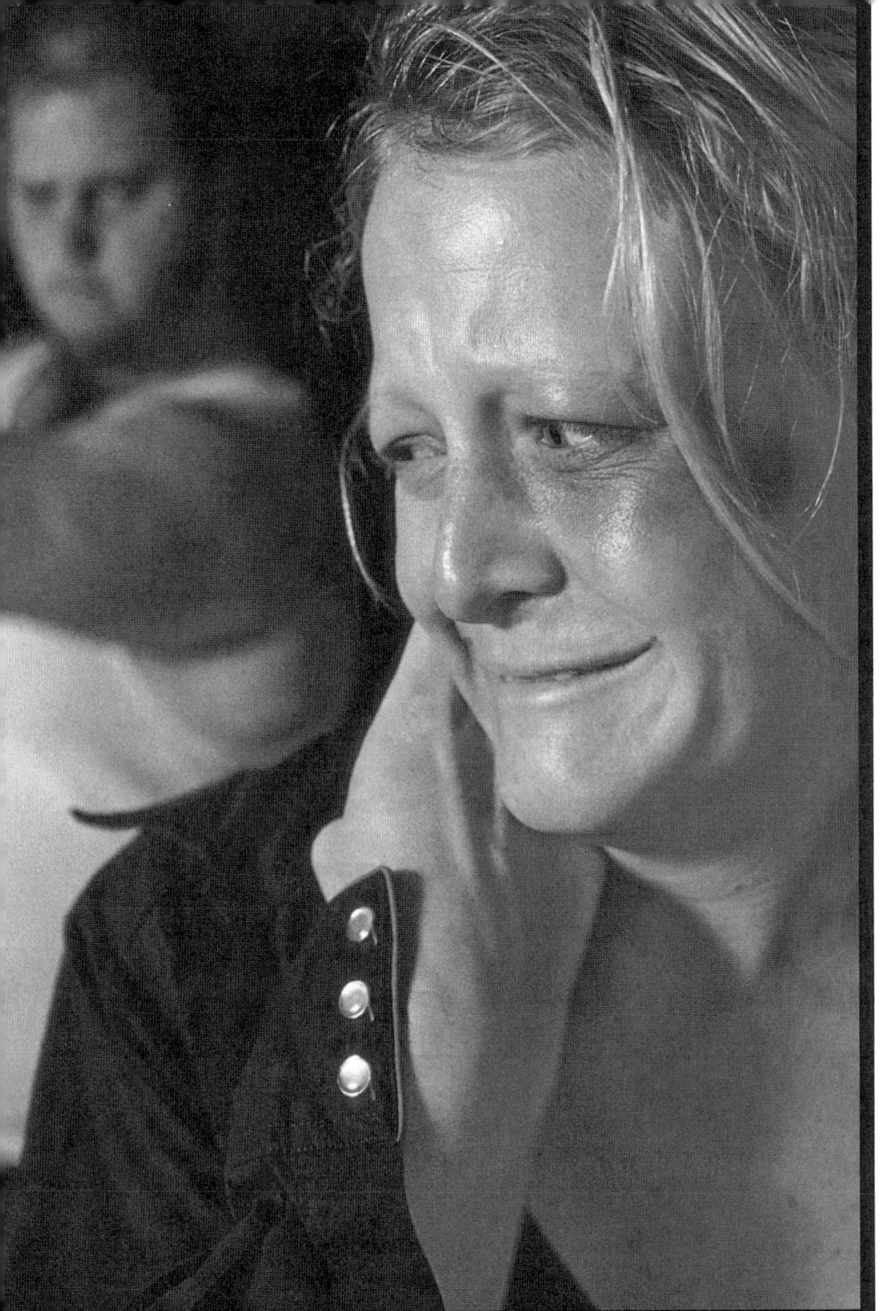

Purestock/Getty Images

## "I Felt Guilty"

The trauma of rape is described by Tammi, a 20-year-old woman who was raped while walking to the parking lot of a college:

*It happened about 10 p.m. I had been doing some research at the library and I was in a hurry to get home because I wanted to see a movie on TV. I was standing next to my car, looking in my purse for my keys. I didn't see the man or hear him until all of a sudden he grabbed me from behind and had me on the ground before I knew what had happened. He held a knife to my throat and told me to do what he said and I wouldn't get hurt. I was too scared to move anyway because I could feel the knife pressing against my neck. He was disgusted that I had on jeans and made a derogatory remark about the way girls dress today. He made me take off my pants and perform oral sex on him. Then he raped me. He kept asking me if I liked it, but I was too scared to answer him. He got angry because I wouldn't answer him and he hit me in the breast with his fist. I started crying and he got off of me and let me get dressed. He told me if I told anyone he would come back and rape me again. He said that he knew who I was and where I lived. I started crying harder and shaking all over. He patted me and told me to grow up, that he'd done me a favor, and that I was old enough to enjoy sex with a man. He finally left and I got into my car and went home.*

*I felt so dirty I took a shower and scrubbed myself all over and got into bed. At 12:30 my roommate came home and I told her what had happened. She insisted I call the police, so I did. Two policemen came to our apartment. They asked such things as where did it happen, and what did he look like, and what time did it happen. They acted like I made it up when they found out it happened two hours ago. The young cop asked me if I had an orgasm and if he had ejaculated. I didn't know what to say as I didn't know, since this was my first encounter with sex. I don't think they believed that either. They told me to come down to the station the next day if I wanted to press charges, but that since I had taken a shower and waited so long I probably didn't have a case. No one told me to go to the hospital to be treated for V.D. or that they could give me something to prevent pregnancy until I talked to a friend the next day. She went with me to the emergency room of a hospital and they told me they didn't treat rape victims. I started crying and she took me home. I was pretty shook up. For three or four days I stayed in bed. I cut all my classes. Finally, I went back to school and everything seemed to be fine until I saw a story about rape on TV. I got so upset my roommate called the Rape Crisis Center and had me talk to them about my feelings. I called them eight or nine times in all.*

*I felt guilty. I thought it was my fault because my mother had been against my leaving home to go to college and against my having an apartment. She had also warned me never to go out alone at night. I didn't tell her I had been raped because I was afraid she'd make me leave school and come back home. So instead of blaming the guy, I blamed myself for being so dumb and naive. It took about three months to get my head together. I feel I have now, but I still am uneasy if a guy comes on too strong, or stops to talk to me in an isolated place, or even if he gets too close in an elevator. I haven't dated since it happened. I guess I shut everyone out and went on my own head trip, but I've started going places with my girlfriends lately and I think I have it together now.*

## Introduction

In April 1999, two teenage boys shot and killed 12 students and a teacher and wounded a number of other students at Columbine High School in Littleton, Colorado. The boys then committed suicide. During a three-week period in October 2002, two snipers randomly shot people in the region around Washington, D.C., killing 10 and wounding three others. In October 2006, a man went into an Amish school in Pennsylvania and shot 10 girls before killing himself. Five of the girls died. In April 2007, a student went on a violent rampage at Virginia Tech University. He killed 32 people, wounded numerous others, and then killed himself. In October 2011, a man walked into a hair salon in Seal Beach, California, and shot and killed his ex-wife (with whom he was in a custody dispute over their son) and seven other people in the salon. In late February 2012, a high school student in Chardon, Ohio, shot five students, killing three of them, in the school's cafeteria. In June, 2016, a heavily armed man walked into a gay nightclub in Orlando, Florida, killed 50 and wounded another 53. In 2017, a man walked into a Baptist church in Sutherland Springs, Texas, shot and killed 16 people and injured 20 more. In 2019, a man killed 23 people in a mass shooting at a Walmart store in El Paso. These incidents are just a sampling of what one of our students called "the horror stories that keep popping up in the news." In addition to such dramatic and terrifying incidents, Americans are confronted by stories of violence daily in the news media.

Because social problems involve *intergroup conflict,* violence enters into nearly every social problem at some point. The conflict often becomes violent, as illustrated by gangs of straight youths who beat up homosexuals, by race riots, by murders when a drug dealer tries to move in on someone else's market, and so on.

In this chapter we deal with various kinds of interpersonal and intergroup violence, all of which concern Americans and all of which are widely believed to detract from the quality of life. We begin by discussing the meaning, the kinds, and the amount of violence in the nation. We show the ways that violence detracts from the quality of life and identify the various sociocultural factors that contribute to the problem. We discuss ways in which violence can be minimized or eliminated from human life.

We then discuss rape. Although some people have thought of rape as a form of sexual deviance, it is essentially an act of violence. The victim may be further victimized by the reactions of family, friends, police officers, and male jurors.

## What Is Violence?

In general, **violence** implies *use of force to kill, injure, or abuse others.* It occurs between two or more individuals as *interpersonal violence,* or it involves identifiable groups in the society and erupts as *intergroup violence* between two or more different races, religions, or political groups. In intergroup situations the violence ultimately means confrontation between individuals whose actions are legitimated by their group affiliation. Interpersonal violence often occurs between people who knew each other prior to the violent confrontation. Intergroup violence, however, is likely to involve people who were strangers prior to the confrontation.

**violence**
the use of force to kill, injure, or abuse others

### How Much Violence Is There?

It is difficult to estimate the amount of violent behavior in the United States. Much is never reported, and for some kinds of violence—riots, gang beatings, violent demonstrations, and terrorist activities—there is no systematic effort to record all incidents. But evidence indicates that there is and always has been a considerable amount of violence in the United States.

For example, the following incidents were reported over a period of a couple of months in a western city:

A distraught man walked into the emergency room of a hospital and began shooting randomly, killing two people and wounding two others.

Militant antiabortion protestors tried to shut down an abortion clinic, resulting in a violent confrontation that required police intervention and numerous arrests.

A confrontation between two rival youth gangs resulted in a number of injuries, including knife wounds.

Several women who were out jogging were caught and raped by a man who may be a serial rapist.

A brawl erupted between police and members of a religious sect after a police officer attempted to arrest a member of the sect for a routine traffic violation.

A university decided to cancel an annual festival that had taken place for more than 50 years because a weekend of rioting caused more than 100 injuries.

Violence comes in numberless forms and occurs in all settings. Violence is no respecter of age. Both children and the elderly are victims of abuse and murder. In 2018, the highest rate of violent victimization, 33.8 per 1,000, occured to those between 12 and 17 years of age (Hullenaar and Ruback 2020). A national study of elder abuse reported that 4.6 percent suffered emotional abuse, 1.6 percent endured physical abuse, 0.6 percent had been sexually abused, and 5.1 percent suffered from neglect (Acierno et al. 2010).

There is no safe haven from violence. Workplace violence has decreased considerably over the past two decades but is still about one-third the rate that occurs in nonworkplace situations (Harrell 2011). The police, security guards, and bartenders have the highest rates of nonfatal workplace violence. Similarly, violence in the family setting has declined, but the family is one of the most violent institutions in society (see Chapter 12).

Violence occurs in all societies, but the United States is one of the most violent nations in the Western world. Violence is so common and so pervasive that about 61 percent of American children are victims of, or witnesses to, some kind of violence at one or more points in their childhood (Finkelhor et al. 2009).

## Interpersonal Violence

As noted earlier, violence afflicts people of all ages and in all situations. For example, although rates of violence (other than rape and sexual assault) on college campuses are lower than those in noncollege situations, a good many studies report that dating violence is a serious and widespread problem among college students (Shorey, Stuart, and Cornelius 2011). A study of 1,530 undergraduates reported that one in four had been involved in a physically abusive dating relationship that included at least two acts of physically violent behavior (Miller 2011). Another study found that students who had hearing disabilities, were homosexual, or were part of a racial/ethnic minority had even higher rates of victimization than did white, heterosexual students (Porter and Williams 2011).

In general, the young are more likely to be victims of, or witnesses to, interpersonal violence. Adolescents aged 18–20 years have the highest rates of assault victimization, and those aged 12–14 years have the second highest rates (U.S. Department of Justice 2011). A survey of 104 fourth- and fifth-grade children in an impoverished inner-city area found that 89 percent had heard the sound of gunfire; 65 percent had been slapped, punched, or hit by someone; 65 percent had seen someone beaten up or mugged; 16 percent had seen someone killed; and 11 percent had been shot at. Bullying is not included in the crime data. But we identify it as a form of violent behavior. A survey of 66 studies of bullying found that one in three children is involved in some form of bullying and one in five is involved in cyberbullying (Zych, Ortega-Ruiz, and Del Rey 2015). Much of the violence experienced by children occurs in the school setting (see Chapter 11).

Violence occurs in intimate relationships (dating, cohabitation, marriage) at every age. A national survey reported that 43.6 percent of American women have suffered some kind of sexual violence, and 21.2 percent have been the victims of attempted or completed rape from an intimate partner (Smith et al. 2018). The survey also found victimization among men, although at a much lower rate: 24.8 percent of men said they had suffered from sexual violence and 2.6 percent said they had experienced attempted or completed rape from an intimate partner.

Rates of intimate partner violence are higher among dating teens than they are among adults (Office of Juvenile Justice and Delinquency Prevention 2006). A national survey reported that about 20 percent of boys and girls experience physical and/or sexual abuse when dating, and more than 60 percent were involved in psychological abuse (Mumford and Taylor 2014). Rates of victimization are similar for males and females, although girls are more likely than boys to claim self-defense as one of their motivations (Mulford and Giordano 2008). Girls are also more likely to suffer negative long-term consequences such as depression, attempted suicide, and drug use. Violent males, on the other hand, injure their dates more severely and more often. About one in five female high school students reports having been physically and/or sexually abused by a dating partner. Overall, women in the 16- to 24-year-old age group have rates of victimization by an intimate partner that are nearly three times the national average.

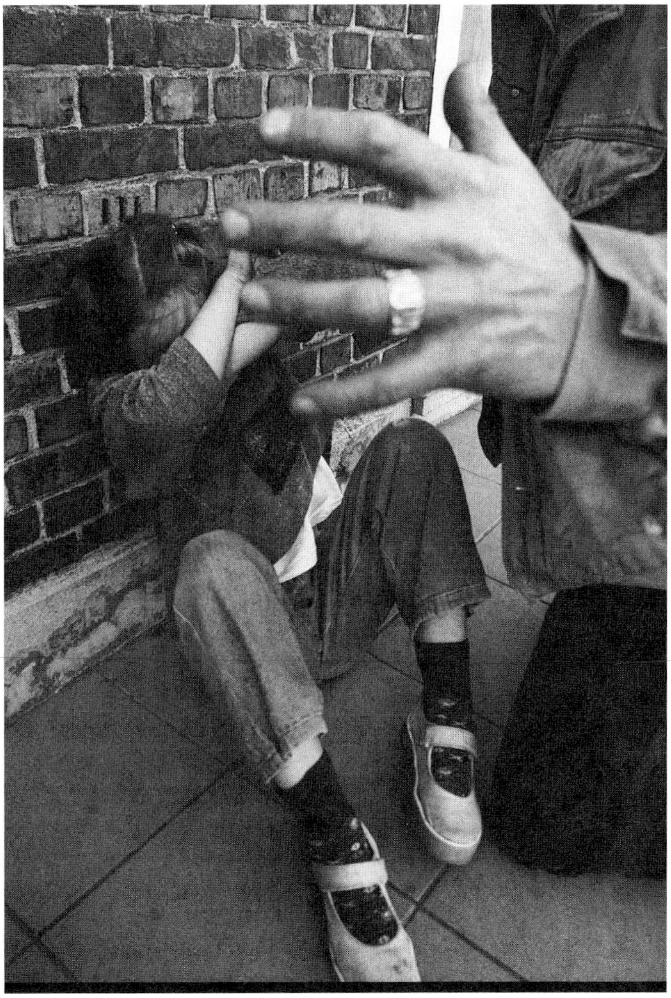

Violence claims victims of both sexes, all racial and ethnic groups, and all ages.

Laurent Hamels/Photoalto/PictureQuest

Rates of victimization for females and males are also similar among adults. A national survey found that violence occurred in nearly a fourth of the relationships of those aged 18–28 years, and both partners were violent in about half of them (Whitaker, Haileyesus, Swahn, and Saltzman 2007). Although the rates are about the same, there is a difference between the violence of men and that of women (Hamberger and Larsen 2015). Women's physical violence tends to be a response to an abusive partner. And in emotional abuse, women tend to use yelling and shouting, while men are more likely to use threats of various kinds. As a result, abused women are likely to be more severely traumatized than are abused men.

The rates of abuse do vary by race/ethnicity, with Black women having the highest rates of victimization. A small survey of Chinese American women reported that 8 percent had experienced severe intimate partner violence in their lifetime (Hicks 2006). Among those ever married, the rate was higher, and nearly a third of those abused had physical injuries that affected their work or education.

Intimate partner violence is a problem in other nations. A New Zealand study reported that domestic conflict (ranging from minor emotional abuse to severe assault) occurred in nearly 70 percent of intimate relationships, with men and women equally likely to be both the perpetrators and the victims of the violence (Fergusson, Horwood, and Ridder 2005).

### Intergroup Violence

How much intergroup violence is there? Ted Gurr (1969:576) attempted to estimate the amount of civil strife in the United States from June 1963 through May 1968, a time of intense conflict. He identified more than 800 events that were either civil rights demonstrations, Black riots and disturbances, or white terrorism against Blacks and civil rights workers. There were more than 2 million participants and more than 9,400 casualties. The most common type of violence was interracial.

In 1995, antigovernment militants used a truck bomb to destroy a federal building in Oklahoma City, killing 168 and wounding more than 500. Americans became aware of the problem of **domestic terrorism** (we discuss international terrorism in Chapter 14). *Domestic terrorism* is the use, or threatened use, of violence by people operating entirely within the United States to intimidate or coerce the government and/or citizens in order to reach certain social or political aims. The FBI classifies domestic terrorism groups into four types: racially motivated violent extremism, antigovernment/antiauthority extremis, animal rights/environmental extremism, and abortion extremism (McGarrity 2019). So racial minorities, the government, and law enforcement are the most common targets. In 2020, a report from the Department of Homeland Security said that white supremacists are the deadliest of the terror threats.

**domestic terrorism**
the use, or threatened use, of violence by people operating entirely within the United States to intimidate or coerce the government and/or citizens in order to reach certain social or political aims

To get a sense of the world of right-wing groups in our nation, consider some of the groups that have arisen in recent years. The Aryan nation is a white-supremacist group. The Survivalists are expecting, and preparing for, the breakdown of the economy and the government by preparing to defend and support themselves in the resulting chaos. The Patriots stress the rights of states and the people over the federal government. Posse Comitatus is a tax-resistance group that is also anti-Semitic. Various militias (more than a dozen scattered throughout the nation) accumulate weapons to promote and defend the kind of society they believe the Constitution was meant to create (Witt 2004).

These groups tend to be sustained by various conspiracy theories. That is, they believe that they are a line of defense against sinister and powerful forces that are determined to quash individual freedom and impose a social order that is detrimental to the well-being of group members.

Group members adhere to the theories even though the ideas appear bizarre to outsiders. For example, a theory called QAnon arose in 2017. It affirmed the existence of a group of people who were Satan-worshippers and pedophiles, engaged in a global child-trafficking scheme, and working to get rid of President Trump. Supporters of QAnon showed up at political rallies, openly espousing their strange beliefs.

As long as such groups operate, there is a strong potential for violence. Many groups not only have sophisticated weapons but also engage in regular training exercises in their use. Their members are deadly serious about what they see as their mission and are prepared to engage in violent measures to achieve it.

## Violence and the Quality of Life

You can get a feel for how violence detracts from the quality of life by looking at both objective and subjective evidence. As will be evident, the negative impact of violence on the quality of life can be severe and long term.

## Human Injury and Destruction

Violence results in *human destruction* and is, therefore, a *contradiction* to American values of well-being and freedom from fear. Violent crime, riots, and other forms of interpersonal and intergroup violence can lead to both injury and death. Labor-management and interracial confrontations are the kinds of intergroup conflict most likely to result in deaths and serious injuries. One of the worst riots in modern U.S. history occurred in Los Angeles in 1992 following the acquittal of white police officers who had severely beaten a Black man who had resisted arrest (Pringle 1997). Three days of rioting left 55 people dead, 2,300 injured, and 1,093 buildings damaged or destroyed. The injured or killed in such situations include spectators or people who are traveling through the area.

People who are injured as the result of violence may suffer various kinds of long-term health problems. Abused children have a higher rate of health problems in adulthood than do nonabused children (Thompson, Kingree, and Desai 2004; Corso, Edwards, Fang, and Mercy 2008). Most women who end up in prison because of substance abuse and mental disorders were sexually abused earlier in their lives (Karlsson and Zielinski 2020). A substantial number of battered women sustain brain injuries (Valera and Berenbaum 2003). Women abused during pregnancy are at greater risk of miscarriage (Morland et al. 2008). A substantial number of homeless women have fled from violent husbands (Jasinski, Wesely, Wright, and Mustaine 2010), choosing to face the health-debilitating life of the streets rather than the domestic violence. Long-term victims of violence are far more likely than others to rate their health as poor and may develop a *stress-related somatic disorder,* which involves pain, fatigue, negative moods, problematic cognitive functioning, and sleep disturbance (Crofford 2007; Boynton-Jarrett, Ryan, Berkman, and Wright 2008).

## Psychological Disruption and Dehumanization

Victims of violence endure various kinds of *psychological trauma.* Sexual and/or physical abuse at the hands of a parent, other close relative, or an intimate partner is especially traumatic. Adolescent experiences of violence in intimate relationships can result in depression, running away from home, thoughts of suicide, dropping out of school, teenage pregnancy, and becoming a perpetrator as well as a victim of violence (Hagan and Foster 2001; Spano, Rivera, and Bolland 2010). Similarly, adult victims of intimate partner violence are more likely than others to suffer depression, impaired ability to function normally at home and work, problems of drug abuse, lower self-esteem, lower life satisfaction, and thoughts of suicide (Calder, McVean, and Yang 2010; Smith, Elwyn, Ireland, and Thornberry 2010; Randle and Graham 2011; Crowne et al. 2011; Gehring and Vaske 2017).

Depending on the relationship between victim and abuser, *the victim may come to see himself or herself as a bad person who somehow deserves the abuse.* For example, you—like the rest of us—want to believe that your parents are good, loving people. So if they abuse you, you may feel that it is because you deserve it. The outcome of the abuse, then, can include such problems as low self-esteem or even self-hatred, emotional instability, behavior problems, and disturbed relationships with an inability to trust or relate in a healthy way to others (Litrownik et al. 2003; McMullin, Wirth, and White 2007). Even if parents do not abuse their children, the *children may be harmed by witnessing violence between the parents.* Being exposed to such violence raises the probability that the child will engage in delinquent behavior and develop a depressive or anxiety disorder, a substance abuse problem, or other kinds of mental health impairment (Herrenkohl et al. 2013; Huang et al., 2015).

**posttraumatic stress disorder**
an anxiety disorder associated with serious traumatic events, involving such symptoms as nightmares, recurring thoughts about the trauma, a lack of involvement with life, and guilt

Moreover, *the consequences can be long term, enduring even after the individual is no longer in the abusive situation.* Both adolescents abused by parents or peers and women abused by husbands or boyfriends may develop **posttraumatic stress disorder** (Dutton, Boyanowsky, and Bond 2005; Lawyer et al. 2006). This disorder involves emotional and physical difficulties after a traumatic experience. The difficulties can last for years—even a lifetime. They include such symptoms as nightmares, recurring thoughts about the traumatic experience, a lack of involvement with life, and feelings of guilt.

Both violent victimization and exposure to violence can produce posttraumatic stress disorder and other emotional problems (Scarpa 2003; Hannan Orcutt, and Miron 2017). For example, the Oklahoma City bombing resulted in the disorder among some people who were exposed to, though not directly involved in, the violence (Sprang 1999). Although Oklahoma City residents were most likely to be adversely affected, even people who lived hundreds of miles away reported emotional problems six months afterward. Research into the effects of mass shootings reported adverse emotional effects on the survivors and members of the communities (Lowe and Galea 2017). In survey of California adults, nearly half of those who had been exposed to violence said the experience created problems of social functioning for them (Aubel et al. 2020). Finally, a study of Palestinian adolescents, who regularly are exposed to violence, found that they had significantly high levels of aggression, mental health symptoms, and problems of family and social functioning (Al-Krenawi and Graham 2012).

Interpersonal violence not only traumatizes the victim, it also perpetuates the violence. Children of couples who engage in violent behavior are more likely to have a violent marriage of their own (Murshid and Murshid 2018). Parents who abuse their children typically were beaten as children. Thus, the *dehumanization process* continues. In addition, as a study of women who were sexually assaulted as children showed, childhood sexual abuse means that the victims are more likely to be revictimized in adulthood, engage in unhealthy or no sexual activity, and experience little or no gratification from sexual activity (Lemieux and Byers 2008). They also have higher rates of disrupted marriage.

Intergroup violence is no less disruptive and dehumanizing than interpersonal violence. For example, adolescents exposed to the ongoing violence between Catholics and Protestants in Northern Ireland have more mental health problems and lower self-esteem than youths more insulated from the conflict (Muldoon and Wilson 2001).

## Violence as Seductive Self-Destruction

Throughout American history, groups have resorted to violence either to bring about certain changes or to try and maintain the status quo. In either case, violence often has been defined as the "only way" to reach the desired goals but instead has facilitated the victory of the opposition. Because expectations and outcome often have been contradictory, violence has frequently been a kind of *seductive self-destruction.*

A survey of violence associated with the labor movement concluded that when laborers resorted to violence, it was almost always harmful to the union (Taft and Ross 1969). In general, violence did not bring the advantages the workers had wanted. Historian Richard Hofstadter (Hofstadter and Wallace 1970) agreed with this conclusion, pointing out that one of the more effective tactics of labor was the series of sitdown strikes in the 1930s. These strikes were designed to avoid rather than instigate violence.

Hofstadter also made the point that violence has seemed more effective in maintaining the status quo than in bringing about change, at least in the short run. The long history of violence by whites against Blacks to maintain Blacks in a subordinate status was seductively self-destructive. Whites did not keep Blacks subjugated; nor did management, which employed violence far more than workers did, prevent unionization of workers.

Violence, in sum, can appeal to people as a means either to bring about or to resist certain changes, but violence typically turns out to be counterproductive. Not only does the group using violence fail to achieve its goals, but it also may ensure victory for its opponents. Nonviolence, in contrast, not only avoids the destructiveness of violent protest but, as Chenoweth and Stephan (2011) document in their study of civil resistance movements in many nations, is more than twice as effective as violence in bringing about the desired change.

### Economic Costs

Violence carries a high price tag. The costs of interpersonal violence include maintaining the criminal justice system and family service agencies, obtaining needed medical care, and lost productivity. Intergroup violence involves medical costs of individuals and the cost of repairing damaged property. Pringle (1997) estimated $1 billion loss from damages in the 1992 Los Angeles riot. According to the Global Peace Index, the direct and indirect economic cost of violence in the world is about $8.3 trillion (Dudley 2019). Looking at the ranking of individual countries, the United States has the highest cost ($1.6 trillion), followed by China ($1 trillion) and India ($496 billion).

## Contributing Factors

Violence has been linked with a *human need to be aggressive.* Many psychologists argue that **aggression** is related to *frustration.* Certainly, the frustrations produced by firings and other stressors in businesses have contributed to a rise in the level of violence in the workplace.

**aggression**
forceful, offensive, or hostile behavior toward another person or society

But frustration-generated aggression does not adequately explain violence, for aggression can be channeled into such outlets as competitive sports, hobbies, or hard physical labor. To fully explain violence, let's look at various sociocultural factors that contribute to the problem.

### Social Structural Factors

*Norms.* *Group norms legitimate various kinds of violent behavior* (Reitzel-Jaffe and Wolfe 2001). If you have abusive friends, you are more likely to be abusive in your own relationships. In some families, children observe their parents using violence to settle disagreements or they are taught to employ violence in defending themselves or asserting their rights. This may be based on the *fallacy of non sequitur:* "If I hit you, you will stop doing the things I dislike." It does not follow that violence stops further violence. In fact, the violence is likely to elicit more violence.

fallacy

This tendency for the norms that justify violence to perpetuate rather than stop further violence is seen in urban ghettoes. A study of Black youth living in impoverished areas found support for the existence and impact of a "code of the street" (first formulated by Elijah Anderson) that develops among poor youth (Stewart and Simons 2009). The "code" is a set of norms that governs behavior on the streets, including the norm of using violence to deal with any perceived lack of respect. Those who do not respond appropriately (namely, violently) to any instance of disrespect lose face with their peers. Because lack of respect can involve even such apparently minor acts as eye contact that lasts too long, there are frequent occasions where violence is justified.

The point is underscored by another norm that involves children—*the norm of physical punishment.* In the short term, physical punishment may lead children to conform to adult expectations. But what happens subsequently? Studies using national samples have concluded that over time, *the use of physical punishment increases the likelihood of aggressive behavior, delinquency, and antisocial behavior by children and is also associated with violent crime in adulthood* (Straus, Sugarman, and Giles-Sims 1997; Straus 2001; Sheehan and Watson 2008). The more severe the abuse, the more severe the adult crimes are likely to be. Thus, child molesters are likely to have been physically and sexually abused themselves as children (Cohen and Galynker 2009).

Historically, American norms have legitimated official violence—against radicals and striking laborers, for instance. This official violence is supported by attitudes that approve the use of violence for social control. Throughout the nation's history, groups defined as radical or as a threat to social order also have been defined as legitimate objects of suppression by violence.

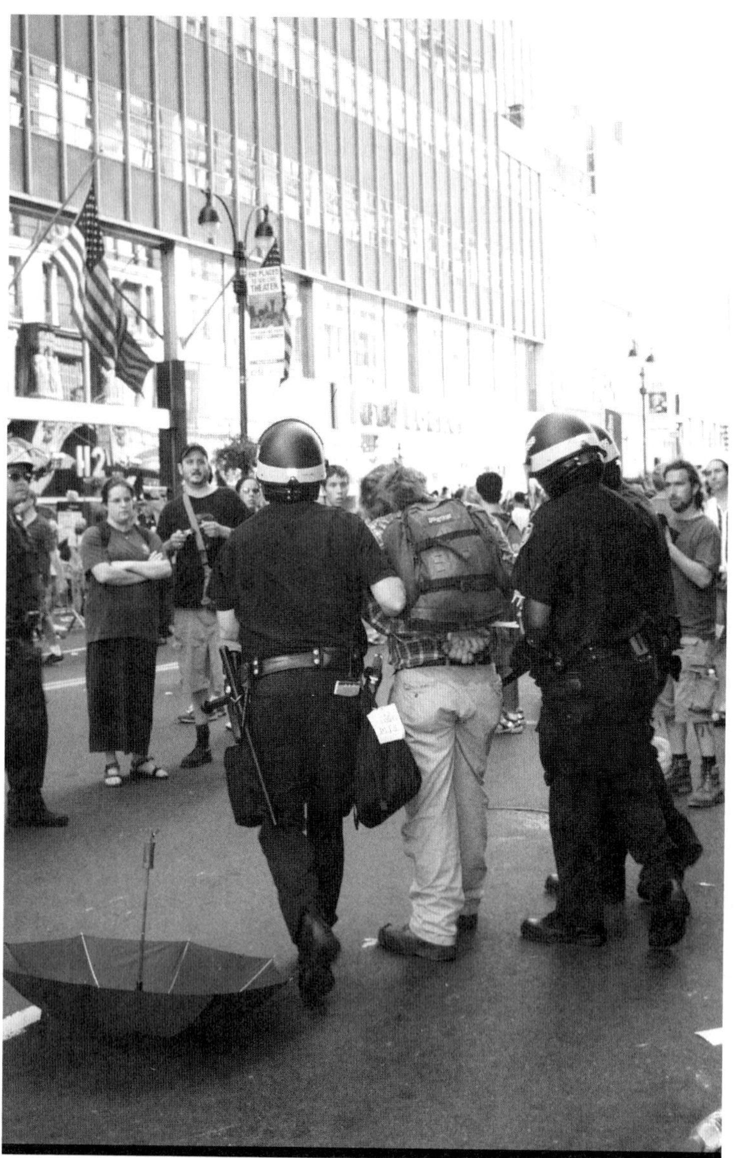

Riots are one form of violence that erupts periodically in the United States.

Jill Braaten/McGraw Hill

An example is the violence of the Chicago police against young antiwar demonstrators during the Democratic Convention of 1968. The committee that investigated the situation called it a "police riot." The police injured many innocent bystanders, including some reporters and news photographers (Hofstadter and Wallace 1970:382). One witness said the police acted like "mad dogs" looking for something to attack. Many people were horrified by the brutality of the police, but public opinion polls showed that the majority of people supported the police. This support came not only because some of the young people had baited the police by taunting them with obscenities, but also because Americans tend to expect and approve violence in the name of social order.

Approval of violence was clear in the Trump presidency. At his rallies, Trump castigated the press, supported people who attacked protesters, and even threatened to use violence himself against people who criticized him.

*Political Arrangements.* Certain political factors affect the level of violence in American society. United States history is characterized by the *exclusion of minorities from the core benefits of and participation in American life.* (*Exclusion* here means both lack of access to economic opportunities and denial of access to the political power by which grievances can be redressed.) This exclusion was maintained and continues to exist to some extent because of political action or inaction. The exclusion has been an important factor in race riots and other interracial violence.

In more recent years, the antiabortion movement has been associated with violence. In 1998, Dr. Barnett Slepian, a physician who performed abortions, became the seventh person killed in the United States by antiabortionists (Gegax and Clemetson 1998). In addition, arson and bombing of abortion clinics and violent confrontations between anti- and pro-abortion groups have characterized the struggle over abortion. Although there has been a decline in the violence in recent years, newspapers continue to report incidents of death threats, stalking, vandalism, protestors shouting at those entering abortion clinics, and arson. Those who support abortion believe their rights of choice are threatened and that women's health is jeopardized by the antiabortion movement. Those who oppose abortion feel that the rights of the unborn have been legislated away by court decisions and that politicians seem to ignore their cause. Thus, they resort to militant and even violent actions to influence the political process and bring about new laws that restrict a woman's right to have an abortion.

In essence, then, *political arrangements virtually guarantee a certain amount of violence* in a society that has groups with diverse and strong beliefs, interests, and demands, and in which violence is defined as a legitimate way to pursue group interests. If Blacks make political gains, the Ku Klux Klan or other white-supremacist groups may become more militant and violent. Violence against Asian immigrants has occurred both from white supremacists and from people who feel economically threatened (such as the commercial fishermen in Texas who tried to stop Vietnamese immigrants from fishing). The government can never fully satisfy all the diverse interests of the people. Whatever decisions are made are likely to generate adverse reactions and even violence from people who feel cheated, deprived, or oppressed by these decisions.

*The Politics of Gun Control.* Government policy on *gun control* bears on violence in the United States. Gun control is highly controversial, with strong arguments on both sides of the issue (including the debate about whether the Second Amendment guarantees citizens the right to own firearms). Let's begin with some data. Although the proportion of households with guns in the United States has declined in recent decades, Americans are still one of the *most heavily armed people on Earth*. A 2018 estimate put the number of guns at 393 million, more than one for every individual in the nation, and close to half of all privately owned guns in the world (Yablon 2018)! And Americans have the highest rate of firearm deaths in the world–six times the rate in Canada and 15 times the rate in Germany.

The *government's ability to guarantee security* to the citizenry affects the number of handguns. The less confidence that citizens have in the federal government, the more likely they are to own firearms (Jiobu and Curry 2001). The important point here, incidentally, is not whether the government protects citizens well by some objective standard but whether the citizens perceive a secure social order. In addition to giving people a (false) sense of security, gun ownership makes people feel more powerful as they cope with life (Mencken and Froese 2019).

The significance of the number of guns is also underscored by their role in violence. Although the government no longer publishes data on the kind of weapons used in crime, Table 4.1 shows the latest figures available (from 2011). The relative proportions of different weapons shown was roughly the same for many years, with guns being the most common weapon used in violent crimes.

We should not overlook here the use of guns as instruments of coercion. Millions of American women have had an intimate partner use a gun to gain control over them (Sorenson and Schut 2018). They may not have been shot, but they are victims nonetheless.

**TABLE 4.1**
Weapon Usage in Selected Crimes

| Type of Weapon | Percent in Which Weapon Used: Violent Crime | Rape/Sexual Assault | Robbery | Assault |
|---|---|---|---|---|
| Firearm | 9 | 7 | 29 | 6 |
| Knife | 5 | 2 | 10 | 4 |
| Other | 7 | * | 2 | 8 |

*Less than 0.5%
SOURCE: Bureau of Justice website.

Although gun owners may feel more secure and powerful because of their weapons, our society as a whole suffers from the proliferation of guns. A study of firearm deaths in all 50 states from 1981 to 2010 found that the more guns in an area, the more homicides and suicides there will be (Siegel, Ross, and King 2013). For each 1 percent increase in household gun ownership, the researchers found a 0.9 percent increase in the homicide rate. Another study reported that the murder rate of law enforcement officers was three times higher in states with high firearm ownership than in those with low ownership (Swedler et al. 2015). And the suicide rates of men are higher in those states with high rates of firearm ownership (Siegel and Rothman 2016).

Since 1960, more than a million Americans have died from gun-related homicides, suicides, and accidents. The rate of children killed by guns is higher in the United States than in any other industrialized nation. On an average day in the United States, 20 children and adolescents sustain firearm injuries that require hospitalization (Mitka 2014). Access to guns has also been shown to be an important factor in the killing of intimate partners, gang violence, and school rampage shootings (Braga 2003; Campbell et al. 2003; Newman et al. 2004). And don't overlook the large number of injuries. For every person killed, nearly three others are wounded by firearms.

In addition to numbers, there is the sheer horror and senselessness of the incidents. A man goes to a school and wounds and kills children whom he does not know. A man and a boy are snipers who kill people they have selected at random. A man walks into his place of employment and starts shooting at everyone, including those who had no part in whatever grievances he has. The point is, the victims of the violence are frequently innocent adults and children who just happened to be where the assailant chose to carry out the attack or attacks.

In spite of tragic incidents like these and in spite of the relationship between the number of gun-involved crimes and gun-control legislation, the issue of gun control is hotly debated. Many people insist, in spite of the evidence presented above, that the widespread existence of guns does not contribute to the amount of violence in the nation. One argument is that it is people, not guns, that kill; if a gun is not available, a person will find a different weapon. Professionals dispute the relationship between the number of guns and the amount of violence. Some argue that this society is a violent one and that violence will not be reduced simply by controlling the sale and possession of guns. Many Americans agree that the effort at control would be frustrating at best and counterproductive at worst. As a popular slogan puts it, when guns are outlawed, only outlaws will have guns. This slogan illustrates the *fallacy of appeal to prejudice.* However, evidence, not emotional slogans, is needed to make a reasonable decision about the issue.

fallacy

## VIOLENTLY OPPOSED TO VIOLENCE

At one time, most of the states had laws prohibiting abortions except when necessary to protect the mother's life. Initially, physicians led the way in calling for a reform of abortion laws. Some lawyers also pressed for change. Abortion should be allowed, they argued, when the mother's mental health or life was jeopardized by the pregnancy or when the pregnancy resulted from rape or incest. Women's groups joined the movement, ultimately resulting in the 1973 Supreme Court decision to legalize abortion.

The Right-to-Life movement then began to work vigorously to reverse the effects of the 1973 decision. Members have pressed for such changes as a constitutional amendment to ban abortions and legislative action to stop funding welfare abortions. Some members became more aggressive, picketing abortion clinics or trying to block people from entering the clinics. Beginning in the 1980s, the efforts have included acts of violence. Arson, bombing of clinics, and even murders have occurred. Some members of the movement—probably a very small number—have resorted to violence to oppose what they define as violence against human life.

Arrange an interview with workers in one or more abortion clinics in your area. Ask them what effect the activities of the Right-to-Life movement have had on their work. Do they fear violence? How do they respond to the charge that they are violently ending human life?

Also interview some members of the Right-to-Life movement. Ask them if they approve of bombing clinics. Is violence against a clinic justifiable? Why? How far would they go in opposing abortions? What answer do they give to people who charge that they are trying to impose their morals on others?

involvement

In the first place, guns are the weapon most frequently used in homicides. Contrary to the argument that killers would simply find alternative weapons, the gun is the deadliest of weapons; the fatality rate for shootings is about five times higher than the rate for stabbings. Moreover, murder frequently is an act of passion that the killer himself or herself might later regret. At least in some cases, without the gun there would be no murder.

Second, guns are the most frequent weapons used in armed robberies. A gun often seems essential for armed robbery, because without it the offender is unable to produce the necessary threat of force. The fatality rate in armed robberies involving guns is about four times as high as the rate involving other weapons.

Some citizens believe that firearms are necessary to defend their home. This argument has little substance. Many murders occur in homes, but seldom do they involve strangers. The most frequent kind of offender-victim relationship in homicide in homes is that of husband and wife. There is also the possibility of accidental injury or death because of a gun in the home. Children who live in homes with one or more guns are more likely than others to be both victims and perpetrators of violence (Ruback, Shaffer, and Clark 2011). A study of shootings in Philadelphia found that individuals who possessed a gun were 4.5 times more likely to be shot in an assault than those without a gun (Branas et al. 2009).

Finally, it may be true that people, rather than guns, do the killing; but it is also true that people with guns are more likely to kill than are people without guns. Berkowitz (1981) conducted research that suggests that the mere presence of a gun increases aggressiveness, so that although it is true that "the finger pulls the trigger," it also appears that "the trigger may be pulling the finger." In the research, each student was paired with a partner, ostensibly another student but actually a confederate of the researcher. The two were to come up with ideas to improve record sales and boost the image of a popular singer. Each student was to explain his or her ideas to the partner, who would then administer electric shocks—1 shock if the partner thought the ideas were good and up to 10 shocks if the partner thought the ideas were relatively poor. Some of the students became angry after being given seven shocks. Those students then evaluated their partners. They were taken to the room containing the electric-shock machine and a telegraph key that administered the shocks. Some saw nothing but the key lying on a table. Others saw a badminton racket and shuttlecocks, and a third group saw a shotgun and a revolver. Those students who saw the firearms gave their partners a greater number of shocks and administered each for a longer period of time.

The evidence suggests, then, that gun control could reduce some kinds of violence (murder and armed robbery) and minimize the destructiveness of other kinds (assaults and arguments). Public opinion polls show that most Americans favor the *registration of firearms.* There are two important reasons for the existence of political inaction in the face of the evidence and the will of the people. One is that the evidence is still ambiguous; legislators are not convinced of the value of control. The other reason is the strong *lobbying efforts* of the National Rifle Association (NRA). The NRA has a large, paid staff and thousands of local clubs in every state. It spends millions of dollars a year on direct lobbying efforts. Consequently, as of this writing, little has been done to reduce the number of guns in American society.

*The Stratification System.* In an effort to put violence in the United States in historical perspective, Graham and Gurr (1969) identified certain *political and economic inequalities* between various groups that have been associated with violence. The early Anglo-Saxon settlers gained the political and economic leverage necessary to resist *efforts by subsequent groups of immigrants to share fully in the nation's opportunities.* Difficult economic times have been particularly fertile for fueling violence, as illustrated by the mob violence against African Americans in the South during inflationary shifts in the price of cotton (Beck and Tolnay 1990).

Inequalities also have been identified as factors in urban riots. In the 1992 riot in Los Angeles, inequality *formed the motivating basis for many of the participants.* Using interviews with 227 African Americans living and/or working in the area at the time of the riot, researchers compared participants with nonparticipants (Murty, Roebuck, and Armstrong 1994). Participants tended to be younger males with lower incomes and lower amounts of education. They also had more arrest records than nonparticipants. But *nonparticipants as well as participants indicated general acceptance of the rioting.* It wasn't that they approved of rioting as such but that they believed collective violence is the only way to get the larger society to address their grievances (poverty, discrimination, unemployment, and police brutality).

At an interpersonal level, in both the United States and the European countries, rates of violence against an intimate partner are higher among those in the lower socioeconomic strata (Reichel 2017). Child abuse is far higher for children whose families are economically insecure than for those who are insecure (Conrad-Hiebner and Byram 2020). Thus, boys whose fathers have a history of unemployment are more likely to engage in violent behavior than are sons of fully employed fathers. Violent behavior here refers to beating up or hurting someone on purpose (other than a brother or sister). Of course, unemployed fathers are more likely to be found in the lower socioeconomic strata. Unemployment generates strains in the family life of lower- and working-class youths. In turn, these strains seem to be conducive to greater violent behavior. Thus, both children and adults who live in economic deprivation are more prone to violent behavior and aggression, including murder (Benson, Fox, DeMaris, and Van Wyk 2003; Pollock, Mullings, and Crouch 2006; Schneider, Hacknett, and McLanahan 2016).

Clearly, then, *certain kinds of inequality are related to violence.* Inequality generates frustrations and rage in individuals when they find themselves powerless to resolve their situation, and the probability of violence goes up. Some people may engage in the collective violence of riots and public disorder. Others may vent their rage by fighting on their own. In any case, the violence is the consequence of a stratification system that leaves some Americans in the gutters of the economy.

*Role of the Mass Media.* *The mass media expose Americans to an enormous amount of violence.* It would be interesting to record the number of violent incidents that impinge upon your life in a week of reading, listening to the radio, and watching television. Concern about violence on television began in the 1950s when it became evident that there was a high degree of violence in everything from children's shows to late-night adult entertainment. From time to time, television executives have promised to scale back the amount of violence, but the level remains high.

Children who watch television regularly, play video games, or attend movies are likely to be exposed to thousands of violent deaths and a staggering number of violent incidents during their childhood. Even Disney films portray a great deal of violent behavior. A study of 45 animated feature films produced by Disney between 1937 and 2006 found 561 incidents of child maltreatment among the 1,369 child characters in the films (Hubka, Hovdestad, and Tommyr 2009). In addition, 62 percent of the main child characters in the films suffered maltreatment at least once.

What are the consequences of all this violence? Some observers argue that it results in an increase of violent behavior. Others argue that watching violence on television provides a kind of **catharsis,** *a discharging of aggressive emotions* through vicarious participation in violence. For example, a man who has become extremely hostile toward his wife can discharge his aggression and avoid violence against his wife by watching violent acts on television.

**catharsis**
discharge of socially unacceptable emotions in a socially acceptable way

But displacement of aggression and vicarious discharge of aggression are not the same thing. Contrary to the idea of catharsis, portrayal of violence in motion pictures and on television increases the level of violence in society. And there is evidence to support this conclusion. Those who watch violence on TV can be *socialized into the norms, attitudes, and values that support and foster violence.* In other words, the more that people—particularly children and adolescents—watch violent TV programs, the more likely they are both to approve of and to engage in violent behavior (Anderson et al. 2015; Dillon and Bushman 2017; Khurana et al. 2019). Moreover, as a study of third- to fifth-grade children found, there is likely to be a decrease in prosocial behavior as well as an increase in violence, and the violent behavior includes both verbal and physical violence (Gentile, Coyne, and Walsh 2011). Researchers have also found that aggressive attitudes and behaviors increase from reading violent comic books, listening to songs with violent lyrics, and playing violent video games (Kirsh and Olczak 2002; Polman, de Castro, and van Aken 2008; Willoughby, Adachi, and Good 2012; Hummer 2015).

How much violence on TV does someone have to watch before being socialized into the violence? How long does it take for the violent shows to have their effect? In order to answer the questions, some researchers have looked for possible effects over a period of years. For example, Johnson et al. (2002) assessed 707 individuals over a 17-year period. The researchers found a significant association between the amount of time spent watching television as adolescents and young adults and subsequent aggressive behavior. But the effects can occur in a much shorter period of time. A study of youths 10–15 years of age who had used the Internet in the previous six months identified a portion of the youth who had engaged in seriously violent behavior (Ybarra et al. 2008). Of those who had been violent, 38 percent were exposed to violence online. Those who reported seeing violence between real people (rather than cartoon or computer-generated characters) were significantly more likely than others to engage in seriously violent behavior. Another study looked at the effects on both Japanese and American students of playing violent video games (Anderson et al. 2008). Among both the Japanese and the Americans, those who played the games habitually early in the school year became more physically aggressive later in the school year.

The consensus among researchers, then, is that viewing violence in the media socializes some individuals into a more violent way of life. As Murray (2008) states in his review of 50 years of research on the effect of TV violence on children, the conclusion is "inescapable" that the effects of media violence on children are both real and strong, increasing aggressive attitudes, values, and behavior.

Another consequence of media violence is that the viewer can develop a jaundiced view of the world (Anderson et al. 2015). People may believe that there is even more violence than actually occurs, and may become distrustful and fearful of others. They may also become less concerned about the victims of violence. In an experiment with fourth- and fifth-grade students, Molitor and Hirsch (1994) found that those who watched violence were afterward less likely to be concerned about two other children who engaged in a violent confrontation. The subjects watched a TV monitor that supposedly showed two children in an adjacent room. The subjects were told to get help if anything happened. Those who had watched clips from a violent movie were less likely to, or slower to, get help when the children on the monitor became violent with each other.

Finally, note the possibility that even watching violent sports can increase aggression. Researchers who investigated the rate of violent assaults on women in the Washington, D.C. area reported an increase in admissions to hospital emergency rooms following victories by the Washington Redskins' football team (White, Katz, and Scarborough 1992). They speculate that viewing the success of violence—even in a sporting event—may give some fans a sense of license to try and dominate their own surroundings by the use of force.

Admittedly, even with all the research we have noted, it is difficult to state unequivocally that exposure to the mass media leads to specific effects because of the many other factors that operate within people's lives. However, the evidence is growing and overwhelmingly supports the position that mass media violence is associated with aggressive attitudes and behavior. The evidence suggests that mass media violence teaches people how to be violent and tends to create violent behavior in viewers.

## Social Psychological Factors

*Attitudes.* *Certain attitudes legitimate violence.* One is the attitude of approval of violence itself. To be sure, people have a tendency to be selective about what circumstances justify violence. But most Americans accept violence as, at times at least, a problem solver. In particular, many Americans accept intimate partner violence if the circumstances warrant it (Sacks et al. 2001). A study of high school students reported that 77 percent of the females and 67 percent of the males endorsed some form of sexual coercion, including unwanted kissing, genital contact, and sexual intercourse (Office of Juvenile Justice and Delinquency Prevention 2006:4).

**relative deprivation**
a sense of deprivation based on some standard used by the individual who feels deprived

One explanation of violence is **relative deprivation,** which means that people have a *sense of deprivation in relation to some standard.* Here, the attitudes people have toward their deprivation are more important than any objective assessment of that deprivation. This observation goes back at least as far as de Tocqueville (1955), who pointed out that the French were experiencing real economic gains prior to the Revolution. An observer could have told the French that, objectively, they were better off at the time of their revolt than they had been at other times in the past. Yet what if the people used a different standard than their past to measure their deprivation? They might then perceive themselves to be less well off than they *should* be and rebel, which is precisely the idea of relative deprivation.

Davies (1962) used the notion of relative deprivation to explain revolutions. He constructed a *"J-curve" theory of revolution.* In essence, the theory states that a *widening gap between what people want and what they get leads to a revolutionary situation.* People do not revolt when the society is generally impoverished. Rather, people develop a revolutionary state of mind when they sense a threat to their expectations of greater opportunities to satisfy needs.

You will always experience a gap between your expectations and the satisfaction of your needs. Some degree of gap is tolerable, and although over time both your satisfactions and your expectations tend to increase, something may happen to suddenly increase the gap. Expectations continue to rise while actual need satisfactions remain level or suddenly fall. The gap then becomes intolerable, and a revolutionary situation is created.

According to Davies' theory, the deprivation of people in a revolutionary situation is relative. Actual satisfaction of their needs may be higher at the time of a revolution than earlier, but their expectations are also higher. The people may be better off in terms of their past, but worse off in terms of their expectations. Their attitudes rather than their objective condition make the situation revolutionary.

Relative deprivation has been identified as a factor in racial militancy and the approval of violent protest by northern Blacks. Interviews with 107 riot-area residents of Detroit in 1967 showed that those who were most militant in their attitudes and who believed the riots helped the Black cause were those who felt relatively deprived rather than relatively satisfied (Crawford and Naditch 1970).

A survey of 6,074 young adults found that those who saw themselves as economically deprived compared to their friends, neighbors, and Americans generally were more likely to engage in violent behavior (Stiles, Liu, and Kaplan 2000). The sense of deprivation led to negative feelings about themselves, which motivated them to use violent means to cope with their situation.

Finally, *attitudes about firearms help maintain the large number of guns in American homes.* In a Pew Research Center survey, 52 percent of Americans said it is more

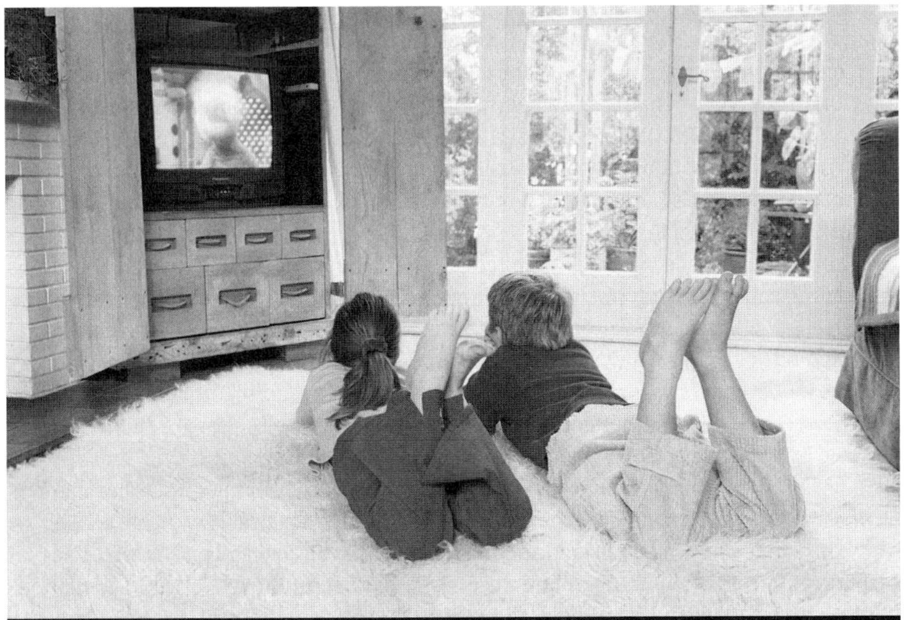

Television, including children's programs, exposes children to an enormous amount of violence.

Daniel Pangbourne/Digital Vision/Getty Images

important to control gun rights than it is to control gun ownership; in fact, support for gun control laws has actually fallen since 1990 (Kohut 2015). Such attitudes support the continued proliferation of guns in the nation, and this means the continued problem of gun-related violence.

**retributiveness** paying people back for their socially unacceptable behavior

*Values.* Attitudes that justify violence are often reinforced by certain values. In American society, people are likely to agree on the values of **retributiveness** and self-defense.

Retributiveness, or retributive justice, is summarized by the notion of "an eye for an eye and a tooth for a tooth." It is a value of punishment, of paying people back for their antisocial behavior. This value comes into play when people insist on the death penalty and other harsh forms of punishment.

Self-defense as a value means an *affirmation of the right to violence, including killing, in order to defend yourself or your family.* Some people would extend the value to include the defense of your home as well. In part, these values are maintained through the mass media which, as we have seen, justify various kinds of violent behavior.

## Solutions: Public Policy and Private Action

We already have discussed some steps for reducing violence, because whatever effectively deals with the problem of crime also reduces the level of violence. In addition, the various norms, attitudes, and values that support violence need to be changed. Early intervention in the lives of children can teach them alternatives to violence and aggression in solving their problems and gaining their goals in life. In families, schools, and churches, children need to learn how to employ nonviolent methods to survive and to find fulfillment. For example, a violence prevention program called Peace Builders has been shown to decrease aggression and increase social competence in children in kindergarten through fifth grade (Vazsonyi, Belliston, and Flannery 2004). Such programs cost relatively little and reach children at an early age.

American norms and attitudes about when violence is legitimate also need to change. In particular, no one should be taught that he or she deserves violent treatment from another person. Many women abused by a male partner remain in the relationship for years in the belief that they somehow brought the violence on themselves. Or they are convinced that they will eventually change the partner into a nonviolent individual. Women who break away from such relationships have learned to reject the notion that they deserve abuse or that they are responsible for helping their partner to change (Rosen and Stith 1995).

Second, *gun-control measures* may reduce the violence in our society. Homicide is the leading cause of death in Colombia, South America; but when two cities—Cali and Bogotá—banned the carrying of firearms on weekends, holidays, and election days, the homicide rates went down (Villaveces et al. 2000). In another study, researchers found, in states that passed laws making gun owners responsible for storing firearms so that they were inaccessible to children, unintentional shooting deaths of children younger than 15 declined by 23 percent (Cummings, Grossman, Rivara, and Koepsell 1997). Similarly, the 1994 federal ban on assault weapons contributed to lower gun murder rates and murders of police officers by criminals armed with assault weapons (Roth and Koper 1999). A study of suicide rates in states reported that the rates went down when the states passed such gun-control laws as background checks, gun locks, and open carrying regulations (Anestis and Anestis 2015). Finally, there were 13 mass shootings in Australia between

1979 and 1996, leading that nation to pass new gun-control laws (Chapman, Alpers, and Jones 2016).

Third, violence in the mass media should be reduced. The reduction is needed in cartoons as well as other kinds of programming. An experiment with third- and fourth-grade children found that cutting back on the amount of time children spent watching television and playing video games reduced the amount of aggressive behavior (Robinson et al. 2001).

Not only should violence be reduced, but the programs should include a greater amount of modeling of desirable behavior. *Television could become a medium for promoting more prosocial behavior.* After all, if the depiction of violence leads some people to become more aggressive, it is reasonable to expect that the depiction of prosocial behavior will increase the amount of such behavior in the society. Indeed, one researcher found such an effect from the words of popular songs (Greitemeyer 2009). Three separate studies showed that listening to songs with prosocial lyrics led to more empathy for others and fostered helping behavior. Other research found that playing prosocial video games led people to be more likely to help someone after a mishap and to intervene in a harassment situation (Greitemeyer and Osswald 2010).

Finally, violence will lessen as we deal with some of the inequalities in our society. We discuss this further when we consider poverty and other problems in Part 3.

*Follow-Up.* Would you like to see a ban on corporal punishment of children become a matter of public policy? Why or why not?

## The Violence of Rape

We know of no society that completely lacks rape or that fails to punish it. The definition of rape, however, varies. The American legal code distinguishes between two kinds of rape: forcible and statutory. **Forcible rape** is defined as the "carnal knowledge of a female forcibly and against her will" (Federal Bureau of Investigation 2002:454). The victim of forcible rape can be of any age, and attempts or assaults to rape are included. **Statutory rape** refers to sexual intercourse with a female who is under the legal age for consenting.

**forcible rape**
the carnal knowledge of a female forcibly and against her will

**statutory rape**
sexual intercourse with a female who is below the legal age for consenting

Rape is an extremely *traumatic experience* for victims. For the perpetrators, rape is typically an expression of violent aggression against women, not an act of sexual passion.

How prevalent is rape in the United States? It is difficult to say because an unknown number of rapes are *never reported.* In 2019, only a third of raped women reported the crime to the police (Morgan and Truman 2020). Adult victims are often reluctant to report a rape because of fear that the rapist will try to get even with them or will attack them again. They also fear publicity, embarrassment, and the way they may be treated by police and prosecutors (Monroe et al. 2005).

An increasing proportion of rape victims do report the crime to the police. Still, we get a more accurate picture of the amount of rape in the victimization studies. In 2014, there were 284,350 rapes (Truman and Langton 2015). In addition, there were perhaps that many attempts to rape that were successfully fought off.

Not everyone is equally likely to be a victim of rape or sexual assault (attacks, including verbal threats, that involve unwanted sexual contact between the victim and the offender). Table 4.2 shows how the rates vary by various demographic factors. Mixed-race and Black women have the highest rates, followed by white, Hispanic, and Asian women. Rates also vary by age, with higher rates in younger age groups. These data do not include rapes of those under the age of 12, but one survey found that 21.6 percent of

**TABLE 4.2**
Demographics of Rape and Sexual Assault Victims

| | | Victimizations per 1,000 Females Aged 12 or Older | | | |
|---|---|---|---|---|---|
| Marital Status | | Race/Hispanic Origin | | Age | |
| Never married | 4.1 | White | 2.2 | 12–17 | 4.1 |
| Married | 0.6 | Black | 2.8 | 18–34 | 3.7 |
| Widowed | 0.8 | Hispanic | 1.4 | 35–64 | 1.5 |
| Divorced/Separated | 4.4 | Asian | 0.7 | 65 or older | 0.2 |
| | | Two or more races | 5.1 | | |

SOURCE: Planty et al. 2016.

women who reported being raped said that their first experience of rape occurred before the age of 12 (Tjaden and Thoennes 2006).

Contrary to popular belief, there is little interracial rape, and most rapes *do not involve strangers*. Of those women who have been rape victims, 51.1 percent identified the perpetrator as a current or former intimate partner, 12.5 percent identified a family member, and 2.5 percent identified a "person of authority" such as a boss, teacher, coach, clergyman, doctor, or therapist (Black et al. 2011). Only 13.8 percent of rapists were strangers to the victim.

**incest**
exploitative sexual contact between relatives in which the victim is under the age of 18

Finally, there is the problem of sexual assault on children, including **incest,** which refers to exploitative sexual contact between relatives in which the victim is under 18 years of age. With regard to sexual assault on children generally, a national study reported that more than 285,000 children, 17 years old or younger, were sexually abused in one year (Finkelhor, Hammer, and Sedlak 2008). The bulk of them were female (89 percent) and between the ages of 12 and 17 (71 percent). About 4 percent were five years old or younger. Most of the victims were non-Hispanic whites (64 percent). Non-Hispanic African Americans accounted for another 18 percent. And 71 percent were assaulted by a relative or someone they knew.

With regard to incest, there is very little research. A pioneering study by Russell (1986) reported that 19 percent of the women interviewed had been victims of *incestuous abuse*. A survey of some university students in Turkey found that 6.3 percent reported incest (Aydin, Altindag, and Ozkan 2009). A study of young girls in Internet chat rooms reported that 38 percent had had sex with a relative (Atwood 2007). None of these studies had a random or representative sample, so it is not possible to say how many females are victimized by incest. It is clear, however, that incest is not rare.

According to the victims' reports, the most common type of incest is that between a father and his daughter; the incest is painful, often begins before the girl is 10 years old, and may continue for years on a regular basis. The victims' suffering does not end when the abuse stops, but results in the same kind of long-term, devastating psychological consequences as rape, including posttraumatic stress disorder (Aydin et al. 2009; Celbis et al. 2020).

## Rape and the Quality of Life

Regardless of the background characteristics of the victim, the consequences for the quality of life are similar: Rape is a highly traumatic experience, and fear of rape probably causes uneasiness in most women at some time.

## Emotional and Physical Trauma

Rape victims suffer *intense emotional trauma.* Rape contradicts the ideal of healthy, voluntary, and nonviolent relationships. The emotional trauma that results from rape is incompatible with the desired quality of life.

Children who are sexually abused are likely to experience both short-term and long-term negative consequences. They are at risk for anxiety disorders, stress disorder, and posttraumatic stress disorder (Maniglio 2013). Female victims, compared to those who are not sexually abused, have higher rates of bodily pain, poorer general health, and higher rates of depression (Coles et al. 2015).

Adult victims of rape experience what Burgess and Holmstrom (1974) delineated as the *rape trauma syndrome.* The syndrome involved two phases of reaction of the victim: *an initial, acute phase of disorganization and a long-term phase of reorganization.* The acute phase, which lasted for a few weeks after the incident, involved both physical and emotional reactions. The *physical reactions* included soreness and bruises resulting from the violence of the offender; tension headaches, fatigue, and disturbance of sleep; various gastrointestinal disturbances such as nausea, stomach pains, and lack of appetite; and genitourinary problems such as vaginal itching and pain. The *emotional reaction* during the acute phase ranged "from fear, humiliation, and embarrassment to anger, revenge, and self-blame. Fear of physical violence and death was the primary feeling described" (Burgess and Holmstrom 1974:983). Although it may seem surprising that victims should feel guilty or blame themselves, such feelings are common (see "I Felt Guilty," at the beginning of this chapter). A young woman reported strong guilt feelings in these terms:

> I'm single but I'm not a virgin and I was raised a Catholic. So I thought this might be some kind of punishment to warn me I was doing something against the Church or God.

Another victim remarked, "My father always said whatever a man did to a woman, she provoked it" (Burgess and Holmstrom 1974:983).

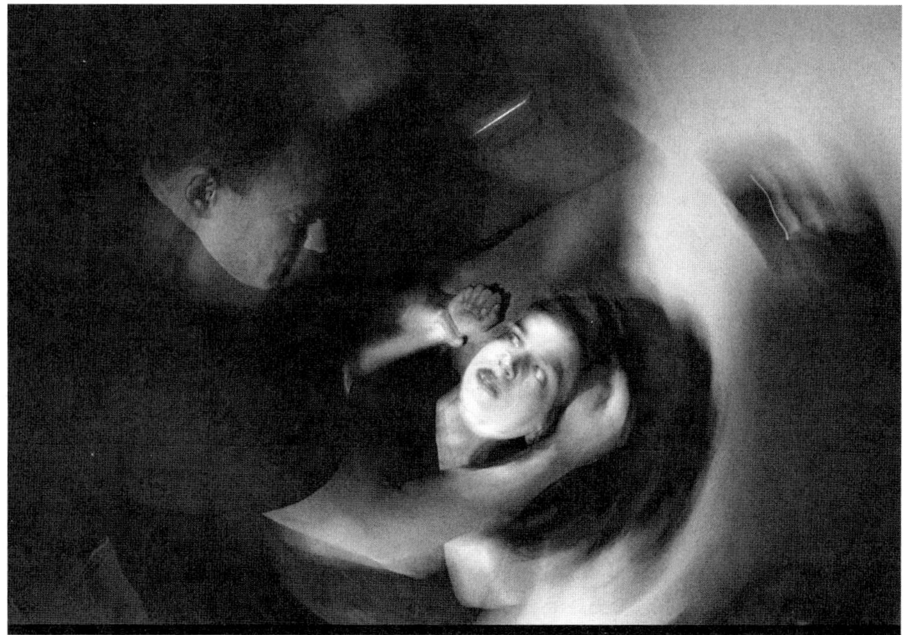

Rape is one of the most traumatic experiences a woman endures.
William Fritsch/Brand X Pictures

The long-term phase of reorganization included *motor and emotional consequences.* Common motor consequences included actions such as changing residence, changing telephone numbers, and visiting family and friends to gain support. Among the emotional consequences were nightmares; the development of various phobias, such as the fear of being indoors, outdoors, alone, in a crowd, or hearing but not seeing people walking behind one; and sexual fears. One victim reported that five months after the incident she could still get hysterical with her boyfriend: "I don't want him near me; I get panicked. Sex is OK, but I still feel like screaming" (Burgess and Holmstrom 1974:984).

In a follow-up study of 81 victims, reinterviewed from four to six years after they were raped, Burgess and Holmstrom (1979) found that less than a full recovery was reported by 71 percent of the victims who had never had sexual relations, 27 percent of those inactive at the time of the rape, and 35 percent of those sexually active when they were attacked. More than two-thirds of the victims said they had decreased sexual activity, and many of them said that they experienced pain and discomfort and had difficulty reaching an orgasm when they resumed sexual activity.

Subsequent studies confirm and extend the findings of Burgess and Holmstrom (Stein et al. 2004). Virtually every area of a woman's life is negatively affected by the experience of rape (Black et al. 2011). Among other things, victims are more likely than others to experience problems of physical and mental health, feelings of fear, anxiety about safety, sleep problems, activity limitations, missed days at work, and posttraumatic stress disorder. Although the number of male victims is considerably smaller and male rape has received less attention, a survey of nearly 60,000 men found similar consequences for male rape victims: poorer mental health and life satisfaction, activity limitations, and lower levels of emotional and social support (Choudhary, Coben, and Bossarte 2010).

Finally, most women experience at least some trauma because of the *fear of rape* (Mesch 2000). As one female student told us: "Every woman knows that she is a potential victim of a rapist." Such a fear takes a toll on free movement and peace of mind.

### Physical Abuse

Although most female victims who report being injured have relatively minor kinds of physical injuries, rapists may use weapons, beat or choke the victim, and use strength or threats to subdue her (DiMaio 2000). Some victims require medical treatment for their physical injuries. The *force and brutality so commonly involved in rapes* lead us to conclude that rapes are acts of violence rather than sexual passion. The rapist is not someone with an overwhelming sex drive; he is, typically, a man who feels compelled to assault and humiliate women. He uses rape as a weapon to express his hatred of females. Physical abuse, therefore, is an inevitable consequence for the female victim.

## Contributing Factors

Most of the factors that contribute to other kinds of violence also contribute to rape as a particular form of violence. Other factors distinctively associated with rape tend to *encourage offenders* and to *oppress the victims.*

## Social Structural Factors

*Norms.* Certain *traditional norms about sex roles* may be factors in rape. That is, in the traditional roles, males are aggressive and females are submissive. The more strongly that men adhere to traditional rather than egalitarian roles, the more likely they are to have victim-callous rape attitudes (Whatley 2005). For some men, it may be acceptable to rape an assertive woman so that she learns her "proper place."

In general, it seems *the more that men are integrated into a culture where the norms support male dominance and superiority,* the more likely they are to find rape acceptable (Locke and Mahalik 2005). The locker-room talk of athletes tends to treat women as objects, encourage sexist attitudes, and promote rape (McMahon 2007). Such talk seems to correlate with behavior, for *athletes* tend to have high rates of sexually aggressive behavior (Carter, Khan, and Brewer 2018).

The *college norm of heavy drinking at parties* is also a factor in rape (Mohler-Kuo, Dowdall, Koss, and Wechsler 2004). About 5 to 6 percent of women in colleges and universities report being rape victims, and the majority were raped while they were intoxicated (Mohler-Kuo et al. 2004; Holloway and Bennett 2018). The researchers concluded that a female student's chances of being raped are far greater on campuses in which the student body as a whole has a high rate of binge drinking and in which individuals consume large amounts of alcohol. Nor is this true only for those who "can't hold" their liquor. As shown in the research of Testa and Hoffman (2012), heavy drinking in college is a significant risk factor for sexual victimization for both experienced and inexperienced drinkers.

*Family. Negative family experiences can foster the development of a rapist.* Three researchers who compared a sample of rapists with a sample of child sexual abusers found such problems in the family of origin of both groups (Simons, Wurtele, and Durham 2008). Nine out of 10 men in each group reported inadequate bonding with their parents and frequent exposure to violence in the media when they were growing up. Among the child sexual abusers, 65 percent had been exposed to pornography before the age of 10, and 73 percent had been victims themselves of childhood sexual abuse. Among the rapists, 7 out of 10 reported having been physically and/or emotionally abused as children, and 78 percent witnessed parental violence.

The great majority of the sexual offenders, in short, had abusive experiences as children. As with other social problems, both the quality of family life and exposure to violent media are important variables in understanding sexual offenders.

*Mass Media.* As with violence in general, the mass media also play a role in the problem of rape. Men who watch sports on TV, particularly aggressive sports, are more likely than others to accept the rape myths discussed below (Custers and McNallie 2017). Reading men's magazines is associated with a greater likelihood of engaging in coercive sexual behavior (Hust et al. 2019). Watching violent pornography is a factor in the sexual aggression of men (Davis et al. 2006). This conclusion is supported by a series of pioneering experiments (Donnerstein 1980; Donnerstein and Linz 1984; Weisz and Earls 1995) that showed men who watch movies that portray sexual violence, including those shown in theaters around the country, are more likely to engage in bizarre or antisocial behavior. Even a few minutes of watching a sexually violent movie can lead to antisocial attitudes and behavior. The men in the experiments were more likely afterward to accept the myths about rape (that, for instance, a woman really wants to be raped; see the list in the following section), to indicate a willingness to commit

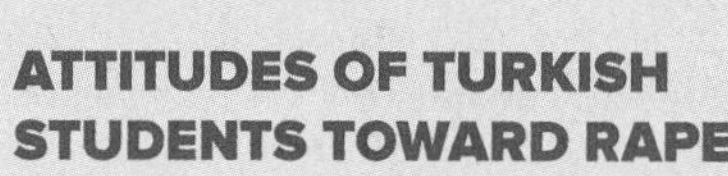

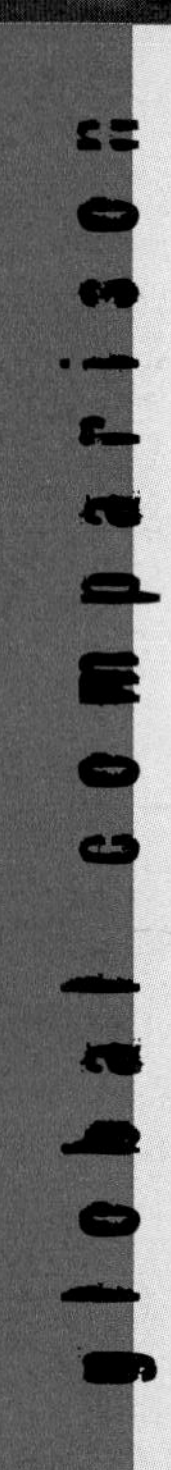


## ATTITUDES OF TURKISH STUDENTS TOWARD RAPE

Is it rape if the woman lures him on? Is it rape if she agrees to go with him to his apartment? Is it rape if the woman is his wife? Should the rape be reported to the police regardless of the circumstances? Americans have had differing opinions about the appropriate answer to such questions. People in other nations also differ in their attitudes about rape.

Four researchers who investigated the attitudes of Turkish university students toward rape found a high degree of condemnation by both male and female students but also some interesting variations depending on gender and the circumstances. The sample consisted of 432 females and 368 males from a number of universities in Istanbul.

Each student was presented with three different rape scenarios. The first was of a young man and woman who knew each other for two years and had been dating for six months. On a date that involved drinking and dancing until 2 a.m., they went to his house for a cup of coffee. They kissed and stroked each other, but the woman didn't want to go any further. She asked to go, but he ignored her and engaged in physically forced sex.

The second scenario was of a woman who was followed home by a stranger after shopping at the supermarket. She heard him as she was walking down the dark and empty street toward her house. She walked faster, but he caught up with her, put a knife to her throat, and raped her.

The third scenario also involved a stranger, but rape myth information was added. The young woman was returning home alone at 1 a.m. wearing a miniskirt, a low-cut blouse, and high boots. She was raped after getting off a bus and walking to her house.

The students were asked, for each of the scenarios, whether the rape should be reported to the police, whether a crime was committed, and what kind of punishment (if any) should be meted out to the offender. Figure 4.1 shows the proportion of students who agreed that the rape should be reported. Nearly all the students agreed that the rape by a stranger should be reported. The great majority agreed that the rape by a stranger of the woman wearing the provocative clothing should be reported, though slightly more women than men agreed. And a majority would report the date rape,

rape, to engage in aggressive behavior against a woman in a laboratory situation, and to have less sensitivity to the trauma of rape for women. In another experiment, men who watched a film that was sexually degrading to women were more likely than other men to believe that a rape victim found the experience pleasurable and "got what she wanted" (Milburn, Mather, and Conrad 2000). Finally, an experiment in which young men played a video game that included violence against women and depicted them as sex objects, raised the men's level of rape-supportive attitudes (Beck et al. 2012).

### Social Psychological Factors

*Attitudes.* Are the following statements true or false?

Rape tends to be an unplanned, impulsive act.

Women frequently bring false accusations of rape against men.

Most women fantasize about being raped and find erotic pleasure in the fantasy.

A woman who is raped is usually partly to blame for the act.

It is not possible for a man to rape a healthy woman unless she is—consciously or unconsciously—willing.

What are your answers? If you said that any of the previous statements is true, you have accepted one of the *myths about rape.* In point of fact, many people—even a minority of college women—accept one or more of these beliefs (Holcomb, Holcomb, Sondag, and Williams 1991; Carmody and Washington 2001). Overall, however, men are more likely to accept rape myths and to blame the victim than are women (Grubb and Harrower 2009). And men, older people, political conservatives, and people from the lower though significantly more of the women than the men agreed. More women than men also agreed that the date rape was a crime (22.6 percent of the men said "no"). And in all three scenarios, women would mete out greater punishment than would the men. Thus, in Turkey, as in most societies, men are less likely than women to view rape as a serious, violent crime when they can use circumstances to justify the rape.

SOURCE:
Golge, Yavuz, Muderrisoglu, and Yavuz 2003.

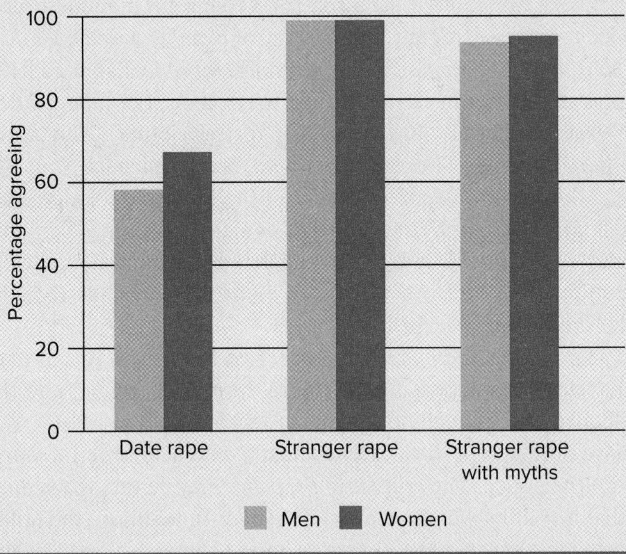


**FIGURE 4.1** Proportion Agreeing Victim Should Report Rape to Police.

socioeconomic strata are more inclined to commit rape and are less likely to be sympathetic toward rape victims (Chiroro, Bohner, Viki, and Jarvis 2004). They thereby not only lend support to those who rape but also help perpetuate injustice in the efforts to prosecute rapists.

It is important, then, to deal with the attitudes expressed in the myths. In contrast to the notion that rape is impulsive, significant proportions of convicted rapists have admitted that they intended to find a victim prior to the rape and that they looked for women who they thought could not or would not resist the attack (Stevens 1994). As for the fantasy myth, only a small proportion of women report that they fantasize about being forced to have sex.

The myth that women frequently bring false charges of rape against men has no factual basis. There is a good deal of evidence that women frequently do not report rape to the authorities, but no evidence that they frequently make false accusations.

Let's look in more detail at the other two myths, for they are more difficult to answer definitively. First, the humiliating treatment to which a rape victim is often subjected during a trial follows from the *attitude that the victim was somehow to blame* for provoking the offender. This is the *fallacy of personal attack* at its worst. Instead of receiving help and support, the victim of violence becomes the defendant of her own integrity. The attitude that "the victim was asking for it" ignores three things. One, women are socialized to make themselves attractive to men by their dress and mannerisms. Two, provocative dress cannot be considered sufficient justification for inflicting the physical and emotional brutality of rape upon a woman. As Horos (1974:12) argued,

fallacy

> Does a woman's dress or mannerisms give any man the right to rape her? Because you carry money in your pocket, does it mean that you're asking to be robbed? Perhaps this myth

arose because rape is the only violent crime in which women are never the perpetrators, but always the victims.

Three, provocative dress is not even involved in all rapes. The victim may be an elderly woman in a long robe, a woman wearing a coat, or a young girl in modest school clothes. In any case, to focus on dress is simply another way of *blaming a victim for an injustice.*

fallacy

*The attitude that a healthy woman can always prevent rape* also may help acquit an offender and oppress the victim. This attitude may reflect the *fallacy of retrospective determinism.* In essence, people may be saying to the victim: "The situation could have had no other outcome. The man is not to blame because you allowed it to happen—and you allowed it to happen because of the kind of person you are."

This attitude ignores the *paralyzing fear* that can grip a woman. Perhaps a third or more of rape victims exhibit *tonic immobility,* which is an involuntary, reflexive response to a fearful situation, a response in which the victim "freezes" as though paralyzed (Galliano, Noble, Travis, and Puechl 1993).

This attitude also ignores the *amount of force* used by rapists. Recall that rape typically involves the use of a weapon. Furthermore, beating, choking, and the threat of death may be effective even though no weapon is visible.

We already have pointed out the lack of sympathy and help a victim may experience in encounters with the police. The *attitude of the police* may be that the woman provokes the attack and that a healthy woman cannot be raped. In addition, the police may suspect the woman is merely using the charge of rape to punish a man or get attention for herself. To be sure, there are rare cases in which a woman charges rape to retaliate against a man or fulfill some pathological need.

Furthermore, the police know that not all victims of rape are respectable citizens with backgrounds free of suspicious behavior. In part, then, the attitudes of the police reflect a genuine need for caution. Nevertheless, a past police record, provocative clothing, or minimal resistance do not give a man license to forcibly rape a woman.

Considerable improvement has occurred in recent decades in the treatment of rape victims. Yet it is still true that the police, along with legal and medical personnel, can fail to give victims needed services (Campbell et al. 2001). Victims who go to formal authorities for help receive more negative reactions than those who rely on informal sources such as friends and family (Ullman and Filipas 2001).

*Justification and Values.* Finally, we raise the question of the social psychology of the offender. What kind of man is a rapist? When the rapists themselves were asked about their behavior, they either had no explanation at all or gave reasons that justified or minimized the negative significance of rape (Mann and Hollin 2007). Among the things they said are that it was an impulsive act; that the victims were seductive; that women say "no" but they really mean "yes"; that most women eventually relax and enjoy the experience; that women who are "nice" will not get raped; and that the act was at best a minor offense that did not merit the penalty the offender was now suffering. In other words, the men appeared to accept the rape myths. As we noted earlier, men who accept the myths are more likely to be sexually aggressive and to approve of rape.

Other offenders, however, admitted their guilt and viewed their behavior as morally wrong. They claimed that the rape was either the result of their use of alcohol or drugs, or the result of their emotional problems. They also tended to try to present an image of themselves as "nice" guys whose "true" self should not be judged on the basis of the rape.

*Macho values also seem to be a factor in the tolerance of, and proneness to, rape.* In a classic experiment, young men were asked to listen to the tape of a simulated rape and imagine themselves in the role of the rapist (Mosher and Anderson 1986). The tape described an encounter between a man and a woman stranded on a lonely road because of a flat tire. The man forced the woman to have sex with him. Some of the listeners found the tape repugnant, but others found it interesting and sexually arousing. In particular, those with macho values (real men engage in violence and find danger exciting) were more likely to have a positive reaction to the tape.

Finally, whatever else he may or may not be, the rapist and the man who accepts the myths about rape have a high level of hostility toward women (Marshall and Moulden 2001). Every rape involves aggression.

## Solutions: Public Policy and Private Action

Four lines of attack can be pursued in dealing with the rape problem. First, *programs of prevention* need to be established (Bryant-Davis 2004). We have noted the high rate of date rape. Many colleges and universities have established programs to make students aware of date and acquaintance rape. Research has shown that rape-education programs can change attitudes of both men and women (Fonow, Richardson, and Wemmerus 1992).

Some cities also have set up prevention programs. These programs include a variety of services such as self-defense training, public education activities, and support services to professionals in the sexual assault field. The programs may prepare and provide booklets on prevention and self-defense and work with the mass media to gain a wide audience for their educational materials.

The idea of self-defense presents women with a dilemma. On the one hand, the woman who does not struggle may find the police or some jury members unsympathetic to her case. On the other hand, the research on physical resistance has come up with mixed results in terms of recommendations. Some earlier researchers claimed that forceful fighting and screaming reduced the severity of the sexual abuse, but others argued that resistance only increased the likelihood of physical injury. A more recent meta-analysis concluded that any kind of resistance—verbal or physical—made it less likely that the rape would be completed (Wong and Balemba 2018). Unfortunately, the analysis did not deal with the issue of physical injury.

Second, *sex-role norms, legal processes, and attitudes* need to be changed. Some changes will occur only through a painfully slow process of education, for even knowledgeable and well-educated people can be deeply ignorant about rape. A male graduate psychology student told us, "There is a simple way for women to avoid the trauma of rape. They should just decide to relax and enjoy it." Such attitudes encourage offenders and oppress the victims. The fact that a graduate student could hold this kind of attitude illustrates the point that changing attitudes is going to be a painfully slow process. But changing such attitudes, including attitudes about the various rape myths, will reduce the amount of sexual assault (Lanier 2001).

Third, *rapists need treatment.* Rapists tend to be psychologically disturbed in some way. As such, they need therapy, some kind of rehabilitation, and not simply punishment. Punishment may remove the rapist from society for a period of time, but it will not deter him from future offenses.

The fourth line of attack is to *provide help for the victims* of rape (Kalmuss 2004). The victims clearly need a good deal of help, including emotional support. But a study of 103 women who had been victimized found that their romantic partners provided relatively little support and aid and often tended to blame the victim for the rape (Ahrens, Cabral, and Abeling 2009). Counselors and friends were more helpful than romantic partners.

An important source of help for rape victims are the *rape crisis centers* that have been established throughout the nation. The centers offer assistance in dealing with authorities, information about available legal and medical care, and counseling to facilitate recovery from the emotional trauma. The centers also frequently have prevention programs and offer courses in self-defense.

The centers may also offer the services of a rape victim advocate. A study of 81 rape victims in two urban hospitals reported that those who had the help of a rape victim advocate were more likely to have police reports taken and less likely to be treated negatively by police officers (Campbell 2006). They also reported less distress with the legal and medical systems, and they received more medical services such as emergency contraception and sexually transmitted disease prophylaxis. *Rape victim advocates should be available* in all areas.

The attitudes of authorities seem to be changing in the direction of greater sympathy for the victims of rape. A number of cities have established *rape squads* of male/female police teams with the specific responsibility of dealing with rape cases. The female member of the team interviews the victim while the male helps gather evidence. Various states have reformed their laws on rape, and hospitals are beginning to open rape reception centers instead of refusing to treat victims. Ultimately, the aim is prevention rather than sympathetic treatment of victims. Meanwhile, the new types of services for the victims and potential victims are a welcome help for women. They suggest that men finally may be realizing that the rape victim should be helped and not oppressed further by humiliating encounters with the authorities.

*Follow-Up.* With volunteers from your class, explore, and then report back to the class, any programs you have on campus for educating students about date rape and for aiding victims when date rape occurs.

## Summary

Violence is a problem that concerns most Americans. Generally, violence refers to the use of force to kill, injure, or abuse others. Interpersonal violence occurs between individuals or a number of individuals. Intergroup violence involves identifiable groups, such as different races or religions.

In estimating the amount of violence, we find an impressive amount based on self-reports, newspaper accounts, and police statistics. The United States has one of the highest homicide rates in the world. Virtually all Americans are exposed to a vast amount of violence in the mass media.

The meaning of violence can be summed up in terms of human destruction and injury, psychological disruption and dehumanization, economic costs, and "seductive self-destruction." These factors all diminish the quality of life, and their impact can be both severe and long term.

Violence has been linked with a human need for aggression, yet this explanation is not sufficient. Various sociocultural factors contribute to the problem. One structural factor is group and societal norms, which make violence more likely among members of those groups. An important factor in intergroup violence is exclusion from the political process. People who are unable to exert power through legitimate political means may resort to violence. An important factor in interpersonal violence is the lack of adequate gun control. Inequality is related to violence; political and economic inequalities between groups in a society increase the likelihood of violence.

Among the social psychological factors in violence are a number of attitudes that legitimate violence. The majority of Americans agree that physical force is sometimes justified, including the use of force in intimate relationships. A frequent explanation of violence involves the notion of relative deprivation, which means that attitudes toward deprivation rather than the objective condition are the critical factor.

Certain values support violence, including retributiveness and self-defense. Such values can be internalized, along with attitudes, through exposure to the mass media. The extent to which the mass media socialize people into violent attitudes and behavior is a matter of controversy. However, the bulk of the evidence indicates that violence portrayed and conveyed in the mass media is related to aggressive attitudes and behavior.

Rape is a form of interpersonal violence that afflicts tens of thousands each year. Fear of rape is one of the more common fears of women. All rapes involve both physical and emotional trauma. The rape trauma syndrome involves several weeks of acute symptoms and disorganization, and a long period of painful emotional readjustment.

The more men agree with traditional norms about sex roles, and the more they are integrated into a culture whose norms support male dominance and superiority, the more likely they are to be sexually aggressive and to minimize the harm of rape.

The mass media contribute to the problem of violence against women in general and rape in particular through portrayals of sexual violence. These portrayals increase the tendency of males to engage in antisocial attitudes and behavior. Studies of offenders show that they had negative family experiences and are psychologically disturbed. All have extremely high levels of aggression.

## Key Terms

**Aggression**
**Catharsis**
**Domestic Terrorism**
**Forcible Rape**
**Incest**
**Posttraumatic Stress Disorder**
**Relative Deprivation**
**Retributiveness**
**Statutory Rape**
**Violence**

## Study Questions

1. How would you define violence? How much violence is there in America?
2. What are the physical and emotional consequences of being a victim of violence?
3. What social structural factors contribute to the level of violence in America?
4. What role do the mass media play in violent behavior?
5. How common is rape?
6. Discuss the physical and emotional consequences of being a victim of rape or attempted rape.
7. Why do men rape?
8. What can be done about the violence, including rape, in American society?

## Internet Resources/Exercises

1. Explore some of the ideas in this chapter on the following sites:

**http://www.vpc.org** Site of the Violence Policy Center, with an emphasis on gun control in order to reduce violence in America.

**http://www.ncadv.org** The National Coalition Against Domestic Violence offers surveys, discussions of public policy, and ways for victims to get help.

**http://www.rapecrisis.com** Has information, services, and links for sexual assault victims and their families.

2. Investigate a group involved in domestic terrorism, such as a right-wing militia, the Earth Liberation Front, or the Animal Liberation Front. How does the group justify its stance? How do law enforcement officials and other observers define the activities of the group? What social structural and social psychological factors do you think contribute to the existence and work of the group?

3. Find stories of rape victims. Compare their accounts with the discussion in the text about the rape trauma syndrome. How does the text's description of the syndrome capture or fail to fully capture the victims' experiences?

## For Further Reading

Bourke, Joanna. *Rape: Sex, Violence, History.* Glebe, Australia: Counterpoint, 2007. A historian examines such issues as the history of sexual aggression, laws about sexual psychopathology in the United States and Britain, how military culture affects views of sexual assault, how rapists respond to their offense, and the ways in which popular culture informs our discussion of rape.

Gottesman, Ronald, ed. *Violence in America: An Encyclopedia.* New York: Charles Scribner's Sons, 1999. Covers every aspect of violence, summing up what researchers have found, including not only violence against people but also violence against animals and property.

Harding, Kate. *Asking For It: The Alarming Rise of Rape Culture–and What We Can Do About It.* New York: De Capo Lifelong Books, 2015. Argues that American culture is more supportive of the rapist than the victim, and offers various ideas on how to take a more realistic and helpful approach to sexual abuse and still honor the rights of the accused.

Hirsch, Jennifer S., and Shamus Khan. *Sexual Citizens: A Landmark Study of Sex, Power, and Assault on Campus.* New York: Norton, 2020. An extensive and in-depth study, including victims' stories, of the problem of sexual assault in colleges and universities.

Kleck, Gary. *Point Blank: Guns and Violence in America.* New York: Aldine Transaction, 2005. A thorough look at the major issues involving guns, gun control, and violence, including suggestions for a national weapons policy.

Newman, Katherine, Cybelle Fox, David Harding, Jal Mehta, and Wendy Roth. *Rampage: The Social Roots of School Shootings.* New York: Basic Books, 2004. An extensive investigation of school shootings, including various factors that help explain why students resort to such violence.

Scheper-Hughes, Nancy, and Phillipe I. Bourgois, eds. *Violence in War and Peace: An Anthology.* Malden, MA: Blackwell, 2004. Two anthropologists put together a collection of essays that explore social, literary, and philosophical theories of violence, ranging from violence in everyday life to genocide to war.

## References

Acierno, R., et al. 2010. "Prevalence and correlates of emotional, physical, sexual, and financial abuse and potential neglect in the United States." *American Journal of Public Health* 100:292–97.

Ahrens, C. E., G. Cabral, and S. Abeling. 2009. "Healing or hurtful: Sexual assault survivors' interpretation of social reactions from support providers." *Psychology of Women Quarterly* 33:81–94.

Al-Krenawi, A., and J. R. Graham. 2012. "The impact of political violence on psychosocial functioning of individuals and families." *Child & Adolescent Mental Health* 17:14–22.

Anderson, C. A., et al. 2008. "Longitudinal effects of violent video games on aggression in Japan and the United States." *Pediatrics* 122:1067–72.

——. 2015. "SPSSI research summary on media violence." *Analyses of Social Issues and Public Policy* 15:4–19.

Anestis, M. D., and J. C. Anestis. 2015. "Suicide rates and state laws regulating access and exposure to handguns." *American Journal of Public Health* 105:2049–58.

chapter 4 review

Atwood, J. D. 2007. "When love hurts: Preadolescent girls' reports of incest." *American Journal of Family Therapy* 35:287-313.

Aubel, A. J., et al. 2020. "Exposure to violence, firearm involvement, and socioemotional consequences among California adults." *Journal of Interpersonal Violence,* online article.

Aydin, Y. E., A. Altindag, and M. Ozkan. 2009. "Childhood traumatic events and dissociation in university students." *International Journal of Psychiatry in Clinical Practice* 13:25-30.

Beck, E. M., and S. E. Tolnay. 1990. "The killing fields of the deep south: The market for cotton and the lynching of blacks, 1882-1930." *American Sociological Review* 55 (August):526-39.

Beck, V. S., et al. 2012. "Violence against women in video games." *Journal of Interpersonal Violence* 27:3016-31.

Benson, M. L., G. L. Fox, A. DeMaris, and J. Van Wyk. 2003. "Neighborhood disadvantage, individual economic distress, and violence against women in intimate relationships." *Journal of Quantitative Criminology* 19:207-35.

Berkowitz, L. 1981. "How guns control us." *Psychology Today* (June):12-13.

Black, M. C., et al. 2011. *The National Intimate Partner and Sexual Violence Survey.* Atlanta, GA: Centers for Disease Control and Prevention.

Boynton-Jarrett, R., L. M. Ryan, L. F. Berkman, and R. J. Wright. 2008. "Cumulative violence exposure and self-rated health." *Pediatrics* 122:961-70.

Braga, A. A. 2003. "Serious youth gun offenders and the epidemic of youth violence in Boston." *Journal of Quantitative Criminology* 19:33-54.

Branas, C. C., et al. 2009. "Investigating the link between gun possession and gun assault." *American Journal of Public Health* 99:2034-40.

Bryant-Davis, T. 2004. "Rape is: A media review for sexual assault psychoeducation." *Trauma Violence and Abuse* 5:194-95.

Burgess, A. W., and L. L. Holmstrom. 1974. "Rape trauma syndrome." *American Journal of Psychiatry* 131 (September):981-86.

——. 1979. "Rape: Sexual disruption and recovery." *American Journal of Orthopsychiatry* 49 (4):648-57.

Calder, J., A. McVean, and W. Yang. 2010. "History of abuse and current suicidal ideation." *Journal of Family Violence* 25:205-14.

Campbell, J. C., et al. 2003. "Risk factors for femicide in abusive relationships." *American Journal of Public Health* 93:1089-97.

Campbell, R. 2006. "Rape survivors' experiences with the legal and medical systems." *Violence against Women* 12:30-45.

Campbell, R., S. M. Wasco, C. E. Ahrens, T. Sefl, and H. E. Barnes. 2001. "Preventing the 'second rape.'" *Journal of Interpersonal Violence* 16:1236-59.

Carmody, D. C., and L. M. Washington. 2001. "Rape myth acceptance among college women." *Journal of Interpersonal Violence* 16:424-36.

Carter, D. M., R. Khan, and G. Brewer. 2018. "Sexual aggression in sport." *Journal of Forensic Practice* 20 (3):211-14.

Celbis, O., et al. 2020. "Evaluation of incest cases." *Journal of Child Sexual Abuse* 29:79-89.

Chapman, S., P. Alpers, and M. Jones. 2016. "Association between gun law reforms and intentional firearm deaths in Australia, 1979-2013." *Journal of the American Medical Association* 316:291-99.

Chenoweth, E., and M. J. Stephan. 2011. *Why Civil Resistance Works.* New York: Columbia University Press.

Chiroro, P., G. Bohner, G. T. Viki, and C. I. Jarvis. 2004. "Rape myth acceptance and rape proclivity." *Journal of Interpersonal Violence* 19:427-42.

Choudhary, E., J. Coben, and R. M. Bossarte. 2010. "Adverse health outcomes, perpetrator characteristics, and sexual violence victimization among U.S. adults males." *Journal of Interpersonal Violence* 25:1523-41.

Cohen, L. J., and I. I. Galynker. 2009. "Psychopathologyi and personality traits of pedophiles." *Psychiatric Times* 26. Psychiatric Times website.

Coles, J., et al. 2015. "Childhood sexual abuse and its association with adult physical and mental health." *Journal of Interpersonal Violence* 3:1929-44.

Conrad-Hiebner, A., and E. Byram. 2020. "The temporal impact of economic insecurity on child maltreatment." *Trauma, Violence, & Abuse* 21:157-78.

Corso, P. S., V. J. Edwards, X. Fang, and J. A. Mercy. 2008. "Health-related quality of life among adults who experienced maltreatment during childhood." *American Journal of Public Health* 98:1094-1100.

Crawford, T., and M. Naditch. 1970. "Relative deprivation, powerlessness, and militancy: The psychology of social protest." *Psychiatry* 33 (May):208-23.

Crofford, L. J. 2007. "Violence, stress, and somatic syndromes." *Trauma, Violence, & Abuse* 8:299-313.

Crowne, S. S., et al. 2011. "Concurrent and long-term impact of intimate partner violence on employment stability." *Journal of Interpersonal Violence* 26:1282-1304.

Cummings, P., D. C. Grossman, F. P. Rivara, and T. D. Koepsell. 1997. "State gun safe storage laws and child mortality due to firearms." *Journal of the American Medical Association* 278 (October 1):1084-86.

Custers, K., and J. McNallie. 2017. "The relationship between television sports exposure and rape myth acceptance." *Violence Against Women* 23: 813-29.

Davies, J. C. 1962. "Toward a theory of revolution." *American Sociological Review* 27 (February):5-19.

Davis, K. C., J. Norris, W. H. George, J. Martell, and J. R. Heiman. 2006. "Men's likelihood of sexual aggression." *Aggressive Behavior* 32:581-89.

de Tocqueville, A. 1955. *The Old Regime and the French Revolution*. New York: Anchor Books.

Dillon, K. P., and B. J. Bushman. 2017. "Effects of exposure to gun violence in movies on children's interest in real guns." *JAMA Pediatrics* 171:1057-62.

DiMaio, V. J. 2000. "Homicidal asphyxia." *American Journal of Forensic and Medical Pathology* 21 (March):1-4.

Donnerstein, E. 1980. "Pornography and violence against women: Experimental studies." *Annals of the New York Academy of Sciences* 347:227-88.

Donnerstein, E., and D. Linz. 1984. "Sexual violence in the media: A warning." *Psychology Today* (January):14-15.

Dudley, D. 2019. "Cost of violence around the world estimated at $14 Trillion a year, with U.S. facing biggest bill." *Forbes,* June 12. Forbes website.

Dutton, D. G., E. O. Boyanowsky, and M. H. Bond. 2005. "Extreme mass homicide: From military massacre to genocide." *Aggression and Violent Behavior* 10:437-73.

Federal Bureau of Investigation. 2002. *Crime in the United States: 2002*. FBI website.

Fergusson, D. M., L. J. Horwood, and E. M. Rider. 2005. "Partner violence and mental health outcomes in a New Zealand birth cohort." *Journal of Marriage and the Family* 67:1103-19.

Finkelhor, D., H. Hammer, and A. J. Sedlak. 2008. "Sexually assaulted children: National estimates and characteristics." *NISMART,* August, U.S. Department of Justice.

Finkelhor, D., H. Turner, R. Ormrod, S. Hamby, and K. Kracke. 2009. "Children's exposure to violence." *Juvenile Justice Bulletin,* October.

Fonow, M. M., L. Richardson, and V. A. Wemmerus. 1992. "Feminist rape education: Does it work?" *Gender and Society* 6 (March):108-21.

Galliano, G., L. M. Noble, L. A. Travis, and C. Puechl. 1993. "Victim reactions during rape/sexual assault." *Journal of Interpersonal Violence* 8 (March):109-14.

Gegax, T. T., and L. Clemetson. 1998. "The abortion wars come home." *Newsweek,* November 9.

Gehring, K. S., and J. C. Vaske. 2017. "Out in the open." *Journal of Interpersonal Violence* 32:3669-92.

Gentile, D. A., S. Coyne, and D. A. Walsh. 2011. "Media violence, physical aggression, and relational aggression in school age children." *Aggressive Behavior* 37:193-206.

Golge, Z. B., M. F. Yavuz, S. Muderrisoglu, and M. S. Yavuz. 2003. "Turkish university students' attitudes toward rape." *Sex Roles* 49:653-61.

Graham, H. D., and T. R. Gurr, eds. 1969. *The History of Violence in America*. New York: Bantam.

Greitemeyer, T. 2009. "Effects of songs with prosocial lyrics on prosocial thoughts, affect, and behavior." *Journal of Experimental Social Psychology* 45:186-90.

Greitemeyer, T., and S. Osswald. 2010. "Effects of prosocial video games on prosocial behavior." *Journal of Personality and Social Psychology* 98:211-21.

Grubb, A. R., and J. Harrower. 2009. "Understanding attribution of blame in cases of rape." *Journal of Sexual Aggression* 15:63-81.

Gurr, T. R. 1969. "A comparative study of civil strife." In *The History of Violence in America,* ed. H. D. Graham and T. R. Gurr, pp. 572-632. New York: Bantam.

Hagan, J., and H. Foster. 2001. "Youth violence and the end of adolescence." *American Sociological Review* 66:874-99.

Hamberger, L. K., and S. E. Larsen. 2015. "Men and women's experience of intimate partner violence." *Journal of Family Violence* 30:699-717.

Harrell, E. 2011. *Workplace Violence, 1993-2009*. Washington, DC: Department of Justice.

Hannan, S. M., H. K. Orcutt, and L. R. Miron. 2017. "Childhood sexual abuse and later alcohol-related problems." *Journal of Interpersonal Violence* 32:2118-38.

Herrenkohl, T. I., et al. 2013. "Developmental impacts of child abuse and neglect related to adult mental health, substance use, and physical health." *Journal of Family Violence* 28:191–99.

Hicks, M. H. 2006. "The prevalence and characteristics of intimate partner violence in a community study of Chinese American women." *Journal of Interpersonal Violence* 21:1249–69.

Hofstadter, R., and M. Wallace, eds. 1970. *American Violence*. New York: Vintage.

Holcomb, D. R., L. C. Holcomb, K. A. Sondag, and N. Williams. 1991. "Attitudes about date rape: Gender differences among college students." *College Student Journal* 25 (December):434–39.

Holloway, K., and T. Bennett. 2018. "Alcohol-related rape among university students." *Victims & Offenders* 13:471–86.

Horos, C. V. 1974. *Rape*. New Canaan, CT: Tobey.

Huang, C., et al. 2015. "Children's exposure to intimate partner violence and early delinquency." *Journal of Family Violence* 30:953–65.

Hubka, D., W. Hovdestad, and L. Tommyr. 2009. "Child maltreatment in Disney animated feature films: 1937-2006." *The Social Science Journal* 46:427–41.

Hullenaar, K., and B. B. Ruback. 2020. "Juvenile violent victimization, 1995–2018." *Juvenile Justice Bulletin,* December. OJJDP website.

Hummer, T. A. 2015. "Media violence effects on brain development." *American Behavioral Scientist* 54: 1709–1806.

Hust, S. J., et al. 2019. "Rape myth acceptance, efficacy, and heterosexual scripts in men's magazines." *Journal of Interpersonal Violence* 34:1703–33.

Jasinski, J. L., J. K. Wesely, J. D. Wright, and E. E. Mustaine. 2010. *Hard Lives, Mean Streets: Violence in the Lives of Homeless Women*. Boston, MA: Northeastern University Press.

Jiobu, R. M., and T. J. Curry. 2001. "Lack of confidence in the federal government and the ownership of firearms." *Social Science Quarterly* 82:77–88.

Johnson, J. G., P. Cohen, E. M. Smailes, S. Kasen, and J. S. Brook. 2002. "Television viewing and aggressive behavior during adolescence and adulthood." *Science* 295:2468–71.

Kalmuss, D. 2004. "Nonvolitional sex and sexual health." *Archives of Sexual Behavior* 33:197–209.

Karlsson, M. E., and M. J. Zielinski. 2020. "Sexual victimization and mental illness prevalence rates among incarcerated women." *Trauma, Violence, & Abuse* 21:326–49.

Khurana, A., et al. 2019. "Media violence exposure and aggression in adolescents." *Aggressive Behavior* 45:70–81.

Kirsh, S. J., and P. V. Olczak. 2002. "The effects of extremely violent comic books on social information processing." *Journal of Interpersonal Violence* 17:1160–78.

Kohut, A. 2015. "Despite of lower crime rates, support for gun rights increases." Pew Research Center website.

Lanier, C. A. 2001. "Rape-accepting attitudes." *Violence against Women* 7:876–85.

Lawyer, S. R., K. J. Ruggiero, H. S. Resnick, D. G. Kilpatrick, and B. E. Saunders. 2006. "Mental health correlates of the victim-perpetrator relationship among interpersonally victimized adolescents." *Journal of Interpersonal Violence* 21:1333–53.

Lemieux, S. R., and E. S. Byers. 2008. "The sexual well-being of women who have experienced child sexual abuse." *Psychology of Women Quarterly* 32:126–44.

Litrownik, A. J., R. Newton, W. M. Hunter, D. English, and M. D. Everson. 2003. "Exposure to family violence in young at-risk children." *Journal of Family Violence* 18:59-73.

Locke, B. D., and J. R. Mahalik. 2005. "Examining masculinity norms, problem drinking, and athletic involvement as predictors of sexual aggression in college men." *Journal of Counseling Psychology* 52:279–83.

Lowe, S. R., and S. Galea. 2017. "The mental health consequences of mass shootings." *Trauma, Violence, & Abuse* 18:62–82.

Maniglio, R. 2013. "Child sexual abuse in the etiology of anxiety disorders." *Trauma, Violence, and Abuse* 14: 96–112.

Mann, R. E., and C. R. Hollin. 2007. "Sexual offenders' explanation for their offending." *Journal of Sexual Aggression* 13:3-9.

Marshall, W. L., and H. Moulden. 2001. "Hostility toward women and victim empathy in rapists." *Sexual Abuse* 13:249–55.

McGarrity, M. C. 2019. "Confronting the rise of domestic terrorism in the homeland." FBI website.

McMahon, S. 2007. "Understanding community-specific rape myths." *Affilia: Journal of Women and Social Work* 22:357–70.

McMullin, D., R. J. Wirth, and J. W. White. 2007. "The impact of sexual victimization on personality." *Sex Roles* 56:403-14.

Mencken, F. C., and P. Froese. 2019. "Gun culture in action." *Social Problems* 66:3-27.

Mesch, G. S. 2000. "Women's fear of crime." *Violence and Victims* 15:323-36.

Milburn, M. A., R. Mather, and S. D. Conrad. 2000. "The effects of viewing R-rated movie scenes that objectify women on perceptions of date rape." *Sex Roles* 43: 645-64.

Miller, L. M. 2011. "Physical abuse in a college setting." *Journal of Family Violence* 16:71-80.

Mitka, M. 2014. "Firearm-related hospitalizations: 20 US children, teens daily." *Journal of the American Medical Association* 311:664.

Mohler-Kuo, M., G. W. Dowdall, M. P. Koss, and H. Wechsler. 2004. "Correlates of rape while intoxicated in a national sample of college students." *Journal of Studies on Alcohol* 65:37-45.

Molitor, F., and K. W. Hirsch. 1994. "Children's toleration of real-life aggression after exposure to media violence." *Child Study Journal* 24 (3):191-207.

Monroe, L. M., et al. 2005. "The experience of sexual assault." *Journal of Interpersonal Violence* 20:767-76.

Morgan, R. E., and J. L. Truman. 2020. "Criminal victimization, 2019." Bureau of Justice Statistics website.

Morland, L. A., et al. 2008. "Intimate partner violence and miscarriage." *Journal of Interpersonal Violence* 23:652-69.

Mosher, D. L., and R. D. Anderson. 1986. "Macho personality, sexual aggression, and reactions to guided imagery of realistic rape." *Journal of Research in Personality* 20 (March):77-94.

Muldoon, O. T., and K. Wilson. 2001. "Ideological commitment, experience of conflict and adjustment in Northern Irish adolescents." *Medicine, Conflict, and Survival* 17:112-24.

Mulford, C., and P. C. Giordano. 2008. "Teen dating violence." *NIJ Journal,* Issue 261:34-40.

Mumford, E. A., and B. G. Taylor. 2014. "National survey on teen relationships and intimate violence." NORC website.

Murray, J. P. 2008. "Media violence." *American Behavioral Scientist* 51:1212-30.

Murshid, N. S., and N. Murshid. 2018. "Intergenerational transmission of marital violence." *Journal of Interpersonal Violence* 33:211-27.

Murty, K. S., J. B. Roebuck, and G. R. Armstrong. 1994. "The black community's reactions to the 1992 Los Angeles riot." *Deviant Behavior* 15:85-104.

Newman, K., C. Fox, D. Harding, J. Mehta, and W. Roth. 2004. *Rampage: The Social Roots of School Shootings.* New York: Basic Books.

Office of Juvenile Justice and Delinquency Prevention. 2006. "Teen dating violence awareness and prevention week." *OJJDP's E-Mail Information Resource.*

Planty, M., et al. 2016. "Female victims of sexual violence, 1994-2010." Bureau of Justice Statistics website.

Pollock, J. M., J. L. Mullings, and B. M. Crouch. 2006. "Violent women." *Journal of Interpersonal Violence* 21:485-502.

Polman, H., B. O. de Castro, and M. A. G. van Aken. 2008. "Experimental study of the differential effects of playing versus watching violent video games on children's aggressive behavior." *Aggressive Behavior* 34:256-64.

Porter, J., and L. M. Williams. 2011. "Intimate violence among underrepresented groups on a college campus." *Journal of Interpersonal Violence* 26:210-24.

Pringle, P. 1997. "Remembering while building for the future." *San Diego Union-Tribune,* April 27.

Randle, A. A., and C. A. Graham. 2011. "A review of the evidence on the effects of intimate partner violence on men." *Psychology of Men and Masculinity* 12:97-111.

Reichel, D. 2017. "Determinants of intimate partner violence in Europe." *Journal of Interpersonal Violence* 32:1853-73.

Reitzel-Jaffe, D., and D. A. Wolfe. 2001. "Predictors of relationship abuse among young men." *Journal of Interpersonal Violence* 16:99-115.

Robinson, T. N., M. L. Wilde, L. C. Navracruz, K. F. Haydel, and A. Varady. 2001. "Effects of reducing children's television and video game use on aggressive behavior." *Archives of Pediatric and Adolescent Medicine* 155:17-23.

Rosen, K. H., and S. M. Stith. 1995. "Women terminating abusive dating relationships." *Journal of Social and Personal Relationships* 12 (February):155-60.

Roth, J. A., and C. S. Koper. 1999. *Impacts of the 1994 Assault Weapons Ban: 1994-96.* Washington, DC: National Institute of Justice.

Ruback, R. B., J. N. Shaffer, and V. A. Clark. 2011. "Easy access to firearms: Juveniles' risks for violence offending and violent victimization." *Journal of Interpersonal Violence* 26:2111-38.

Russell 1986. *The Secret Trauma: Incest in the Lives of Girls and Women*. New York: Basic Books.

Sacks, J. J., T. R. Simon, A. E. Crosby, G. Shelley, and M. P. Thompson. 2001. "Attitudinal acceptance of intimate partner violence among U.S. adults." *Violence and Victims* 16:115-26.

Scarpa, A. 2003. "Community violence exposure in young adults." *Trauma, Violence, and Abuse* 4:210-27.

Schneider, D., K. Harknett, and S. McLanahan. 2016. "Intimate partner violence in the Great Recession." *Demography* 3:471-505.

Sheehan, M. J., and M. W. Watson. 2008. "Reciprocal influences between maternal discipline techniques and aggression in children and adolescents." *Aggressive Behavior* 34:245-55.

Shorey, R. C., G. L. Stuart, and T. L. Cornelius. 2011. "Dating violence and substance use in college students." *Aggression & Violent Behavior* 16:541-50.

Siegel, M., and E. F. Rothman. 2016. "Firearm ownership and suicide rates among US men and women, 1981-2013." *American Journal of Public Health,* published online.

Siegel, M., C. S. Ross, and C. King. 2013. "The relationship between gun ownership and firearm homicide rates in the United States, 1981-2010." *American Journal of Public Health* 103:2098-105.

Simons, D. A., S. K. Wurtele, and R. L. Durham. 2008. "Developmental experiences of child sexual abusers and rapists." *Child Abuse and Neglect* 32:549-60.

Smith, C. A., L., J. Elwyn, T. O. Ireland, and T. P. Thornberry. 2010. "Impact of adolescent exposure to intimate partner violence on substance use in early adulthood." *Journal of Studies on Alcohol and Drugs* 71:219-30.

Smith, S. G., et al. 2018. "The national intimate partner and sexual violence survey." Centers for Disease Control and Prevention website.

Sorenson, S. B., and R. A. Schut. 2018. "Nonfatal gun use in intimate partner violence." *Trauma, Violence, & Abuse* 19:431-42.

Spano, R., C. Rivera, and J. M. Bolland. 2010. "Are chronic exposure to violence and chronic violent behavior closely related to developmental processes during adolescence?" *Criminal Justice and Behavior* 37:1160-79.

Sprang, G. 1999. "Post-disaster stress following the Oklahoma City bombing." *Journal of Interpersonal Violence* 14 (February):169-83.

Stein, M. B., et al. 2004. "Relationship of sexual assault history to somatic symptoms and health anxiety in women." *General Hospital Psychiatry* 26:178-83.

Stevens, D. J. 1994. "Predatory rapists and victim selection techniques." *Social Science Journal* 31 (4):421-33.

Stewart, E. A., and R. L. Simons. 2009. *The Code of the Street and African-American Adolescent Violence*. National Institute of Justice website.

Stiles, B. L., X. Liu, and H. B. Kaplan. 2000. "Relative deprivation and deviant adaptations." *Journal of Research in Crime and Delinquency* 37 (February):64-90.

Straus M. A. 2001. "New evidence for the benefits of never spanking." *Society* 38:52-60.

Straus, M. A., D. B. Sugarman, and J. Giles-Sims. 1997. "Spanking by parents and subsequent antisocial behavior of children." *Archives of Pediatrics and Adolescent Medicine* 151 (August):761-67.

Swedler, D. I., et al. 2015. "Firearm Prevalence and Homicides of Law Enforcement Officers in the United States." *American Journal of Public Health* 105:2042-48.

Taft, P., and P. Ross. 1969. "American labor violence: Its causes, character, and outcome." In *The History of Violence in America,* ed. H. D. Graham and T. R. Gurr, pp. 281-395. New York: Bantam.

Testa, M., and J. H. Hoffman. 2012. "Naturally occurring changes in women's drinking from high school to college and implications for sexual victimization." *Journal of Studies on Alcohol and Drugs* 73:26-33.

Thompson, M. P., J. B. Kingree, and S. Desai. 2004. "Gender differences in long-term health consequences of physical abuse of children." *American Journal of Public Health* 94:599-604.

Tjaden, P., and N. Thoennes. 2006. "Extent, nature, and consequences of rape victimization: Findings from the national violence against women study." NIJ website.

Truman, J. L., and L. Langton. 2015. "Criminal Victimization, 2014." Bureau of Justice Statistics website.

Ullman, S. E., and H. H. Filipas. 2001. "Correlates of formal and informal support seeking in sexual assault victims." *Journal of Interpersonal Violence* 16:1028-47.

U.S. Department of Justice. 2011. *Criminal Victimization, 2010*. U.S. Department of Justice website.

Valera, E. M., and H. Berenbaum. 2003. "Brain injury in battered women." *Journal of Consulting and Clinical Psychology* 71:797-804.

Vazsonyi, A. T., L. M. Belliston, and D. J. Flannery. 2004. "Evaluation of a school-based universal violence prevention program." *Youth Violence and Juvenile Justice* 2:185-206.

Villaveces, A., et al. 2000. "Effect of a ban on carrying firearms on homicide rates in two Colombian cities." *Journal of the American Medical Association* 283 (March 1):1205-09.

Weisz, M. G., and C. M. Earls. 1995. "The effects of exposure to filmed sexual violence on attitudes toward rape." *Journal of Interpersonal Violence* 10 (March):71-84.

Whatley, M. A. 2005. "The effect of participant sex, victim dress, and traditional attitudes on causal judgments for marital rape victims." *Journal of Family Violence* 20:191-200.

Whitaker, D. J., T. Haileyesus, M. Swahn, and L. S. Saltzman. 2007. "Differences in frequency of violence and reported injury between relationships with reciprocal and nonreciprocal intimate partner violence." *American Journal of Public Health* 97:941-47.

White, G. F., J. Katz, and K. E. Scarborough. 1992. "The impact of professional football games upon violent assaults on women." *Violence and Victims* 7 (2):157-71.

Willoughby, T., P. J. C. Adachi, and M. Good. 2012. "A longitudinal study of the association between violent video game play and aggression among adolescents." *Developmental Psychology* 48:1044-57.

Witt, H. 2004. "9 years after Oklahoma City blast, militias remain shadowy groups in U.S." Knight Ridder/Tribune News Service, April 18.

Wong, J. S., and S. Balemba. 2018. "The effect of victim resistance on rape completion." *Trauma, Violence, & Abuse* 19:352-65.

Yablon, A. 2018. "Just how manyh guns do Americans own?" The Trace website.

Ybarra, M. L., et al. 2008. "Linkages between Internet and other media violence with seriously violent behavior by youth." *Pediatrics* 122:929-37.

Zych, I., R. Ortega-Ruiz, and R. Del Rey. 2015. "Systematic review of theoretical studies on bullying and cyberbullying." *Journal of Aggression and Violent Behavior* 23:1-21.

CHAPTER

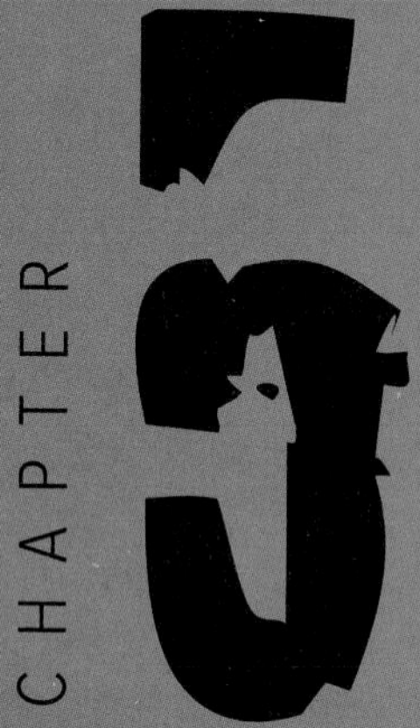

# Sexual Deviance

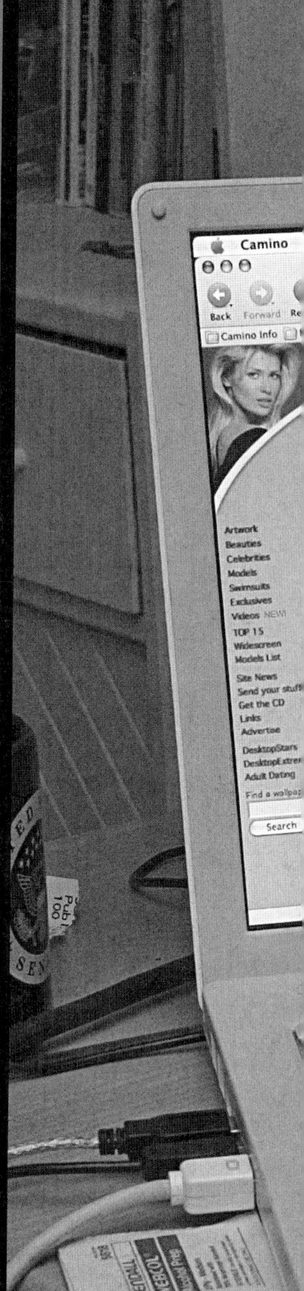


OBJECTIVES

1. Learn the meaning and some of the types of sexual deviance.
2. Be able to discuss why cybersex is a problem.
3. Understand factors that make prostitution and pornography social problems.
4. Show how prostitution affects a woman's quality of life.
5. Know how pornography affects people's behavior.
6. Identify ways to address the problems of prostitution and pornography.

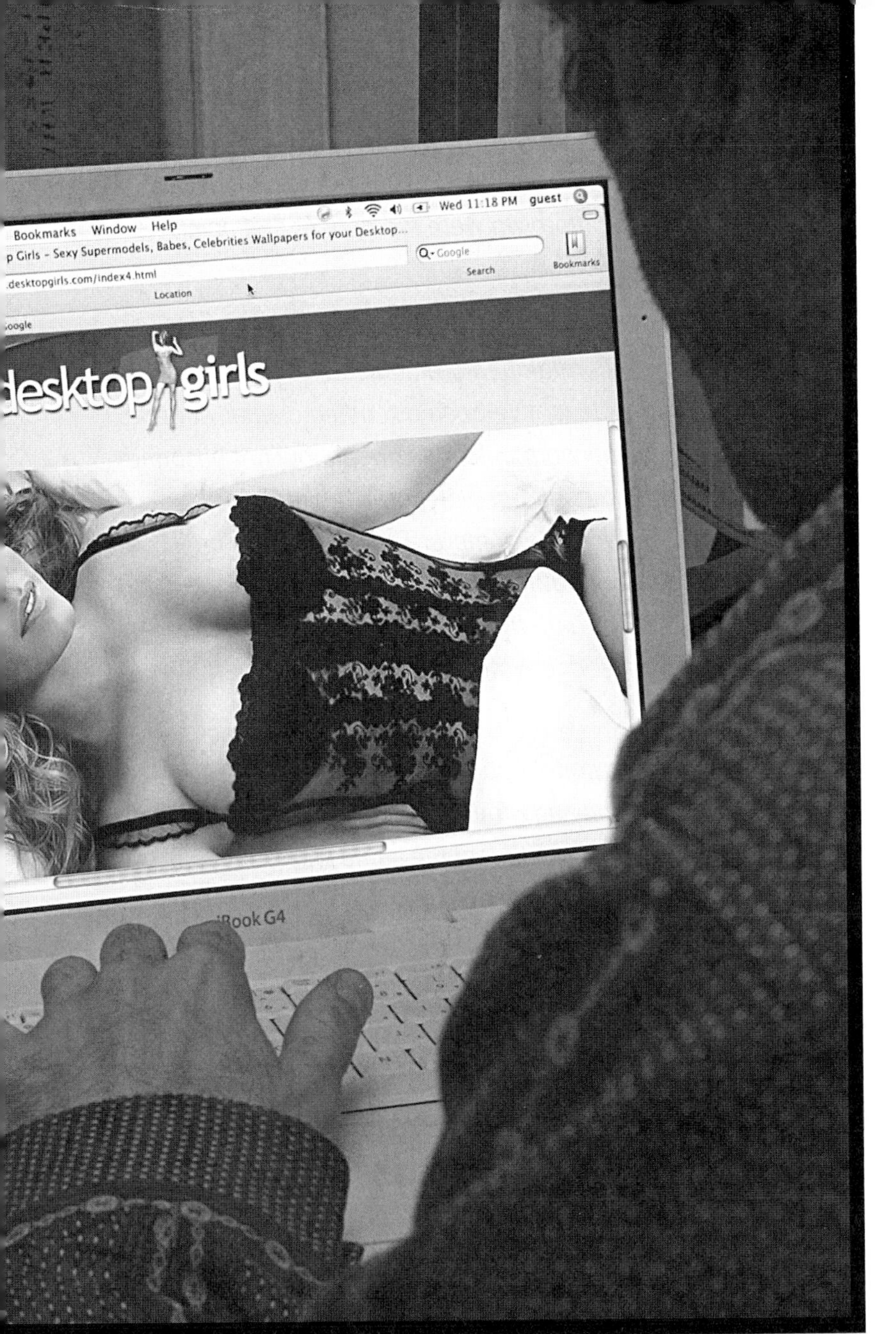

John Flournoy/McGraw Hill

## "My Husband Is a Porn Addict"

Kathy is a 26-year-old woman who has been married for four years. She was quite happy in her marriage for the first two years. Then she happened to catch her husband viewing pornographic sites on his computer. The last two years have been a struggle for her:

*When I accidentally caught Jake watching porn, I was shocked. I had no idea he was into that kind of thing. I knew he liked sex a lot. But so do I. Or at least, I did. Our sex life hasn't been much to talk about these past couple of years. It's really tough for me to feel aroused by him when I know how much time he's spending watching that stuff on his computer.*

*That's the thing that shocked me the most—the amount of time he spends at it. I didn't realize it at first because he would watch it late at night after I was asleep or when I was out of the house. However, one night I caught him watching porn when he thought I was in the shower. After a quick shower, I decided to sneak up on him before I dressed and invite him to go to bed, but I stopped dead in my tracks when I saw his computer screen. He tried to convince me that it was all harmless. That it only increased his desire for me and made our sex life better.*

*That didn't make sense to me. "You mean you have to watch other naked women to feel sexy toward me?" I asked him. He couldn't give me a satisfactory answer. Then I asked him how long and how often he had been watching the porn. He tried to weasel out of a direct answer, but he finally admitted that he had been into it for years—even before we were married. At that point, I realized that my husband is a porn addict!*

*Previously, I had thought that all porn addicts were perverts, but I've discovered that a lot of seemingly normal men are addicted to porn. And some of them are a lot worse than Jake. I've been attending a small support group for wives of porn addicts. One woman told us about how her husband was into the violent stuff and would act it out with her. She got tired of the above, and refuses to have sex with him any more. They'll probably get divorced soon. Another woman said that her husband convinced her to watch with him. He said it would spice up their sex life. She tried, but she couldn't take it. And when she refused to watch any more, he got verbally and emotionally abusive.*

*Jake hasn't gone that far. But to be honest about it, that doesn't make it any easier for me. I feel like he's having affairs. He's investing himself emotionally in other women. And I just can't feel the same way about him while he's doing it. At this point, I think I still love him. I certainly love the man I thought I married. But I'm not sure how much longer I can stay married to a porn addict.*

## Introduction

There's an old story about an expert who was scheduled to give an after-dinner speech on sex. At the appointed time, he arose and said: "Ladies and gentlemen. Sex. It gives me great pleasure." Then he sat down.

Clearly, sex is a source of great pleasure to humans. It is also a source of pain and controversy. Whether it is one or the other depends on whom you're talking to and what kind of sex you're talking about. In this chapter, we look at what is meant by sexual deviance. Then we expand on two kinds of sexual deviance that are regarded as social problems: prostitution and the use of pornography.

### Examples of Sexual Deviance

What is sexual deviance? The answer depends on which society you are talking about. All societies regulate sex, but not all regulate it in the same way. Studies of sexual norms show that there are variations both within and between societies (Bolin and Whelehan 2003; Higgins and Browne 2008). In the United States, for example, lower-class women are more likely than middle-class women to believe that men's sex drive is a biological necessity, thereby limiting the lower-class women's prerogative to refuse sex. And in contrast to the United States, some other societies consider the behavior that Americans have historically regarded as deviant (such as homosexuality and extramarital sex) to be acceptable. Of course, people everywhere take their own norms seriously, but the point is that sexual behavior, like all other behavior, is social. No particular type of sexual behavior is "natural" or "normal" in contrast to other types.

Nevertheless, there are certain kinds of sexual behavior that are considered deviant in most societies. Some of these behaviors characterize only a very small proportion of the population. For example, it is likely that *exhibitionism* (exposing one's genitals to a stranger) and *voyeurism* (spying on people who are having sexual relations) are practiced by only a small proportion of people. We don't know the figures for America, but two Swedish researchers reported that 3.1 percent of a national sample admitted to exhibitionism and 7.7 percent had engaged in voyeurism (Langstrom and Seto 2006).

Another type of sexual behavior considered deviant in most societies is **promiscuity,** sex between an unmarried individual and an excessive number of partners. Both men and women say that they prefer sex to occur in the context of an intimate relationship and that the emotional satisfaction of sex is strongly associated with being in a committed, exclusive relationship (Waite and Joyner 2001). An experiment that used college students as subjects reported that the students considered people who are promiscuous less desirable as potential dating or marriage partners (Perlini and Boychuk 2006).

**promiscuity**
undiscriminating, casual sexual relationships with many people

*Extramarital sex* also varies from American norms. From a list that included such events as divorce, gambling, having a baby outside of marriage, abortion, suicide, and cloning humans, the item that the fewest people regarded as morally accepted was an extramarital affair (Bowman 2004:48). Behavior doesn't always reflect attitudes, however, and in point of fact a substantial number of Americans engage in extramarital sex. There is a generation gap in the amount of extramarital sex, however (Wolfinger 2017). In 2016, 20 percent of those aged 55 and above, but only 14 percent of those under 55 years of age, admitted to having extra-marital sex. The higher rate among older adults has held since about 2004. Still, the majority of Americans practice fidelity, though not as many as say they disapprove of infidelity.

Still another form of deviant sex is **cybersex,** sexual activity conducted via the Internet. A forerunner of cybersex was telephone sex, which involved a per-minute charge to engage in a sexual conversation with someone (Ross 2005). Telephone sex never attracted as many customers, however, as has cybersex.

**cybersex**
sexual activity conducted via the Internet

Cybersex can be carried on in a number of ways. In one form, the individual uses online pornographic sites for sexual pleasure or for exhibitionism. Some people do this by posting nude pictures of themselves. A number of websites cater to people who want to expose their nude bodies on the Internet (Jones 2010). It is probably more common, however, to engage in **sexting**, sending erotic or nude photos or videos of oneself to a particular person or to a number of others via a cell phone or the Internet. The purpose of sexting is to enhance sexual desire and/or to ultimately have sexual intercourse.

**sexting**
sending erotic or nude photos or videos of oneself to a particular person or to a number of others via a cell phone or the Internet

Another way to use the Internet for sexual pleasure is to search for sexual partners. In a survey of 5,187 people who used a website for married people wanting partners for extramarital sex, the researchers found that males and females were equally likely to cheat but that females were more likely than males to engage in sexting (Wysocki and Childers 2011).

The Internet is also used to enhance sexual desire. A small number of people literally become addicted to Internet pornography (Weinstein and Lejoyeux 2010). Others, however, use it occasionally, either alone or with a partner, as a form of arousal. Some users report that they are more open to new sexual experiences and find it easier to talk about what they want sexually as a result of watching sex online. Others say that they have less sex with the partner who uses online sex sites or that they are less aroused by real sex after watching sexual acts online (Grov, Gillespie, Royce, and Lever 2011).

In a second form of cybersex, two or more people engage in sexual talk while online in order to gain sexual pleasure. A Swedish study found that those who engaged in this form of cybersex also tended to have more offline sexual partners (Daneback, Cooper, and Manisson 2005).

A third form of cybersex is the online game in which the participants can do such things as create their own characters (who can resemble themselves) and have those characters engage in whatever kinds of sexual behavior they desire (Biever 2006). In some of the games, people can go beyond the online sex and use the site to date those with whom their characters have had sex.

Is such online sex just harmless fun? In one study, 41 percent of a sample of people engaged in cybersex did not consider what they did to be cheating on a relationship partner at all (Ross 2005). But the story at the beginning of this chapter gives one woman's account of the harm done to her marriage by a husband involved in cybersex. And a survey of 91 women and 3 men whose partners had been heavily involved in cybersex found a good deal of hurt—feelings of betrayal and rejection, jealousy, and anger—as well as adverse effects on their children (Schneider 2003).

Finally, many Americans view *strip clubs* as a form of deviant sex. In both male and female strip clubs, patrons can watch people strip and engage in erotic dancing and, in some cases, chat with the strippers. For women, the shared experience of being at the club with friends and bonding with other women may be more important to them than the show itself (Montemurro, Bloom, and Madell 2003). For men, on the other hand, regular attendance at strip clubs is associated with their sexuality and masculinity. Katherine Frank (2003, 2005) found a variety of motivations among men for going to strip clubs, including a desire to express a masculine self free of obligations and commitments, experience adventure, feel desirable, and have a sexualized interaction with a woman that is without risk.

Let's look in greater detail at prostitution and pornography. Both have been strongly condemned and vigorously defended.

## Prostitution

**prostitution**
having sexual relations for remuneration, usually to provide part or all of one's livelihood

**Prostitution** is a paid sexual relation between the prostitute and his or her client. Male prostitutes are often young boys—mostly from impoverished homes. They have run away or been thrown out of their homes and offer themselves as sexual partners to gay men. Many regard themselves as heterosexuals; in any case, they view what they do as a job that gives them a source of income (Bimbi 2007). Whatever their age, male prostitutes secure clients in a variety of ways: through agencies, personal ads, working on the streets, or via one of the websites throughout the nation that offer their services (Logan 2010). Because research on male prostitution is sparse, our focus here is on the female prostitute and her clientele.

**fellatio**
oral stimulation of the male genitalia

**cunnilingus**
oral stimulation of the female genitalia

Although not every prostitute agrees to perform every sexual act, prostitutes are available for a variety of sexual services. These include **fellatio** (oral stimulation of the male genitalia), **cunnilingus** (oral stimulation of the female genitalia), and various other sexual practices that an intimate partner may not want to engage in. In a survey of 1,342 men arrested for solicitation in four western cities, fewer than one in six said that vaginal sex is the most common type they have with a prostitute (Figure 5.1). While most prostitutes basically offer anonymous and impersonal sex acts, a few (not streetwalkers) specialize in a more intimate and emotional experience for the client (Bernstein 2007). Such a prostitute may function as a girlfriend for the time she spends with her client.

How much prostitution exists in the United States? Official records depend on arrests. The FBI website indicates 26,713 arrests for prostitution in 2019, but an unknown number

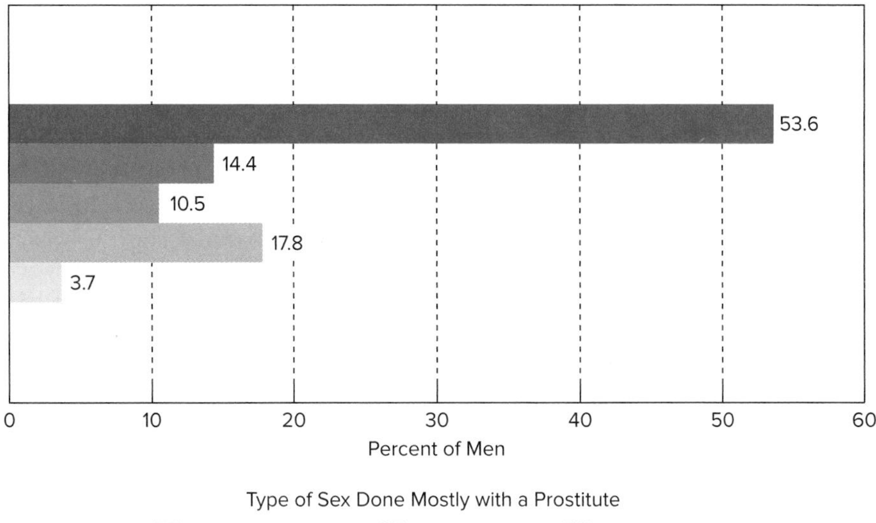


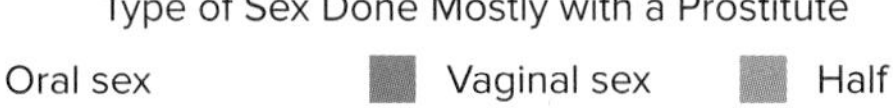


**FIGURE 5.1**
What Men Want from Prostitutes.
Source: Della Giusta, Di Tommaso, Shima, and Strom 2009.

of these were repeat offenders and not all prostitutes are arrested. Part of the problem of estimating is that there are *various kinds of female prostitutes,* from streetwalkers to high-paid call girls to brothel workers to prostitutes who use the Internet to solicit customers (Roane 1998). Some work full time, and others use prostitution to supplement their incomes. Some work for decades, and others quit after a short time. We don't know how many prostitutes there are but it's likely that at any point in time there are hundreds of thousands of them at work.

Hundreds of thousands is a reasonable figure in light of the amount of prostitution in other parts of the world. The proportions range from 0.7 percent to 4.3 percent among nations in sub-Saharan Africa, from 0.2 percent to 2.6 percent among nations in Asia, from 0.1 percent to 1.4 percent in western Europe, and from 0.2 percent to 7.4 percent among nations in South America (Vandepitte et al. 2006). If we assume there are 200,000 to 300,000 prostitutes in the United States, the comparable figure would be somewhere between 0.1 percent and 0.2 percent of the female population, which is comparable to that of other industrial nations.

We will discuss below some of the reasons why women opt to be prostitutes, but we must not ignore the fact that a substantial number of prostitutes are the victims of *human trafficking.* Human trafficking is a form of forced labor or slavery (U.S. Department of State 2020). Traffickers seize women, girls, and boys and force them to engage in prostitution.

A study of trafficking in Ohio identified 1,032 victims over a five-year period (Anderson, Kulig, and Sullivan 2019). A Florida study found that those seized were more likely than others to have been sexually abused prior to the enforced prostitution (Reid et al. 2017).

Who uses the services of a prostitute? Again, it is impossible to give exact figures. Yet considering the number of prostitutes available and the number of times they can have sex each day, it is clear that a substantial portion of the male population has some experience with a prostitute. One researcher estimates that 16 percent of American men pay for sex at some point in their lives (Westerhoff 2009). Although men of any age may use a prostitute, the typical customer, or "john," is a married, middle-aged, well-educated white male (Della Giusta, Di Tommaso, Shima, and Strom 2009; Farley et al. 2011). Only a small proportion of the men limit their use of prostitutes to one time. A study of men who used the Internet to secure a prostitute found that nearly two-thirds were between 40 and 60 years old, 85 percent were white, nearly 80 percent had a college degree, 66.3 percent were married, and 27 percent used a prostitute one or more times a week (Milrod and Monto 2012). And in a sample of 1,342 men arrested for solicitation, nearly one out of eight said they had sex with a prostitute at least once a month (Della Giusta et al. 2009).

Surveys of men in various other nations have found that roughly 9 to 10 percent admit that they used the services of a prostitute in the past year (Carael, Slaymaker, Lyerla, and Sarkar 2006). The proportion varied considerably by region, however: 13 to 15 percent in central Africa, 10 to 11 percent in eastern and southern Africa, 5 to 7 percent in Asia and Latin America. Keep in mind that these numbers represent those who said they had sex with a prostitute in the past year; the proportion who ever used a prostitute would be considerably higher.

Why do men pay for sex? The survey of 1,342 men arrested for solicitation asked them to indicate which of 13 possible reasons applied to them (Della Giusta et al. 2009). They could agree with more than one of the reasons. The most frequently chosen reasons (and the proportion agreeing with them) were these: wanting to be with a woman who "likes to get nasty" (52 percent), approaching a prostitute is exciting (43 percent), wanting to be in control during sex (42 percent), preferring a variety of sexual partners (41 percent), wanting a different kind of sex than he has with his regular partner (41 percent), and feeling awkward when trying to meet a woman (41 percent). In the study of men who used the Internet to find a prostitute, the top three motives with which they agreed strongly were the following: "I like to be with a woman who really likes sex" (84.4 percent); "I like to be with a woman who likes to act very uninhibited and horny" (71.7 percent); and "I like to have a variety of sexual partners" (45.3 percent) (Milrod and Monto 2012). These reasons suggest that the men (most of whom are married or living with someone) desire some kinds of sexual experiences that they don't have with their regular partner.

## Prostitution and the Quality of Life

Prostitutes may prefer their profession to other perceived options. This preference is not so much evidence of the high quality of life for prostitutes as it is testimony to the *low quality of life endured by the women before they decided to become prostitutes.*

In Prince's (1986) interviews of 300 prostitutes, all of the streetwalkers named money as the major advantage of their work. Brothel workers and call girls were more likely to name such things as time flexibility, adventure, and learning about themselves and others. Whatever the advantages, however, there are serious problems with the quality of life.

*Physical Problems.* In the first place, *prostitution contradicts our value of physical well-being.* Americans cherish good health and value the youthful physique. Most prostitutes, however, face certain occupational hazards that may lead to physical problems. In the past, *venereal disease* was a prominent problem. Today it is less frequent because many prostitutes get regular medical checkups and also carefully examine each customer for signs of venereal disease. Juvenile prostitutes, however, may be resistant to medical help because they fear attracting the attention of authorities.

Another common physical problem "is a chronic pelvic congestion characterized by a copious discharge from the cervix and vaginal lining, and a sensation of tenderness and fullness of the side walls of the pelvis" (Winick and Kinsie 1971:70). The congestion results from the prostitute's avoidance of orgasm. She may try to get relief through narcotic drugs.

Finally, prostitutes face the hazard of contracting acquired immune deficiency syndrome (AIDS) (Yuen et al. 2016). They run the risk both from their clients and from the tendency of some to become intravenous drug users. Once they have the virus, of course, they help spread it. Rates of infection are particularly high among male prostitutes. A study of young male prostitutes in San Francisco reported that 12 percent of them were infected (Bacon et al. 2006). Fewer than half of the prostitutes required their clients to use condoms, and only 41 percent of those infected were even aware of their condition. Even higher rates have been found in other nations. A survey of Cambodian prostitutes reported an infection rate of 54 percent (Ohshige et al. 2000). A study of prostitutes in Vancouver, Canada, reported a 26 percent rate of infection (Shannon, Bright, Gibson, and Tyndall 2007). Rates are even higher in some African nations, and are particularly high among the street prostitutes who use drugs (Needle et al. 2008).

A different problem is the *physical abuse that threatens the prostitute* (Raphael and Shapiro 2004). The abuse is most likely to come from customers. A survey of 325 prostitutes in Miami reported that over 40 percent had experienced violence in the preceding year: 24.9 percent had been beaten, 12.9 percent had been raped, and 13.8 percent had been threatened with a weapon (Surratt, Inciardi, Kurtz, and Kiley 2004). Prostitutes may also suffer abuse from the police. A study of sex workers in Baltimore, Maryland, reported 78 percent had had one or more abusive encounters with the police (Footer et al. 2019).

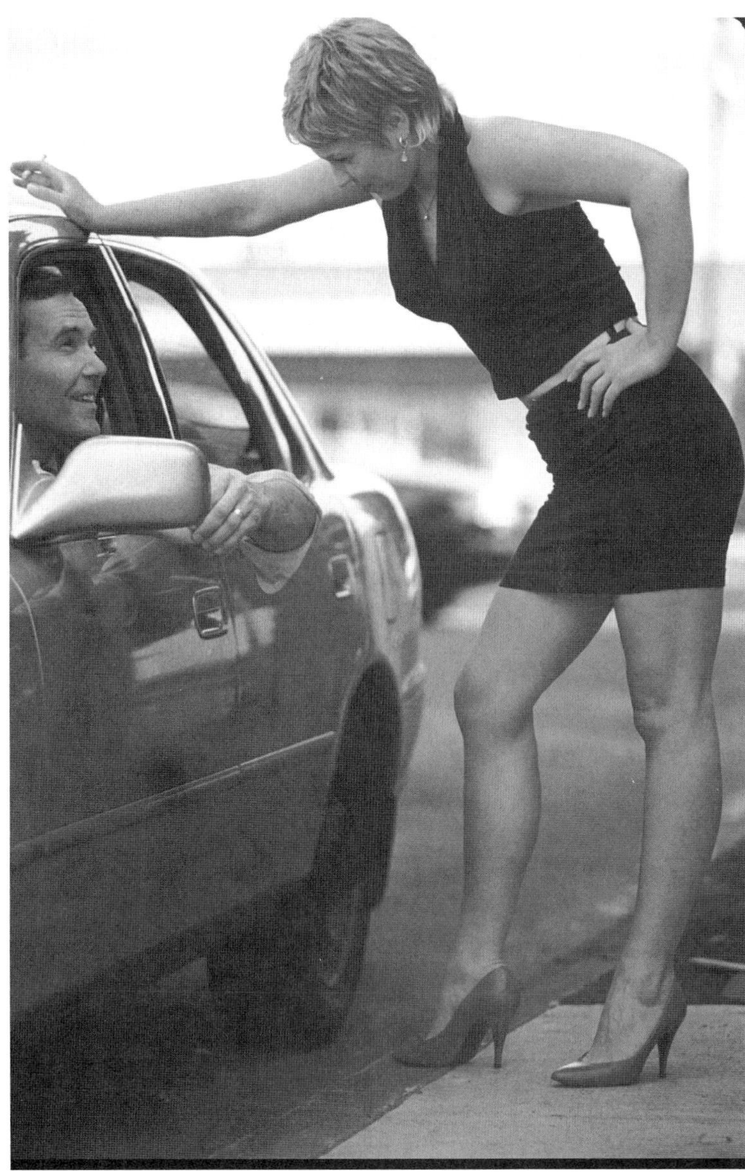

There are different kinds of prostitution, with different consequences for the prostitute.
Ingram Publishing/SuperStock

A prostitute may also suffer abuse at the hands of her husband or boyfriend and her **pimp** (one who earns all or part of his or her living by acting as a manager for the prostitute) (Dalla 2000). The highly paid call girl, who serves a more affluent clientele, is not likely to endure physical abuse, but the streetwalker must be constantly alert.

**pimp**
one who earns all or part of his or her living by acting as a manager or procurer for a prostitute

The constant threat of abuse is one reason a prostitute needs a pimp. Ironically, Norton-Hawk (2004) found that, among the 50 jailed prostitutes she interviewed, pimp-controlled prostitutes were more likely to be victims of customer violence than were those without pimps. The pressure to make extra money to support the pimp may lead these prostitutes to take more risks, exposing themselves to a greater chance of violence.

At the same time, the pimp himself inflicts physical abuse (Williamson and Cluse-Tolar 2002). Sometimes the pimp will beat a prostitute when he begins his relationship with her to establish his dominance and to ensure the woman's loyalty. If the prostitute does not behave in a way the pimp deems appropriate, he may continue to abuse her. One prostitute explained the pimp's behavior in terms of the master-slave relationship. The master seems to have total power but lives in fear because of the uncertainty of how the slave will react to his or her bondage. Like the master with his slave, the pimp fears the loss of his property.

We do not know how frequently prostitutes endure physical abuse from customers or their pimps, but the threat of abuse is constant. It is unlikely that any prostitute can ply her trade for many years without suffering abuse (Nixon et al. 2002). A study of 130 prostitutes in San Francisco reported that 82 percent had been physically assaulted, 83 percent had been threatened with a weapon, and 68 percent had been raped while working as a prostitute (Farley and Barkan 1998). It is estimated that street prostitutes are 60 to 100 times more likely to be murdered than are other women (Salfati, James, and Ferguson 2008). Such violence in their lives, along with the drug use that is common, is a major reason for the higher rate of mortality among prostitutes (Potterat et al. 2004). Compared with other women of their age, prostitutes are nearly twice as likely to die.

*Psychological and Emotional Problems.* A psychological problem reported by prostitutes arises from the contradiction between the value of sexual fulfillment and the role of the prostitute. The problem is a psychological counterpart to the previously mentioned physical ailment that can result from the prostitute's avoidance of orgasm. Far from achieving sexual fulfillment, the prostitute often becomes *virtually asexual* with respect to her own sexual functioning (Dalla 2001). Again, however, we have to distinguish between different kinds of prostitutes. A majority of streetwalkers believe they should avoid orgasms, but only a third of brothel workers and 4 percent of call girls believe it.

There is also a contradiction between the value of *human dignity* and the prostitute's role. The continual exposure to violence, along with other aspects of the prostitute's work, may lead to various kinds of emotional trauma (including depression and posttraumatic stress disorder), drug use and abuse, feelings of isolation and worthlessness, attempted suicide, and sexually transmitted diseases including AIDS (Norton-Hawk 2002; Burnette, Schneider, Timko, and Ilgen 2009; Krumrei-Mancuso 2016). Emotional problems are intensified by the fact that prostitutes generally do not form a cohesive group among themselves because they are competing for customers. They mainly have contempt for their customers and do not establish bonds with them. They often cannot form close relationships with people not connected with "the life" because of the stigma attached to their role. Therefore, prostitutes are barred from a sense of community with anyone.

One way prostitutes cope with this problem is to seek *refuge in drugs* (Dalla 2000; Degenhardt, Day, Conroy, and Gilmour 2006). A considerable number of prostitutes need help with addiction (Valera, Sawyer, and Schiraldi 2001). In many cases, the prostitutes were drug users before they began to engage in sex work (Bletzer 2005). Once they started working as prostitutes, however, their drug use tended to escalate.

When the drugs no longer are sufficient to make their existence bearable, prostitutes may try to end their lives. The rate of *attempted suicide* is quite high among prostitutes (Ling, Wong, Holroyd, and Gray 2007). In Prince's (1986) study, 68 percent of the streetwalkers, 25 percent of the call girls, and 19 percent of the brothel workers admitted trying to kill themselves.

There is, then, ample evidence of psychological and emotional problems among prostitutes. Moreover, these problems are built into the role of the prostitute, making escape

global comparison

## CHILD PROSTITUTES

In the United States, women may become prostitutes because, among other reasons, they come from impoverished backgrounds. In some other countries, the relationship between poverty and prostitution takes a different twist—children sell themselves, or are sold by their parents, into prostitution in order to survive. The United Nations estimates that 1.2 million children are trafficked across international borders every year, most of them destined for prostitution.

We should note that not all child prostitution comes out of impoverished settings. Cultural norms also play a role. For example, in Thailand girls sometimes go into prostitution because it appears to be the only choice they have in order to fulfill the norms of their culture. Those norms dictate that the young should repay their parents for the sacrifices the parents have made and should help improve their parents' financial standing. They have the obligation to do so even if the family is relatively well off. But females have little opportunity to make enough money to enhance the family's income and status. Consequently, some of them opt for prostitution as a "bearable" way to fulfill their cultural obligations.

Most child prostitution, however, is tied up with poverty and the need to survive. The close link between child prostitution and survival is illustrated by the account of a 17-year-old Chilean prostitute, who told how the first effort she and her brothers made to get food was to go out and beg, or pick up leftovers at the market. Then they started selling celery, but when they couldn't sell enough to get the food needed by the family, "my mom almost beat us to death." After that, the girl began to sell herself. A Chilean sociologist has estimated that as many as 50,000 children in Chile engage in prostitution in order to survive.

Southeast Asia is another area with child prostitutes. No one knows just how many, but estimates run into the hundreds of thousands and as high as a million. One-fifth of prostitutes in Thailand begin their work between the ages of 13 and 15, and girls as young as 8 are in the brothels of Thailand, Cambodia, India, China, Taiwan, and the Philippines. Many of the girls were sold to the brothel owners by their parents in order to get money for food or other essentials for their families. Once sold, the girls are considered the property of the brothel owners and must work until they pay off their purchase price—or until they get AIDS.

In some cases, the family may run its own prostitution business. A mother with four daughters in Manila looked for clients for the two youngest daughters, ages 8 and 12. When the 12-year-old resisted, the mother held her down while the men raped her.

The clients of child prostitutes come from many different nations, including America. Why do they want children? No doubt they have various motivations, but one seems to be the fear of AIDS. The AIDS virus is spreading rapidly among prostitutes in Asia. The younger the prostitute, so the reasoning goes, the less likely she is to have AIDS. As a result, hundreds of thousands of Asian girls are living in sexual slavery.

SOURCES: *Chicago Tribune,* March 17, 1996; *New York Times,* April 14, 1996; Kuo 2000; Willis and Levy 2003; Bower 2005; Mathews 2006.

difficult. For some women, prostitution seems to be more desirable than other available options, but the psychological and emotional quality of the prostitute's life is low.

*Exploitation.* Quality of life is further diminished by the *contradiction between the roles of the prostitute and the people with whom she must deal and the ideal of "I-Thou" relationships* in which people relate to each other as person to person and not as person to thing. The role of prostitute involves exploitation. Pimps, madams, bellboys, taxi drivers, lawyers, disreputable medical examiners, abortionists, police officers receiving hush money—the prostitute must deal with them all, and they all treat her as a "thing" rather than as a person by using her to make or to supplement their own living. The women offer their sexual services to men, pay their fines to men, and return to the streets only to be arrested again by men—all to satisfy the public's sense of "decorum."

Arresting prostitutes satisfies the public because the appearance of police safeguarding morality is maintained. The prostitute is exploited by many different people, all of whom regard her as an object to serve their own interests.

Perhaps the most exploited of prostitutes are those whom we discussed earlier, the sex slaves forced unwittingly into prostitution by traffickers who kidnap them or who lure them into another country with the promise of work or husbands (van Hook, Gjermeni, and Haxhiymeri 2006). In some cases, the women fled into another country trying to fend off extreme poverty and even starvation. Once there, however, they were forced into prostitution as the only way to survive.

There are probably hundreds of thousands of sex slaves throughout the world. Asian nations have particularly high rates of sex slaves, but there are tens of thousands of them in the United States (Field 2004). Federally funded human trafficking task forces found more than 2,000 incidents of sex trafficking between January 2008 and June 2010 (Banks and Kyckelhahn 2011). Although most sex slaves in the United States are from a Latin American or Southeast Asian background, the task forces reported that 83 percent of the victims in the incidents they identified were American citizens. Like sex slaves in other nations, those in the United States are typically deceived and forced into prostitution by those exploiting them for personal gain.

## Contributing Factors

If the quality of life for the prostitute is so low, and if many Americans believe the very presence of prostitutes offends traditional morals, why does prostitution continue?

*Social Structural Factors.* Social structural factors help explain both why men seek prostitutes and why women enter into the life. American society has traditionally held to the norm of sex only within marriage. In addition, sex has not been openly discussed through much of the nation's history. These two factors—*rejection of nonmarital sex and no open discussion of sex*—were set forth by Winick and Kinsie (1971) as crucial determinants of the amount of prostitution in a society. They pointed out that among the Tokopia of the Solomon Islands, both nonmarital sex and open discussion of sex are accepted, and there is practically no prostitution. They hypothesize that in societies in which social norms forbid either or both of these conditions, there will probably be prostitution. This line of reasoning is supported by the fact that open discussions about sex have become more acceptable, and nonmarital sex (especially premarital) has become more widely accepted in American society. At the same time, although roughly the same number of men appear to use the services of prostitutes, fewer are young men, and the number of visits by each man may have declined.

In addition to traditional norms about nonmarital sex and discussion of sex, the *institution of marriage* does not provide the kinds of sexual experiences that some men desire (Monto 2004). Nor, we would add, should it. A wife is a human partner, not a sex slave who must fulfill her husband's every fantasy regardless of her own needs. Of course, most married men are content with their experiences in marital sex. But some men go to prostitutes to experience variety, to compensate for a lack of gratification with their mates, or to avoid concern about pregnancy (Brents, Jackson, and Hausbeck 2010). Married men who give and receive oral sex report that they are happier with their sex lives and their marriages, but it appears that wives are less into oral sex than are their husbands. Consequently, as shown in Figure 5.1, the desire for fellatio is an important reason some men use prostitutes (Monto 2001).

Men may also go to prostitutes because their wives do not desire sexual relations as often as they do. The prostitute then provides a sexual outlet that does not require the time and emotion that would be involved in an extramarital affair.

The nature of the economy also facilitates male use of prostitution. Men who spend a great deal of time away from home (e.g., traveling salesmen and truck drivers) are a major source of business for brothels. A study of Chinese men who used prostitutes reported that one type of client was the man who was required to work far away from his wife or girlfriend (Pochagina 2006). To the extent that *the economy requires travel,* there will likely be clientele for the prostitute.

Structural factors help explain why women enter the life. They tend to come from a *low position in the stratification system.* They may have existed in a situation of poverty, abuse, and family instability in their early years (McCarthy, Benoit, and Jansson 2014). They usually have little education and few job skills, and resort to prostitution out of what they regard as economic necessity (Dalla 2000; Kramer and Berg 2003). A study of women working in Nevada brothels found that three-fourths were sex workers because of financial considerations (Brents et al. 2010). Young, homeless male and female prostitutes also resort to this way of life in order to survive (Tyler and Johnson 2006). Some of these youth view prostitution as nothing more than a desperate attempt to get the necessities of life. They see no other alternative. Pimps take advantage of their desperation by looking for runaway girls in bus stations, arcades, and malls (Albanese 2007). They act like concerned new friends, buying the girls food and clothing and eventually having sex with them. After that, they use the girls' emotional and financial dependence to force them into prostitution, using drugs and threats if necessary. The pimp is no longer a friend; he is the boss, the man who tells the prostitute how much money she must earn for him each day. An example of how pimps work is the man who recruited Canadian girls, took them to Hawaii, and then seized their passports so they could not leave (Albanese 2007). He drugged and handcuffed them, and told them to comply with his demands or he would send photos of them engaging in sex to magazines or to their families.

Studies of prostitutes in other nations reveal a similar pattern: Prostitutes tend to come from impoverished backgrounds and feel compelled to engage in prostitution in order to survive. Often, perhaps most of the time, it is not only a matter of the individual's survival but also that of her family (Wong, Holroyd, Gray, and Ling 2006). In some cases, it may not be a matter of sheer survival, but of the level of income available to women. In Tijuana, Mexico, sex workers can earn 5 times as much as average professionals and 10 times what most people earn (Kelly 2008).

In addition to their position in the socioeconomic system, prostitutes frequently come from backgrounds of *disturbed family experiences and participation in groups with norms that accept prostitution.* Prince (1986) reported that the prostitute's relationship with her father seems to be the most important family factor. In particular, the prostitutes tended to describe a father who abandoned the family, who lost contact after a divorce, or who treated the girl abusively or with indifference. About 9 out of 10 of the streetwalkers said that they did not have a close or happy relationship with either their mother or father while growing up. The call girls tended to have a good relationship with their mother, but fewer than half had one with their father. Among the brothel workers, the proportions reporting good relationships were 43 percent with their mother and 39 percent with their father.

Similarly, interviews with 33 parents of teenage prostitutes reported that the parents were stressed from a history of failed intimate relationships and financial hardships (Longres 1991). They also raised their daughters in neighborhoods conducive to easy entry into prostitution.

In many cases, the disturbed family experiences go beyond mere deprivation. Prostitutes come disproportionately from families involved in physical and/or sexual abuse, alcoholism, and use of other drugs (Dalla 2001; Nixon et al. 2002; Lung, Lin, Lu, and Shu 2004). A study of 72 Australian prostitutes found that all but one of them had traumatic experiences that typically began in early childhood, including child sexual abuse (Roxburgh et al. 2006). A study of Mexican brothel workers reported that a number of the women became prostitutes to support themselves so they could escape from an abusive, violent relationship with a husband or lover (Kelly 2008). Abuse, exploitation, and deprivation continue to lead many young women to run away from home. Faced with the urgency of getting food and shelter, and possessing little or no money, they are lured into prostitution in an effort to survive. Even if they do not run away, early sexual abuse increases the chances of their becoming prostitutes.

*Social Psychological Factors.* Although "respectable" people are frequently thought to abhor prostitution, the bulk of the prostitute's clientele are so-called respectable people. Their psychological and social adjustment may be somewhat less than that of others. A study of 1,672 men arrested for trying to hire a street prostitute reported that they, compared to men generally, were less likely to be married, less likely to be happily married if they were married, and more likely to report being generally unhappy (Monto and McRee 2005). But, as the researchers pointed out, the differences tended to be small, suggesting that the customers differed from others by degree rather than by significant amounts.

A study of Chinese men found eight different motivations for using prostitutes (Pochagina 2006). First, some young men with no sexual experience or who have difficulty forming a lasting intimate relationship engage prostitutes. Second, because there are millions more men than women in China, some men gain sexual satisfaction through prostitutes. Third, some men who find it difficult to find sexual satisfaction with a wife or girlfriend use prostitutes. Fourth, others use prostitutes when age, appearance, or psychological makeup make them unable to form a meaningful sexual relationship. Fifth, some men engage prostitutes as a way to bolster their self-esteem. Sixth, others turn to prostitutes when they are required to work away from wives or girlfriends. Seventh, some use prostitutes to reduce tension in their lives. And finally, some are married but are looking for diversity while on a trip or a vacation.

Other social psychological factors that maintain prostitution include the tolerant attitudes of officials and public acceptance of the ideology that male sexuality needs the outlet. With regard to the former, it is often noted that prostitution could not continue if the authorities were determined to eliminate it. Although this is an overstatement, it is true that police seldom make a determined effort to stop all prostitution. Of course, as long as there is a demand for the services of prostitutes, it is unlikely that the police can eliminate the practice even if they wished to do so.

Tolerance about prostitution is partly rooted in the ideology about male sexuality. Some people believe that prostitution brings more benefits than problems to their communities. For example, they believe that prostitutes keep their sons from early marriage, prevent premarital pregnancies in their daughters, and decrease the amount of rape and other violent crime. Such beliefs reflect the ideology that male sexuality, in contrast to female sexuality, must find expression and that traditional values about marriage, the family, and the purity of women are contingent on men's having a sexual outlet. People who accept this ideology will tolerate prostitution.

## Solutions: Public Policy and Private Action

Prostitutes and civil rights activists argue that prostitution should be legalized, or at least decriminalized. To legalize it would make it a legitimate business like any other and would gain the maximum benefits for communities, for law enforcement, and for those involved in the business (Weitzer 2012). Decriminalization, on the other hand, would mean that while people could no longer be prosecuted as criminals, the trade could still be regarded as a misdemeanor subject to fines or as a practice requiring special permits.

There are a number of reasons for advocating legalization. The United States is one of relatively few nations in the world that define prostitution as illegal. In most nations, prostitution is either legal with restrictions (e.g., prostitutes must register and have regular health exams) or legal and regulated (e.g., age limits, no forced prostitution, registration, and regular health exams) (Westerhoff 2009).

In addition, advocates for legalization argue that prostitution should be neither a sin nor a crime. Rather, it falls into the realm of work, choice, and civil rights (Miller and Jayasundara 2001). Women who choose prostitution as their work have their civil rights violated because of existing laws. Moreover, as Weitzer (2007:31) points out, legalized prostitution "can be organized in a way that increases workers' health, safety, and job satisfaction." Indeed, in those Nevada counties where prostitution is legal, prostitutes are able to work without fear of arrest and are better able to protect their health (Brents and Hausbeck 2005). In general, compared to streetwalkers, indoor prostitutes (those who work in such places as bars and brothels or who work as call girls on their own or through an escort service) earn more money, are safer from violence, and are less likely to abuse drugs or to contract a sexually transmitted disease (Weitzer 2007). Nevertheless, the majority of Americans oppose legalization and regulation of prostitution, so it is unlikely that there will be a widespread change in public policy in the near future.

Even decriminalization will not completely solve the problem. If prostitution were decriminalized, there would still need to be regulation of the business (Kuo 2002). One reason for regulation is health. Current efforts to suppress prostitution are based in part on the effort to control the spread of venereal disease (Ness 2003). There is also the issue of the prostitute's own health–regular checkups are needed.

In addition, because of potential abuse from customers, prostitutes may still feel the need for pimps. If the prostitutes work in brothels, thereby avoiding the need for pimps, they will still be treated as objects rather than as people and will confront the various psychological and emotional problems inherent in the life.

The problem can also be attacked by lessening the demand rather than punishing the supply. In many cities the police have begun to arrest johns and even to publish their names. Some states have a First Offender Prostitution Program, which allows men arrested for solicitation to pay a fine and attend a class in which they hear a lecture about the law, watch slides that depict the effects of venereal disease, and listen to ex-prostitutes tell how much they despised their customers. In return, the arrest for soliciting sex is removed from their records. Although such programs may be effective, the fact is that most states and municipalities ignore laws that allow them to arrest pimps, traffickers, and customers and focus instead on the prostitutes themselves (Miller and Jayasundara 2001).

Finally, a good part of the problem of prostitution could be resolved if women from lower socioeconomic positions had opportunities to gain some measure of success in other kinds of work. The problem could also be alleviated if women with drug habits and/or women who come from abusive homes had other ways to support themselves and to get the help they need to deal with their problems.

*Follow-Up.* Set up a debate in your class on the question "Should prostitution be decriminalized? Yes or no."

## Pornography, Erotica, and Obscenity

One person's pornography is another person's literature. It is no surprise, then, that this subject generates strong feelings and great disagreement. What exactly are we talking about when we speak of pornography and how extensively does it penetrate society?

### Nature and Extent of the Problem

What comes to mind when you see or hear the word *pornography?* What, if anything, do you think should be done about materials that you would personally label as pornographic? Read the following materials, then return to these questions and see whether your answers have changed in any way.

*Definitions.* People tend to label as pornographic any kind of *sexual materials that they find personally offensive.* Researchers who asked a sample of over 2,000 people to rate 20 different samples from sexual media, found a range of responses from some who saw very little of what they would call pornography to those who labeled even the slightest hint of sexual content as pornographic (Willoughby and Busby 2016). Clearly, the definition of pornography cannot be left to individual tastes. Rather, we need to differentiate between pornography, erotica, and obscenity (Hyde and DeLamater 2007). Generally, social scientists define **pornography** as *literature, art, or films that are sexually arousing.* You can further distinguish between so-called soft-core pornography, which is suggestive but does not depict actual intercourse or genitals, and hard-core pornography, in which sexual acts and/or genitals are explicitly depicted.

**pornography**
literature, art, or films that are sexually arousing

Some people are aroused by sexual acts that others would consider degrading, such as forced sex or sex involving children. **Erotica** refers to *sexually arousing materials that are not degrading or demeaning to adults or children.* Erotica, for example, may involve a depiction of a husband and wife engaged in sex play and intercourse. To be sure, some people will find this erotica offensive and degrading. Yet for many, including scholars who research this area, there is an important distinction between erotica and pornography. A woman being raped is pornographic. Two mutually consenting adults engaged in sexual intercourse is erotica, not pornography.

**erotica**
sexually arousing materials that are not degrading or demeaning to adults or children

**Obscenity** is the legal term for pornography that is defined as unacceptable. It refers to those materials that are *offensive by generally accepted standards of decency.* A 1957 Supreme Court decision, *Roth v. the United States,* attempted to establish precise guidelines for deciding when a book, movie, or magazine would be considered obscene (Francoeur 1991): The dominant theme of the material as a whole must appeal to a prurient (lewd) interest in sex; the material must be obviously offensive to existing community standards; and the materials must lack any serious literary, artistic, political, or scientific value. The 1973 *Miller v. California* decision reaffirmed the position that obscenity is not protected by the First Amendment.

**obscenity**
materials that are offensive by generally accepted standards of decency

However, the decisions did not resolve a number of vexing questions: Who decides what is a prurient interest? What is the "community" whose standards must be followed? Who decides whether something has literary, artistic, political, or scientific value? What about the Internet? Should the government regulate Internet content to protect children from pornographic materials? The struggle between opposing positions continues in both public forums and the courts.

*Extent of the Problem.* Erotica, pornography, and obscenity appear in many places—books, magazines, videos, telephone messages, and the Internet. It's difficult to know just how much is available overall. In one year, however, Americans spent $13.3 billion on X-rated magazines, videos, DVDs, live sex shows, strip clubs, adult cable shows, and computer pornography (Weitzer 2010). In addition, a good deal of pornography is available free in the more than 260 million pages of pornography on the Internet (Paul 2004). A large-scale survey of Internet users found that 75 percent of the men and 41 percent of the women had viewed or downloaded pornographic materials (Albright 2008). And 87 percent of the men and 31 percent of the women in a sample of students from six colleges admitted to using pornography (Carroll et al. 2008). As much as 20 percent of the pornographic Internet pages involve child pornography (Klein, Davies, and Hicks 2001). A study of 1,501 young users of the Internet reported that about one in five had gotten a sexual solicitation, and dozens said they had been asked to meet with or telephone the solicitor, or had received mail, money, or other gifts (Bowker and Gray 2005).

Free or easily accessible pornography on the Internet has led to a dramatic decline in the numbers of pornographic videos and DVDs that Americans rent each year (Richtel 2007). Still, hundreds of millions are rented. Pornographic magazines are also readily available. A study of magazines and videos available in a New York township reported that 25 percent of the magazines and 26.9 percent of the videos contained some kind of sexual violence (Barron and Kimmel 2000).

Moreover, as technology continues to advance, new outlets for pornography appear. The increasing capabilities of cell phones have opened the way for mobile porn (Tanner 2006). Sex magazines like *Playboy* and *Penthouse* now have mobile divisions in their organizations. And an estimated 20 percent of mobile Google searches involve pornography.

Lebeque (1991) reviewed the 3,050 magazine and book titles surveyed in the 1986 Attorney General's Commission on Pornography to see whether the titles themselves fulfilled the criteria for an act of **paraphilia** (the need for a socially unacceptable stimulus in order to be sexually aroused and satisfied). Paraphilia is a disorder listed and described by the American Psychiatric Association. Using their criteria, Lebeque found that 746 (one-fourth of all the titles) fit the definition of paraphilia. **Sadomasochism** is the most common kind of paraphilia. It includes such behavior as being tied up, gagged, whipped, or beaten and using verbal abuse as part of a sexual encounter.

**paraphilia**
the need for a socially unacceptable stimulus in order to be sexually aroused and satisfied

**sadomasochism**
the practice of deriving sexual pleasure from the infliction of pain

**pedophile**
an adult who depends on children for sexual stimulation

We cannot say exactly how much of this type of material is consumed by Americans. Much child pornography used by **pedophiles** (adults who depend on children for sexual stimulation) is underground. We do know that Americans spend hundreds of millions of dollars every year to buy erotic and pornographic magazines and billions of dollars to rent or buy hundreds of millions of X-rated videos, and that a substantial number subscribe to porn television stations (Schlosser 1997; Paige 1998). Moreover, consumption has increased in recent decades. Comparing the 2000s with the 1970s, a national survey reported a 16 percent increase in consumption among young men and an 8 percent increase among young women (Price et al. 2016).

Like prostitution, pornography is a global problem, not merely an American one. For example, a study of a random sample of Norwegians found that 82 percent of those responding admitted that they had read pornographic magazines (Traeen, Nilsen, and Stigum 2006). A slightly higher proportion, 84 percent, had seen pornographic films, and 34 percent had looked at pornography on the Internet. Significantly more men than women made use of the pornography (this is also true in the United States).

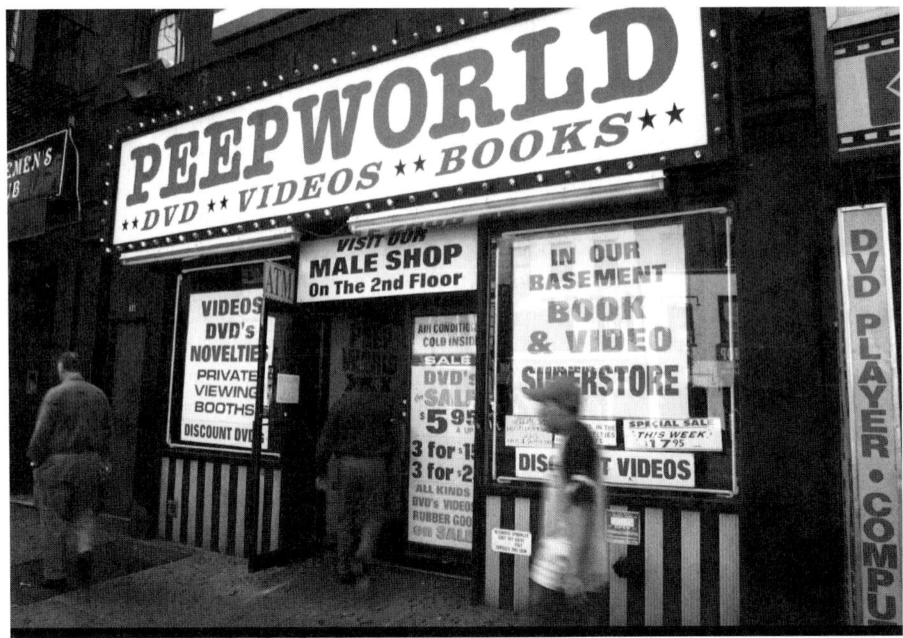


Erotic and pornographic materials are easily accessible, including the violent pornography that increases male aggression.
Gary He/McGraw Hill

## Pornography, Erotica, Obscenity, and the Quality of Life

With most social problems, there is some consensus about the ways in which a particular problem affects the quality of life. Researchers in the area of pornography, erotica, and obscenity, however, proceed from different premises (Francoeur 1991). Some assume that pornographic materials provide people with an outlet for sexual feelings and needs. The materials are like a safety valve, allowing people to reduce sexual tension without harming others. A different premise is that the materials do just the opposite: They offer models of behavior that lead people to act in sexually aggressive and offensive ways that are harmful to others. Thus, researchers, like the general population, are divided in their assumption about and approaches to the problem.

It is our position that pornography and obscenity do have adverse effects on the quality of life, including the quality of relationships. For example, the extensive use of pornography produces negative attitudes about the value of marriage, reduces marital quality, and wives who discover such use by their husbands struggle with the meaning of their marriage, their own worth and desirability, their sense of security in the relationship, and their satisfaction with lovemaking (Arkowitz and Lilienfeld 2010; Perry 2018). The romantic partners and wives of men who consume pornography report lower sexual and relationship quality (Poulsen, Busby, and Galovan 2013; Perry 2016; Wright et al. 2019). Pornography consumers are more likely to have an extramarital affair and to divorce, and less likely to be happy (Doran and Price 2014; Perry and Schleifer 2018). Young adults who use pornography are more likely to engage in risky sexual behavior and use drugs (Carroll et al. 2008). Women who watch online porn report such things as a lowered body image, partners who are critical of their bodies, and pressure to perform the kinds of acts seen in pornographic films (Albright 2008). Ironically, they also have less actual sex. In fact, there is evidence that pornography has contributed to the rise in various sexual issues of men—erectile dysfunction, delayed ejaculation, decreased sexual satisfaction, and lower sexual desire (Park et al. 2016).

There is also evidence of a relationship between pornography and abusive behavior. Research on rural women in Ohio identified pornography as a major factor in intimate abuse (DeKeseredy and Hall-Sanchez 2016). Another study found that physically abused wives are significantly more likely to be sexually abused when their husbands are into pornography (Shope 2004). There is a higher rate of recidivism among those child molesters who continue to consume pornography (Kingston et al. 2008). Finally, there is evidence that exposure to televised pornography has potential negative effects on children, including the modeling of the behavior; interference with normal sexual development; emotional problems such as anxiety, guilt, confusion, and shame; stimulation of premature sexual activity; and the development of harmful attitudes and beliefs about sex and sexual relationships (Benedek and Brown 1999). Consider a few other consequences.

*Exploitation of Children.* Although the use of pornography continues to be defended and cast in positive terms by some, on one point most agree—child pornography is exploitation. Films and pictures that depict sexual acts with children clearly victimize the children (Hyde and DeLamater 2007). Because of their developmental level, children are unable to give truly informed consent to engage in such activities. When persuaded or coerced into doing so, they run the risk of severe emotional trauma.

Such exploitation is a contradiction with the value of *a child's right to dignity and protection.* Unfortunately, those who are responsible for protecting children—parents and other adult relatives—are frequently the ones who are the exploiters. When a porn magazine ran an ad for young girl-child models, dozens of parents responded. An 11-year-old girl was accepted and told to have sex with a 40-year-old man. She ran to her mother and said she couldn't do it, but her mother told her she had to do it because they needed the money.

*Degradation of Women.* American ideology says that all people should be treated with dignity and respect, but much pornography contradicts that ideal. This degradation seems clear in obscenity or pornography that portrays, for example, rape or men urinating on women. Even if there is no violence, however, pornography generally is degrading to women because it depicts them as sex objects whose bodies can be used for male pleasure (Yao, Mahood, and Linz 2010).

Pornography also reinforces certain **stereotypes.** Mayall and Russell (1993) analyzed pornographic magazines, books, films, videos, games, and cards to see how women of various ethnic groups were portrayed. Generally, they found that Asian women were depicted as pliant dolls, Latin women as sexually voracious but also completely submissive, and African American women as dangerous sexual animals.

**stereotype**
an image of members of a group that standardizes them and exaggerates certain qualities

Degradation also occurs because most pornography and obscenity involve male dominance, female subjection, and, frequently, verbal and physical aggression against the women (Sun et al. 2008). And these characteristics are found in films made by both male and female directors. Even if no aggression is involved, most women are likely to react negatively to the porn because of the dominance-subjection relationship. Thus, when erotic and pornographic slides were shown to a group of female undergraduates, they reacted positively to the erotica (Senn and Radtke 1990) but disliked the pornography and strongly disliked the pornography that included violence. Measures of mood before and after watching the slides showed that the pornography led to significant mood disturbance.

*Violence.* One of the more controversial aspects of the problem is whether the use of pornographic and obscene materials leads to violent behavior. Some researchers find little or no relationship between the use of pornography and violent behavior (Ferguson and Hartley 2009). Far more, however, find a definite connection. Research supporting

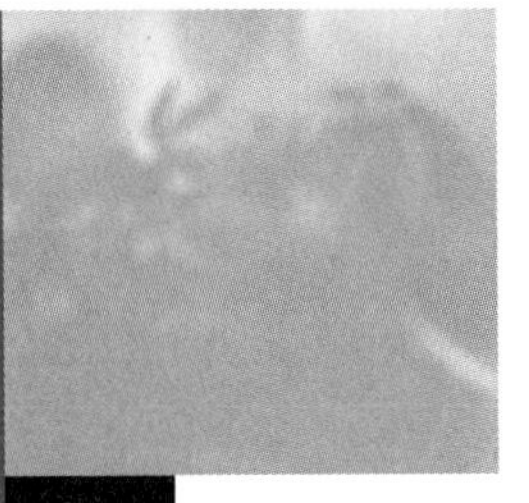

*involvement*

## SEXY OR DISGUSTING?

Looking at an erotic picture of a scantily clad young woman, a man responded: "That is the sexiest thing I've ever seen." A woman evaluated the same picture with: "I think it's disgusting." Do men and women always react so differently to erotic materials? Take a survey of a number of students at your school. Enlist the aid of at least one other student of the opposite sex, or make this a class project.

Interviewers should interview a minimum of 10 subjects of their own gender. Ask the following three questions:

1. Do you see any positive value to magazines like *Playboy?* What? (List as many as respondents can think of.)
2. Do you see any negative consequences from such magazines? What? (Again, list as many as possible.)
3. Have you ever looked at, or do you now look at, such magazines? Why or why not?

Analyze your results. What positive values do students see in such materials? What negative consequences? Do men and women differ in their opinions? If so, how? Did nonreaders have very strong opinions? Did nonreaders differ from readers? How? Finally, if the positive values and negative consequences identified by your respondents represented the thinking of all Americans, including researchers, what recommendations would you make about the availability of such materials?

the latter includes the work of Boeringer (1994), who distinguished between different types of pornography in his testing of 477 college men. Those who watched pornography that included violence and rape were more likely to be sexually aggressive. Those who watched soft-core pornography were less likely to approve of or engage in rape, but more likely to use sexual force and other kinds of coercion.

Boeringer's research is consistent with that of others who have found an association between pornography–both the violent and the nonviolent kind–and aggressive attitudes and behavior on the part of both male and female users of the pornography (Shope 2004; Kernsmith and Kernsmith 2009; Hald, Malamuth, and Yuen 2010; Mancini, Reckdenwald, and Beauregard 2012; Foubert and Bridges 2016). In fact, two researchers who gathered data from 100 female victims of sexual violence reported that 28 percent of the victims said the abuser used pornography and 12 percent said that the abuser imitated the pornography during the abusive incident (Bergen and Bogle 2000).

Violent pornography, then, *contradicts our value on human well-being as well as the norm that sexual behavior should be voluntary and not coerced.* Violent pornography affects not only the women who are directly involved, the existence of violent pornography is a threat to all women. Every time a woman sees a store that sells such materials, she is reminded that she is a potential victim.

### Contributing Factors

Clearly one of the big factors in maintaining the supply of pornographic and obscene materials is the demand. By the nature of the industry, it is not easy to know who the customers are. An analysis of hundreds of users of Internet pornography reported that the strongest predictors were weak religious ties and an unhappy marriage (Stack, Wasserman, and Kern 2004). Some women are consumers of pornography, but the majority of consumers are men. Social structural and social psychological factors help guarantee a continuing supply of materials for those men.

*Social Structural Factors.* From an institutional perspective, *the economy and the legal system both work to maintain the supply of materials.* Economically, the porn business is extremely profitable. The profit margin on magazines is high; a store with a brisk business can bring in hundreds of thousands of dollars in gross sales a year. Overall, Americans spend billions of dollars on pornographic materials each year, and a considerable proportion of the money is spent on child pornography (Hyde and DeLamater 2007).

The legal system presents an extremely difficult issue: *Does any effort to suppress materials, to exercise censorship, violate First Amendment rights?* As we noted earlier, a continuing series of court cases following the 1957 case have attempted to define what is obscene. The reason for the ongoing cases is that the battle over pornography and obscenity involves a *conflict of values.* Some people value openness in sexual matters. They believe that the worst thing that could happen would be to pass any laws infringing on the constitutional right of free speech, and they point out some of the extremes to which people go as they try to guard their own version of morality–such as the removal of a copy of Goya's masterpiece *The Nude Maja* from a classroom wall at Pennsylvania State University on the grounds that it made some of the female students uncomfortable (Strossen 1995) or the order of Attorney General John Ashcroft in 2002 to cover the bare breast of the statue *Spirit of Justice* in the Justice Department's Great Hall.

Others contend that society must be responsible and responsive to the needs of people whose quality of life is depressed by the materials. They argue, for instance, that to protect the right of pornographers in the name of free speech is a violation of the more basic right of women to freedom from exploitation and inequality.

fallacy

Each side tends to use the *fallacies of dramatic instance and personal attack.* For example, those who argue for regulation may cite a newspaper article about sexual violence by someone who read pornographic magazines and call their opponents the destroyers of personal and social morality. Those who stand for openness, on the other hand, may offer Nazi Germany as an example of a repressive society and argue that Americans are heading in the same direction when they suppress materials simply because some people find them offensive. They may call their opponents prudes or narrow-minded people who are willing to sacrifice the basic rights of all Americans to alleviate their own fears.

In essence, *the legal system has helped both sides.* By its ongoing effort to specify what is obscene, the Supreme Court has made the production and distribution of some offensive materials a criminal matter. In the effort to maintain the right of free speech, on the other hand, the courts have allowed the continued production and distribution of materials that women find offensive and degrading, as well as some materials (violent pornography) that increase the aggressiveness of men against women.

*Social Psychological Factors.* *Americans are divided in their attitudes toward pornographic materials.* They are divided, among other things, along the lines of age and according to whether they are users or nonusers. In the survey of students from six colleges, 67 percent of the young men and 49 percent of the young women agreed that using pornography is acceptable behavior (Carroll et al. 2008). In a national survey of a larger age span, however, 41 percent said that magazines showing adults having sexual relations should be banned from their communities, 48 percent said it is appropriate for stores to remove magazines like *Playboy* and *Penthouse* from their newsstands, and 8 out of 10 Americans want Internet obscenity laws vigorously enforced (Pierce 2002). Finally, a 2018 Gallup poll found that 43 percent of Americans believe pornography is morally acceptable. So a substantial minority have no problem with pornography, and a small majority have varying degrees of opposition to it. Perhaps this ambivalence reflects a conflict between the value of personal freedom and a particular ideology of sexual morality. Or perhaps it reflects the more tolerant attitude toward sexual openness among the young. In any case, because a substantial number of Americans have tolerant attitudes about the use of pornography, the supply is likely to remain large and available.

## Solutions: Public Policy and Private Action

A number of steps can be taken to reduce the flow of pornographic materials in general and violent pornography in particular. One is to provide *education at an early age about the ways in which pornography degrades women.* If boys understand how such materials affect females, they may be less prone to consume them.

A second step is the *mobilization of groups to picket, boycott, and protest in other ways the sale of materials they find offensive.* Boycotts against stores that sold materials offensive to people in a community have led to the removal of the materials. Economic pressure may be effective where other attempts at persuasion fall short.

Third, citizens can mobilize to press for *stricter enforcement of existing obscenity laws.* They can urge more stringent regulation or even a ban of porn cable programs and dial-a-porn telephone services. Such efforts, however, will likely be stymied unless people distinguish between erotica, pornography, and obscenity. Efforts at regulation should begin with those materials most clearly offensive—violent pornography.

Fourth, government at all levels can take action, including the passage of legislation. Local governments have engaged in a number of successful campaigns to reduce the amount of pornography in their communities. For example, New York City officials closed down an entire block of businesses in Manhattan, including porn movie houses, bookstores, and strip joints (Kirby 1996). The city helped bring in retail stores and more wholesome forms of entertainment to the area.

Congress enacted laws in the late 1990s to punish people who make obscene materials available to minors via the Internet. The laws ran into problems in the courts because they violated the First Amendment right of free speech. The challenge, therefore, is to enact laws that regulate obscenity without violating the First Amendment. Children, who have access to some of the worst pornography available, need protection. One such law was the 2000 Children's Internet Protection Act that required libraries receiving federal technology funds to install pornography-blocking software on their computers. The American Civil Liberties Union and a number of librarian groups challenged the law as a violation of free speech, but it was upheld by the Supreme Court in 2003.

Clearly, laws are needed that address the problem of pornography without raising allegations of First Amendment violations. Knee (2004) has suggested enacting laws that make illegal the giving or receiving of payment to perform sex acts. Such laws, he argues, would put some of the largest pornographers out of business because they could no longer pay people to perform in hard-core pornographic films.

Fifth, businesses and corporations can help by reducing the supply. Small businesses can refuse to stock and sell pornographic magazines. Video rental chains can refuse to stock and rent pornographic videos and DVDs. And large corporate enterprises such as cable companies can block offensive sites. A number of cable companies have already begun to purge Internet bulletin boards and websites that feature child pornography from their systems (Hakim 2008).

Finally, there is a need for *research on the customers of pornographic materials.* What needs do such materials fulfill? Why and how are they used? Answering such questions will point to ways for reducing the demand. This approach is crucial. For as long as there is demand, there will be a supply—whether legal or not.

*Follow-Up.* Apart from legislation, what other effective ways can you think of to protect children from pornography on the Internet?

## Summary

Sexual gratification is an important part of American life. Some kinds of sex are considered "deviant" rather than "normal." Deviant sex includes such things as exhibitionism, voyeurism, promiscuity, extramarital affairs, cybersex, and strip clubs. Prostitution and pornography are two additional ways of gaining sexual gratification that deviate from the norm. Both involve contradictions and incompatibility with the desired quality of life, and both are sustained by multilevel factors. At any one time, hundreds of thousands of prostitutes are at work in the nation. The prostitute's quality of life is diminished by physical problems inherent in "the life," as well as by psychological, emotional, and economic problems, including fear, alienation, isolation, and exploitation.

Prostitution is maintained because of (1) norms about nonmarital sex and open discussion of sex; (2) lack of sexual gratification in marriage; and (3) characteristics of the economy, such as jobs that require men to travel and discrimination against women in job opportunities and income. The tolerance of prostitution on the part of both the public and officials is rooted in American ideology about sexuality–the notion that male sexuality, in contrast to female sexuality, must find expression.

It is important to distinguish between pornography, erotica, and obscenity. Such materials are available in multiple forms and are widely consumed in America. Pornographic and obscene materials have a negative impact on the quality of life by exploiting children; degrading women; and in the case of violent pornography, increasing aggressive attitudes and behavior of men toward women.

The materials continue to be widely available for a number of reasons: They are extremely profitable; efforts to suppress them raise the issue of First Amendment rights; and public attitudes are divided, perhaps reflecting concern over censorship.

## Key Terms

Cunnilingus
Cybersex
Erotica
Fellatio
Obscenity
Paraphilia
Pedophile
Pimp
Pornography
Promiscuity
Prostitution
Sadomasochism
Sexting
Stereotype

## Study Questions

1. What is meant by sexual deviance?
2. Name and explain six kinds of sexual deviance.
3. What problems do prostitutes face?
4. Why do women and men become prostitutes?
5. What factors help maintain prostitution in American society?
6. How would you differentiate between pornography, erotica, and obscenity?
7. How do pornographic and obscene materials affect men? Women? Children?
8. Discuss the factors that contribute to the problem of pornography.

## Internet Resources/Exercises

1. Explore some of the ideas in this chapter on the following sites:

**http://www.prostitutionresearch.com** Has numerous materials on various aspects of prostitution; sponsored by the San Francisco Women's Centers.

**http://www.asacp.org** Home page of the Association of Sites Advocating Child Protection, an organization devoted to eliminating child pornography from the Internet.

**https://aclu.org** The American Civil Liberties Union site posts warnings on the abridgment of free speech.

2. Good arguments can be made both against and in defense of prostitution. Use the prostitution and ACLU sites listed above, along with a search engine to find additional materials on prostitution, and construct a list of arguments on both sides of the issue. The results can be used for a class debate.

3. Pornography, including child pornography, is a global problem. Search the Internet for materials that discuss the extent of the problem. Compare what you find with materials in the text on pornography in the United States.

## For Further Reading

Albert, Alexa. *Brothel: Mustang Ranch and Its Women.* New York: Random House, 2001. Interviews with prostitutes at a legal house of prostitution in Nevada, telling how they came to be there and how they feel about what they do.

Hall, Ann C., and Mardia J. Bishop, eds. *Pop-Porn: Pornography in American Culture.* New York: Praeger, 2007. An examination of the way in which soft-core porn has spread throughout the culture, including the marketing of sexually arousing women's lingerie and clothing, reality television, and the statements and lifestyles of famous people.

Hardy, Kate, Sarah Kingston, and Teela Sanders, eds. *New Sociologies of Sex Work*. Burlington, VT: Ashgate, 2010. An examination of various facets of prostitution in nations throughout the world, including such topics as public policy, sexual tourism economies, and the organization of sex workers.

Moran, Rachel. *Paid For: My Journey Through Prostitution*. New York: W.W. Norton & Company, 2015. The experiences of a former prostitute, who left home at age 14 and entered prostitution in order to survive, including the emotional damage the trade caused her.

Raphael, Jody. *Listening to Olivia: Violence, Poverty, and Prostitution.* Boston: Northeastern University Press, 2004. Tells the life story of an American prostitute, from the time she first entered the life until she left it.

Wilson, Gary. *Your Brain on Porn: Internet Pornography and the Emerging Science of Addiction.* Richmond, VA: Commonwealth Publishing, 2015. Combines neuroscience with the experiences of porn consumers to portray the addictive nature of pornography.

Wortley, Richard. *Internet Child Pornography: Causes, Investigation, and Prevention*. New York: Praeger, 2012. An in-depth study of the role of the Internet in spreading child pornography, including profiles of the consumers.

## References

Albanese, J. 2007. "Commercial sexual exploitation of children." *NIJ Special Report,* December.

Albright, J. M. 2008. "Sex in America online." *Journal of Sex Research* 45:175–86.

Anderson, V. R., T. C. Kulig, and C. J. Sullivan. 2019. "Estimating the prevalence of human trafficking in Ohio, 2014-2016." *American Journal of Public Health,* AJPH website.

Arkowitz, H., and S. O. Lilienfeld. 2010. "Sex in bits and bytes." *Scientific American Mind,* July/August, pp. 64–65.

Bacon, O., et al. 2006. "Commercial sex work and risk of HIV infection among young drug-injecting men who have sex with men in San Francisco." *Sexually Transmitted Diseases* 33:228–34.

Banks, D., and T. Kyckelhahn. 2011. *Characteristics of Suspected Human Trafficking Incidents, 2008–2010.* Washington, DC: Government Printing Office.

Barron, M., and M. Kimmel. 2000. "Sexual violence in three pornographic media." *Journal of Sex Research* 37:161–68.

Benedek, E. P., and C. F. Brown. 1999. "No excuses: Televised pornography harms children." *Harvard Review of Psychiatry* 7 (November–December):236–40.

Bergen, R. K., and K. A. Bogle. 2000. "Exploring the connection between pornography and sexual violence." *Violence and Victims* 15:227–34.

Bernstein, E. 2007. *Temporarily Yours: Intimacy, Authenticity and the Commerce of Sex*. Chicago, IL: University of Chicago Press.

Biever, C. 2006. "The irresistible rise of cybersex." *New Scientist* 190:67.

Bimbi, D. S. 2007. "Male prostitution: Pathology, paradigms and progress in research." *Journal of Homosexuality* 53:7–35.

Bletzer, K. V. 2005. "Sex workers in agricultural areas." *Culture, Health and Sexuality* 6:543–55.

Boeringer, S. B. 1994. "Pornography and sexual aggression: Associations of violent and nonviolent depictions with rape and rape proclivity." *Deviant Behavior* 15 (3):289–304.

Bolin, A., and P. Whelehan. 2003. *Perspectives on Human Sexuality*. New York: McGraw-Hill.

Bower, B. 2005. "Childhood's end." *Science News* 168:200–01.

Bowker, A., and M. Gray. 2005. "The cybersex offender and children." *FBI Law Enforcement Bulletin* 74:12–17.

Bowman, K. H. 2004. *Attitudes about Homosexuality*. American Enterprise Institute website.

Brents, B. G., and K. Hausbeck. 2005. "Violence and legalized brothel prostitution in Nevada." *Journal of Interpersonal Violence* 20:270–95.

Brents, B. G., C. A. Jackson, and K. Hausbeck. 2010. *The State of Sex: Tourism, Sex, and Sin in the New American Heartland*. New York: Routledge.

Burnette, M. L., R. Schneider, C. Timko, and M. A. Ilgen. 2009. "Impact of substance-use disorder treatment on women involved in prostitution." *Journal of Studies on Alcohol and Drugs* 70:32-40.

Carael, M., E. Slaymaker, R. Lyerla, and S. Sarkar. 2006. "Clients of sex workers in different regions of the world." *Sexually Transmitted Infections* 82:26-33.

Carroll, J. S., et al. 2008. "Generation xxx." *Journal of Adolescent Research* 23:6-30.

Dalla, R. L. 2000. "Exposing the 'Pretty Woman' myth: A qualitative examination of the lives of female streetwalking prostitutes." *Journal of Sex Research* 37:333-43.

Dalla, R. L. 2001. "Et tu Brute? A qualitative analysis of streetwalking prostitutes' interpersonal support networks." *Journal of Family Issues* 22:1066-85.

Daneback, K., A. Cooper, and S. Manisson. 2005. "An Internet study of cybersex participants." *Archives of Sexual Behavior* 34:321-28.

Degenhardt, L., C. Day, E. Conroy, and S. Gilmour. 2006. "Examining links between cocaine use and street-based sex work in New South Wales, Australia." *Journal of Sex Research* 43:107-14.

Dekeseredy, W. S., and A. HallSanchez. 2016. "Adult pornography and violence against women in the heartland." *Violence against Women,* published online.

Della Giusta, M., M. L. Di Tommaso, I. Shima, and S. Strom. 2009. "What money buys: Clients of street sex workers in the US." *Applied Economics* 41:2261-77.

Doran, K., and J. Price. 2014. "Pornography and marriage." *Journal of Family and Economic Issues* 35:489-98.

Farley, M., and H. Barkan. 1998. "Prostitution, violence, and posttraumatic stress disorder." *Women's Health* 27:37-49.

Farley, M., et al. 2011. "Comparing sex buyers with men who don't buy sex." Paper presented at Psychologists for Social Responsibility annual meeting, July 15.

Ferguson, C. J., and R. D. Hartley. 2009. "The pleasure is momentary . . . the expense damnable?: The influence of pornography on rape and sexual assault." *Aggression and Violent Behavior* 14:323-29.

Field, K. 2004. "Fighting trafficking in the United States." *CQ Researcher* 14:284-85.

Footer, K. H., et al. 2019. "Police-related correlates of client-perpetrated violence among female sex workers in Baltimore City, Maryland." *American Journal of Public Health,* AJPH website.

Foubert, J. D., and A. J. Bridges. 2016. "Predicting bystander efficacy and willingness to intervene in college men and women." *Violence against Women,* published online.

Francoeur, R. T. 1991. *Becoming a Sexual Person.* 2nd ed. New York: Macmillan.

Frank, K. 2003. "'Just trying to relax': Masculinity, masculinizing practices, and strip club regulars." *Journal of Sex Research* 40:61-75.

——. 2005. "Exploring the motivations and fantasies of strip club customers in relation to legal regulations." *Archives of Sexual Behavior* 34:487-504.

Grov, C., B. J. Gillespie, T. Royce, and J. Lever. 2011. "Perceived consequences of casual online sexual activities on heterosexual relationships." *Archives of Sexual Behavior* 40:429-39.

Hakim, D. 2008. "Net providers to block sites with child sex." *New York Times,* June 10.

Hald, G. M., N. M. Malamuth, and C Yuen. 2010. "Pornography and attitudes supporting violence against women." *Aggressive Behavior* 36:14-20.

Higgins, J. A., and I. Browne. 2008. "Sexual needs, control, and refusal." *Journal of Sex Research* 45:233-45.

Hyde, J. S., and J. DeLamater. 2007. *Understanding Human Sexuality.* New York: McGraw-Hill.

Jones, M. T. 2010. "Mediated exhibitionism: The naked body in performance and virtual space." *Sexuality & Culture* 14:253-69.

Kelly, P. 2008. *Lydia's Open Door: Inside Mexico's Most Modern Brothel.* Berkeley, CA: University of California Press.

Kernsmith, P. D., and R. M. Kernsmith. 2009. "Female pornography use and sexual coercion perpetration." *Deviant Behavior* 30:589-610.

Kingston, D. A., P. Fedoroff, P. Firestone, S. Curry, and J. M. Bradford. 2008. "Pornography use and sexual aggression." *Aggressive Behavior* 34:341-51.

Kirby, J. A. 1996. "Big Apple excises X-rated rot." *Chicago Tribune,* April 19.

Klein, E. J., H. J. Davies, and M. A. Hicks. 2001. "Child pornography: The criminal-justice system response." National Center for Missing and Exploited Children website.

Knee, J. A. 2004. "Is that really legal?" *New York Times,* May 2.

Kramer, L. A., and E. C. Berg. 2003. "A survival analysis of timing of entry into prostitution." *Sociological Inquiry* 73:511-28.

Krumrei-Mancuso, E. J. 2016. "Sex work and mental health." *Archives of Sexual Behavior,* published online.

Kuo, L. 2002. *Prostitution Policy: Revolutionizing Practice through a Gendered Perspective.* New York: New York University Press.

Kuo, M. 2000. "Asia's dirty secret." *Harvard International Review* 22:42–45.

Langstrom, N., and M. C. Seto. 2006. "Exhibitionistic and voyeuristic behavior in a Swedish national population survey." *Archives of Sexual Behavior* 11:23–35.

Lebeque, B. 1991. "Paraphilias in U.S. pornography titles: 'Pornography made me do it' (Ted Bundy)." *Bulletin of the American Academy of Psychiatry and Law* 19 (1):43–48.

Ling, D. C., W. C. W. Wong, E. A. Holroyd, and S. A. Gray. 2007. "Silent killers of the night: An exploration of psychological health and suicidality among female street sex workers." *Journal of Sex and Marital Therapy* 33:281–99.

Logan, T. D. 2010. "Personal characteristics, sexual behaviors, and male sex work." *American Sociological Review* 75:679–704.

Longres, J. F. 1991. "An ecological study of parents of adjudicated female teenage prostitutes." *Journal of Social Service Research* 14 (1-2):113–27.

Lung, F. W., T. J. Lin, Y. C. Lu, and B. C. Shu. 2004. "Personal characteristics of adolescent prostitutes and rearing attitudes of their parents." *Psychiatry Research* 125:285–91.

Mancini, C., A. Reckdenwald, and E. Beauregard. 2012. "Pornographic exposure over the life course and the severity of sexual offenses." *Journal of Criminal Justice* 40:21–30.

Mathews, D. 2006. "The Rescue Foundation." *New Internationalist* 390:33.

Mayall, A., and D. E. Russell. 1993. "Racism in pornography." *Feminism and Psychology* 3 (2):275–81.

McCarthy, B., C. Benoit, and M. Jansson. 2014. "Sex work." *Archives of Sexual Behavior* 43:1379–90.

Miller, J., and D. Jayasundara. 2001. "Prostitution, the sex industry, and sex tourism." In *Sourcebook on Violence against Women,* ed. C. M. Renzetti, J. L. Edleson, and R. K. Bergen, pp. 459–80. Thousand Oaks, CA: Sage.

Milrod, C., and M. A. Monto. 2012. "The hobbyist and the girlfriend experience." *Deviant Behavior* 33: 792–810.

Montemurro, B., C. Bloom, and K. Madell. 2003. "Ladies night out: A typology of women patrons of a male strip club." *Deviant Behavior* 24:333–52.

Monto, M. A. 2001. "Prostitution and fellatio." *Journal of Sex Research* 38:140–45.

——. 2004. "Female prostitution, customers, and violence." *Violence against Women* 10:160–88.

Monto, M. A., and N. McRee. 2005. "A comparison of the male customers of female street prostitutes with national samples of men." *International Journal of Offender Therapy and Comparative Criminology* 49:505–29.

Needle, R., et al. 2008. "Sex, drugs, and HIV." *Social Science and Medicine* 67:1447–55.

Ness, E. 2003. "Federal government's program in attacking the problem of prostitution." *Federal Probation* 67:10–12.

Nixon, K., L. Tutty, P. Downe, K. Gorkoff, and J. Ursel. 2002. "The everyday occurrence: Violence in the lives of girls exploited through prostitution." *Violence against Women* 8:1016–43.

Norton-Hawk, M. A. 2002. "Lifecourse of prostitution." *Women, Girls, and Criminal Justice* 3:1–9

——. 2004. "Comparison of pimp- and non-pimp-controlled women." *Violence against Women* 10:189–94.

Ohshige, K., et al. 2000. "Cross-sectional study on risk factors of HIV among female commercial sex workers in Cambodia." *Epidemiology of Infections* 124 (February):143–52.

Paige, S. 1998. "Babylon rides high-tech wave." *Insight on the News,* September 28.

Park, B. Y., et al. 2016. "Is internet pornography causing sexual dysfunctions?" *Behavioral Science* 6:17–27.

Paul, P. 2004. "The porn factor." *Time*, January 19.

Perlini, A. H., and T. L. Boychuk. 2006. "Social influence, desirability and relationship investment." *Social Behavior and Personality* 34:593–602.

Perry, S. L. 2016. "Does viewing pornography reduce marital quality over time?" *Archives of Sexual Behavior.* Published online.

Perry, S. L. 2018. "Pornography use and marital quality." *Personal Relationships* 25:233–48.

Perry, S. L., and C. Schleifer. 2018. "Till porn do us part?" *The Journal of Sex Research* 55:284–96.

Pierce, J. 2002. "Poll: 8 of 10 want Internet obscenity laws enforced." *American Center for Law and Justice Newsletter,* March 18.

Pochagina, O. 2006. "The sex business as a social phenomenon in contemporary China." *Far Eastern Affairs* 34:118–34.

Potterat, J. J., et al. 2004. "Mortality in a long-term open cohort of prostitute women." *American Journal of Epidemiology* 159:778-85.

Poulsen, F. O., D. M. Busby, and A. M. Galovan. 2013. "Pornography use associated with couple outcomes." *Journal of Sex Research* 50:72-83.

Price, J., et al. 2016. "How much more xxx is Generation X consuming?" *Journal of Sex Research* 53:12-20.

Prince, D. A. 1986. "A psychological profile of prostitutes in California and Nevada." Unpublished PhD dissertation, United States International University, San Diego, CA.

Raphael, J., and D. L. Shapiro. 2004. "Violence in indoor and outdoor prostitution venues." *Violence against Women* 10:126-39.

Reid, J. A., et al. 2017. "Human trafficking of minors and childhood adversity in Florida." *American Journal of Public Health* 107 (2):306-11.

Richtel, M. 2007. "For pornographers, Internet's virtues turn to vices." *New York Times,* June 2.

Roane, K. R. 1998. "Prostitutes on wane in New York streets but take to Internet." *New York Times,* February 23.

Ross, M. W. 2005. "Typing, doing, and being: Sexuality and the Internet." *Journal of Sex Research* 42:342-52.

Roxburgh, A., et al. 2006. "Posttraumatic stress disorder among female street-based sex workers." *BMC Psychiatry* 24:6-24.

Salfati, C. G., A. R. James, and L. Ferguson. 2008. "Prostitute homicides." *Journal of Interpersonal Violence* 23:505-43.

Schlosser, E. 1997. "The business of pornography." *U.S. News and World Report,* February 10.

Schneider, J. P. 2003. "The impact of compulsive cybersex behaviours on the family." *Sexual and Relationship Therapy* 18:329-54.

Senn, C. Y., and H. L. Radtke. 1990. "Women's evaluations of and affective reactions to mainstream violent pornography, nonviolent pornography, and erotica." *Violence and Victims* 5 (3):143-55.

Shannon, K., V. Bright, K. Gibson, and M. W. Tyndall. 2007. "Sexual and drug-related vulnerabilities for HIV infection among women engaged in survival sex work in Vancouver, Canada." *Canadian Journal of Public Health* 98:465-69.

Shope, J. H. 2004. "When words are not enough." *Violence Against Women* 10:56-72.

Stack, S., I. Wasserman, and R. Kern. 2004. "Adult social bonds and use of Internet pornography." *Social Science Quarterly* 85:75-88.

Strossen, N. 1995. "The perils of pornophobia." *Humanist,* May-June, pp. 5-7.

Sun, C., A. Bridges, R. Wosnitzer, E. Scharrer, and R. Liberman. 2008. "A comparison of male and female directors in popular pornography." *Psychology of Women Quarterly* 32:312-25.

Surratt, H. L., J. A. Inciardi, S. P. Kurtz, and M. C. Kiley. 2004. "Sex work and drug use in a subculture of violence." *Crime and Delinquency* 50:43-59.

Tanner, J. C. 2006. "XXX adult content: Coming to a phone near you?" *America's Network,* June, pp. 26-32.

Traeen, B., T. S. Nilsen, and H. Stigum. 2006. "Use of pornography in traditional media and on the Internet in Norway." *Journal of Sex Research* 43:245-54.

Tyler, K. A., and K. A. Johnson. 2006. "Trading sex: Voluntary or coerced?" *Journal of Sex Research* 43:208-16.

U.S. Department of State. 2020. "Trafficking in persons report." U.S. Department of State website.

Valera, R. J., R. G. Sawyer, and G. R. Schiraldi. 2001. "Perceived health needs of inner-city street prostitutes." *American Journal of Health Behavior* 25:50-59.

van Hook, M. P., E. Gjermeni, and E. Haxhiymeri. 2006. "Sexual trafficking of women." *International Social Work* 49:29-40.

Vandepitte, J., et al. 2006. "Estimates of the number of female sex workers in different regions of the world." *Sexually Transmitted Infections* 82:8-25.

Waite, L. J., and K. Joyner. 2001. "Emotional satisfaction and physical pleasure in sexual unions." *Journal of Marriage and the Family* 63:247-64.

Weinstein, A., and M. Lejoyeux. 2010. "Internet addiction or excessive Internet use." *American Journal of Drug and Alcohol Abuse* 36:277-83.

Weitzer, R. 2007. "Prostitution: Facts and fictions." *Contexts* 6 (Fall):28-33.

——. 2010. "Sex work: Paradigms and policies." In *Sex for Sale: Prostitution, Pornography, and the Sex Industry,* ed. R. J. Weitzer, pp. 1-46. New York: Routledge.

——. 2012. *Legalizing Prostitution: From Illicit Vice to Lawful Business.* New York: New York University Press.

Westerhoff, N. 2009. "Why do men buy sex?" *Scientific American Mind* 20:70–75.

Williamson, C., and T. Cluse-Tolar. 2002. "Pimp-controlled prostitution." *Violence against Women* 8:1074–92.

Willis, B. M., and B. S. Levy. 2003. "Child prostitution increasing." *Southern Medical Journal* 96:69.

Willoughby, B. J., and D. M. Busby. 2016. "In the eye of the beholder." *Journal of Sex Research* 53:678–88.

Winick, C., and P. M. Kinsie. 1971. *The Lively Commerce*. Chicago, IL: Quadrangle.

Wolfinger, N. H. 2017. "America's generation gap in extramarital sex." Institute for Family Studies website.

Wong, W. C. W., E. A. Holroyd, A. Gray, and D. C. Ling. 2006. "Female street sex workers in Hong Kong." *Journal of Women's Health* 15:390–99.

Wright, P. J., et al. 2019. "Associative pathways between pornography consumption and reduced sexual satisfaction." *Sexual and Relationship Therapy* 34:422–39.

Wysocki, D. K., and C. D. Childers. 2011. "'Let my fingers do the talking': Sexting and infidelity in cyberspace." *Sexuality & Culture* 15:217–39.

Yao, M. Z., C. Mahood, and D. Linz. 2010. "Sexual priming, gender stereotyping, and likelihood to sexually harass." *Sex Roles* 62:77–88.

Yuen, W. W., et al. 2016. "Psychological health and HIV transmission among female sex workers." *AIDS Care* 7:816–24.

PART 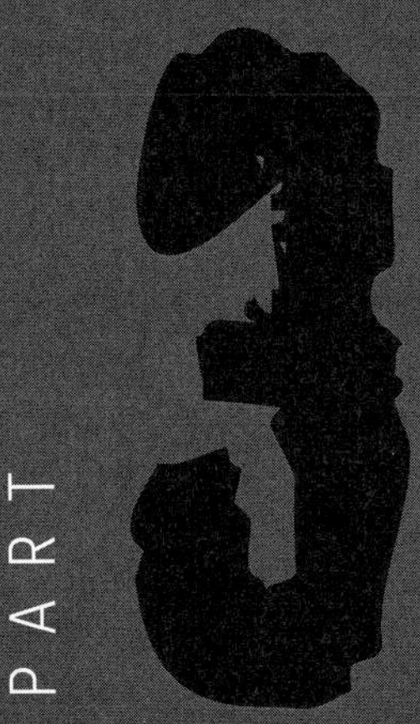

# Problems of Inequality

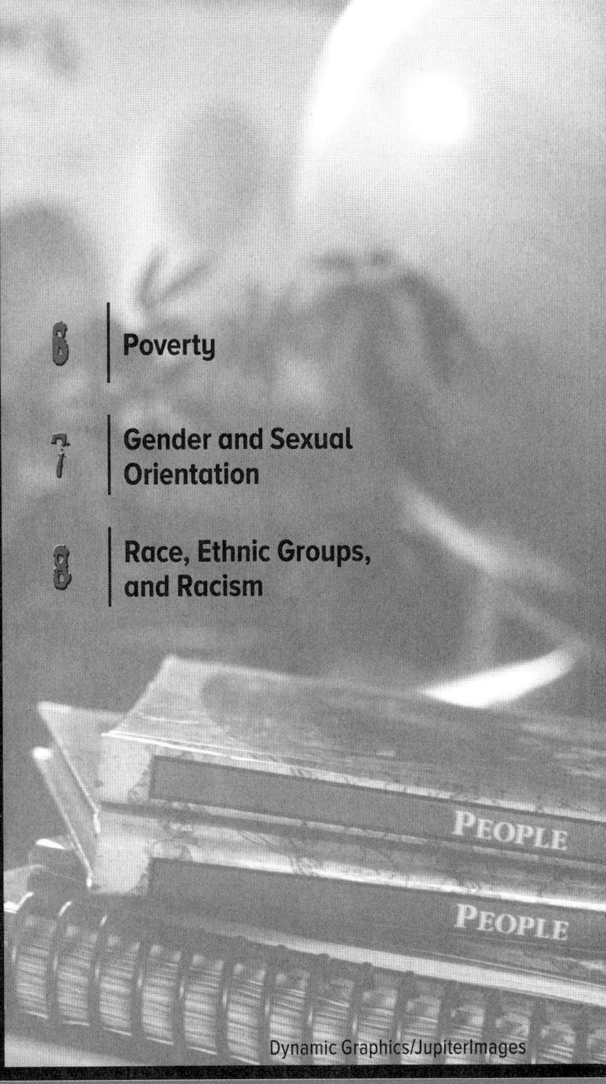




Dynamic Graphics/JupiterImages

The next three chapters address inequalities in the distribution of things that Americans value. These inequalities are so significant that major segments of the population suffer from serious deprivations. We look first at the unequal distribution of wealth in the United States and discuss the problems of the poor in some detail. Then we examine inequalities experienced by three groups in the population: women, the gay/lesbian community, and racial/ethnic minorities.

The people we focus on in this part are largely victims of inequality because of the circumstances of their birth. That is, they did not choose the socioeconomic status of the family into which they were born, or their gender, or their sexual orientation, or their race or ethnicity. And in contrast to the problems discussed in Part 2, in which people were acting in ways that are contrary to and disapproved of by the vast majority of Americans, those who cope with the problems discussed in this part are more likely to face inequitable treatment by a society whose norms and values they affirm and strive to follow.

CHAPTER

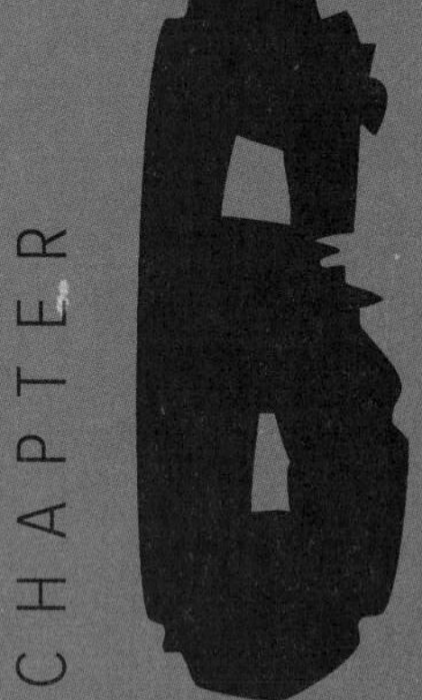

# Poverty

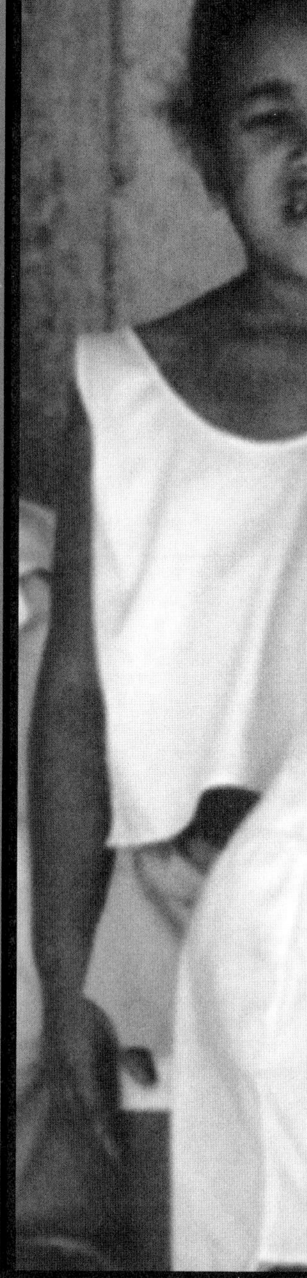

OBJECTIVES

1. Define and discuss the extent of poverty in the United States.
2. Identify the people most likely to be poor.
3. Show how poverty affects basic human rights and needs.
4. Discuss the way in which social institutions contribute to the problem of poverty.
5. Explain how both the attitudes toward the poor and the attitudes of the poor contribute to the perpetuation of poverty.

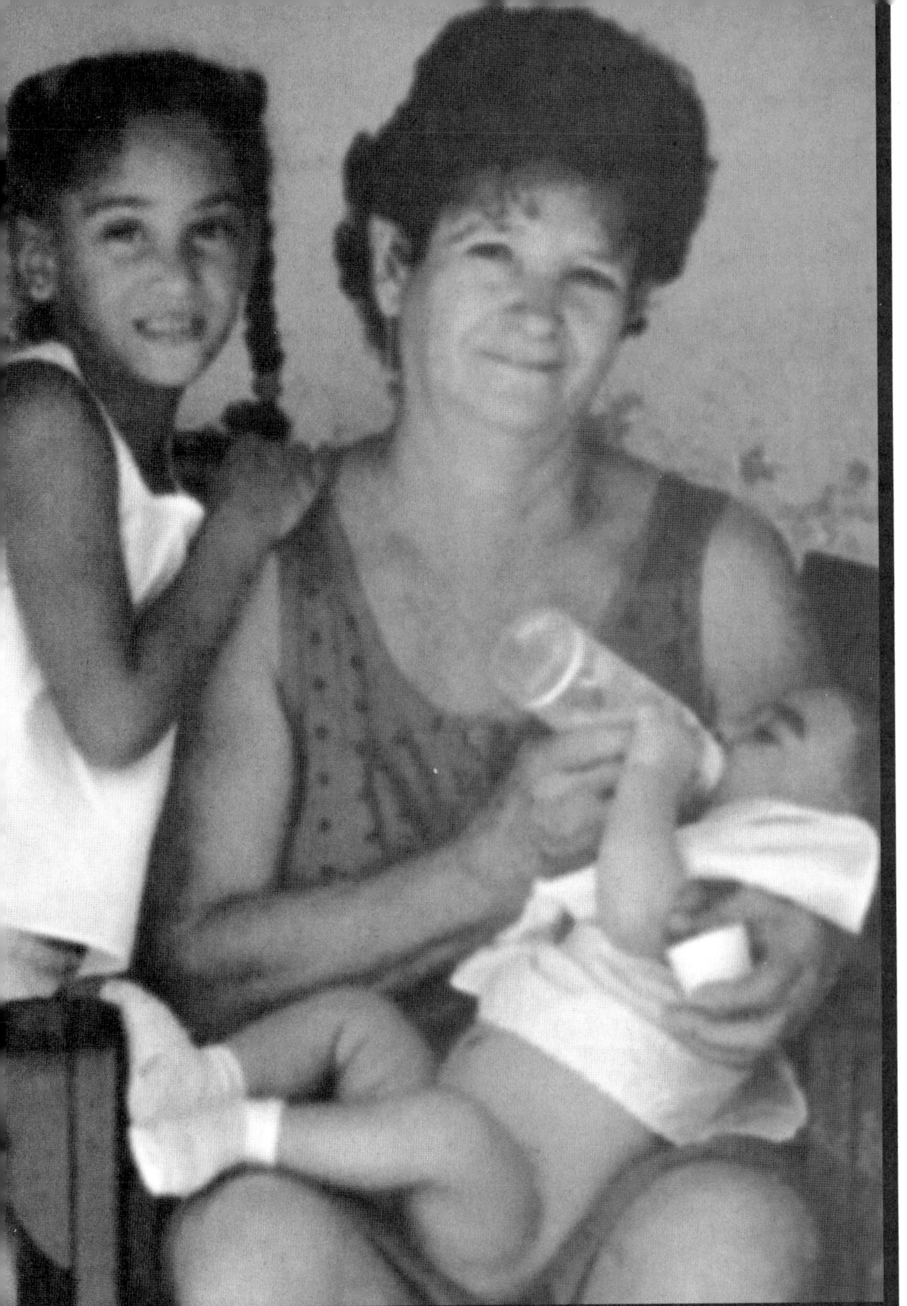

Source: USDA

### "We Feel Like Deadbeats"

Marlene is in her late 30s, married, the mother of two, and poor. Poverty is something new in her life. For some years, her married life resembled the middle-class home in which she was raised. Then an accident forced her to go on long-term disability leave, her husband's business failed, and for the past three years they have lived deep in poverty. Savings, credit, friends, and relatives helped for a while, but now they have reached "the year I lost 25 pounds without even trying":

*We've hit bottom. We have no insurance. We are continually harassed by collection agents. They tell us we're deadbeats. Actually we feel like deadbeats. The first time I really got angry was a few months ago when I saw a guy with a toy attached to his car window. I knew that toy cost around $15, and I could feel the anger rising in me as I thought about how much food I could buy with $15.*

*I thought about my kids, who now are getting used to strange combinations of vegetables and rice or noodles, and how much they would enjoy the meal I could buy. And all of a sudden I was enraged at someone I didn't even know for spending so much money on a joke. Then it made me mad that $15 seemed like so much money. Then it made me mad that I had gotten mad.*

*I started watching the expensive cars go by when I was walking or taking a bus. It's like they were advertising the fact that they made it and I haven't. I've never had that kind of car, but it bothered me that other people did. Suddenly I began to take their arrogance personally. And when I read about a guy paying*

*$20,000 for a watch, I wondered if he was part of the human race. How could he do that when there were hungry kids living just a few miles away?*

*I've gotten to the point where I see that without money, a person just doesn't matter. I thought I was a pretty knowledgeable person, but I had no idea of the violent, demoralizing effect of poverty. I had no idea how it would feel to have no food in the house, no gas to drive to buy food, no money to buy gas, and no prospect of money. My husband and I believe we'll pull out of this. But I have a dread in my bones that the worst is not over yet, and that even when it is over, it will never be altogether in the past for any of us.*

## Introduction

A wealthy car dealer who was elected to Congress sought to lower taxes on the rich and retain tax breaks for corporations, and he questioned the value of unemployment checks for workers who lost their jobs (Whoriskey 2011). He explained his own wealth as the result of working hard all his life. No doubt the man did work hard. But he didn't mention all his initial advantages: the fact that his father had owned a car dealership, that he had attended an elite university, and that a few years after graduation he married an heiress to an oil fortune.

He sees himself as an example of the fulfillment of the American dream. But his attitudes about wealth and poverty are part of an American myth—that through persistent hard work anyone can succeed. The pursuit of the American dream is far more complex than the simple faith in persistent hard work suggests. In this chapter we examine that segment of the population for whom the American dream has been elusive and see how the difficulties of the poor are related to the behavior of the nonpoor. To understand why the poor are poor, it is important to understand why the rich are rich.

We discuss what is meant by poverty, identify who the poor are and how many there are, and examine how poverty affects the quality of life. After we identify the structural and social psychological factors that contribute to poverty, we consider what has been done and what might be done to address the problem.

## What Is Poverty?

Poverty in the United States is old and new. It is old in the sense that it has always existed, and it is new in the sense that it was not *commonly defined* as a problem until more recently. As late as the 1950s, economists assumed that, economically, Americans were consistently improving. They were producing more and incomes were increasing. The question about poverty was not *whether* but *when* it would be eliminated. Although sociologists have always identified poverty as a problem, the Gallup poll showed that not until 1965 did the public begin to identify it as one of America's serious problems (Lauer 1976). An influential factor in creating an awareness of the problem was a book by Michael Harrington (1962), *The Other America.* Harrington portrayed the plight of millions of impoverished people in affluent America.

What, exactly, is poverty? **Poverty** is a state in which income is insufficient to provide basic necessities such as food, shelter, medical care, and clothing. *Absolute poverty* means that the insufficiency is so severe that it is life-threatening. *Relative poverty* means that the insufficiency is substantially greater than that of most others in the society.

**poverty**
a state in which income is insufficient to provide the basic necessities of food, shelter, clothing, and medical care

Why did Americans generally fail to identify poverty as a social problem until the 1960s? One reason is that the poor were largely invisible to many Americans. Another reason is many people failed to make the distinction between absolute and relative poverty; they insisted that even the lowest-income groups in America were not really poor because they fared better than the starving people in other countries.

To be sure, many of America's poor have more food, more clothing, better shelter, and so on than the poor in other nations; but the standard for evaluating America's poor cannot be the starving people in other nations. Rather, poverty in the United States must be evaluated in terms of the *standard of living* attained by the majority of Americans. To tell a poor American whose family suffers from malnutrition that people in other nations are starving to death is not consoling, particularly when the poor person knows that millions of Americans throw away more food every day than that person's family consumes.

In discussing poverty in the United States, then, we are talking about people who are better off than some others in the world but who have much less than most Americans. But less of what? And how much less? The federal government answers these questions in terms of *income.* In the 1960s, the Department of Agriculture developed an "economy food plan" for temporary or emergency use when a family's financial resources were minimal. At the time, the poor spent an estimated one-third of their total budget on food. The government, therefore, simply multiplied the cost of the economy food plan by 3 and came up with the dividing line between "poor" and "nonpoor." In 1964, that meant a family of four with an income below $3,000 per year was officially classified as at the **poverty level.** By 2019, a family of four (two adults and two children) with an annual income less than $25,750 was officially poor.

**poverty level**
the minimum income level that Americans should have to live on, based on the Department of Agriculture's calculations of the cost of a basic diet called "the economy food plan"

This method of defining poverty is considered woefully inadequate by many social scientists. For one thing, it ignores the cost-of-living differences between various areas. For another, it puts millions of Americans above the poverty level even though they cannot afford what most of us would regard as a minimal standard of living.

Finally, the official poverty level uses a nutritionally inadequate food plan as a primary criterion, bases any increases on the **consumer price index,** and maintains the ratio of food to nonfood costs at one-third. But Americans now spend an average of about 10 percent of their income on food (U.S. Census Bureau website). The relative costs of other items, such as housing, have increased considerably since the 1960s. Thus, you could argue that the poverty level should be eight times the cost of food, which would raise substantially the proportion of Americans who are poor.

**consumer price index**
a measure of the average change in prices of all types of consumer goods and services purchased by urban wage earners and clerical workers

Because of the clear inadequacies of the existing definition, the Census Bureau released a new Supplemental Poverty Measure in 2011 (Aguilera 2011). This measure takes into account such factors as regional differences in the cost of living, child care expenses for working parents, and government benefits such as food stamps. The Supplemental Poverty Measure changes the proportion of the poor in various groups (such as age groups, racial/ethnic groups), raising the rates in some groups and lowering them in others. But it tends to increase somewhat the rate for the nation as a whole.

For example, an analysis of the 2013 numbers found that the Supplemental rate was 0.9 percent higher than the official rate (Short 2014). But the Supplemental rate for those under 18 was lower than the official rate for that group, It was also lower for

African Americans than was the official rate. For other groups, the Supplemental rate increased the proportion who were poor.

Many scholars would argue that even the Supplemental Poverty Measure underestimates the number of people who should be considered poor. For whether the official or the new measure is used, the definition *excludes many people who define themselves, and whom most of you would define, as poor.* It isn't known yet whether the Supplemental Poverty Measure will replace the official measure, but as of this writing government and scholarly writings use the official measure, so that is what we shall use in the remainder of this chapter.

Consider now three questions concerning the *extent of poverty* in the United States: How many poor are there? Who are the poor? Are the majority of the poor better off or worse off now than they were in the past?

## Extent of Poverty

The proportion of Americans officially defined as poor has fluctuated over time. The rate declined substantially from 1960 through the 1970s, then rose again and has fluctuated ever since (Figure 6.1). By 2019, 34 million Americans were officially in poverty, representing 10.5 percent of the population. The United States has one of the highest rates of poverty among the rich industrial nations of the world.

A caution—one dealt with in the previous section—is that the official figures minimize the number of poor. Many of you would probably consider yourselves poor if your income were just above the official poverty level. The Census Bureau defines "near" poverty as between 100 and 125 percent of the poverty threshold

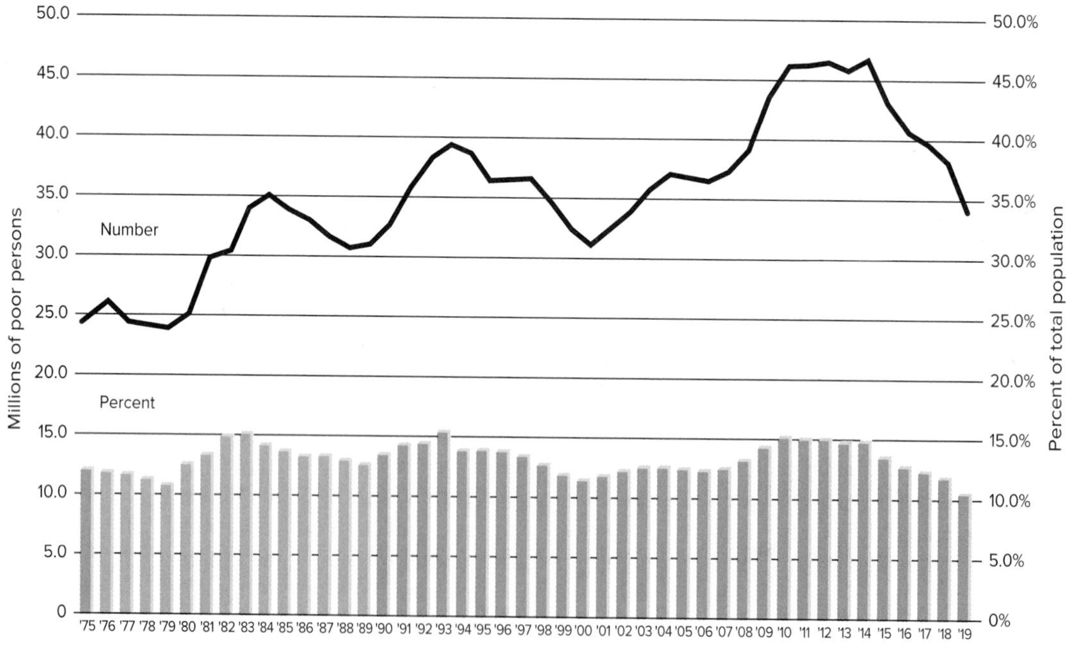


**FIGURE 6.1** The Number and Proportion of the Poor, 1970–2019.

Source: Semega et al. 2020.

(Hokayem and Heggeness 2014). People in that range will likely have an ongoing struggle with making ends meet and satisfying their basic needs. In 2012, there were nearly 15 million Americans living in "near" poverty.

One other caution: Most of those in poverty are an ever-changing group. That is, there are people who are not now poor but will be and people who are not now poor but have been. In other words, there is always movement into and out of poverty, so the number of poor at any given time does not reveal the total number of people who will be affected by the problem during their lifetime. For example, during the four-year period from 2009 to 2012, 34.5 percent of the population had at least one period of poverty that lasted two or more months (Proctor, Semega, and Kollar 2016). Only 2.7 percent of Americans lived in poverty for the entire 48 months. Such figures indicate that poverty will be a part of the experience of a majority of Americans at some point in their lives.

## Who Are the Poor?

Wealth and poverty are *not distributed equally* among various social groups. Most Americans are neither wealthy nor impoverished, but the chances of being in one of these categories are greater for certain social groups. For example, the probability of being poor is greater for families headed by a female, for racial and ethnic minorities, and for those under 18 years of age (see Figure 6.2). Single-parent families headed by mothers are the most impoverished group in the nation. About a fourth of American children live in those single-mother families, which is why the United States has one of the highest rates of children in poverty among developed nations (Kramer 2019).

Among those racial/ethnic minorities for whom the Census Bureau regularly collects and publishes data, African Americans have the highest poverty rate (18.8 percent in 2019). If we

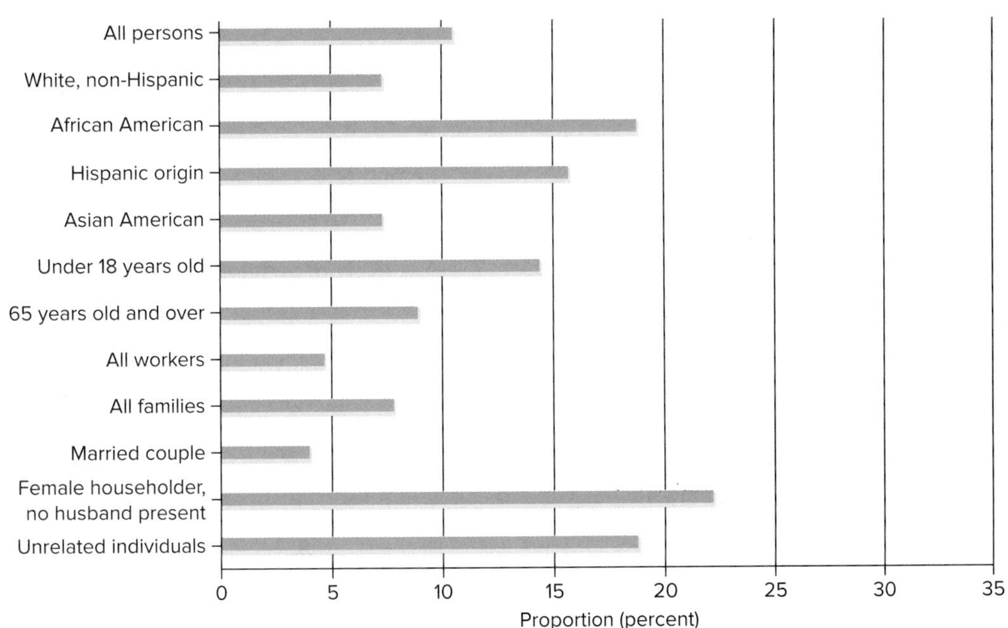


**FIGURE 6.2** Proportion of Poverty for Different Kinds of People.

Source: Semega et al. 2020.

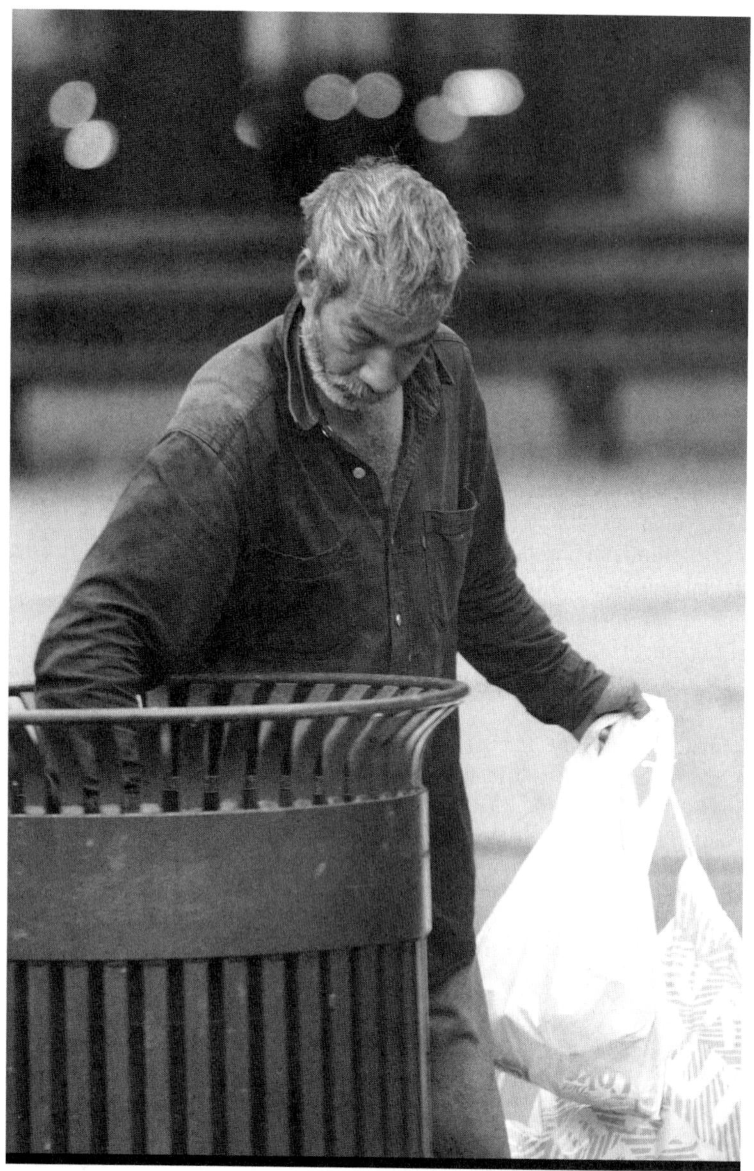

A homeless person digs through garbage in an attempt to survive.

Gary He/McGraw Hill

look at absolute numbers rather than rates, the racial/ethnic group with the largest number of poor is non-Hispanic whites (because the white population is so much larger than that of other races). In 2019, for example, the number (and rates) of poverty were as follows: non-Hispanic whites, 14.2 million (7.3 percent); African Americans, 8.1 million (18.8 percent); Asian Americans, 1.5 million (7.3 percent); and Hispanics, 9.6 million (15.7 percent) (Semega et al. 2020).

Note that above we pointed out that African Americans have the highest poverty rate of any racial/ethnic minority for whom the Census Bureau regularly collects and publishes data. However, the Census Bureau website lists the latest available numbers at 18.5 percent of Native American families and 23.0 percent of all individual Native Americans living in poverty. In general, Native Americans continue to have the highest rates of poverty of any ethnic/racial group. Even the proliferation of tribal casinos has not sufficed to dramatically improve their lot (Davis, Roscigno, and Wilson 2016).

In short, the *number* of poor whites is substantially higher than the number of poor Hispanics or poor African Americans or poor Native Americans, but the *rate of poverty* among whites is substantially lower than that among the other groups (see Figure 6.2). These data are the basis for what sounds like a paradoxical statement: If you are white, you are less likely to be poor than if you are nonwhite, but if you are poor, you are more likely to be white than nonwhite.

Figure 6.2 also shows the high rate of poverty among youths under age 18. This *high rate of poverty among children* is something new in American history, and it is the highest rate among the industrial countries of the world (Duncan and Magnuson 2011). One out of every five American children below the age of 18 lives in poverty. The highest rate occurs among non-Hispanic Black children living in small cities (10,000 to 50,000 population)—47 percent (Forum on Child and Family Statistics 2020).

Finally, the rate of poverty is higher outside (13.3 percent) than inside (10.0 percent) metropolitan areas (Semega et al. 2020). Extensive rural poverty is one reason many Americans are unaware of the seriousness of the problem. The rural poor are even less visible than those in urban **ghettoes.**

**ghetto**
an area in which a certain group is segregated from the rest of society; often used today to refer to the impoverished area of the inner city

Although people move into and out of poverty, there is also a core of people who remain in poverty, an underclass that experiences unemployment, substandard housing, chronic hunger, and **malnutrition** (Hoefer and Curry 2012). Insufficient food increases depression and suicide attempts and it inhibits cognitive and psychological development (Alaimo, Olson, and Frongillo 2001, 2002). The underclass is only a minority of the poor, but it presents the nation with poverty's most serious challenge—how to deal with those who seem caught in the throes of poverty on a more or less permanent basis.

**malnutrition** inadequate food, in amount or type

*The Working Poor.* An additional fact about the identity of the poor is important. Contrary to popular opinion, people are not poor simply because of their *unwillingness to work.* A good many of the poor do not work, to be sure, but they include people who can't find a job, the disabled, the elderly, and single parents who would have to pay more for child care than they would earn in the jobs available to them. Many of those who are not working both want, and intend, to find a job at some point that will enable them to support themselves and their families. As a young single mother told us:

> I know the stereotype of a welfare mother. Well, that's not me. I don't sit around watching TV. I work 40 hours a week, go to college at night, and have worked and paid taxes since I was a teenager. I don't intend to be on welfare all my life, but I just don't have a choice right now.

Who are those Americans who are working but still poor? In 2019, 18.7 million people living in poverty had some kind of work experience during the year (Semega et al. 2020). Among those 2.3 million worked full time during the year, and another five million worked year-round but not full time. African Americans and Hispanics were more than twice as likely as whites and Asians to be among the working poor. Finally, the working poor tended to have less education than the nonpoor and were more likely than other workers to be in a service occupation.

Even though they work millions of Americans suffer all the usual consequences of poverty. For example, two-thirds of low-income Americans find it hard to pay for the food they need (Jacobe 2008). In some cases, they may forgo certain food purchases to pay for other necessities; the combination of work income and government assistance is insufficient for their needs, and they must make frequent trips to free food distribution organizations (Berner, Ozer, and Paynter 2008).

*The Homeless.* The homeless are those who live in their cars or on the streets because they cannot afford any kind of housing. The very lack of a stable, identifiable residence makes it difficult to know exactly how many Americans are homeless. The National Alliance to End Homelessness (2020) estimates that there were 567,715 homeless people in 2019. This represents a decline from previous years. And most of the homeless stay in a shelter or in transitional housing; only a third are on the street or in abandoned buildings. A majority of the homeless are individuals, but 30.2 percent were families and 6.2 percent were youth or children on their own.

The chronically homeless will die on the streets. Those who are not chronically homeless may spend anywhere from months to a few years on the street. Those who are homeless for a shorter period of time are likely to be younger, earn income, have family support, and lack a history of arrest or addiction (Caton et al. 2005).

Many homeless women are on the streets because they fled from domestic violence. One study concluded that one out of four homeless women left her home because of the abuse she suffered (Jasinski et al. 2010). These women decided that living on the streets would be preferable to the ongoing violence in their homes. Tragically, many find that their lives on the streets offer no more safety from violence than did their lives in homes. A survey of homeless young people in Columbus, Ohio, reported that among those who were in an intimate relationship, about a third experienced verbal and/or physical abuse (Slesnick et al. 2010).

High rates of mental illness, addictions, and victimization exist among the homeless (National Coalition for the Homeless 2009). At least a fourth of the homeless struggle with some kind of serious mental illness: As many as 4 out of 10 homeless adults are addicted to alcohol, and a fourth or more have problems with other kinds of drugs. The homeless suffer a disproportionate rate of street crimes, including assault, robbery, and theft (Ellsworth 2019). They are also vulnerable to being victimized by hate crimes (National Coalition for the Homeless 2016). A number of homeless people are beaten or even killed each year. Most victims and perpetrators are male.

People are not homeless, then, simply because they prefer the streets to gainful employment. Some, like the children and the mentally ill, cannot support themselves. Others are victims of the economy. Home and rental costs have soared in recent decades. Millions of Americans now spend half or more of their income on housing. This means that the homeless, who often work for minimum or near-minimum wages, can't get any kind of housing even if they could spend half their income on it. People who work for the federal minimum wage would need two or three times that much just to rent a home in an urban area. Some states have minimum wage requirements higher than the federal level, but none are sufficient to cover housing costs. Thus, families throughout the nation are at risk of homelessness if they are supported by a single, low-wage worker. Any kind of unexpected, additional financial burden can result in eviction from rental property or the loss of a home (Desmond and Kimbro 2015; West and Mottola 2016).

## The Changing Nature of Poverty

How has the lot of the poor changed over time in the United States? Certainly the proportion of Americans who are poor is lower than it was in the past—but are those who are poor now in better or worse condition than the poor of other generations? Although we have no systematic evidence on the question, it seems reasonable that poverty is more difficult when the proportion becomes smaller. It is one thing to be poor when the majority of people, or even a substantial minority, share your poverty. It is another thing to be poor when most people are living comfortably or in affluence.

Still, if the poor were making gains relative to the rich, poverty might be less stressful than in the past. Unfortunately, they are not. Table 6.1 shows the percentage of income received by people in various income brackets. In 2019, for example, those at the top 20 percent got 51.9 percent of the income, which is two and a half times the amount they would have gotten if there had been perfect equality (no "top" or "bottom"). Moreover, their share of the total income has increased since 1970. Note, in contrast, what has happened to the bottom 40 percent. Their share of income has dropped substantially. In other words, the poor have lost ground relative to the rest of the population for nearly five decades.

**TABLE 6.1**
Distribution of Money Income of Households, Ranked According to Income Received, 1929–2019 (percent of aggregate income)

| | 1929 | 1941 | 1950 | 1960 | 1970 | 1980 | 1990 | 2000 | 2019 |
|---|---|---|---|---|---|---|---|---|---|
| Lowest 40% | 12.5 | 13.6 | 16.4 | 17.0 | 17.6 | 16.7 | 15.4 | 14.1 | 11.4 |
| Next 40% | 33.1 | 37.6 | 40.8 | 41.8 | 41.4 | 41.8 | 40.4 | 38.3 | 36.8 |
| Highest 20% | 54.4 | 48.8 | 42.8 | 41.3 | 40.9 | 41.6 | 44.3 | 47.4 | 51.9 |
| Top 5% | 30.0 | 24.0 | 17.3 | 15.9 | 15.6 | 15.3 | 17.4 | 20.8 | 23.0 |

SOURCES: U.S. Census Bureau 1961, 1976, 2012; Semega et al. 2020.

Although, as Table 6.1 shows, the richest are getting a smaller proportion of income than they did before World War II, it is important to keep in mind that money income is only a part of the wealth of the rich, and for many it is not the most important part. Net wealth is all assets minus all liabilities. Assets include real estate, savings and checking accounts, investments, and retirement accounts. Liabilities include all indebtedness—mortgages, unpaid loans and bills, and so forth. The inequality in the distribution of wealth is greater than that in income. The Board of Governors of the Federal Reserve System (2020) put a dollar figure on wealth and came up with the following:

- The top 1 percent have $31.39 trillion.
- The top 90 to 99 percent have $40.31 trillion.
- The top 50 to 90 percent have $31.05 trillion.
- The bottom 50 percent have $1.9 trillion.

In brief, the United States has a greater gap between the rich and the poor than does any other industrial nation.

We should also note that the rich fare better than others both in a good economy and in a recession. During the severe recession from 2007 to 2009, the share of wealth of the top 20 percent increased by 2.2 percent, whereas that of the bottom 80 percent decreased by 2.2 percent.

In sum, in terms of income there has been a redistribution, but it has not benefitted the poor. Rather, the middle- and upper-middle groups are the beneficiaries of income redistribution. Since the late 1960s, the upper 20 percent have made gains in both income and total wealth at the expense of the lower 80 percent. Much of this gain is due to good luck rather than hard work, for "the majority of new wealth arises from short-term speculative investments, such as hedge funds" (Anderson 2009:72). The result is a dramatic accumulation and concentration of wealth at the top. Since 1980, there are hundreds of new billionaires and millions of new millionaires. And the pay for CEOs has jumped from roughly 30 to 40 times that of the average worker in past years to 361 times that of the average worker in 2017 (AFL-CIO 2018). When you try, therefore, to assess the meaning of poverty in the United States, you must recognize that although the proportion of the poor is less than it was in the twentieth century, the lot of the poor is worse when compared with the rest of society. Americans who are poor today may have more possessions than the poor of 1920, but they are worse off relative to others in the society than were their counterparts in 1920.

## Poverty and the Quality of Life

Some sense of the trauma of living in poverty, even if you assume that it is only a temporary state, may be seen in the account of Marlene (see "We Feel Like Deadbeats," at the beginning of the chapter). In essence, the trauma arises from the fact that the poor get less of everything considered important and necessary for a decent life (less money, food, clothing, and shelter). The *deprivation of the poor is pervasive* (Samaan 2000; Rank 2001). Compared to infants of the nonpoor, infants of the poor are more likely to die. Their children are more likely to fail in school even when they are intelligent. Their children are more likely to drop out of school. They are more likely to become mentally ill. They are more likely to lose their jobs and to drop out of the labor force. They are more likely to experience hostility and distrust rather than neighborliness with those around them. They are less likely to participate in meaningful groups and associations. They are more likely to get chronic illnesses. In the face of more health problems, they are less likely to own health insurance (a problem only partly relieved by Medicaid). In the ultimate deprivation, they are likely to die at a younger age. Thus, poverty diminishes the quality of a person's life in many ways.

## The Right to Life and Happiness

*The position of the poor in the economy contradicts the American value of the right to life and the pursuit of happiness.* The inadequacy of their financial resources deprives the poor of freedom to pursue a full and happy life. Some people argue that lack of money should not be equated with lack of happiness, that many of the poor are carefree, spontaneous, and even better off without the worries that accompany possession of money. It's generally only people with money who use this argument. There is, in fact, a positive correlation between income and *perceived happiness.* Surveys of attitudes both in the United States and in 55 other nations show that the proportion of people who describe themselves as very happy is lower among those in the lower-income than those in the middle- and upper-income groups (Pew Research Center 2006; Ball and Chernova 2008; Alderson and Katz-Cerro 2016). Poverty brings *more despair than happiness and more fear than fullness of life.*

*Discontent and Despair.* When deprivation was widespread during the Great Depression of the 1930s, unrest was also widespread. People marched and demonstrated, demanding food and expressing a willingness to fight rather than starve. In a 1932 Chicago demonstration there were "no bands" and "no quickstep," only "rank after rank of sodden men, their worn coat collars turned up, their caps . . . pulled down to give as much protection as possible" as they marched in driving rain (Hutchinson 1962:274).

The multitude of problems and frustrations of poverty—crowded, dilapidated housing in crime-ridden neighborhoods; inadequate health care; constant financial strain; poor-quality and inadequate food; lack of opportunities for betterment; and so on—are so overwhelming that the impoverished individual may suffer from chronic depression. Low-income mothers, for example, are likely to be depressed, which adversely affects the development of their children (Petterson and Albers 2001). The children are stressed not only by the negative emotions of their parents, but by high rates of family turmoil and disruption, violence, and the lack of order and routine in their lives (Evans, Brooks-Gunn, and Klebanov 2011).

Despair is not the lot of all the poor, but it is much more frequent among the poor than among the nonpoor. When the despair comes, it can be devastating, and it can strike even the young. Consider Elaine, a teenager whose mother was a chronic alcoholic. Elaine lived in poverty with her grandmother in an urban apartment. She watched television 10 or more hours a day, even though the television only increased her depression because it continually reminded her of how much she lacked. Despite her superior intelligence, Elaine always felt extremely ashamed in school:

> "If I only had some clothes." Today Elaine . . . [is] dressed in neatly ironed jeans that are badly frayed at the cuffs and worn thin. On top she wears a stained cheerleader's sweater, out in one elbow, which she has had since she was thirteen. Despite its holes and stains, Elaine wears the sweater every day. It reminds her, she says, of a time when she was happy (Williams and Kornblum 1985:8).

global comparison

## POVERTY IN THE WORLD SYSTEM

Gross inequalities exist not only within most nations but also between the nations of the world. There are various ways in which we could characterize the inequalities: average family income, average life span, expenditures for health care or education, and so on. Figure 6.3 shows one measure—the gross national income per capita. Keep in mind that a high figure does not mean that everyone in the society is rich, nor does a low figure mean that everyone is poor. Every society has inequality. And the extent of the inequality, as measured by the gap in income between the richest 10 percent and the poorest 10 percent, has increased in recent decades.

As Figure 6.3 illustrates, the inequality between nations is as dramatic as the inequality within nations. Switzerland's national income of $85,500 per capita is 143 times higher than the $600 figure for Ethiopia. People in richer nations have seven or more times as many physicians per 1,000 population as those in poorer nations. The infant mortality rates in the poorer nations range from 5 to 30 times higher than those in the richer nations. More than a billion people suffer from hunger and malnutrition in the poorer nations, and the life expectancy of people in the richer nations is generally 15 to 20 years higher than in the poorer nations. A child born in the United States in 2010 could expect to live to age 78; a child born in Afghanistan, Angola, or Mozambique could expect to live less than 45 years.

In other words, the people of poorer nations suffer the kinds of deprivations that afflict the very poorest people in the United States. The number of the poor throughout the world is staggering. More than 1 billion of the earth's population live on $1 a day or less, particularly in South Asia and sub-Saharan Africa. Those who earn $2 a day or more are in the top half of the income distribution! And the disparity between the rich and the poor nations is increasing. The richest 10 percent of people in the world now get over half of all the income, whereas the poorest 50 percent get less than 10 percent. Even though many of the poor live in agricultural societies, hundreds of millions have inadequate shelter, food, and medical care. They lack safe drinking water and educational opportunities for their children. And millions die every year simply because they are too poor to survive.

SOURCES: Lauer 1991; Gardner and Halweil 2000; Bowles, Durlauf, and Hoff 2006; U.S. Census Bureau 2012.

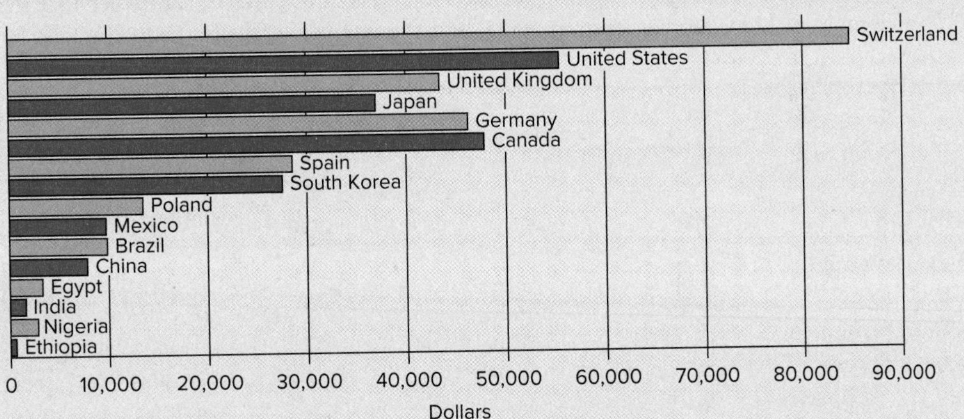


**FIGURE 6.3** Gross National Income Per Capita for Selected Countries.
Source: World Bank website, 2020.

The despair that always threatens to overcome the poor is manifested in what Rainwater's (1967) classic study called *survival strategies*—ways of living that enable the poor to adapt to their "punishing and depriving milieu." The *expressive strategy* involves manipulating others and making oneself appealing through means such as bettering someone in a rap session, gaining the affection of a female, wearing dramatic clothes, or winning a gambling bet. The *violent strategy* involves actions such as fighting, shoplifting, or making threats. It is a dangerous strategy for everyone, and not many of the poor adopt it. The *depressive strategy,* which involves withdrawal and isolation, characterizes a great number of the poor as they grow older. An individual may alternate among the strategies as he or she grows older, but all three strategies have the same purpose—to enable the individual to cope with a punitive situation. As such, they dramatize the despair that always hovers near the poor.

*Freedom from Fear.* We mentioned in Chapter 5 that freedom from fear is a condition of the right to life and the pursuit of happiness. The poor live in a *capricious world.* The chronic uncertainty of their lives means they have much to fear. We discuss this topic further under the subheading "Dilemmas of Poverty" later in this chapter. Here we look at two kinds of fear that affect the poor more than others—the *fear of being the victim of a crime* and the *fear of being harassed by law enforcement officers.*

As Table 6.2 shows, the poor are more likely than other people to be victims of crime. The table shows rates for property crimes, but the poor are also more victimized more than others by violent crime. In 2019, the rate (per 1,000 people age 12 and older) of being victimized by a crime was 37.8 percent of those with less than $25,000 annual income. For those with $200,000 or more annual income the rate was 18.0 (Morgan and Truman 2020). The poor are, of course, aware of the high crime rates in the areas where they live, and so they typically express a greater fear of walking alone at night than do the well-to-do.

The fear of being harassed by law enforcement officers is particularly a problem for the homeless (National Coalition for the Homeless 2006). We noted earlier that the number of homeless has been growing, and the number of shelter beds available for

| | Victimizations per 1,000 Households | | | |
|---|---|---|---|---|
| Household Income Level | Total | Burglary | Auto Theft | Theft |
| Less than $7,500 | 168.7 | 44.4 | 4.0 | 120.4 |
| $7,500—14,999 | 170.4 | 47.2 | 5.9 | 117.3 |
| $15,000—24,999 | 144.9 | 32.8 | 8.3 | 103.7 |
| $25,000—34,999 | 133.9 | 27.1 | 7.4 | 99.4 |
| $35,000—49,999 | 120.5 | 21.6 | 5.9 | 93.1 |
| $50,000—74,999 | 115.4 | 19.1 | 5.9 | 90.4 |
| $75,000 or more | 119.3 | 16.7 | 5.1 | 97.5 |

**TABLE 6.2**

Property Crime Victimizations, by Income

SOURCE: U.S. Department of Justice 2011.

them is inadequate. Faced with the growing numbers, many cities have now criminalized the problem of the homeless by prohibiting such things as sleeping, camping, eating, sitting, or begging in public places and using the ordinances to punish the homeless. Some cities even use laws against loitering or having open containers against the homeless. Finally, there have been sweeps of areas where the homeless live. The homeless are driven out and their personal property may be destroyed.

## The Right to Dignity as a Human Being

For the poor, the *right to dignity as human beings* is violated by the *contradiction between the American ideal of the worth of every individual and the pattern of interaction between the poor and the nonpoor.* At best, the poor tend to be treated paternalistically. At worst, they tend to be subjected to contempt and rejection, and blamed for their plight (Cozzarelli, Wilkinson, and Tagler 2001). Ironically, they may be defined as even less deserving in societies with a high degree of inequality (Heiserman and Simpson 2017). This loss of dignity is manifested in a number of myths about the poor, myths that employ the *fallacy of personal attack* to discredit the poor and legitimate an unwillingness to support programs to help them.

fallacy

*"The poor are lazy."* It's a myth that the poor are lazy; they are willing to work, and in fact, most male heads of poor families do work. To say that the poor are lazy justifies the nonpoor's contempt and disavowal of personal or societal responsibility for dealing with poverty. No evidence supports the myth, but it is still prevalent, and it robs the poor of human dignity.

*"People on welfare have it good."* The expressive style of coping may have helped create the myth that people on welfare often live at higher standards than do people who work. A few "con artists" may manage to get a substantial living by *welfare fraud,* but the majority of people on welfare (and the majority of the poor in general) live in circumstances that would be repugnant to most Americans. What dignity is there, for instance, in not being able to buy adequate food for your children, or in living in a rat-infested apartment, or in huddling inside your apartment at night in fear of thieves and drug addicts?

And what kind of dignity is there in trying to survive on welfare payments that may mean an income far below the poverty level? Many nonpoor Americans have a distorted notion of how much help people receive from welfare. The amount received varies depending on which state you live in, the number in your household, and the working status of household members (Dautovic 2020). In any case, the amount received is barely sufficient just to survive. For example, the Supplemental Nutrition Assistance Program (previously known as food stamps) allowed $680 a month for a family of four. That works out to be about $2.40 per meal per person, which is hardly having "it good."

*"Welfare is draining us."* One myth by which the poor are humiliated is that they are social leeches. This myth asserts that the cost of maintaining the poor is depriving the nonpoor by raising taxes and reducing the standard of living. As we noted, however, the poor receive a lower share of national income now than they did in the early twentieth century. Historically, welfare payments have done little to reduce the inequity, and the standard of living for middle- and upper-class Americans is higher than ever. A large number of Americans now possess two or more automobiles and television sets, items that were luxuries in the not-too-distant past.

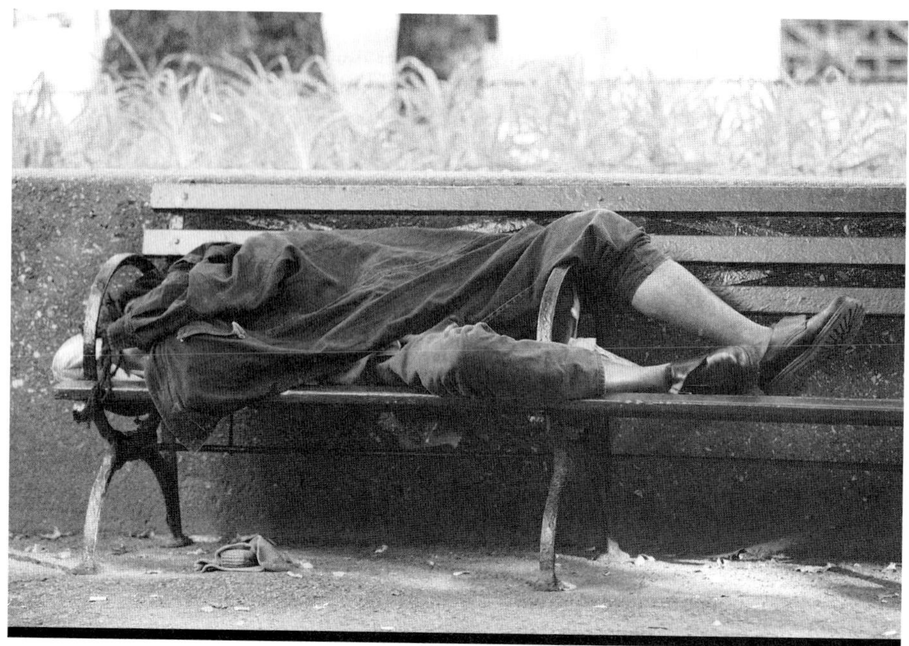

The poor, especially the homeless, lose their dignity as human beings.

Gary He/McGraw Hill

*"Welfare turns people into lazy, dependent deadbeats."* "Welfare bums" is the term used by some Americans to show their contempt for people who rely on welfare rather than on their own earnings. Even with the change to "workfare" (discussed later in this chapter), people who receive government aid are still regarded by many Americans as lazy and unmotivated, preferring a "free ride" at the expense of Americans who work (Lauter 2016).

This myth ignores certain important facts. First, most of the people on welfare are not able-bodied workers. Well over half of welfare recipients are children, the aged, the disabled, or mothers of small children (some of whom work).

Second, as shown by a number of studies, the able-bodied workers generally prefer to work rather than to be on welfare. In-depth interviews with 47 recipients of Temporary Assistance to Needy Families (TANF), previously Aid to Families with Dependent Children (AFDC), found that the recipients were eager for welfare reform and were supportive of work requirements (Seccombe, Walters, and James 1999).

Third, there is very little long-term dependency among welfare recipients. In fact, as we pointed out earlier, there is a *good deal of movement in and out of poverty.* Only one of four children who spend most of their growing-up years in poverty is still poor at age 25 to 29.

## Poverty and Health

The circumstances under which the poor are required to live cause higher rates of mental and physical illness among the poor than among the rest of the population (Chen, Matthews, and Boyce 2002; Price, Khubchandani, and Webb 2018). The *homeless are particularly prone to ill health.* A substantial proportion of the homeless suffer from various physical ailments, hunger, malnutrition, drug addiction, and mental illness (Stratigos and

## FROM RICHES TO RAGS

In a now-famous experiment, a reporter had his skin darkened and his hair shaved close, and then he began traveling through four southern states to see what it was like to be a Black man. It was a revelation to him. Some nights, he reported, he was so upset by the way people treated him that he cried himself to sleep.

There are times when the only way to understand what a social problem means for the victims is to "walk a mile in their shoes." This project will involve you in a personal experience of poverty, but you will find it easier to do if you work with someone else.

First, try to live for two weeks on a poverty-level food budget. In the latest figures from the U.S. Census Bureau, find the current poverty-level income threshold. (Remember, this is the most you can have to be classified as living in poverty.) Use the figure given for a nonfarm family of two, and divide it by three to get a yearly food budget comparable to the way the poverty level was originally defined. Divide that figure by 26 to get the two-week budget. For example, in 2019 the poverty level for two people under the age of 65 was $16,240—about $5,413.33 for food. For the two weeks of the experiment, that amounts to $208.20 for food for you and your partner.

As a second part of your experiment, dress in some shabby clothing. Try to achieve a poor though clean look. Then, go to a public place and ask directions. Also go into a department store and ask for help in finding some relatively expensive clothes.

Record your experiences. Describe in detail your experiences and feelings about grocery shopping, cooking, and eating on a poverty budget. Discuss the reactions you received when asking for directions and when seeking to look at some expensive clothing. Compare the way people related to you with the way you normally experience relationships.

The problem of poverty has received less attention from the mass media in subsequent decades than it did in the 1960s. As a final part of your project, you might share your experience by writing an article that reminds people of the great numbers of poor in the United States. Submit it to the features editor of a local newspaper or a general magazine.



Katsambas 2003; Lee and Greif 2008). It isn't clear, however, whether addiction and mental illness are the *causes* or the *result* of homelessness (Wasserman and Clair 2010). In either case, the health needs of the homeless are unlikely to be met. A national study found that 73 percent of homeless respondents reported at least one unmet health need, including medical and surgical care, medications, mental health care, and dental care (Baggett, O'Connell, Singer, and Rigotti 2010).

Even the poor who are not homeless suffer a disproportionate amount of ill health. Compared to those of the nonpoor, the health problems of the poor are manifested in higher rates of physical illness, infant mortality, clinical depression and other problems with mental health, and difficulty with such daily living tasks as cooking, shopping, managing money, walking, eating, and dressing (Belle 2003; Wheaton and Clarke 2003; Okechukwu et al. 2012; Stewart et al. 2016). Even a short time in poverty damages people's health, and getting out of poverty does not repair all the damage done (McDonough and Berglund 2003). There can be long-term negative consequences for both adults and children. Thus, those who were poor from birth through age 5 are nearly three times as likely as those who were well-to-do to report poor health as adults (Duncan and Magnuson 2011). An Australian study found that children who spent time in poverty in their early years had a greater risk of problems with anxiety and depression when they were examined at age 14 and again at age 21 (Najman et al. 2010).

One possible reason for the long-range consequences may be that people develop poor health habits while they are in poverty (skipping medical checkups and eating cheap but unhealthy food) that tend to persist even if their income rises above the poverty level. Another reason is the higher proportion of the poor who lack health insurance. In 2019, 25.8 percent of the poor had no health insurance (Cohen et al. 2020). The lack of insurance, combined with insufficient medical care facilities in poor areas, means that many of the poor get no medical help until their situation becomes critical or unbearable (Kirby and Kaneda 2005).

Some of the health problems of the poor result from poor nutrition, which, in turn, is related to inadequate income. In 2019, an estimated 10.5 percent of American households were food insecure at least some time during the year (Coleman et al. 2020). That means nearly 13 million American households did not have enough food for an active, healthy life for all household members.

The consequences of inadequate food or of malnutrition are serious (Alaimo, Olson, Frongillo, and Briefel 2001). Food-insecure adults tend to suffer from depression as well as various physical problems (Wu and Schimmele 2005). Food-insecure children are vulnerable to a variety of physical and mental problems. In recent decades, American children have suffered from pellagra, scurvy, rickets, parasitic worms, and mental retardation as a result of prolonged malnutrition. Children who receive an inadequate amount of protein can suffer a variety of maladies, including an inability to concentrate and to learn in school (Kar, Rao, and Chandramouli 2008). Even mild undernutrition can have long-term adverse effects on children's development. Opponents of the welfare system sometimes ask how many children have starved to death in America. The answer is few, if any; but this is little solace to the mother who watches her child grow up with mental or physical deficiencies because of inadequate diet.

Clearly, poverty contradicts the value of good health. The relationship between poverty and health, in fact, is another of the *vicious circles* that often characterize social problems. Because health problems put additional strains on a family's meager financial resources, illness can be perpetuated. Poverty can generate stress that leads to illness that intensifies the stress, and the circle continues.

## Dilemmas of Poverty

**autonomy**
the ability or opportunity to govern oneself

Americans *value* ***autonomy*** *and equal opportunity.* They want to control their own destinies and they want opportunities for advancement. These values are *contradicted* by the realities of poverty. People at the lower end of the stratification system have little control over their lives and have few, if any, opportunities compared to people at the upper end. Poverty is an ongoing series of *dilemmas.* Even when a poor person can choose between options, all the options may have undesirable aspects.

Consider the problems of existing on a poverty budget. Even Americans with incomes that are low but somewhat above the poverty level have to deal with frustrating dilemmas. Matters that would be an inconvenience to people with higher incomes—car problems, illness, appliance breakdowns—can become a crisis for low-income families (Shipler 2004). In fact, anything that adds to the expense of living presents a dilemma to the poor. An unexpected spell of cold weather that raises heating bills means less food for poor parents and their children (Bhattacharya, DeLeire, Haider, and Currie 2003).

Even if a poor family is able to spend the full third of its income on food, how adequate would the food be? What kind of a diet would you have if you existed on the food budget allocated to the poor? The exercise in the Involvement box challenges you to try eating on a poverty-level food budget for two weeks. If you conduct this experiment by yourself rather than with a partner, the 2019 poverty level figure of $12,060 for one person under the age of 65 will allot you $11.04 per day for food. Keep in mind that this figure is for people who are at the top of the poverty scale. Since most of the poor are not at the top, most have less money for food. How much of what you like to eat now would you be able to have? Another way to look at it is that the poor person's food budget for a whole day could be spent at one meal at a fast-food hamburger restaurant. For some of the poor, the choice may be between adequate nutrition and clothes, or between adequate nutrition and medical care. Most students do not face such limited choices.

One of the key dilemmas of the poor is the *choice between security and change.* Should poor individuals maintain whatever security they have or take some risks in order to change their lot? For instance, the ghetto child may be told that the only way to escape poverty is to stay in school and use the education to get a good job, but the only security the child's family may have against utter deprivation is for the child to drop out of school and earn money to add to the family income. At the same time, perhaps the only way the child can be *psychologically secure* is to accept the negative judgments of his or her peers about school. The low value that many of the poor place on intellectual achievement threatens ostracism to any young person who is serious about education. Furthermore, the child has grown up in an unpredictable world and has felt the powerlessness of the individual to change his or her lot in life. Why should the child risk years of schooling (which involves a loss of income) when the payoff is vague and uncertain?

Adults also face dilemmas and the *frustrations of powerlessness.* Consider, for example, the single mother living in poverty who wants to better her lot and that of her children, but who neither has a car nor the resources to get one. In essence, her problem with transportation means that she has restricted access to opportunities for education or work that could lift her and her children out of poverty (Blumenberg and Agrawal 2014). Or consider the incident shared with us by a woman who grew up in poverty in a ghetto area: "When I was a girl, I was given a part in the school play. I was as happy as I could be, and proud to think of my parents watching me perform. But on the night of the play my father got drunk instead of coming to school. I was terribly upset at the time, but later on I realized why he had gotten drunk. He was ashamed to come to the play in the clothes he had, and he didn't have enough money to buy anything new. He didn't know what to do; so he got drunk."

It is easy enough to condemn the man, but remember, the poor live with an agonizing mixture of ambition and powerlessness, of the need for security and the need for change. The security is meager, but the risk of change may appear to be great.

## Contributing Factors

It is true that there always have been poor people. It is also true that poverty is a global problem and that the poor of other nations are worse off in absolute terms than are the poor of America. But why is there any poverty at all in affluent America? In part, this is because a number of structural and social psychological factors that operate to create poverty also tend to perpetuate it.

## Social Structural Factors

The structural factors that bear upon the problem of poverty include the institutional arrangements of government, the economy, the family, and education. We examine each in turn.

*Political Decision Making.* Poverty continues in America, in large part, because of the *distribution of power.* The people who control the wealth are among the most powerful, whereas the poor are among the most powerless in America. As a result, governmental decisions typically reflect the interests of the well-to-do rather than of the poor. Thus, Hacker and Pierson (2010) pointed out that the dramatically disproportionate increase since the 1970s in income received, and wealth accumulated, by the wealthiest of Americans can be explained by a number of government actions: lowered business and corporate taxes, deregulation of financial markets and executive pay, and the weakening of groups such as labor unions that work for the middle class and the poor. All of these actions clearly reflect the interests and enhance the power of the wealthy.

Another problem relates to the location of governmental and nongovernmental agencies that help the poor. These agencies are not always found in the areas where the need is greatest (Allard 2008). It is much more difficult for the poor who live in the more impoverished areas or in areas where racial/ethnic minorities are the majority to get help than it is for those who live in more affluent or white areas.

In addition, the political structure is detrimental to the poor because of the *multiple decision-making centers.* The term *"multiple decision-making centers"* refers to the federal, state, and local governmental levels and also to the multiple branches—executive, legislative, and judicial—at each level. All these facets of government have certain decision-making powers, and all have different constituencies. Most categories or organizations of citizens can exercise influence at some point, but there are also many points at which a program or a policy initiative can be stopped. However, some categories of the population have little influence at any point in this complex, and one such category is the poor.

The political arrangements, therefore, mean that programs designed to help the poor are particularly vulnerable to variation, veto, sabotage, or atrophy through neglect. One such example is the 1967 Medicaid program that was intended to ensure adequate health care for the poor. The program was to be operated by the states, which would set up their own schedules of benefits and definitions of eligibility. The federal government would pay half or more of the costs of the program. States could choose not to participate or to provide fewer benefits than other states. Some states were unwilling to assume any financial responsibility for health care of the poor, so they did not participate. Others set up programs with limited benefits. The majority of the poor are still not covered by Medicaid.

Many other programs have been set up to help the poor. Unfortunately, the failure of these programs to sufficiently reduce or eliminate poverty led to a backlash in the 1990s. The largest assistance program for poor families with children—Aid to Families with Dependent Children—was replaced in 1996 with Temporary Assistance to Needy Families (TANF), which included limited help and work requirements. The exact requirements for receiving help were left to the various states. The amount of help was, and continues to be, so small in many cases that the combined value of TANF benefits and food stamps leave the family far below the poverty level. In fact, since TANF was created in 1996, the benefits have tended to decline. By 2020, if a family had no other source of income, it would be far below the poverty line in all the states (Safawi and Floyd 2020). For example, in 2020, the poverty threshold for a family of three was $21,720. If you lived in Illinois, your TANF benefits would be $6,396. If you lived in Texas, you would have received $3,636. The amount varies from state to state, but in all states it leaves the people far below the poverty line.

Hundreds of thousands of the poor received even less help when government at all levels faced budget crises because of the severe recession that began in 2007. Many states made deep cuts in TANF benefits (Schott and Pavetti 2012). The cuts affected more than a million children who were already living far below the poverty level, and included eliminating the assistance that had been given to families with physical or mental health problems. Some states also cut assistance for child care, making it difficult for poor parents who had jobs to keep them.

*Class Composition of Government.* Regardless of the intentions of the various programs and policies, the work of interest groups and the middle-class composition of government make it unlikely that the poor will greatly benefit or that the middle strata will be greatly hurt by government action. Consider housing. The federal government loses more in revenue by allowing people to deduct mortgage interest from income taxes than it spends on housing programs for low-income Americans. In other words, in the area of housing the well-to-do benefit far more from government programs than do the poor.

Another fact that underscores the *class composition of the government* is that the nonpoor generally benefit as much from the programs designed to help the poor as the poor themselves do. Programs that would help the poor at the expense of other groups are unlikely to be implemented or even proposed. Medicaid helps some of the poor, but it also makes a number of physicians wealthy. Job-training programs help some of the poor, but they also provide high-salaried positions for a number of middle-class administrators.

*Who Benefits from Government?* Given the multiple decision-making centers and the class composition of government, it is not surprising that the middle and upper classes benefit far more from government programs than do the lower class generally and the poor in particular. Some of the poor do not even benefit from programs that were created specifically to help them. One reason is the cumbersome and often bewildering application process. Similarly, other kinds of programs never reach the intended recipients because of inadequate staffing of government offices, complex application processes, and inadequate communication of the availability of the programs. In a survey of low-income parents in Los Angeles County, 51 percent said they were never informed about child care services for which they were eligible, and 52 percent said that the lack of child care caused them to lose a job (National Coalition for the Homeless 2000).

Some benefits do filter down to the poor, but the primary beneficiaries of government decisions and programs are (and always have been) the well-to-do. Two researchers who analyzed the rapidly growing income of the super-rich over the past few decades identified the crucial role of government action (or inaction) in the economy: an increasingly conservative Congress; declining union membership; lower tax rates for those in the higher income brackets; more open trade policies; and asset bubbles in the stock and real estate markets (Volscho and Kelly 2012). In the light of this, it is ironic that the people on welfare are castigated as "freeloaders," whereas the well-to-do have used their power since the beginning of the Republic to secure handouts from the federal government; but the handouts that the well-to-do secure are referred to as **subsidies,** or tax benefits to stimulate business. From extensive gifts of land to the railroads, to guaranteed

**subsidy**
a government grant to a private person or company to assist an enterprise deemed advantageous to the public

prices for various farm products, to tax concessions and research money for industry, the federal government has been engaged in a long history of acts that have benefited the well-to-do. In many cases the benefits received by the well-to-do are not as obvious as those given to the poor, even though they are greater.

Consumer advocate Ralph Nader (1990) identified four areas of abuse in the American "corporate welfare state." The first area of abuse is *bailouts,* the federal government's guaranteed loans or guaranteed restitution for corporate mismanagement. In the 1970s, the government guaranteed loans to Lockheed Corporation and Chrysler Corporation to prevent bankruptcy. In the 1990s, hundreds of billions of dollars were needed to deal with the ravages of fraud and speculation in the savings and loan industry and cleanup costs for nuclear weapons plants managed by private firms. In 2007, the federal government stepped in to rescue the economy from the home-loan fiasco (massive numbers of loans to unqualified home buyers). In 2020, the economic strains caused by the COVID-19 pandemic (see Chapter 13) required assistance to both corporations and small businesses. Bailouts occur regularly, and the question of whether they are all needed is debatable.

*Resource depletion* is a second area of abuse. The government has leased at "bargain-basement prices" the rights to minerals and timber. In Alaska, taxpayers paid to build the roads into some timberland that would reap huge profits for those companies that had been given the low-cost lease.

A third area of abuse is *taxpayer-funded research and development.* The government has funded research, including studies in government labs, and then given patent rights to private business. The National Cancer Institute developed the application of the drug AZT to the problem of AIDS. A private drug firm then secured an exclusive patent to market AZT without paying royalties to the government and without agreeing to any price restraints on the drug.

Finally, *subsidies to profit-making businesses* is the fourth area of abuse. The federal government has subsidized everything from private golf clubs to farm crops to giant corporations. **Corporate welfare** refers to government benefits given to corporations that are not available to individuals or to other groups. Federal, state, and local governments all contribute to the welfare, which takes the form of such benefits as tax exemptions and tax reduction, training grants, investment credits, infrastructure (roads, water and sewer lines, etc.) improvements, and low-rate loans. Corporate welfare has been on the increase in recent decades. Thus, in the 1950s, corporate taxes were 28 percent of all federal taxes collected, whereas by 2019 they were only 7 percent (Center on Budget and Policy Priorities 2020).

**corporate welfare**
governmental benefits given to corporations that are unavailable to other groups or to individuals

Why is it immoral to feed the hungry and moral to pay for private golf clubs? Is the president of an airline, whose high salary is possible partly because of government subsidies, more moral than the child who has no father and receives paltry sums of money through welfare? If the government can pay millions of dollars to rescue a corporation from bankruptcy, why is it wrong to rescue people from poverty? The answer is that the poor are powerless to secure what the well-to-do secure with relatively little difficulty. Ironically, through the structure and functioning of government, the well-to-do and powerful give to each other that which they say is immoral to give to the poor.

Probably few people in the middle class are aware of how many benefits they receive from government programs. For example, a young man attends a public school, rides on a free school bus, and eats a free or subsidized (and therefore cheap) lunch. If he later spends time in the armed forces, he may pursue a subsidized college education. He then may buy a farm or a home with a loan that is subsidized and guaranteed by the federal government. He may go into business for himself with a low-interest loan from the Small

Business Administration (SBA). The young man may marry and have children who are born in a hospital that was built in part with federal funds. His aged parents may have serious and expensive health problems, which are largely covered by the federal Medicare program. This program enables him to save his own money, which he banks in an institution protected and insured by the federal government. His community may benefit economically from an industrial project underwritten by the government, and his children may be able to go to a college because of financial assistance from the government. Then the man, like many good Americans, may rebel against federal programs and high taxes and assert that this country was built on rugged individualism, unaware that his whole existence is enriched and subsidized by various government programs.

The interests of the middle and upper strata are also reflected in the *tax structure.* Presumably, the tax structure is an equalizing mechanism that takes disproportionately from the rich in order to benefit the poor. This equalization has not happened. Both wealthy individuals and corporations continue to be adept at finding loopholes in federal tax laws that reduce their tax burden. For example, in 2018 the corporate tax rate was 21 percent. But 379 profitable corporations paid 11.3 percent (Institute on Taxation and Economic Policy 2019). And 91 corporations, including Amazon, Chevron, and IBM, paid no taxes at all in 2018!

For individuals, the wealthy tend to pay higher rates of federal income tax than do the middle class and the poor. However, most state and local tax systems severely penalize the poor (Institute on Taxation and Economic Policy 2015; Newman and O'Brien 2011). This is particularly true for states that rely for their revenue more on sales tax than on progressive property and income taxes. Nationwide, the richest Americans pay 5.4 percent of their income in state and local taxes, compared to about 9 percent for middle-income families and 10.9 percent for the poor. Even when federal taxes are added in, the proportion of income paid in taxes declines consistently from the poorest to the wealthiest.

Although the wealthy do enjoy advantages, we do not mean to imply that they pay no taxes. Most do, in fact, pay a considerable amount in taxes. The question is whether they have paid a proportionately larger amount of their income than the nonwealthy. The answer depends on whether only federal taxes or the total taxes paid–federal, state, and local taxes–are included. When all taxes are considered, the poor have paid a higher proportion of their income than have the nonpoor.

*Poverty and the Economy.* The American economy works for the rich and against the poor in various ways. A capitalist economy, which is supported by government policies, allows *concentration of wealth.* The fact that the share of income of the richest Americans has declined during this century (see Table 6.1) is misleading unless you recognize that a large part of the wealth of the very rich does not come from personal income. *Stocks, bonds, and real estate are important sources of wealth* for those at the top of the socioeconomic ladder. This is why it is important to consider wealth and not merely income when assessing the amount of inequality.

A second way the economy works against the poor is by *entrapping them in a vicious circle.* Consider, for example, a woman whose job pays her only poverty-level wages. She cannot get a better-paying job because she lacks education or skills. She cannot afford to quit to gain the skills or advance her education because she has a family to support. There is no union, and she is unwilling to risk her job and perhaps her physical well-being to try and organize her fellow workers or even to support a move to unionization. Meanwhile, her debts mount, she may accumulate medical bills, and the rate of inflation may far surpass any wage increase she gets. As she sinks more deeply into debt, she is less and less able to risk the loss of the income she has. Ultimately, she may reach the point of despair that we described earlier. Perhaps she will cling to the hope that at least some of her children can escape the poverty that has wrung the vigor out of her own life.

A third way the economy hurts the poor is by *guaranteeing that a certain proportion of the population will be unable to find employment or unable to find jobs that pay more than poverty-level wages* (Rank, Yoon, and Hirschl 2003). Although most of the poor are not unemployed, a substantial number of families are poor because the family head is either squeezed out of the job market or can find only low-paying jobs. This "squeezing out" can occur when companies close down or downsize, recessions occur, and technological changes make jobs obsolete. Some of these people will spend time on welfare as they struggle against economic forces that are beyond their control.

The low-paying jobs that keep the working poor impoverished are most likely to be found in the service industry, particularly in food preparation and service jobs (Bureau of Labor Statistics 2020). A disproportionate number of those who fill such jobs are young (under the age of 25), female, and work part-time. In 2019, 392,000 workers earned the minimum wage—$7.25 per hour. But federal regulations do not cover all workers. An additional 1.2 million Americans worked for less than the minimum. To understand the impact of working at such jobs, consider the following: If an individual worked full-time (40 hours per week) year-round (52 weeks), that individual's income would put him or her a little above the poverty line; but if that individual were responsible for one or more other people, the family would be in poverty. Clearly, no one can be an adequate breadwinner for a family and work for the federal minimum wage.

*Immigrants are prime targets for companies that pay low wages.* A New York reporter went into a Brooklyn garment factory that had a sign posted in Chinese: "Earnestly, urgently looking for workers" (Lii 1995). Because the reporter spoke Chinese, the owner assumed that she was an immigrant seeking her fortune in America. She accepted the job and took her place in a long line of Chinese women bending over sewing machines and working diligently in silence. At the end of seven days and 84 hours of work, she was told that in three weeks she would be paid $54.24—which came to 65 cents an hour! She walked away "from the lint-filled factory with aching shoulders, a stiff back, a dry cough and a burning sore throat."

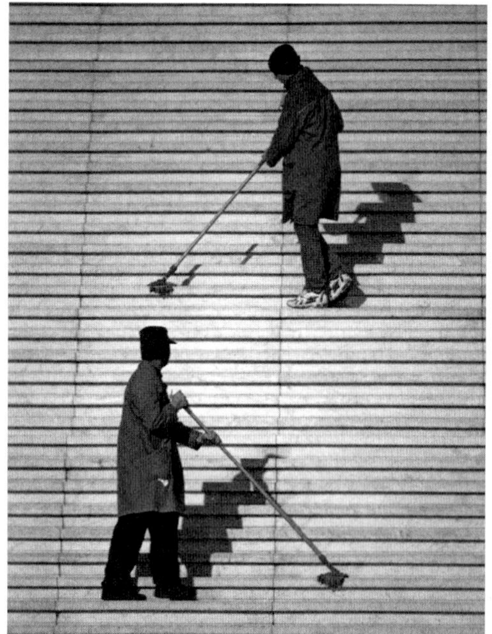

Immigrants are prime targets for low-paying jobs.
C. Zachariasen/PhotoAlto

Similar stories could be told of Asians and Hispanics in various parts of the country. Both legal and illegal immigrants are exploited. Lacking language skills and/or legal status and desperate for income, they may fall prey to managers who pay only the minimum wage or less.

One way to deal with low-paying jobs is to *unionize* the workers. Unfortunately, as we point out in Chapter 10, unions have had their own problems in recent years in organizing the workforce. The problem of low-paying jobs is likely to continue for some time.

The same economy that allows low-paying labor furthers the disadvantage of the poor in regard to the purchase of consumer goods and services, including everything from groceries to health care (Brookings Institution Metropolitan Policy Program 2005; Talukdar 2008). Thus, one study showed that low-income families in Philadelphia paid at least $500 more than other families for the same kind of car and $400 more per year for insurance for the car. Similarly, a study of the cost of being poor in Gary, Indiana, reported that stores in the poor neighborhoods charged more for food and clothes than did stores in other areas (Barnes 2005). Why don't the poor simply go to the other stores, then? They may have neither the time nor the resources to travel to cheaper but distant stores. And some who did found themselves being watched with suspicion in grocery stores when they used food stamps or treated discourteously when shopping for clothes.

To be sure, it is more costly to do business in ghetto neighborhoods than elsewhere because of greater losses through theft and higher insurance premiums. Although higher prices may be legitimate from a business perspective, they do contribute to keeping the poor impoverished.

*Patterns of Family Life.* One aspect of family life that tends to perpetuate poverty is the size of the family. The rate of poverty among large families is two to three times that of two-person families.

Even in small families, however, the family is likely to perpetuate its own poverty because of *certain social-class differences in family life* (Heymann 2000; Pittman and Chase-Lansdale 2001; Lareau 2003). Family life among the poor can discourage intellectual achievement (and, therefore, the higher levels of education that are vital for upward mobility). Among the factors that are important for a child's intellectual growth are parents' willingness to give time to the child, parental guidance, parental aspirations for the child's achievement, provision of intellectual stimulation, and the use of external resources such as nursery schools and advice from experts. Children who live in poverty for a period of time are less likely to receive this kind of family help than are those who are not poor (Evans 2004; Evans et al. 2011).

The advantages that accrue to the children of the well-to-do are underscored in a long-term study of a sample of schoolchildren in Baltimore (Alexander, Entwisle, and Olson 2007). The children were monitored from the time they were in first grade until they were 22 years old. Those from the middle and upper social strata had varied kinds of summer learning experiences that gave them an advantage in academic progress over their peers from poorer families. The experiences were not only summer classes or programs, but also the parents working with their children to enhance their knowledge and skills. The additional learning in the summer led to higher academic achievement, which, in turn, led to a greater likelihood of being in a college-preparatory track and actually attending a four-year college. The poorer children, by contrast, had lower test scores and were, therefore, less likely to be in a college-preparatory program. They were also less likely to complete high school. Nationally, dropout rates from high school in 2014 were 11.6 percent for those in the lowest income bracket compared to 4.7 percent of those in the high-middle bracket and 2.8 percent for those in the highest bracket (Kena et al. 2016).

Why? Can't poor parents provide the same kind of motivation and help as the nonpoor? In theory, yes. But consider the circumstances of living in poverty. The atmosphere of the impoverished home is unlikely to be conducive to learning. In a poor family, *interaction of children with adults generally, and parents in particular, tends to be minimal* (Heymann 2000). The home of the poor child is likely to be crowded, busy, and noisy. There are likely to be many people, including a number of children, living in the home, though it is less likely that there are two parents. No single child gets much attention. The children watch television, listen to music, and see movies, but do little reading. Moreover, they have little sustained interaction with adult members of their families.

Evidence also shows that consistent mothering by one person facilitates development of children's ability to express themselves verbally. Children in poor families are less likely to have such a relationship in their early years. Instead, responsibility for child care tends to be assumed by a number of people, including adults and other children. TANF policy, which requires single mothers to find work and become self-supporting, exacerbates the problem.

The interaction that does occur may hinder rather than facilitate intellectual growth because there is a *greater proportion of nonverbal compared to verbal interaction* among the poor. The emphasis on the nonverbal rather than the verbal and on the physical rather than the mental is why children from poor homes tend to move their lips while reading and to use their fingers while counting.

Because the verbal ability of poor adults is generally low, increasing the amount of verbal interaction between adults and children would not resolve the problem. Many language differences have been found between the lower and the middle and upper socioeconomic strata. These language differences involve grammatical distinctions; pronunciation, stress, and intonation; range of vocabulary; and style and taste in the selection and use of words and phrases. Differences in these linguistic features mean differences in how the world is experienced and communicated. In general, poor parents are equipped with neither the financial resources nor the intellectual tools necessary to maximize the intellectual growth of their children. The parents' own opportunities to acquire these resources and tools are minimal, and hence the family environment they provide will tend to perpetuate the limitations in their children.

Another aspect of family life that bears crucially on the problem of poverty is the *high rate of divorce.* Recall that persons in female-headed families have the highest rates of poverty in the nation (see Figure 6.2). Divorce is likely to have negative economic consequences for women and may be particularly severe for women with children. One study, for example, found that the financial status of mothers and their children fell by 37 percent, compared to a drop of 16 percent for the nonresident fathers (Stirling and Aldrich 2008). Among those with low incomes, the poverty rate for fathers was 28 percent, while that for mothers was 73 percent! Indeed, nearly half the increase in child poverty in recent years is due to changing family structure (more children born to single women and greater numbers of single-parent families because of separation, death, or divorce).

*The Education of the Poor.* In general, the lower the income, the lower the educational achievement of children (Kena et al. 2016). As noted previously, family patterns contribute significantly to this pattern. In addition to the way parents interact with their children at home, parental involvement in the school is less among the lower- than the higher-income families. Among other things, parents in the highest income bracket are twice as likely to attend a class event and volunteer at school as those in the lowest income bracket. Even the educational expectations of both poor children and their parents tend to be lower than those in the middle and upper classes (Goyette 2008). These expectations are reflected in lower levels of educational achievement. This educational disadvantage in turn exacerbates the worst aspects of poverty, depressing well-being and shutting people out of many economic opportunities.

Unfortunately, the educational environment itself contributes in a number of ways to the low academic achievement of the poor. Chapter 11 considers the problem of the inequitable distribution of quality education and shows that schools in poor neighborhoods tend to have meager facilities and inexperienced or inadequate teachers. Here we focus on the ways *school personnel affect poverty-level students* at the interpersonal level.

Children of poor families may experience **discrimination** when they attend school with children of nonpoor families. Teachers come primarily from middle-class backgrounds. They may find it difficult to understand and relate in a helpful way to children from poor homes. They may also *have different expectations for students from different socioeconomic backgrounds,* and the expectations of teachers can significantly retard or stimulate intellectual growth and performance (Sparks 2010). Hence, when middle-class teachers expect students from poor families not to perform well, this expectation can lead the children to perform below their capabilities.

**discrimination**
arbitrary, unfavorable treatment of the members of some social group

In essence, the poor are less likely than the nonpoor to have gratifying and encouraging experiences in school. They are, therefore, more likely to drop out. Children from lower socioeconomic levels, compared to those from the middle and upper strata, also tend to be more dissatisfied with school, report more interpersonal problems (such as not being popular), feel more difficulty in expressing themselves well, and are more likely to express difficulties concentrating and studying. It is not surprising, then, that the majority of school dropouts are from the lower strata.

In sum, the poor are less likely than the nonpoor to perform well in school or to seek more than minimal education—not necessarily because of innate ability, but because of sociocultural factors. Even when ability levels of poor and nonpoor are equated, the poor are less likely to pursue higher education.

## Social Psychological Factors

fallacy

Some attitudes and values held by both the nonpoor and the poor help perpetuate poverty. For example, many nonpoor accept the *fallacy of retrospective determinism* with regard to poverty: They believe that poverty is inevitable—"There have always been poor people, and there always will be poor people." This kind of attitude may manifest itself

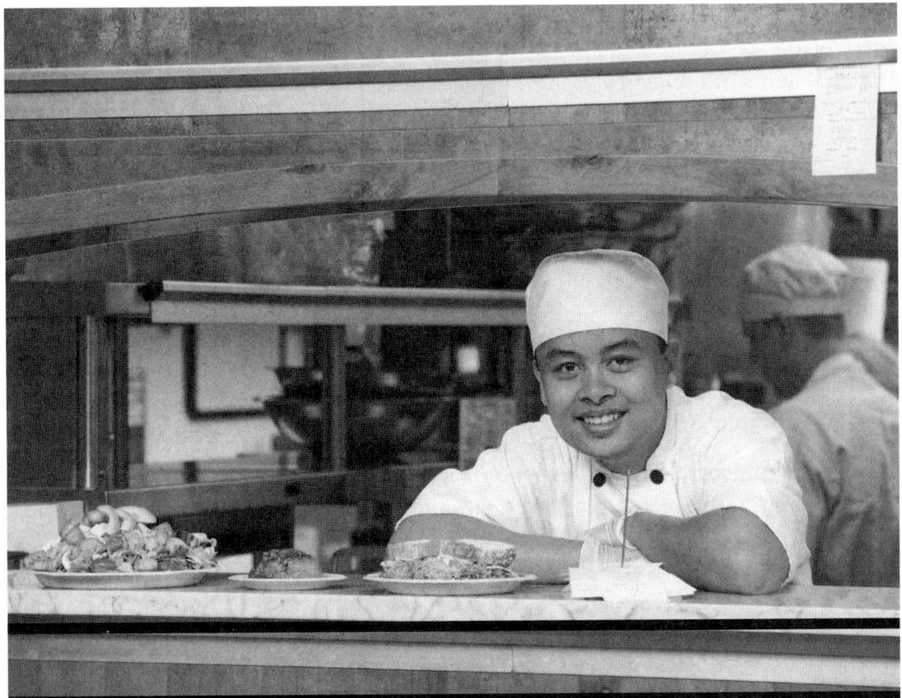

People with menial jobs may be poor even though they work full-time.
Tetra Images/Alamy Stock Photo

as opposition to government antipoverty programs, pitting the nonpoor against the poor as various interest groups vie for funds.

*Disparagement and Discrimination.* As we pointed out earlier, *the nonpoor tend to disparage the poor.* Throughout history, and in virtually all societies, the poor have been considered disreputable in some sense. Such attitudes seriously undermine self-respect among the poor and at the same time perpetuate the political and economic processes that maintain poverty. You might think that people's disparagement of the poor would lessen during times of more general hardship, but there is no evidence that beliefs about the causes of poverty and attitudes toward the poor or toward welfare change even when the entire society is in an economic recession.

**self-fulfilling prophecy**
a belief that has consequences (and may become true) simply because it is believed

Negative attitudes toward the poor may become **self-fulfilling prophecies.** If a man is poor because he is out of work, he may find that when he secures work, hostility is directed toward him because he comes from an impoverished background. We once lived in a community in which a manufacturing company placed a full-page advertisement in the local newspaper, pointing out that a program to bus inner-city workers to the plant had failed. The ad asked what was wrong with the workers. Why were the jobs still open? The company implied that what many people think is actually true: The poor are too lazy to work and will not accept an opportunity even if it is offered to them. A subsequent investigation showed that the chronically unemployed, who were all Black, were unwilling to work because of pressures, hostility, and racial bias.

The tendency to disparage the poor is also at the root of opposition to government programs designed to alleviate poverty. A national poll that asked whether welfare programs help people get started again or just create dependency found significant differences by political affiliation (Ekins 2019). Those who believed the programs do nothing more than encourage dependency included 27 percent of Democrats, 36 percent of independents, and 68 percent of Republicans.

*The Ideology of Wealth and Poverty.* Many Americans *believe strongly in an ideology of individualism, attributing both wealth and poverty to the qualities of individuals rather than to the social system.* A *New York Times* survey reported that 80 percent of the respondents believed that people can start out poor, work hard, and become rich (Scott and Leonhardt 2005). This is in accord with an individualist ideology of wealth and poverty, which argues that each individual is responsible for his or her own status because the system itself allows opportunities to all. Clearly, such an ideology allows no basis for political action that would alleviate poverty. It is understandable, therefore, that Americans, compared to those in some European nations, are less concerned about establishing a minimum income level for all citizens (Osberg and Smeeding 2006).

## Solutions: Public Policy and Private Action

There have, of course, been attempts to resolve the problem of poverty. The so-called War on Poverty initiated in the 1960s was a multifaceted attack on the problem. The Economic Opportunity Act of 1964 set up several programs intended to benefit the poor, including the Job Corps (to train young people who have little education or skills), the College Work Study Program (to help college students from low-income families), and the Community Action Program.

The failure of the War on Poverty to eliminate the problem is used by some Americans to disparage any government efforts and to insist that, ultimately, the poor themselves must take advantage of the opportunities in the land to lift themselves from poverty. This argument not only ignores the fact that the war was often more rhetoric than support but also ignores the genuine gains that were made. The poverty rate fell from more than 22 percent in 1959 to a low of 11 to 12 percent in the 1970s. The subsequent rise occurred with the cutback in government programs. Without the programs that exist now, the rate would be much higher than it is. You must also realize that some programs will fail; the study of human behavior is not sufficiently scientific to be able to put together an infallible solution to a problem. Some programs have worked well. Head Start and other early childhood education programs have provided impoverished children with skills that have enabled them to reach higher levels of academic achievement and success (West et al. 2010). Kenworthy (1999) examined the effects of social welfare programs in 15 affluent nations, including the United States, and found that the programs have reduced poverty rates in all of them.

To eliminate poverty, some attitudes and ideologies among people generally, and political leaders in particular, must be altered. Typically, the more information people have and the more they are exposed to impoverished individuals, the more positive their attitudes are likely to be toward the poor (and, therefore, the more likely they are to support programs that help the poor). Three researchers who studied attitudes toward the homeless found that people who were most exposed to homelessness—including everything from television shows and articles to having been in or worked in a homeless shelter—had the most favorable attitudes (Lee, Farrell, and Link 2004). Whatever governments and community organizations can do to increase exposure is likely to increase support for programs that help.

The attitudes and ideologies of political leaders are also crucial, and the commitment of the federal government is essential. Unfortunately, federal commitment varies enormously from one administration to another. New policies and programs are needed, but the emphasis in the early 2000s was on cutting back old programs.

Because single mothers have the highest rate of poverty in the nation, strategies to help them must have priority. The welfare reform of 1996 assumed that if single mothers were deprived of long-term support they would marry and their husbands' income would lift them out of poverty. Unfortunately, unmarried women with children are not appealing as mates for men who could support them (Graefe and Lichter 2007). One way to help the mothers who work but are still in poverty would be to create a system of fringe benefits for low-wage workers. The benefits could include an increase in the Earned Income Tax Credit, tax credits for child care expenses, and a tax credit for housing expenses.

Some of the poor also could be helped by raising the minimum wage. An individual worker cannot support a family above the poverty level by working full time at the minimum wage level.

Another important step is *to continue to search for antipoverty programs, including welfare programs,* that work. It appears that workfare, introduced in the 1980s, is going to be the policy for the foreseeable future. Under the TANF program, the federal government does not provide long-term aid to the poor. Instead, states are given block grants to run their own programs. Each state has considerable flexibility, but certain guidelines must be followed. Generally, the guidelines are that no family will be given welfare payments for more than five years, and if the head of a family does not find work within two years, the family will lose benefits.

How effective has workfare been so far? First, the program has greatly reduced welfare rolls and moved many former recipients into work (Grogger and Karoly 2005).

Second, however, *the reduction in welfare benefits has been far greater than the reduction of poverty.* The earnings from the kinds of jobs available to those moving out of welfare (who are likely to have minimal skills) are frequently no more than the benefits they were receiving from welfare. Thus, they are working, but they are no better off financially than they were while on welfare. Some are even worse off because the jobs they secure offer no benefits such as health care, assistance in child care, and leave for maternity or even for family or personal illness (Collins and Mayer 2010).

Most disturbing is the fact that, for whatever reasons, the TANF average caseload fell from 4.4 million families in 1996 to 2.2 million in 2020 (Office of Family Assistance 2020). In essence, then, TANF is helping far fewer families than previous programs. It is not surprising, then, that studies of workers who have participated in TANF programs show that *the majority are not able to escape from poverty* even though they follow through to the end of the process that is supposed to rescue them (Cancian et al. 2003; Blalock, Tiller, and Monroe 2004). Moreover, there are some recipients, particularly those with less than a high-school education and a poor work history, who are unable to secure a job within the time limits set by the state (Taylor, Barusch, and Vogel-Ferguson 2006). They are left with nothing.

In addition, another problem has plagued the poor under workfare. Although one of the goals was to strengthen family life by encouraging parents to be responsible breadwinners, workfare has had no effect on the living arrangements of poor white children, has increased the proportion of Hispanic children living with a married parent, but has actually decreased the proportion of Black children living with any parent (Bitler, Gelbach, and Hoynes 2004). And a study of low-income single mothers who moved from welfare to work found that the conditions of employment (long hours, erratic work schedules, lengthy commutes, etc.) resulted in a variety of emotional and interpersonal problems among the children (Dunifon, Kalil, and Bajracharya 2005).

In short, workfare may not even be a solution for all the able-bodied workers who have been on welfare, much less for those who are not able to work. A writer who tried to survive by working for a month at low-paying jobs put it this way:

> I lost almost four pounds in four weeks, on a diet weighted heavily toward burgers and fries. How former welfare recipients and single mothers will (and do) survive in the low-wage workforce, I cannot imagine. . . . I couldn't hold two jobs and I couldn't make enough money to live on with one. (Ehrenreich 1999:52)

What, then, is to be done at the level of public policy? A number of steps need to be taken at both the federal and state levels of government, including the following:

- Provide benefits for as long as it takes (rather than the current limits) to enable families to escape poverty.
- Spend all unused TANF money (billions of unspent dollars are available to the states), or replace TANF with more effective programs.
- Simplify the process of getting available benefits such as food stamps, child care, health care, and transportation so that the poor are both aware of and able to get the help they need.
- Set a federal minimum wage that enables workers to be self-supporting and able to afford housing.

- Expand educational and training programs so that workers can secure better-paying jobs.
- Provide more supportive services for low-income families.

Finally, various forms of private action can help the poor. One example is Habitat for Humanity, which has built more than 100,000 homes for poor people in the United States and other countries. Interested Americans can volunteer to help in the construction or can donate money to support others who do the work. Other programs include the work of various civic and religious groups in repairing and renovating homes, providing food for the hungry, offering health care to the poor, and giving scholarships to poor children. Such programs reach a portion of the poor, but they cannot replace the broader public policies that are needed to help the millions of poor Americans.

*Follow-Up.* Think about actions that you as a private citizen have taken to help alleviate the problem of poverty. What more could you do in the future?

## Summary

Poverty may not be as bad in America as it is in some parts of the world, but America's poverty must be evaluated in terms of the standard of living attained by the majority of Americans. The government's definition of poverty is based on the cost of a basic diet called the "economy food plan." It is revised to account for inflation and varies according to location (farm or nonfarm), size of the family, and sex and age of the head of the family. In 2015, a family of two adults and two children with an annual income or $24,036 or less was officially poor. This official definition is challenged as inadequate or unrealistic because it sets the poverty level quite low.

The proportion of people who are poor varies over time. Poverty is not equally distributed among the population, however. Your chances of being poor are greater if you are in a female-headed family, are a member of a minority group, are under 18 years of age, and are living in a rural area. Contrary to popular opinion, poverty is not basically a problem of unemployment. Many of the poor work, and some work full time. Some of the poor are homeless. Homelessness is associated with many other problems, such as mental and physical health.

The quality of life for the poor can be characterized as pervasive deprivation: The poor get less of everything that is valued in American society, including rights to life and the pursuit of happiness. Poverty brings despair and fear, including the fear of being victimized by crime. Various myths that disparage the poor diminish their dignity as human beings. Their health is poorer than that of most Americans, and their poverty and ill health can become a vicious circle. The individual living in poverty is forced to choose between limited, undesirable alternatives.

Among the structural factors that contribute to poverty, the distribution of power is of prime importance. People who control the wealth are the most powerful, and their interests are typically reflected in governmental decisions. Both the structure and the functioning of American government tend to work to the detriment of the poor. Multiple decision-making centers, the middle-class composition of the bureaucracy, and the complexities of getting aid all work to the detriment of the poor. Ironically, the well-to-do and powerful give to each other through government actions what they say is immoral to give to the poor. The economy works against the poor in three ways: by allowing the concentration of wealth, by entrapping the poor in a vicious circle, and by guaranteeing that a certain proportion of the population will be unable to find employment or jobs that pay more than poverty-level wages.

The family environment tends to perpetuate poverty when there are many children in the family. Even when there are few children, poor families tend to transmit poverty by anti-intellectual attitudes and patterns of interaction that inhibit intellectual development. Disrupted families are also an important source of poverty, and many widows and divorced women spend a part of the time after disruption in poverty. Educational arrangements themselves contribute to the problem because quality education is much less likely to be available to poor children than to nonpoor children. Also, poor children tend not to have gratifying and encouraging experiences in school or to pursue higher education even when they have the ability to do so.

Attitudes and values of both the poor and the nonpoor contribute to the poverty problem. The attitudes and values of the nonpoor legitimate their disparagement of and discrimination against the poor. The American value of individualism and ideology of equal opportunity combine to justify negative attitudes toward the poor and programs designed to help them.

## Key Terms

**Autonomy**
**Consumer Price Index**
**Corporate Welfare**
**Discrimination**
**Ghetto**
**Malnutrition**
**Poverty**
**Poverty Level**
**Self-Fulfilling Prophecy**
**Subsidy**

## Study Questions

1. What do we mean by "poverty"? How many Americans are poor?
2. Who is most likely to be poor in America?
3. How have the problems of poverty and the lot of the poor changed over time in our country?

4. Explain the various ways in which poverty affects the basic rights and needs of people.
5. What is meant by the "dilemmas of poverty"?
6. How do social institutions contribute to the problem of poverty?
7. How do attitudes and ideologies help perpetuate poverty?
8. What are some steps that could be taken to eliminate or at least minimize poverty?

## Internet Resources/Exercises

1. Explore some of the ideas in this chapter on the following sites:

**http://www.census.gov** The U.S. Census Bureau offers regular reports and the latest data on poverty in the United States.

**http://ssc.wisc.edu/irp** The University of Wisconsin's Institute for Research on Poverty offers a wealth of information, including a newsletter with reports from their researchers.

**http://www.ipr.northwestern.edu** The Institute for Policy Research offers a variety of publications on poverty that can be downloaded free.

2. TANF requirements vary from state to state. Choose four states and get information on their TANF programs. Also gather, if possible, any data on the effectiveness of the programs (numbers of people moved off welfare, numbers of those out of poverty, etc.). Which of the programs do you think is most effective? In which state or states would a poor person get the most help?

3. European nations tend to have lower rates of poverty than the United States. Investigate what various European nations are doing to alleviate poverty and ensure at least a minimally adequate income for all citizens.

## For Further Reading

Danziger, Sheldon H., and Robert H. Haveman, eds. *Understanding Poverty.* Cambridge, MA: Harvard University Press, 2002. Various experts address the causes and consequences of poverty, antipoverty policies, and efforts by local communities and neighborhoods to ameliorate the problem.

Desmond, Matthew. *Evicted: Poverty and Profit in the American City.* New York: Crown, 2016. Puts a face on one kind of experience of poor-the loss of housing-with stories of landlords and tenants in impoverished areas of Milwaukee. Shows through both stories and data the traumatic effects on individuals, families, and the entire community.

Edwards, John, Marion Crain, and Arne L. Kalleberg, eds. *Ending Poverty in America: How to Restore the American Dream.* New York: The New Press, 2007. A collection of articles by a diverse group of social scientists, business people, and community organizers on varied facets of the problem of poverty. Includes suggestions on the kinds of public policies that could solve the problem.

Jensen, Eric. *Teaching with Poverty in Mind: What Being Poor Does to Kids' Brains and What Schools Can Do about It.* Alexandria, VA: Association for Supervision & Curriculum Development, 2009. Discusses the nature of poverty, how poverty affects the behavior of children, including academic behavior, and what can be done in schools and in the classroom to foster academic success among the children of the poor.

Lareau, Annette. *Unequal Childhoods: Class, Race, and Family Life.* Berkeley, CA: University of California Press, 2003. A participant observation study of 12 families in which there were children who were 9 or 10 years old. Shows how parenting and daily routines differ between the middle-class families and those that are working-class or poor.

Rank, Mark Robert. *One Nation, Underprivileged: Why American Poverty Affects Us All.* New York: Oxford University Press, 2004. A leading poverty researcher explores the basic causes of poverty, the extent of poverty, and the reasons poverty is an issue of vital concern to the nation.

Shipler, David K. *The Working Poor: Invisible in America.* New York: Alfred A. Knopf, 2004. A thorough study of people who are working but still poor or nearly poor by the official poverty level. The author spent as many as seven years working with some of his subjects; he well understands their struggles.

## References

AFL-CIO. 2018. "Executive paywatch." AFL-CIO website.

Aguilera, E. 2011. "New scale shows greater poverty." *San Diego Union-Tribune,* November 8.

Alaimo, K., C. M. Olson, and E. A. Frongillo Jr. 2001. "Food insufficiency and American school-aged children's cognitive, academic, and psychosocial development." *Pediatrics* 108:44–53.

——. 2002. "Family food insufficiency, but not low family income, is positively associated with dysthymia and suicide symptoms in adolescents." *Journal of Nutrition* 132:719–25.

Alaimo, K., C. M. Olson, E. A. Frongillo Jr., and R. R. Briefel. 2001. "Food insufficiency, family income, and health in U.S. preschool and school-aged children." *American Journal of Public Health* 91:781–86.

Alderson, A. S., and T. Katz-Gerro. 2016. "Compared to whom? Inequality, social comparison, and happiness in the United States." *Social Forces* 95:25–54.

Alexander, K. L., D. R. Entwisle, and L. S. Olson. 2007. "Lasting consequences of the summer learning gap." *American Sociological Review* 72:167–80.

Allard, S. W. 2008. "Rethinking the safety net: Gaps and instability in help for the working poor." *Focus,* Summer/ Fall.

Anderson, R. 2009. "The emerging class of the lucky-rich." *Contexts* 8:72–73.

Baggett, T. P., J. J. O'Connell, D. E. Singer, and N. A. Rigotti. 2010. "The unmet health needs of homeless adults." *American Journal of Public Health* 100:1326–33.

Ball, R., and K. Chernova. 2008. "Absolute income, relative income, and happiness." *Social Indicators Research* 88:497–529.

Barnes, S. L. 2005. *The Cost of Being Poor.* New York: State University of New York Press.

Belle, D. 2003. "Poverty, inequality, and discrimination as sources of depression among U.S. women." *Psychology of Women Quarterly* 27:101–13.

Berner, M., T. Ozer, and S. Paynter. 2008. "A portrait of hunger, the social safety net, and the working poor." *Policy Studies Journal* 36:403–20.

Bhattacharya, J., T. DeLeire, S. Haider, and J. Currie. 2003. "Heat or eat? Cold-weather shocks and nutrition in poor American families." *American Journal of Public Health* 93:1149–54.

Bitler, M. P., J. B. Gelbach, and H. W. Hoynes. 2004. "Has welfare reform affected children's living arrangements?" *Focus* 23:14–20.

Blalock, L., V. R. Tiller, and P. A. Monroe. 2004. "'They get you out of courage': Persistent deep poverty among former welfare-reliant women." *Family Relations* 53:127–37.

Blumenberg, E., and A. W. Agrawal. 2014. "Getting around when you're just getting by." *Journal of Poverty* 18:355–78.

Board of Governors of the Federal Reserve System. 2020. "Distribution of household wealth in the US. since 1989." FRS website.

Bowles, S., S. N. Durlauf, and K. Hoff, eds. 2006. *Poverty Traps.* Princeton, NJ: Princeton University Press.

Brookings Institution Metropolitan Policy Program. 2005. *The Price Is Wrong.* Brookings Institution website.

Bureau of Labor Statistics. 2020. "Characteristics of minimum wage workers, 2019." Bureau of Labor Statistics website.

Cancian, M., et al. 2003. "Income and program participation among early TANF recipients." *Focus* 22:2–10.

Caton, C. L. M., et al. 2005. "Risk factors for long-term homelessness." *American Journal of Public Health* 95:1753–59.

Center on Budget and Policy Priorities. 2020. "Policy basics." CBPP website.

Chen, E., K. A. Matthews, and W. T. Boyce. 2002. "Socioeconomic differences in children's health." *Psychological Bulletin* 128:295–329.

Cohen, R. A., et al. 2020. "Health insurance coverage." National Center for Health Statistics website.

Coleman, A., et al. 2020. "Household food security in the United States in 2019." U.S. Department of Agriculture website.

Collins, J. L., and V. Mayer. 2010. *Both Hands Tied: Welfare Reform and the Race to the Bottom in the Low-Wage Labor Market.* Chicago, IL: University of Chicago Press.

Cozzarelli, C., A. V. Wilkinson, and M. J. Tagler. 2001. "Attitudes toward the poor and attributions for poverty." *Journal of Social Issues* 57:207–27.

Dautovic, G. 2020. "Straight talk on welfare statistics." Fortunly website.

Davis, J. J., V. J. Roscigno, and G. Wilson. 2016. "American Indian poverty in the contemporary United States." *Sociological Forum* 31:5-28.

Desmond, M., and R. T. Kimbro. 2015. "Eviction's fallout: Housing, hardship, and health." *Social Forces* 94:295-324.

Duncan, G. J., and K. Magnuson. 2011. "The long reach of early childhood poverty." *Pathways,* Winter, pp. 22-27.

Dunifon, R., A. Kalil, and A. Bajracharya. 2005. "Maternal working conditions and child well-being in welfare-leaving families." *Developmental Psychology* 41:851-59.

Ehrenreich, B. 1999. "Nickel-and-dimed: On (not) getting by in America." *Harper's Magazine,* January, pp. 37-52.

Ekins, E. 2019. "Welfare, work, and worth national survey." Cato Institute website.

Ellsworth, J. T. 2019. "Street crime victimization among homeless adults." *Victims & Offenders* 14:96-118.

Evans, G. W. 2004. "The environment of childhood poverty." *American Psychologist* 59:77-92.

Evans, G. W., J. Brooks-Gunn, and P. K. Klebanov. 2011. "Stressing out the poor." *Pathways,* Winter, pp. 16-21.

Forum on Child and Family Statistics. 2020. *America's Children in Brief: Key National Indicators of Well-Being, 2020.* Washington, DC: Government Printing Office.

Gardner, G., and B. Halweil. 2000. *Underfed and Overfed: The Global Epidemic of Malnutrition.* Washington, DC: Worldwatch Institute.

Goyette, K. 2008. "College for some to college for all: Social background, occupational expectations, and educational expectations over time." *Social Science Research* 37:461-84.

Graefe, D. R., and D. T. Lichter. 2007. "When unwed mothers marry." *Journal of Family Issues* 28:595-622.

Grogger, J., and L. A. Karoly. 2005. *Welfare Reform: Effects of a Decade of Change.* Cambridge, MA: Harvard University Press.

Hacker, J. S., and P. Pierson. 2010. *Winner-Take-All Politics: How Washington Made the Rich Richer—and Turned Its Back on the Middle Class.* New York: Simon and Schuster.

Harrington, M. 1962. *The Other America.* Baltimore, MD: Penguin.

Heiserman, N., and B. Simpson. 2017. "Higher inequality increases the gap in the perceived merit of the rich and poor." *Social Psychology Quarterly* 80:243-53.

Heymann, J. 2000. "What happens during and after school: Conditions faced by working parents living in poverty and their school-aged children." *Journal of Children and Poverty* 6:5-20.

Hoefer, R., and C. Curry. 2012. "Food security and social protection in the United States." *Journal of Policy Practice* 11:59-76.

Hokayem, C., and M. L. Heggeness. 2014. "Living in near poverty in the United States: 1966-2012." U.S. Census Bureau website.

Hutchinson, P. 1962. *The Christian Century Reader.* New York: Association Press.

Institute on Taxation and Economic Policy. 2015. *Who Pays? A Distributional Analysis of the Tax System in All 50 States.* ITEP website.

——. 2019. "Corporate tax avoidance in the first year of the Trump tax law." ITEP website.

Jacobe, D. 2008. "Food prices a hardship for 64% of low-income Americans; One in five of those making less than $30,000 a year call the situation 'severe.'" *Gallup Poll News Service,* April 24.

Jasinski, J. L., J. K. Wesely, J. D. Wright, and E. E. Mustaine. 2010. *Hard Lives, Mean Streets: Violence in the Lives of Homeless Women.* Boston, MA: Northeastern University Press.

Kar, B. R., S. L. Rao, and B. A. Chandramouli. 2008. "Cognitive development in children with chronic protein energy malnutrition." *Behavioral and Brain Functions* 4:31.

Kena, G., et al. 2016. "The condition of education 2016." National Center for Education Statistics website.

Kenworthy, L. 1999. "Do social-welfare policies reduce poverty? A cross-national assessment." *Social Forces* 77 (March):1119-39.

Kirby, J. B., and T. Kaneda. 2005. "Neighborhood socioeconomic disadvantage and access to health care." *Journal of Health and Social Behavior* 46:15-31.

Kramer, S. 2019. "U.S. has world's highest rate of children living in single-parent households." Pew Research Center website.

Lareau, A. 2003. *Unequal Childhoods: Class, Race, and Family Life.* Berkeley, CA: University of California Press.

Lauer, R. H. 1976. "Defining social problems: Public opinion and textbook practice." *Social Problems* 24 (October):122–30.

——. 1991. *Perspectives on Social Change.* 4th ed. Boston, MA: Allyn and Bacon.

Lauter, D. 2016. "How do Americans view poverty?" *Los Angeles Times,* August 14.

Lee, B. A., and M. J. Greif. 2008. "Homelessness and hunger." *Journal of Health and Social Behavior* 49:3–19.

Lee, B. A., C. R. Farrell, and B. G. Link. 2004. "Revisiting the contact hypothesis: The case of public exposure to homelessness." *American Sociological Review* 69:40–63.

Lii, J. H. 1995. "Week in sweatshop reveals grim conspiracy of the poor." *New York Times,* March 12.

McDonough, P., and P. Berglund. 2003. "Histories of poverty and self-rated health trajectories." *Journal of Health and Social Behavior* 44:198–214.

Morgan, R. E., and J. L. Truman. 2020. "Criminal victimization, 2019." Bureau of Justice Statistics website.

Nader, R. 1990. "Corporate state is on a roll." *Los Angeles Times,* March 5.

Najman, J. M., et al. 2010. "Family poverty over the early life course and recurrent adolescent and young adult anxiety and depression." *American Journal of Public Health* 200:1719–23.

National Alliance to End Homelessness. 2020. "The state of homelessness in America." NAEH website.

National Coalition for the Homeless. 2000. *Welfare to What II?* Washington, DC: NCH.

——. 2006. "A dream denied: The criminalization of homelessness in U.S. cities." NCFH website.

——. 2009. "Who is homeless?" NCH website.

——. 2016. "No safe street." NCH website.

Newman, K. S., and R. L. O'Brien. 2011. "Taxing the poor: How some states make poverty worse." *Pathways,* Summer, pp. 22–26.

Office of Family Assistance. 2020. "TANF caseload data, 2020." OFA website.

Okechukwu, C. A., et al. 2012. "Household food insufficiency, financial strain, work-family spillover, and depressive symptoms in the working class." *American Journal of Public Health* 102:126–33.

Osberg, L., and T. Smeeding. 2006. "'Fair' inequality? Attitudes toward pay differentials." *American Sociological Review* 71:450–73.

Petterson, S. M., and A. B. Albers. 2001. "Effects of poverty and maternal depression on early child development." *Child Development* 72:1794–813.

Pew Research Center. 2006. "Are we happy yet?" Pew Research Center website.

Pittman, L. D., and P. L. Chase-Lansdale. 2001. "African American adolescent girls in impoverished communities." *Journal of Research on Adolescence* 11:199–224.

Price, J. H., J. Khubchandani, and F. J. Webb. 2018. "Poverty and health disparities: What can public health professionals do?" *Health Promotion Practice* 19:170–74.

Proctor, B. D., J. L. Semega, and M. A. Kollar. 2016. "Income and poverty in the United States: 2015." U.S. Census Bureau website.

Rainwater, L. 1967. "Crisis of the city: Poverty and deprivation." *Washington University Magazine* (Spring):17–21.

Rank, M. R. 2001. "The effect of poverty on America's families." *Journal of Family Issues* 22:881–903.

Rank, M. R., H. Yoon, and T. A. Hirshi. 2003. "As American as apple pie: Poverty and welfare." *Contexts* 2:41–49.

Safawi, A., and I. Floyd. 2020. "TANF benefits still too low to help families, especially black families, avoid increased hardship." Center on Budget and Policy Priorities website.

Samaan, R. A. 2000. "The influences of race, ethnicity, and poverty on the mental health of children." *Journal of Health Care for the Poor and Underserved* 11 (February):100–10.

Schott, L., and L. Pavetti. 2012. "Many states cutting TANF benefits harshly despite high unemployment and unprecedented need." Center on Budget and Policy Priorities website.

Scott, J., and D. Leonhardt. 2005. "Class in America: Shadowy lines that still divide." *New York Times,* May 15.

Seccombe, K., K. B. Walters, and D. James. 1999. "'Welfare mothers' welcome reform, urge compassion." *Family Relations* 48 (April):197–206.

Semega, J., et al. 2020. "Income and poverty in the United States: 2019." U.S. Government Publishing Office.

Shipler, D. K. 2004. *The Working Poor: Invisible in America.* New York: Alfred K. Knopf.

Short, K. 2014. "The supplemental poverty measure: 2013." U.S. Census Bureau website.

Slesnick, N., et al. 2010. "Prevalence of intimate partner violence reported by homeless youth in Columbus, Ohio." *Journal of Interpersonal Violence* 25:1579–93.

Sparks, S. D. 2010. "Raising expectations is aim of new effort." *Education Week* 30:16–17.

Stewart, M., et al. 2016. "Respiratory health inequities experienced by low-income children and parents." *Journal of Poverty* 20:278–95.

Stirling, K., and T. Aldrich. 2008. "Child support: Who bears the burden." *Family Relations* 57:376–89.

Stratigos, A. J., and A. D. Katsambas. 2003. "Medical and cutaneous disorders associated with homelessness." *Skinned* 2:168–72.

Talukdar, D. 2008. "Cost of being poor: Retail price and consumer price search differences across inner-city and suburban neighborhoods." *Journal of Consumer Research* 35:457–71.

Taylor, M. J., A. S. Barusch, and M. B. Vogel-Ferguson. 2006. "Heterogeneity at the bottom: TANF closure and long-term welfare recipients." *Journal of Human Behavior in the Social Environment* 13:1–14.

U.S. Census Bureau. 2012. *Statistical Abstract of the United States*. Washington, DC: Government Printing Office.

U.S. Department of Justice. 2011. *Criminal Victimization, 2010*. U.S. Department of Justice website.

Volscho, T. W., and N. J. Kelly. 2012. "The rise of the super-rich." *American Sociological Review* 77:679–99.

Wasserman, J. A., and J. M. Clair. 2010. *At Home on the Street: People, Poverty and a Hidden Culture of Homelessness*. Boulder, CO: Lynne Rienner.

West, J., et al. 2010. "Head Start children go to kindergarten." ACF-OPRE Report. Administration for Children & Families website.

West, S., and G. Mottola. 2016. "A population on the brink: American renters, emergency savings, and financial fragility." *Poverty & Public Policy* 8:56–71.

Wheaton, B., and P. Clarke. 2003. "Space meets time: Integrating temporal and contextual influences on mental health in early adulthood." *American Sociological Review* 68:680–706.

Whoriskey, P. 2011. "Wealth-gap divide: Lawmakers, constituents." *San Diego Union-Tribune*, December 27.

Williams, T., and W. Kornblum. 1985. *Growing Up Poor*. Lexington, MA: DC Heath.

World Bank. 2020. "World development indicators." World Bank website.

Wu, Z., and C. M. Schimmele. 2005. "Food insufficiency and depression." *Sociological Perspectives* 48:481–504.

CHAPTER

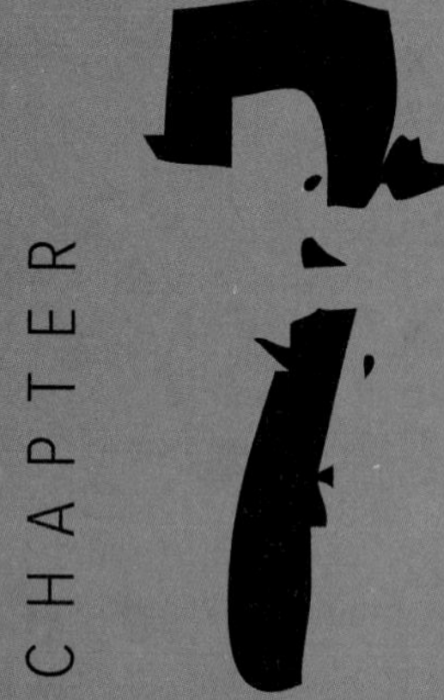

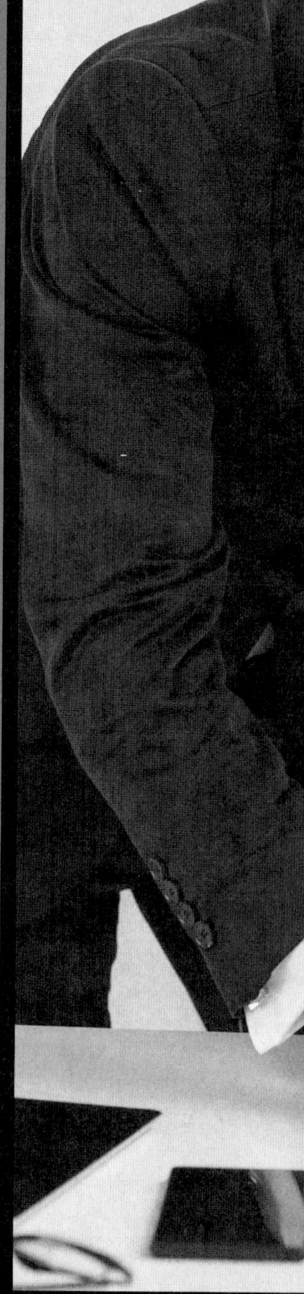

# Gender and Sexual Orientation

OBJECTIVES

1 Discuss the issue of biological versus social bases for gender differences.

2 Show how inequalities between the sexes affect women's lives.

3 Explain the social structural and social psychological factors that contribute to gender inequality.

4 Learn various explanations of homosexuality.

5 Identify how homophobia affects the quality of life of homosexuals and how to address the problem of homophobia.

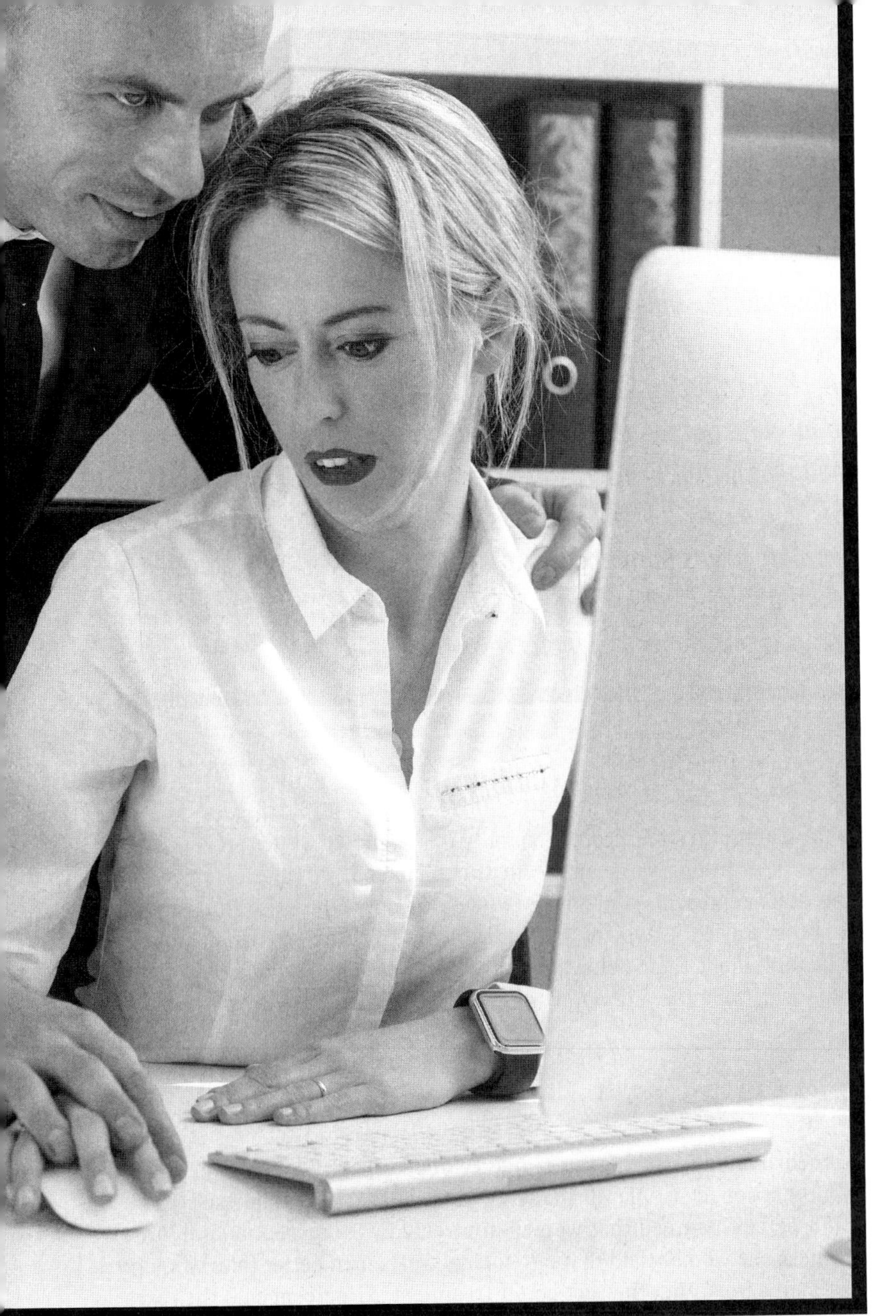

Kaspars Grinvalds/Shutterstock

### "I Didn't Need the Extra Hassles"

Sandra, a high-ranking university administrator in her 50s, started her graduate work when the youngest of her two children began school. In a sense she has it all—family and a successful career—but, as she notes, it has at times been a "journey of outrage":

*When I had the chance to go to graduate school, I was deliriously happy. Most of the other students were younger, but I could tell they accepted me and enjoyed having me around. I'm sure part of it was my enthusiasm for the program. I soon discovered, however, that I was embarking on a journey of outrage as well as one of a new career. My first inkling was when one of my fellow students hit on me one day in the library. He wanted to take me out somewhere. I must admit that I was rather flattered, since I was 10 years older than he was. So I just smiled and reminded him that I was married. He smiled back and said, "I don't mind." I told him that I did mind and that I had to get on with my studying.*

*I could have easily shrugged it off. But every time I tried to study in the library, he would sit at a table nearby and stare at me. I complained to the librarian, but he said that the student had broken no rules. I reminded him that this was really threatening to a woman. How could I be sure that the guy wouldn't try to do something crazy? The librarian looked sympathetic but helpless. I did the only thing I could. I stopped studying at the library and studied at home whenever I could find a quiet moment. Shortly after that, one of the faculty members started making overtures to me. This was really threatening, because I knew he could blackball me. I had to do a dance around him for three years. He did a good job of quenching a lot of my enthusiasm for school.*

*I could tell countless stories, but one more will illustrate why I call all this a journey of outrage. I came up for tenure in my first academic position. They turned me down. I hadn't published a whole lot, but I had published as much as a male colleague who got tenure. A friend told me that they rejected me because they thought my productivity would decline because of my family commitments. So all the way along, I faced one outrage after another. And just because I'm a woman. It was hard enough to do graduate work and start a career while raising a family. I didn't need the extra hassles. And what makes them so outrageous is that if I were a man they wouldn't have happened.*

## Introduction

What does it take for a group to suffer from inequality in the United States? It isn't size, because while one of the groups we examine in this chapter is comparatively small (homosexuals), the other represents a majority (women comprise nearly 51 percent of the population). In other ways, the two groups are similar in the extent to which biological versus social factors affect their behavior. Moreover, both have a long history of suffering from both discrimination and oppression.

## Gender Inequality

Are American women treated with the same dignity and respect as American men? A 2019 Gallup poll questioned people on the issue (Ray 2019). Less than half of the women surveyed (48 percent) agreed that women are treated with respect and dignity. Moreover, 59 percent of the women said that our society treats men better than women. Only 34 percent of men agreed that they get better treatment; 51 percent said the sexes are treated the same. Gender inequality is not as great as it was in the past, but it continues to vex the lives of many women.

**innate**
existing in a person from birth

**sex**
an individual's biological identity as male or female

**gender**
the meaning of being male or female in a particular society

**gender role**
the attitudes and behavior that are expected of men and women in a society

Because women suffer from inequality as a result of an **innate** characteristic (their sex), women are called the *largest minority* in America even though they are a slight majority of the population. As we discuss gender inequality, we use a number of important terms. **Sex** refers to an individual's biological identity as male or female. **Gender** is the meaning of being male or female in a particular society, and **gender role** refers to the attitudes and behavior that are expected of men and women in a society.

The terminology indicates that *some aspects of men and women are determined by social rather than biological factors.* This social aspect is the first issue we examine. Contrary to the argument that gender inequalities are the necessary outcome of biological differences, we show that the problems are sociocultural in origin and how they affect the quality of life for women. Finally, we look at structural and social psychological factors that contribute to gender inequality and suggest some ways to address the problems.

## Biology or Society?

There are numerous differences in the attitudes, behavior, and personalities of the sexes (Marano and Strand 2003; Goldman et al. 2004; Schmitt, Realo, Voracek, and Allik 2008; Redmond and McGuinness 2020). Among other aspects, men and women differ in their attention span, their aspirations, the strategies they use in competitive games, the amount they smile, their vulnerability to particular diseases and to addictions, the structure and functioning of their brains, their sexual interests, their satisfaction with their jobs, and the extent to which they are agreeable and conscientious. The question we want to examine here is, what accounts for those differences? Are they rooted in biology or in society? The questions are important because people who hold to a strong biological position are likely to fall into the *fallacy of retrospective determinism,* arguing that whatever has happened to women in American society is inevitable because people are determined by their own biological makeup to behave and function in certain ways.

fallacy

*Gender and Biology.* The "damsel in distress" and "white knight" of folklore illustrate the longstanding notion that men are the independent and women the dependent creatures. An empirical basis for asserting the natural subservience of women is claimed by people who draw on research in the areas of sociobiology (the use of biological factors to explain social phenomena), the brain, and human hormones (Wilson 2000; Pfaff 2002). These researchers claim, on the basis of various kinds of evidence, that human behavior must be understood in terms of *innate biological differences between the sexes.* Some stress humans' continuity with other animals and argue that male and female behavior reflect the imperatives of the evolutionary process–the struggle to survive and to perpetuate one's kind.

People who draw on research on the brain and hormones also stress the biological differences but do not necessarily talk about them in terms of evolutionary imperatives. Rather, the differences are used to explain such factors as the higher levels of aggression among males, the greater verbal abilities of females, and the tendency of women to be more stressed than men by emotional conflict (Brizendine 2006).

Clearly, there are differences between males and females in both the structure and functioning of the brain (Kreeger 2002), but the implications of these differences are controversial. First, many of the differences are relatively small or even trivial (Hyde 2005). Second, research continues to modify some of the conclusions about differences. For example, it is not true, as many have believed, that boys are inherently better at math than are girls. An analysis of hundreds of studies comparing how males and females perform in math concluded that there are no differences (Lindberg, Hyde, Petersen, and Linn 2010). The two sexes have equal capacity for doing math and science.

Thus, the implications for behavior of the differing brain and hormonal structures of males and females are uncertain and controversial. It is best, we believe, to accept the conclusion of a biologist that social interaction affects biological processes as well as vice versa, so that mind, body, and culture interact with each other (Fausto-Sterling 1992). Behavior is always a function of multiple factors, and no one can say with certainty how much of any particular behavior is biologically driven and how much is socially formed.

*Men's Issues.* In the late 1980s, a *men's movement rapidly gained momentum.* In the University of California reference system, the number of books related to men and masculinity

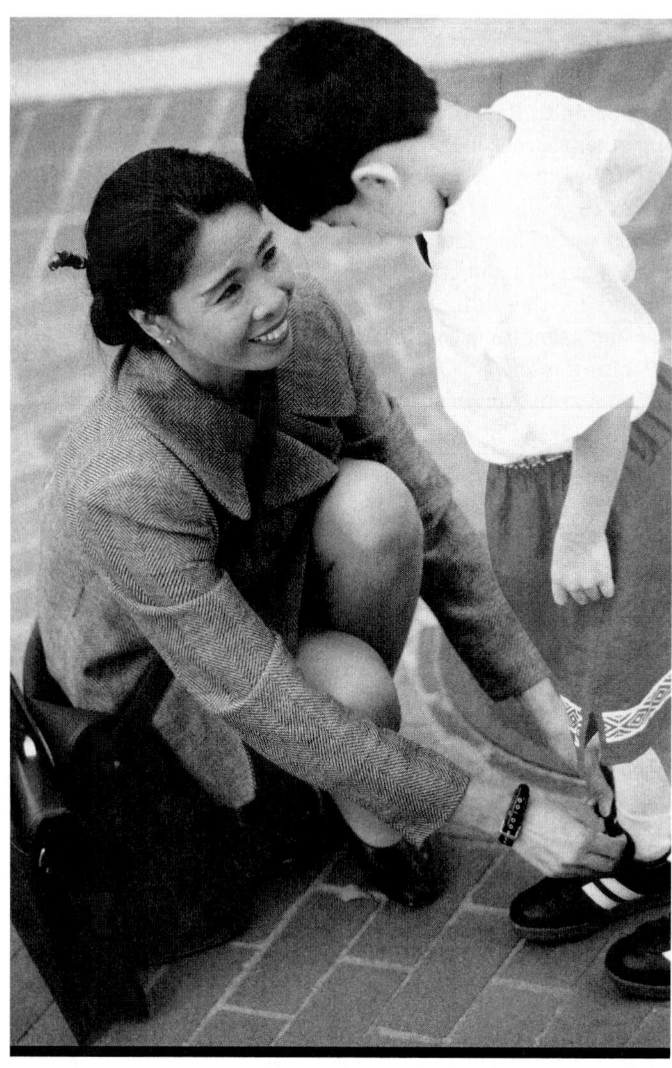

Nurturing is a significant part of the traditional role of women.

EyeWire Collection/Getty Images

increased sevenfold between 1989 and 1995 (Newton 1998). During the period, the number of scholarly essays in the area tripled and the number of popular magazine articles increased tenfold.

We look briefly at this movement for two reasons. First, we don't want to give the impression that men have all the advantages and none of the problems. Men's issues are as legitimate as women's. Second, the men's movement illustrates our point that gender behavior is sociocultural and not merely biological.

Issues of concern to men include the following (Newton 1998; Blais and Dupuis-Deri 2012; Bote 2020):

- The meaning of masculinity in a time of changing gender roles.
- The meaning of being a father and a husband in the face of feminist assertions and cultural expectations.
- The rights of divorced and single fathers.
- Perceived discriminatory treatment by lawyers and the courts in divorce and child custody hearings.
- Reverse bias in hiring and promotions when women are chosen over men who are more qualified.

Some segments of the men's movement take the position that men, not women, are the truly oppressed group today (Ferber 2000). They argue that men have been "demasculinized," that women and the women's movement are responsible, and that men must reclaim their masculinity and their rightful authority.

Others in the movement are concerned with more specific issues such as fatherhood (Ranson 2001). In the past, fathers were thought of as breadwinners who had limited time to spend with their children. Today fathers are expected to be much more involved in their children's lives, but they are also expected to be successful in the workplace. How can they meet the competing demands? What do they do when parenting and work requirements contradict each other? What is the role of the wife and mother in all this?

Clearly, such questions arise not out of biology but out of the social milieu. Men's issues, like women's, are a reflection of the sociocultural context–or, to put it another way, gender roles result from sociocultural, not merely biological, factors.

## Gender Inequality and the Quality of Life

Although men as well as women have problems and complaints, our focus is on the inequality faced by women. Epstein (2007) pointed out that the world is "made up of great divides" such as nationality, wealth, race, and class. Where you stand in such categories has a profound effect on your life. But the "most fundamental social divide," she argued, is sex. Your life is significantly affected and shaped by whether you are male or female. In this section we will see the basis for such a claim as we examine *the contradictions between the ideology of equal opportunities and the reality of life for women.* Keep in mind that the gender inequalities we discuss are not merely an American problem, but are pervasive in the world. The United States is neither the best nor the worst when it comes to gender equality. Rather, it ranked 53rd out of 153 countries studied in terms of their degree of gender equality in the areas of economic participation and opportunity, educational attainment, health and survival, and political empowerment (World Economic Forum 2020). The three countries with the greatest equality were Iceland, Norway, and Finland; the three with the greatest inequality were Iraq, Pakistan, and Yemen.

*Career Inequality.* After World War II, the ideal pattern for women was to marry and become a homemaker and stay-at-home mother. Both the ideal and the reality have changed. The proportion of married women in the labor force rose from 23.8 percent in 1950 to 58.2 percent in 2018; the proportion of women who were in the labor force and had children under 6 years of age increased even more dramatically, from 11.9 percent in 1950 to 64.7 percent in 2018 (Bureau of Labor Statistics 2019). It might appear that this means increasing equality in the labor market. Such a conclusion would be further buttressed by unemployment rates (Table 7.1), which measure the number of people who desire employment but are out of work. Until the 1990s, the rates were nearly always higher for women than for men, a contradiction of the *ideology of equal opportunity.* Since 1990, however, the rates have tended to be roughly equal or to be higher for men than for women.

Yet equal economic opportunities only begin at the point of employment. What about women's opportunities for advancement? What about their income? Are they also equal to those of men?

Unfortunately, the ideology of equal opportunity is *contradicted by the discriminatory treatment of women in various occupations.* Women experience discrimination in hiring, in on-the-job training, in promotions, and in the way they are treated by supervisors and coworkers (Knoke and Ishio 1998; Yoder and Berendsen 2001; Gorman and Kmec 2009). And this is not only an American problem. A study of 22 industrialized

**TABLE 7.1**
Unemployment Rates, by Sex, 1948 to 2019
*(persons 16 years and over)*

| Year | Male | Female |
|---|---|---|
| 1948 | 3.6 | 4.1 |
| 1950 | 5.1 | 5.7 |
| 1960 | 5.4 | 5.9 |
| 1970 | 4.4 | 5.9 |
| 1980 | 6.9 | 7.4 |
| 1990 | 5.6 | 5.4 |
| 2000 | 3.9 | 4.1 |
| 2010 | 10.6 | 8.6 |
| 2015 | 5.3 | 5.2 |
| 2019 | 3.7 | 3.6 |

SOURCES: U.S. Census Bureau, *Statistical Abstract of the United States*, various editions, and Bureau of Labor Statistics website.

nations reported that while developed welfare states (such as Sweden) have a high proportion of women in the labor force, those women tend to be concentrated in female-typed occupations and are less likely to be in managerial occupations (Mandel and Semyonov 2006). The consequences of discrimination in pursuing a meaningful career include increased physical and emotional health problems (Pavalko, Mossakowski, and Hamilton 2003).

Consider the following facts about the amount and kind of discrimination women encounter. In many occupational categories, women are found disproportionately in the lower-echelon jobs. Although far more women than men are teachers, the proportion of women in top administrative jobs in education (superintendents, assistant superintendents, principals, and assistant principals) is low (Wrushen and Sherman 2008). Increasing proportions of admissions to medical schools are female, but women may be encouraged to pursue the traditional "female" specialties such as pediatrics, psychiatry, and preventive medicine. Moreover, although women compose nearly half of all medical students, only 35 percent of full-time medical faculty, 19 percent of full professors in medical schools, and 13 percent of medical department chairs and deans are women (Association of American Medical Colleges 2011).

Table 7.2 illustrates the fact that many occupations continue to be male or female dominated, what social scientists call a *segregated labor market.* Such segregation has detrimental consequences for women. The occupations that have a high proportion of women tend to be lower in status and lower in pay (Cohen and Huffman 2003). In some cases, the occupations are also less desirable from the point of view of meaningful work.

In other words, in a segregated labor market, people tend to evaluate jobs and careers in terms of the predominant gender of the workers as well as the education and skills required. An apparently obvious solution would be for women to choose male-dominated occupations if they want to maximize their status and their income. Unfortunately, women do not gain the same prestige as men when they enter predominantly male occupations. Many women in male-dominated careers feel that they not only must prove their competence but must do so by performing their job even better than a man would. On the other hand, when men come into a predominantly female occupation, they tend to get more pay, better positions, and high respect (Barnett and Rivers 2020).

Finally, women face career discrimination because they are more likely than men to experience conflict between their work and their home responsibilities, a conflict that is intensified if the woman has more responsibility for child care (Hill, Hawkins, Maartinson, and Ferris 2003). Women continue to find childbearing costly to their careers, and those in a male-dominated occupation where long hours are the norm for workers may drop out of the labor force entirely (Cha 2013; Kahn, Garcia-Manglano, and Bianchi 2014). It's true that fathers are more involved with child care and household chores than they were in the past. Nevertheless, even when the mother is working part- or full-time, she continues to bear more responsibility for family and home. The Bureau of Labor Statistics (2020) time use survey found that on an average day 85 percent of women and 71 percent of men spent time on household chores; women spent 2.5 hours and men averaged 1.9 hours on the chores. In addition, on an average day men had 5.5 hours of leisure activities, while women had 4.9 hours. And in households with children under the age of six, women spent 1.1 hours on physical care, while men spent spent 27 minutes.

*Income Inequality.* Slower advancement means that women tend to cluster in the lower levels of virtually all occupational categories and are, therefore, accorded less prestige and lower salaries than men. The demand of the women's movement for *equal*

| Occupation | Percent Female | Occupation | Percent Female |
|---|---|---|---|
| Total | 47.0 | | |
| *Managerial and Professional* | | *Service* | |
| Chief executives | 27.6 | Dental assistants | 94.9 |
| Managers, medicine/health | 69.7 | Firefighters | 3.3 |
| Architects | 24.5 | Chefs and head cooks | 20.0 |
| Civil engineers | 13.9 | Waiters and waitresses | 71.3 |
| Computer programmers | 20.3 | Child care workers | 93.4 |
| Physicians and surgeons | 40.8 | Pest control workers | 6.7 |
| College/university teachers | 47.4 | Police officers/sheriffs | 17.6 |
| Elementary school teachers | 80.5 | *Natural Resources and Construction* | |
| Librarians | 79.9 | Farming, fishing, forestry | 25.2 |
| Lawyers | 36.4 | Carpenters | 2.8 |
| Writers and authors | 63.5 | Electricians | 2.2 |
| Social workers | 81.9 | Highway maintenance | 3.6 |
| *Sales and Office* | | *Production and Transportation* | |
| Cashiers | 71.2 | Bakers | 60.4 |
| Secretaries | 93.2 | Machinists | 5.6 |
| Receptionists | 89.3 | Laundry/dry cleaning | 75.4 |
| Postal clerks | 55.1 | Painting workers | 8.9 |
| Bank tellers | 84.7 | Pilots/flight engineers | 7.5 |
| Wholesale sales reps | 27.2 | Taxi drivers/chauffeurs | 16.8 |

SOURCE: Bureau of Labor Statistics website.

**TABLE 7.2**
Employed Persons by Sex and Selected Occupation, 2019

*pay for work of equivalent value* reflects the fact that women are not rewarded equally with men even when they are equally prepared, equally qualified, and equally competent (Newcomb 2018). There is a "glass ceiling," a term used to refer to the arbitrary and often invisible barriers that limit women's advancement. The glass ceiling on income exists in all occupational categories (Cotter, Hermsen, Ovadia, and Vanneman 2001; Bureau of Labor Statistics 2020).

Overall, from the 1950s until the late 1970s, women received about 60 percent of the income men received. Then the gap began to close, although the disparity is still large: By 2018, the median earnings of women who worked full-time year-round was 81 percent of that for men (Bureau of Labor Statistics website). As Figure 7.1 shows, the disparity holds for all races.

Even when taking into account such factors as education, occupational category, hours worked, experience, and performance ratings, there is still a substantial wage gap that is not explained (Dey and Hill 2007; Castilla 2008; Fernandez-Mateo 2009). For example, Roth (2003) examined a group of Wall Street securities professionals who were similar to each other in terms of such factors as education and ability. She found significant gender differences in earnings that could not be explained by anything other than discrimination. Similarly, a study of University of Michigan law school graduates reported that 15 years after graduation the men earned 52 percent more than the women, 17 percent more than women with similar characteristics, and 11 percent more than

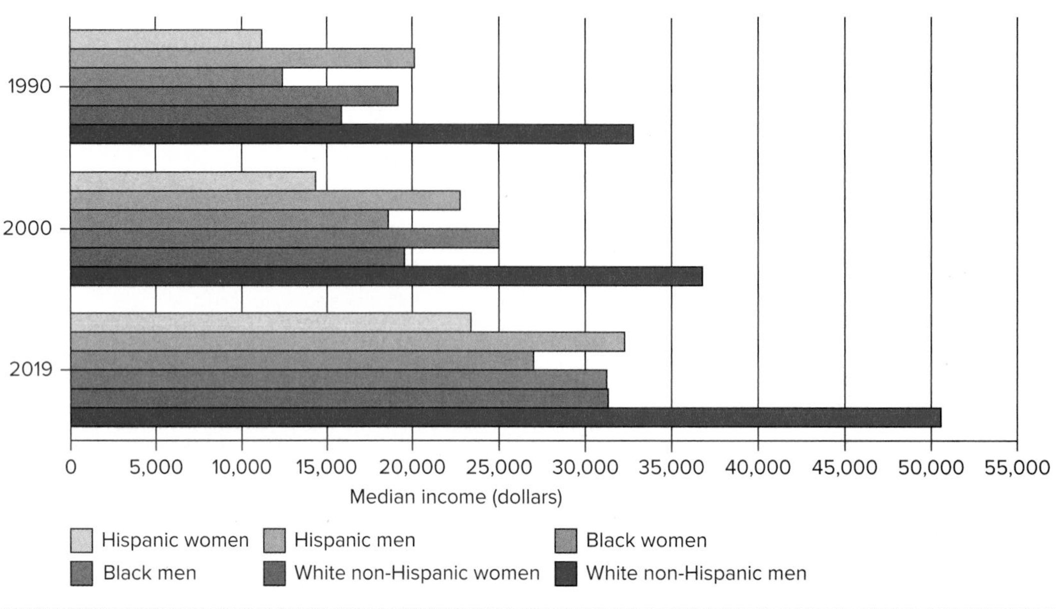


**FIGURE 7.1** Median Income of Persons, 1990–2019.
Source: U.S. Census Bureau website.

women with similar characteristics in the same job settings (Noonan, Corcoran, and Courant 2005). In the medical field, female registered nurses far outnumber male nurses, but the males are paid more and the income gap has persisted for decades (Muench et al. 2015). And a study of physicians who teach at medical schools reported an average gender gap of $20,000 a year even after controlling for age, experience, specialty, faculty rank, and productivity (Jena, Olenski, and Blumenthal 2016).

*The Beauty Myth.* The "beauty myth" involves a *contradiction between the belief in the dignity of all humans,* on one hand, and the *ideology about a particular group,* on the other hand. According to the beauty myth, a woman must be beautiful to be acceptable and attractive (Sullivan 2001). It's a destructive myth. Nevertheless, women (including adolescents) spent billions of dollars a year on millions of procedures in an effort to appear more beautiful (Lee et al. 2017; Elflein 2019). In 2019, Americans opted for 1.47 million surgical (e.g., breast augmentation and liposuction) and 3.12 million nonsurgical (e.g., botox and hair removal) procedures.

But beauty is a trap. Women who see themselves as homely cannot enjoy their accomplishments because they are haunted by their failure to be beautiful, and women who are beautiful and successful may attribute their success to their beauty rather than to their abilities.

A particularly destructive aspect of the beauty myth is the current ideal of a slender figure for women. Bombarded by media depictions of thinness as the ideal, many women develop *a problem of body image.* They become dissatisfied with the shape and size of their bodies. White and Hispanic women are slightly more likely than Black women to experience body dissatisfaction, but the problem occurs among all races (Grabe and Hyde 2006; Boroughs, Krawczyk, and Thompson 2010). It develops quite early in girls' lives. A study of 55 preschool girls concluded that girls may become emotionally invested in the thin ideal as early as 3 years of age (Harriger, Calogero, Witherington, and Smith 2010).

Body dissatisfaction can result in a variety of negative consequences for well-being. It can lead to lowered self-esteem, problematic sexual functioning (including risky sexual behavior), depression, and anxiety (Davison and McCabe 2005; Gillen, Lefkowitz, and Shearer 2006). It also leads some women, in an effort to get thinner, to succumb to eating disorders, such as *anorexia nervosa (a form of self-starvation)* and *bulimia (repeated binge eating followed by vomiting or laxatives).* The disorders are associated with a variety of physical and emotional health problems. For example, anorexia nervosa is associated with the loss of the menstrual period, anemia, loss of hair and bone density, and kidney failure (Torpy and Glass 2006). Eating disorders are also associated with depression (Stice and Bearman 2001).

In extreme cases, some young women have died from these eating disorders. A woman can go to such an extreme because the disorders involve a disturbed body image (Miyake et al. 2010). That is, the woman does not see herself as thin even when others see her as emaciated.

Body image is an issue for men also (Grogan and Richards 2002). For men, a well-toned, muscular body provides confidence and a sense of power in social situations. Like women, men may engage in unhealthy dieting behaviors in an effort to realize their ideal (Markey and Markey 2005). But the problem of body image is more severe among women, who expressed more dissatisfaction than did men about their body shape (Demarest and Allen 2000).

*Harassment and Violence.* A different form of assault on dignity is the **sexual harassment** to which so many women have been subjected. Sexual harassment refers to unwelcome sexual advances, requests for sexual favors, and other verbal or physical conduct of a sexual nature that results in some kind of punishment when the victim resists or that creates a hostile environment. Although both men and women may be sexually harassed, the proportion of women who experience it is higher. For example, a survey of sexual harassment and assault experienced by reservists during military service found that 60 percent of females (compared to 27.1 percent of males) reported being victims of sexual harassment, and 13.1 percent of the females (compared to 1.6 percent of the males) reported a sexual assault (Street, Gradus, Stafford, and Kelly 2007). A national survey of college students found that 35 percent of females and 29 percent of males had been physically harassed (touched, grabbed, pinched in a sexual way), while 57 percent of females and 48 percent of males had been verbally harassed (American Association of University Women 2006). A national study of middle school and high school students found that 56 percent of the girls and 40 percent of the boys had been sexually harassed (American Association of University Women 2012). Nearly a third experienced electronic harassment by such means as texting, e-mail, and Facebook, and many of them were also harassed in person.

**sexual harassment**
unwelcome sexual advances, requests for sexual favors, and other sexual behavior that either results in punishment when the victim resists or creates a hostile environment or both

Sexual harassment, then, occurs in all kinds of settings, among all ages, and both personally and electronically. It happens to female graduate students (Rosenthal, Smidt, and Freyd 2016). It happens to women in positions of authority as well as those in subordinate positions (McLaughlin, Uggen, and Blackstone 2012). And it happens to workers in all occupations from professionals (e.g., lawyers, professors, scientists) to blue-collar workers (e.g., autoworkers) who report experiences of sexual harassment (Bronner, Peretz, and Ehrenfeld 2003; Menard, Phung, Ghebrial, and Martin 2003; Hinze 2004; Settles, Cortina, Malley, and Stewart 2006). Overall, estimates are that at least half of all women will be harassed at some point during their academic or working lives, resulting in such things as lowered job satisfaction, physical and mental health

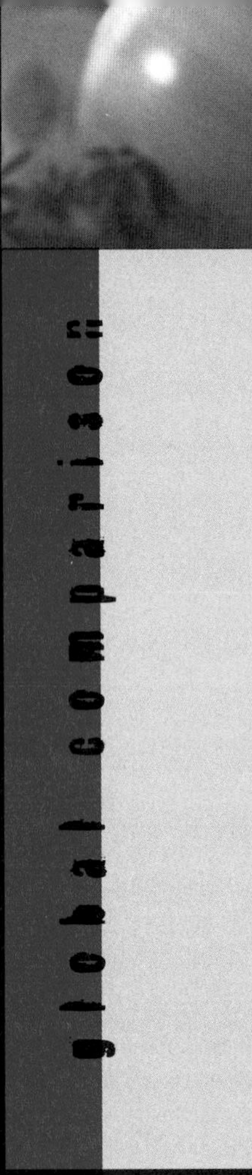


## OCCUPATIONAL SEX SEGREGATION IN DEVELOPING COUNTRIES

As noted in the text, occupational sex segregation is detrimental to the interests of women in the job market. In a highly segregated job market, women's income and status, compared to those of men, both tend to be depressed. Although researchers have found such segregation not only in the United States but also in other industrial nations, little has been done to examine it in developing countries. Chang's (2004) work, however, not only examined the patterns and extent of sex segregation in a number of developing nations but also identified the effects of government policies on the segregation.

Occupational sex segregation exists in all countries, though the extent of the segregation varies considerably (Figure 7.2). Interestingly, Chang found that government policies were the strongest predictor of variations in the extent of segregation. In particular, the lower levels of segregation occurred in nations that have maternity leave legislation. When women must be given maternity leave, increased numbers of them are able to enter the otherwise male-dominated managerial and production occupations.

On the other hand, a surprising finding was that those nations whose governments had enacted antidiscrimination legislation had the highest levels of segregation! Because Chang did not have data both before and after the legislation, it is possible that the legislation did reduce the amount of segregation. But because the levels were so high prior to the legislation, those nations still had higher levels of segregation than the others. It is also possible that antidiscrimination legislation is less effective because it is difficult to enforce and may not be enforced because of cultural restrictions on male-female interaction.

Finally, Chang found that the levels of occupational sex segregation in the developing nations that she studied were higher than the levels found by other researchers in the developed nations. With increasing development, the amount of segregation—and, consequently, the detrimental consequences for women—may diminish. But no nation yet has achieved sexual equality in the job market.

problems, and postraumatic stress symptoms (Chan, Lam, Chow, and Cheung 2008; Woods, Buchanan, and Settles 2009; Harnois and Bastos 2018).

The harassment is so pervasive and the results so stressful that the Me Too (or #MeToo) movement arose in 2006. It gained momentum in 2017 when a number of actresses went public with their experiences of harassment in the film industry. Me Too is an effort both to publicize the problem and to encourage women generally to be open about their experiences and thereby help bring about change.

The perpetrator of harassment is most likely to be someone in a position of authority over the victim (Uggen and Blackstone 2004). In fact, perhaps the most destructive harassment occurs in the *sexual exploitation of women by men of authority in the helping professions.* Such male power figures include psychiatrists and other therapists, physicians, lawyers, clergymen, and teachers or mentors. Women are particularly vulnerable to sexual pressures in dealing with such power figures. A therapist, for example, may convince a woman that he can provide her with the kind of sexual experience she needs to work through her problems. A clergyman may convince a woman that there is some kind of divine sanction to their relationship. Although we don't know the number of women exploited in this way, increasing attention is being paid to the problem. Indeed, some professional organizations have explicitly condemned such behavior in their codes of ethics.

Finally, violence is the ultimate assault on the dignity of women. Hundreds of thousands of violent acts are committed against women every year, and about a fifth of all violence against women comes from an intimate partner. The problem is worldwide. A

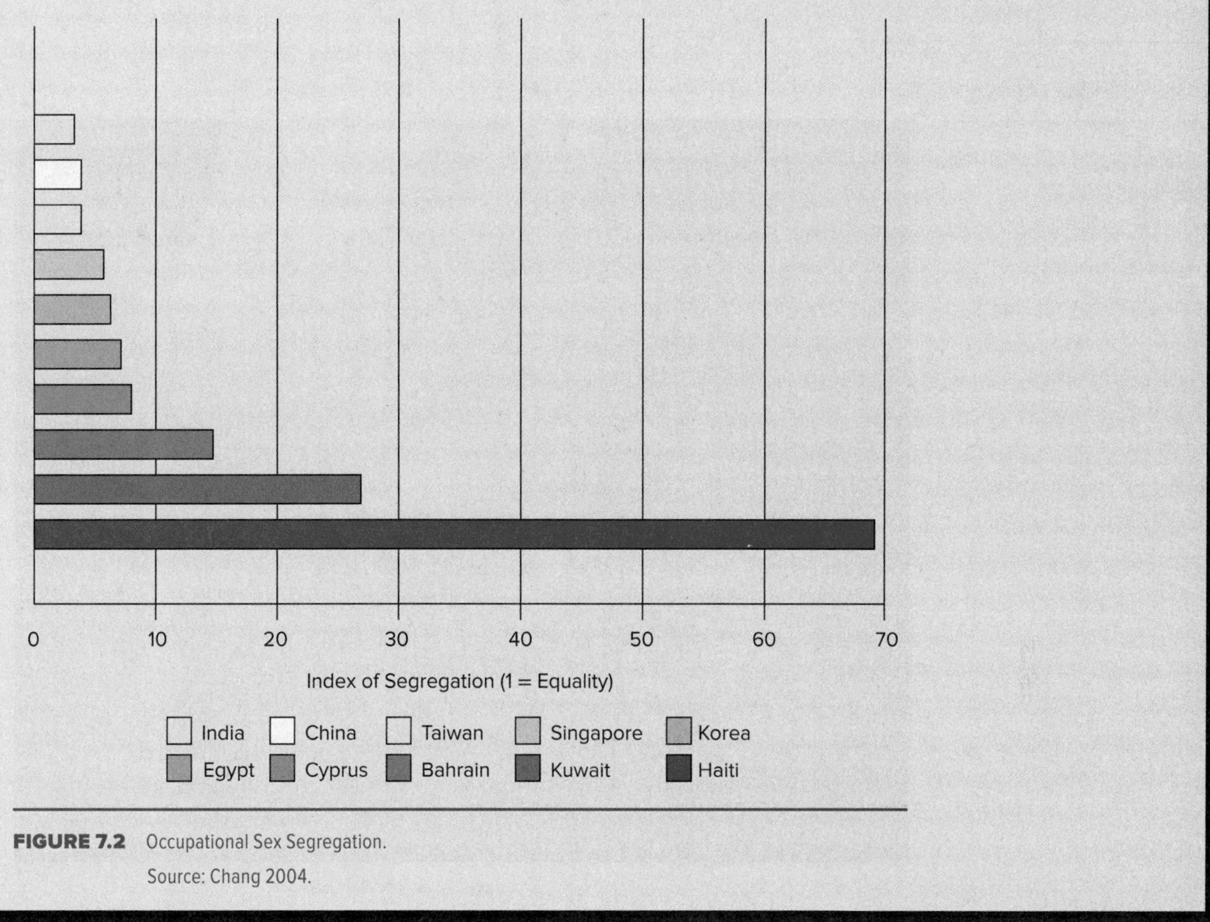


**FIGURE 7.2** Occupational Sex Segregation.
Source: Chang 2004.

United Nations global survey found that during their lifetime, 67.2 percent of women reported physical or sexual violence and 81.6 percent reported psychological violence by their current husband (Fokir 2011). And a fourth of women reported such violence by someone other than their husband.

## Contributing Factors

As with all social problems, many factors contribute to gender inequality. As we examine these factors, it will be clear that the problem is not simply one of men versus women but of a plexus of factors that together create and maintain this inequality.

*Social Structural Factors.* The *normative role of the female* is an important factor in gender inequality because *gender roles specify certain kinds of behavior as appropriate, and other kinds as inappropriate, for men and women.* What, then, is the *traditional role for the American female,* and how does this role contribute to inequality?

In essence, Americans have advocated the *traditional homemaker role of females and the parallel traditional breadwinner role of males.* Certainly, not all females conform to the traditional role. Working-class and African American women, in particular, have been likely to work outside the home. For the bulk of middle- and upper-class whites, however, the wife has been expected to provide a home for her husband and children and to find her fulfillment in caring for her family. The role assumes, then, that a woman will marry and have children and will focus on pleasing her husband and caring for her children.

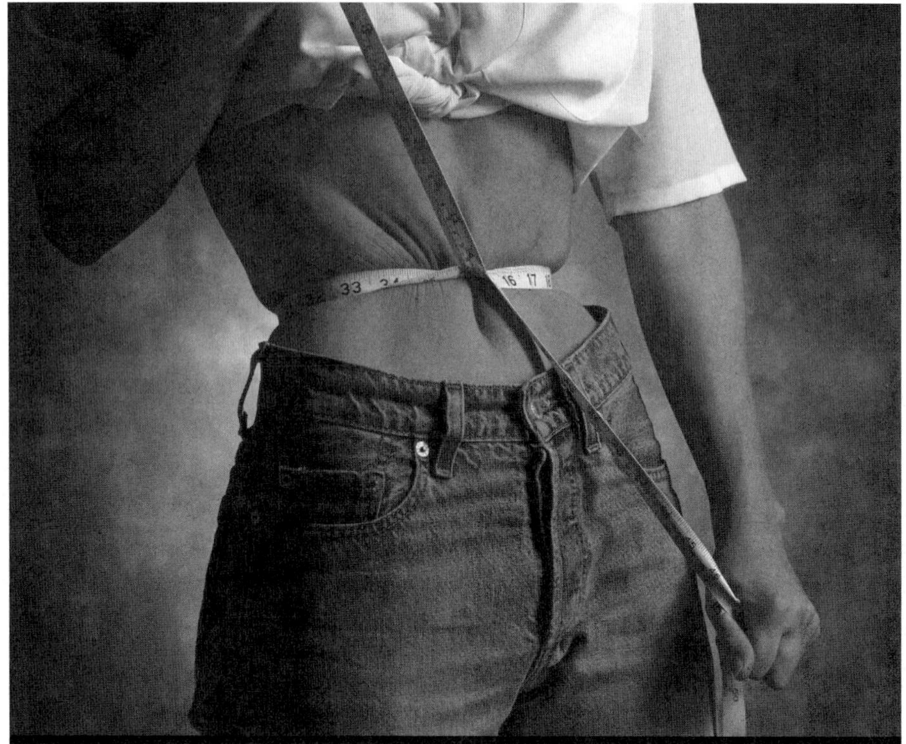

The beauty myth can result in a body image problem.

Colin Anderson/Brand X Pictures/Getty Images

In the 1960s and 1970s women's attitudes toward this traditional role changed considerably. By 2019, 56 percent of American women preferred working to homemaking (Brenan 2019). That proportion grows to 64 percent among women with a college degree. Even among women who have children under the age of 18, 45 percent prefer to work.

But the traditional view still receives considerable support, particularly among very conservative religious groups that affirm the subordinate role of the wife. This perspective is well illustrated by the Protestant pastor who summed up the role by saying the wife is the manager of the home and the husband is the manager of the wife.

The traditional role obviously discourages women from pursuing higher education or a career. In a social context in which being female means taking care of a home and family and submitting to one's husband, it may be difficult to secure an advanced degree or to commit oneself to a career.

The research on women's aspirations suggests that if females are treated the same as males, if parents hold similar expectations for their girls and boys and encourage them equally, women will achieve the same levels of education and probably the same levels of work and careers. A great many women would like to work or pursue a career but do not because it conflicts with other role obligations. Only a minority of women prefer either a career without marriage or marriage and children without a career.

The ability to opt for multiple roles is crucial because a *restrictive role for women can lead to illness.* For both men and women, both marriage and employment increase well-being (see Chapter 10). Multiple roles not only promote well-being, including physical health, but also tend to lengthen a woman's life (Rose et al. 2004; Bryant and Constantine 2006). To be a wife, a mother, and also have a career, then, tends to enhance the emotional and physical well-being of women.

Even though women who go to work have better physical and mental health, working does not solve all their problems. Such women are still likely to have more health problems than their male counterparts. A number of factors bear on the question of how much married women with children will benefit by working outside the home or pursuing a career, including the nature of the work and the division of labor in the home. As far as the nature of the work is concerned, mothers are healthier when they have high-quality jobs, and when they prefer to work rather than to be a stay-at-home mother (Usdansky, Gordon, Wang, and Gluzman 2011). During the preschool years of their children, mothers may benefit more from part-time than full-time work (Buehler and O'Brien 2011). Indeed, a study of women in 28 countries found that homemakers are slightly happier than those who work full-time, but not happier than those who work part-time (Treas, van der Lippe, and Tai 2011).

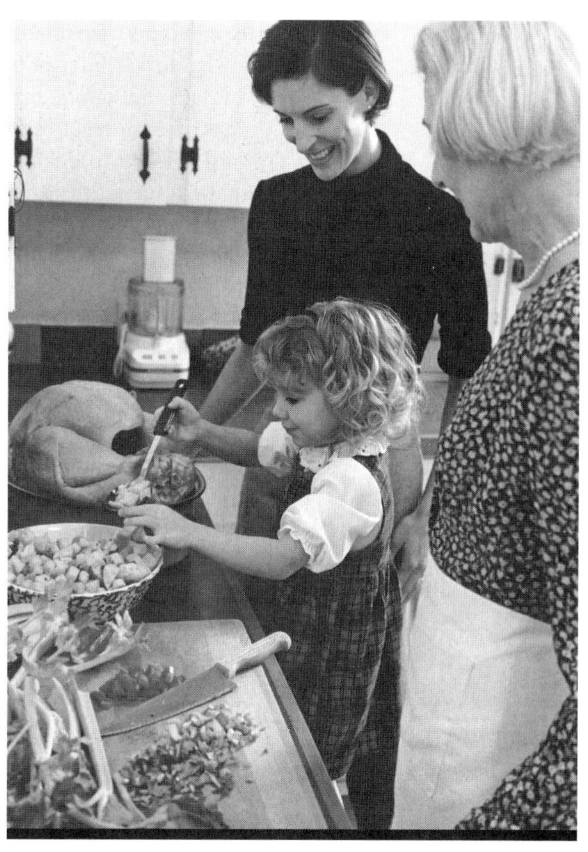

Many children are reared in accord with gender stereotypes.

Ryan McVay/Getty Images

With regard to the division of labor in the home, the likelihood is that having a job outside the house means "in addition" rather than "instead of" taking care of the home. There has been a trend toward greater sharing of household responsibilities, but employed women still spend substantially more hours than their husbands doing housework (Kulik 2011). Surveys of how Americans spend their time show that by 2019, the average amount of time spent on household activities (housework, meal preparation and cleanup, and lawn and garden care) each day was 1.85 hours for women and 1.28 hours for men (Bureau of Labor Statistics 2020). On an average day, 85 percent of women and 71 percent of men spent some time on those activities. And on an average day, women with children under age 6 spent 1.1 hours, while fathers spent only 27 minutes, providing physical care. The result of this inequity in the household division of labor is a higher level of stress and a greater likelihood of depression for the woman (Frisco and Williams 2003). Mothers are also stressed by their greater likelihood of sleep deprivation as they care for the needs of their family (Maume, Sebastian, and Bardo 2010). In short, working outside the home may have positive health benefits for mothers, but the benefit would increase measurably if fathers would assume an equitable share of housework and child care.

A second important social structural factor in gender inequality is the *socialization that occurs at home, in school, and through the mass media.* In the home, parents tend to treat their sons and daughters differently from the beginning, with the result that children become aware of gender-role differences while they are still toddlers (Martin 2014). The differential treatment continues in the kinds of toys and play activities parents, probably unaware of the effects, provide for their children. For example, a Barbie doll can create the desire in young girls for a thinner body (Dittmar, Halliwell, and Ive 2006). And girls who played with Barbie dolls also believed they had fewer future career options than boys did (Sherman and Zurbriggen 2014). By the early school years, children already have a sense of which occupations are "feminine" and which are "masculine," as well as the relative status of the various occupations (Teig and Susskind 2008). Some girls who otherwise might have pursued a career in science, engineering, or math may already have their interest in such a career undermined by stereotypes of what is feminine and what is masculine in the world of work (Shapiro and Williams 2012).

Parents also react differently to sons and daughters in the emotional realm. Fathers reward girls but punish boys for expressing sadness and fear (Bayrakdar-Garside and Klimes-Dougan 2002). When children misbehave in ways that could lead to injury, mothers are angry with their sons but disappointed with their daughters, whereas once an injury occurs, mothers attribute their sons' risky misbehavior to factors beyond their control and daughters' risky misbehavior to factors they can influence (Morrongiello and Hogg 2004).

The school may reinforce the parental pattern. Girls get higher scores than boys on most academic and cognitive tests (Francis and Skelton 2005). Nevertheless, teachers can, like parents, treat boys and girls in terms of traditional gender roles. For example, various studies have found that teachers expect girls to behave better, that they treat boy underachievers as bright but bored and overlook girl underachievers (perhaps they don't consider it as important for girls to achieve academically), and that in physical education boys get more attention and feedback (praise, criticism, technical information) than do girls (Jones and Myhill 2004; Myhill and Jones 2006; Nicaise, Cogerino, Bois, and Amorose 2006).

The *mass media are an important source of gender-role socialization.* Children's books (including picture books for the very young, elementary reading books, the Sunday comics in newspapers, TV ads, Halloween costumes, and Valentine cards all still tend to portray males and females in traditional dominant-submissive roles (Diekman and Murnen 2004; Kahlenberg and Hein 2010; McCabe, Brewster, and Tillman 2011; Mager and Helgeson 2011; Murnen, Greenfield, Younger, and Boyd 2016). An analysis of music videos found that they reinforced the image of women as sex objects and as tending to be subordinate to men (Wallis 2011). Some popular magazines and books also reinforce the power differences between men and women, portray women as sex objects, and perpetuate the ideal of thinness (Zimmerman, Haddock, and McGeorge 2001; Krassas, Blauwkamp, and Wesselink 2001). An analysis of 100 top income-grossing films found that middle-aged men were more likely than their female counterparts to play leadership roles and to have occupational power (Lauzen and Dozier 2005).

Such portrayals in the media have an impact. Men who watch television programs that portray women as sex objects are more likely to engage in sexual harassment (Galdi, Maass, and Cadinu 2014). Girls and women exposed to the thinness ideal on television and in magazines have an increased likelihood of lowered self-esteem, depression, eating disorders, and approval of cosmetic surgical procedures such as liposuction and breast augmentation (Botta 2003; Vaughan and Fouts 2003; Bessenoff 2006).

fallacy

Another practical consequence of media portrayal of the sexes is that people who engage in the *fallacy of circular reasoning* find support for their arguments. Consider the following exchange we once had with an older man who made the statement: "Everyone knows that men are rational and women are emotional." We asked the man how he knew that. "Everyone knows that. Look around you. Look at television." When the man was told that television is fiction, he replied: "But it is based on fact, on what is real about people. And men are really rational and women are really emotional."

*A third social structural factor is the economics of gender inequality.* Situations that continue in the nation are *likely profitable* for someone, and gender inequality is no exception. The kind of gender inequalities we have discussed are beneficial for men in a variety of ways. They increase men's job opportunities, incomes, and power. It has

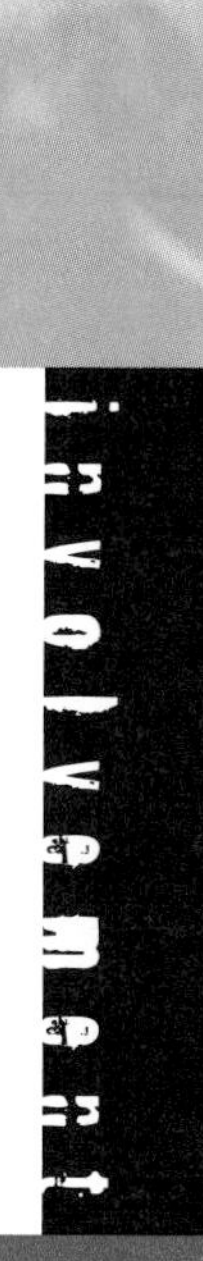


## YOU ARE WHAT YOU READ

Someone has said, "You are what you read." As noted in this chapter, one factor in perpetuating gender-role inequality is the books that you read as a child. Conduct your own research into children's literature. The librarian at a local public library can help you make a selection. Decide on what age level you want to investigate first. Then find five books written for this age level before 1975 and five of the most recent.

Compare the books in terms of the number of male and female characters and the gender roles portrayed. How do the earlier books differ from the more recent ones? To what extent do you believe that the later books overcome gender inequality? Identify two or three aspects of traditional gender roles in the earlier books that are either maintained or eliminated in the later ones.

If the entire class does this project, assign people to cover different age levels (beginning with picture books for preschool children) and see whether there are any differences by age.

been said that the hand that rocks the cradle rocks the world (which suggests that real power belongs to women). In most people's experience, however, the hand that holds the biggest purse holds the most power—and this hand typically belongs to a man.

Furthermore, the present amount of income inequality between men and women means that men benefit by having to work less to earn the same amount of money. In essence, a woman might work seven days or more to earn what a man makes in five days (because, as noted earlier, the median income of women of all races is less than that of their male counterparts).

Since the end of World War II, women and men have been engaged in an ongoing struggle over the extent of women's participation in the workplace. That the struggle is one for the better positions is illustrated by the relative ease with which women can secure menial and low-paying jobs. Such jobs must be done by someone if other jobs are to be highly paid and employers are to maintain high levels of profit. Who will take such jobs?

As we shall see in the next chapter, racial and ethnic minorities also are likely to cluster in these low-level jobs, which means that **sexism** *and racism are functional substitutes* with respect to such work. Where racial or ethnic minorities are available, they provide that labor. Where they are not available, women provide it. This doesn't mean that women are equal to men in the labor market where racial or ethnic minorities are available for low-paying jobs. Rather, the point is that women are the next-to-the-lowest group on the hierarchy rather than the lowest.

**sexism**
prejudice or discrimination against someone because of his or her sex

*One other social structural factor in gender inequality is religion.* Justification for gender inequality is found in both the teachings and the practices of many religious groups (Crandall 2006). In those groups, which are found in all the world's major religions, the leaders assert or imply that men are superior to women and/or that women should be subservient.

In recent decades, a number of Christian theologians, both male and female, have argued that biblical teachings have been misinterpreted by generations of people who used them to justify and maintain patriarchal systems (Meyers 1988; Clifford 2001). Nevertheless, many religious people, but particularly the most conservative ones (known as fundamentalists), justify sexism on religious grounds (Haggard et al. 2019). Religious conservatism and social conservatism tend to go hand in hand. Thus,

85 percent of religious liberals, but only 59.6 percent of religious conservatives, disagree that men are better suited emotionally to politics than are women (McConkey 2001); and 81.2 percent of the liberals, but only 68.1 percent of the conservatives, disagree that it is more important for wives to help their husband's careers than to have careers themselves.

Sexism in religion is also seen in the fact that women generally do not hold the most honored positions—minister, priest, rabbi. It is true that an increasing number of women are assuming places of leadership (Fiedler 2010), and a number of Protestant denominations technically allow women to hold top positions. Nevertheless, very few women have actually held these positions (Sandstrom 2016). Lay religious leaders are also likely to be men, even though women may be more numerous and more consistently involved in the activities of the group. In some fundamentalist groups, women are not even allowed to speak before a group or lead public worship.

*Social Psychological Factors.* While American attitudes toward gender roles have become more *egalitarian,* some attitudes detrimental to women's continued progress still exist. In particular, some believe that there is no longer any discrimination, that women have opportunities equal to those of men, and that those who continue to complain are troublemakers or "radical feminists."

Such attitudes fly in the face of the realities of women's lives. We have already discussed the amount of sexual harassment with which women must deal. We have also noted the fact that discrimination in the workplace, in spite of the progress made, continues to depress the income of women. And women continue to face *negative attitudes in the workplace* with regard to their competence and commitment to the job.

Many women feel compelled to perform better than men in order to prove themselves and be accepted. For example, there is evidence that women must work harder to prove that they have the ability because men expect women—including women in supervisory and managerial positions—to be less competent than men and this bias enters into the evaluation of women (Martell, Parker, and Emrich 1998; Heilman 2001).

As we noted earlier, many women also fear that they will be penalized in their careers if they become mothers. In fact, some employers do place women into two categories: achievers and mothers. Those who opt for motherhood may find themselves on the "mommy track" of their career. The mommy track means that working mothers follow a modified career line in which they continue their work but do not advance as rapidly as men or those women without children. Thus, for example, women lawyers who take time off to attend to child care are less likely to become partners in their firms and earn less even if they do become partners (Noonan and Corcoran 2004).

*Ideology is also a factor in gender inequality.* Many Americans still believe that a woman's place is in the home and that when she leaves the home to pursue higher education or a career, she leaves her post as one of the guardians of the social order. The ideology that *women's abdication of the home* can only result in *social disorganization* was expressed by those who insisted that women return to their homes after World War II. They identified working women as a primary cause of delinquency and argued that for women to continue in the labor force would mean instability in the social institutions of the nation. More recently, in the surveys of religious people noted earlier, 81.2 percent of religious liberals, but only 44.2 percent of conservatives, disagreed that everyone is better off if the man is the achiever outside the home and the woman cares for her home and family (McConkey 2001:162). A study of 349 American adults found two nonreligious ideologies that foster prejudice against working women (Christopher and Wojda

2008). The "social dominance orientation" includes the belief of superior-inferior groups (with men, of course, being superior). Right-wing authoritarianism includes deference to established authority, which means that women and men fulfill complementary roles but that women need to be protected and cared for by men. Adults in the research with a social dominance orientation tended to have a "hostile sexism," viewing women in negative, disparaging terms; those with a right-wing authoritarian ideology tended to have a "benevolent sexism," viewing women in the traditional terms of those whose proper place is in the home.

Many books and magazines also continue to extol the virtues of the stay-at-home mother and to warn mothers of the dangers of going to work while they have children in the home (Johnston and Swanson 2003). Some books portray employed mothers as tired, busy, and guilty, whereas other books laud the bliss of stay-at-home mothers. And although some Americans believe that women's magazines promote a feminist agenda, the image of women that comes from an examination of those magazines is a person who is focused on consumption, is beautiful, and is domestic.

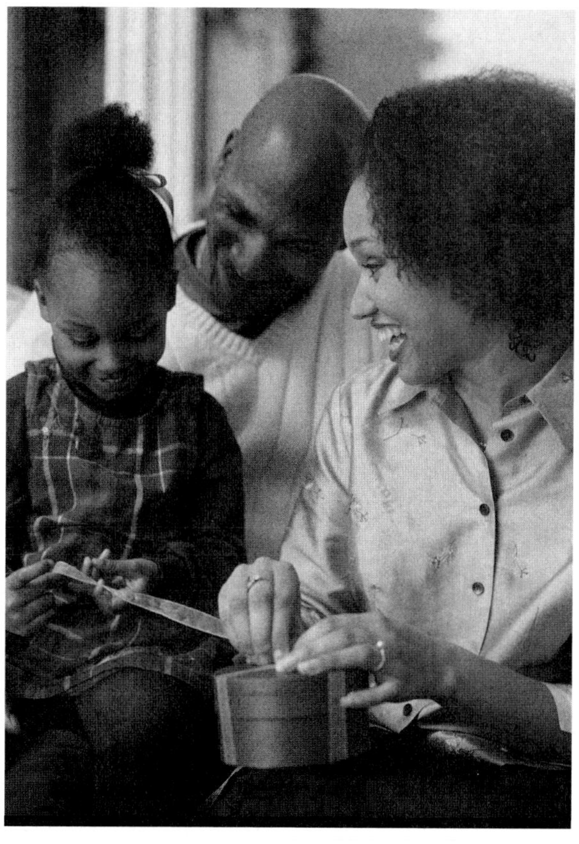

Working mothers have children as happy and healthy as do stay-at-home mothers.

Ryan McVay/Getty Images

Is it true, as an important part of the ideology asserts, that children are harmed when their mothers work? Many Americans agree with the idea that a mother with small children (and, in some cases, with any children) should remain at home. A review of research conducted throughout the 1990s, however, concluded that there was little relationship between maternal employment and child outcomes (Perry-Jenkins, Repetti, and Crouter 2000). In fact, maternal employment may be beneficial for the children of single mothers and lower-income families.

There are circumstances, however, that might foster negative consequences. For one thing, the effects *depend in part on how family members define the mother's working.* Agreement that it is a good thing for the mother to work minimizes any negative effects and can even have positive outcomes for the children in terms of their educational and career aspirations. Disagreement can create some serious problems.

A second important circumstance is the nature of the mother's work, including the pay, the hours worked, and the time of day spent working. In general, children of working mothers do as well academically as those of nonworking mothers (Goldberg, Prause, Lucas-Thompson, and Himsel 2008). However, research on welfare-reliant single mothers found that when the number of hours worked increased, the children were more likely to skip school and less likely to perform above average (Gennetian, Lopoo, and London 2008). And a national study of single mothers found that part-time, low-wage work and working nonstandard hours can both lead to poorer home environments (Lleras 2008).

The consequences of maternal employment also may vary by age of the child. Available research indicates no negative consequences for infants at least 2 years old. In some cases, day care may even be better than home care because it offers the children various kinds of enrichment not available in their homes. For infants under the age of 2, however, the research is contradictory and not always encouraging for those who prefer to work. Some research suggests that babies cared for by others are less securely attached to their mothers. Such children may have to cope with problems of insecurity for years or even a lifetime. In addition, there is evidence of some detrimental effects on cognitive development for children whose mothers go to work during the first year of their lives (Baum 2003). Such children score lower on measures of cognitive development than do children whose mothers stayed at home.

In sum, the evidence is that children over the age of 2 will probably not be harmed by a mother working and may even be helped by it, as long as the family defines the work as appropriate activity and the children have adequate supervision and care. For infants 2 years and under, more research is needed. But it is *a myth that there are inexorable, undesirable consequences for the children when the mother works.*

## Solutions: Public Policy and Private Action

fallacy

Like other social problems, gender inequality is so pervasive and so entrenched that pessimists may commit the *fallacy of retrospective determinism* and argue that the nation will never be rid of it. Whether a perfectly equitable society is achievable may be debatable, but it is clear that progress can be made.

What kind of action can address the problems of women? What kind of public policy is needed, and what other forms of private initiative in addition to consciousness-raising groups can help?

Clearly, the federal government needs to be involved. Federal antidiscriminatory laws have helped American women. But the Council on Contemporary Families (2003) compared American husbands and the American government to their counterparts in Germany, France, Italy, and Japan. The council concluded that American husbands do more housework and child care than do husbands in the other nations, but the U.S. government does the least of all the governments to help employed wives. In France, women workers have a government-mandated and protected benefit of a fully paid leave 6 weeks prior to and 10 weeks after the birth of a child. Both parents can also receive some additional paid leave until the child's third birthday. The United States needs more and better *child care centers* and more extensive *family leave laws* (laws that allow people time off from their jobs without penalty when a child is born, adopted, or seriously ill). The right to parental leave in the United States covers only about half of the private sector workforce and is generally short and often unpaid. Some other nations offer universal, paid leaves of 10 months or more.

The importance of such measures is underscored by the fact that millions of women in the labor force have children under the age of 6. The well-being of employed mothers is dependent on adequate child care. Employed mothers who have no problems in arranging for child care and whose husbands participate in child care have very low depression levels, whereas those who have difficulties and who have sole responsibility for child care tend to have very high levels of depression.

The children of satisfied mothers are better adjusted whether the mothers stay at home or work away from home. Women who prefer, or who feel the need, to work will not be satisfied to stay at home; but the option of working is closed to many women unless child care centers are available. Such centers are a part of the "bill of rights" of the National Organization for Women (NOW).

As more women become politically involved and are elected to public office, the government is more likely to enact measures that help women. As Swers (2002) has found, women legislators engage in more, and more intense, action in behalf of women's interests than do men. And this finding is true in both political parties.

*Changes in education* are crucial in order to alter notions of the "proper" roles of the sexes and to attack the ideology that restricts women's sphere of appropriate activity to the home. Education needs to aid people's understanding about the capabilities of women. Educators need to treat males and females equally from kindergarten through graduate training; they need to teach people how to parent so that females are no longer socialized into a subordinate role; and they need to help people develop new norms about women's participation in all sectors of the economy.

In addition, educational institutions should find ways to increase the amount of mentoring women receive. A study of chemists reported that the women believed they had received less mentoring than the men at every level of their training–the undergraduate, graduate, and postdoctoral levels (Nolan, Buckner, Marzabadi, and Kuck 2008). Such differences in mentoring can easily carry over into different degrees of advancement and achievement in one's career.

Still another form of action involves changing the policies and practices of organizations. A controversial proposal to eliminate income inequalities is the notion of *comparable worth* (Barko 2000). In essence, the idea is that women should receive equal pay not just for equal work but for work that is judged to be of comparable worth. The basis for such a proposal is the fact that women are overrepresented in such areas as nursing and clerical work, whereas men are overrepresented in such jobs as pilot and truck driver. The occupations in which women are overrepresented tend to pay less than those in which men are overrepresented, even though they may require similar amounts of training. The argument is that when jobs are of comparable worth, they should pay equal salaries. Otherwise gender inequality in income will continue indefinitely.

Why, for example, should beginning engineers (mostly men) earn 30 to 70 percent more than beginning teachers (mostly women) (Barko 2000)? Is a truck driver (probably a man) 45 percent more valuable than a child care worker (a college graduate and probably a woman)? Proponents of comparable worth raise such questions. They argue that experts can examine jobs in terms of their difficulty, responsibility, and education and experience requirements; rate the jobs accordingly; and equalize the pay for equivalent work.

Although both federal laws and laws in most states reflect a basic principle of comparable worth by prohibiting gender-based differences in pay, the inequality persists. But at least there is a legal basis for unions and individuals to pursue cases against organizations whose policies and/or practices perpetuate inequality.

Action by work organizations is also needed to deal with the problem. The majority of employers responded in the 1990s to the problem by instituting grievance procedures and sensitivity training (Dobbin and Kelly 2007). Victims now have legal redress, and employers are held responsible for harassment that occurs in their places of work. Among other changes, employers have been encouraged to avoid legal problems by making policy statements to employees, setting up grievance procedures for alleged victims, and educating employees on appropriate behavior between the sexes. Such procedures are designed to correct one of the basic reasons for the continuation of harassment: people's ignorance of the problematic nature and consequences of harassment and of the recourse available to victims. Harassment also can be reduced if work organizations assume the responsibility for training all employees to be supportive of women's dignity and intolerant of harassment.

Legal change can be effective in reducing inequality. Antidiscrimination laws have brought about significant changes on the nation's college and university campuses. Among other changes, discrimination in official policies and practices and admissions quotas have been abolished. Accordingly, students are to be treated equally in terms of rules and services; married women, for instance, are no longer excluded from financial aid because they are married, and sexual harassment is explicitly forbidden. As we noted earlier, covert discrimination still occurs, and the problems of women on the campus are by no means fully resolved, but gains have been made as a result of legal change.

Finally, business and industry can take the important step of *ensuring women equal career opportunities.* In particular, the business world can reject the "Mommy Track" notion and allow women to be mothers without sacrificing a professional career. Many companies now have such things as paid parental leave when a child is born, but too many female workers do not have such benefits. The business world needs to explore ways to ensure women that they will not have to choose between fulfilling their work and their family responsibilities and opportunities.

*Follow-Up.* Set up a class debate on this topic: Comparable worth offers the most promising solution for ending gender inequality in the United States.

## The LGBTQ Community

**heterosexual**
having sexual preference for persons of the opposite sex

**homosexual**
having sexual preference for persons of the same sex; someone who privately or overtly considers himself or herself a homosexual

**homophobia**
irrational fear of homosexuals

In American society, the fulfillment of intimacy needs is often framed in terms of a **heterosexual** relationship. In this section, we will look at people who find fulfillment in other kinds of relationships, such as the **homosexual**. We will see the problems homosexual individuals encounter because of irrational fears and disdain, as illustrated by **homophobia**, and we will look at factors that perpetuate the problems.

### The LGBTQ Community: Definitions and Numbers

Not everyone who engages in a homosexual act can be considered a homosexual. Boys commonly engage in homosexual activity during adolescence, but most of them become exclusively heterosexual. We define a homosexual as an individual who has both a sexual preference for those of the same sex and who also defines himself or herself as homosexual. *Gay* is a synonym for homosexual, though some use it to refer primarily to males. The shorthand way to designate those who engage in some form of homosexual behavior is LGBTQ.

**lesbian**
a female homosexual

**bisexual**
having sexual relations with either sex or both together

**transgender**
having a gender identity different from one's anatomy

Female homosexuals are called **lesbians**. Some people are **bisexual,** finding gratification with both sexes and having no strong preference for either, but bisexuals are not as common as those who are exclusively heterosexual or homosexual. **Transgender** refers to those who have a gender identity that differs from their anatomy. The body may be male, but the person feels like a woman, or the body is female but the person feels like a man. Finally, some people add the "Q" (which stands for "queer") to the acronym to refer to people who are questioning their sexual identity or who feel that none of the other categories quite fit who they are.

Homosexuality is found throughout the world. It is difficult to estimate the proportion of people who are homosexual. In some societies, homosexuality is still a crime and homosexuals must keep their sexual orientation secret. Many studies have examined only small populations, such as college students, that are not representative of the nation as a whole. Moreover, as noted earlier, many people are either bisexual or have a homosexual experience at some point but prefer heterosexual relations. For example, a survey of same-sex activity among American teenagers and young adults (ages 15 to 21) who had never married or cohabited reported that 11 percent of females and 4 percent of the males had had some same-sex experience (McCabe, Brewster, and Tillman 2011). Most of those who reported same-sex experience also preferred it exclusively, but some of those who acknowledged same-sex activity indicated they preferred only heterosexual relationships.

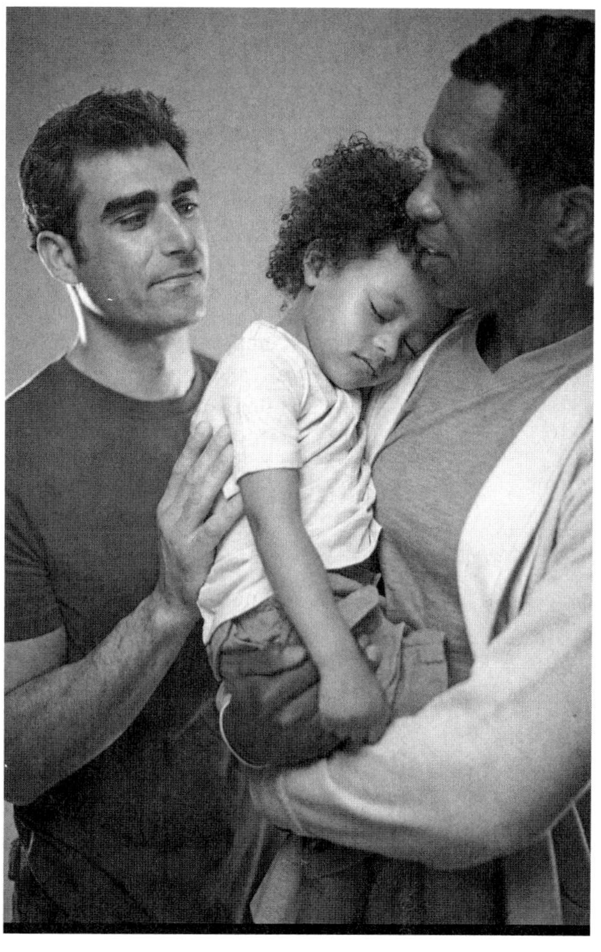

Many homosexuals lead well-adjusted lives even when faced with negative social reaction.

Image Source/Getty Images

One of the most comprehensive studies of sexual behavior in recent decades was the National Health and Social Life Survey, conducted by researchers at the University of Chicago (Laumann, Michael, Gagnon, and Michaels 1994). Using a sample of 3,432 American men and women between the ages of 18 and 59, the researchers found that 2.7 percent of sexually active men and 1.3 percent of sexually active women had a homosexual experience in the past year. Further, they reported that 9.1 percent of men and 4.3 percent of women have had a homosexual experience since puberty, and 7.7 percent of men and 7.4 percent of women said they felt some degree of same-sex *attraction* or interest. More recently, a researcher used various sources of data and estimated that about 5 percent of men are gay (Stephens-Davidowitz 2013). And a national study of U.S. adults that were asked about any same-sex experience since age 18 reported a doubling of the proportion from the early 1990s (3.6 percent of women and 4.5 percent of men) to the early 2010s (8.7 percent of women and 8.7 percent of men) (Twenge, Sherman, and Wells 2016). Bisexual behavior also increased, from 3.1 to 7.7 percent. The increase could represent increasing homosexual behavior or increasing willingness to acknowledge homosexual behavior or both.

At any rate, it is safe to say that a minimum of 3 to 4 percent of American men and 2 to 3 percent of American women prefer to be exclusively homosexual. The proportions are not high, but in absolute terms we are talking about 10 million Americans at a minimum.

It is even more difficult to estimate the number of transgender individuals. Estimates range from 0.7 percent to just under 3 percent (Regnerus 2018). Two incidents brought transgenderism into focus in recent years. One was when the Olympic decathlon champion Bruce Jenner announced in 2015 that he identified himself as a female. He changed his name to Caitlyn and his appearance to female. The other incident was the public restroom battles that began in 2007 centering on the issue of whether someone, for example, who is anatomically a male can use the women's room. We'll discuss the matter further in the following sections.

## Why Are Some People Homosexual?

Enormous pressures exist in American society for people to be heterosexual. Few of you have grown up without hearing the word "homosexual" or a slang term meaning homosexual applied to someone in a disparaging way. Moreover, books, television, and observation all reinforce the expectation of heterosexual relations. Why, then, do some people prefer homosexual relations?

*Biological Explanations.* A number of observers believe that *homosexuality is genetically programmed into some people.* Balthazart (2012), for example, has forcefully argued that homosexuality is not an individual's free choice but is the result of "embryonic endocrine/genetic phenomena" that fashion the individual's sexual desires and needs. A number of other researchers have reported differences between homosexuals and heterosexuals in brain structure or genetic makeup (Mustanski, Chivers, and Bailey 2002; Safron et al. 2017). While biological factors may contribute in some way to homosexuality, there is no single genetic cause to homosexuality (Reardon 2019).

Some behavioral studies lend support to the biological explanation. Both gay men and lesbians recall having different preferences and behaviors in childhood from those of most of their peers. The difference is confirmed in research with parents of gay men, who also recall much atypical gender behavior in their sons, including a lack of interest in sports (Aveline 2006).

Subsequent studies lend further support (Landolt et al. 2004). Studies of lesbians report that, as children, they preferred masculine roles and "boy's games" (Bering 2010). Similarly, among a sample of adults who still had home videos from their childhood, both lesbian and gay adults were more gender nonconforming than heterosexual adults in the home videos they watched as children (Rieger, Linsenmeier, Gygax, and Bailey 2008). In short, gender nonconformity in children is a strong predictor of homosexuality.

Additional evidence emerges in studies of twins (Dawood et al. 2000). In a study of male twins in which at least one brother was gay, two researchers found that in 52 percent of 56 sets of identical twins, both brothers were gay, compared to 22 percent of 54 sets of fraternal twins (Bailey and Pillard 1991). They also looked at 57 families in which a gay son had an adoptive brother and found that only 11 percent of the adoptive brothers were also gay.

The point is that the chances that both siblings will turn out to be homosexual increases dramatically according to the amount of genes they share. At the same time, as the researchers acknowledge, the fact that not all the identical twins were homosexual suggests that sociocultural factors play a role. Let's look at some of those factors.

*Sociocultural Explanations.* Some social scientists argue that homosexuality is a *learned pattern of behavior* rather than the natural outgrowth of an innate drive. Because there are strong pressures toward heterosexuality, these social scientists look for factors in family life or in patterns of interaction that differ for homosexuals and heterosexuals.

Some researchers have tried to identify troubled relationships in the family as a cause of homosexuality. But the issue of problematic family experiences remains

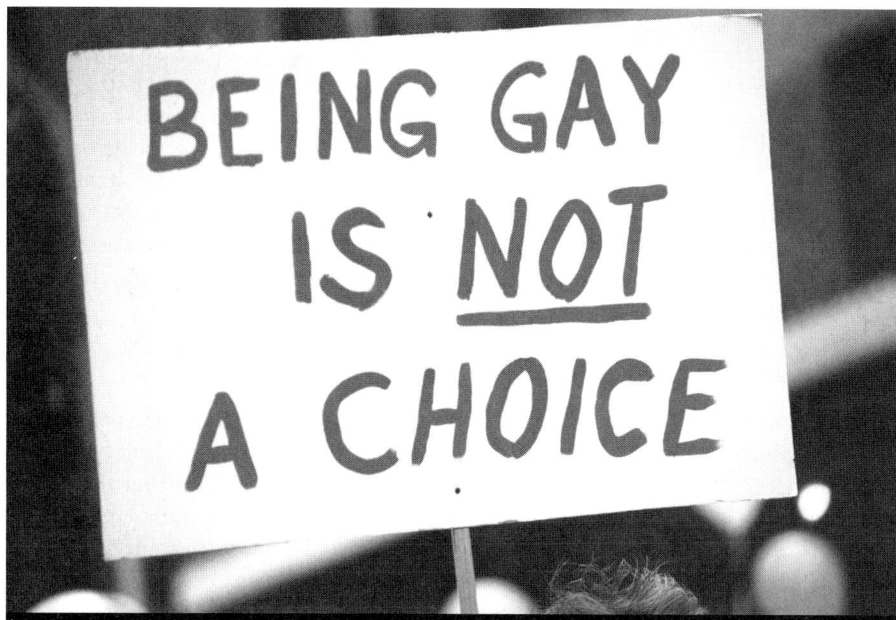


Gay activists parade to protest the negative societal reaction they must often endure.
Jack Star/PhotoLink/Getty Images

clouded. Most studies rely on the recollections of adults. Earlier ones, conducted from the 1950s through the 1970s, tended to find deficiencies in the family life of homosexuals, whereas subsequent studies tend to find no differences between homosexual and heterosexual backgrounds. Thus, we cannot say with certainty whether family experiences contribute to the development of homosexuality.

One family factor that is intriguing but has not so far been convincingly explained either biologically or socioculturally is birth order in a family with two or more sons. There is a correlation between sexual orientation and the number of older brothers (Cantor, Blanchard, Paterson, and Bogaert 2002; McConaghy et al. 2006). Each older brother that a man has raises his odds of being homosexual by about 33 percent. This fraternal birth order effect accounts for the sexual orientation of about one of every seven gay men.

A sociocultural factor that may be important, however, is the *norms of one's peers during adolescence.* Some young males engage in homosexual activities with adults to earn money. It may be a purely financial transaction for the boys that is approved by group norms. The same norms, on the other hand, define the adult homosexuals as "queers." The boys do not regard themselves as homosexuals and do not continue homosexual activity when they become adults.

By contrast, if an adolescent participates in a *homosexual clique,* homosexuality may be defined as preferable, and the individual may accept a homosexual identity as he or she internalizes the norms of the group. Some, perhaps a majority, of young male prostitutes engage in sex with adults not merely for money, but because, as an older study reported (Earls and David 1989), their own orientation is homosexual.

What can you conclude from all this information? The overall evidence suggests that *there are both genetic and sociocultural factors involved in the development of homosexuality* (Bailey et al. 2016). The genetic component is strong, but if homosexuality were purely genetic in origin, then all sets of identical twins would be homosexual and all brains of homosexuals would differ from those of heterosexuals. If homosexuality were purely sociocultural in origin, on the other hand, then differences in gender orientation would not be observable from an early age, and the findings of the twin studies could not be explained. However, we do not yet know the precise way in which genetic and sociocultural factors combine to lead to a homosexual identity.

## The LGBTQ Community and the Quality of Life

Homosexuality is a pattern of behavior involving social contradictions that both homosexuals and heterosexuals define as incompatible with the desired quality of life. Homosexuals point to two contradictions in particular. One is that the *American ideology of equality contradicts American attitudes and behavior toward homosexuals.* The other is that the stereotyped homosexual role (see the discussion of myths in the following section) contradicts the actual homosexual role. People who condemn homosexuals are frequently condemning the stereotyped rather than the actual role.

fallacy

*Myths about Homosexuality.* A contradiction exists between the ideal of the *dignity of human beings and the prevalent ideology about homosexuals.* This contradiction is manifested in a *number of myths about homosexuality,* myths that involve the *fallacies of personal attack and appeal to prejudice.* Perhaps the most common myth is that homosexuals have characteristics that are normal for the opposite sex—males are "effeminate" and females are "masculine." While it is true, as noted earlier, that gender nonconformity among children is a strong predictor of homosexuality, that nonconformity does not persist for the majority of homosexuals. As Taywaditep (2001) pointed out, most gay men who are gender nonconforming as children "defeminize" during adolescence. They may do so to avoid social stigma or because it is a natural part of growing up. In any case, the majority of adult homosexuals are not gender nonconforming in their mannerisms and behavior.

A second myth about homosexuals is that they fear, and are incapable of, having heterosexual relationships. Homosexuality is commonly attributed to unsatisfactory heterosexual experiences that cause fear of relationships with the opposite sex.

Although experiences with people of the opposite sex may be a factor in the development of homosexuality, there does not seem to be any evidence that homosexuals are incapable of relating to the opposite sex. By definition, a homosexual prefers sexual relations with those of his or her own sex exclusively. However, homosexuals do make and maintain good relationships with people of the opposite sex. In fact, while we have not done systematic research on the matter, in our work with couples in long-term marriages we have often been told that single, heterosexual women enjoy rewarding and close friendships with gay men.

Still another myth is that a homosexual is attracted to, and will make advances to, anyone of his or her own sex, children as well as adults. The homosexual, however, is as selective as a straight person (Bailey et al. 2016). The great bulk of gay men, like heterosexual men, prefer mature partners. They are not drawn to sex with children.

Finally, there is the myth that homosexuals do not form the same kinds of long-term attachments as heterosexuals. When homosexuality was even more of a stigma than it is today, it would have been difficult to maintain such a relationship without rousing suspicions. But researchers have found that homosexuals want essentially the same things as heterosexuals in intimate relationships. There are few differences between homosexual and heterosexual couples at any stage of the relationship from dating to long-term commitment (Roisman et al. 2008). And that includes a long-term relationship with the same partner; long-term homosexual couples resemble long-term heterosexual couples in virtually everything except their sexual orientation (Gottman et al. 2003). In short, *homosexual couples have the same hopes, the same needs, the same desires, the same levels of satisfaction, and the same levels of commitment as heterosexual couples* (Patterson 2000; Joyner, Manning, and Prince 2019). And they also have the same kinds of relational problems, including instances of verbal and physical abuse (He 2020).

Homosexuals may want, like heterosexuals, to be parents (Drexler 2012). They do so by adoption or by finding a woman who is willing to be inseminated with the sperm of one or both of them and bear them a child.

Independent of desire and satisfaction is the question of the *well-being of children raised in a homosexual family.* A national study of gay and lesbian parents found more similarities than differences between them and heterosexual parents (Johnson and O'Connor 2002). Where they did find differences, moreover, the gay and lesbian parents had, in a number of areas, more positive child-rearing practices: They were, compared to the heterosexual parents, more responsive to their children, more child-oriented, and more egalitarian in sharing household tasks between the partners. In sum, the research available so far indicates that the overall well-being of children raised in a homosexual family is as high as that of children raised in heterosexual families (Patterson 2000; Wainwright and Patterson 2006, 2008). In both their psychological and social adjustment the children of homosexuals do as well or better than children with heterosexual parents (Mechcatie and Rosenberg 2018). And contrary to what some people believe, children raised by a homosexual pair are no more likely to be homosexual themselves than are children raised by a heterosexual pair (Fulcher, Sutfin, and Patterson 2008).

*Equality of Opportunity.* The American ideology of *equality of opportunity contradicts the norms about the hiring of homosexuals and about their rights to equal treatment in such things as* housing. Until the start of this century, the homosexual was a criminal under state **sodomy** laws. Legally, the term "sodomy" was ambiguous. Depending on the state, it referred to anal intercourse, mouth-genital sex, or sex with animals. Sodomy laws were established to prevent what people considered to be "unnatural" kinds of sexual behavior. In practice, however, the laws were used mainly to prosecute homosexuals. The laws were not always enforced, and were finally overturned by the Supreme Court in 2003. But homosexuals and lesbians have had to contend with a number of barriers to equal opportunity within both the government and the business sectors.

**sodomy**
intercourse defined as "unnatural"; particularly used to refer to anal intercourse

The lack of equal opportunity is not based on any lack of ability or inferior performance by homosexuals. In fact, homosexuals may *suffer discrimination in spite of proven adequate or even superior performance.* They may experience harassment, stalled careers, or other sanctions if their sexual orientation is known.

Tilesik (2011) sent fictitious pairs of résumés to 1,769 postings of available jobs in seven different states. In each pair, one of the résumés included experience in a gay campus organization, and the other listed experience in an organization that had nothing to do with sexual orientation. Otherwise, the two applicants had the same experience and qualifications. The researcher found that employers in some of the states—those with stronger antigay attitudes and weaker antidiscrimination laws—were significantly more likely to reject the gay applicants. And a study of physicians' experiences in the practice of medicine found that among physicians who were lesbian, gay, bisexual, or transgender, 10 percent said they were denied referrals from heterosexual colleagues, 15 percent reported being harassed by a colleague, and 22 percent said they were socially ostracized (Eliason, Dibble, and Robertson 2011).

In addition to the workplace, homosexuals are sometimes the victims of discrimination in the housing market. A Canadian study looked at inquires about renting available apartments and found significant discrimination of same-sex couples relative to heterosexual couples (Lauster and Easterbrook 2011).

**sanctions**
mechanisms of social control for enforcing a society's standards

*Negative Sanctions.* **Sanctions** are rewards (positive sanctions) or punishments (negative sanctions) designed to influence behavior. Homosexuals are subjected to *numerous negative sanctions,* including ridicule, suppression, physical abuse, and ostracism. Negative sanctions contradict the American ideology that every citizen has a right to life, liberty, and the pursuit of happiness. All the sanctions, of course, are aimed at changing the homosexual into a heterosexual. Transgender people experience many of the same kind of negative sanctions. Transgender youth are punished for public displays of affection and for violating gender norms (Snapp et al. 2015). And transgender adults report arrests and incarceration and abuse while in the custody of law enforcement (Stotzer 2014).

Transgender rights became the focus of national attention after an Illinois transgender girl athlete demanded the right to use the girl's locker room to change (Stolberg et al. 2016). The federal Department of Education's support of the girl raised the issue elsewhere, including the use of public rest rooms by transgender people. The federal government ordered all public schools to let transgender people use the bathroom of their choice, leading to a series of lawsuits by states that wanted to require students to use bathrooms in accord with their anatomy. As of this writing, the controversy continues.

Negative sanctions can come from parents or caretakers, other family members, friends, acquaintances or strangers (Balsam, Rothblum, and Beauchaine 2005). Rejection by parents may be one of the reasons for the high rate of homelessness among gay and lesbian youth. A representative sample of public school students in Massachusetts in grades 9 through 12 reported that 25 percent of lesbian/gay students, compared to 3 percent of heterosexual students, were homeless (Corliss, Goodenow, Nichols, and Austin 2011). Lesbian/gay youth also experience a disproportionate amount of other kinds of victimization (Button, O'Connell, and Gealt 2012). One study of 528 gay, lesbian, and bisexual youth found that because of their sexual orientation nearly 80 percent had been verbally abused, 11 percent had been physically abused, and 9 percent had been sexually victimized (D'Augelli, Grossman, and Starks 2006). A study using a national probability sample of gay, lesbian, and bisexual adults reported that 20 percent had been victimized by a personal or property crime because of their sexual orientation, 50 percent had suffered verbal harassment, and more than 10 percent reported an experience of employment or housing discrimination (Herek 2009).

The verbal abuse includes such things as being *labeled perverts or called mentally ill.* The physical abuse may be sufficiently severe to result in injuries or even death (D'Augelli and Grossman 2001). In fact, FBI (2019) statistics show that 16.7 percent of the thousands of hate crimes in 2018 were based on bias against people because of their sexual orientation.

*Fear.* Homosexuals *live with a certain amount of fear.* One of the freedoms cherished by Americans is the freedom from fear. For the homosexual, this ideal is contradicted by the norms and laws that apply to gay people as well as by the experience of being abused. Lesbian/gay youth are 2.4 times more likely than heterosexuals to miss school out of fear (Friedman et al. 2011). And, depending on the community in which they function, the fear continues into adulthood.

In other words, the homosexual is subject to fear of exposure if he or she decides to remain secretive and to fear of negative sanctions if he or she decides to come out. Not every homosexual goes around constantly haunted by fear. Nevertheless, all homosexuals must come to terms with realistic fears. The fears reflect the realities of life in a culture that still practices various ways of disparaging and rejecting homosexuals. The harassment may come from parents or other family members. It may come from bullying by fellow students in elementary school (Hart et al. 2018). It may come from fellow students in college, who show their contempt for certain kinds of behavior by saying "that's so gay" or "no homo" (Winberg et al. 2019). It may come from colleagues at work who still regard homosexuality as a perverse choice. The sources are endless, and they can tarnish one's life from childhood to death.

*Psychological and Emotional Problems.* You might expect that it is difficult for those in the LGBTQ community to avoid psychological and emotional problems as they wrestle with the contradictions that impinge upon their lives. In fact, a number of studies have identified problems that result from the *stress generated by the societal reaction to an individual's homosexuality.* Among other things, homosexuals and transgender people have higher rates than heterosexuals of isolation, depression, anxiety, substance abuse, eating disorders, posttraumatic stress disorder, and suicide proneness (Bostwick, Boyd, Hughes, and McCabe 2010; Langhinrichsen-Rohling, Lamis, and Malone 2011; McCallum and McLaren 2011; Baams, Grossman, and Russel 2015; Miller and Grollman 2015; Mustanski, Andrews, and Puckett 2016; Parker and Harriger 2020).

It is important to underscore the point that these psychological and emotional problems are the result of stress imposed by the social environment rather than because of any innate flaws in homosexuals themselves. For example, those who are in legally recognized relationships (marriages or civil unions) have fewer and less severe mental health problems and higher levels of general well-being than those homosexuals who are single (Riggle, Rostosky, and Horne 2010). Homosexuals in states that have laws and policies that protect homosexuals against hate crimes and employment discrimination have significantly fewer psychiatric disorders (Hatzenbuchler, Keyes, and Hasin 2009). And homosexuals who have strong social support in the form of a social network have fewer mental health issues than those with little social support (Teasdale and Bradley-Engen 2010).

In spite of the greater prevalence of psychological and emotional problems, homosexuals generally function quite well in society. Three conclusions follow from the varied evidence we have presented in this section. First, there is no basis, in other words, for claiming that a homosexual orientation per se is associated with clinical symptoms of mental illness. As the American Psychiatric Association has underscored by removing homosexuality from its list of mental disorders, the notion that gays are inherently disturbed individuals who need therapy in order to change their sexual preference is no longer tenable. Second, the stress induced by societal reaction to the individual's homosexuality creates emotional and psychological problems (Meyer 2003). Third, many homosexuals come to terms with the societal reaction, cope with the problems, and lead well-adjusted and productive lives.

## Contributing Factors

Without the societal reaction to the LGBTQ community among Americans, we could not speak of their behavior as a social problem. In this section we look at some of the multilevel factors that account for this societal reaction and that create stress for homosexuals and transgender people.

*Social Structure Factors.* In the United States, *normative sexual behavior* is heterosexual. The norms of society define homosexuality as deviant, but such norms do not reflect universal standards or innate biological imperatives. In fact, even when heterosexual relations are dominant, a society may not disapprove of or *punish homosexuality.* In her study of a variety of primitive societies, Brown (1952) found that 14 of 44 of the societies for which data were available did not punish male homosexuality, and 8 of 12 did not punish female homosexuality.

Many modern societies refrain from formally punishing homosexual acts that are conducted in private between consenting adults. These acts, for example, are not considered a crime in Japan, Korea, Mexico, Argentina, Uruguay, Egypt, and the Sudan.

The United States is the only large Western nation that allows the punishment of adults who privately engage in consensual homosexual acts. This attitude reflects the English heritage of America, particularly the views of the Puritans, who saw homosexuality as one symptom of the moral corruption of England in the 17th century (Mitchell 1969). Changes have since occurred in England. In 1967 the House of Commons reformed the laws on homosexuality and removed private, consensual homosexual acts between adults from the criminal statutes.

The changes in England were facilitated by the support of prominent Anglican and Catholic clergymen. In the United States, many religious leaders, particularly fundamentalist Christians, stress that homosexuality is a "vice" condemned by various biblical teachings. In general, although most religious people are becoming more tolerant, the more conservative people are in their faith, the more negative their views on homosexuality. For example, a national survey by the Barna Group (2018) found that 76 percent of very conservative Christians, but only 24 percent of other Christians agreed that homosexuality is morally wrong.

Gay Christians and Jews have formed a number of organizations, including Evangelicals Concerned, and Dignity (Roman Catholic), in an effort to win acceptance for themselves. Some religious leaders have spoken out in support of homosexuals. And some theologians have constructed a religious justification for homosexuality (Lowe 2009). Nevertheless, by and large, religious groups continue to view homosexuality in negative terms.

The result is that trying to attend church or a synagogue can be a stressful experience for a homosexual. It may only intensify a sense of guilt. At the least, it underscores the fact that official religion is likely to be as much a problem as a comfort.

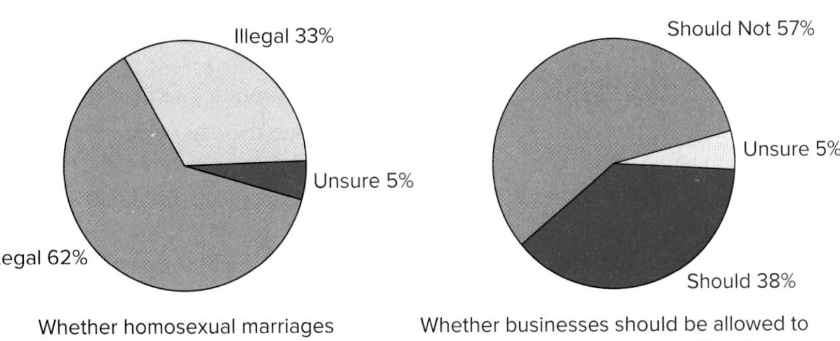


**FIGURE 7.3**
Attitudes about Homosexuality.
Source: Polling Report 2020.

*Social Psychological Factors.* The homosexual's stressful environment is maintained by social psychological factors that support and reinforce norms and institutional arrangements. Attitudes about homosexuality and homosexual behavior generally have been negative throughout most of our history. Even though homosexual marriages are now legal, a third of Americans still believe they should not be (Figure 7.3). So a majority support gay rights, but a substantial minority still resists them. At the same time, many people distinguish between the formal rights and the informal privileges (such as public displays of affection) (Doan, Loehr, and Miller 2014). Some who support the formal rights are not as accepting of the informal privileges. And a study of health care providers found a preference for treating heterosexual over homosexual patients (Sabin, Riskind, and Nosek 2015). Finally, attitudes about the rights of transgender individuals are ambivalent. For example, when transgenders use public restrooms, should they use the ones that correspond to their birth gender or those that reflect their gender identity? As a national poll and some instances of legislation show, Americans are sharply divided on the answer. In the national poll, 48 percent said they should use the restroom that corresponds with their birth gender and 45 percent said they should use the ones that correspond to their gender identity (McCarthy 2017).

In sum, the LGBTQ community still has to deal with many negative attitudes. But we expect the shift to positive attitudes will continue. That shift has been considerable. Up until the late 1980s, three-fourths or more of Americans believed that homosexual relationships were always wrong. It's not clear why negative attitudes changed so rapidly and dramatically. But they have. By 2020, 82 percent of Americans agreed that those in the LGBTQ community should be protected under civil rights laws and 70 percent said they would be open to having a gay president of the nation (Poling Report 2020).

Various other studies confirm this pattern of increasing acceptance and approval. Research comparing college students living in a residence hall in 1985 with those living there in 2001 found the 2001 group more accepting of lesbians, more likely to have contact with lesbians, and more likely to say their parents had positive views about lesbians (Newman 2007). Those who continue to hold negative attitudes are more likely to be found among older age groups, political conservatives, and fundamentalist Protestants (Wood and Bartkowski 2004). Negative attitudes are also more likely among those who believe that homosexuality is a choice or the result of nurture rather than a genetically based predisposition (Smith, Zanotti, Axelton, and Saucier 2011).

We should note that the increasing acceptance of homosexuality has occurred in many other nations (Poushter and Kent 2020). For instance, from 2002 to 2019, attitudes of acceptance increased from 69 to 85 percent in Canada; 33 to 54 percent in South Africa; 25 to 44 percent in South Korea; and 15 to 37 percent in India.

There are, of course, many nations where acceptance remains low. But the global trend is toward acceptance. How do those who continue to hold negative attitudes justify them? Some believe their attitudes are legitimated by the ideology that homosexuals are "sick." For the professional, this attitude means that people who prefer homosexual relations suffer from an emotional disorder and need to be treated in the same way as any other emotionally disturbed individual. We heard a therapist analyze homosexuals as people who can never be happy because heterosexual relations are basic to human development and well-being. This view implies that *those who prefer homosexual relations should be identified, treated, and cured.*

fallacy

Some nonprofessionals view homosexuals as not only sick but also perverse *(the fallacy of personal attack).* Just as some Americans believe that alcoholics could stop drinking "if they only wanted to," they also believe that homosexuals could change their sexual behavior "if they only wanted to." In other words, some Americans view homosexuality as a personal problem, not a social one. They believe that the norms, institutional arrangements, attitudes, values, and ideology that work together to condemn and oppress homosexuals are legitimate.

## Solutions: Public Policy and Private Action

An important way to deal with the oppression and discrimination experienced by homosexuals is to *change the legal status of homosexuals.* In the early 1980s, the gay rights movement began to focus on national policies, giving priority to such things as extending the Civil Rights Act to prohibit discrimination based on sexual orientation. Gay rights advocates continue to press for antidiscrimination laws and policies in all spheres of life. In other words, homosexuals are striving to acquire the status of a recognized and protected minority group in American life. That effort was greatly helped by the Supreme Court's decision to make same-sex marriage legal in all states. The challenge now is to work on people's attitudes and practices that still denigrate and discriminate against those in the LGBTQ community.

To help the LGBTQ community combat the problems that still exist, there must be additional research and educational programs. People need to understand the nature of homosexuality and the perspectives of homosexuals. They need to understand what it means to be a transgender person. Fortunately, some helpful efforts already exist. There are college seminars on homosexuality as well as gay and lesbian programs. Articles in the print media and television and movie programs are powerful tools for combating antigay attitudes. Such educational efforts help people recognize that prejudice and discrimination achieve nothing but trauma. They also help young homosexual and transgender people to receive the social support from friends and family that will enable them to deal with the challenges and stresses in their lives. Educational efforts helped bring about dramatic changes in attitudes in the past (Loftus 2001). But those efforts must continue until the LGBTQ community is as fully accepted as heterosexuals in American society.

*Follow-Up.* Investigate whether your school has any classes or seminars on homosexuality. Ask the instructors about the content of the classes, the assigned reading materials, and how effective the courses are in developing understanding of and tolerance for homosexual lifestyles.

## Summary

Because they have suffered some of the same problems as minorities, women have been called America's "largest minority." In fact, they compose a slight majority of the population. Until recently, much of professional and popular opinion viewed the disadvantages of women as rooted in biology rather than in society. But the bulk of evidence points to sociocultural rather than biological factors for most differences between men and women.

Gender inequality means that women do not have the same opportunities for work and career as do men. Women's income is also less than men's. And women are victimized by the beauty myth and by harassment and violence.

The normative role of the female in American society is an important structural factor perpetuating women's problems. That role is reinforced by socialization at home, at school, and through the mass media. Discrimination is also practiced because it is economically profitable to men. Finally, some religious groups help maintain women's subordination by both their teachings and their practices.

Among social psychological factors in gender inequality are attitudes, such as the belief that women now have equal opportunities with men, and the ideology that asserts that wives and mothers who work outside the home pose a threat to their own families and to the well-being of the entire society.

Homosexuality, the sexual orientation of 2 to 3 percent of American women and 3 to 4 percent of American men, is also associated with inequality. Both biological and social factors are involved in sexual orientation. But some Americans view homosexuality as nothing more than a perverse choice.

The quality of life for homosexuals is diminished by such things as the myths that detract from their human dignity, negative sanctions, fear, and problems resulting from societal rejection and oppression. Social structural factors that tend to perpetuate the problem include societal norms and the legal and religious policies and practices that support those norms. Social psychological factors include a number of attitudes and the ideology that homosexuals are either sick or perverse.

## Key Terms

Bisexual
Gender
Gender Role
Heterosexual
Homophobia
Homosexual
Innate
Lesbian
Sanctions
Sex
Sexism
Sexual Harassment
Sodomy
Transgender

## Study Questions

1. What is the evidence for both biological and social factors as the basis for sex differences?
2. To what extent do women have equal economic opportunities with men?
3. How does the "beauty myth" affect the lives of women?
4. How does socialization affect the role of women?
5. Discuss the stance of religion on women's role in society.
6. What are the attitudes and ideologies that tend to perpetuate gender inequality?
7. What steps can be taken to reduce gender inequality?
8. What is meant by homosexuality and homophobia?
9. What is the evidence for biological and sociocultural factors in someone becoming homosexual?
10. What kind of negative sanctions do homosexuals face?
11. What attitudes and ideologies help you understand the problems homosexuals face?

## Internet Resources/Exercises

1. Explore some of the ideas in this chapter on the following sites:

**http://www.infoplease.com/ipa/A0001523** This site has information about most of the issues related to gender, to the LGBTQ community, and to the problem of abuse.

**http://www.now.org** The site of the National Organization for Women has information on a wide range of issues affecting women, including economic justice, abortion and reproductive rights, ending discrimination, and stopping violence.

**http://www.glaad.org/** Defends gays and lesbians against defamation; offers publications and other resources as well as ongoing reporting of news about homosexuals from media around the nation.

2. Use a search engine to explore "gender equality." Find materials on the problem of equality and inequality between men and women in other nations. How would you compare the United States with those other nations? In what kinds of nations do women seem to have the most equality? The most inequality?

3. Explore the Internet for sites that condemn homosexuality and those that assert that sexual orientation can be changed. How would you respond to these sites using the materials in your text?

## For Further Reading

Cruse, Sheryle. *Thin Enough: My Spiritual Journey Through the Living Death of an Eating Disorder.* Birmingham, AL: New Hope, 2006. A woman shares her torturous struggle with anorexia and bulimia, and her use of self-discipline and faith to overcome her eating disorders.

Flexner, Eleanor. *Century of Struggle: The Woman's Rights Movement in the United States.* New York: Atheneum, 1972. An excellent and thorough history of the struggle of American women–both white and African American–from colonial times to 1920.

Hesse-Biber, Sharlene Nagy, and Gregg Lee Carter. *Working Women in America: Split Dreams.* New York: Oxford University Press, 2004. An examination of every facet of the issue of women working, including the impact of globalization, the problems of the glass ceiling and sexual harassment, and the management of multiple roles.

Robertson, Mary. *Growing Up Queer: Kids and the Remaking of LGBTQ Identity.* New York: NYU Press, 2019. A participant-obsservational study of youth at an LGBTQ center that probes such things as how youth deal with their status in society, the kinds of family experiences they have, and how they understand their sexual and gender identities.

Stiers, Gretchen A. *From This Day Forward: Commitment, Marriage, and Family in Lesbian and Gay Relationships.* New York: St. Martin's Press, 2000. Interviews with 90 gay men and lesbians, who offer their perspectives on making a commitment, getting married, and having a family in a homosexual relationship.

Wharton, Amy S. *The Sociology of Gender.* New York: Blackwell, 2004. An overview of gender issues, including theory and research on gender at the individual, interactional, and institutional levels.

Williams, Joan. *Unbending Gender: Why Family and Work Conflict and What to Do about It.* New York: Oxford University Press, 2000. A discussion of the contradictions between the economy and family life, and policy suggestions for resolving the problems. Williams advocates what she calls "reconstructive feminism."

## References

American Association of University Women. 2006. "Drawing the line survey." AAUW website.

——. 2012. "Crossing the line: Sexual harassment at school." AAUW website.

Association of American Medical Colleges. 2011. *Women in Academic Medicine.* AAMC website.

Aveline, D. 2006. "Did I have blinders on or what?" *Journal of Family Issues* 27:777–802.

Baams, L., A. H. Grossman, and S. T. Russel. 2015. "Minority stress and mechanisms of risk for depression and suicidal Ideation among lesbian, gay, and bisexual youth." *Developmental Psychology* 51:688–96.

Bailey, J. M., and R. C. Pillard. 1991. "A genetic study of male sexual orientation." *Archives of General Psychiatry* 48 (December):1089–98.

Bailey, J. M., et al. 2016. "Sexual orientation, controversy, and science." *Psychological Science in the Public Interest,* vol.17. Thousand Oaks, CA: Sage.

Balsam, K. F., E. D. Rothblum, and T. P. Beauchaine. 2005. "Victimization over the life span." *Journal of Consulting and Clinical Psychology* 73:477–87.

Balthazart, J. 2012. *The Biology of Homosexuality.* New York: Oxford University Press.

Barko, N. 2000. "The other gender gap." *American Prospect,* June 19, pp. 61–67.

Barna Group. 2018. "Gen Z and morality." Barna Group website.

Barnett, R. C., and C. Rivers. 2020. "Men are doing increasingly well in female-dominated fields." Psychology Today website.

Baum, C. L., II. 2003. "Does early maternal employment harm child development?" *Journal of Labor Economics* 21:409–48.

Bayrakdar-Garside, R., and B. Klimes-Dougan. 2002. "Socialization of discrete negative emotions." *Sex Roles* 47:115–28.

Bering, J. 2010. "Is your child a 'prehomosexual'?" *Scientific American,* September 15.

Bessenoff, G. R. 2006. "Can the media affect us? Social comparison, self-discrepancy, and the thin ideal." *Psychology of Women Quarterly* 30:239–51.

Blais, M., and F. Dupuis-Deri. 2012. "Masculinism and the antifeminist countermovement." *Social Movement Studies* 11:21–39.

Boroughs, M. S., R. Krawczyk, and J. K. Thompson. 2010. "Body dysmorphic disorder among diverse racial/ethnic and sexual orientation groups." *Sex Roles* 63:725–37.

Bostwick, W. B., C. J. Boyd, T. L. Hughes, and S. E. McCabe. 2010. "Dimensions of sexual orientation and the prevalence of mood and anxiety disorders in the United States." *American Journal of Public Health* 100:468–75.

Bote, J. 2020. "Shooting suspect was a men's rights activist. What does that mean?" USA Today website.

Botta, R. A. 2003. "For your health? The relationship between magazine reading and adolescents' body image and eating disturbances." *Sex Roles* 48:389–99.

Brenan, M. 2019. "Record-high 56% of U.S. women prefer working to home-making." Gallup Poll website.

Brizendine, L. 2006. *The Female Brain*. New York: Morgan Road Books.

Bronner, G., C. Peretz, and M. Ehrenfeld. 2003. "Sexual harassment of nurses and nursing students." *Journal of Advanced Nursing* 42:637–44.

Brown, J. S. 1952. "A comparative study of deviations from sexual mores." *American Sociological Review* 17 (April):135–46.

Bryant, R. M., and M. G. Constantine. 2006. "Multiple role balance, job satisfaction and life satisfaction in women school counselors." *Professional Counseling* 9:265–71.

Buehler, C., and M. O'Brien. 2011. "Mothers' part-time employment." *Journal of Family Psychology* 25:895–906.

Bureau of Labor Statistics. 2019. "Women in the labor force: A databook." Bureau of Labor Statistics website.

——. 2020. "Characteristics of minimum wage workers, 2019." Bureau of Labor Statistics website.

Button, D. M., D. J. O'Connell, and R. Gealt. 2012. "Sexual minority youth victimization and social support." *Journal of Homosexuality* 59:18–43.

Cantor, J. M., R. Blanchard, A. D. Paterson, and A. F. Bogaert. 2002. "How many gay men owe their sexual orientation to fraternal birth order?" *Archives of Sexual Behavior* 31:63–71.

Castilla, E. J. 2008. "Gender, race, and meritocracy in organizational careers." *American Journal of Sociology* 113:1479–526.

Cha, Y. 2013. "Overwork and the persistence of gender segregation in occupations." *Gender & Society* 27:158–84.

Chan, D. K., C. B. Lam, S. Y. Chow, and S. F. Cheung. 2008. "Examining the job-related, psychological, and physical outcomes of workplace sexual harassment." *Psychology of Women Quarterly* 32:362–76.

Chang, M. L. 2004. "Growing pains: Cross-national variation in sex segregation in sixteen developing countries." *American Sociological Review* 69:114–37.

Christopher, A. N., and M. R. Wojda. 2008. "Social dominance orientation, right-wing authoritarianism, sexism, and prejudice toward women in the workforce." *Psychology of Women Quarterly* 32:65–73.

Clifford, A. M. 2001. *Introducing Feminist Theology*. Maryknoll, NY: Orbis Books.

Cohen, P. N., and M. L. Huffman. 2003. "Occupational segregation and the devaluation of women's work across U.S. labor markets." *Social Forces* 81:881–908.

Corliss, H. L., C. S. Goodenow, L. Nichols, and S. B. Austin. 2011. "High burden of homelessness among sexual-minority adolescents." *American Journal of Public Health* 101:1683–89.

Cotter, D. A., J. M. Hermsen, S. Ovadia, and R. Vanneman. 2001. "The glass ceiling effect." *Social Forces* 80:655–82.

Council on Contemporary Families. 2003. "U.S. husbands first, U.S. government last in support for working wives." *Work and Family Newsbrief*, June, p. 4.

Crandall, B. 2006. *Gender and Religion*. Charleston, SC: BookSurge.

D'Augelli, A. R., A. H. Grossman, and M. T. Starks. 2006. "Childhood gender atypicality, victimization, and PTSD among lesbian, gay, and bisexual youth." *Journal of Interpersonal Violence* 21:1462–82.

D'Augelli, A. R., and A. H. Grossman. 2001. "Disclosure of sexual orientation, victimization, and mental health among lesbian, gay, and bisexual older adults." *Journal of Interpersonal Violence* 16:1008–28.

Davison, T. E., and M. P. McCabe. 2005. "Relationships between men's and women's body image and their psychological, social, and sexual functioning." *Sex Roles* 52:463–75.

Dawood, K., R. C. Pillard, C. Horvath, W. Revelle, and J. M. Bailey. 2000. "Familial aspects of male homosexuality." *Archives of Sexual Behavior* 29:155–64.

Demarest, J., and R. Allen. 2000. "Body image: Gender, ethnic, and age differences." *Journal of Social Psychology* 140:465–72.

Dey, J. G., and C. Hill. 2007. *Behind the Pay Gap*. Washington, DC: AAUW Educational Foundation.

Diekman, A. B., and S. K. Murnen. 2004. "Learning to be little women and little men: The inequitable gender equality of nonsexist children's literature." *Sex Roles* 50:373–85.

Dittmar, H., E. Halliwell, and S. Ive. 2006. "Does Barbie make girls want to be thin? The effect of experimental exposure to images of dolls on the body image of 5- to 8-year-old girls." *Developmental Psychology* 42:283–92.

Doan, L., A. Loehr, and L.R. Miller. 2014. "Formal rights and informal privileges for same-sex couples." *American Sociological Review* 79:1172-95.

Dobbin, F., and E. L. Kelly. 2007. "How to stop harassment: Professional construction of legal compliance in organizations." *American Journal of Sociology* 112:1203–43.

Drexler, P. 2012. "Gay parents raising kids: how will they fare?" Psychology Today website.

Earls, C. M., and H. David. 1989. "A psychological study of male prostitution." *Archives of Sexual Behavior* 18 (5):401–20.

Elflein, J. 2019. "Cosmetic surgery: Statistics and facts." Statista website.

Eliason, M. J., S. L. Dibble, and P. A. Robertson. 2011. "Lesbian, gay, bisexual, and transgender (LGBT) physicians' experiences in the workplace." *Journal of Homosexuality* 58:1355–71.

Epstein, C. F. 2007. "Great divides: The cultural, cognitive, and social bases of the global subordination of women." *American Sociological Review* 72:1–22.

Fausto-Sterling, A. 1992. *Myths of Gender: Biological Theories about Women and Men*. New York: Basic Books.

Federal Bureau of Investigation. 2019. "Hate crime statistics." FBI website.

Ferber, A. L. 2000. "Racial warriors and the weekend warriors: The construction of masculinity in mythopoetic and white supremacist discourse." *Men and Masculinities* 3:30–56.

Fernandez-Mateo, I. 2009. "Cumulative gender disadvantage in contract employment." *American Journal of Sociology* 114:871–923.

Fiedler, M. E. 2010. *Breaking Through the Stained Glass Ceiling*. New York: Seabury Books.

Fokir, M. A. 2011. "Violence against women survey: 2011." United Nations website.

Francis, B., and C. Skelton. 2005. *Reassessing Gender and Achievement*. London: Routledge & Kegan Paul.

Friedman, M. S., et al. 2011. "A meta-analysis of disparities in childhood sexual abuse, parental physical abuse, and peer victimization among sexual minority and sexual nonminority individuals." *American Journal of Public Health* 101:1481-94.

Frisco, M. L., and K. Williams. 2003. "Perceived housework equity, marital happiness, and divorce in dual-earner households." *Journal of Family Issues* 24:51–73.

Fulcher, M., E. L. Sutfin, and C. J. Patterson. 2008. "Individual differences in gender development." *Sex Roles* 58:330–41.

Galdi, S., A. Maass, and M. Cadinu. 2014. "Objectifying media: their effect on gender role norms and sexual harassment of women." *Psychology of Women Quarterly* 38:398–413.

Gennetian, L. A., L. M. Lopoo, and A. S. London. 2008. "Maternal work hours and adolescents' school outcomes among low-income families in four urban counties." *Demography* 45:31–53.

Gillen, M., E. Lefkowitz, and C. Shearer. 2006. "Does body image play a role in risky sexual behavior and attitudes?" *Journal of Youth and Adolescence* 35:230–42.

Goldberg, W. A., J. Prause, R. Lucas-Thompson, and A. Himsel. 2008. "Maternal employment and children's achievement in context." *Psychological Bulletin* 134:77–108.

Goldman, N., et al. 2004. "Sex differentials in biological risk factors for chronic disease." *Journal of Women's Health* 13:393–403.

Gorman, E. H., and J. A. Kmec. 2009. "Hierarchical rank and women's organizational mobility." *American Journal of Sociology* 114:1428–74.

Gottman, J., et al. 2003. "Correlates of gay and lesbian couples' relationship satisfaction and relationship dissolution." *Journal of Homosexuality* 45:23–44.

Grabe, S., and J. S. Hyde. 2006. "Ethnicity and body dissatisfaction among women in the United States." *Psychological Bulletin* 132:622–40.

Grogan, S., and H. Richards. 2002. "Body image: Focus groups with boys and men." *Men and Masculinities* 4:219–32.

Haggard, M. C. 2019. "Religion's role in the illusion of gender equality." *Psychology of Religion and Spirituality* 11:392–98.

Hamois, C. E., and J. L. Bastos. 2018. "Discrimination, harassment, and gendered health inequalities." *Journal of Health and Social Behavior* 59:283–99.

Harnois, C. E., and J. L. Bastos. 2018. "Discrimination, harassment, and gendered health inequalities: Do perceptions of workplace mistreatment contribute to the gender gap in self-reported health?" *Journal of Health and Social Behavior* 59:283–99.

Harriger, J. A., R. M. Calogero, D. C. Witherington, and J. E. Smith. 2010. "Body size stereotyping and internalization of the thin ideal in preschool girls." *Sex Roles* 63:609–20.

Hart, T. A., et al. 2018. "Childhood maltreatment, bullying victimization, and psychological distress among gay and bisexual men." *The Journal of Sex Research* 55:604–16.

Hatzenbuchler, M. L., K. M. Keyes, and D. S. Hasin. 2009. "State-level policies and psychiatric morbidity in lesbian, gay, and bisexual populations." *American Journal of Public Health* 99:2275–81.

He, X., et al. 2020. "Domestic violence." *Georgetown Journal of Gender and Law* 21:253–98.

Heilman, M. E. 2001. "Description and prescription: How gender stereotypes prevent women's ascent up the organizational ladder." *Journal of Social Issues* 57:657–74.

Herek, G. M. 2009. "Hate crimes and stigma-related experiences among sexual minority adults in the United States." *Journal of Interpersonal Violence* 24:54–74.

Hill, E. J., A. J. Hawkins, V. Maartinson, and M. Ferris. 2003. "Studying 'working fathers.'" *Fathering* 1:239–62.

Hinze, S. W. 2004. "'Am I being over-sensitive?' Women's experience of sexual harassment during medical training." *Health* 8:101–27.

Hyde, J. S. 2005. "The gender similarities hypothesis." *American Psychologist* 60:581–92.

Jena, A. B., A. R. Olenski, and D. M. Blumenthal. 2016. "Sex differences in physician salary in US public medical schools." *JAMA Internal Medicine* 176:1294–1304.

Johnson, S. M., and E. O'Connor. 2002. *The Gay Baby Boom*. New York: New York University Press.

Johnston, D. D., and D. H. Swanson. 2003. "Invisible mothers: A content analysis of motherhood ideologies and myths in magazines." *Sex Roles* 48:21–33.

Jones, S., and D. Myhill. 2004. "Seeing things differently: Teachers' constructions of under-achievement." *Gender and Education* 16:531–46.

Joyner, K., W. Manning, and B. Prince. 2019. "The qualities of same-sex and different-sex couples in young adulthood." *Journal of Marriage and Family* 81:487-505.

Kahlenberg, S. G., and M. M. Hein. 2010. "Progression on Nickelodeon? Gender-role stereotypes in toy commercials." *Sex Roles* 62:830–47.

Kahn, J. R., J. Garcia-Manglano, and S. M. Bianchi. 2014. "The Motherhood penalty at midlife." *Journal of Marriage and Family* 76:56–72.

Knoke, D., and Y. Ishio. 1998. "The gender gap in company job training." *Work and Occupations* 25 (May):141–67.

Krassas, N. R., J. M. Blauwkamp, and P. Wesselink. 2001. "Boxing Helena and corseting Eunice: Sexual rhetoric in Cosmopolitan and Playboy magazines." *Sex Roles* 44:751–71.

Kreeger, K. Y. 2002. "Deciphering how the sexes think." *Scientist*, January 21, pp. 28–33.

Kulik, L. 2011. "Developments in spousal power relations: Are we moving toward equality?" *Marriage & Family Review* 47:419–35.

Landolt, M. A., et al. 2004. "Gender nonconformity, childhood rejection, and adult attachment: A study of gay men." *Archives of Sexual Behavior* 33:117–28.

Langhinrichsen-Rohling, J., D. A. Lamis, and P. S. Malone. 2011. "Sexual attraction status and adolescent suicide proneness." *Journal of Homosexuality* 58:52–82.

Laumann, E. O., R. T. Michael, J. H. Gagnon, and S. Michaels. 1994. *The Social Organization of Sexuality*. Chicago: University of Chicago Press.

Lauster, N., and A. Easterbrook. 2011. "No room for new families?" *Social Problems* 58:389–409.

Lauzen, M. M., and D. M. Dozier. 2005. "Maintaining the double standard: Portrayals of age and gender in popular films." *Sex Roles* 52:437–46.

Lee, K., et al. 2017. "Adolescent desire for cosmetic surgery." *Plastic and Reconstructive Surgery* 139:1109–18.

Lindberg, S. M., J. S. Hyde, J. L. Petersen, and M. C. Linn. 2010. "New trends in gender and mathematics performance." *Psychological Bulletin* 136:1123–35.

Lleras, C. 2008. "Employment, work conditions, and the home environment in single-mother families." *Journal of Family Issues* 29:1268–97.

Loftus, J. 2001. "America's liberalization in attitudes toward homosexuality, 1973 to 1999." *American Sociological Review* 66:762–82.

Lowe, M. E. 2009. "Gay, lesbian, and queer theologies." *Dialog: A Journal of Theology* 48:49–61.

Mager, J., and J. G. Helgeson. 2011. "Fifty years of advertising images." *Sex Roles* 64:238–52.

Mandel, H., and M. Semyonov. 2006. "A welfare state paradox: State interventions and women's employment opportunities in 22 countries." *American Journal of Sociology* 111:1910–49.

Marano, H. E., and E. Strand. 2003. "Points of departure." *Psychology Today,* July/August, pp. 48–49.

Markey, C., and P. Markey. 2005. "Relations between body image and dieting behaviors." *Sex Roles* 53:519–30.

Martell, R. F., C. Parker, and C. G. Emrich. 1998. "Sex stereotyping in the executive suite." *Journal of Social Behavior and Personality* 13 (1):127–38.

Martin, C. L. 2014. "Gender early socialization." Encyclopedia on early childhood website.

Maume, D. I., R. A. Sebastian, and A. R. Bardo. 2010. "Gender, work-family responsibilities, and sleep." *Gender & Society* 224:746–68.

McCabe, J., K. L. Brewster, and K. H. Tillman. 2011. "Patterns and correlates of same-sex sexual activity among U.S. teenagers and young adults." *Perspectives on Sexual and Reproductive Health* 43:142–50.

McCallum, C., and S. McLaren. 2011. "Sense of belonging and depressive symptoms among GLB adolescents." *Journal of Homosexuality* 58:83–96.

McCarthy, J. 2017. "Americans split over new LGBT protections, restroom policies." Gallup Poll website.

McConaghy, N., et al. 2006. "Fraternal birth order and ratio of heterosexual/homosexual feelings in women and men." *Journal of Homosexuality* 51:161–74.

McConkey, D. 2001. "Whither Hunter's culture war? Shifts in evangelical morality, 1988–1998." *Sociology of Religion* 61:149–74.

McLaughlin, H., C. Uggen, and A. Blackstone. 2012. "Sexual harassment, workplace authority, and the paradox of power." *American Sociological Review* 77:625–47.

Mechcatie, E., and K. Rosenberg. 2018. "No detrimental effects in children of same-sex parents." *American Journal of Nursing* 118:55.

Menard, K. S., A. H. Phung, M. F. Ghebrial, and L. Martin. 2003. "Gender differences in sexual harassment and coercion in college students." *Journal of Interpersonal Violence* 18:1222–39.

Meyer, I. H. 2003. "Prejudice, social stress, and mental health in lesbian, gay, and bisexual populations." *Psychological Bulletin* 129:674–97.

Meyers, C. 1988. *Discovering Eve: Ancient Israelite Women in Context.* New York: Oxford University Press.

Miller, L. R., and E. A. Grollman. 2015. "The social costs of gender nonconformity for transgender adults." *Sociological Forum* 30:809–31.

Mitchell, R. S. 1969. *The Homosexual and the Law.* New York: Arco.

Miyake, Y., et al. 2010. "Brain activation during the perception of distorted body images in eating disorders." *Psychiatry Research: Neuroimaging* 181:183–92.

Morrongiello, B. A., and K. Hogg. 2004. "Mothers' reactions to children misbehaving in ways that can lead to injury." *Sex Roles* 50:103–18.

Muench, U., et al. 2015. "Salary differences between male and female nurses in the United States." *Journal of the American Medical Association* 313:1265–67.

Murnen, S. K., C. Greenfield, A. Younger, and H. Boyd. 2016. "Boys act and girls appear." *Sex Roles* 74:78–91.

Mustanski, B. S., M. L. Chivers, and J. M. Bailey. 2002. "A critical review of recent biological research on human sexual orientation." *Annual Review of Sex Research* 13:89–140.

Mustanski, B., R. Andrews, and J. A. Puckett. 2016. "The effects of cumulative victimization on mental health among lesbian, gay, bisexual, and transgender adolescents and young adults." *American Journal of Public Health* 106:527–33.

Myhill, D., and S. Jones. 2006. "'She doesn't shout at no girls': Pupils' perceptions of gender equity in the classroom." *Cambridge Journal of Education* 36:99–113.

Newcomb, A. 2018. “Women’s earnings lower in most occupations.” U.S. Census Bureau website.

Newman, B. S. 2007. “College students’ attitudes about lesbians.” *Journal of Homosexuality* 52:249–65.

Newton, J. 1998. “White guys: Hegemonic masculinities.” *Feminist Studies* 24:11–20.

Nicaise, V., G. Cogerino, J. E. Bois, and A. J. Amorose. 2006. “Students’ perceptions of teacher feedback and physical competence in physical education classes.” *Journal of Teaching in Physical Education* 25:36–57.

Nolan, S. A., J. P. Buckner, C. H. Marzabadi, and V. J. Kuck. 2008. “Training and mentoring of chemists.” *Sex Roles* 58:235–50.

Noonan, M. C., and M. E. Corcoran. 2004. “The mommy track and partnership: Temporary delay or dead end?” *The Annals of the American Academy of Political and Social Science* 596:130–50.

Noonan, M. C., M. E. Corcoran, and P. M. Courant. 2005. “Pay differences among the highly trained.” *Social Forces* 84:831–51.

Parker, L. L., and J. A. Harriger. 2020. “Eating disorders and disordered eating behaviors in the LGBT population.” *Journal of Eating Disorders* 8:51.

Patterson, C. J. 2000. “Family relationships of lesbians and gay men.” *Journal of Marriage and Family* 62:1052–69.

Pavalko, E. K., K. N. Mossakowski, and V. J. Hamilton. 2003. “Does perceived discrimination affect health? Longitudinal relationships between work discrimination and women’s physical and emotional health.” *Journal of Health and Social Behavior* 44:18–33.

Perry-Jenkins, M., R. L. Repetti, and A. C. Crouter. 2000. “Work and family in the 1990s.” *Journal of Marriage and the Family* 62:981–98.

Pfaff, D., ed. 2002. *Hormones, Brain and Behavior.* San Diego, CA: Academic.

Poling Report. 2020. The Polling Report website.

Poushter, J., and N. Kent. 2020. “The global divide on homosexuality persists.” Pew Research Center website.

Ranson, G. 2001. “Men at work: Change—or no change?—in the era of the ‘new father.’” *Men and Masculinities* 4:3–26.

Ray, J. 2019. “Respect for U.S. women hits new low before midterms.” Gallup Poll website.

Reardon, S. 2019. “Massive study finds no single genetic cause of same-sex sexual behavior.” Scientific American website.

Redmond, P., and S. McGuinness. 2020. “Explaining the gender gap in job satisfaction.” *Applied Economics Letters* 27:1415–18.

Regnerus, M. 2018. “The future of American sexuality and family.” Public Discourse website.

Rieger, G., J. A. W. Linsenmeier, L. Gygax, and J. M. Bailey. 2008. “Sexual orientation and childhood gender nonconformity.” *Developmental Psychology* 44:46–58.

Riggle, E. D. B., S. S. Rostosky, and S. G. Horne. 2010. “Psychological distress, well-being, and well-being in same-sex couple relationships.” *Journal of Family Psychology* 24:82–6.

Roisman, G. I., E. Clausell, A. Holland, K. Fortuna, and C. Elieff. 2008. “Adult romantic relationships as contexts of human development.” *Developmental Psychology* 44:91–101.

Rose, K. M., et al. 2004. “Women’s employment status and mortality.” *Journal of Women’s Health* 13:1108–18.

Rosenthal, M. N., A. M. Smidt, and J. J. Freyd. 2016. “Still second class.” *Psychology of Women Quarterly* 40:364–77.

Roth, L. M. 2003. “Selling women short: Gender differences in compensation on Wall Street.” *Social Forces* 82:783–802.

Sabin, J. A., R. G. Riskind, and B. A. Nosek. 2015. “Health care providers’ implicit and explicit attitudes toward lesbian women and Gay Men.” *American Journal of Public Health* 105:1831–41.

Safron, A., et al. 2017. “Neural correlates of sexual orientation in heterosexual, bisexual, and homosexual men.” *Scientific Reports,* February 1.

Sandstrom, A. 2016. “Women relatively rare in top positions of religious leadership.” Pew Research Center website.

Schmitt, D. P., A. Realo, M. Voracek, and J. Allik. 2008. “Why can’t a man be more like a woman? Sex differences in big five personality traits across 55 cultures.” *Journal of Personality and Social Psychology* 94:168–82.

Settles, I. H., L. M. Cortina, J. Malley, and A. J. Stewart. 2006. “The climate for women in academic science.” *Psychology of Women Quarterly* 30:47–58.

Shapiro, J. R., and A. M. Williams. 2012. “The role of stereotype threats in undermining girls’ and women’s performance and interest in STEM fields.” *Sex Roles* 66:175–83.

Sherman, A. M., and E. L. Zurbriggen. 2014. “Boys can be anything.” *Sex Roles* 70:195–208.

Smith, S. J., D. C. Zanotti, A. M. Axelton, and D. A. Saucier. 2011. "Individuals' beliefs about the etiology of same-sex sexual orientation." *Journal of Homosexuality* 58:1110–31.

Snapp, S. D., et al. 2015. "Messy, butch, and queer: LBGTQ youth and the school-to-prison pipeline." *Journal of Adolescent Research* 30:57–82.

Stephens-Davidowitz, S. 2013. "How many American men are gay?" *New York Times,* Dec. 8.

Stice, E., and S. K. Bearman. 2001. "Body-image and eating disturbances prospectively predict increases in depressive symptoms in adolescent girls." *Developmental Psychology* 37:597–607.

Stolberg, S. G., et al. 2016. "New front line in culture war: the bathroom." *New York Times,* May 22.

Stotzer, R. L. 2014. "Law enforcement and criminal justice personnel interactions with transgender people in the United States." *Journal of Aggression and Violent Behavior* 9:263–77.

Street, A. E., J. L. Gradus, J. Stafford, and K. Kelly. 2007. "Gender differences in experiences of sexual harassment." *Journal of Consulting and Clinical Psychology* 75:464–74.

Sullivan, D. A. 2001. *Cosmetic Surgery: The Cutting Edge of Commercial Medicine in America.* New Brunswick, NJ: Rutgers University Press.

Swers, M. L. 2002. *The Difference Women Make: The Policy Impact of Women in Congress.* Chicago, IL: University of Chicago Press.

Taywaditep, K. J. 2001. "Marginalization among the marginalized: Gay men's anti-effeminacy attitudes." *Journal of Homosexuality* 42:1–28.

Teasdale, B., and M. S. Bradley-Engen. 2010. "Adolescent same-sex attraction and mental health." *Journal of Homosexuality* 57:287–309.

Teig, S., and J. E. Susskind. 2008. "Truck driver or nurse? The impact of gender roles and occupational status on children's occupational preferences." *Sex Roles* 58:848–63.

Tilesik, A. 2011. "Pride and prejudice: Employment discrimination against openly gay men in the United States." *American Journal of Sociology* 117:586–626.

Torpy, J. M., and R. M. Glass. 2006. "Anorexia nervosa." *Journal of the American Medical Association* 295:2684.

Treas, J., T. van der Lippe, and T. C. Tai. 2011. "The happy homemaker? Married women's well-being in cross-national perspective." *Social Forces* 90:111–32.

Twenge, J. M., R. A. Sherman, and B. E. Wells. 2016. "Changes in American adults' reported same-sex sexual experiences and attitudes, 1973-2014." *Archives of Sexual Behavior* 45:1713.

Uggen, C., and A. Blackstone. 2004. "Sexual harassment as a gendered expression of power." *American Sociological Review* 69:64–92.

Usdansky, M. L., R. A. Gordon, X. Wang, and A. Gluzman. 2011. "Depression risk among mothers of young children." *Journal of Family and Economic Issues* 32:1-12.

Vaughan, K. K., and G. T. Fouts. 2003. "Changes in television and magazine exposure and eating disorder symptomatology." *Sex Roles* 49:313–20.

Wainwright, J. L., and C. J. Patterson. 2006. "Delinquency, victimization, and substance use among adolescents with female same-sex parents." *Journal of Family Psychology* 20:526–30.

——. 2008. "Peer relations among adolescents with female same-sex parents." *Developmental Psychology* 44:117–26.

Wallis, C. 2011. "Performing gender: A content analysis of gender display in music videos." *Sex Roles* 64:160–72.

Wilson, E. O. 2000. *Sociobiology: The New Synthesis.* Cambridge, MA: Harvard University Press.

Winberg, C., et al. 2019. "Hearing "That's so gay" and "No homo" on campus and substance use among sexual minority college students." *Journal of Homosexuality* 66:1472–94.

Wood, P. B., and J. P. Bartkowski. 2004. "Attribution style and public policy attitudes toward gay rights." *Social Science Quarterly* 85:58–74.

Woods, K. C., N. T. Buchanan, and I. H. Settles. 2009. "Sexual harassment across the color line." *Cultural Diversity and Ethnic Minority Psychology* 15:67–76.

World Economic Forum. 2020. "The global gender gap report." World Economic Forum website.

Wrushen, B. R., and W. H. Sherman. 2008. "Women secondary school principals." *International Journal of Qualitative Studies in Education* 21:457–69.

Yoder, J. D., and L. L. Berendsen. 2001. "Outsider within the firehouse." *Psychology of Women* 25:27–36.

Zimmerman, T. S., S. A. Haddock, and C. R. McGeorge. 2001. "Mars and Venus: Unequal planets." *Journal of Marital and Family Therapy* 27:55–68.

CHAPTER

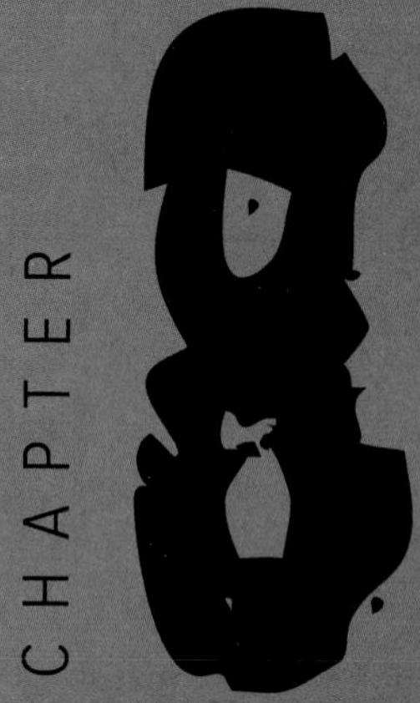

# Race, Ethnic Groups, and Racism

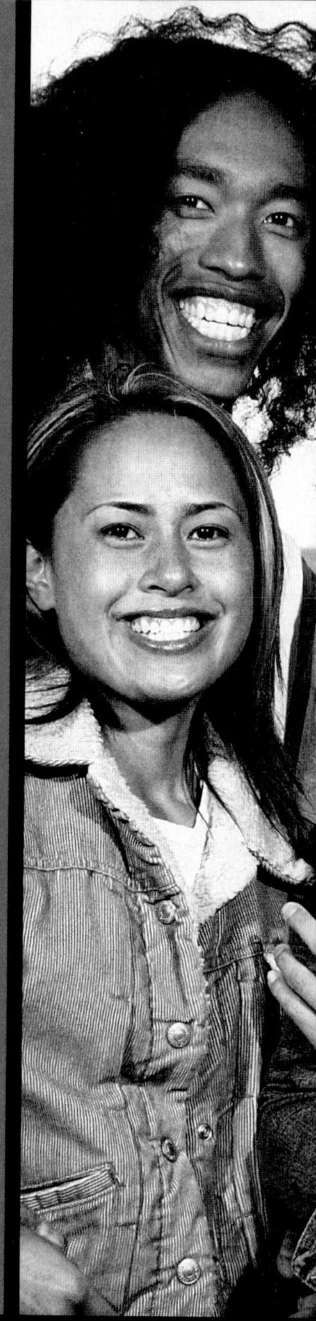

## OBJECTIVES

1. Discuss the meanings of the terms *race, ethnic group,* and *racism.*
2. Understand the extent and origin of the problems of minorities.
3. Identify the ways in which the problems of minorities negatively affect the quality of life for them.
4. Know the social structural and social psychological factors that contribute to the problems of minorities.
5. Show some ways to address the problems of minorities.

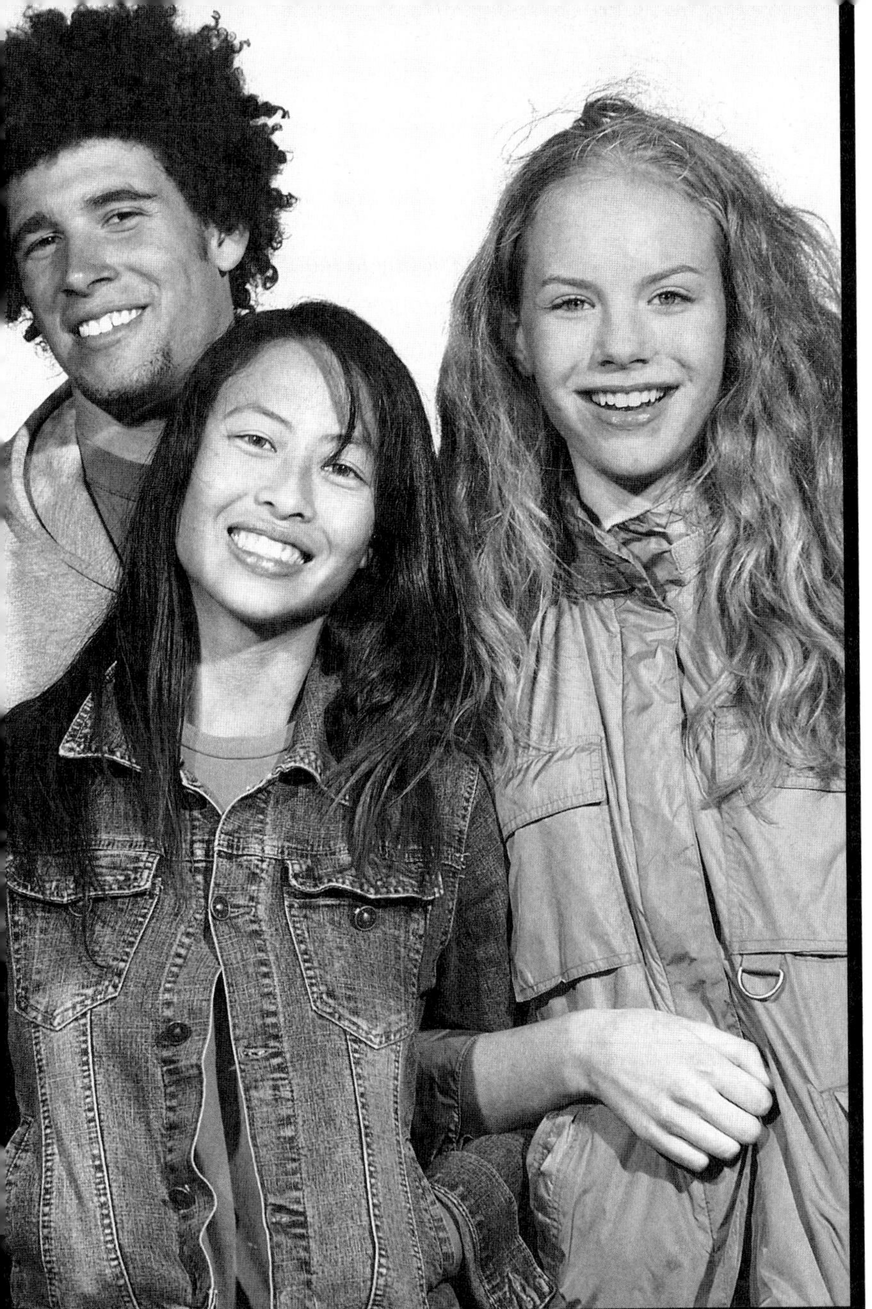
Plush Studios/Blend Images LLC

### Will It Ever End?

Daryl is in his 50s, Black, and a college administrator. He was a teenager when the civil rights movement began to have a strong impact. Daryl has lived in two different worlds, because he spent his early years in the segregated South, but, as he recounts, there are some disturbing continuities:

*I can remember going into a department store and finding the drinking fountain that said "colored only" on it. We couldn't drink out of the same fountains or go into the same bathrooms as the whites. I've achieved a place in society that neither my grandfather nor my father could have ever dreamed of being.*

*But it hasn't been easy. I guess I could forget those segregated water fountains if white people didn't keep reminding me that I'm different. I served in the army for a time in Germany. I married a white, German woman. We came back to this country so I could pursue a graduate degree. We took a trip down South in 1969 so I could show my wife where I grew up. We drove around my old neighborhood, then went into a restaurant in the suburbs. It was the last time we tried that. I had come back here to pursue my graduate degree, not to get into conflict with a lot of hostile people. They couldn't tolerate an interracial couple. Their glares made us both extremely uncomfortable during dinner. We wound up eating hurriedly and getting out.*

*I've had a lot of other incidents to contend with, sometimes with my wife and sometimes just on my own. You'd think it would be over by now, wouldn't you? But recently I attended a conference of Black college administrators in a resort area. There was a convention of doctors there at the same time. One morning I came down into the lobby to meet a friend and saw one of our female administrators in a heated argument with a doctor. I stepped in and broke it up. It turned out that she was just standing at the desk when he came up and started making remarks to her about how hostile and arrogant Blacks are. He said Blacks keep causing trouble because we cry about discrimination when we have just as many opportunities as anyone else.*

*Instead of going out for a pleasant morning with an old friend, I wound up calling a meeting of our officers and trying to decide what to do about the incident. I don't think white people realize what it's like to be vulnerable to those kinds of things just because of the color of your skin. And I really wonder sometimes if it will ever end.*

## Introduction

Are people with white skin biologically inferior? Are they inherently less capable, less deserving, or less willing to work to get ahead than others? These questions may sound absurd to some of you, but millions of Americans who are minorities confront such questions about themselves. Throughout American history, minorities have been treated as if they were somehow inferior human beings, but racial inequalities are rooted in sociocultural rather than biological factors. We are all one species—human.

Before discussing the race problem (which is a shorthand phrase for the problem of relationships between people of diverse racial and ethnic backgrounds), we explore the meaning of race. Then we look at the origin and distribution of America's minorities, what the "race problem" means for them, what factors contribute to the problem, and how the problem can be attacked.

## The Meaning of Race, Ethnic Groups, and Racism

**race**
a group of people distinguished from other groups by their origin in a particular part of the world

**biological characteristic**
an inherited, rather than learned, characteristic

We define **race,** in accord with the U.S. Census Bureau, as a group of people who are distinguished from other groups by their origin in a particular part of the world (Grieco and Cassidy 2001). As such, they tend to share a particular *skin color* (Blacks originated in Africa; whites in Europe, the Middle East, or North Africa; etc.). Many people use the single **biological characteristic** of skin color to identify races, but there are so many shades of skin color that classifying someone as a member of one or another race solely on skin color is arbitrary.

In addition, if race were a purely biological phenomenon, a number of other biological characteristics could be used: blood type, the presence or absence of the Rh factor in the blood, or the ability to taste the chemical phenylthiocarbamide. In each case the groups would be composed of different people. For instance, people who can taste the chemical (as opposed to those who cannot taste it) include large numbers of

Europeans, Americans, American Indians, and Chinese. The point is that any biological basis for distinguishing among people is arbitrary and results in different groupings, which is why geneticists view race as more of a sociological than a biological phenomenon (Lewis 2002).

All human beings belong to one biological species—*Homo sapiens.* The breakdown of that species into subcategories is arbitrary. As Jefferson Fish (1995:55) aptly summed it up, "The short answer to the question 'What is race?' is: There is no such thing. Race is a myth. And our racial classification scheme is loaded with pure fantasy." Nevertheless, people continue to identify different races primarily on the basis of skin color, and the inequalities people experience follow directly from that identification. We follow the categories of the U.S. Bureau of the Census, which uses people's self-identification to place them into one of the following: white or non-Hispanic white, Black or non-Hispanic Black, Asian/Pacific Islander, American Indian/Eskimo/Aleut, other, and two or more races. In addition, the Census Bureau collects data on one ethnic group—Hispanic origin, which includes people of any race.

The term **ethnic group** refers to people who have a shared historical or cultural background that leads them to identify with each other. Although the Census Bureau routinely gathers data only for Hispanics, numerous ethnic groups have been involved in the growth of the nation. Many, such as the Irish and the Polish, have faced problems of acceptance. At present, Hispanics are the largest ethnic group struggling with integration into American society.

**ethnic group**
people who have a shared historical and cultural background that leads them to identify with each other

Keep in mind that *all people have more shared than different characteristics, and no group is biologically superior to another.* Nevertheless, **racism,** the belief that some racial groups are inherently inferior to others, has been common and is used to *justify discrimination and inequality.* We'll explore various forms of racism throughout this chapter.

**racism**
the belief that some racial groups are inherently inferior to others

## Extent and Origin of Races and Racism in America

As Table 8.1 and Figure 8.1 show, the composition of the American population is changing. Racial minorities and Hispanics make up a substantial proportion of the total population of the nation, and their proportion continues to grow. According to the Census Bureau, from 2010 to 2019 the white population increased 4.3 percent, compared to 11.6 percent for Blacks, 29.3 percent for Asian Americans, and 20 percent for Hispanics. By 2019, 40 percent of Americans identified themselves as something other than non-Hispanic white (Budiman 2020a). By the middle of the 21st century, if not sooner, racial minorities will comprise half or more of the total population.

The increase in the minority population reflects not only differing birthrates among various groups but also changing immigration patterns. In 1960, 75 percent of the foreign-born population was from Europe and 9.4 percent was from Latin America; by 2019, only 10.4 percent was from Europe, while 31.4 percent were from Asia and 50.3 percent was from Latin America (U.S. Census Bureau website).

In addition to the changing proportions of various racial/ethnic groups, the United States is becoming more diverse in the sense that an increasing number of Americans identify themselves as multiracial. According to the Census Bureau, more than 11 million Americans claim to be of two or more races.

As we discuss the quality of life of the racial and ethnic groups, it is important to keep in mind the diversity within groups. Among Hispanics, for example, there are

**TABLE 8.1**
U.S. Resident Population, by Race and Hispanic Origin, 1980 and 2019

| | Number (1,000) | | Percent Distribution | |
|---|---|---|---|---|
| Race | 1980 | 2019 | 1980 | 2019 |
| All races | 226,546 | 328,340 | 100.0 | 100.0 |
| White | 194,713 | 250,447 | 85.9 | 76.3 |
| Black | 26,683 | 43,984 | 11.8 | 13.4 |
| Hispanic origin | 14,609 | 60,572 | 6.4 | 18.5 |
| Asian/Pacific Islander | 3,729 | 19,366 | 1.7 | 5.9 |
| American Indian, Eskimo, Aleut | 1,420 | 4,267 | 0.6 | 1.3 |

Note: Persons of Hispanic origin may be of any race and are included in the figures for the other races.
SOURCE: Humes, Jones, and Ramirez 2011, and U.S. Census Bureau website.

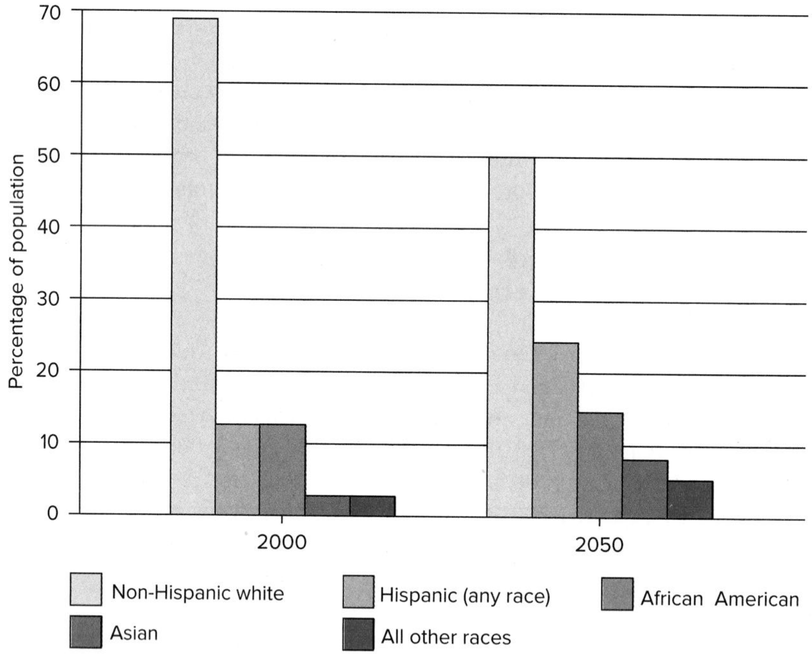


**FIGURE 8.1**
Composition of U.S. Population, 2000–2050.

Source: "Projected population of the United States," U.S. Census Bureau website.

clear and often considerable differences between Mexicans, Puerto Ricans, Cubans, and other Hispanics in such matters as their citizenship status, educational attainment, marriage and divorce rates, employment status, and household income (U.S. Census Bureau 2010; Krogstad and Noe-Bustamante 2020). Similarly, although Asians as a group are among the more educated and higher-income groups in the nation (including whites), some of the immigrants from Southeast Asia, such as the Vietnamese, have lower education levels and higher unemployment and poverty rates.

## Racism in American History

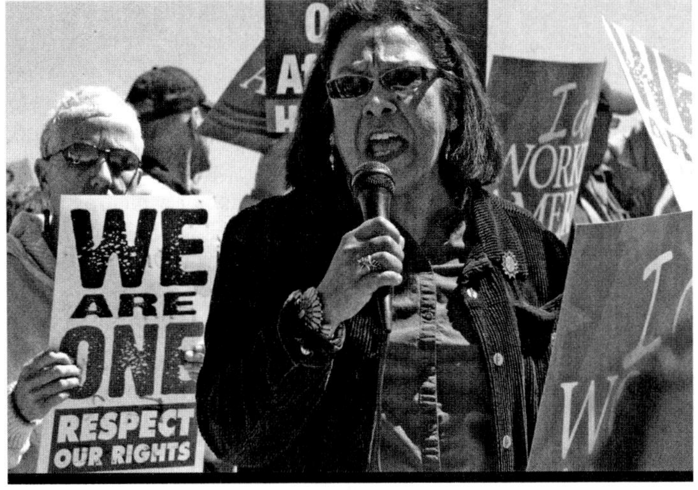


Minorities continue to use nonviolent protest to gain equal rights.

Susan See Photography

Why do problems exist among the various races and ethnic groups in the United States, the supposed "melting-pot" nation of the world? In part, the problems stem from historical circumstances. For example, the high rates of poverty and other problems among American Indians cannot be separated from events that began with the European colonization of the Americas. The colonists decimated both the population and the culture of the various Indian groups. Indians were defrauded of, or forced off, their traditional lands. Solemn treaties between tribes and the American government were repeatedly broken by the latter with little or no compensation to the Indians. And granting tribes a certain autonomy on reservations is a mixed bag at best. They are free from much federal law, but they are also isolated to a considerable extent from the mainstream of the nation's economy.

Similarly, the problems of African Americans cannot be separated from their historical experience of slavery and segregation. The first African Americans to arrive, in 1619, were indentured servants, not slaves. However, states soon passed laws that legitimated slavery, and *those brought here as slaves were legally defined as property, not as persons.* Their enslavement was justified by various kinds of "evidence" of the inherent inferiority of the Black race.

The system of slavery ultimately gave way to a castelike system. In a caste system, people are categorized into groups according to some characteristic over which they have no control, such as their race or the status of their parents. The groups have differing amounts of power, status, and access to those things that are valued. In the United States, whites formed one caste and African Americans another, with the whites having the bulk of the power, status, and financial resources. Of course, there were also differences within the two races. But even lower-class whites could be better off than higher-class Blacks. That is, the two races were like two separate class systems, with the great majority of African Americans in the lower levels of their class system, and with the Black upper class at roughly the same level as the white middle class in terms of material advantages. Segregation in such things as housing, schools, and public accommodations helped maintain the system.

Finally, in the 1950s, Black leaders, including Martin Luther King Jr., led a civil rights movement designed to break down segregation and give African Americans all the rights and privileges enjoyed by whites. They fought the notion of inferiority, rejected discrimination and prejudice, and insisted upon nothing less than full equality of opportunity for all of America's citizens. Their efforts resulted in many significant gains.

Nevertheless, severe problems of racial and ethnic inequality continue to tarnish the American dream of freedom and justice for all. The problems are dramatically illustrated by the Black Lives Matter movement, which began in 2013. The movement emphasizes the problem of police brutality and other violence against Blacks (Gramlich 2020). Many of the instances the movement cites involve the death of an unarmed Black person. Between 2013 and 2020, police killed or injured a Black whose only "weapon" was a hairbrush, a set of keys, a pill bottle, or a candy bar! Most Americans, and people throughout the world, were shocked to see, on May 25, 2020, a video of a policeman with his knee on the neck of an unarmed Black man, George Floyd, who was prone and helpless on the ground. Floyd could not breathe. He died, his only offense being an allegation by a store clerk that he had passed a counterfeit $20 bill.

In sum, despite our *ideology of equal opportunity for all,* racism or ethnic hostility confronts many people who hope to take advantage of the American dream. The United States is not a melting pot. Someone has suggested that a more apt metaphor is a salad bowl, since the various groups tend to retain their identity even as they mix together in the society.

Even the salad bowl metaphor overstates the case, however. For *racial and ethnic segregation persist* in the nation. There may be less, and different patterns of, segregation in metropolitan areas, but segregation is not disappearing (Roscigno, Karafin, and Tester 2009; Rothstein 2018; Rotberg 2020). The predominant pattern is still segregation. Unfortunately, segregated children who grow up in segregated areas are likely to define this as both normal and desirable and perpetuate the pattern of segregation—a pattern that works against the American dream of equal opportunity and freedom from discrimination.

## Immigration

In 2020, more than 40 million people living in the United States were born in another country (Budiman 2020b). Immigrants were 13.7 percent of the total population. Immigration illustrates well the ongoing struggles of minorities to gain full acceptance into American society. Historically, every racial and ethnic group that has come to the United States in large numbers has faced suspicion, nonacceptance, discrimination, and harassment. Whether the Chinese laborers who worked on the railroads in the West, or the Irish who swarmed into the East coast, or the Vietnamese who fled to this country in hopes of finding freedom, or any of the many other groups, none were greeted with welcoming, open arms by those already living here.

Two major concerns regarding immigrants have always been the economic threat they seem to pose (they take away "our" jobs) and the danger of cultural corrosion (they will change our way of life because their ways are not our ways). A national poll reported that a third of Americans see immigrants as a burden to the nation because they take "our jobs" and they take advantage of the health care system (Jones 2016). In response to these concerns, advocates of immigration point out that the immigrants typically do jobs that most Americans don't want to do anyway. In addition, immigrants can have a very positive effect on the economy, thereby benefiting all Americans. Indeed, immigrants comprised a significant proportion of the industrial workforce from 1880 to 1920 and, thus, were a disproportionate part of the laborers who fueled the industrial revolution in the United States (Hirschman and Mogford 2009). As far as the concern about cultural corrosion is concerned, immigration advocates note that American culture has always included influences from a variety of sources. Moreover, American culture has had a greater impact on immigrants than immigrant culture has had on American society.

In recent decades, the *major concern has been with unauthorized immigrants,* frequently called "illegals." Hundreds of thousands of people enter the country illegally every year, primarily to find work and the income and opportunities that they cannot get in their own countries. Early in this century, the number of unauthorized immigrants exceeded that of legal immigrants (Passel and Cohn 2008). By 2017, there were 10.5 million unauthorized immigrants in our nation, accounting for 3.2 percent of the total population (Budiman 2020b). This represents a decrease from 2007, when the estimate was 12.05 million. More stringent efforts to halt immigration and to deport those discovered, along with reduced opportunities in the United States as a result of a severe recession, account for the lower number.

Unauthorized immigration is a racial/ethnic problem because most entrants are Hispanics, Asians, or Africans. The largest number of unauthorized immigrants (58 percent) are from Mexico, although from 2009 to 2014 more Mexicans left than entered; there was a net loss of 140,000 Mexicans (Gonzalez-Barrera 2015). Despite the decrease in numbers and lack of evidence about serious detrimental effects of the unauthorized immigrants (see the discussion below), anti-Mexican attitudes were widespread by 2015. Millions of Americans supported the plan of one of the presidential candidates to deport all illegals and to build a wall across the entire U.S.-Mexican border. Some unauthorized immigrants travel back and forth between the United States and their native country, but many have remained here for 10 or more years.

*Is Unauthorized Immigration a Threat?* Many Americans define unauthorized immigration as a threatening situation. Some argue, particularly those who live in areas of high unemployment, that the immigrants take away jobs from natives (Esses, Brochu, and Dickson 2011). Others believe that their taxes are higher because they are paying for social benefits (such as health care and in-state tuition at state schools) received by unauthorized immigrants (Berg 2009).

Responding to the perceived threats, a majority of state legislatures have passed or introduced anti-immigration legislation. Arizona led the way in 2010, with a law that authorized deportation of all undocumented immigrants. To facilitate the process, the law included the following provisions: local police are to make immigration checks; immigrants who are authorized must carry papers with them; it is illegal for an unauthorized immigrant to live, or to look for work, in the state; and it is illegal for anyone to knowingly shelter, transport, or hire unauthorized immigrants.

Interestingly, not only states with a large number of unauthorized immigrants, like Arizona, but states with a relatively small number, like Alabama, have enacted such legislation. In Alabama, the new law became effective in 2011. It eliminated all state and local services (driver's licenses, tuition help, enrolling in college, securing employment, etc.) to anyone who was undocumented (Symmes 2012). The law was popular with the residents, and many of the unauthorized immigrants left the state. But some Alabamans soon began to question its effects. Businesspeople couldn't find enough people to do the low-wage work that the unauthorized immigrants had done; they wanted the immigrants back. In addition, a couple of police stops that questioned foreign employees (who were, it turned out, authorized) led to concern about backlash and withdrawal of foreign firms with plants in the state. The combination of disruption of businesses, potential loss of industrial plants, and the high costs of enforcing the law resulted in the legislature working on modifications in early 2012. Nevertheless, state legislatures continued to propose legislation that would restrict the freedom of the immigrants to live at peace in their states. In 2016 alone, 19 states considered legislation that the American Civil Liberties Union called "misguided, mean-spirited, and, in many instances, unconstitutional" (ACLU 2016).

The point is, as with all social problems there are conflicting positions about how to deal with unauthorized immigration. Some—including businesspeople, advocates of the free market, and ethnic advocacy groups—want a policy of amnesty and eventual citizenship for unauthorized immigrants. Others—including cultural conservatives, unions, and people concerned about employment and taxes—advocate deportation and greater border security to prevent the unauthorized from entering the country.

*The Myths of Unauthorized Immigration.* There are legitimate points made by both sides of the issue of unauthorized immigration, but we need to frame the debate in light of the increasing amount of evidence about the actual impact immigrants have on our society. Weeks and Weeks (2010) studied the impact of unauthorized immigration from Latin America on states in the South. The researchers identified a number of myths people hold about the impact of such immigration. One myth is the idea that tighter border security will reduce the numbers. Actually, before the recent state and federal efforts to make the borders more secure, many of those from Mexico would travel back and forth to be with family on holidays and special family occasions. Their long-range plans might include eventually settling back in their own country. With the tightening of the borders, however, many no longer take the risk of traveling back and forth, but choose to remain in this country. They have children here (thereby making the children legal American citizens), work here, and become more Americanized over time.

A second myth is the assertion that the unauthorized are an economic drain on our resources. On the contrary, as the situation in Alabama illustrates, the immigrants are a needed labor supply; some agricultural business has relocated to Mexico because of the lack of workers in this country. Other researchers have come to the same conclusion about the economic impact. Overall in the nation, unauthorized immigrants have *not* increased the number of Americans living in poverty, and the states in which the new laws have been passed have, at this point, suffered adverse economic consequences rather than lessened their economic burden (Peri 2011; Esses, Brochu, and Dickson 2011).

A third myth is that the culture is diluted and altered by the large number of unauthorized immigrants. Many believe that the immigrants don't bother to learn English, that they expect bilingual education in the schools for their children, and that they promote foreign ideas about political and social life. In point of fact, most of the immigrants do learn English and are far more affected by American culture than American culture is affected by them.

Finally, some Americans fear that the influx of unauthorized immigrants is bringing unknown numbers of "undesirable" people into the country, such as criminals and even terrorists. The inevitable consequence, it is believed, is an increase in crime and violence. However, Sampson (2008) showed that as immigration numbers increased after the 1990s, the number of homicides decreased. He estimated the probability of violence in differing kinds of neighborhoods in Chicago and concluded that some of the safest places in our nation are areas of cities with concentrations of immigrants. And Light and Miller (2018) researched the effects of unauthorized immigrants in all 50 states and the District of Columbia. They found no increase in violence because of the immigrants; in fact, in most cases there was a decrease rather than an increase in violent crimes.

## Race, Ethnicity, and the Quality of Life

What does it mean to be a minority in America? How does being a minority affect the *quality of life?* We will look at four areas in which all Americans are supposed to have equal rights:

1. Certain rights as citizens.
2. Equal economic opportunities.

3. The right to life, liberty, and the pursuit of happiness.
4. The right to dignity as a human being.

In each of the four areas, being white is a distinct advantage. Although the advantage is not as great as it was in the past, discrimination is still a part of the life experiences of minorities. In a national survey, 71 percent of African Americans and 52 percent of Hispanics said they have regularly or occasionally experienced discrimination or have been treated unfairly because of their race or ethnicity (Krogstad 2016).

## The Rights of Citizenship

The mass media often remind you of the *rights and privileges attached to your citizenship:*

1. This is a nation governed by laws rather than by individuals.
2. As a citizen, you have both the privilege and the responsibility of participating in the political process to ensure that laws reflect the will of the people.
3. The people do not exist to serve the government; the government exists to serve the people, and to serve all equally.

All these statements break down when we consider minority groups.

*The Right to Vote.* If you don't like the way things are going, it is said that you can express your disapproval at the polls. Indeed, voting is the responsibility of every citizen because one way that Americans are presumably able to change things is by exercising their right to vote. However, this right and privilege, basic as it is to our notions of government, has often eluded African Americans and was long withheld from American Indians.

When the Fifteenth Amendment to the Constitution was ratified in 1870, all male Americans over age 21 had the right to vote, regardless of their race, creed, color, or prior condition of servitude. The subsequent history of African American voting is one of ongoing efforts to negate or suppress the right to vote (Brown, Batt, and Kim 2020). Immediately after the Fifteenth Amendment passed steps were taken to keep African Americans from voting. The southern states passed laws that effectively **disfranchised** Black voters. Some of the laws required literacy and property tests. Others imposed a poll tax. Such laws excluded poor whites as well as African Americans, however, so loopholes were created. One loophole was the "understanding clause," which allowed a registrar to enroll any individual who could give a "reasonable" explanation of a part of the state constitution that was read to him. Similarly, the "grandfather clause" exempted from the literacy test those who descended from pre-1865 voters.

**disfranchise**
to deprive of the right to vote

Intimidation also was used to keep African Americans from registering and voting. Sometimes the threat of violence or actual violence (including even murder) discouraged African Americans. The pressure of economic intimidation also was applied. They faced the possibility of losing their jobs or of being refused supplies at local stores.

Nor is all of this disfranchisement mere history now. From time to time, a report appears in the news media about efforts to keep various minorities from voting. Rather than intimidation, however, a tactic more likely to be used is drawing voting district lines in a way that neutralizes the power of minority votes (by, for example, splitting areas with heavy concentrations of minorities into separate districts so that whites are in the majority in each of the areas). Various other measures may be used at the state and local level. Laws have been enacted in recent years that make it more difficult to register and/or to vote. Registration has become a more rigorous process with particular kinds of required identification. With regard to voting, beginning in 2001, more than a thousand voter ID laws have been proposed and hundreds have been adopted in various states (Hicks et al. 2015). Proponents of such laws claim they are necessary to prevent voter fraud. As of this writing, however, there is no evidence of significant voting fraud, and what fraud we know about is likely to occur with absentee ballots rather than with people who come to the polls to vote (Fogarty et al. 2015). Proponents still argue that the laws are necessary as a preventive measure. Opponents counter that the laws essentially function to disfranchise certain segments of the population—in particular the poor, seniors, and racial and ethnic minorities, all of whom are less likely than others to have a government-issued photo ID card (Rosenfeld 2007). As of this writing, the issue of whether photo ID laws violate the constitutional right to vote is still a matter of contention.

*The Rule of Law.* Another right and privilege of citizenship is to live in a land governed by laws rather than by individuals. The laws, however, have failed to fully protect minority rights in the areas of *housing and school desegregation.*

With regard to housing, the laws forbid discrimination in the sale, rental, or financing of any housing. Legally, a home that is for sale should be available to anyone who can afford it. However, some white property owners have "restrictive covenants" in their deeds that bar racial minorities from purchasing their homes (San Francisco Bureau 2001), and a certain amount of *racial steering* (diverting minorities away from predominantly white neighborhoods) still occurs. A study of 20 major metropolitan areas found racial steering of African Americans and discrimination against Hispanics in access to rental housing (Ross and Turner 2005). According to the National Fair Housing Alliance (2020), there are over 4 million incidents of housing discrimination every year. And a survey of the literature on housing discrimination concluded that both institutional (such as banks, real estate agents, and insurance companies) and individual (such as landlords and homeowners) factors contribute to the problem (Roscigno et al. 2009). The result is continuing residential segregation. To be sure, the extent to which residential areas are segregated has declined over the past few decades. Nevertheless, by 2010 non-Hispanic whites lived in areas in which 75 percent of the other residents were also non-Hispanic whites (Farley 2011). Another way to look at it is that African Americans account for about 14 percent of urban residents, but are only 8 percent of the residents in areas in which the majority is white.

Even if minorities don't encounter obstacles in obtaining the kind of housing they prefer, they may find themselves at a disadvantage in the financing process. In the study of 20 major metropolitan areas, the researchers reported that Hispanics got less help in obtaining financing (Ross and Turner 2005). Lending agents may reject minority applicants at a higher rate than that for whites (the rejection rate for high-income minorities is often as high as that for low-income whites) and may exact higher interest rates from minorities than from whites (Williams and Nesiba 2005; Faber 2018).

Ironically, during the early 2000s minorities appeared to be getting help in housing by securing subprime mortgages. These mortgages became available as government regulations eased. They were a high risk for investors. They were also a high risk for those obtaining them, because most were adjustable-rate mortgages. When the housing market changed in 2006, refinancing became more difficult and many homeowners could no longer afford to pay their mortgages. Minorities were particularly affected by the situation because mortgage brokers tended to target them as customers for the risky subprime loans (Rugh and Massey 2010).

Finally, *segregated educational facilities* were declared illegal in the now-famous 1954 Supreme Court decision in the *Brown v. Board of Education of Topeka* case. Such facilities were ruled unconstitutional on the grounds that they are *inherently unequal,* but the desegregation process has been agonizingly slow. In recent years, moreover, there has been a reversal of the gains that were made in the years immediately after the Supreme Court decision, such that segregation is as much a problem now as it was in the 1950s (Orfield and Jarvie 2020). Desegregation peaked around 1988, when 37 percent of Black students attended schools that had a majority of white students. But by 2018, only 19 percent of Black students were in schools that had a majority of white students, and 40 percent of Blacks were in intensely segregated (90–100 percent) nonwhite schools. The segregation would be less if all children attended nearby public schools, but a large number go to private, magnet, and charter schools and thereby increase the segregation in local, public schools (Saporito and Sohoni 2006). African Americans and Hispanics tend to be more segregated than Asians, but all minorities still experience segregated schooling to some extent.

*Equality before the Law.* All Americans are supposed to stand as *equals before the law.* Most people, of course, quickly recognize that not all Americans are treated equally. The wealthy are rarely accorded the harsh treatment endured by the poor. Probably few people are aware of the extent to which minorities receive unequal treatment in virtually every aspect of civil and criminal proceedings (Butterfield 2000).

For example, police are more likely to be verbally abusive and to use excessive force against Hispanics and African Americans (Weitzer and Tuch 2004; Durose, Smith, and Langan 2007). In a national survey, 45 percent of Black respondents, compared to 19 percent of Hispanics and 9 percent of whites, said they had been unfairly stopped by the police because of their race (Parker, Horowitz, and Anderson 2020). Hispanic and Black youth are more likely to be detained by the police and the courts than are white youth (Demuth and Steffensmeier 2004). For example, although white, Black, and Hispanic youth report using drugs at similar rates, Black youth are detained at nearly five times the rate, and Hispanic youth at twice the rate, of white youth (Bell, Ridolfi, Finley, and Lacey 2009). A study of youths on probation found that the officers consistently described Black youths differently from white youths in their written reports, attributing Blacks' offenses to negative attitudes and personality traits and whites' offenses to the social environment (Bridges and Steen 1998).

Federal courts mete out harsher penalties for Black and Hispanic than for white perpetrators (Demuth and Steffensmeier 2004; Alexander 2010). Minorities are more likely than whites to be stopped while driving and to be imprisoned, even for the same offense (Daniels 2004; Rojek, Rosenfeld, and Decker 2012). As a result, there is a disproportionate number of African Americans and Hispanics in jails and prisons. Two researchers estimated that for men born between 1965 and 1969, 3 percent of whites and 20 percent of African Americans served time in prison by their early thirties (Pettit and Western 2004). It is estimated that about 1 in 3 Black males, 1 in 6 Hispanic males, and 1 in 17 white males will spend time in prison over their lifetime (Bonczar 2003). Put another way, the number of years that Black, Hispanic, and white males can expect to spend in prison or jail over their lifetime are 3.09, 1.06, and 0.5, respectively (Hogg et al. 2008).

Finally, a disproportionate number of minorities, particularly African Americans, are given the death penalty. Although only a minority of those who receive a death sentence are actually executed, minorities convicted of killing whites are more likely than other capital offenders to be executed (Jacobs, Qian, Carmichael, and Kent 2007). As we noted in Chapter 3, 42 percent of prisoners on death row at the end of 2018 were African Americans.

## The Right to Equal Economic Opportunities

Among other factors, racial and ethnic discrimination means that minorities are more likely to be poor, unemployed, or–if they work–underemployed. Minorities also receive, on average, less income than whites.

*Employment.* A group might have *unequal access to employment* in at least five ways. First, the group might have a higher rate of unemployment than other groups. Second, a greater proportion of the group might be *underemployed.* Third, members of the group might be clustered at the lower levels of occupational categories (i.e., even if the proportion of minorities in a category is the same as that of whites, the minorities cluster at the lower levels). Fourth, members of the group might have less job security than whites. And, fifth, a disproportionate number of the group might become disillusioned and drop out of the labor market.

All five kinds of inequality apply to minorities in the United States (Herring 2002; Coleman 2004; Fullerton and Anderson 2013). And the *inequality is maintained by practices at the job candidate, job entry, and job promotion stages.* At the job candidate stage, many of the better jobs are still discovered through informal methods such as friends as much as through a formal recruitment process. Those without such an informal network of people who can exercise influence in the job market will be at a great disadvantage. Immigrants dramatize the extent of the disadvantage. Consider, for example, the plight of the Asian immigrant women who work sewing in sweatshops. An estimated 70 percent of the workers in Los Angeles' garment industry are immigrants (Davis 2017). A 2016 Department of Labor investigation of those shops found rampant cheating of the workers, some of whom were earning as little as $4.50 per hour while working at a rapid pace without the protection of air conditioning from the summer heat.

Even with a formal recruitment process, minorities are disadvantaged when tacit hiring preference is given to whites. Three researchers had white and racial minority applicants with equal qualifications apply for waiter/waitress jobs in a number of fine dining restaurants in New York City (Bendick, Rodriguez, and Jayaraman 2010). Although the overt treatment of all the applicants was courteous, the minorities were only 54 percent as likely as the whites to receive a job offer.

Among the most accessible data on inequality in employment are unemployment rates (Figure 8.2; in this and other figures and tables in this chapter, all groups are included for which data are available). The unemployment rates for African Americans have been double or more those of whites since 1948, and unemployment rates for Hispanics (available since 1973) have been between one and a half and two times those of whites. American Indians tend to have the highest unemployment of all groups–about 46 percent in 2004 (Center for Community Change 2005). And in addition to higher rates, the unemployment spells of minorities are longer than those of non-Hispanic whites (Palumbo 2010). In short, minorities are far more likely to be out of work and looking for a job, and are likely to be out of work for a longer period of time, than are non-Hispanic whites.

Underemployment (working fewer hours than desired or at a job for which the worker is overqualified) is also more common among minorities, and it is detrimental to the well-being of workers (see Chapter 10). A 2016 report from the Bureau of Labor Statistics put the proportion of workers who are involuntarily working part-time at

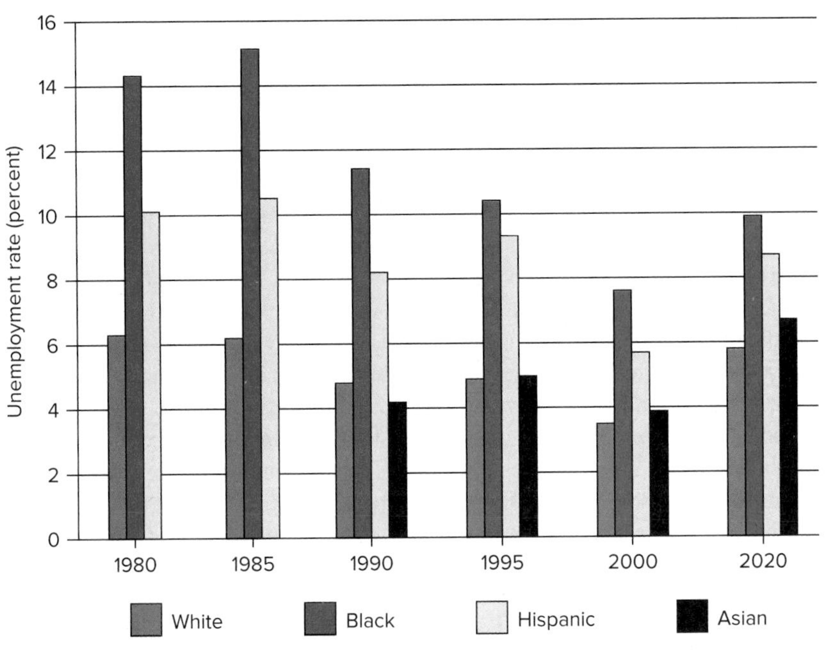


**FIGURE 8.2** Unemployment Rates, 1980–2020.

Source: Various editions of the *Statistical Abstract of the United States* and the Bureau of Labor Statistics website.

**TABLE 8.2**
Employed Persons, by Race and Occupation, 2019

| Occupation | Percent of Total That Is | | |
|---|---|---|---|
| | African American | Hispanic | Asian |
| Total | 12.3 | 17.6 | 6.8 |
| Managerial and professional | 9.6 | 10.1 | 8.7 |
| Service occupations | 17.1 | 25.0 | 5.9 |
| Sales and office occupations | 13.0 | 17.1 | 5.2 |
| Natural resources, construction, maintenance | 7.7 | 31.9 | 2.2 |
| Production, transportation, material moving | 16.9 | 23.0 | 5.0 |

3.6 percent for whites, 5.6 percent for Blacks, and 69 percent for Hispanics (Young and Mattingly 2016).

Table 8.2 offers additional evidence on the problem of *discrimination in job opportunities*. As with most economic data, among the minority groups for which figures are given here, Asian Americans are found disproportionately in the highest group (managerial and professional). But African Americans and Hispanics are more likely to be found in the lower-prestige and lower-income categories (if there were perfect equality, the proportion for each job category in the table would be the same as the group's proportion of the labor force: 12.6 percent Black and 17.8 percent Hispanic in 2019). Moreover, a detailed inspection of each of the categories shows that minorities tend to cluster in the lower levels of those categories.

For example, in the managerial and professional category, the proportion of African Americans and Hispanics who are chief executives, physicians, and lawyers are less than half the two groups' proportion of the population. On the other hand, their proportion in some of the less prestigious and less rewarding occupations in that category—such as tax examiners, community and social service specialists, and teacher assistants—is greater than their proportion of the total population.

Furthermore, once in a job or a career line, minorities are likely to find advancement more difficult for them than for their white peers. A study of female workers found that African Americans and Hispanics experienced less job mobility than did whites (Alon and Tienda 2005b). And a researcher who investigated promotion experiences reported that, compared to white men, Black men had to work longer periods of time after leaving school and Hispanics had to have more years with their current employer before getting a promotion (Smith 2005). And Black and Hispanic women, compared to white men, needed more job-specific experience and more overall work experience in order to get a promotion.

Clearly, *race and ethnic background are factors in all aspects of employment.* And that includes the loss of work and change of job or career. Here, again, minorities may suffer more than their white counterparts. For one thing, minorities are more vulnerable to losing their jobs (Wilson 2005). For another thing, minorities are less likely than whites to benefit when finding new employment. Among workers displaced from some high-technology industries, African Americans and Hispanics suffered greater earnings losses than did whites, whether their new jobs were within or outside the high-tech sector (Ong 1991).

*Income and Wealth.* Wealth includes all the assets of a family—housing equity, investments, insurance, and so on. Great disparity exists between the races in wealth. The Census Bureau does not regularly publish data on wealth, so the following median net worth of households are for 2016 (the latest available as of this writing): non-Hispanic whites, $143,600; African Americans, $12,920; Asian Americans, $210,000; and Hispanics, $21,420. Thus, non-Hispanic white households had 11.1 times the wealth of Black households and 6.7 times the wealth of Hispanic households. Moreover, over time the wealth gap has tended to increase (Thomas et al. 2020).

An important component of wealth is income. Table 8.3 shows the extent to which minorities are concentrated more heavily than whites in the lower income brackets. Some people believe that minorities have made significant progress. However, although the income of all racial groups has been increasing, the gap between whites and minorities other than Asian Americans is greater than it was in the 1970s (Figure 8.3). In 2019, Black household income was 59.7 percent and Hispanic household income was 73.8 percent that of non-Hispanic whites (Semega et al. 2020).

In general, income inequality is widespread across occupations and is certainly a consequence of discrimination. Black income is lower than that of whites even for those workers with the same education, occupation, experience, authority, and number of hours worked (Coleman 2003). The gap increases in the higher-income occupational categories (Grodsky and Pager 2001). Rank (2009) summed up the consequences of the "economic racial divide" for African Americans: Compared to whites, they are far more likely to experience poverty and far less likely to achieve affluence, less likely to be able to buy a home at an early age or to accumulate a large amount of equity in a home, and more likely to have low levels of wealth across all phases of their lives.

**TABLE 8.3**
Money Income of Households, 2019: Percent Distribution by Income Level, by Race, and Hispanic Origin

| Income | Percentage of Households | | | |
|---|---|---|---|---|
| | White | Black | Hispanic | Asian |
| Under $15,000 | 7.8 | 17.2 | 10.7 | 6.8 |
| $15,000 to $24,999 | 7.5 | 11.5 | 8.8 | 5.1 |
| $25.000 to $34,999 | 8.0 | 11.4 | 10.5 | 5.1 |
| $35,000 to 49,999 | 11.5 | 13.7 | 114.1 | 8.6 |
| $50,000 to $74,999 | 16.7 | 16.8 | 19.5 | 13.6 |
| $75,000 to $99,999 | 12.7 | 9.8 | 12.2 | 12.5 |
| $100,000 to $149,999 | 16.3 | 10.8 | 13.0 | 17.9 |
| $150,000 to $199,999 | 8.7 | 4.7 | 5.9 | 12.5 |
| $200,000 and over | 10.8 | 4.6 | 5.3 | 18.3 |

SOURCE: Semega et al. 2020.

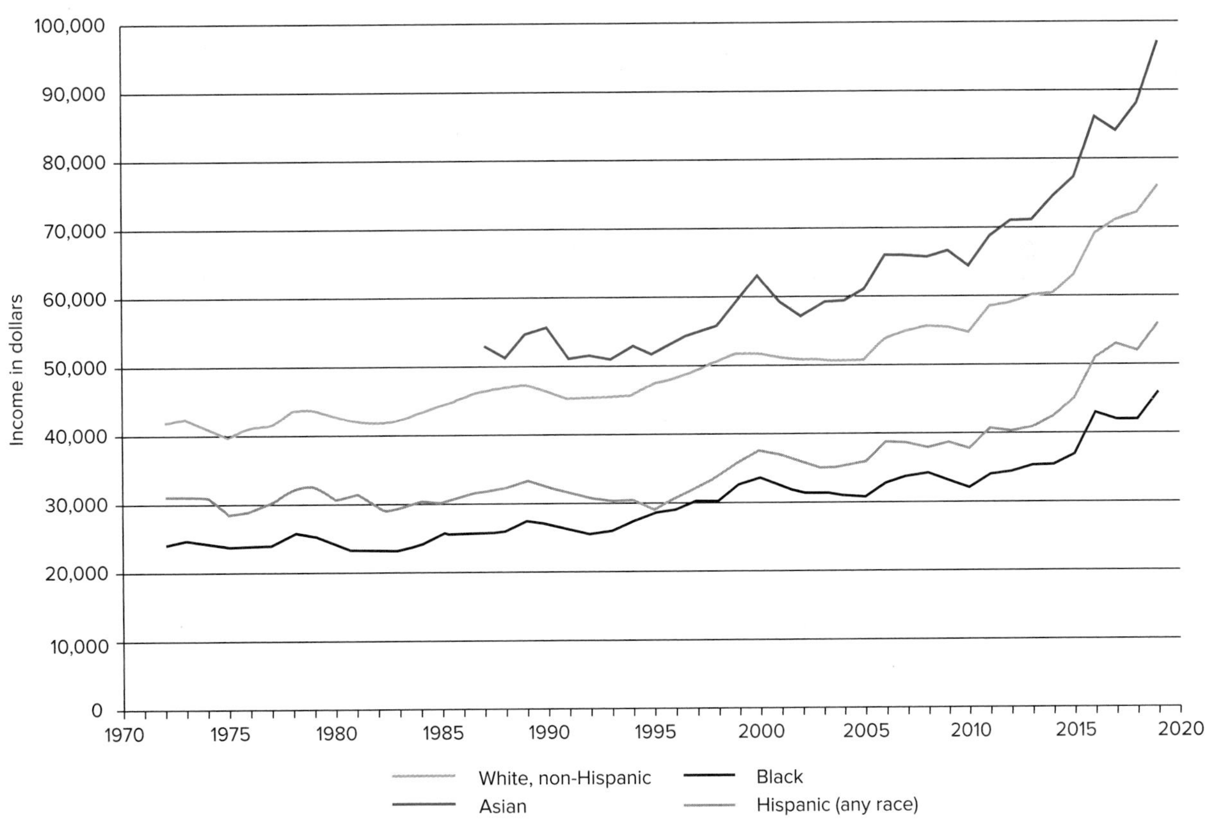


**FIGURE 8.3** Median Household Income, by Race and Hispanic Origin, 1972–2019.
Source: Semega et al. 2020. (Data on Asian income only available after 1986.)

## The Right to Life and Happiness

The right to "life, liberty, and the pursuit of happiness" was affirmed in the Declaration of Independence. However, those rights are not distributed equally in the United States. In particular, although the differences between whites and the racial/ethnic minorities are declining, there is still less reported happiness and life satisfaction among African Americans and Hispanics than among whites (Coverdill et al. 2011). The lower levels for minorities, in turn, are related to significant inequalities in life chances and in freedom from fear.

**life chances**
the probability of gaining certain advantages defined as desirable, such as long life and health

*Life Chances.* Insurance companies and government agencies compile large amounts of information on **life chances,** which include probability of divorce, disease, suicide, mental illness, and premature death. The life chances of whites are generally better than those of minorities (Williams, Neighbors, and Jackson 2003; Spence, Adkins, and Dupre 2011; Herne, Bartholomew, and Weahkee 2014; Buchmueller et al. 2016; Sancar, Abbasi, and Bucher 2018). For example, compared to whites, minorities tend to have (1) lower levels of physical and mental health; (2) a higher rate of infant deaths and deaths from tuberculosis, AIDS, homicide, and suicide; (3) a lower median family income; (4) lower-level jobs; (5) proportionately fewer full-time and white-collar jobs; and (6) fewer people with health insurance and fewer who receive old age and survivor insurance benefits. Many of the differences are striking. Black and Puerto Rican women have particularly high rates of infant mortality (Ely and Driscoll 2020). A Black baby's life expectancy is nearly five years less than that of a white baby, and this gap has changed little in more than half a century (Carr 2005). The risk of a Black youth being murdered is four times that of a white youth (Snyder and Sickmund 2006). And Native Americans have rates of alcohol abuse and alcohol-related rates of death that are five or more times as great as the rates for whites (Landen et al. 2014).

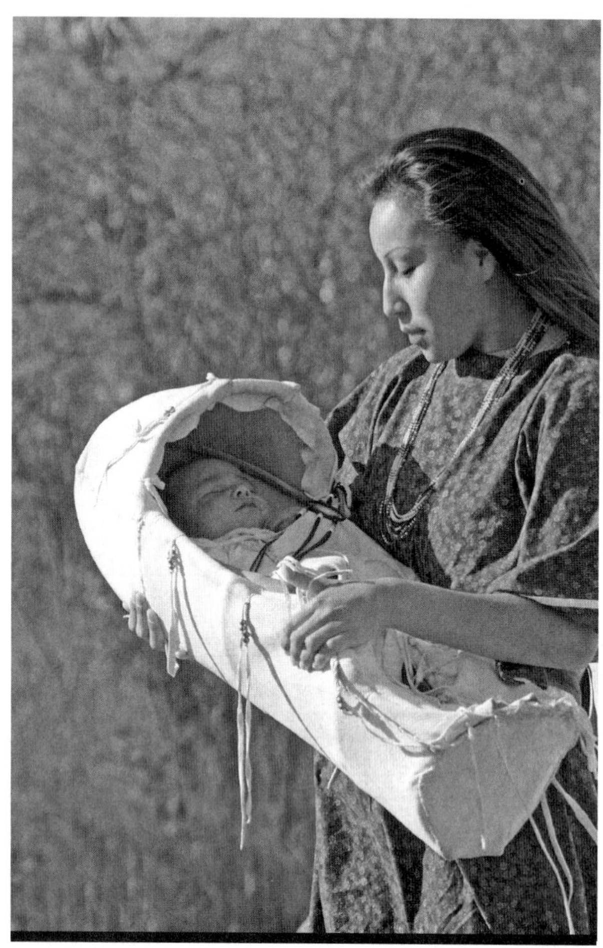

Native Americans are the poorest minority group in the United States.

Nancy Greifenhagen/Nancy G. Western Photography/Alamy

Disadvantages with respect to life chances are rooted in a number of factors. Racism and perceived discrimination are major contributors to problems of both physical and mental health (Flores et al. 2008; Chou, Asnaani, and Hofmann 2012; Gibbons et al. 2014; Hunter et al. 2016). Minorities are more likely to live near hazardous waste facilities and be exposed to toxic materials (Mohai and Saha 2007; Downey and Hawkins 2008). Finally, minorities are disadvantaged in life chances because of their lower economic levels (Meckler 1998; McLaughlin and Stokes 2002). People who live in poverty or who try to survive at low income levels have higher rates of physical and emotional problems. Impoverishment combined with racism takes a dreadful toll on poor African Americans in high rates of cirrhosis of the liver, homicide, accidents, and drug and alcohol abuse.

Minorities are also more likely to be victims of both property and violent crimes (Morgan and Truman 2020). In an interesting examination of the higher rates of violent crime in neighborhoods with a high percentage of minorities, Hipp (2011) raised the question of whether the minorities increased the rates or the rates increased the number of minorities. He found that whites are more likely than minorities to move out of neighborhoods with high rates of crime, whereas minorities are more likely than whites to move into neighborhoods that already have a high rate of crime. For some people, the only financially practical choice is to move into a house in a high-crime neighborhood or to be homeless.

Of all the racial/ethnic groups, American Indians/Alaska Natives are the most deprived in terms of life chances. They are more likely than others to be poor and unemployed (Castor et al. 2006). They have higher rates of criminal victimization than any other group (Pavkov et al. 2010). They have disproportionately high rates of sexual assault (Arnold 2014). A survey of Indian and Alaska Native women in New York City found that 65 percent had experienced some form of interpersonal violence, including childhood physical abuse (28 percent), rape (48 percent), or domestic violence (40 percent) (Evans-Campbell, Lindhorst, Huang, and Walters 2006). The women reported high levels of emotional trauma resulting from the violence. In addition to abuse, American Indians have serious problems of neglect, alcoholism, fetal alcohol syndrome, mental and physical disabilities, depression, school problems, and delinquency (Grant et al. 2004).

*Freedom from Fear.* One of the four basic freedoms proclaimed by President Franklin Roosevelt was freedom from fear. No one should have to live in constant fear of offending someone who claims to be superior. Yet, for decades Black mothers and fathers taught their children to fear offending white people. Richard Wright related an incident from his own childhood that illustrates the point (Bernard 1966). A group of white boys threw broken bottles at him and some of his friends, and the two groups fought. Wright was badly cut. He went home and sat on his steps to wait for his mother to come home from work. Rather than sympathy, he received a severe beating. Had a white mother treated her son in this way, you might have questioned her love; but Wright's mother was teaching him what she regarded as a most important lesson—to avoid such encounters at all costs. She was teaching him what it meant to be Black in America: that he would always be the loser in battles with whites.

Violence and threats of violence against people because of some characteristic of a group to which the people belong are now called *hate crimes* (Harlow 2005). The characteristic may be religion or sexual orientation or being a member of a gang, but the majority of hate crimes are motivated by the victim's race or ethnicity. Such crimes remind minorities that some people despise them and are willing to use violent means to intimidate them. You need only read the daily papers to realize that the victims of hate crimes include African Americans, Hispanics, Jews, Asians, and Indians. The crimes range from verbal abuse to physical violence and even murder. People who survive hate crimes are likely to suffer severe emotional problems (McDevitt, Balboni, Garcia, and Gu 2001). In recent years, the incidents have included chaining a Black man to the rear of a truck and dragging him to his death, shooting Jewish children at a day care center, and brutally beating a Hispanic boy with a metal pipe.

Many hate crimes are committed by members of the hundreds of racist and neo-Nazi groups in the nation who proclaim the superiority of the white race and the threats posed by the varied minorities. Some hate crimes are committed by local groups of vigilantes. The FBI recorded 4,930 victims of hate crimes in 2019. The crimes included intimidation, assault, and even death, and were all perpetrated because of the victim's race or ethnicity. That figure is far below the number that comes from victimization studies. A 2012 victimization report put the number of hate crimes at 293,800 (Wilson 2014). Over half the victimizations were motivated by the race or ethnicity of the victim.

The cherished rights of Americans to move about as they please, to live according to their means, and to enjoy the use of all public facilities has not yet been fully extended to minorities. Minorities who try to break down old barriers are still subject to threats of violence and efforts at intimidation. Freedom from fear is an unmet promise rather than a reality.

### The Right to Dignity as a Human Being

Most of the material already discussed in this chapter illustrates how minorities are directly *deprived of their dignity as human beings.* A majority of Hispanics and African Americans believe they have experienced some kind of discrimination during their lives. What kind of discriminatory behavior do they encounter? Much of it is what Eddings (1995) called **stealth racism,** which involves hidden or subtle acts of prejudice and discrimination, acts that may be apparent only to the victim. Examples of stealth racism include taxis that never stop for minorities; suspicious stares from clerks in stores; the assumption that the minority individual is in a subordinate role (like the couple who came out of an expensive restaurant and asked an African American man to get their car, not realizing he was a senior editor at a national magazine); the sense of being unwelcome (such as when looking for a new home in a well-to-do neighborhood); and the surprise expressed when the minority person is articulate and sophisticated.

**stealth racism**
hidden or subtle acts of prejudice and discrimination that may be apparent only to the victim

Some of the incidents are irritating and demeaning. For instance, a Black woman returning a rented video is ignored by the clerks until she speaks up and asks for help. Or consider the problem of "dwb"—driving while Black. There is evidence that Black drivers are far more likely to be stopped by police than are white drivers, and are more likely to have their cars searched (Kowalski and Lundman 2007). Stealth racism can also be hazardous for the victims, such as when Black and Hispanic women are less likely than white women to get the proper care in the early stages of breast cancer (Bickell et al. 2008). At that point, the right to dignity may mean the right to life-saving measures.

The right to dignity also includes the right to truthful representation of one's group. Two often-heard myths violate this right.

*The Myth of Success around the Corner.* A common American myth is that *success is "just around the corner" for anyone who is willing to work for it.* The implication is that the minorities can end their impoverishment merely by being willing to work as hard as other people. "If they want to get ahead," it is said, "let them work for it and earn it." The point, of course, is that if they do not get ahead, it is their own fault. The *fallacy of personal attack* is used to defend an unjust social order. The reasoning is that if the minorities have as many opportunities as everyone else and yet remain in the lower levels of society, something is wrong with the minorities.

fallacy

Unfortunately, many people do believe that minorities have the same opportunities as whites. The minorities themselves overwhelmingly reject the notion. In national polls, e.g., more than eight in ten African Americans assert that they are treated less fairly than whites in matters of hiring, pay, and promotions (Newport 2020).

Many whites believe not just that minorities have an equal opportunity, but that minorities now possess an advantage. These whites see themselves as hampered in their access to the best education and the most desirable jobs and careers because of their race

(Cohen 2003; Flynn 2003). They believe they have lost out, or potentially could lose out, to people less qualified than they are simply because the other people are part of a minority. In other words, they see themselves as victims of *reverse discrimination,* with their own opportunities becoming restricted as minority opportunities have opened. They cite cases in which minorities (including women) have been given preference over white males even when the white males have seniority or somewhat better qualifications. According to such beliefs, if minorities do not achieve success, it is clearly their own fault.

Associated with the myth that success is readily available to those willing to work for it is the notion that African Americans prefer welfare to hard work. This notion is also a distortion of the truth. African Americans did not appear on welfare rolls in large numbers until the late 1940s. Furthermore, few able-bodied men of any race are receiving welfare. Poor African Americans are, like anyone else, eager to escape their poverty. There is no evidence that minorities prefer welfare to work or that they are failing to take advantage of work opportunities available to them. Quite simply, the notion that success is just around the corner for anyone willing to work for it is a myth.

*The Myth of Inferiority.* The insidious myth that minorities are *inherently inferior* is still around. The argument about inferiority takes a number of different forms. One argument is that minorities are, and always have been, biologically inferior. This argument can take the form of the *fallacy of circular reasoning.* An individual argues that African Americans are inferior because their IQs are lower than those of whites. "But," one could reply, "they are only lower for those who live in deprived conditions." "No," is the response, "they are lower because they are inferior people."

fallacy

The theory of biological inferiority has also been claimed in a few scientific circles. The most recent attempt to argue for innate inferiority is *The Bell Curve,* by Herrnstein and Murray (1994). Herrnstein, a psychologist, and Murray, a political scientist, claimed that about 60 percent of IQ is genetic. Differences in achievement, therefore, are both inevitable and unchangeable. The work of Herrnstein and Murray has been criticized and refuted on various grounds. One is the lack of any evidence of a gene that is conclusively linked to intelligence, so that it is not possible to prove any genetic link of intelligence with race (Sternberg, Grigorenko, and Kidd 2005). Another is the fact that African Americans made gains of from four to seven IQ points on non-Hispanic whites between 1972 and 2002, indicating that the gap reflected social rather than genetic differences (Dickens and Flynn 2006).

The argument of a second form of the inferiority myth is that minorities are *culturally inferior.* Whatever may or may not be true biologically, it is argued, the culture of a particular people is obviously inferior and the people therefore are unfit to rise above their low status.

African Americans, Hispanics, and American Indians are all perceived to have cultural characteristics that make them different and less committed to such traditional American values as education and hard work; but most people in America tend to have the same aspirations for themselves and their families. Thus, a study of the life goals of graduating high school seniors found similar educational and occupational aspirations among the white, Black, Hispanic, and Asian youths (Chang et al. 2006). The aspirations were high for all groups. And a Pew Research survey reported that 86 percent of Hispanic parents, 79 percent of Black parents, and 67 percent of white parents said that it is extremely or very important that their children get a college degree (Stepler 2016). The fact that minorities have not achieved such aims cannot be attributed to cultural inferiority nor to cultural values that differ from those of white America.

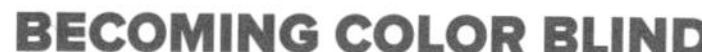

involvement!

### BECOMING COLOR BLIND

We were once involved in arranging an exchange of ministers and choirs between a Black and a white church. After the Black pastor had spoken at the white church, one of the members said to us, "You know, the longer that man preached, the less I thought of him as Black." It was her way of saying that the contact had broken down some of the prejudice she had harbored all her life.

Social scientists have long known that interracial contact is one way to deal with prejudice. Arrange for a visit with a group of a race other than your own. It might be a local church, a student organization on campus, or some kind of community organization. Talk with some of the members and explore how they feel about the current racial situation. Ask them about their aspirations for themselves and their children. Discuss their outlook on the future. Do they feel that the situation for their race has improved or worsened in the 2000s? Why?

What insights into the life of the other race did you gain from the visit? Do they have any needs and aspirations that are fundamentally different from your own? How does America's race problem look from their point of view? Can you see the basis for their point of view?

If possible, you might arrange some kind of exchange visit with the group. As the people from the different races mingle with each other, note any changes in prejudicial attitudes and any increases in mutual understanding.

## Contributing Factors

The problems of minorities in America are well described by the title of Gunnar Myrdal's classic work *An American Dilemma* (Myrdal 1944). The author, a Swedish social economist, came to the United States in 1938 to direct an analysis of the problem. The book that resulted defined the problem as a moral issue and stated that the *dilemma involved a contradiction between the American creed and our racial behavior.* The creed proclaims the primacy of individual dignity, equality, and the right of all citizens to the same justice and the same opportunities, but the racial behavior systematically denies minorities the same rights and benefits accorded to whites.

The problem also involves *contradictory value systems.* Some people define the segregated and deprived state of African Americans as a problem, but others define efforts to "mix" the races as the real problem. The latter vigorously resist efforts of the former to alter the existing structure of segregated relationships. They fear an integrated society for various reasons. They argue that such a society will lack the strength and vigor of the present society.

Finally, the problem involves *contradictions in the social structure.* Minorities today are hampered by the changed economy, for our economy has developed to the point where the demand for unskilled and semiskilled labor is relatively small. Unlike the immigrants earlier in our history, therefore, people cannot better their lot today by going to work in vast numbers in the factories, where few or no skills are required.

### Social Structural Factors

The tables in this chapter show that minorities occupy a *low position in the stratification system.* This finding raises the question of whether the main problems facing minorities are due to social class, racial or ethnic identity, or both. The answer seems to be both. Minorities share some characteristics with lower-class whites, but, as you have seen, even those who achieve higher socioeconomic levels still face various disadvantages and assaults on their dignity.

The disadvantages are not always due to biased individuals. The term **institutional racism** was coined to refer to the fact that established policies and practices of social institutions tend to perpetuate racial discrimination. In other words, whether or not the people involved are prejudiced or deliberate in their discriminatory behavior, the normal practices and policies themselves guarantee that minorities will be shortchanged. Policies and practices are set by those in power, and minorities typically have lacked the power necessary to control institutional processes. We examine institutional racism in four important areas: the media, education, the economy, and government.

**institutional racism** policies and practices of social institutions that tend to perpetuate racial discrimination

*Mass Media.* *The portrayal of minorities in the media has tended to perpetuate various negative stereotypes.* The problem was particularly severe in the past when movies and radio and television programs—such as the *Amos 'n Andy* radio show—portrayed African Americans as lazy, inferior, stupid, and dishonest. After the mid-1960s, the portrayals changed, and various racial minorities appeared more frequently and in more positive roles.

*Racial and ethnic minorities still do not receive equitable treatment in the media,* however. Hispanics appear far less on TV programs than their proportion in the population (Mastro 2017). They are more likely to appear in service positions rather than high-status jobs and often have accented and inarticulate speech. African Americans fare better in terms of the number who appear on TV (Watson 2020). But, compared to whites, Black men are more disrespected and less aggressive, while Black women are less likely to be seen in professional occupations.

Other media also contribute to the problem of negative stereotypes. A content analysis of best-selling video game magazines and video game covers found that minority males were underrepresented and were more likely than whites to be shown as athletic or aggressive or thugs, and less likely than whites to be shown in military combat or using technology (Burgess et al. 2011). Even college textbooks can be misleading. In her examination of economics textbooks, Clawson (2002) found Black faces "overwhelmingly portrayed" among the poor (recall that, in terms of numbers, there are far more poor whites than poor Blacks).

One thing that could help would be for more minorities to be in positions of influence in the media. The minority cause is not helped by the proportion of minorities who work in newsrooms of newspapers. According to the Pew Research Center (2016), the proportion of Black workers in newsrooms actually declined from 5.4 percent in 2003 to 4.7 percent in 2014, and the proportion of Hispanic workers declined from 4.4 percent in 2005 to 4.2 percent in 2015. In sum, some progress has been made, but the mass media as a whole continue to either neglect minorities or reinforce negative stereotypes.

*Education.* Four primary and secondary educational practices that perpetuate discrimination are *segregated schools, so-called IQ testing, so-called ability-grouping of children, and differential treatment of children based on racial or ethnic identity.* All these practices discriminate against people in the lower socioeconomic strata, and because most minorities are disproportionately in the lower strata, they suffer disproportionately from such practices. The discrimination begins early in the school career. A study of fifth-grade students reported that 15 percent of the children perceived racial or ethnic discrimination, and 80 percent of the discrimination occurred at school (Coker et al. 2009). And those who perceived discrimination were more likely than others to have symptoms of depression and other mental disorders.

Schools continue to be more segregated than integrated. As noted earlier in this chapter, by 2018 only 19 percent of Blacks were in schools that had a majority of white students. This was a significant decline from the early 1990s, when desegregation was at its peak. The resegregation of schools was due, in part, from the assumption that schools districts no longer need court oversight; once released from that oversight, school districts become increasingly segregated again (Reardon 2012). Attending a segregated school depresses the achievement of minorities (Quillian 2014; Quinn 2015). Among other things, segregated minority schools tend to offer a poorer education because of inadequate resources and, in some cases, lower expectations of the students' interests and abilities. For example, a study of three Los Angeles high schools with a high proportion of minority students found that while the school had an ample number of computers, the computer science program itself was poor (Margolis et al. 2008). In part, the quality of the program reflected the fact that teachers, counselors, and even some of the students had low expectations about both minority student interest and minority student ability in the field of computer science.

IQ testing also works to the disadvantage of minorities. A child may do poorly on an IQ test, for example, because little in his or her home environment has served as preparation for tests constructed by middle-class educators. Then, when placed in a group of lower ability, a child may accept the label of mediocrity or even inferiority.

At the college level, efforts are made to recruit more minority students than have attended in the past. Some of the efforts have been successful, but minorities (other than Asian Americans) still lag considerably behind non-Hispanic whites. By 2019, the proportion of adults 25 years and older who had a college degree was 40.1 percent of non-Hispanic whites, 26.1 percent of African Americans, 58.1 percent of Asian Americans and 18.8 percent of Hispanics (U.S. Census Bureau website).

Finally, as noted previously, teachers may treat minority students differently from white students. In her qualitative study of white student teachers, Marx (2006) found the future teachers' knowledge of the history and culture of the varied origins of the minority students to be sparse at best. For example, they thought that speaking Spanish in the home was a sign of low intelligence and that the cultural context in which minority students were raised was at best an obstacle to be overcome and at worst a sign of innate inferiority.

Differential treatment also occurs in discipline. Schools with a larger proportion of Black students tend to have more punitive disciplinary practices and to implement zero tolerance policies (Welch and Payne 2010). Nationally, 51 percent of students in elementary and high schools are white, but white students account for only 33 percent of expulsions and 29 percent of those with multiple suspensions (Brenchley 2012). Black students are 18 percent of the total, but they make up 35 percent of students suspended once and 39 percent of students expelled. Such differences do not simply reflect differing behavior patterns but teacher and administrator attitudes. Morris (2005) studied an urban school intensively and drew a number of informative conclusions about discipline. First, teachers and administrators tended to view Black girls' behavior as "unladylike," and attempted to discipline them into dress and manners more acceptable to the adults. Second, school officials tended to define the behavior of Hispanic boys as threatening, so that the boys were often disciplined in strict, punitive ways. And third, school officials tended to see the behavior of white and Asian American students as both nonthreatening and gender appropriate; discipline for these students was likely to be less strict and punitive.

It is difficult to learn if your school makes you feel more vulnerable to disciplinary action simply because of your race. It is also difficult to learn if your school's

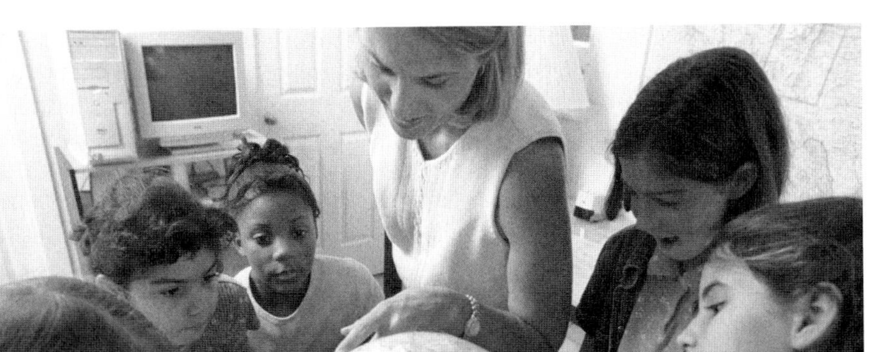

Minority students tend to have higher academic achievement in integrated classrooms.
Dynamic Graphics Group/Creatas/Alamy Stock Photo

cultural values and teaching methods are contrary to the cultural values of your family and community. Such an incongruity helps explain why 25 to 60 percent of all American Indian students drop out of high school each year (Klug and Whitfield 2002).

*The Economy.* Institutional racism has pervaded the economy in at least three ways: **exploitation** *of minority labor, exclusion of minorities from full participation in the economy, and exploitation of minority consumers.* Some gains have been made, of course. For example, racial/ethnic segregation in employment has declined since the 1960s (Tomaskovic-Devey et al. 2006). Nevertheless, as we noted earlier, minorities tend to secure the lower-paying jobs, a tendency that was reinforced by the shift from an industry- to a service-based economy (Jaret 1991). And even in the same occupational categories, a gap exists between minority and white income (McCall 2001).

**exploitation**
use or manipulation of people for one's own advantage or profit

As for participation in the economy, minorities come out best during economic booms and worst when the economy falters. Even in the best of times, they lag considerably behind non-Hispanic whites in terms of employment and income. In the worst of times, their unemployment rate goes up more than that of non-Hispanic whites. For example, in 2019, the COVID-19 pandemic led to shutdowns in businesses that resulted in surging rates of unemployment. But there was a strong racial/ethnic disparity in the rates (Bureau of Labor Statistics website). From the third quarter of 2019 to the third quarter of 2020, the unemployment rate increased from 3.4 to 7.9 percent for whites, 5.6 to 13.2 percent for African Americans, 2.8 to 10.6 percent for Asian Americans, and 4.2 to 11.2 percent for Hispanics. Moreover, African Americans tend to be the first fired when the economy sinks into recession (Couch and Fairlie 2010). Once unemployed, they are much less likely to be reemployed than are white workers with equivalent characteristics and experience (Moore 2010).

Minorities also fail to participate fully in the economy as entrepreneurs, a fact that is closely related to credit practices and policies. Lending institutions traditionally demand credit history, some kind of collateral, and some evidence of potential success before they lend money to prospective businesspersons, whether or not they are white. These are standard practices, defined as necessary and practical when giving credit, but applying them to minorities, who may have poor credit records because of exploitation and who may have nothing to use as collateral because of poverty, means that the standard practices only ensure continued white domination of the economy.

Insisting on comparable "sound" business practices when the prospective customers are minorities results in exploitation of the minority consumer. It is true that the poor are greater credit risks and that businesses in ghetto areas must pay higher insurance premiums because of the greater probability of theft and property damage; yet it is also true that these higher costs of doing business exploit the minority consumer, who must then pay more than others for the same quality of goods.

The most serious exploitation may be in housing, however. African Americans are often forced to pay more than whites for the same quality of housing. In fact, ghetto housing is sometimes costlier in terms of square footage and is frequently costlier in terms of quality square footage than is housing in suburban areas. When minorities attempt to find better housing, they may find themselves, as noted earlier, steered into some areas and kept away from other areas by real estate agents.

*Economic deprivation of minorities* has meant economic gains for whites. When minorities are kept in a subordinate position, whites are able to secure a higher occupational status, lower rates of unemployment, and higher family income (Tomaskovic-Devey and Roscigno 1996). At least some of those who resist equal opportunities are not unaware of such implications.

*Government.* The government is supposed to protect and help all citizens equally. But minorities do not always benefit from the government as much as whites do. In part, this reflects the fact that minorities are not as well represented in Congress as are whites. Malhotra and Raso (2007) tested the proposition that African Americans and Hispanics are not as well served as are whites by the equal representation of each state in the Senate. They concluded that both groups are underrepresented because they tend to be concentrated in a few high-population states.

If minorities are to make headway in their efforts to achieve equality of opportunity, they must be able to secure *political power* and find help in the courts. However, minorities have barely begun to infiltrate positions of political power in spite of the election of the nation's first Black president in 2008. There have been gains. The 117th Congress, which took office in January 2021, was 12 percent African American and 9 percent Hispanic. It was more diverse than any previous Congress in America's history. The numbers of minorities in elected offices have risen dramatically since 1970. And with the election of Barack Obama, they have reached the highest office in the land. But the bulk of minorities are in local and state positions. Overall, then, the record of minority participation in the political process shows only modest gains over the past half century.

## Social Psychological Factors

We said previously that ideology affects social interaction. Why does the ideology of equal opportunity not alter the superior/inferior kind of interaction between whites and minorities that results from the social structure? It might, except for the many ideologies in any society. Some of the ideologies of America have helped shape and sustain the traditional interaction patterns between the races. In fact, some values, attitudes, and ideologies among both whites and minorities tend to perpetuate the race problem. We examine those of the whites first.

*Majority Perspectives.* The initial low position of minorities in America stems from the circumstances of their arrival—as indentured servants, slaves, or unskilled laborers. The *ideology necessary to legitimate the enslavement or subordination of minorities was already present.* The first white settlers in America believed in their own racial superiority and certainly considered themselves superior to the "savages" who were native to America. Similarly, the English, on first making contact with Africans, considered them very "puzzling" creatures and tried to determine why the people were Black. In one explanation, Blacks were said to be the descendants of Ham, whom the Bible says God had cursed. Actually, as stated in the ninth chapter of Genesis, the curse was pronounced by Noah, not God, and it was against Ham's son, Canaan. The fact that many people have accepted the argument underscores the power of the *fallacy of the appeal to prejudice,* for those who accepted the argument undoubtedly acted out of prejudice rather than knowledge of the Bible. In any case, Africans were a different kind of people, and the difference was seen to be undesirable.

fallacy

A number of white groups entered the country in low-status, low-power positions (and were to some extent the objects of prejudice), but none of them were so looked down upon as the minorities. A number of additional factors worked against minorities but not against whites: (1) the economy needed less and less unskilled labor, (2) their skin color was a "visible" disability, (3) the political system no longer offered jobs for votes so freely, and (4) their smaller households probably did not have several wage earners.

**Prejudice,** a "rigid, emotional attitude toward a human group" (Simpson and Yinger 1965:15), is an attitude that is widespread in the white majority (Bonilla-Silva, Goar, and Embrick 2006). Prejudice against any group legitimates different treatment of group members, generates resistance to programs designed to help the group (such as affirmative action programs that increase the number of minorities in higher education and the workplace), creates the desire to live in areas with few or none of the group members, and resists such things as interracial dating and marriage that would break down the racial barriers (Loury 2005; Iceland and Wilkes 2006; Kreager 2008; Lewis, Emerson, and Klineberg 2011). White prejudice, then, helps perpetuate white dominance.

**prejudice**
a rigid, emotional attitude that legitimates discriminatory behavior toward people in a group

Prejudice is an individual characteristic, but its causes lie outside the individual—no one is born with prejudice. Simpson and Yinger (1965:49–51) identified a number of sources of prejudice. The sources included personality needs; the usefulness of prejudice for certain groups (low-status whites, for instance, who have been better off than African Americans); group tradition (children learn to hate without knowing precisely why); and certain attributes possessed by the minority group. "Group attributes" are questionable as a source, however. They may serve as a useful rationalization for prejudice, but they do not generally cause that prejudice.

Prejudice does not necessarily have so rational a basis as a consistent set of beliefs about or a well-defined image of the target group. Social psychologists have known for a long time that certain groups can be defined as undesirable even when the attributes of those groups are vague. This insight is expressed in an old poem:

I do not love thee, Dr. Fell,
the reason why I cannot tell.

But this I know and know quite well,
I do not love thee, Dr. Fell.

fallacy

*One consequence of prejudice is that it facilitates fallacious thinking.* To the prejudiced person, certain *fallacies of non sequiturs* come easily: They are on welfare, therefore they don't want to work; they have more children than they can properly care for, therefore they show themselves to be immoral; they don't speak proper English, therefore they are intellectually inferior; and so forth. The "they," of course, is whichever minority group the speaker wants to castigate. The same arguments have been used about many different groups.

Such prejudicial thinking continues in spite of decades of efforts to combat it. There is, consequently, *a racial divide in attitudes about America's racial situation.* When polls are taken related to the issue of racial equality (e.g., are people treated equally in the justice system and do people have equal opportunities for success), typically a majority of whites but a minority of African Americans believe that racial equality exists in this nation (Brown 2019).

Prejudicial thinking is reflected in interracial behavior, including such things as interaction in classrooms and stores, encounters on the streets, and the process of securing housing (Emerson, Yancey, and Chai 2001; Krysan 2008; Lynn et al. 2011). Discriminatory behavior in these varied settings is the result of, and is justified by, the stereotypes created by prejudice (Frederico 2006). Even positive stereotypes can be used to maintain white dominance. For example, Asian Americans are frequently viewed as the "model minority." In this view, they succeed because of their strong family life, their hard work, and their high value on education. Although the stereotype has some validity, it has been used to dismiss the need for programs that help minorities by providing more educational and work opportunities (Yu 2006). The idea is, if Asian Americans can do it, why can't the other minorities? The argument that if one does it, all can, is another example of a *non sequitur.*

The insidious nature of prejudice is illustrated by the way it legitimates and helps perpetuate the interaction patterns occurring in institutions. In the schools, for instance, a Black child may perform poorly because, in part, he or she senses a teacher's hostility, born of prejudice. The teacher labels the child as having mediocre ability and places him or her in an appropriate group. The child may accept the teacher's definition of his or her ability, and that definition may be further reinforced through IQ tests and subsequent teachers' reactions. Thus, prejudice further reduces the chances of academic success for a poorly prepared child, and the normal policies and practices of the school, such as IQ testing and grouping by ability, reinforce an official definition of the child's ability. If a child rebels against this hostile and repressive environment and becomes a "behavior problem," the teacher will conclude that his or her initial hostility is fully justified.

*Minority Perspectives.* In the face of disparaging attitudes and ideologies, minorities can get trapped in a vicious circle. By experiencing disparagement, deprivation, and powerlessness, members of a minority group may develop attitudes of alienation and cynicism about society. We have already noted that far more minorities than whites agree that minorities suffer from discrimination. They are also less satisfied than whites with the treatment they receive in American society. In a 2016 poll, 65 percent of African Americans, compared to 27 percent of whites, agreed that it is a lot more difficult to be Black than white (Maniam 2016).

Such attitudes can lead minorities to despair of being able to make significant advances in their lives. They may accept their low position rather than struggle against it. In turn, remaining deprived and powerless confirms their perspective. How does this situation compare with our earlier observation that African Americans place an even higher value on education than whites do? Matthew's (2011) research answers the question. In essence, whites tend to equate success with personal factors such as effort, whereas African Americans tend to see structural barriers that can negate their efforts. In other words, African Americans are more likely to believe that education will not pay off for them as it does for whites, that they will be treated unfairly in the workplace regardless of their education. In other words, many minorities who might otherwise aspire to higher education will not go through the struggle to get it because they are convinced that they still live in a racist society in which they face unfair treatment.

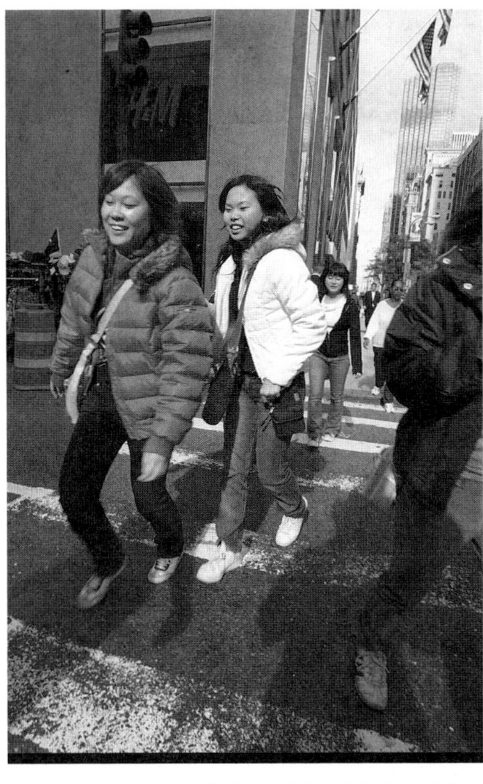

Asian-Americans are often viewed as the "model minority."

©Lars A. Niki

For Hispanics, the attitudes and values underlying their high dropout rates come from their peer groups. As a study of Mexican American students found, Mexican American students are much less involved in informal and extracurricular activities at school than are white students (Ream and Rumberger 2008). They tend, instead, to form street-oriented friendships that place little or no value on formal schooling. As a consequence, Hispanics have considerably lower levels of educational attainment than whites, African Americans, or Asian Americans.

Finally, for minorities in ghetto areas, there is the additional problem of a *lack of role models* (Parker and Reckdenwald 2008). This lack contributes to the amount of violence in ghetto areas as well as depriving the youth of people they could emulate in order to have a more meaningful life. An ironic reason for the lack is the civil rights legislation of the 1960s that gave middle- and upper-class African Americans the opportunity to move out of segregated and impoverished areas. As a result, ghetto youth no longer see people who get a good education, work at good jobs on a regular basis, and thereby become examples of what can be accomplished. Instead, those who remain in the ghettoes see a pervasive hopelessness, cynicism, and rejection of educational and occupational aspirations. They live in a climate of low expectations, and many social psychologists argue that the expectations are crucial, virtually guaranteeing continued deprivation unless the expectations are somehow changed.

## Solutions: Public Policy and Private Action

Minority groups themselves have launched attacks on the forces that discriminate against them to the detriment of their desired quality of life. The result has been *intergroup conflict* as minorities strive to alter values, attitudes, ideologies, and social structural arrangements.

Resolution of the problem requires more than the actions of the minorities, however. What kind of actions may be taken, keeping in mind that any action will probably involve some conflict (verbal debate at the very least)?

global comparison

## PREJUDICE IN EUROPE

Prejudice is found everywhere. It varies from one country to another as well as within countries. In the United States, the fear of economic competition (for jobs and income) has often fanned the flames of prejudice and led to racial tensions and riots. The threat—real or not—of economic competition is also a factor in prejudice in other nations, such as those in Europe. And wherever it is found, it leads to discrimination and conflict (Zick, Pettigrew, and Wagner 2008).

Quillian (1995) studied prejudice in a number of European countries. He found that the average prejudice scores varied from one country to another (Figure 8.4). He also looked at the extent to which the people in each nation defined the threat from people of other races and nationalities as being due to such things as adding to problems of delinquency and violence, leading to lower educational quality, and creating a drain on social security benefits.

Quillian's analysis showed that perceived threat explained most of the variations in average prejudice scores in the 12 European nations. He found that such individual characteristics as education, age, and social class had little impact on prejudice and explained none of the variations between countries. Rather, the economic conditions in each country and the size of the racial or immigrant group were the significant factors, and the more problematic the economy, the more the minorities are perceived to be an economic threat and the higher the level of prejudice.

SOURCE: Quillian 1995.

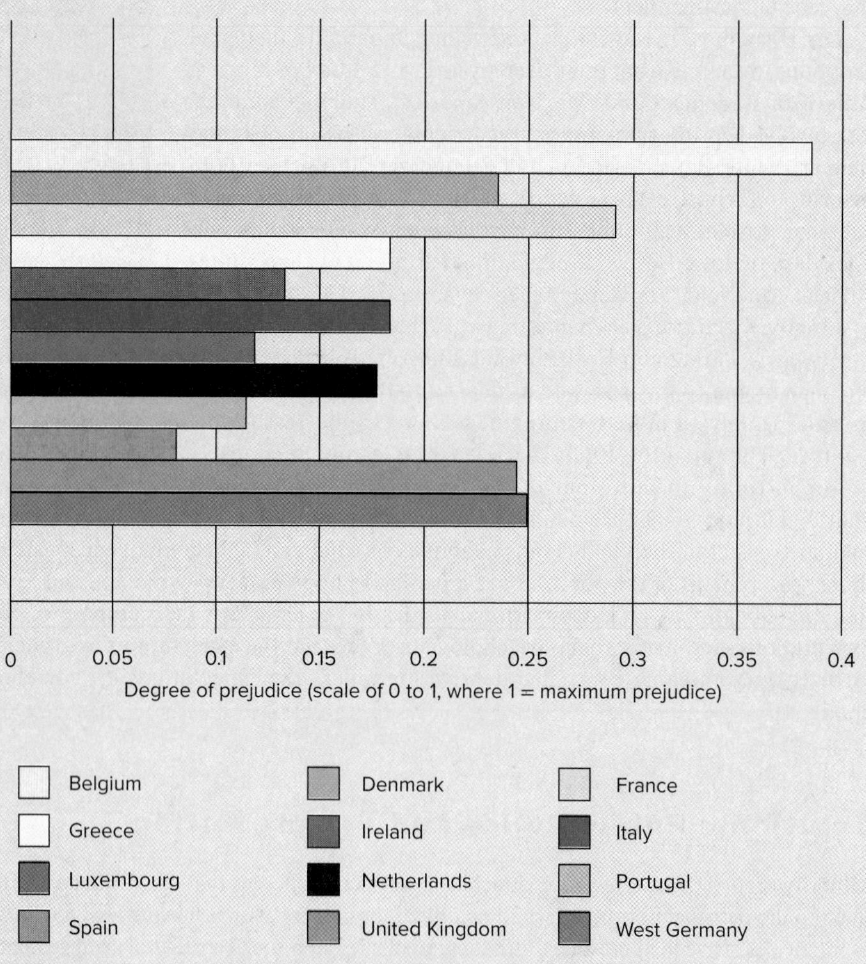


**FIGURE 8.4** Racial Prejudice in Europe.

Source: Adapted from Quillian 1995.

First, attitudes and ideologies can be changed through a policy of persistent education in schools and the mass media. Many efforts have already been initiated, of course, but throughout the country there still are extensive prejudice and adherence to ideologies that disparage minorities. Educational efforts, incidentally, should attack not only the negative attitudes and ideologies about minorities but also the unrealistic ideas that many whites have about the consequences of an integrated society. Many are unaware that school desegregation brings benefits to whites as well as to minorities (Mickelson 2001). Private initiatives that bring whites and minorities together in social and religious settings also can reduce prejudice (Vora and Vora 2002).

Second, minorities need to continue to mobilize for political action that will shape public policy. It is imperative to exercise expanded influence in the government at all levels. Political action is particularly important in the area of employment (Herring 2002). Even though job discrimination is against the law, it continues to occur. New policies and programs are needed to increase workplace equality. Local and state governments could help with the auditing of companies to ferret out instances of discrimination. Funding can be restricted and contracts withheld from firms that repeatedly discriminate against racial and ethnic minorities.

Third, equal educational opportunities must be guaranteed to all minorities. In the late 1980s, Asian Americans protested about discrimination when their numbers were restricted in the California University system. Asian Americans were qualifying in disproportionate numbers for university admission; officials restricted their entry to maintain room for other racial groups. But why should people who are performing well be penalized?

The problem of other groups—notably African Americans and Hispanics—is different. Too few are seeking and gaining entrance to higher education. Programs are needed to keep minorities in school (Hispanics have particularly high dropout rates) and encourage them to seek the highest possible level of attainment. Among other factors, having a higher proportion of faculty and administrators who are minorities and increasing the contact of student affairs officers with minority students help raise the retention rate (Opp 2002). Educators can also recruit those minority students who are in higher education to help analyze the situation and develop strategies for redressing the problem (Hobson-Horton and Owens 2004).

Fourth, legislation must be continually introduced and backed up by the commitment of the federal government to enforce the law. Many beneficial changes have occurred in the wake of such legislation and commitment. Some observers despair of the law having any force, but they often expect too much from law. Laws can change attitudes and alter behavior, but only by increments. A law is passed, people find ways to circumvent it, and a new law is passed to address the contradiction between the intended and the actual results of the first law. Over time the intent of the law is increasingly realized.

Programs must attack institutional racism directly. For example, *affirmative action programs* attempted to increase minority participation in business, industry, education, and service agencies. In essence, affirmative action was a preemptive policy, preventing discrimination before it ever occurred. In spite of considerable evidence that such programs can be effective (Davidson and Lewis 1997; Button and Rienzo 2003; Alon and Tienda 2005a; Fischer and Massey 2007), they have been dismantled and their legality denied in the courts. Some new programs that achieve the same aims are needed.

One aspect of the race problem that has broad implications is *residential segregation.* The majority of American Indians live on reservations. Most Hispanics live in their own segregated neighborhoods, or "barrios." African Americans are concentrated in the inner cities of metropolitan areas. Residential segregation virtually guarantees segregated social life and education (unless there is busing), and it inhibits the kind of intergroup contact that can break down myths, prejudice, and racist ideologies. Any program, therefore, that helps reduce residential segregation, has the potential to ease America's race problem.

*Follow-Up.* Think about the relationships you have had with people of other racial groups. What factors made some of these relationships more positive than others?

## Summary

America's Black, American Indian, Asian, Pacific Islander, and Hispanic minorities compose a substantial and growing proportion of the population. Inequalities between the majority white race and minority races are primarily the result of sociocultural factors. Skin color is a minor biological characteristic, but it is a major sociocultural factor.

The meaning of the problem and the diminished quality of life it imposes on minorities may be summed up in terms of citizenship rights; economic opportunities; the rights of life, liberty, and the pursuit of happiness; and the right to dignity as a human being. In each of these four areas, it is a distinct advantage to be white. Minorities have been deprived of basic citizenship rights, such as the right to vote and the right to be governed by and be equal before the law. Economically, minorities have suffered discrimination in employment opportunities and income. With respect to the value Americans place on life and happiness, minorities have been disadvantaged in terms of life chances. They often have lived in fear and been treated as though their lives were of less value than the lives of whites. Their right to dignity has been violated by the myth of "success around the corner" and the myth of inferiority.

An important social structural factor that contributes to the problem is institutional racism. Minorities are kept clustered in the lower levels of the stratification system and are exploited by the normal policies and practices of institutions, including the mass media, education, the economy, and government. Social psychological factors of attitudes, values, and ideologies of both the white majority and the minorities compound the structural discrimination. Whereas the social structural factors lead to devaluation of minorities, the social psychological factors can lead, in addition, to self-defeating behavior on the part of minorities.

## Key Terms

**Biological Characteristic**
**Disfranchise**
**Ethnic Group**
**Exploitation**
**Institutional Racism**
**Life Chances**
**Prejudice**
**Race**
**Racism**
**Stealth Racism**

## Study Questions

1. What do social scientists mean by "race"?
2. Discuss the extent and origin of races, ethnic groups, and racism in America.
3. How do prejudice and discrimination affect minorities' rights of citizenship?
4. Do minorities have equal economic opportunities?
5. In what sense do prejudice and discrimination violate minorities' rights to life and happiness and to dignity as human beings?
6. How is their position in the stratification system a factor in the problems of minorities?
7. Discuss the ways in which social institutions diminish minorities' quality of life.
8. What are the social psychological aspects of the white majority that are involved in the problems of minorities?
9. What kinds of attitudes on the part of minorities exacerbate the race problem in America?
10. Discuss some of the institutional changes that are needed to address the problems of America's minorities.

## Internet Resources/Exercises

1. Explore some of the ideas in this chapter on the following sites:

**http://www.naacp.org** Site of the National Association for the Advancement of Colored People, with the latest news on racial issues and a variety of other resources.

**http://www.census.gov** The U.S. Census Bureau site, with special reports and comprehensive statistics on racial and ethnic groups.

**http://www.hrw.org** Information on race problems throughout the world by the Human Rights Watch.

2. Find a Hispanic site—a Hispanic magazine or journal, a Hispanic advocacy group, or a Hispanic news site—and make a list of the concerns expressed over the last year or so on the site. To what extent do those concerns reflect and/or address the inequalities identified in the text?

3. Compare the situation of African Americans with that of Asian Americans. Gathering materials from

sites for each of the groups, compare both their grievances and their achievements. On the basis of your findings, what kinds of recommendations would you make to each group?

## For Further Reading

Bowser, Benjamin P., and Raymond G. Hunt, eds. *Impacts of Racism on White Americans.* 2nd ed. Thousand Oaks, CA: Sage, 2002. Various chapters show that, far from disappearing, racism is still strong in America, and there are both advantages and disadvantages for white Americans in racist practices.

Cafferty, Pastora San Juan, and David W. Engstrom, eds. *Hispanics in the United States: An Agenda for the Twenty-First Century.* New Brunswick, NJ: Transaction, 2002. A comprehensive overview of the quality of life of Hispanics in the United States and their role in various social institutions.

Carens, Joseph H. *Immigrants and the Right to Stay.* Cambridge, MA: MIT Press, 2010. A proposal by the author to grant amnesty to unauthorized immigrants who have been in this country a long time, including a chapter on the responses of other scholars.

Ehrlich, Howard J. *Hate Crimes and Ethnoviolence: The History, Current Affairs, and Future of Discrimination in America.* Boulder, CO: Westview Press, 2009. An expert in ethnoviolence discusses such matters as the social conditions that give rise to and justify hate crimes, and the need to include verbal and emotional as well as physical assaults as crimes.

Feagin, Joe R. *Racist America: Roots, Current Realities and Future Reparations.* New York: Routledge, 2001. A sociological analysis of racism that shows how it is embedded in the system, including a discussion of the historical roots of racism in our European heritage.

Gallagher, Charles A. *Rethinking the Color Line.* 6th ed. New York: Sage Publications, 2018. Explores the ways in which racism and ethnicity affect all aspects of American culture and life, including wealth, drug use, immigration, health, etc.

## References

Alexander, M. 2010. *The New Jim Crow: Mass Incarceration in the Age of Colorblindness.* New York: New Press.

Alon, S., and M. Tienda. 2005a. "Assessing the 'mismatch' hypothesis: Differences in college graduation rates by institutional selectivity." *Sociology of Education* 78:294–325.

——. 2005b. "Job mobility and early career wage growth of white, African-American, and Hispanic women." *Social Science Quarterly* 86:1196–1217.

American Civil Liberties Union (ACLU). 2016. "Nationwide, anti-immigration legislation by state." American Civil Liberties Union website.

Arnold, S. B. 2014. "Reproductive rights denied." *American Journal of Public Health* 104:1892–93.

Bell, J., L. J. Ridolfi, M. Finley, and C. Lacey. 2009. *The Keeper and the Kept.* San Francisco, CA: The W. Haywood Burns Institute.

Bendick, M., R. E. Rodriguez, and S. Jayaraman. 2010. "Employment discrimination in upscale restaurants." *Social Science Journal* 47:802–18.

Berg, J. A. 2009. "White public opinion toward undocumented immigrants." *Sociological Perspectives* 52:39–58.

Bernard, J. 1966. *Marriage and Family among Negroes.* Englewood Cliffs, NJ: Prentice-Hall.

Bickell, N. A., et al. 2008. "A tracking and feedback registry to reduce racial disparities in breast cancer care." *Journal of the National Cancer Institute* 100:1717–23.

Bonczar, T. P. 2003. *Prevalence of Imprisonment in the U.S. Population, 1974-2001.* Washington, DC: Government Printing Office.

Bonilla-Silva, E., C. Goar, and D. G. Embrick. 2006. "When whites flock together." *Critical Sociology* 32:229–53.

Brenchley, C. 2012. "Answering questions of fundamental fairness." U.S. Department of Education blog site.

Bridges, G. S., and S. Steen. 1998. "Racial disparities in official assessments of juvenile offenders." *American Sociological Review* 63 (August):554–70.

Brown, A. 2019. "Key findings on American's views of race in 2019." Pew Research Center website.

Brown, A. J. Batt, and E. J. Kim. 2020. "Beyond the 19th: A brief history of the voter suppression of Black Americans." *Social Education* 84:204–08.

Buchmueller, T. C., et al. 2016. "Effect of the affordable care act on racial and ethnic disparities in health insurance coverage." *American Journal of Public Health.* Published online.

Budiman, A. 2020a. "Americans are more positive about the long-term rise in U.S. racial and ethnic diversity than in 2016." Pew Research Center website.

——. 2020b. "Key findings about U.S. immigrants." Pew Research Center website.

Burgess, M. C. R., et al. 2011. "Playing with prejudice: The prevalence and consequences of racial stereotypes in video games." *Media Psychology* 14:289–311.

Butterfield, F. 2000. "Report indicates 'juvenile injustice.'" *San Diego Union-Tribune,* April 26.

Button, J. W., and B. A. Rienzo. 2003. "The impact of affirmative action: Black employment in six Southern cities." *Social Science Quarterly* 84:1-14.

Carr, D. 2005. "Black death, white death." *Contexts* 4:43.

Castor, M. L., et al. 2006. "A nationwide population-based study identifying health disparities between American Indians/Alaska Natives and the general populations living in select urban counties." *American Journal of Public Health* 96:1478-84.

Center for Community Change. 2005. "Issues: The Native American project." CCC website.

Chang, E., C. Chen, E. Greenberger, D. Dooley, and J. Heckhausen. 2006. "What do they want in life? The life goals of a multi-ethnic, multi-generational sample of high school seniors." *Journal of Youth & Adolescence* 35:302-13.

Chou, T., A. Asnaani, and S. G. Hofmann. 2012. "Perception of racial discrimination and psychopathology across three U.S. ethnic minority groups." *Cultural Diversity and Ethnic Minority Psychology* 18:74-81.

Clawson, R. A. 2002. "Poor people, black faces." *Journal of Black Studies* 32:352-61.

Cohen, C. 2003. "Winks, nods, disguises—and racial preference." *Commentary* 116:34-39.

Coker, T. R., et al. 2009. "Perceived racial/ethnic discrimination among fifth-grade students and its association with mental health." *American Journal of Public Health* 99:878-84.

Coleman, M. G. 2003. "Job skill and black male wage discrimination." *Social Science Quarterly* 84:892-906.

——. 2004. "Racial discrimination in the workplace." *Industrial Relations* 43:660-89.

Couch, K. A., and R. Fairlie. 2010. "Last hired, first fired? Black-white unemployment and the business cycle." *Demography* 47:227-47.

Coverdill, J. E., C. A. Lopez, and M. A. Petrie. 2011. "Race, ethnicity and the quality of life in America, 1972-2008." *Social Forces* 89:783-805.

Daniels, L. A., ed. 2004. *The State of Black America 2004.* New York: National Urban League.

Davidson, R. C., and E. L. Lewis. 1997. "Affirmative action and other special consideration admissions at the University of California, Davis, School of Medicine." *Journal of the American Medical Association* 278 (October 8):1153-58.

Davis, C. 2017. "'Made in America'" ATTN website.

DeMuth, S., and D. Steffensmeier. 2004. "The impact of gender and race-ethnicity in the pretrial release process." *Social Problems* 51:222-42.

Dickens, W. T., and J. R. Flynn. 2006. "Black Americans reduce the racial IQ gap." *Psychological Science* 17:913-20.

Downey, L., and B. Hawkins. 2008. "Race, income, and environmental inequality in the United States." *Sociological Perspectives* 51:759-81.

Durose, M. R., E. L. Smith, and P. A. Langan. 2007. "Contacts between police and the public, 2005." *Bureau of Justice Statistics Special Report,* April.

Eddings, J. 1995. "A persistent stealth racism is poisoning black-white relations." *U.S. News and World Report,* October 23.

Ely, D. M., and A. K. Driscoll. 2020. "Infant mortality in the United States, 2018." National Vital Statistics Report website.

Emerson, M. O., G. Yancey, and K. J. Chai. 2001. "Does race matter in residential segregation?" *American Sociological Review* 66:922-35.

Esses, V. M., P. M. Brochu, and K. R. Dickson. 2011. "Economic costs, economic benefits, and attitudes toward immigrants and immigration." *Analyses of Social Issues and Public Policy,* 12 (1):133-37.

Evans-Campbell, T., T. Lindhorst, B. Huang, and K. L. Walters. 2006. "Interpersonal violence in the lives of urban American Indian and Alaska Native women." *American Journal of Public Health* 96:1416-22.

Faber, J. W. 2018. "Segregation and the geography of creditworthiness." *Housing Policy Debate* 28:215-47.

Farley, R. 2011. "The waning of American apartheid?" *Contexts* 10:36-43.

Fischer, M. J., and D. S. Massey. 2007. "The effects of affirmative action in higher education." *Social Science Research* 38:531-49.

Fish, J. M. 1995. "Mixed blood." *Psychology Today,* November-December, pp. 55-61.

Flores, E., et al. 2008. "Perceived discrimination, perceived stress, and mental and physical health among Mexican-origin adults." *Hispanic Journal of Behavioral Science* 30:401-24.

Flynn, G. 2003. "The reverse-discrimination trap." *Workforce* 82:10 6-7.

Fogarty, B. J., et al. 2015. "News attention to voter fraud in the 2008 and 2012 US elections." Research & Politics website.

Frederico, C. M. 2006. "Ideology and the affective structure of whites' racial perceptions." *Public Opinion Quarterly* 70:327-53.

Fullerton, A. S., and K. F. Anderson. 2013. "The role of job insecurity in explanations of racial health inequalities." *Sociological Forum* 28:308-25.

Gibbons, F. X., et al. 2014. "Effects of perceived racial discrimination on health status and health behavior." *Health Psychology* 33:11-19.

Gonzalez-Barrera, A. 2015. "More Mexicans leaving than coming to the U.S." Pew Research Center website.

Gramlich, J. 2020. "20 striking findings from 2020." Pew Research Center website.

Grant, B. F., et al. 2004. "The 12-month prevalence and trends in DSM-IV alcohol abuse and dependence." *Drug and Alcohol Dependence* 74:223-34.

Grieco, E. M., and R. C. Cassidy. 2001. "Overview of race and Hispanic origin." U.S. Census Bureau website.

Grodsky, E., and D. Pager. 2001. "The structure of disadvantage: Individual and occupational determinants of the black-white wage gap." *American Sociological Review* 66:542-67.

Harlow, C. W. 2005. "Hate crime reported by victims and police." *Bureau of Justice Statistics Special Report*. Washington, DC: Government Printing Office.

Herne, M. A., M. L. Bartholomew, and R. L. Weahkee. 2014. "Suicide mortality among American Indians and Alaska Natives, 1999-2009." *American Journal of Public Health* 104:336-42.

Herring, C. 2002. "Is job discrimination dead?" *Contexts* 1:13-18.

Herrnstein, R. J., and C. Murray. 1994. *The Bell Curve: Intelligence and Class Structure in American Life*. New York: Free Press.

Hicks, W. D., et al. 2015. "A principle or a strategy? Voter identification laws and partisan competition in the American States." *Political Research Quarterly* 68:18-33.

Hipp, J. R. 2011. "Violent crime, mobility decisions, and neighborhood racial/ethnic transition." *Social Problems* 58:410-32.

Hirschman, C., and E. Mogford. 2009. "Immigration and the American industrial revolution from 1880 to 1920." *Social Science Research* 38:897-920.

Hobson-Horton, L. D., and L. Owens. 2004. "From freshman to graduate: Recruiting and retaining minority students." *Journal of Hispanic Higher Education* 3:86-107.

Hogg, R. S., et al. 2008. "Years of life lost to prison." *Harm Reduction Journal* 5:4-8.

Humes, K. R., N. A. Jones, and R. R. Ramirez. 2011. *Overview of Race and Hispanic Origin: 2010*. U.S. Census Bureau website.

Hunter, C. D., et al. 2016. "The roles of shared racial fate and a sense of belonging with African Americans in black immigrants' race-related stress and depression." *Journal of Black Psychology*. Published online.

Iceland, J., and R. Wilkes. 2006. "Does socioeconomic status matter? Race, class, and residential segregation." *Social Problems* 53:248-73.

Jacobs, D., Z. Qian, J. T. Carmichael, and S. L. Kent. 2007. "Who survives on death row? An individual and contextual analysis." *American Sociological Review* 72:610-32.

Jaret, C. 1991. "Recent structural change and US urban ethnic minorities." *Journal of Urban Affairs* 13 (3):307-36.

Jones, B. 2016. "Americans' views of immigrants marked by widening partisan, generational divides." Pew Research Center website.

Klug, B. J., and P. T. Whitfield. 2002. *Widening the Circle: Culturally Relevant Pedagogy for American Indian Children*. New York: Routledge/Falmer.

Kowalski, B. R., and R. J. Lundman. 2007. "Vehicle stops by police for driving while black." *Journal of Criminal Justice* 35:165-81.

Kreager, D. A. 2008. "Guarded borders: Adolescent interracial romance and peer trouble at school." *Social Forces* 87:887-910.

Krogstad, J. M. 2016. "Roughly half of Hispanics have experienced discrimination." Pew Research Center website.

Krogstad, J. M., and L. Noe-Bustamante. 2020. "Key facts about U.S. Latinos for national Hispanic heritage month." Pew Research Center website.

Krysan, M. 2008. "Does race matter in the search for housing?" *Social Science Research* 37:581-603.

Landen, M., et al. 2014. "Alcohol-attributable mortality among American Indians and Alaska Natives in the United States, 1999-2009." *American Journal of Public Health* 104:343-49.

Lewis, R. 2002. "Race and the clinic: Good science?" *Scientist* 16 (February 18):16.

Lewis, V. A., M. O. Emerson, and S. L. Klineberg. 2011. "Who we'll live with: Neighborhood racial composition preferences of whites, blacks and Latinos." *Social Forces* 89:1385-1408.

Light, M. T., and T. Miller. 2018. "Does undocumented immigration increase violent crime?" *Criminology* 56:370-401.

Loury, G. C. 2005. "Racial stigma and its consequences." *Focus* 24:1-6.

Lynn, M., et al. 2011. "Examining teachers' beliefs about African American male students in a low-performing high school in an African American school district." *Teachers College Record.* TCR website.

Malhotra, N., and C. Raso. 2007. "Racial representation and U.S. Senate apportionment." *Social Science Quarterly* 88:1038–48.

Maniam, S. 2016. "Sharp differences over who is hurt, helped by their race." Pew Research Center website.

Margolis, J., R. Estrella, J. Goode, J. J. Holme, and K. Nao. 2008. *Stuck in the Shallow End: Education, Race, and Computing.* Cambridge, MA: MIT Press.

Marx, S. 2006. *Revealing the Invisible: Confronting Passive Racism in Teacher Education.* New York: Routledge.

Mastro D. 2017. "Race and ethnicity in US media content and effects." Oxford Research website.

Matthew, E. M. 2011. "Effort optimism in the classroom." *Sociology of Education* 84:225–45.

McCall, L. 2001. "Sources of racial wage inequality in metropolitan labor markets." *American Sociological Review* 66:520–41.

McDevitt, J., J. Balboni, L. Garcia, and J. Gu. 2001. "Consequences for victims: A comparison of bias- and non-bias-motivated assaults." *American Behavioral Scientist* 45:697–713.

McLaughlin, D. K., and C. S. Stokes. 2002. "Income inequality and mortality in U.S. counties." *American Journal of Public Health* 92:99–104.

Meckler, L. 1998. "Blacks in America get sick more than whites, die sooner." *San Diego Union-Tribune,* November 27.

Mickelson, R. A. 2001. "Subverting Swann: Tracking as second generation segregation in Charlotte, North Carolina." *American Educational Research Journal* 38:215–52.

Mohai, P., and R. Saha. 2007. "Racial inequality in the distribution of hazardous waste: A national-level reassessment." *Social Problems* 54:343–70.

Moore, T. S. 2010. "The local of racial disadvantage in the labor market." *American Journal of Sociology* 116:909–42.

Morgan, R. E., and J. L. Truman. 2020. "Criminal victimization, 2019." Bureau of Justice Statistics website.

Morris, E. W. 2005. "'Tuck in that shirt!' Race, class, gender, and discipline in an urban school." *Sociological Perspectives* 48:25–48.

Myrdal, G. 1944. *An American Dilemma.* New York: Harper and Bros.

National Fair Housing Alliance. 2020. "Report housing discrimination." NFHA website.

Newport, F. 2020. "Americans and the role of government." Gallup Poll website.

Ong, P. M. 1991. "Race and post-displacement earnings among high-tech workers." *Industrial Relations* 30 (Fall):456–68.

Opp, R. D. 2002. "Enhancing program completion rates among two-year college students of color." *Community College Journal of Research and Practice* 26:147–63.

Orfield, G., and D. Jarvie. 2020. "Black segregation matters." The Civil Rights Project at UCLA website.

Palumbo, T. 2010. "Dynamics of economic well-being: Spells of unemployment, 2004–2007." *Household Economic Studies.* U.S. Census Bureau website.

Parker, K. F., and A. Reckdenwald. 2008. "Concentrated disadvantage, traditional male role models, and African-American juvenile violence." *Criminology* 46:711–35.

Parker, K., J. M. Horowitz, and M. Anderson. 2020. "Amid protests, majorities across racial and ethnic groups express support for the Black Lives Matter movement." Pew Research Center website.

Passel, J. S., and D. Cohn. 2008. "Undocumented immigration now trails legal inflow, reversing decade-long trend." Pew Research Center website.

Pavkov, T. W., et al. 2010. "Tribal youth victimization and delinquency." *Cultural Diversity and Ethnic Minority Psychology* 16:123–34.

Peri, G. 2011. "The impact of immigration on native poverty through labor market competition." *NBER Working Paper No. 17570.* National Bureau of Economic Research website.

Pettit, B., and B. Western. 2004. "Mass imprisonment and the life course: Race and class inequality in U.S. incarceration." *American Sociological Review* 69:151–69.

Pew Research Center. 2016. "State of the news media." Pew Research Center website.

Quillian, L. 1995. "Population, perceived threat, and prejudice in Europe." *American Sociological Review* 60:586–611.

——. 2014. "Does segregation create winners and losers?" *Social Problems* 61:402–26.

Quinn, D. M. 2015. "Kindergarten black-white test score gaps." *Sociology of Education* 88:120–39.

Rank, M. R. 2009. "Measuring the economic racial divide across the course of American lives." *Race and Social Problems* 1:57–66.

Ream, R. K., and R. W. Rumberger. 2008. "Student engagement, peer social capital, and school dropout among Mexican American and non-Latino white students." *Sociology of Education* 81:109–39.

Reardon, S. F. 2012. "Brown fades: the end of court-ordered school desegregation and the resegregation of American public schools." *Journal of Policy Analysis and Management* 31:876-904.

Rojek, J., R. Rosenfeld, and S. Decker. 2012. "Policing race." *Criminology* 50:993-1024.

Roscigno, V. J., D. L. Karafin, and G. Tester. 2009. "The complexities and processes of racial housing discrimination." *Social Problems* 56:49-69.

Rosenfeld, S. 2007. "Turning back the clock on voting rights." *Social Policy* 38:52-66.

Ross, S. L., and M. A. Turner. 2005. "Housing discrimination in metropolitan America." *Social Problems* 52:152-80.

Rotberg, I. C. 2020. "Crosswords: Integration and segregation in suburban school districts." *Phi Delta Kappan* 101:44-49.

Rothstein, R. 2018. "The Fair Housing Act at 50." *Social Education* 82:68-72.

Rugh, J. S., and D. S. Massey. 2010. "Racial segregation and the American foreclosure crisis." *American Sociological Review* 75:629-51.

Sampson, R. J. 2008. "Rethinking crime and immigration." *Contexts* 7:28-33.

San Francisco Bureau. 2001. "New program hits racist property deeds." *Sun Reporter,* May 24, p. 3.

Sancar, F., J. Abbasi, and K. Bucher. 2018. "Mortality among American Indians and Alaska natives." *Journal of the American Medical Association* 319:112.

Saporito, S., and D. Sohoni. 2006. "Coloring outside the lines: Racial segregation in public schools and their attendance boundaries." *Sociology of Education* 79:81-105.

Semega, J., et al. 2020. "Income and poverty in the United States: 2019." U.S. Government Publishing Office.

Simpson, G. E., and M. Yinger. 1965. *Racial and Cultural Minorities.* New York: Harper and Row.

Smith, R. A. 2005. "Do the determinants of promotion differ for white men versus women and minorities?" *American Behavioral Scientist* 9:1157-81.

Snyder, H. N., and M. Sickmund. 1999. *Juvenile Offenders and Victims: 1999 National Report.* Washington, DC: Office of Juvenile Justice and Delinquency Prevention.

Spence, N. J., D. E. Adkins, and M. E. Dupre. 2011. "Racial differences in depression trajectories among older women." *Journal of Health and Social Behavior* 52:444-59.

Stepler, R. 2016. "Hispanic, black parents see college degree as key for children's success." Pew Research Center website.

Sternberg, R. J., E. L. Grigorenko, and K. K. Kidd. 2005. "Intelligence, race, and genetics." *American Psychologist* 60:46-59.

Symmes, P. 2012. "Hunted in Alabama." *Newsweek,* February 13, pp. 26-27.

Thomas, M., et al. 2020. "Race and the accumulation of wealth." *Social Problems* 67:20-39.

Tomaskovic-Devey, D., and V. J. Roscigno. 1996. "Racial economic subordination and white gain in the U.S. South." *American Sociological Review* 61 (August):565-89.

Tomaskovic-Devey, D., et al. 2006. "Documenting desegregation: Segregation in American workplaces by race, ethnicity, and sex, 1966-2003." *American Sociological Review* 71:565-88.

U.S. Census Bureau. 2010. "Hispanic population in the United States." U.S. Census Bureau website.

Vora, E. A., and J. A. Vora. 2002. "Undoing racism in America." *Journal of Black Studies* 32:389-404.

Watson, A. 2020. "Minorities in media in the U.S." Statista website.

Weeks, G. B., and J. R. Weeks. 2010. *Invisible Forces: Latin American Migration to the United States and Its Effects on the South.* Albuquerque, NM: University of New Mexico Press.

Weitzer, R., and S. A. Tuch. 2004. "Race and perceptions of police misconduct." *Social Problems* 51:305-25.

Welch, K., and A. A. Payne. 2010. "Racial threat and punitive school discipline." *Social Problems* 57:25-48.

Williams, D. R., H. W. Neighbors, and J. S. Jackson. 2003. "Racial/ethnic discrimination and health." *American Journal of Public Health* 93:200-208.

Williams, R., and R. Nesiba. 2005. "The changing face of inequality in home mortgage lending." *Social Problems* 52:181-208.

Wilson, G. 2005. "Race and job dismissal." *American Behavioral Scientist* 48:1182-99.

Wilson, M. M. 2014. "Hate crime victimization, 2004-2012." Bureau of Justice Statistics website.

Young, J. R., and M. J. Mattingly. 2016. "Underemployment among Hispanics." *Monthly Labor Review,* December.

Yu, T. 2006. "Challenging the politics of the 'model minority' stereotype." *Equity and Excellence in Education* 39:325-33.

Zick, A., T. F. Pettigrew, and U. Wagner. 2008. "Ethnic prejudice and discrimination in Europe." *Journal of Social Issues* 64:233-51.

PART

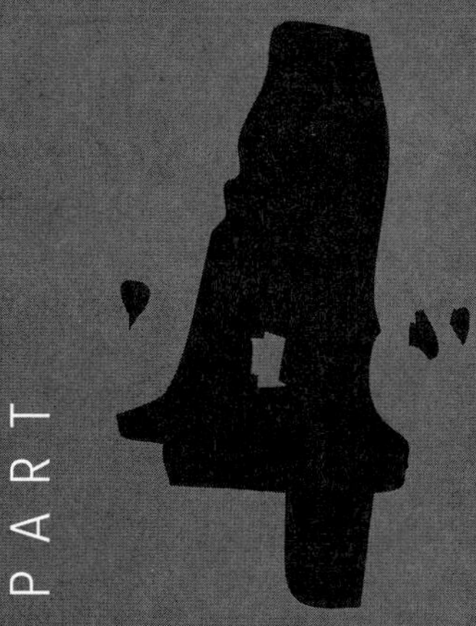

# Problems of Social Institutions



Dynamic Graphics/JupiterImages

Social institutions exist in every society to solve the problems and meet the needs of people. The government should protect people, secure social order, and maintain an equitable society. The economy should provide the basic necessities of life. Education should fulfill people and train them to function well in society. The family should nurture its members and provide them with emotional stability and security. The health care system should maintain emotional and physical well-being.

Unfortunately, social institutions create as well as solve problems. In this section, you'll learn how the government and the political system fail in some of their functions; how the economy, including work, is detrimental to the quality of life for some people; how education fails to fulfill its functions for some individuals; how family life can detract from, rather than enhance, well-being; and how the health care system does not adequately meet the physical and emotional needs of some Americans.

Society cannot exist without social institutions, but not everyone benefits equally from those institutions. Some even become victims. Institutions need reshaping in order to maximize the well-being of all Americans.

CHAPTER

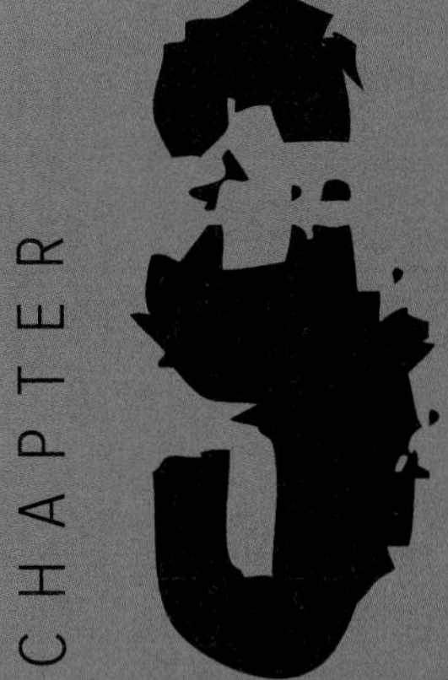

# Government and Politics

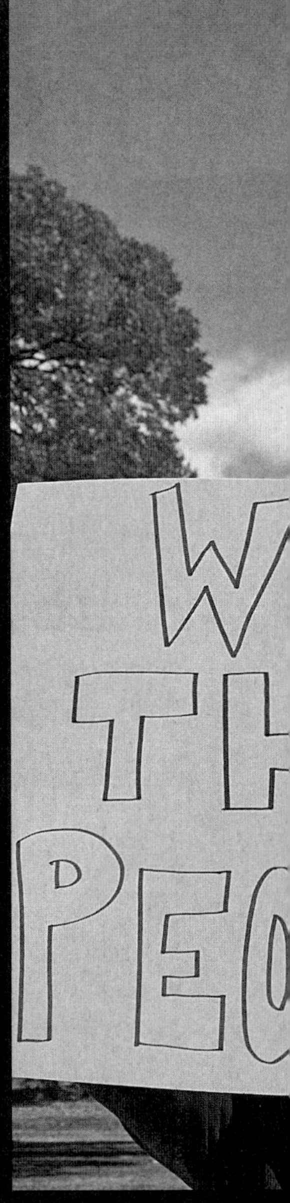



OBJECTIVES

1 Know the functions of government.

2 Identify reasons why government and politics are problems.

3 Discuss how the problems of government and politics affect the quality of life.

4 Explain how size, organization, economics, the media, and interest groups contribute to the problems of government and politics.

5 Show the way in which attitudes and ideologies contribute to the problems of government and politics.

6 Suggest ways to deal with the problems of government and politics.

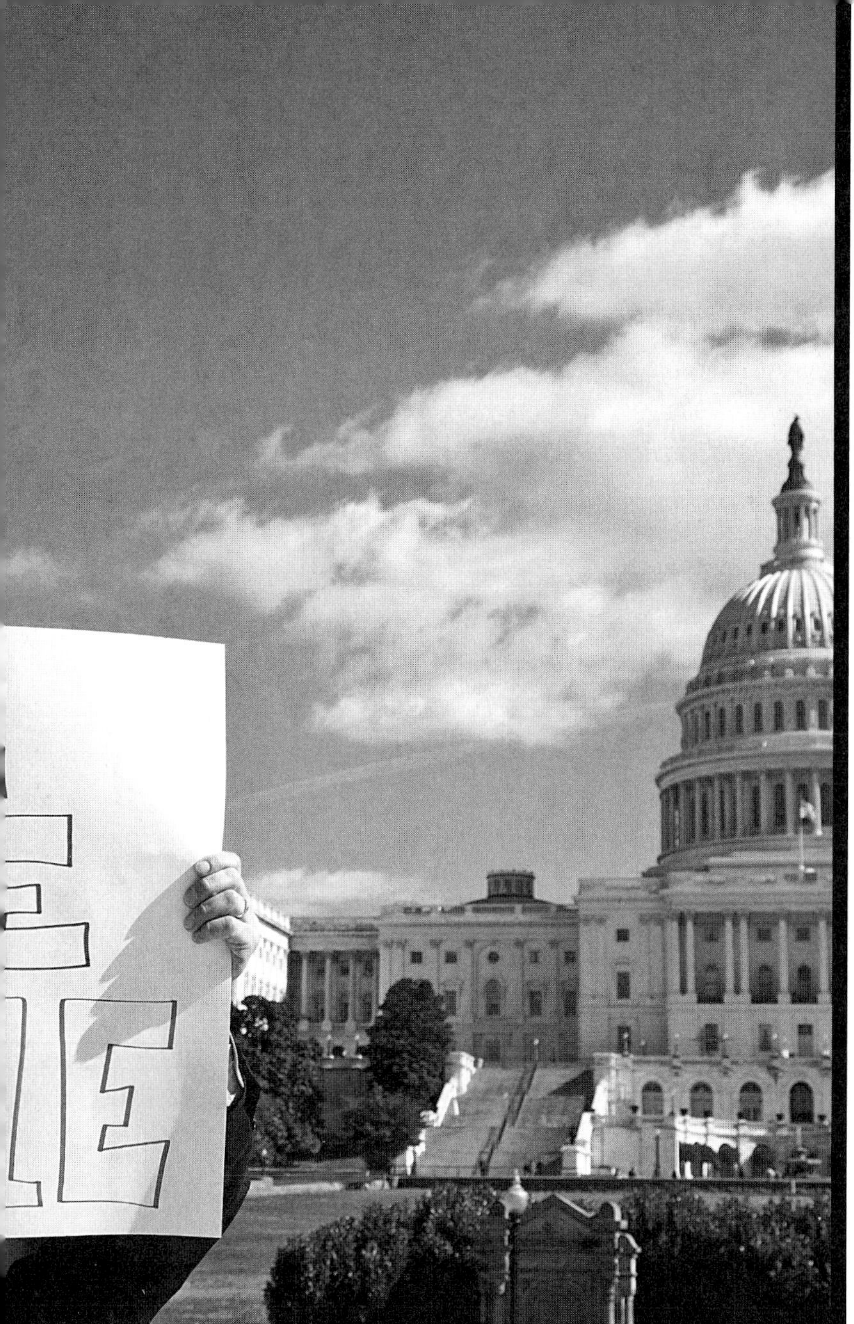

fStop/Alamy Stock Photo

### "Why Isn't There Help for People Like Me?"

Jacquelyn is the single mother of two preschool children. Shortly before her second child was born, her husband, Ed, lost his job. He was unable to find another one. About the time they had exhausted their savings, he announced that he couldn't take it anymore and disappeared. Jacquelyn, who only has a high school education, is struggling to survive:

*We lost our home. The kids and I are living in a cheap apartment. We're barely getting by. I don't have enough money to even buy my kids any new toys. And when I go to the grocery store, I see other mothers putting all kinds of good food into their baskets that I can't afford. My parents give us a little, but my dad is on disability and they have a hard time meeting their own bills. I married Ed right out of high school. So I've never worked, and I don't have any skills. I can't even use a computer.*

*I remember that we were promised the government would give us a safety net. Well, where is it? I'm in a job training program now, but who's going to take care of my kids while I work? And how am I going to pay for someone to take care of my kids? How much do they think I'm going to make from the kinds of jobs they're training me for?*

*What I'd like to know is, why isn't there some real help for people like me? The government tells me I have to get a job in a couple of years or I won't get any more welfare. Why doesn't the government find Ed and make him help support his kids? For all I know, he's found work somewhere else and has plenty of money.*

*Or why doesn't the government make sure that I get a job that will pay me enough so I can give my kids a decent life? Our country goes all over the world helping people in need, and forgets about people like me. I'd like to see some of those politicians take my place for a while. Maybe then they would realize how some of us die a little bit every day from worrying about what's going to happen to us and our kids and how we're going to survive.*

## Introduction

What adjectives would you use to describe American government? How about American politics? If you are like many students we have taught, you probably came up with such adjectives as "huge," "inefficient," "corrupt," and "self-serving." However, we have also had students who described government and politics as "effective" and "helpful."

Let's follow-up with another question: What role does government play in social problems? Some students see government as a major contributor to social problems. Others see it as the only hope for resolving them. Most students agree that the government should take a leading role in attacking various problems.

Each of these responses has some validity. Throughout this book, we note various ways in which the government and politics enter into both the causes and the resolution of social problems. In this chapter, we concentrate on the ways in which government and politics are themselves problems. We begin by examining the functions of government—what people believe they can legitimately expect from government. We then look at four specific ways in which government and politics are problems, how those problems affect people's quality of life, and various structural and social psychological factors that contribute to the problems. Finally, we explore possible ways to attack the problems of government and politics.

## Why Government?

**anarchism**
the philosophy that advocates the abolition of government in order to secure true freedom for people

Can you imagine a society without any government? Some people can. **Anarchism** is a philosophy that advocates the abolition of government in order to secure true freedom for people. According to anarchists, people are free only when they can cooperate with each other to achieve their ends without the restraints of government and law. To be sure, history provides abundant examples of governments that have deprived people of freedom. Nevertheless, we agree with the student who said, "When I look at the way that governments have exploited and oppressed people throughout history, I am sympathetic to the idea of anarchism. But I still think we need government."

The question is, why do we need government? What do people expect from their government? What functions does it fulfill? We shall discuss four important functions. Keep in mind that government at all levels—federal, state, and local—is involved in fulfilling these functions.

### Protect the Citizenry

The first function of government is to protect the citizenry. Americans expect government to protect them from foreign aggressors. This function will be explored in greater detail in Chapter 14. They also expect the government to protect them from various threats to their well-being, *threats that come from sources more powerful than any individual* (Sypnowich 2000). For example, people look to government for protection from environmental hazards, unsafe or unfair business practices, and corporate exploitation of consumers. In recent years, many Americans have looked to government to stop the flow of illegal immigrants into the nation. As noted in the last chapter, hundreds of thousands enter illegally each year, and some Americans believe that they take away jobs from citizens and use services that increase taxes and costs to citizens. In addition, some fear that terrorists will be among those who sneak into the country. Some state and local governments have enacted, or are considering enacting, laws that punish employers who hire illegals and landlords who rent to them.

Protection at the federal level comes in the form not only of laws but of regulatory agencies. A **regulatory agency** is an organization established by the government to enforce statutes that apply to a particular activity. For instance, the Securities and Exchange Commission (SEC) monitors the trading of stocks and bonds, whereas the National Labor Relations Board (NLRB) monitors employer-employee issues. Although many people complain about the irrational and autocratic procedures of the regulatory agencies, they were established mainly in response to demands from citizens who felt the need for protection.

**regulatory agency**
an organization established by the government to enforce statutes that apply to a particular activity

An example of the way the protective function works is seen in the Food and Drug Administration's (FDA) monitoring of prescription drugs. In the early 1960s, the world was shocked at the news of babies being born without arms or legs. The tragedy took place, for the most part, in Europe and Australia and was linked to mothers' ingestion of the drug thalidomide. Thalidomide had been used as a tranquilizer and to treat nausea in pregnant women (Colborn, Dumanoski, and Myers 1997), but it was eventually shown that the drug also caused terrible deformities in children who were exposed to it while in the womb. Although Americans didn't avoid the tragedy altogether, they did escape the large number of cases that occurred in other nations because a physician at the FDA delayed approval of

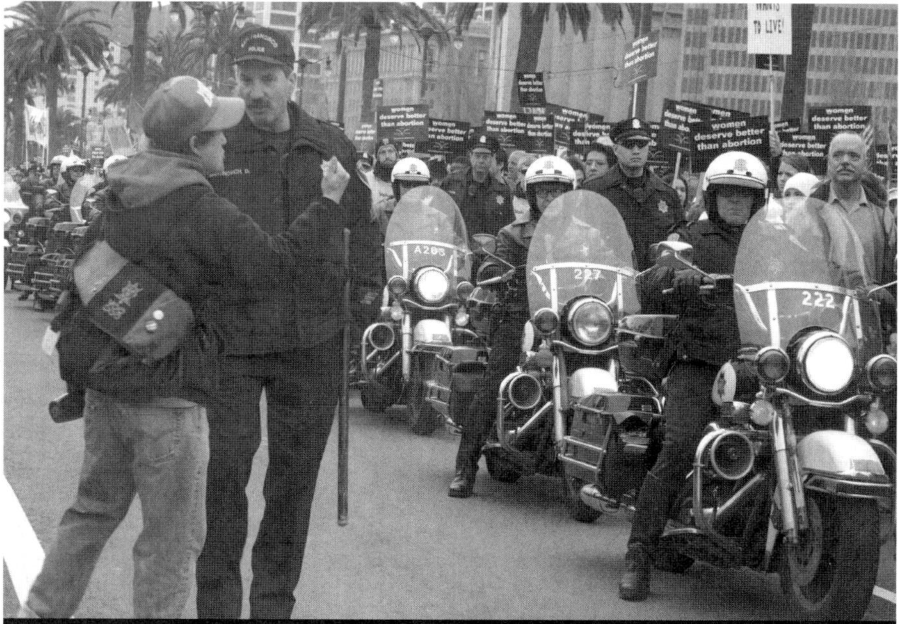


The police are one way the government performs its function of regulating behavior and maintaining civil order.
John Flournoy/McGraw Hill

the drug, insisting on more safety data before the agency would agree to its use. The action of the agency protected a great many children from serious handicaps.

## Secure Order

A second function of government is to *secure order.* In contrast to anarchists, many observers argue that government is necessary to control individuals so that society does not degenerate into chaos and violence. By regulating people's behavior in the economy and other areas of social life, government helps prevent the destructive disorder that would result from a situation in which individuals acted to benefit themselves (Durkheim 1933).

Although there may be disagreement about whether government is necessary for social order, there is no disagreement about the importance of that order. Imagine what it would be like to live in a society in which there were no consensual rules about such matters as traffic, education of the young, or the right to private property. *Order is essential to both emotional and physical well-being.*

## Distribute Power Equitably

A third function of government is to distribute power equitably so that every citizen has *an equal opportunity for life, liberty, and the pursuit of happiness.* In other words, a person's freedom and aspirations should not be constricted because of his or her sex, race, age, religion, or socioeconomic background. A person should not have more power than others simply because he is male rather than female, white rather than nonwhite, and so on.

We have shown in previous chapters that such factors have and do affect people's life chances. In fact, a survey of a number of nations in the world has shown a direct relationship between the way the government functions and the reported happiness of the citizenry (Ott 2011). One way for a government to function well is to redress inequities. In our nation, a good example involves the right to vote (Burns, Peterson, and Cronin 1984). In the early years of the nation, the right to vote was limited to white, male adults who were property owners and taxpayers. Thus, in the first election for which a popular vote was recorded (1824), less than 4 percent of the population voted. In response to public demands, federal and state governments took action to broaden voting rights. For example, a number of constitutional amendments assisted in gradually enlarging the franchise. The Fifteenth Amendment, ratified in 1870, gave Black males the right to vote, although state and local governments found numerous ways to subvert this right. In 1920 women gained the right to vote as a result of the Nineteenth Amendment. Finally, the Twenty-sixth Amendment, ratified in 1971, extended the right to vote to 18-year-olds.

## Provide a Safety Net

Finally, government functions *to provide a safety net, a minimum standard of living below which it will not allow citizens to fall.* Even if opportunities abound, some people—because of such things as the economy and life circumstances—are not able to achieve what most Americans define as a minimal standard of living. In addition, as Americans discovered in the Great Depression that followed the stock-market crash in 1929, there are times when opportunities are severely limited. It was in response to the hardships of the Depression that, in the 1930s, President Franklin Roosevelt initiated the New Deal, which featured programs like the Social Security system. Since that time, Americans (and, for that matter, people throughout the world) have come to expect government actions to provide a safety net that secures a minimum standard of living (Ray and Dugan 2020).

Differences exist over what should be included in the safety net. Currently, safety-net benefits include, for example, Social Security and Medicare for the retired, short-term financial aid for the unemployed, subsidized lunches for poor schoolchildren, and health insurance for children who otherwise would be uninsured (Felland et al. 2003).

## Problems of Government and Politics

The problems discussed in this section reflect the fact that *political parties and government bureaucracy play a central role in the way representative democracy functions in the United States.* **Political parties** are organized groups that attempt to control the government through the electoral process. A **bureaucracy** is an organization in which there are specific areas of authority and responsibility, a hierarchy of authority, management based on written documents, worker expertise, management based on rules, and full-time workers. The government bureaucracy includes those government employees whose jobs do not depend on elections or political appointment.

**political party**
an organized group that attempts to control the government through the electoral process

**bureaucracy**
an organization in which there are specific areas of authority and responsibility, a hierarchy of authority, management based on written documents, worker expertise, management based on rules, and full-time workers

### Inequalities in Power

*The actual distribution of power in American society contradicts the expectation that the government should ensure equity.* But exactly how is power distributed? This question is not easy to answer.

*Pluralism or Power Elites?* Who holds the most power in the United States? Many social scientists believe that America is a *pluralistic society* in terms of the distribution of power. **Pluralism** means that power is distributed more or less equally among **interest groups,** which are groups that attempt to influence public opinion and political decisions in accord with the particular interests of their members. Thus, an interest group such as the National Rifle Association (NRA) exercises power in the political sphere to protect its members' insistence on the right to own firearms. The National Organization for Women (NOW) exercises power to protect and advance the rights of women.

In contrast to the pluralist view, the **power elite model** asserts that power is concentrated in a small group of political, economic, and military leaders (Mills 1956). In essence, the top leaders in government, in business, and in the military determine the major policies and programs of the nation—and they do this in a way that furthers their own interests and solidifies their power. A variation, held by Marxists and some others, is that capitalists wield the power, including power over the government (Barry 2002). Most of the people who hold to the power elite view argue that interest groups have some power, but mainly in their capacity to lobby members of Congress, whereas the great bulk of individuals is an unorganized, powerless mass controlled by the power elite.

**pluralism**
the more or less equal distribution of power among interest groups

**interest group**
a group that attempts to influence public opinion and political decisions in accord with the particular interests of its members

**power elite model**
a model of politics in which power is concentrated in political, economic, and military leaders

Evidence can be gathered in support of both the pluralist and the power elite positions. Domhoff's (1990) analysis of decision making, for example, concludes that the upper class generally rules the nation. Many observers found support for the power elite model in the ties between political leaders and the oil industry during the George W. Bush administration. President Bush himself owned an oil company. Vice President Cheney was head of Halliburton, an energy and construction firm. And Condoleezza Rice, the national security adviser, had been on the Chevron board of directors for a decade. Critics charged that the U.S. Middle East policy, including the war on Iraq, was shaped by the administration's close ties to the oil industry. Further evidence of the ties was the awarding of billions of dollars of government contracts to Halliburton for various projects in rebuilding Iraq and servicing U.S. troops still in Iraq (Burger and Zagorin 2004).

One of the most blatant examples of the power elite was the Trump presidency (Citizens for Responsibility and Ethics in Washington 2020). Reporters documented literally thousands of cases of conflict of interest that personally profited the president, his family, and wealthy people generally. For example, the Trump administration passed a tax relief bill in 2017 that they said would be a boon to the middle class. Actually, it turned out to be a huge gift to the rich, and the president acknowledged that when he told a gathering of the wealthy at his exclusive Florida resort: "You all just got a lot richer."

*Power and Inequality.* Although there is some validity to both the pluralist and the power elite positions, neither seems to capture fully the realities of power distribution. *People are not powerless, particularly when they organize.* Mothers Against Drunk Driving (MADD) has influenced the passage of new legislation on drinking while driving, helping to reduce the number of deaths caused by drunk drivers.

At the same time, *there clearly are power inequities;* otherwise the poor, women, and minorities, among others, would not have had to struggle for so long against their various disadvantages. It is true that women and minorities have made some inroads into the power elite (Zweigenhaft and Domhoff 2006). There are more women and more minorities (particularly more African Americans) among corporate CEOs and directors, in the higher ranks of the military, and in national political and governmental positions. Nevertheless, the struggle for equality has been torturously slow. In spite of its efforts, for example, the National Organization for Women could not get the Equal Rights Amendment (ERA) ratified; and in spite of the work of numerous civil rights organizations, African Americans and other minorities have made only modest headway in their efforts to achieve equity in the economy.

In other words, regardless of which model of power distribution most accurately reflects the realities of social life, the government clearly has not maintained an equitable distribution of power. The longstanding deprivations of certain groups show that Americans have not yet achieved the ideal of liberty and justice for all.

## The Failure of Trust

*An important part of the task of securing order is building trust* (Levi 1998). Trust in this context means having confidence that others will fulfill their responsibilities. Citizens need to trust each other, and they need to trust the government. Trust is essential if people are to cooperate and work together in maintaining the norms and the laws of society. If citizens distrust their government, they are more apt to resist and even ignore government policies and laws.

How much do Americans trust their government? Over the last half century, public confidence in all the major institutions has declined markedly. By 2020, as Figure 9.1 shows, only the military and the medical system had half or more of Americans express "a great deal" or "quite a lot" of confidence in the nation's institutions. And only 13 percent expressed such confidence in Congress.

Why do Americans view government with more skepticism than they do other social institutions? Unfortunately, researchers who survey people on their level of confidence do not probe into the reasons for their responses. It is probable that such factors as the breaking of campaign promises, incompetence, and the lack of responsiveness to people's interests and needs lead to distrust. Scandals and corruption also contribute to distrust. Scandals and corruption have never been absent from American political life,

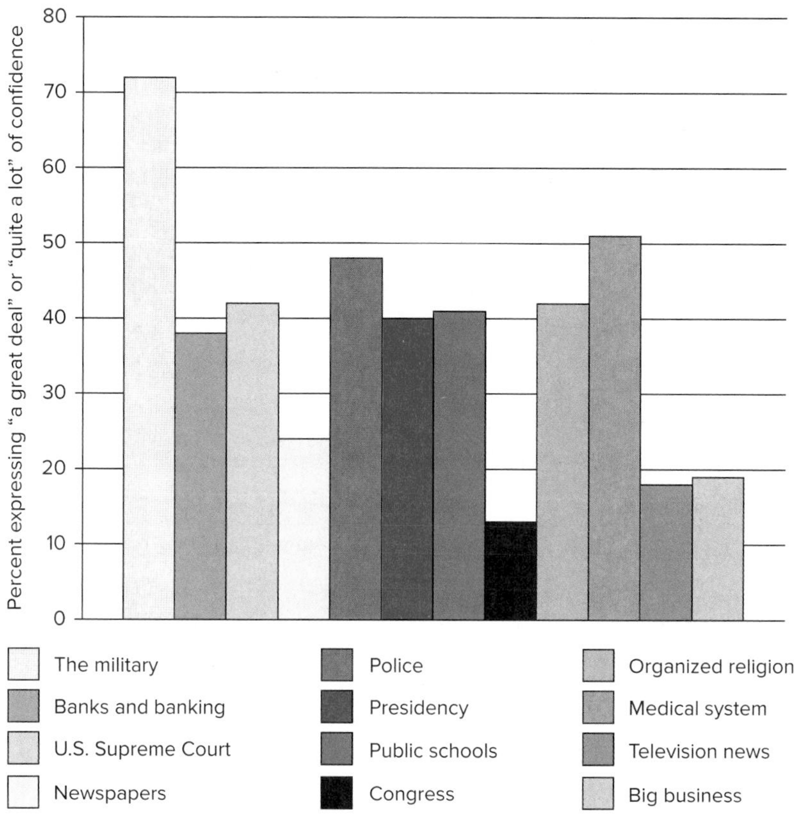


**FIGURE 9.1**
Public Confidence Levels in Selected Institutions, 2020.
Source: Gallup Poll website.

but the Watergate scandal of the Nixon administration seems to have had a particularly strong impact on people. Public confidence in government began to decline dramatically after the media exposed the break-in at the office of the Democratic National Committee and the attempts to cover up the involvement of President Nixon and officials in his administration.

Other events in the 1960s and 1970s–including the growing disillusionment with the Vietnam War and with the truth of official reports about the war–also contributed to the decline in confidence. Moreover, Americans have continued to learn about instances in which the government has not been truthful. What are people to think, for example, when they hear that the Central Intelligence Agency (CIA) admitted lying about the nature of unidentified flying objects (UFOs) in order to keep secret its growing fleet of spy planes, or that the Bush administration created an Office of Strategic Influence that would create news items, some of which would be false, in order to gain support for government decisions (Broad 1997; Wilson 2002)? Or that everyone could keep the health insurance they had once Obamacare passed? Or any of the thousands of lies chronicled during the Trump administration on everything from the trivial (it didn't rain during the inaugural speech) to the momentous (downplaying the COVID-19 virus and refuting scientific evidence with "alternative" facts) (Dale 2021). It's not surprising that in response to the question of how much of the time you can trust the federal government to do what is right, 2 percent of Americans in 2016, compared to 16 percent in 1958, said "just about always," whereas 42 percent in 2016, compared to 23 percent in 1958, said only "some of the time" (American National Election Studies 2020).

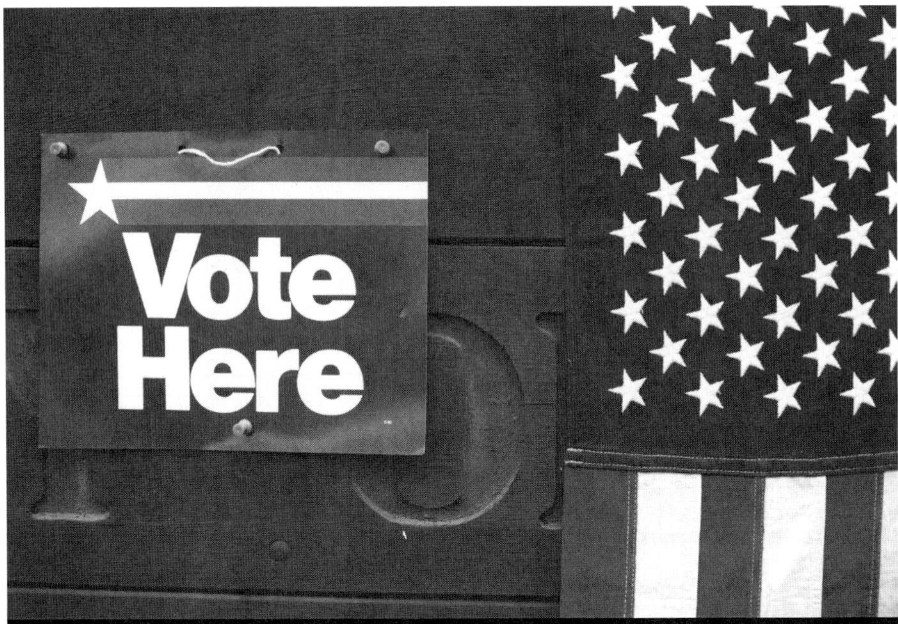


Despite efforts by some states to make it easier to register to vote, Americans seem reluctant to go to the polls at election time.

S. Meltzer/PhotoLink/Getty Images

Whatever the reasons for the distrust, it has produced at least four consequences we need to examine: the emergence of the Tea Party, the lack of citizen participation in the political process, altered voting patterns, and political alienation.

*Emergence of the Tea Party.* In 2009, Tea Party protests erupted around the nation. The dominant type of person in the movement was older, male, lower middle-class, and far-right Republican (Hood, Kidd, and Morris 2015). Economic anxiety and, to some extent, racial resentments characterized the participants (Patenaude 2019). As part of their protests, some Tea Party members dressed like 18th-century American revolutionaries. They claimed that the government, including many politicians in their own party, no longer worked in a way that was acceptable to them. They called for reduced government interference in people's lives and a no-compromise approach to governing. Buttressed by funds from wealthy conservatives and by support from far-right commentators in the media, they were able to influence a number of races in the 2010 elections (Skocpol and Williamson 2012). Members of Congress aligned with the Tea Party were able to force out the Republican Speaker of the House from office in 2015, and their no-compromise approach has contributed to governmental gridlock (see below). The future power of the Tea Party, however, is in doubt. Gallup polls show that support for it declined from 32 percent in 2010 to 17 percent in 2015 (Norman 2015). The point is, however, that whatever the fate of the Tea Party, extremist groups will continue to emerge in a society whose government is not trusted by the people.

*Lack of Citizen Participation.* If the approach of the Tea Party was to protest and work for candidates who support its viewpoint, the approach of others who distrust the government is to simply drop out. After all, why participate in the political process if you lack confidence in the government? Why vote if you believe that no matter who is elected the government will not function as it ought?

Although it is not the only reason for not voting, the *failure of trust is certainly one reason* for the relatively low proportion of Americans who vote (Jamieson, Shin, and Day 2002). It is not true, as some people believe, that low voter turnout is a new phenomenon

| Percentage of Voting-Age Population Casting Votes For: | | | Percentage of Voting-Age Population Casting Votes For: | | |
|---|---|---|---|---|---|
| Year | President | U.S. Representatives | Year | President | U.S. Representatives |
| 1932 | 52.5 | 49.7 | 1976 | 53.5 | 48.9 |
| 1936 | 56.9 | 53.5 | 1980 | 52.8 | 47.6 |
| 1940 | 58.9 | 55.4 | 1984 | 53.3 | 47.8 |
| 1944 | 56.0 | 52.7 | 1988 | 50.3 | 44.9 |
| 1948 | 51.1 | 48.1 | 1992 | 55.1 | 50.8 |
| 1952 | 61.6 | 57.6 | 1996 | 49.0 | 45.8 |
| 1956 | 59.3 | 55.9 | 2000 | 51.2 | 47.2 |
| 1960 | 62.8 | 58.5 | 2004 | 55.5 | 51.4 |
| 1964 | 61.9 | 57.8 | 2008 | 57.1 | 53.3 |
| 1968 | 60.9 | 55.1 | 2012 | 61.8 | 44.1 |
| 1972 | 55.2 | 50.7 | 2016 | 63.0 | n.a. |

**TABLE 9.1**
Participation in Presidential Elections, 1932–2016

SOURCE: U.S. Census Bureau website.

in American politics. Rather, the proportion of people voting has fluctuated over time. Between 1840 and 1908, the proportion who voted in presidential elections varied from about 65 to 82 percent of eligible voters (U.S. Census Bureau 1975:1071–72). The proportion then began to fall. As Table 9.1 shows, the proportion continued to vary between 1932 and 2016 but was never more than 63 percent for president or 58.5 percent for representatives. Voting proportions for representatives in nonpresidential year elections (these years are not shown in the table) are even lower, ranging from about 33 to 38 percent since 1974. In general, then, *about half to two-thirds of the voting-age population participates in national elections, and the proportion is much lower for state and local elections.*

The proportion of people who vote varies considerably by a number of demographic factors. More women than men tend to vote—63 percent of women and 59 percent of men in 2016 (Igielnik 2020). Older people tend to vote more than the young. By race/ethnicity, in the 2016 election, the proportion voting was as follows: white non-Hispanic, 65.3 percent; African American, 59.6 percent; other races, 49.3 percent; and Hispanic, 47.6 percent (File 2017).

At one time, many politicians believed that an important reason for low participation was the *difficulty of registering to vote.* In 1993, therefore, Congress passed the National Voter Registration Act, which required states to register voters at driver's license and motor vehicle bureaus, welfare offices, and military recruiting stations. The new law made it easier to register but has not had a significant impact on voting participation. In fact, when asked why they did not vote, the most common reason given by a national sample was that the individual was "too busy" or had a schedule conflict (U.S. Census Bureau website). Clearly, more than ease of registration is needed to bring more people to the polls.

*Altered Voting Patterns.* A third consequence of the failure of trust is altered voting patterns. That is, whereas some people neglect to vote, others *change the way they would have voted under conditions of high levels of trust.* In particular, third parties are likely to benefit when people do not trust the government. A study of the third-party nominees such as George Wallace, John Anderson, and Ross Perot concluded that lower citizen trust levels strongly predicted a vote for them (Hanenberg and Rojanapithayakorn 1998). The number of votes received by third-party candidates has varied from as few as 9,000 (for the People's Party in 1972) to as many as 19.7 million (for H. Ross Perot

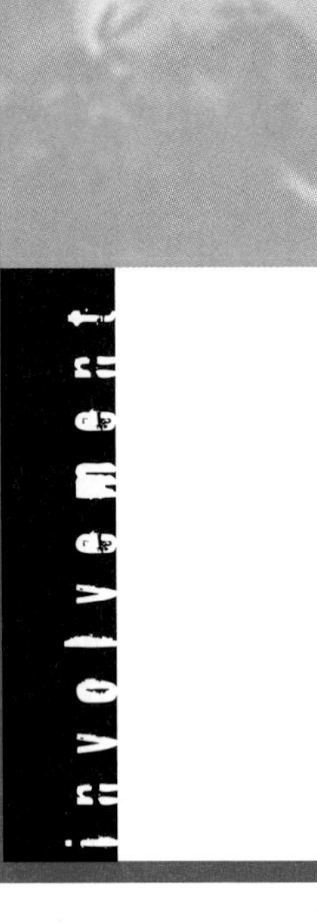


## WHY DON'T PEOPLE TRUST THE GOVERNMENT?

As noted in the text, researchers who have surveyed people about their confidence in American institutions have not asked about the reasons for their responses. Why do most people have little confidence in the government, whereas others still have a good deal of confidence?

Conduct your own survey. Ask 10 people how much confidence they have in the federal, state, and local governments. Have them respond to one of four choices: a great deal, quite a lot, some, or very little. Then ask them why they responded as they did. Use follow-up questions until you feel you fully understand their reasoning.

We hope that you found people whose responses fell into each of these four categories. Why did they respond as they did? Can you categorize their responses (e.g., "Politicians are self-serving." "The whole system is flawed.")? How do your respondents' answers differ by level of government? What conclusions would you draw about Americans' views of their government if your respondents are typical?

If the entire class participates in this project, assign different social categories for the interviews. Assign the following kinds of respondents to various class members: males, females, whites, African Americans, Hispanics. Tabulate all the results and note any gender, racial, and ethnic differences.

of the Independent Party in 1992) (U.S. Census Bureau website). When the number of people voting for third-party candidates is large, it can change the outcome. An analysis of the 2000 election concluded that the 2.5 million votes cast for Ralph Nader were crucial to the election of George Bush over Al Gore for the presidency (Magee 2003). In elections with no third-party candidates, distrustful voters are more likely to vote against the incumbent—whatever the incumbent's party affiliation (Hetherington 1999).

Political scientists and other observers of the political scene disagree on whether a two-party or multi-party system would be best for the nation (Montanaro 2017). But all agree that government and politics would be different under a three-party system. The three-party system might work better than the present two-party system, or it might create the kind of instability and inaction that have plagued some European nations.

If the failure of trust continues to intensify, Americans may well find out how they will be affected by a three-party system. Whether such a system will restore people's confidence in the government or simply plunge them into even deeper disillusionment is something that no one can say with certainty.

**political alienation** a feeling of political disillusionment, powerlessness, and estrangement

*Political Alienation.* The fourth consequence of the failure of trust is **political alienation,** *a feeling of political disillusionment, powerlessness, and estrangement.* Alienated people lose interest in political life (Southwell 2008). They do not necessarily blame individual politicians for the sorry state of affairs in political life. And they are not merely turned off by the mudslinging and broken promises and endless conflict in the political arena. Rather, they are *disillusioned with the entire system,* including the voting process. For example, just after the 2016 election, 24 percent of Americans believed that there is "a lot" of fraud in elections, and only 47 percent believed that the votes were counted properly (Polling Report 2020).

In short, alienated people believe that the system itself is fundamentally flawed (Scher 1997). For such people, it will take more than appeals to civic duty to involve them once again in the nation's political life.

### Waste, Corruption, and Scandals

Americans believe they have a right to expect effectiveness, efficiency, and honesty from the politicians who are running their government. Unfortunately, Americans believe they observe contrary qualities—waste, corruption, and scandals—in those

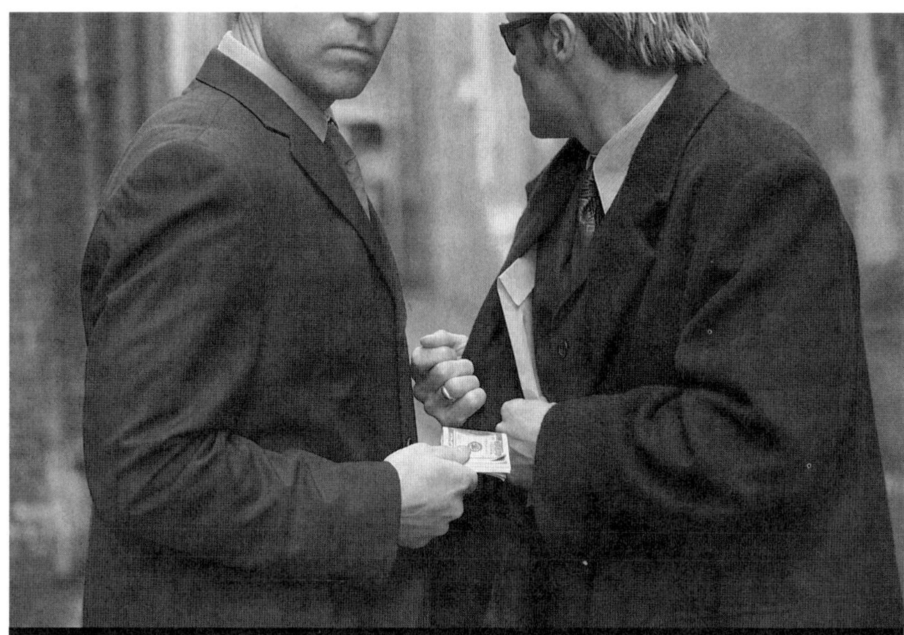

Many Americans think corruption is widespread in politics.
James Lauritz/Getty Images

politicians. In a Gallup poll, half of Americans said they have "somewhat negative" or "very negative" feelings about the federal government (Newport 2020). Moreover, professional assessments of government effectiveness and efficiency do little to change those beliefs. In 2000, for example, various news media reported the results of a study by the Government Performance Review Project of Syracuse University's Maxwell School of Citizenship and Public Affairs (Allen 2000). The researchers looked at the 20 federal agencies that have the most contact with the public and gave them an overall grade of B−. Work done by the agencies includes such activities as cleaning up New York Harbor, administering the national park system, overseeing air traffic, and ensuring that immigrants are in the nation legally. Some agencies did much better than others, but all suffered from such problems as reduced funding in the face of expanded workloads and political interference with their tasks.

Some government tasks, in other words, are not being carried out effectively or efficiently because of political decisions. "Government waste," on the other hand, refers to such things as excessive *paperwork, excessive costs, and unnecessary expenditures.* A number of groups and individuals, including politicians, work on identifying and publicizing examples of wasteful spending by the government. In recent years, for example, the following are a few of the funded projects that some would call waste (Schow 2019). $708 thousand was given to get Zebrafish addicted to nicotine in the U.K. $84 thousand was spent to purchase a statue sculpted by Bob Dylan that was placed in the embassy in Mozambique. And $22 million was designated to help bring Serbian cheese up to international standards.

fallacy

You want to beware of the *fallacy of non sequitur* at this point. It does not follow that, when a particular project sounds pointless or unreasonable, it clearly represents government waste. What one group calls "waste," such as some environmental projects, might be considered important and needed by another group. Nevertheless, no one disputes the fact that waste is a serious problem of government at all levels.

Nor does anyone dispute the *existence of fraud, corruption, and scandals.* A government official estimated that 5 percent of all federal spending in 2005 was lost to fraud, much of it to defense contractors and companies with contracts to rebuild Iraq (Kopecki 2006). In the early 2000s, a number of members of congress were indicted and jailed or forced out of office by various kinds of corrupt practices and ethics violations, including a sex scandal (homosexual overtures to a Congressional page), bribery, exchanging favorable legislation for campaign contributions, using legislative power to enhance their personal wealth, and using their positions to obtain financial benefits for family members (Sloan 2006). For example, one congressman went to prison for amassing personal wealth by agreeing to get government contracts for various businesses in return for monetary payoffs. Another congressman named his wife as his campaign fund-raiser. She had no other clients and no experience in fund-raising. But she received 15 percent of all funds raised for his campaign. And still another congressman had to resign after nearly 12 years in office because he used campaign funds to live in luxury (expensive meals, trips with women with whom he was having affairs, and paying for the tuition of his children's private schools) (Cook and McDonald 2020).

Such things are not new, of course. There is a long history of corruption and scandals in government at every level. In general, the instances of corruption or scandal involve *a politician acting in terms of self-interest or particular interests to the detriment of the politician's constituency or the general public.* The outcome is not only economic waste but also negative attitudes toward the government and lower levels of trust in government officials (Anderson and Tverdova 2003). In fact, public corruption is so threatening to the well-being of government that it is a top-priority item in FBI criminal investigations. According to the agency website, the FBI is investigating more than 2,000 cases of corruption involving public officials in the nation, and in 2010 it recorded more than 900 convictions.

**patronage**
giving government jobs to people who are members of the winning party

A corrupt practice that is less common today than earlier in the nation's history is **patronage,** giving government jobs to people who are members of the winning party. Recall that one of the fundamental characteristics of a bureaucracy is the expertise of workers. Yet politicians have often hired, or used their influence to obtain employment for, relatives, friends, and party workers no matter their level of expertise. This practice is less common than it once was because the bulk of government jobs now come under civil service. But the fundamental principle of rewarding those who support the winners is still carried out in other ways. Thus, states that support the winning presidential candidate, or that have a governor of the same party as the winning candidate, are likely to receive more federal funds than are other states (Larcinese, Rizzo, and Testa 2006). A study of contracts awarded to companies to engage in postwar reconstruction in Afghanistan and Iraq found that campaign contributions and political connections were important factors in securing a contract (Hogan, Long, Stretesky, and Lynch 2006). And a study of states reported that politicians used state-level patronage to increase their chances of maintaining control over various state elective offices (Folke, Hirano, and Snyder 2011).

Corruption may also take the form of "stuffing the ballot box" or other methods of rigging elections. The outcome of the 2000 presidential election was delayed for weeks by disputed votes in Florida (Cannon, Lavelle, and Ragavan 2000; Slevin and Kovaleski 2000). Initially, the news media projected a Democratic victory. Later, they said it was too close to call. After some recounts, the final tally gave George W. Bush an extremely narrow edge over Al Gore. Charges of impropriety quickly surfaced, including flawed ballots, improper instructions, questionable counting methods, and discrimination against nonwhite voters. Democrats took their case to the Florida Supreme Court and, eventually, to the U.S. Supreme Court, whose ruling ensured a narrow victory for George W. Bush. Florida subsequently changed its voting system and abolished the use of punch-card ballots. Americans may never know for certain which candidate was actually preferred by a majority of the Florida voters.

What we do know is that many people were illegally purged from voters rolls (a list sent to election officials included the names of 8,000 Florida residents who had committed misdemeanors rather than the felonies for which they could legitimately be purged) (American Civil Liberties Union 2004). There were also efforts to intimidate Black and Hispanic voters (Miller 2005).

### Gridlock

Frequently, the government seems *mired in inaction,* unable to legislate new policies because of ideological conflict, party differences, or a standoff between the executive and legislative branches of the government. Such a situation is known as **gridlock** (Brady and Volden 1998). Gridlock may reflect the fact that politicians are taking stands in accord with contradictory values and are unable to reach a compromise. However, gridlock also occurs when politicians are engaged in power struggles in which who is in control is more important than what gets done (Chiou and Rothenberg 2003).

**gridlock**
the inability of the government to legislate significant new policies

Gridlock can occur at any level of government. In the late 1990s, a number of states experienced gridlock because they had an increased number of decisions to make after the federal government deferred certain issues to the state level (Levy 1999). For example, in New York the 1999 gridlock prevented passage of the state budget, which was three months late. This delay hampered planning by schools and other nonprofit groups, and important health care proposals languished in political limbo. At the federal level, partisan gridlock in Congress prevented legislation that would fix defects in the No Child Left Behind law, which deals with how schools prepare and evaluate students. Both political parties agreed that changes were needed, but they could not agree on how to fix the problems. By 2012, President Obama began giving states waivers on meeting the existing law's requirements until the gridlock could be broken (Associated Press 2012).

The problem grew more severe during the Trump administration. As one U.S. senator put it, "The Senate has literally forgotten how to function" (Stolberg and Fandos 2018). This is troublesome, because gridlock is likely to maintain or even intensify the failure of trust. A government mired in inaction appears weak to the public it supposedly serves.

## Government, Politics, and the Quality of Life

As with all the problems we are examining, government and politics affect the quality of life of great numbers of people. We consider here the way government action or inaction leads to three problem areas that affect quality of life: unequal opportunities for a high quality of life, inadequate protection of freedoms and rights, and the lack of responsiveness to needs.

### Unequal Opportunities for a High Quality of Life

Today, Americans generally expect government to maintain an equitable distribution of power so that they have an equal opportunity to secure a high quality of life. Politicians themselves acknowledge their role in this quest for a high quality of life. As we wrote this chapter, we searched the Internet for "quality of life and government." The following are among the tens of thousands of items we found:

- The New York City site encouraged citizens to record complaints related to, and point out problems that detract from, their quality of life.
- A Los Angeles news item discussed local government's role in the city's quality-of-life goals.
- A Kansas City report discussed local elections and their consequences for the area's quality of life.
- A Jacksonville, Florida, annual report considered the quality of life in the community.
- An item from Chicago talked about the county government's role in the area's quality of life.
- A report from Philadelphia noted receipt of a grant to combat crimes that depress the city's quality of life.

Clearly, *politicians and citizens alike expect government at all levels to have a role in those matters that affect the quality of life.* Yet government has not measured up to these expectations and maintained a system in which all Americans have an equal opportunity to reap the benefits deemed necessary for a high quality of life. We noted in the previous three chapters various ways in which some groups benefit to the detriment of others: how, for instance, the wealthy benefit more than the poor from tax laws and other government policies and practices and how white males have more opportunities than do women or people of either sex from racial and ethnic minorities.

*These disadvantages mean a lower quality of life for whole groups of people.* For example, African Americans, Hispanics, and people in the lower socioeconomic strata have higher rates of negative mood, such as feelings of sadness, than do whites and people in the higher strata (Blackwell, Collins, and Coles 2002).

The relationship between advantages and quality of life holds true in other nations as well. Surveys of people's sense of their well-being in 55 nations, representing three-fourths of the earth's population, found that the higher the income and the greater the amount of equality in the nation, the higher the people's sense of well-being (Diener, Diener, and Diener 1995).

In essence, then, *the government has failed to maintain a social system in which all individuals, regardless of their social origins, have equal opportunities.* People do not expect equal outcomes. The nation's ideology is that anyone can succeed, but no one expects the government to ensure that every individual achieves the highest quality of life. However, Americans do expect the government to ensure a system in which no one's quality of life is diminished automatically because of his or her sex or social origins.

## Inadequate Protection of Individual Rights

There is also *a contradiction between the value of individual rights and the way government functions to protect them.* As we noted in the last two chapters, government has not always protected the rights of women and of racial and ethnic minorities. In addition, government has threatened or violated certain basic rights that every citizen ideally possesses. For example, for many years the FBI secretly gathered information and kept files on thousands of Americans who openly opposed certain government programs and policies. Some of this information was secured by illegal means, such as breaking and entering or unauthorized taps of telephone lines. Among those under surveillance by the bureau were Martin Luther King Jr. and others in the civil rights movement.

It is important to acknowledge that at least a part of the problem of inadequate protection of individual rights lies in the *dilemma faced by government—how can individual rights and social order both be preserved?* A classic instance of the dilemma is the clash between individual rights and national security. During World War II, the clash was decided in favor of national security, resulting in the internment of around 100,000 Japanese Americans. Even though they were American citizens, they were viewed as a threat because of the war with Japan. Whether this was justified is still a matter of debate (Maki 2019). Some observers affirm the internment as the proper course of action. Others, however, have concluded that Japanese American citizens were deprived of their rights; in fact, lawsuits were instituted in the 1990s to obtain reparations for the injustice.

Individual rights versus national security remains a prominent issue. In the 1990s, various right-wing militias, fringe groups, and Islamic militants engaged in acts of violence against the government. These acts increased the pressure for measures that are likely to violate individual rights such as more covert domestic spying and information gathering by the government. We explore this issue in more detail in Chapter 14.

Additional areas in which individual rights may be threatened or suppressed by government include the criminal justice system, free speech on—and use of—the Internet, drug policies, the rights of immigrants, the rights of homosexuals, police practices, the right to privacy, and religious freedom (see the American Civil Liberties Union website). Consider, for example, the situation of some immigrants. The Immigration and Naturalization Service (INS) uses secret evidence in a small number of cases to deport people considered potential threats. Most of the cases involve Arabs or Muslims who cannot fight the deportation order because they do not have access to the "evidence."

The Freedom of Information Act of 1966 addressed at least some of the problems of individual rights (Unsworth 1999). The act gave the public access to government records and documents. Access is limited to records of the executive branch and only to those materials that have been "declassified" (i.e., that are not a threat to national security). The number of documents declassified has varied depending on the president. Presidents Nixon and Carter expanded declassification, whereas President Reagan restricted it. President Clinton tried to expand it once again. Unfortunately, even if material is declassified, there is no penalty imposed on an agency that refuses to comply with a citizen's request. The issue of the protection of individual rights continues to be a nettlesome one.

## Lack of Responsiveness to Needs

Any satisfying relationship, including the relationship individuals have with organizations, *requires give and take.* If you find school a satisfying experience, for example, it is because you have given your time, money, and energy to complying with the school's requirements and have gained from your classes the knowledge and credentials needed to pursue your goals. People expect the same sort of give and take from government. Yet some Americans perceive the government to be all "take"–in the form of taxes and the demand for compliance with laws and regulations–and no "give"–in the sense of being unresponsive to the needs of the citizenry (see "Why Isn't There Help for People Like Me?" at the beginning of the chapter). Of course, a substantial number of Americans believe that both the "take" and the "give" should be minimal. That is, they accept the ideology that the smaller and less intrusive the government is, the better off people will be. However, three researchers examined data from a number of developed countries around the world over the period from 1981 to 2007 (Flavin, Pacek, and Radcliff 2014). They concluded that the citizenry finds life more satisfying as governmental intervention in the economy increases.

In the United States, there is often considerable opposition to any additional action by the government. The opposition can come from within the government itself, and it may take the form of a refusal to act or a public promise to action without the action ever taking place. For example, in 2005 when Hurricane Katrina devastated the city of New Orleans, officials at all levels, from the president to the governor to the mayor, promised full and rapid aid to victims. Yet the aid was minimal and slow in coming. When President Bush visited New Orleans shortly after the hurricane struck, he promised "one of the largest reconstruction efforts the world has ever seen" (Krugman 2006). The governor of Louisiana and the mayor of New Orleans also issued statements promising aid. However, two researchers who investigated the efforts to rebuild the city and help the citizenry recover described the outcome in terms of "malfeasance, official deviance and the failure to serve and protect a community" (Herron and Smith 2012).

Similar inadequate responses occurred when Hurricane Maria devastated Dominica, St Croix, and Puerto Rico in September 2017. It was the worst natural disaster in recorded history in that area, causing the death of nearly 3,000 people. Two years later, federal data showed that Congress had authorized $42.5 billion in disaster aid for Pureto Rico. But the island had received less than $14 billion (Timm 2019).

Sometimes the government doesn't just fail to respond adequately, it takes action that inflicts harm on people. Perhaps the most egregious example of this was the Flint, Michigan, water crisis (Denchak 2018). Flint is a small city with a high rate of poverty and a large African American population. The governor appointed a manager to cut costs to reduce the city's debt.

In 2013, the manager decided to save money by taking water from the Flint river rather than from Detroit while a new water pipeline from Lake Huron was being built. But officials failed to treat the river water properly.

Thousands of Flint children drank lead-contaminated water for 18 months. The contaminated water also led to an outbreak of Legionnaire's disease. Eventually, a financial settlement was reached for victims. But the impaired health and deaths remain as a grim testament to governmental failure.

Given such incidents, it's understandable that people become cynical. They begin to view *government not as their protector and safety net, but as their competitor for the good things of life, or even as their enemy.* The citizens lose an important source of security and confidence, and the government loses a substantial amount of commitment to civic duty as people ignore or subvert laws and regulations whenever they feel they can do so with impunity.

## Contributing Factors

Although many Americans blame inept or self-serving politicians, the problems of government cannot be reduced to defects in elected officials. You don't want to engage in the *fallacy of personal attack* and claim that the problems of government will be solved when present officials are replaced with better ones. Rather, you must recognize and deal with the varied social structural and social psychological factors that create and help perpetuate the problems of government.

fallacy

### Social Structural Factors

*Size.* "There is no country in the world today where the entire government establishment of 1910 could not comfortably be housed in the smallest of the new government buildings now going up, with room to spare for a grand-opera house and a skating rink" (Drucker 1968:172). This assessment, now more than five decades old, dramatizes the growth of government. Figure 9.2 illustrates that growth. Note that, contrary to the beliefs of many Americans, the federal government has not been growing (at least, in terms of the number of people employed). There are fewer people working for the federal government now than there were in the 1980s. Employment by state and local governments, on the other hand, has increased considerably over the past few decades. In 1982, federal civilian employment stood at 2.85 million; by 2019, the number had dropped to 2.7 million. In contrast, there were 12.99 million state and local government employees in 1982, and 14.9 million by 2019.

Of course, the number of people employed is not the only way to measure size. In addition to those directly employed, there are those who provide goods and services under contracts, grants, and mandates (Light 2020). These add millions more people to the size of government.

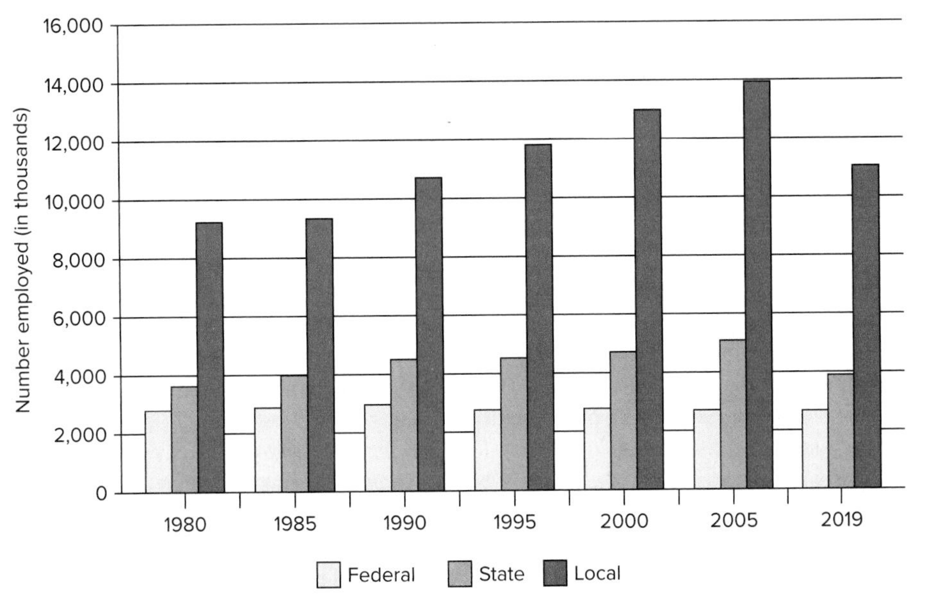


**FIGURE 9.2**
Government Employees, 1980–2019.
Source: U.S. Census Bureau website.

*The growth of government reflects both a growing population and a growing number of functions and services assumed by government.* Government was smaller and simpler in the early years of the nation. There were far fewer people and a more homogeneous population. There were also no income taxes to collect, no services to the poor to regulate, no monitoring and regulating of the conduct of businesses, no governmental health care obligations, no elaborate defense system to support, and so on. Whether the size of government today is necessary may be debatable, but a substantial amount of the growth was either inevitable because of the growing population or a response to public demand for protection or assistance.

Still, *size—both the size of government and size of the population—has consequences for functioning.* Consider the size of government. It is more difficult for large organizations to be efficient and responsive to the needs of people. Questions must be addressed and procedures must be followed that are not necessary when individuals help each other or small community organizations help people locally. When an individual seeks assistance from the federal government, for example, such questions as the following arise: What agency is responsible for helping? Who in the agency should handle the situation? What procedures (including filling out necessary paperwork) must be followed to meet the requirement of accountability? Who in the agency and/or other government organizations must approve the assistance? And so on. In the case of entire groups who need help (the poor, those suffering discrimination, those without health insurance, etc.), the questions and answers become even more complicated and demanding.

The size of the governed population also affects function. It is more difficult to gain compliance and enforce rules when regulating a large number of people. For instance, Ehrenhalt (1997) reported that there were nearly 3.1 million outstanding violations of the New York City housing code in 1996. However, the city's 200 inspectors could make only about 160,000 inspections per year. Most of the violations, therefore, can never be addressed. As Ehrenhalt noted, the city government's failure to respond to these violations is rooted in neither indifference nor ineptness. Rather, there are simply more citizens violating the law "than even the most efficient government can possibly keep track of." It may be that the difficulties of effectively governing large cities is one reason two researchers found in a study of 55 American cities that the larger the size of the city, the less trust the citizens had in their local government (Rahn and Rudolph 2005).

It is also more difficult to adequately represent the people when their number and diversity increase. Consider the fact that the U.S. House of Representatives has remained at 435 members since 1911, which means that now a House member represents on average more than 760,000 citizens. Clearly, the extent to which a representative can function effectively for that number of constituents is limited. In fact, as the size of a district increases, both the accessibility to and the approval of the representative diminishes.

*The Structure of Government.* Two aspects of the structure of government contribute to the problems. The first is the extent to which a government is a political democracy. Frey and Al-Roumi (1999), who define democracy as the extent to which a nation maintains political rights and civil liberties for the citizenry, gathered data on the quality of life from 87 countries of the world. Quality of life was measured by infant mortality rate, literacy rate, and life expectancy. They found *a strong relationship between the level of political democracy and the quality of life in the nations.* It seems that such advantages as competitive elections, the opportunity for all citizens to participate in the political process, and a free press contribute to the government's being more responsive to people's needs and implementing policies that enhance their well-being. To the extent that political democracy is maintained, the government is more of a solution than a problem.

The other aspect of structure is *the way the government is organized to fulfill its functions.* In the United States, the federal system provides a constitutional separation of powers between the national and state governments. In addition, there are county, municipal, and township governments. All have direct authority over individuals. This arrangement creates unity without enforcing uniformity, encourages experimentation, and keeps government close to the people (Burns et al. 2005).

However, there are disadvantages as well. What level of government is best equipped to provide efficient and effective service? What level of government is responsible for dealing with various social problems? Consider, for example, the following questions: Is a safety net for the poor the primary responsibility of the federal government or of state and local governments? Who is going to handle problems of discrimination based on race/ethnicity, gender, age, or sexual orientation? Should there be national standards for education, or should education be completely under the control of local school boards?

An ongoing struggle among various levels of government over responsibility, or the efforts of government at one level to shift responsibility for a problem to government at another level, can result in an inadequate response to people's needs. As we discussed in Chapter 6, the current transfer of major responsibility for poverty from the federal to the state and local level in the form of workfare is having a negative impact on the quality of life of many of America's poor.

Finally, *the government is organized along bureaucratic lines in order to fulfill its various functions.* Look back at the characteristics of a bureaucracy that we discussed earlier, and you will see that it should be a highly efficient and effective form of large-scale administration. If people in a bureaucracy function according to the criteria we listed, the organization should help people expertly and impartially.

In practice, however, bureaucracies never measure up to the ideal. As a result, and in spite of many positive achievements, the very term "bureaucrat" has become a term of disparagement, and a wide variety of government problems are blamed on the bureaucrats. To blame bureaucrats, however, is to substitute the *fallacy of personal attack* for a realistic appraisal.

fallacy

There are various reasons for the disparity between the ideal and the reality. Middle-class bureaucrats may not treat lower-class citizens with the same respect and concern that they do citizens in higher classes. Bureaucrats who try to be impartial in their dealings with people face severe pressure and potential reprisals from individuals who want special consideration. Some government bureaucrats may be in positions for which they have not been properly trained and for which they lack needed expertise.

Other bureaucrats may rigidly follow the rules of the organization even if the rules don't apply well to particular cases. Two business writers once called such bureaucrats the "white-collar gestapo," arguing that they mindlessly enforce a growing number of arbitrary rules and regulations (McMenamin and Novack 1999). Indeed, even though the bureaucratic rules and regulations are supposed to cover all circumstances, you can raise the question of whether this is possible when dealing with a large, heterogeneous population. Perhaps bureaucrats need the flexibility to exercise more discretion.

Furthermore, in spite of the highly bureaucratic nature of government, *the government is not organized in a way to deal effectively with waste and corruption.* One way to stop waste and corruption would be to encourage employees to act as internal watchdogs and report such practices (to be "whistleblowers" in contemporary terminology). From time to time this happens. But in spite of the Whistleblower Protection Act, most government employees fear reprisals if they blow the whistle on

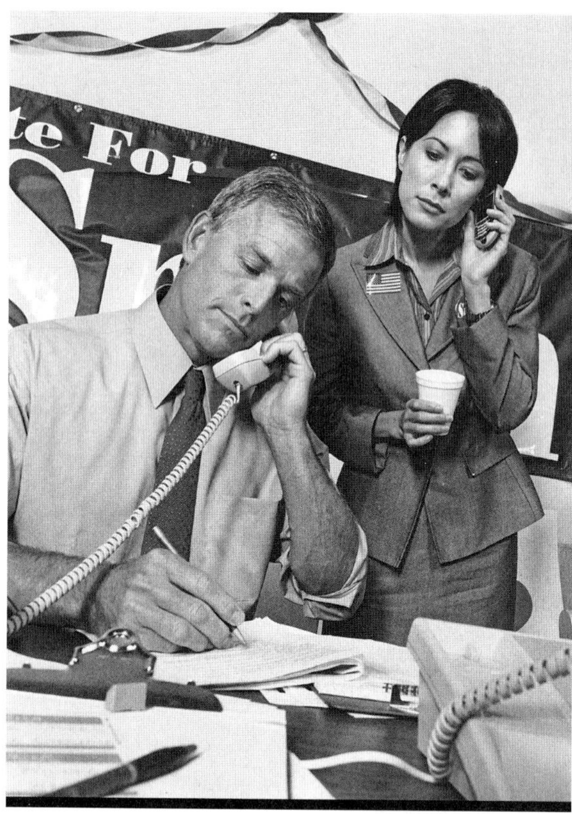


Campaigning for elective office is expensive, and critics argue that the wealthy are at an advantage when they have millions of dollars of their own money to spend in their efforts to be elected.

Digital Vision/Getty Images

corrupt or wasteful practices. Such fears are justified because whistleblowers are as likely to suffer retaliation (including demotion, loss of career, and even threats to their well-being) as to bring about a rectification of the problem they identify (Dehaven-Smith 2011).

*The Economics of Campaigning.* How much would it cost you to become a U.S. senator? It would depend on the state in which you ran, of course, and the amount of opposition you faced. But political advisers can put a price tag—and the price is steep—on every race from the presidency to local offices.

The cost of political office is not only high but has, as shown in Figure 9.3, been on an upward path. The 2020 election was the most expensive ever, with the total amount spent in the congressional and presidential races reaching the $14 billion mark (Goldmacher 2020).

The cost of political office will continue to soar because of the 2010 Supreme Court decision to allow corporations and individuals to spend as much as they want on political advertising as long as the ads are not coordinated with the candidates' campaigns. The controversial ruling led to the creation of so-called Super PACs, organizations that create ads in support of particular candidates (and sometimes are run by former advisers or staff members of those candidates). The Super PACs are often able to pour enough money into particular campaigns to literally buy offices for their preferred candidates.

In light of the costs of running a campaign, *it is evident that people without access to considerable sums of money or money-raising skills are unlikely to win an election.* In recent decades, some very wealthy individuals have invested millions from their own fortunes as they sought political office. Such a use of personal wealth raises the concern that the nation may be entering a time when only the rich can successfully run for office.

In order to gain and remain in office, whether they are personally rich or not, politicians need massive amounts of money. This need makes politicians beholden to the wealthy and to various interest groups. A politician may be able to vote against the interests and preferences of those who support him or her only at the cost of continuing in office. The fact that poor people in a politician's district have pressing needs for various kinds of aid is not likely to take priority over the interests of the wealthy individuals and interest groups that provide the money that keeps the politician in office.

Some measures have been taken to *reform campaign financing,* which became a hotly debated issue in the late 1990s. In the 1970s, Congress set up the Federal Election Commission and limited the amount that individuals can contribute to a campaign. However, wealthy individuals and interest groups circumvent the intent of the law by giving so-called soft money, contributions directly to the party instead of to an individual candidate. Legislation in 2002 banned national parties from raising soft money. But politicians circumvented the law through "527 political organizations," which are political interest groups that are tax-exempt under Section 527 of the Internal Revenue Code and have not been regulated by the Federal Election Commission. Clearly, campaign financing remains problematic.

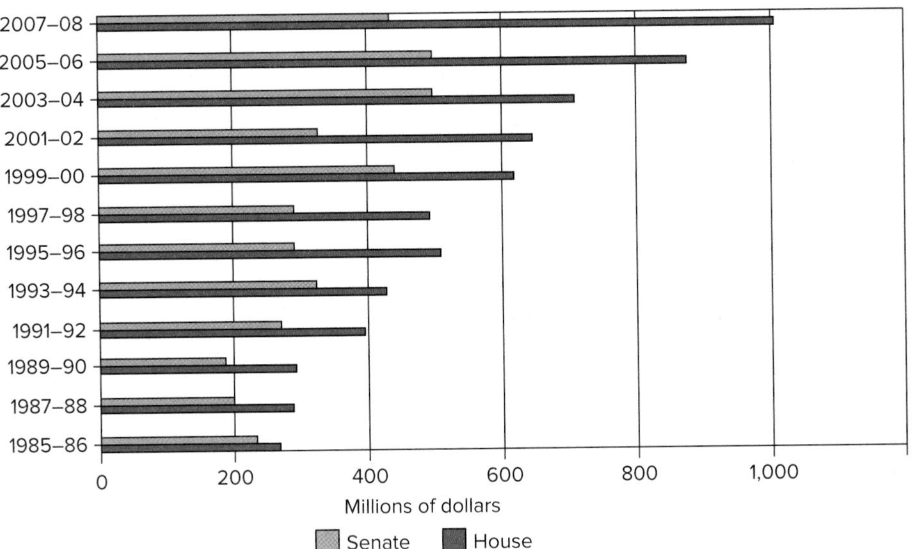


**FIGURE 9.3**
Cost of Congressional Campaigns.
Source: U.S. Census Bureau website.

*The Media.* In the first of the televised presidential debates in 1960, Richard Nixon looked unkempt and nervous in contrast to John F. Kennedy, who appeared crisp and confident. Although Nixon won the debate among radio listeners, Kennedy came out ahead among television watchers. This event began a new era in the relationship between media coverage and election results.

The media have always played a role in American politics, of course—but *both the nature of the coverage and the influence of the media have changed as radio, network television, cable television, and now the Internet have been added to the print media as factors in the political process.* Let's explore the impact of the media on three aspects of political life: elections, political agendas and action, and public trust.

First, the media are important in political campaigns. For one thing, advertising by candidates accounts for a substantial proportion of the enormous costs of campaigns. Television advertising is particularly expensive, but it is necessary *because a substantial proportion of Americans rely on television for their political news* and television ads affect the outcome of elections (Drew and Weaver 2006; Grieco 2020). Relying on television means that voters get less information than is provided by the print media or radio because they depend heavily on "sound bites"—those brief excerpts from the campaign trail that, in the opinion of television editors, capture something informative about the candidate's position or something newsworthy or sensational about the candidate's activities. Sound bites generally consume less than 10 seconds, raising the question of how much accurate information they convey about a candidate's position.

In addition to television, the social media of candidates are an important source of information. Unfortunately, those who get their news from social media are less knowledgeable than those who use other sources (Mitchell et al. 2020). In the 2016 election, about a fourth of U.S. adults turned to social media posts by the two presidential candidates (Shearer 2016). That was far more than the 10 percent who relied on the candidates' websites or the nine percent who relied on e-mails from the candidates. Overall, a third of Americans got most of their election news from at least one of the three sources.

## BUREAUCRACY IN INDONESIA

As noted in the text, bureaucrats are supposed to have expertise and act impartially in accord with written rules—but they do not always function that way. In some areas of Indonesia, for example, people are able to purchase positions in the government bureaucracy; they need money, not expertise, to secure the position (Kristiansen and Ramli 2006). Dwight King (1998a, 1998b) made an intensive study of the Indonesian civil service and found a number of additional reasons the bureaucracy falls short of the ideal.

The Indonesian civil service is organized in 17 ranks. Each employee has a grade and a step ranking within the grade that is based on education and seniority. Employees who perform their duties well advance one step every four years and eventually can qualify for a higher grade. At a certain level, however, the employees must acquire additional education or pass a test in order to continue their advancement.

In spite of this apparently well-organized arrangement, there is often a disparity between an individual's qualifications and the requirements of the position that he or she holds. For instance, an individual who has a graduate degree in liberal arts might be promoted to the head of the agency on public works because no one with an engineering degree is in as high a grade at the time as is the liberal arts graduate. Bureaucrats' educational attainment and civil service grade are more important in determining where they work in the government than is their educational specialization.

In addition, a substantial number of civil servants are promoted even when they have not reached the required grade. Two practices are at work here. One is to promote someone to an "acting" position. The other is to utilize an exception clause in the regulations that allows individuals who have performed in an "extraordinary" way for two years to be promoted even when they are not in the necessary grade.

The point is, voters' knowledge of candidates and their positions comes either from the candidates' brief postings or from the other electronic media. What appears in the media, therefore, affects how people vote. The way the media interpret an incumbent president's performance, for example, strongly influences his or her chances for re-election (Dover 1998). Similarly, a study of House elections and the media concluded that incumbents have an advantage, particularly among less educated voters, because they have had more television coverage and much of that coverage is positive (Prior 2006). In fact, the more television stations in a district, the greater the advantage of the incumbent.

While television continues to be a major source of political information, the Internet has become an increasingly powerful political tool. By the time of the 2010 elections, 24 percent of Americans (compared to 7 percent in 2002) said that the Internet was their main source of campaign news (Smith 2011). The proportion was highest among the young (35 percent of those aged 18–29), the college educated (34 percent), and those in the higher ($75,000 and above) income brackets (32 percent). In the 2008 election, Barack Obama supporters were far more active on the Internet than were supporters of John McCain, which was one of the factors in Obama's election to the presidency.

It was not the first time the Internet played a key role in a campaign. In 2004, bloggers and sites such as the Drudge Report helped George W. Bush defeat John Kerry by raising doubts about such matters as Kerry's status as a war hero (Feld and Wilcox 2008). In fact, the large, active number of political activists on the Internet, and the clear nature

For some functions, the Indonesian government bureaucracy is also hampered by the lack of clearly defined areas of responsibility. For example, three different agencies have responsibility for education: the Ministry of Education and Culture (MOEC), the Ministry of Home Affairs (MOHA), and the Ministry of Religious Affairs (MORA). MOEC is responsible for secondary and higher education, but shares responsibility for primary education with MOHA. MORA is responsible for the Islamic schools, which are mainly at the post-primary level.

This dispersion of responsibility has negative consequences for Indonesian education. First, little effort is made to improve primary education because neither MOEC nor MOHA seeks the resources needed. MOHA secures funding for primary education, but has not sought additional funds because it is responsible for funding, not for quality. MOEC is aware of the need for improvement, but funding is not part of its responsibility.

Second, some schools do not receive the resources they need. For example, MOEC publishes textbooks and sends them to regional warehouses. From there, the regional government is supposed to distribute them to the schools. But the regional governments complain that they do not have the necessary funds to distribute books. Thus, some schools, particularly those in relatively isolated areas, may not receive needed texts and materials.

Third, career advancement for primary school teachers occurs in the context of the contrary decisions of MOEC and regional governments. MOEC evaluates the teachers' performance. Regional governments, however, make promotion and transfer decisions—often independently of MOEC evaluations.

In sum, government bureaucracy in Indonesia is similar to that in other nations: It falls short of the bureaucratic ideal. Yet it does no good to simply complain of "bureaucrats." A different set of people in the same system would make little or no difference in the outcome. It is the way the bureaucracy is organized, not the kind of people in it, that is primarily responsible for the problems.

of the impact they can have, has given rise to the term *"netroots."* Netroots (from Inter*net* and grass*roots*) refers to the networks of those who use the Internet as their primary medium to engage in political discussion and action. It is imperative for a candidate for political office to have (and most do) a netroots coordinator who can both monitor and try to influence information being passed around the Internet.

The second impact of the media is on political agendas and government actions. The influence of the media is not limited to elections. As Cook (1998) argued, *the media are an integral part of the governing of the nation.* Government officials use the media to shape public opinion and gain support for decisions and programs. In turn, officials are influenced in their decision-making process by the information they glean from the media. To a considerable extent, the media help decide what are the issues, problems, and crises to which political leaders must respond.

If the media were impartial and always accurate, their influence would not be a cause for concern. But news networks are owned by corporations, and the news they share tends to reflect the political leanings of the corporate leaders. Consider, for example, the effect on someone for whom MSNBC (a liberal network) or Fox News (a conservative network) is the sole source of news. Clearly, such a person would not have a realistic understanding of political affairs. Fox News is particularly biased. In fact, Common Cause, a nonpartisan watchdog group, and a liberal political advocacy group filed a petition with the Federal Trade Commission arguing that Fox should stop using its slogan of being "fair and balanced" in the news. In fact, the groups maintained, the news on Fox is consistently biased in favor of the Republican Party and right-wing perspectives. That such a biased perspective affects voters is shown in an analysis by two economists, who found that when Fox News becomes available in a town, Republicans gain votes (DellaVigna and Kaplan 2006).

fallacy

This point does not mean that media information is always biased or distorted. It does mean, however, that people must be careful not to engage in the *fallacy of authority* and assume that what comes to them through the media is *ipso facto* accurate and impartial. On the other hand, we must be careful not to overreact by dismissing everything in the media as unreliable. The Trump presidency saw an unprecedented attack on the media, particularly on reporters and TV newspeople whom the president defined as "the enemy of the people" proclaiming a relentless stream of "fake news." For supporters of the president, this campaign against the media intensified distrust in both the media and the government (Lee and Hosam 2020).

*Interest Groups.* The most effective way to influence a massive organization like government is through other organizations. The lone individual has little chance of bringing about change, but an organization can put considerable pressure on politicians. For that reason, *interest groups have become an increasingly important factor in American political life.*

There are at least 30,000 interest groups in the United States. Many have political action committees (PACs) that are registered with the government and legally entitled to raise funds and make contributions to election campaigns and political parties (Table 9.2). The number of political action committees grew considerably after 1980. PACs contribute hundreds of millions of dollars to candidates each presidential election year, a substantial amount of which comes from a relatively few wealthy donors. In 2020, PACs gave $248 million to Democrats and $238 million to Republicans (Center for Responsive Politics 2020).

**lobbyist**
an individual who tries to influence legislation in accord with the preferences of an interest group

Interest groups also hire **lobbyists,** individuals who try to influence legislation in accord with the preferences of the interest groups. *Lobbyists use various means to influence politicians.* They may provide a politician with information that supports the interest group's position on a given issue. They may try to cultivate personal friendships with particular politicians. They may treat a politician to expensive dinners and trips. In

**TABLE 9.2**
Number and Type of Political Action Committees

| | Number | | | |
|---|---|---|---|---|
| Type | 1980 | 1990 | 2000 | 2016 |
| Corporate | 1,206 | 1,795 | 1,523 | 1,621 |
| Labor | 297 | 346 | 316 | 278 |
| Trade, membership, and health | 576 | 774 | 812 | 926 |
| Nonconnected | 374 | 1,062 | 902 | 1,786 |
| Cooperative | 42 | 59 | 39 | 41 |
| Corporation without stock | 56 | 136 | 114 | 92 |
| Total | 2,551 | 4,172 | 3,706 | 5,819 |

SOURCE: Federal Election Commission 2016.

addition, there is always the promise of support through votes and contributions by members of the interest group.

The number of lobbyists in Washington, D.C., declined for the first time in decades in 2011, perhaps a reflection of legislative gridlock and a fragile economy (Eggen 2012). Still, the number of registered lobbyists was 12,600 (not all lobbyists register because the rules are unclear and the penalty for not registering is light), and the various interest groups who hired the lobbyists spent about $3.27 billion on lobbying efforts during the year. The money is not merely to pay the salaries of the lobbyists. One of the lures the lobbyist uses is a substantial contribution to a politician's campaign. The money is also used to wine and dine politicians, provide them with tickets to sporting events and concerts, offer them free trips, and provide them with gifts of various kinds.

The abuses of the practice were dramatized in 2006 when a powerful lobbyist, Jack Abramoff, pleaded guilty to fraud, tax evasion, and conspiring to bribe public officials (Stone 2006). Abramoff gained enormous personal wealth while funneling money and other perks to lawmakers in return for favorable legislation. Linkages with Abramoff cost a number of politicians their positions either through resignation or through defeat at the polls.

Another aspect of lobbying that most Americans find troublesome is the fact that many lobbyists are relatives of lawmakers or members of their staff (Eisler and Kelley 2006). In a poll, 80 percent of Americans agreed that it's wrong for relatives to lobby lawmakers. Nevertheless, an investigation reported 53 cases in one year in which members of the House or Senate appropriations committee or their top aides had relatives who were lobbyists. And of those relatives who attempted to get money in appropriations bills for their clients, 22 were successful.

## Social Psychological Factors

*Public Attitudes.* The American ideal is that government is of the people, by the people, and for the people. This statement means that government originates in the people, involves the people, and effectively represents them. Government is meant to be the people's ally, not their opponent. But consider some of the results of national polls in recent years:

- Only 37 percent of Americans have a great deal, or quite a lot, of confidence in the Supreme Court;
- only 11 percent of Americans have a great deal, or quite a lot, of confidence in Congress;
- 69 percent believe Super PACs should be illegal; and
- only 41 percent are satisfied with "the way things are going in the United States at this time."

While the numbers fluctuate and can even change rapidly, such attitudes reflect the failure of trust. They also help perpetuate the failure of trust. Instead of stimulating people to get involved in government and make necessary reforms, *negative attitudes lead to alienation and withdrawal from political life* (Plane and Gershtenson 2004).

The irony here is that people who believe that the government does not help them become alienated and do not bother to vote. But research shows that members of Congress not only strive to direct resources into their districts but also try to put those resources where they appear to pay off in terms of votes (Martin 2003). In other words, *alienation becomes a self-fulfilling prophecy* because negative attitudes lead to nonparticipation and nonparticipation results in fewer benefits.

In addition to negative attitudes about government and politics, a set of *contrary attitudes* contribute to the problem. Cronin and Genovese (1998) identified a number of these contrary attitudes in their discussion of the "nine paradoxes" of the American presidency:

Americans want strong leaders, but they also fear the abuse of power that a strong leader might bring to the office.

Americans have favorable attitudes toward ordinary people holding political office (thus, the traditional appeal of the candidate who was born in a log cabin), but they also value charisma in their leaders.

Americans want leaders who will unify the people, but they do not want to compromise their own positions in order to forge the unity.

Americans admire leaders with vision, but they also believe that leaders should be responsive to public opinion.

Moreover, Americans tend to approve of such items as lower taxes, reduced government spending, and less government interference in daily life. Yet Americans also resist proposals to reduce government or government spending in those areas from which they benefit or which they support for ideological reasons. In a Gallup poll, 54 percent of Americans said they want the government to do more to solve our country's problems, compared with 41 percent who said the government is trying to do too many things that should be left to individuals and businesses (Newport 2020).

Such contrary attitudes pose *a dilemma for politicians.* In essence, no matter what a politician does, some segment of the population will be disappointed and frustrated. The easiest course of action is to follow his or her conscience when possible and, at other times, follow the desires of those who contribute the funds necessary to stay in office.

*Ideologies.* Americans, for the most part, are suspicious of extreme ideologues and value compromise in resolving political conflicts. Indeed, when politicians of opposing ideologies work together, the result is usually compromise; but under some circumstances, the result may be gridlock. Brady and Volden (1998) studied legislative gridlock in the U.S. Congress. They concluded that members of Congress fall at various points on a liberal-conservative continuum. The median ideology of Congress is also somewhere on this continuum. Recall that the median is the point at which half the cases are above and half are below. For example, if you use −10 as the extreme conservative position, and +10 as the extreme liberal position, then calculate the average of all the members of Congress, you might find that the median position of a particular Congress is −2 (slightly conservative).

Let's say that a new policy is proposed, and that it can be placed at +1 (slightly liberal). It has a good chance of passing because it is not that far from the median. It has an even better chance of passing if the existing policy is more liberal than the proposed one. It has less chance if the existing policy is −2, that is, right at the median.

The situation is compounded by Senate filibusters and presidential vetoes. Taken together, these factors indicate a "gridlock region," an area on the continuum that results in gridlock if a proposed new policy falls in this region. The gridlock reflects the fact that there is a sufficient number of politicians on both sides of opposing ideologies so that the issue cannot be resolved.

## Solutions: Public Policy and Private Action

Many of the factors that contribute to the problems of government pose an ongoing dilemma. For example, you cannot reduce the size of the population served. It is doubtful that the overall size of government can be reduced (the number of federal employees declined in the 1990s, but government employees at other levels increased, so that there was a net increase in the total).

Although selected restructuring might be helpful, it is always a trial-and-error process. For example, some people believe that term limits will enable politicians to function more effectively because they will not be hampered by catering to special interests or their own ambitions to pursue long-term careers. However, in states that have instituted term limits for legislators, the tendency is for more power to go to the governor (Mahtesian 1999). With little time to gain political savvy, legislators are likely to have far less influence than the executive branch of state government. At this point, therefore, it is not clear whether term limits for state legislators make state governments more or less responsive to people's needs.

Campaign finance reform is one of the most needed areas for addressing the problems of government. Individuals and groups with money have the most power in government because politicians are dependent on them to gain, and remain in, office. In recent elections, the candidate who raised the most money was also most likely to win. In spite of reforms in recent years, such as certain limits on contributions to specific candidates, huge amounts of money flow from individuals and interest groups into the political coffers as corporations and rich donors find ways to *circumvent the laws on contribution limits* (Rosen 2000).

A number of states have implemented campaign financing reforms that could serve as a model for the federal government. Maine and Arizona became the first states to have a completely subsidized public finance system for legislative candidates (Francia and Hernson 2003). A number of other states offer partial funding. Candidates who accepted the full funding spent less of their time raising money than did other candidates, including those who had partial public funding. In Europe and other parts of the world, public financing of elections is in place (Aleem 2015). If the United States adopted such a system, it would mean that campaigns would be shorter, less expensive (fewer television ads, etc.), and more likely to focus on issues rather than on personal attacks and extravagant events. To enact such a change, Congress will have to overcome the resistance of interest groups, wealthy individuals, television executives, and others. Without a change, however, politicians will continue to be captive to their sources of money.

Greater citizen participation is another step needed to address the problems of government. The Internet is a powerful tool for building greater citizen participation in political decision making (Leighninger 2011). It facilitates debate and discussion, can be used to gather support for particular points of view, and could increase the number of people who vote. Some observers argue that more citizen participation is not just desirable, but necessary to the health of our democracy (Kenney 2020).

At the state and local levels, a number of cases of citizen participation in the governing process illustrate the value of the practice (Kramer 1999). For example, officials in a county in Florida wanted to attack several social problems, including juvenile crime in a poor community composed mostly of racial and ethnic minorities. At first, they made no progress. But when they worked with citizens of the community and included representatives of the racial and ethnic groups in the discussions, the project was not only successful but became a model for other communities. Only when the people became involved were the government officials able to fully understand the situation and become responsive to the people's needs.

The problem is, given the political alienation of so many citizens, how do you secure more participation? One way you can change attitudes is to encourage citizens to become part of a group that engages in political discussions. The National Issues Forum (NIF) sponsors deliberative forums and study groups on national issues. A study of people who participated in NIF discussions found that, at the end of their participation, they had a much more coherent understanding of issues and much less attitudinal uncertainty about political issues (Gastil and Dillard 1999).

Certainly, politically alienated people have little motivation to join such a group. Thus, to increase citizen participation in the governing process, it is necessary to educate people about the effectiveness of such groups and to publicize efforts at various levels of government that have brought about change.

Other measures that increase citizen participation include easing the registration process and allowing citizen-initiated ballot measures at the state level. Increased numbers of people vote in those states that now permit registration on election day (Brians and Grofman 2001). A comparison of states that allow citizen-initiated ballot measures with those that do not showed considerably higher turnout in the former (as much as 35 to 45 percent higher in presidential elections) (Tolbert, Grummel, and Smith 2001).

Still another measure that can increase voting is *the use of social pressure.* Three researchers carried out an interesting experiment in which they sent a series of mailings to hundreds of thousands of registered voters (Gerber, Green, and Larimer 2008). They found a substantially higher proportion of actual voting among those who received mailings that promised to publicize that they voted to members of their household or to neighbors.

Finally, *face-to-face canvassing increases the number who vote* (Michelson 2003). Voters who are contacted are significantly more likely to vote than those who are not. And this contact may have a long-term payoff. In a field experiment with 25,200 registered voters, researchers found that those people who were urged to vote either through direct mail or face-to-face canvassing not only voted in significantly higher proportions but also were more likely to vote in subsequent elections (Gerber, Green, and Shachar 2003).

*Follow-Up.* What recommendations would you make to government and school officials to increase voter participation?

## Summary

Government is necessary because it fulfills a number of important social functions, functions that reflect people's expectations of their government. First, government is expected to protect the citizenry from foreign aggressors and from threats to individual well-being. Regulatory agencies were established to protect citizens from threats to their well-being. Second, government is expected to secure social order. Third, government is expected to distribute power equitably so that citizens have an equal opportunity for life, liberty, and the pursuit of happiness. Fourth, government is expected to provide a safety net, a minimum standard of living below which it will not allow citizens to fall.

A number of problems of government and politics exist in the United States. There are inequalities in the distribution of power. Social scientists disagree about whether power is distributed in accord with a pluralistic or a power elite model. The failure of trust is a second problem. Americans trust most other institutions far more than they trust the government. This distrust has a number of consequences: it leads to a lack of citizen participation in the political process; it alters people's voting patterns; and it leads to political alienation, a feeling of political disillusionment, powerlessness, and estrangement.

A third problem involves waste, corruption, and scandals in government. Waste refers to such problems as excessive paperwork, excessive costs, and unnecessary expenditures. Corruption and scandals usually involve a politician acting in terms of self-interest or particular interest to the detriment of the politician's constituency or the general public.

Gridlock is a fourth problem. Gridlock means that the government is mired in inaction, unable to legislate significant new policies because of ideological conflict, party differences, or a standoff between the executive and legislative branches. Gridlock is likely to intensify the failure of trust.

Problems in government and politics affect the quality of life in a number of ways. Such problems mean that people have unequal opportunities for a high quality of life. They mean that the freedoms and rights of citizens are not always adequately protected and that the government is not adequately responsive to people's needs.

Various factors contribute to the problems of government and politics. The size of the population served and the size of the government itself both affect how well the government can function. The way the government is organized to fulfill its functions—the separation of powers between the national and state governments and the bureaucratic nature of government agencies—also creates some difficulties in effective functioning. On the other hand, the government is *not* organized so as to deal effectively with waste and corruption.

The costs and financing methods of campaigning have particularly adverse effects. Many social scientists believe that campaign finance issues threaten the democratic process itself and virtually ensure politicians' unresponsiveness to people's needs.

The media also contribute to the problems. They are a substantial part of the cost of campaigns, and they determine the information and perspectives that voters receive about the candidates. The media affect political agendas and actions of those in office, which gives them an integral part of the governing of the nation. They also contribute to the failure of trust.

Interest groups have become an increasingly important part of American political life through contributions, lobbyists, and influence on voting blocs. Interest groups can affect legislation in a way that protects particular interests to the detriment of the general well-being.

Social psychological factors that contribute to the problems include the attitudes of the public and the ideologies of politicians. Negative attitudes of the public lead to alienation and withdrawal from political life; contrary attitudes pose a dilemma for politicians. Ideological positions of politicians can lead to gridlock.

## Key Terms

Anarchism
Bureaucracy
Gridlock
Interest Group
Lobbyist
Patronage
Pluralism
Political Alienation
Political Party
Power Elite Model
Regulatory Agency

## Study Questions

1. What is meant by anarchism, and why does it appeal to some people?
2. What are the functions of government?

3. Explain the different views on the distribution of power in the United States.
4. What is meant by the "failure of trust," and what are the consequences of this failure?
5. Give some examples of waste, corruption, and scandals in government.
6. How can legislative gridlock occur?
7. In what ways do problems of government and politics affect Americans' quality of life?
8. What social structural factors contribute to the problems of government and politics?
9. How do public attitudes affect the political life of the nation?
10. Explain how political ideologies can lead to gridlock in the government.
11. What are some of the important steps to be taken in order to deal with the problems of government and politics?



## Internet Resources/Exercises

1. Explore some of the ideas in this chapter on the following sites:

**http://www.gao.gov** Access reports of the General Accounting Office, the congressional watchdog of federal spending.

**http://www.uspirg.org** Reports plus access to information and programs of state organizations associated with the Public Interest Research Group.

**https://www.usa.gov/statistics** The gateway site to all the statistical data published by the federal government, including data on government at all levels.

2. Go to the PIRG site listed above. Select one of the state PIRGs. Then read their materials on an area of interest to you (higher education, health care reform, government reform, etc.). If you live in the state, write a letter to your representative advocating one or more of the changes or programs in the PIRG materials. If you live in a different state, try to locate materials on the same topic and compare them with the state PIRG materials.

3. Find information on corruption, scandals, or waste in one or more other countries. How does the information you get compare with materials in the text on such problems in America? Do other nations have the same or different kinds of problems? Which nation seems to have the most serious problems?

## For Further Reading

Haidt, Jonathan. *The Righteous Mind: Why Good People Are Divided by Politics and Religion.* New York: Vintage, 2013. A social psychologist draws on a number of disciplines to provide understanding into the polarization that exists today in politics and other areas as well.

Iyengar, Shanto. *Media Politics: A Citizen's Guide.* 2nd ed. New York: W. W. Norton & Company, 2011. A critical examination of the role of the media in American politics, including how politicians use the media to get elected and to stay in office, the role of the FCC, and the impact of the media on framing news and politics.

Kamens, David H. *A New American Creed: The Eclipse of Citizenship and Rise of Populism.* Stanford, CA: Stanford University Press, 2019. Kamens argues that the election of Trump reflected a resurgence of populism, and he explores various trends from the 1930s to the present that produced the resurgence.

Lakoff, George. *Moral Politics: How Liberals and Conservatives Think.* 2nd ed. Chicago: University of Chicago Press, 2002. An examination of the worldviews and ways of thinking of liberals and conservatives, including their differing views of morality and their diverse approaches to such issues as taxes, crime, the death penalty, and the environment.

Light, Paul C. *A Government Ill Executed: The Decline of the Federal Service and How to Reverse It.* Cambridge, MA: Harvard University Press, 2008. Using Alexander Hamilton's seven "tests" of a good government, Light discusses why the federal government increasingly has difficulty passing these tests and suggests what can be done to rectify the situation.

Maisel, Sandy L., and Mark D. Brewer. *Parties and Elections in America: The Electoral Process.* 5th ed. New York: Rowman & Littlefield, 2009. Discusses political parties and the electoral process at all levels (local, state, and national); includes an examination of the role of the media and the issue of campaign financing.

Terry, Janice J. *U.S. Foreign Policy in the Middle East: The Role of Lobbies and Special Interest Groups.* London: Pluto Press, 2005. A case study of the pro-Israel lobby and the way it affects foreign policy, illustrating the power of special interests and lobbyists on the U.S. government.

## References


Aleem, Z. 2015. "7 other nations that prove just how absurd U.S. elections really are." MIC website.

Allen, J. T. 2000. "Making the grade, or not." *U.S. News and World Report,* March 13, p. 24.

American Civil Liberties Union. 2004. "Purged! how a patchwork of flawed and inconsistent voting systems could deprive millions of Americans the right to vote." American Civil Liberties Union website.

American National Election Studies. 2020. "Trust the Federal Government." ANES website.

Anderson, C. J., and Y. V. Tverdova. 2003. "Corruption, political allegiances, and attitudes toward government in contemporary democracies." *American Journal of Political Science* 47:91-109.

Associated Press. 2012. "10 states get No Child Left Behind waivers." Governing magazine website.

Barry, B. 2002. "Capitalists rule OK? Some puzzles about power." *Politics, Philosophy and Economics* 1:155-84.

Blackwell, D. L., J. G. Collins, and R. Coles. 2002. *Summary Health Statistics for U.S. Adults.* Washington, DC: Government Printing Office.

Brady, D. W., and C. Volden. 1998. *Resolving Gridlock: Politics and Policy from Carter to Clinton.* Boulder, CO: Westview Press.

Brians, C. L., and B. Grofman. 2001. "Election day registration's effect on U.S. voter turnout." *Social Science Quarterly* 82:170-83.

Broad, W. J. 1997. "C.I.A. admits government lied about U.F.O. sightings." *New York Times,* August 3.

Burger, T. J., and A. Zagorin. 2004. "Did Cheney okay a deal?" *Time,* June 7, p. 42.

Burns, J. M., et al. 2005. *Government by the People.* 20th ed. Upper Saddle River, NJ: Pearson/Prentice Hall.

Burns, J. M., J. W. Peterson, and T. E. Cronin. 1984. *Government by the People.* 12th ed. Englewood Cliffs, NJ: Prentice-Hall.

Cannon, A., M. Lavelle, and C. Ragavan. 2000. "In the court of last resort." *U.S. News and World Report,* November 27, p. 33.

Center for Responsive Politics. 2020. "What is a PAC?" CRP website.

Chiou, F. Y., and L. S. Rothenberg. 2003. "When pivotal policies meets partisan politics." *American Journal of Political Science* 47:503-22.

Citizens for Responsibility and Ethics in Washington. 2020. "New report: President Trump has 3,400 conflicts of interest." CREW website.

Colborn, T., D. Dumanoski, and J. P. Myers. 1997. *Our Stolen Future.* New York: Plume.

Cook, M., and J. McDonald. 2020. "Duncan Hunter's misconduct detailed in lengthy memo from prosecution." *Los Angeles Times,* March 11.

Cook, T. E. 1998. *Governing with the News: The News Media as a Political Institution.* Chicago, IL: University of Chicago Press.

Cronin, T. E., and M. A. Genovese. 1998. *The Paradoxes of the American Presidency.* New York: Oxford University Press.

Dale, D. 2021. "The 15 most notable lies of Donald Trump's presidency." CNN website.

Dehaven-Smith, L. 2011. "Myth and reality of whistleblower protections." *Public Integrity* 13: 207-20.

DellaVigna, S., and E. Kaplan. 2006. "The Fox news effect: Media bias and voting." *NBER Working Paper No. 12169.* NBER website.

Denchak, M. 2018. "Flint water crisis." NRDC website.

Diener, E., M. Diener, and C. Diener. 1995. "Factors predicting the subjective well-being of nations." *Journal of Personality and Social Psychology* 69:851-64.

Domhoff, G. W. 1990. *The Power Elite and the State: How Policy Is Made in America.* New York: Aldine de Gruyter.

Dover, E. D. 1998. *The Presidential Election of 1996: Clinton's Incumbency and Television.* Westport, CT: Praeger.

Drew, D., and D. Weaver. 2006. "Voter learning in the 2004 presidential election." *Journalism and Mass Communication Quarterly* 83:25-42.

Drucker, P. F. 1968. *The Age of Discontinuity.* New York: Harper and Row.

Durkheim, E. 1933. *The Division of Labor in Society, trans. George Simpson.* New York: Free Press.

Eggen, D. 2012. "Lobbying dips sharply in 2011." *Washington Post,* January 26.

Ehrenhalt, A. 1997. "Big numbers that haunt the government." *Governing Magazine,* January, pp. 7-12.

Eisler, P., and M. Kelley. 2006. "Public wary of links with lobbyists." *USA Today,* October 18.

Federal Election Commission. 2016. "Pac Count–1974 to present." FEC website.

Feld, L., and N. Wilcox. 2008. *Netroots Rising: How a Citizen Army of Bloggers and Online Activists Is Changing American Politics*. Westport, CT: Praeger.

Felland, L. E., et al. 2003. "The resilience of the health care safety net, 1996-2001." *Health Services Research* 38:489-502.

File, T. 2017. "Voting in America." U.S. Census Bureau website.

Flavin, P., A. C. Pacek, and B. Radcliff. 2014. "Assessing the impact of the size and scope of government on human well-being." *Social Forces* 92:1241-58.

Folke, O., S. Hirano, and J. M. Snyder. 2011. "Patronage and elections in U.S. States." *American Political Science Review* 105:567-85.

Francia, P. L., and P. S. Hernson. 2003. "The impact of public finance laws on fundraising in state legislative elections." *American Politics Research* 31:520-39.

Frey, R. S., and A. Al-Roumi. 1999. "Political democracy and the physical quality of life." *Social Indicators Research* 47 (May):73-97.

Gastil, J., and J. P. Dillard. 1999. "Increasing political sophistication through public deliberation." *Political Communication* 16 (1):3-23.

Gerber, A. S., D. P. Green, and C. W. Larimer. 2008. "Social pressure and voter turnout." *American Political Science Review* 102:33-48.

Gerber, A. S., D. P. Green, and R. Shachar. 2003. "Voting may be habit-forming." *American Journal of Political Science* 47:540-50.

Goldmacher, S. 2020. "The 2020 campaign is the most expensive ever." *New York Times,* October 28.

Grieco, E. 2020. "Americans' main sources for political news vary by party and age." Pew Research Center website.

Hanenberg, R., and W. Rojanapithayakorn. 1998. "Expressions of distrust: Third-party voting and cynicism in government." *Political Behavior* 20:17-34.

Herron, J., and M. W. Smith. 2012. "The disaster of Hurricane Katrina: Malfeasance, official deviance, and the failure to serve and protect a community." *International Journal of Interdisciplinary Social Sciences* 6:1833-82.

Hetherington, M. J. 1999. "The effect of political trust on the presidential vote, 1968-96." *American Political Science Review* 93 (June):311-23.

Hogan, M. J., M. A. Long, P. B. Stretesky, and M. J. Lynch. 2006. "Campaign contributions, post-war reconstruction contracts, and state crime." *Deviant Behavior* 27:269-97.

Hood, M. V., Q. Kidd, and I. L. Morris. 2015. "Tea leaves and southern politics." *Social Science Quarterly* 96:923-40.

Igielnik, R. 2020. "Men and women in the U.S. continue to differ in voter turnout rate, party identification." Pew Research Center website.

Jamieson, A., H. B. Shin, and J. Day. 2002. *Voting and Registration in the Election of November 2000.* Washington, DC: Government Printing Office.

Kenney, J. 2020. "Citizen participation in the electoral process." *Pennsylvania Capital Star,* October 115.

King, D. Y. 1998a. "Qualifications of Indonesia's civil servants: How appropriate to the dynamic environment?" *Journal of Political and Military Sociology* 26 (Summer):23-38.

——. 1998b. "Reforming basic education and the struggle for decentralized educational administration in Indonesia." *Journal of Political and Military Sociology* 26 (Summer):83-95.

Kopecki, D. 2006. "On the hunt for fraud." *Business Week,* October 11, p. 11.

Kramer, R. 1999. "Weaving the public into public administration." *Public Administration Review* 59 (January-February):89-92.

Kristiansen, S., and M. Ramli. 2006. "Buying an income: The market for civil service positions in Indonesia." *Contemporary Southeast Asia* 28:207-33.

Krugman, P. 2006. "Broken promises." *New York Times,* August 28.

Larcinese, V., L. Rizzo, and C. Testa. 2006. "Allocating the U.S. federal budget to the states." *Journal of Politics* 68:447-56.

Lee, T., and C. Hosam. 2020. "Fake news is real: The significance and sources of disbelief in mainstream media in Trump's America." *Sociological Forum* 35:996-1018.

Leighninger, M. 2011. "Citizenship and governance in a wild, wired world." *National Civic Review,* Summer, pp. 20-30.

Levi, M. 1998. "A state of trust." In *Trust and Governance,* ed. V. Braithwaite and M. Levi, pp. 77-98. New York: Russell Sage Foundation.

Levy, C. J. 1999. "More power was supposed to grease these skids." *New York Times,* June 27.

Light, P. C. 2020. "The true size of government is nearing a record high." Brookings Institution website.

Magee, C. S. P. 2003. "Third-party candidates and the 2000 presidential election." *Social Science Quarterly* 84:574-95.

Mahtesian, C. 1999. "So much politics, so little time." *Governing,* August, pp. 22-26.

Maki, M. T. 2019. "Japanese internment was wrong." *Los Angeles Times,* February 20.

Martin, P. S. 2003. "Voting's rewards: Voter turnout, attentive publics, and congressional allocation of federal money." *American Journal of Political Science* 47:110-27.

McMenamin, B., and J. Novack. 1999. "The white-collar gestapo." *Forbes,* December 1, pp. 82-91.

Michelson, M. R. 2003. "Getting out the Latino vote: How door-to-door canvassing influences voter turnout in rural central California." *Political Behavior* 25:247-63.

Miller, M. C. 2005. *Fooled Again.* New York: Basic Books.

Mills, C. W. 1956. *The Power Elite.* New York: Oxford University Press.

Mitchell, A., et al. 2020. "Americans who mainly get their news on social media are less engaged, less knowledgeable." Pew Research Center website.

Montanaro, D. 2017. "2-party system? Americans might be ready for 8." PBS website.

Newport, F. 2020. "Americans and the role of government." Gallup Poll website.

Norman, J. 2015. "In U.S., support for Tea Party drops to new low." Gallup Poll website.

Ott, J. C. 2011. "Government and happiness in 130 nations." *Social Indicators Research* 102:3-22.

Patenaude, W. 2019. "Modern American populism." *American Journal of Economics and Sociology* 78:787-834.

Plane, D. L., and J. Gershtenson. 2004. "Candidates' ideological locations, abstention, and turnout in U.S. midterm Senate elections." *Political Behavior* 26:69-93.

Polling Report. 2020. The Polling Report website.

Prior, M. 2006. "The incumbent in the living room." *Journal of Politics* 68:657-63.

Rahn, W. M., and T. J. Rudolph. 2005. "A tale of political trust in American cities." *Public Opinion Quarterly* 69:530-60.

Ray, J., and A. Dugan. 2020. "How well are countries keeping their people safe?" Gallup Poll website.

Rosen, J. 2000. "Talk is cheap—Campaign finance reform meets the Internet." *New Republic,* February 14, pp. 20-24.

Scher, R. K. 1997. *The Modern Political Campaign.* New York: M. E. Sharpe.

Schow, A. 2019. "Here are the most wasteful government projects in 2019." Daily Wire website.

Shearer, E. 2016. "Candidates' Social media outpaces their websites and emails as an online campaign news source." Pew Research Center website.

Skocpol., T., and V. Williamson. 2012. *The Tea Party and the Remaking of Republican Conservatism.* Oxford, UK: Oxford University Press.

Slevin, P., and S. F. Kovaleski. 2000. "Outside Palm Beach, complaints growing." *Washington Post,* November 11.

Sloan, M. 2006. "Election shows corruption still matters." *San Diego Union-Tribune,* December 6.

Smith, A. 2011. "The Internet and political news sources." Pew Research Center website.

Southwell, P. L. 2008. "The effect of political alienation on voter turnout, 1964-2000." *Journal of Political and Military Sociology* 36:131-45.

Stolberg, S. G., and N. Fandos. 2018. "As gridlock deepens in Congress, only gloom is bipartisan." *New York Times,* January 27.

Stone, P. H. 2006. *Heist: Superlobbyist Jack Abramoff, His Republican Allies, and the Buying of Washington.* New York: Farrar, Straus & Giroux.

Sypnowich, C. 2000. "The culture of citizenship." *Politics and Society* 28:531-55.

Timm, J. C. 2019. "Fact check: Trump says Puerto Rico got $92 billion. They've seen only a fraction." NBC online news.

Tolbert, C. J., J. A. Grummel, and D. A. Smith. 2001. "The effects of ballot initiatives on voter turnout in the American states." *American Politics Research* 29:625-48.

Unsworth, M. E. 1999. "Freedom of information: Its ebb and flow." *American Libraries,* June-July, pp. 82-86.

U.S. Census Bureau. 1975. *Historical Statistics of the United States, Colonial Times to 1970.* Washington, DC: Government Printing Office.

Wilson, G. C. 2002. "Truth be told, they do lie." *National Journal,* March 2, p. 636.

Zweigenhaft, R. L., and G. W. Domhoff. 2006. *Diversity in the Power Elite: How It Happened, Why It Matters.* Lanham, MD: Rowman and Littlefield.

CHAPTER 10

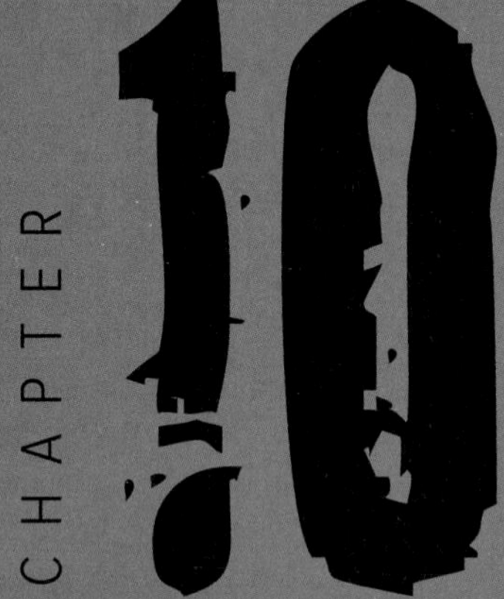

# Work and the Economy

OBJECTIVES

1. Identify various ways in which the economy is changing.
2. Know how work and the workforce are changing, and how problems of work detract from people's quality of life.
3. Understand the ways in which the economic system is detrimental to the well-being of many Americans.
4. Identify the ways in which the government and social roles contribute to the problems of work.
5. Discuss attitudes toward work and workers, including the ideology of the work ethic, as aspects of the work problem in America.
6. Suggest steps that can be taken to reduce the problems and make work more meaningful.

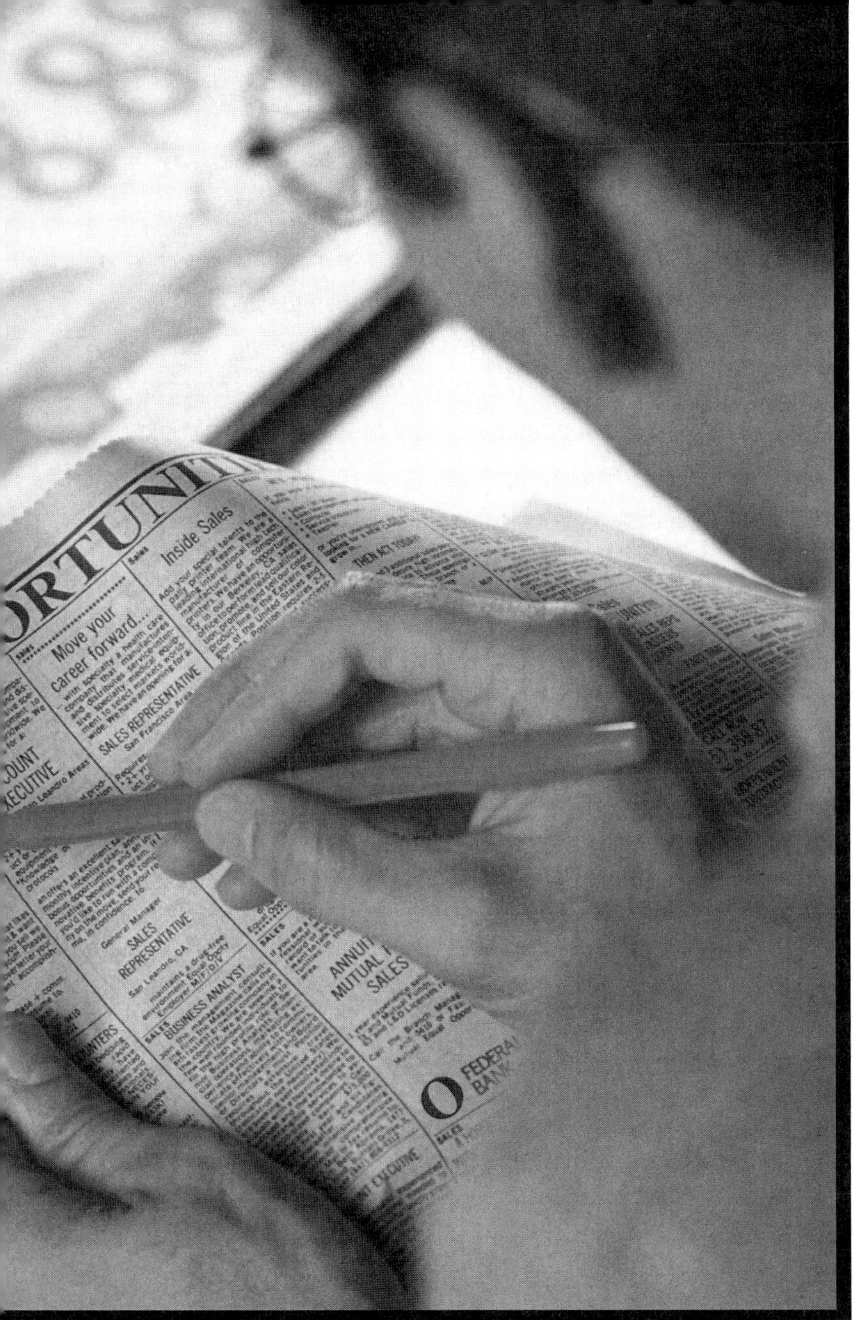


Photodisc/Punchstock

### "I'm Not a Worrier. But . . ."

Some people are optimistic by nature. They tend not to worry even when they are struggling with problems. But, as Ted points out, unemployment can strain even the most optimistic of outlooks. Ted is in his late 40s. He has been out of work for more than a year, a situation that was inconceivable to him only a few months before he lost his job:

*I'm an engineer. I've never been out of work before. In fact, only a few months before I was laid off, I was planning to stay in my job until I retired. A group of us were laid off at the same time. We were all completely taken by surprise. We knew things were slack, but there was no talk of any layoffs. They just called us each in one day and told us they didn't have a job for us anymore.*

*At first, I was kind of cocky about it. I was hurt, because I really liked working there. But I was also sure that I would have another job in a few weeks. Probably even with better pay. I fantasized about writing them a letter and thanking them for giving me the opportunity to advance myself. You know, rub it in, and make them sorry.*

*That was over a year ago. It was about a hundred résumés and applications ago. I'm not a worrier. But I'm really worried now. And every month when the mortgage comes due, I worry a little more. My wife's job keeps us afloat, but we've about exhausted our savings, and we're now thinking about selling our house and moving into an apartment.*

*But you know what the worst part of it is? Just waiting and waiting and not hearing, and feeling more and more useless and more and more helpless. I've lost the chance at jobs for which I'm a perfect fit because they could hire someone younger and cheaper. It's really depressing. I'll keep trying, but it gets harder all the time to make yourself go through the application process, and it gets harder all the time to feel hopeful, to really believe that this could be the place that will finally hire me.*

## Introduction

Many Americans fantasize about becoming independently wealthy so that they can do whatever they please. Moreover, they believe that the American economy offers that possibility. Think about this fantasy for a moment. Do you believe that the American economy offers you the possibility of becoming independently wealthy? If so, what are your chances? If it happens, what will you do? Will you continue to work?

When we pose such questions to social problems classes, virtually everyone agrees that he or she could become independently wealthy. Many do not think the chances of this are very good, however, and nearly all the students say they would continue to work.

**work ethic**
the notion that your sense of worth and the satisfaction of your needs are intricately related to the kind of work you do

In general, the students believe that the American economy is the best economy, and they are committed to it and to the work ethic. The **work ethic** involves the notion that *your sense of worth and the satisfaction of your needs are intricately related to the kind of work you do.*

In this chapter we explore evidence related to these beliefs about work and the economy. We look at the changing nature of the economy, work, and the workforce as well as the diverse meanings people attach to their work. We consider the kinds of problems associated with work, discuss how they affect the quality of life, and note the factors that contribute to and help to perpetuate those problems. Finally, we outline a few approaches to resolving the problems.

## The Economy, Work, and the Workforce in America

All things change. The American economy, the nature of work, and the nature of the workforce are vastly different today from what they were at various times in the past.

### The Changing Economy

**capitalism**
an economic system in which there is private, rather than state, ownership of wealth and control of the production and distribution of goods; people are motivated by profit and compete with each other for maximum shares of profit

Initially, the United States was *an agrarian society,* that is, a society in which agriculture is the dominant form of work and people and animals are the major sources of energy. It has been estimated that as late as 1850, 65 percent of the energy used in American work was supplied by people and animals (Lenski 1966). After the middle of the 19th century, the nation industrialized rapidly. In simple terms, *industrialization is economic development through a transformation of the sources and quantities of energy employed.*

American industrialization, like that of most nations, occurred in the context of **capitalism,** an economic system in which there is private, rather than state, ownership of wealth and control of the production and distribution of goods. In a capitalist system,

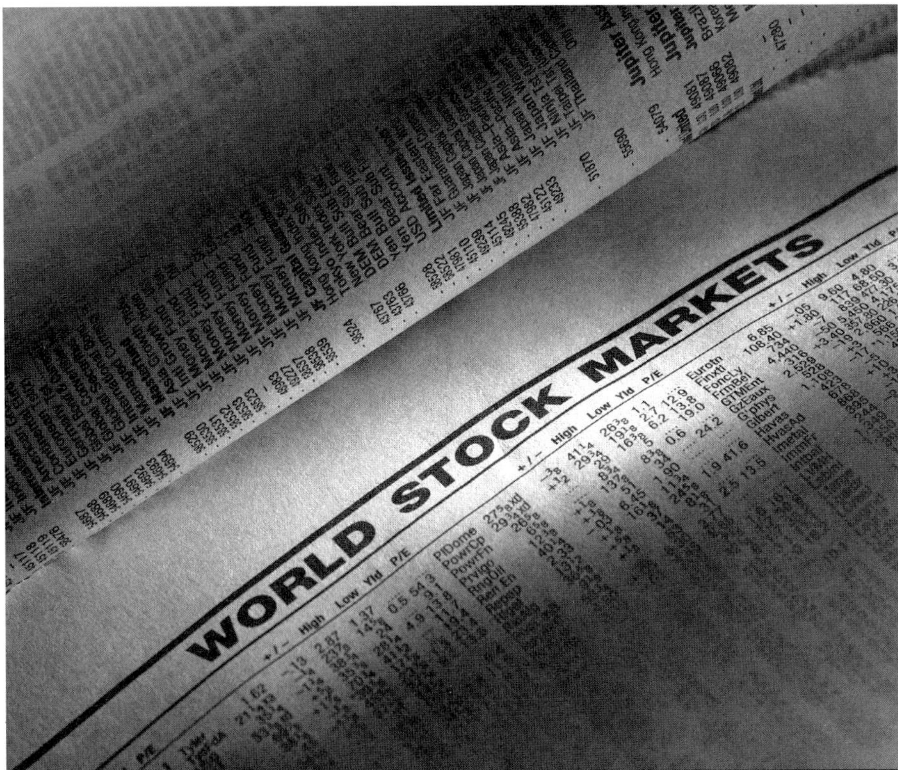


The global economy now drives the U.S. economy.
Steve Allen/Brand X Pictures

people are motivated by profit and they compete with each other to maximize their share of the profits. The premise is that the combination of private ownership and the pursuit of profit benefits everyone, because it motivates capitalists to be efficient and to provide the best goods and services at the lowest possible prices.

In a pure capitalist system, government involvement in the economy is minimal. In the United States, the government role in the economy has grown over the past century. In addition, our economy is affected by various other factors such as the global economy, weather, and wars. *The global economy has become particularly important.* In simplest terms, globalization of the economy means a significant increase in the amount of international trade and investment (Weisbrot 2000). In the United States, for example, trade provides an increasingly large percentage of the gross domestic product, so much so that some observers claim global markets are now necessary to keep the U.S. economy healthy (Griswold 2010). Supermarkets have become more important than superpowers for key economic decisions. When governments try to impose restrictions to protect or enhance the national economy, enterprises simply shift the work to another setting. For instance, when Japan raised postage rates, direct mailers sent their mailings to Hong Kong, which mailed them back to Japan at considerably less cost to the mailers; and when the United States put limits on the number of work permits given to foreign computer programmers, some companies changed the work location to other nations.

Technology has driven down the cost of international communication and travel. Thus, there has been a growth in trade, the flow of capital across national borders, foreign investment, shared research and development, and movement of personnel (including students attending universities in foreign countries). Business enterprises maximize their profits by locating the best markets and the least expensive places for operations. As a result, a particular product may have components made in various parts of the world.

In other words, the economy is now truly global. The amount of international trade in goods and services is enormous. In one month in 2020, for example, the United States exports totaled $176.4 billion, while the imports totaled $240.2 billion (U.S. Bureau of Economic Analysis 2020). Many large U.S. firms, including Exxon, Colgate-Palmolive, and Coca-Cola, obtain the majority of their income from overseas markets. Economists differ on the effects of trade and on whether we should strive for "free" trade agreements or a system of restrictions on what and how much can be imported and exported. The public, on the other hand, looks at trade as good for the economy as a whole, but only one in five believe that trade creates jobs for Americans (Stokes 2015).

*The consequences of globalization, then, are controversial.* On the one hand, researchers have identified positive consequences such as a reduction in occupational sex segregation and gender inequality (Meyer 2003). On the other hand, many observers argue that globalization has led to a growing gap between the world's rich and poor (Amin 2004). Whatever the consequences for the world as a whole, globalization and new technologies combine to present the U.S. economy and the American worker with new challenges. *Globalization means that businesses shift their operations to other nations where the employees work for lower pay than Americans and other business expenses are less, thus lowering the costs of products and services.* The results of this process, called *outsourcing,* are debatable. It is argued that, on the one hand, outsourcing helps American companies stay competitive in the global market, while, on the other hand, it also increases unemployment in the United States (Amadeo 2016). Research has not resolved the issue. For example, two studies (both at Duke University) of outsourcing among engineering firms came to different conclusions (Engardio 2006). One study reported that the companies resort to outsourcing because they need more talent and they shift some of their more complex work to countries such as India and China because they can decrease the time it takes to get their products to market. The other study, however, argued that the outsourcing reflects no shortage of talent in the United States; rather, the only motivation is to reduce costs.

In any case, it is undeniable that one outcome of outsourcing is that well-paid, lower-skilled jobs in the United States are increasingly difficult to find. Indeed, the prospects for lower-skilled workers are more bleak than they were in the early 1990s (Bartik and Houseman 2008). Other kinds of work have also been affected, such as that in science, engineering, and technology. Many of the jobs in these areas have moved to other countries (Hira 2009). One CEO of a large high-tech company even stated that his company could succeed without ever hiring another American.

Globalization has also contributed to what Kalleberg (2009:2) calls "precarious work," work that is "uncertain, unpredictable, and risky from the point of view of the worker." The precarious nature of work is dramatized by the fact that literally tens of millions of Americans lost their jobs involuntarily since the early 1980s.

In the competitive context of the global economy, then, *a number of changes have occurred that are detrimental to the well-being of many American workers* (Caskey 1994; Harrison 1994; U.S. Department of Labor 2000):

**downsizing**
reduction of the labor force in a company or corporation

- Businesses and corporations have used both outsourcing and **downsizing** (reduction of the labor force) to reduce costs and maximize profits.
- An increasing number of jobs are temporary or part-time, with no fringe benefits such as health insurance.
- Unions continue to decline in membership and power.

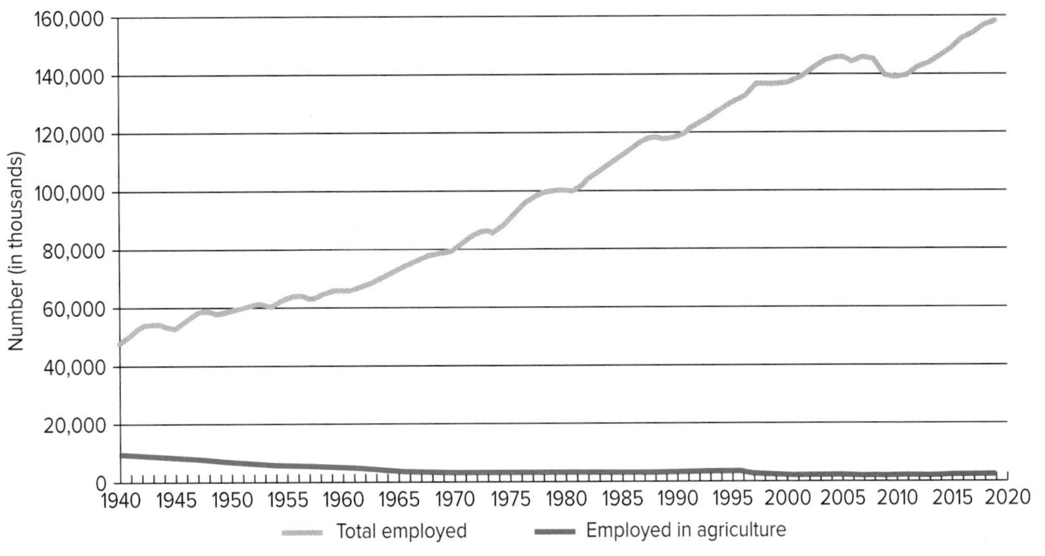


**FIGURE 10.1** Civilian Employment, 1940–2019.

Source: "Employment status of the civilian noninstitutional population," Bureau of Labor Statistics website.

- Corporate tax obligations have been reduced, cutting back on revenues necessary to support social programs.
- When corrected for inflation, the income of many American families has declined.

As a result of such changes, many Americans are not only unable to better their lot in comparison to their parents, but are finding themselves worse off than their parents.

In sum, the nature of the changes in the economy means that many American families are worse off financially than they were in the 1970s. For many, the American dream seems more remote than ever.

## The Changing Workforce

**labor force**
all civilians who are employed or unemployed but able and desiring to work

The **labor force** (defined as all civilians who are employed or unemployed but able and wanting to work) has increased enormously since the founding of the nation. The number of those actually employed has also risen fairly steadily (Figure 10.1). It was the rapid increase since the beginning of the 19th century that made the nation's swift industrial growth possible. The workforce was low in 1800 because all but a small proportion of Americans lived on farms, and the family farmer along with his wife and children is not counted—only those who work for pay outside the home are included in the workforce. Since 1940 the labor force has been growing faster than the population. This growth has been fueled by population growth, by the rapid entry of women into the labor force, and by the fact that more older workers are staying in the labor force beyond the age of 65 (Desilver 2016).

**division of labor**
the separation of work into specialized tasks

The *occupational structure* also has changed with an increasing **division of labor,** or *specialization.* There are now more than 30,000 different occupations. This change is not due to growth in all job categories, however. If you look at the categories of occupations used by the Census Bureau, you will find that since the beginning of the 20th century the proportion of workers in professional, technical, managerial, clerical, and service jobs has increased greatly. The proportion of workers classified as farm workers, on the other

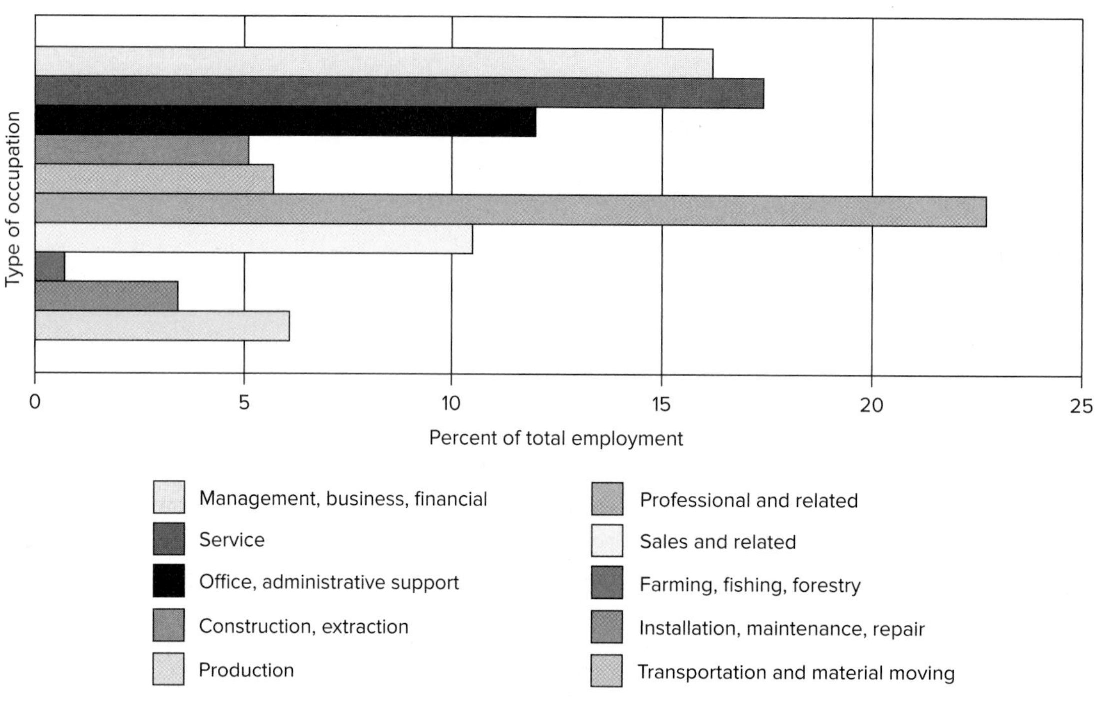


**FIGURE 10.2** Distribution of Occupations.
Source: Bureau of Labor Statistics website.

hand, has declined dramatically. In 1900, 17.7 percent of all employees worked on farms (U.S. Census Bureau 1975:144). As Figure 10.1 shows, the number of agricultural employees continues to decline, comprising less than 2 percent of all employees in 2019.

Jobs requiring more skill and training have tended to increase at a faster rate than others. In other words, there has been a general upgrading of the occupational structure. With increased industrialization and technological development, the need for farmers and unskilled workers has diminished and the need for skilled workers and clerical and other white-collar workers has increased. The United States has moved into a service and, some would argue, an informational society, in which growing numbers of workers are needed outside the manufacturing areas (Figure 10.2). It is increasingly likely that workers will engage in tasks involving *substantive complexity* such as verbal and math skills and abstract thinking rather than motor skills such as lifting, stooping, coördination, or finger dexterity. Unfortunately, many new jobs, particularly those in the service area, do not pay well. According to the Bureau of Labor Statistics, in 2019, 8.05 million workers, representing 5.1 percent of all workers, supplemented their income by working two or more jobs. Thus, many American workers either work longer hours or face a lower standard of living.

## The Changing Composition of the Labor Force

Data from the Bureau of Labor Statistics website show how the demographics of the labor force have changed over time. First, as the general skill level increases, *the educational level of the workforce also increases.* In 1970, 38.7 percent of the labor force had

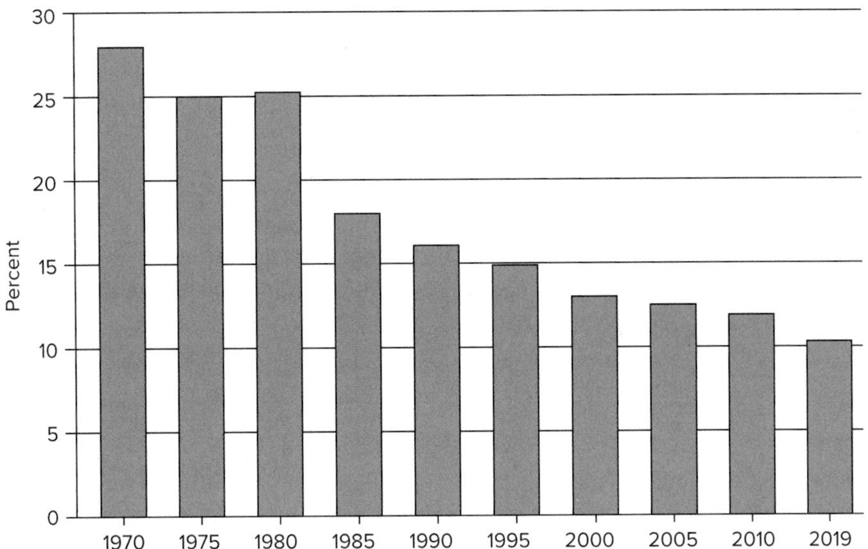


**FIGURE 10.3**
Membership in Labor Unions as a Proportion of the Labor Force, 1970–2019.

Source: Bureau of Labor Statistics website.

less than four years of high school, whereas 12.0 percent had four or more years of college. By 2016, only 4 percent of whites, 7 percent of African Americans, 6 percent of Asian Americans, and 26 percent of Hispanics had less than four years of high school. And the proportions of those with four of more years of college increased to 61 percent of Asian Americans, 43 percent of whites, 28 percent of African Americans, and 20 percent of Hispanics.

Another substantial change in the labor force involves the *proportion of workers who are female.* From 1950 to 2018, the participation rate of men fell from 82.4 percent to 69.1 percent, whereas that of women rose from 32.0 percent to 57.1 percent.

A third change is the increasing number of undocumented immigrants in the workforce. The exact number is not known. But the Bureau of Labor Statistics reports that in 2019 there were 28.4 million "foreign-born" workers in the labor force, composing 17.4 percent of all workers. The foreign-born population includes legally admitted immigrants, refugees, temporary residents such as students and temporary workers, and undocumented immigrants. The majority of the undocumented come in from Mexico and other Latin American nations. They are generally concentrated in the lower-paying occupations, such as farming, cleaning, construction, and food preparation.

Finally, the labor force also became more *unionized* until the 1960s. Since then, however, the proportion of workers who are union members has declined (Figure 10.3). By 2019, only 10.3 percent of wage and salary workers were union members. The type of workers who are unionized has changed as well. Unions no longer involve mainly blue-collar workers. Federal, state, and local government workers comprise a substantial proportion of all union workers: 4 out of 10 government workers are in unions, compared to about 1 out of 12 private-sector employees. Among occupational groups, unionization is highest among government workers in protective services such as the police and firefighters. In private industry, the highest union membership rates are found in public utilities, transportation, and construction.

## The Changing Meaning of Work

When we try to determine the *meaning of work* for Americans, we find ourselves in a morass of contradictions. Some people argue that work is one of the most important activities in an individual's life. They maintain that those who do not have a satisfying job do not have a fully satisfying life. Others insist that work is purely instrumental, a way to attain the goal of *maximum consumption.* There is also disagreement about whether Americans enjoy their work, with some observers claiming that most Americans hate their jobs and others asserting that there is a high rate of *job satisfaction.*

What about the *work ethic,* the notion that work is intrinsically good and useful and that people should therefore continue to work even if they are financially independent? Do Americans still believe this? Or would they gladly abandon work for leisure pursuits if they had the means to do so?

It is difficult to resolve the contradictions, but research and polls do indicate that the work ethic remains strong. A Pew Research Center (2019) survey reported that 60 percent of Americans believe that you can be successful if you are willing to work hard. An earlier Pew Research Center (2016) survey found that about half of Americans describe their job as a career and another 18 percent say it's a step toward a career.

With regard to work satisfaction, public opinion polls from the 1970s up to the present consistently reported that 80 percent or more of workers say they are "satisfied" or "very satisfied" with their jobs. In the Pew Research Center (2016) survey, 49 percent said they were "very satisfied" with their jobs and another 30 percent said they were "somewhat satisfied." In short, a majority of Americans are satisfied with their current jobs.

At the same time, an increasing number of Americans no longer accept the notion that their self-worth is tied in with their work or that they have a moral duty to work. On the contrary, Americans increasingly expect their work to have *meaning,* to be emotionally and intellectually *stimulating,* and to offer an opportunity to feel *good about themselves and the products of their labor.* Income is no longer the most important facet of an individual's work.

In evaluating job quality, an individual is likely to consider not just income, but such nonincome factors as job duties and working conditions, job satisfaction, period of work, job status, and job security (Moen and Yu 2000). *Job duties and working conditions* refer to such matters as whether the job is hazardous, repetitious, stressful, closely supervised, and isolated (versus working with a team). *Job satisfaction* increases when the worker engages in problem solving, has the opportunity to be creative, gains recognition, can fully utilize skills and learn new skills, and has the chance for advancement.

*Period of work* is the extent to which the job involves weekend or shift work, overtime, or flexible work hours. *Job status* includes both social status (being recognized by outsiders as having a more prestigious or less prestigious job) and status within the organization. *Job security* means that workers can be confident of retaining their jobs as long as their performance is satisfactory. Where, for whatever reason, such security is lacking, there will be an increase in distress and burnout among workers (Jiang and Probst 2016).

fallacy

Americans, then, are not rejecting work. They are rejecting meaningless work and low-quality jobs. To say, as we have heard from some students and employers, that Americans today "just don't want to work anymore" is the *fallacy of personal attack.* In a national survey, only 5.1 percent of those not working said it was because they were "not interested in working" (Weismantle 2001). The great majority wants work, but work that is important and that fosters a sense of achievement.

## Work as a Social Problem

Because most Americans want to work and expect their work to provide some degree of personal fulfillment, there are three basic problems associated with work in America today. First, there is the problem of *unemployment and* **underemployment.** People are underemployed if they work full time for poverty wages, work part time when they desire full-time work, or work at jobs that are temporary or below their skill levels. Second, there is the problem of *dissatisfaction and alienation.* Finally, there is the problem of various kinds of *work hazards.*

**underemployment**
working full time for poverty wages, working part time when full-time work is desired, or working at a job below the worker's skill level

### Unemployment and Underemployment

Underemployment is perhaps as serious as unemployment for people who look to work for meaningful activity. Underemployment results in frustration, financial worry, and lowered job satisfaction (Vaisey 2006). Moreover, there is a stigma attached to being underemployed. For example, one research team found that underemployed college graduates who tried to get better jobs had a 30 percent lower callback rate than those who were adequately employed (Nunley et al. 2016).

How many Americans are underemployed? The Bureau of Labor Statistics (2018) reported that in 2017, 5.9 million workers, representing 3.8 percent of all workers, had contingent jobs (the jobs are temporary or the workers do not expect the jobs to last). A disproportionate number of the contingency workers are young and nonwhite.

A substantial number of the underemployed are working part time, which means that they have no benefits (including health insurance). Lacking the kind of social benefits available in countries such as Sweden, such workers *cannot achieve their desired quality of life without working full time* (Reynolds 2004). Another large group of the underemployed are those in temporary jobs. And professionals—lawyers, accountants, engineers, and so on—make up a substantial proportion of the temporary market (Thottam 2004; Bureau of Labor Statistics 2018). Businesspeople claim that temporary work serves the interests of those people who want something other than a permanent work situation. However, *temporary workers are underemployed because most of them are looking for full-time permanent employment* and most dislike the lack of stability and the degradation of being a temporary worker. However, it isn't the workers but the owners who are most likely to benefit from temporary employees. The temps are cheaper, easier to deal with, and easier to get rid of than are full-time employees (Hatton 2011).

With regard to those out of work, reliable data exist on the **unemployment rate.** The rate fluctuates considerably (Table 10.1). By 2019, the overall rate was 3.7 percent, or 3.2 million workers. The statistic does not mean, however, that only 3.2 million Americans were affected by unemployment in that year. Many people are unemployed for only a portion of the year. The length of unemployment may rise during times of economic recession. Thus, between 2007 and 2010, the length of time the unemployed spent looking for work before finding a job increased from 5.2 weeks to 10.4 weeks (Ilg and Theodossiou 2012).

**unemployment rate**
the proportion of the labor force that is not working but is available for work and has made specific efforts to find work

In addition, a good many Americans who want to work are not counted as part of the labor force or the unemployment rate because they are not actively looking for work. In 2011, 6.1 million Americans wanted to work but were not considered unemployed or part of the labor force for various reasons (Theodossiou 2012). They were discouraged by such things as lack of education or training or the inability to find a job, or because other factors such as family responsibilities or health problems prevented them. When

**TABLE 10.1**
Unemployment Rates, 1950–2019

| Year | Total | White | Black | Hispanic | Asian |
|---|---|---|---|---|---|
| 1950 | 5.3 | 4.9 | 9.0 | | |
| 1955 | 4.4 | 3.9 | 8.7 | | |
| 1960 | 5.5 | 4.9 | 10.2 | | |
| 1965 | 4.5 | 4.1 | 8.1 | | |
| 1970 | 4.9 | 4.5 | 8.2 | | |
| 1975 | 8.5 | 7.8 | 14.8 | | |
| 1980 | 7.1 | 6.3 | 14.3 | 10.1 | |
| 1985 | 7.2 | 6.2 | 15.1 | 10.5 | |
| 1990 | 5.5 | 4.7 | 11.3 | 8.0 | 4.2 |
| 1995 | 5.6 | 4.9 | 10.4 | 9.3 | 5.0 |
| 2000 | 4.0 | 2.6 | 5.4 | 4.4 | 2.7 |
| 2005 | 5.1 | 4.4 | 10.0 | 6.0 | 4.0 |
| 2010 | 9.5 | 8.7 | 16.0 | 12.5 | 7.5 |
| 2015 | 4.8 | 4.2 | 8.3 | 5.6 | 3.8 |
| 2019 | 3.7 | 3.4 | 5.6 | 4.2 | 2.8 |

SOURCE: Bureau of Labor Statistics website.

you take into account those who want to work but are not counted in the unemployment rate as well as those who are unemployed for only a part of the year, the number of people affected by unemployment becomes far higher than the official figures.

As Table 10.1 shows, *unemployment does not strike all groups the same.* Typically, the rates are higher for minorities than for whites and are higher for younger than for older workers. In some years, the unemployment rate for workers 16 to 19 years of age is double, triple, or more the rate for the workforce as a whole. At the end of 2020, for example, the overall unemployment rate was 6.7, but it was 16.0 for 16- to 19-year-olds and 11.2 for 20- to 24-year-olds.

Unemployment also varies by occupational category, with rates tending to be higher among blue-collar and service workers. The lowest rates are likely to be found in the higher-status, high-income occupations of the managerial and professional category.

## Dissatisfaction and Alienation

In Chapter 3, we defined *alienation* as a sense of estrangement that is usually measured by an individual's feelings of powerlessness, normlessness, isolation, and meaninglessness. This definition is a subjective approach to alienation. Alienation is an objective phenomenon, according to Karl Marx. In a capitalist society the worker is *estranged from his or her own labor* (because work is something that is coerced and external to the worker rather than a fulfillment of the worker's needs), from other people, and from his or her own humanity. The worker sinks to the level of a commodity and becomes the most wretched of commodities. Because capitalism wrenches the means of production from the control of those intimately involved in production, workers are necessarily alienated whether or not they feel any sense of alienation.

The amount of alienation in the workplace, therefore, depends on whether you take a Marxist or a social psychological approach to the question. For Marxists, all workers in a capitalist society are alienated by definition. For social psychologists, workers are alienated to the extent that they perceive themselves as powerless and isolated. Social psychological studies indicate that some American workers, but by no means the majority, are alienated. In fact, some researchers have found that many workers say they would rather continue their jobs than get the same wages for not working.

Nevertheless, indications are that dissatisfaction is still a problem. First, no matter which polls are used to measure job dissatisfaction, the results translate into tens of millions of dissatisfied American workers. Second, there is evidence of various troublesome issues. For example, workers who have low control over their work situation may experience dissatisfaction and anger (Fitzgerald, Haythornthwaite, Suchday, and Ewart 2003). And, as noted earlier, workers in a situation of insecurity (e.g., where some of the workforce is being laid off or workers are being asked to take unpaid leave) may experience dissatisfaction and anxiety (Berkshire et al. 2011).

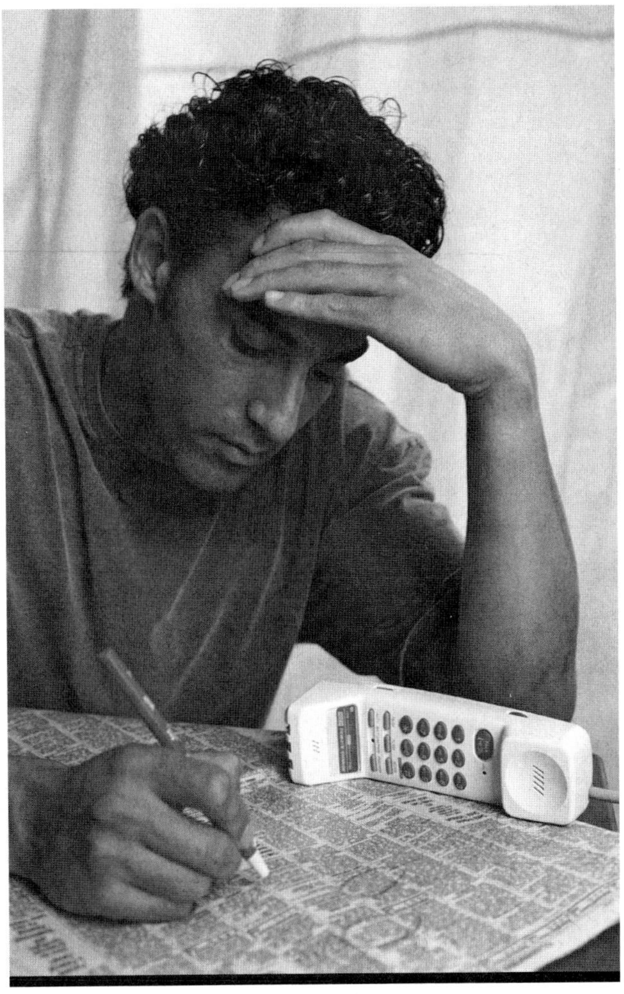

Unemployment is higher for minorities and younger workers.

Jack Star/PhotoLink/Getty Images

## Work Hazards and Stress

The Bureau of Labor Statistics (2020a) reported 2.8 million nonfatal workplace injuries and illnesses in 2019. In addition, there were 4,178 fatalities among wage and salary workers and 1,072 fatalities among self-employed workers. The likelihood of injury, illness, or death varied by occupation. Ten occupations accounted for a third of all cases that resulted in days away from work: nursing assistants, heavy truck drivers, freight and material laborers, light truck drivers, construction workers, maintenance and repair workers, stockers and order fillers, janitors, registered nurses, and retail salespersons.

Not included in the government report are the risks posed to adolescents who work. A national survey of working adolescents revealed that over a third reported a violation of guidelines for hazardous occupations (such as working at a job or using equipment that is prohibited for them), 11 percent reported working past the latest hour allowed on a school night, and 15 percent reported working off the clock (Rauscher, Runyan, Schulman, and Bowling 2008).

We use the term "work hazards" broadly to include *work-induced stress* as well as *work-related injuries and illnesses.* For example, a spot welder on an auto assembly line told about some of the daily hazards to which he is exposed.

> I pulled a muscle in my neck, straining. This gun, when you grab this thing from the ceiling, cable, weight, I mean you're pulling everything. . . . This whole edge here is sharp. I go through a shirt every two weeks, it just goes right through. My overalls catch on fire. I've had gloves catch on fire. (Indicates arms.) See them little holes? That's what sparks do. I've got burns across here from last night (Terkel 1972:224).

*Psychological as well as physical hazards occur in the workplace.* Some occupations are particularly likely to expose workers to stress. For instance, many taxi drivers work under the continual threat of robbery. Salespeople often endure harassment from

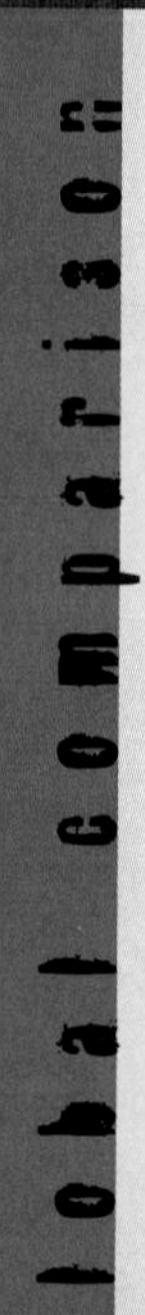


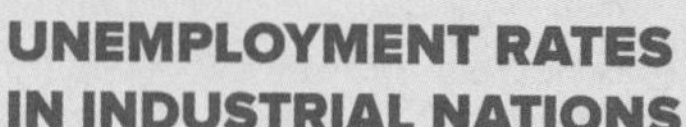

## UNEMPLOYMENT RATES IN INDUSTRIAL NATIONS

Unemployment is a huge and ongoing problem in many underdeveloped nations. For one thing, economic growth lags behind population growth, so that even a robust economy cannot absorb all the new workers coming into the labor force each year. In the developed nations, unemployment tends to be smaller but is still an enduring problem. The unemployment rate varies considerably, however, depending on how the economy is structured. Note in Table 10.2 that some nations have lower rates than the United States, and others have higher rates.

Although the rates are strikingly low in some cases, every nation confronts the problem in which a segment of its population wants but is unable to obtain employment—and in every nation, unemployed people face some of the same problems of stress and self-worth as do Americans. One major difference is that in countries such as Sweden and Japan, more benefits are available for the unemployed, so that unemployment is not as likely to be associated with abject poverty.

| Country | 2000 | 2005 | 2010 | 2020 |
|---|---|---|---|---|
| United States | 4.0 | 5.1 | 9.6 | 4.4 |
| Canada | 6.8 | 6.8 | 8.0 | 6.5 |
| Australia | 6.3 | 5.0 | 5.2 | 5.6 |
| Japan | 4.7 | 4.4 | 5.1 | 2.9 |
| France | n.a. | 8.9 | 9.3 | 9.5 |
| Germany | 7.8 | 11.1 | 7.1 | 3.8 |
| Italy | 10.2 | 7.7 | 8.4 | 11.1 |
| Netherlands | 3.0 | 4.7 | 4.5 | 4.8 |
| Sweden | 4.7 | 7.1 | 8.4 | 6.6 |
| United Kingdom | 5.4 | 4.9 | 7.9 | 4.4 |

**TABLE 10.2**
Unemployment Rates, by Country, 2000–2020
SOURCE: International Labor Organization website.

customers. Many high-tech workers feel ongoing pressure to produce and to make their work the consuming focus of their lives. Psychiatrists and psychotherapists often find their work to be emotionally draining. In other jobs, stress is associated with such conditions as lack of communication and delegation of authority by management, fast-paced work in poor environmental conditions, frequent overtime, conflict between workers, recent reduction of employee benefits, nonstandard work schedules, and downsizing (Grunberg, Anderson-Connolly, and Greenberg 2000; Cho 2018; Schneider and Harknett 2019; Ananat and Gassman-Pines 2021).

## Work and the Quality of Life

Many people thoroughly enjoy their work. They find it meaningful and satisfying, thus providing them with a higher quality of life. They are more likely to enjoy their work when they perceive themselves to be included in the information network and the decision-making processes of their workplace (Barak and Levin 2002).

There are also many people for whom the effect of working is a kind of *emotional and spiritual malaise.* They do not despise their work, but neither are they excited by it. They may simply be apathetic or resigned. Finally, there are some who find their work to be disturbing or frustrating or even destructive to their well-being. The point is, then, that work can have very positive or very negative consequences for the worker (Campione 2008). And one of the areas that work effects is the mental and physical health of the worker.

## Work, Unemployment, and Health

Ironically, both working and not working can adversely affect your health. What are the risks?

*Work and Health.* Work can have a *negative impact on both the emotional and the physical well-being of workers* (Dalgard et al. 2009; Hauke, Flintrop, Brun, and Rugulies 2011; Nixon et al. 2011). Feelings of alienation or high levels of job dissatisfaction or job stress may lead to heavy drinking in an effort to cope (Broome and Bennett 2011) or to burnout (Fragoso et al. 2016). People whose work provides relatively low rewards (including low job security or advancement possibilities) for high levels of effort may increase their risk of cardiovascular disease three- to fourfold (Siegrist 1995). Regardless of the level of effort, job insecurity puts workers under continual stress and can produce various kinds of both physical and mental health problems (Bernhard-Oettel, Sverke, and De Witte 2006; Caroli and Godard 2016; Watson and Osberg 2018). In some high-stress occupations, such as physicians and law enforcement, suicide rates are high (Kulbarsh 2016; American Website for Suicide Prevention website). Finally, exposure to various kinds of hazardous conditions can impair both physical and mental health. A variety of cognitive and physical disabilities have been linked with such work conditions as repetitive loading, and exposure to heat, pesticides, and other toxic chemicals or metals (Ross et al. 2016).

Underemployment also poses health risks. People who are underemployed, in the sense of being overeducated and overqualified for their jobs, are likely to lack job satisfaction, leave their jobs sooner than other workers, and struggle emotionally with their lot in life (Hochberg 2009). Further, they are more likely than adequately employed workers are to report lower levels of health and well-being and exhibit symptoms of depression (Dooley, Ham-Rowbottom, and Prause 2001; Friedland and Price 2003).

The risks to health are related both to job satisfaction and to working conditions. Those who are less satisfied are more likely to exhibit various kinds of physical and mental health problems (see, e.g., Bovier, Arigoni, Schneider, and Gallacchi 2009). And as we noted earlier, 5,250 Americans died from work-related conditions in 2018. A national study of workers reported that, although Americans generally like their jobs, a substantial minority–30 percent–view their work as "just a job" that enables them to "get by" (Pew Research Center 2016). Such a perspective is hardly conducive to physical and mental health. Finally, another national study found that a third of all workers feel chronically overworked (Galinsky et al. 2005). The study also reported that the overworked have higher levels of stress, a higher proportion of depression, and more reports of poor health than do other workers.

There is, in sum, a strong relationship between stressful working conditions and physical and emotional illness. And the stress occurs in all kinds of work. A Protestant minister described his own health problems caused by stress at work. The stresses he experienced could occur in virtually any kind of job, and his story shows that no one is immune.

> I arrived at my new church with an intense anticipation of a rewarding and fruitful ministry. I brought the enthusiasm and recklessness of youth to a job that demanded the caution and wisdom of age. For about a year, the enthusiasm was sufficient. It carried me through some discouragements and minimized any overt criticism. Then I made the mistake of criticizing an older member of the church. The criticism was neither harsh nor malicious, but the member was quite sensitive and quite influential. I also plunged ahead and pushed programs and began projects without first consulting the officers. At the beginning of my second year, criticism erupted and quickly mushroomed.
>
> For about the next five years, I had problems with various people in the church. And I had a series of things go wrong with myself, both emotionally and physically. At one point, it seemed that everything was coming to a head and there would be a final all-out struggle to see whose way would prevail—mine or those that felt I was taking the church down the wrong road. Just before this culminating battle, I lost about 20 pounds from my slender physique. One week I broke out in a rash. I had severe sinus problems. Worst of all, I nearly developed a phobia about being in an enclosed area with a lot of people. I found it torturous to go to a crowded restaurant. One day I had to leave a church conference because my heart was pounding and I felt intense panic. Sometimes I even felt serious anxiety when I led the worship service.
>
> As it turned out, the "final" battle was not really the final one after all. It had only served to trigger the various physical and mental ailments that I endured for the next few years. Ultimately, we were able to work out the differences we had. I think I gained some in wisdom and lost some of my recklessness. The church began to stabilize and then grow, and some of those with whom I had fought became my best friends. After about eight years or so, I finally lost my fear of crowded places. In a way, I suppose you could say it all had a happy ending. But I wouldn't go through that again for anything. It was the only time of my life when the thought of suicide entered my mind as an appealing option.

*Unemployment and Health.* The stress of being forcibly unemployed can be as serious as the stress of working in undesirable conditions or in an unfulfilling job. For most people, *unemployment* is a traumatic experience. Millions of Americans are affected by unemployment every year. Two researchers looked at work in the early 2000s and called it the era of the "disposable worker" (Dixon and Van Horn 2003). They pointed out that nearly a fifth of American workers lost their jobs and that the great majority of these workers had no advance notice, no severance pay, and no career counseling from their employers. Some workers who lose their jobs are unemployed for only a portion of the year. Some find employment, but the work is not meaningful to them. Some have dropped out of the labor force, discouraged by their inability to find employment in their line of work. Some are the victims of downsizing that eliminated their jobs and left them in despair (Junna, Moustgaard, and Martikainen 2021).

Whatever the reason for being out of work, *unemployment is detrimental to both physical and emotional well-being* (Reine, Novo, and Hammarstrom 2004; Burgard, Brand, and House 2007). Unemployment can result in high levels of stress and lowered life satisfaction. It can lead to such problems as depression, lowered self-esteem, anger and resentment, shame and embarrassment, social isolation, serious mental illness, physical health problems, alcohol abuse, criminal behavior, and suicide (Mossakowski 2009; Morin and Kochhar 2010; Pellegrini and Rodriguez-Monguio 2013). A study of women in Texas who gave birth reported that, compared to those who were working, the unemployed gave birth to children with lower birth weights and they experienced higher

**TABLE 10.3**
Impact of a Sustained 1 Percent Rise in Unemployment

| Stress Indicator | Percent Increase |
|---|---|
| Suicide | 4.1 |
| State mental hospital admissions | 3.4 |
| State prison admissions | 4.0 |
| Cirrhosis of the liver mortality | 1.9 |
| Cardiovascular-renal disease mortality | 1.9 |

SOURCE: Brenner 1978.

rates of infant mortality (Scharber 2014). The negative consequences are likely to be more severe for workers who experience a second job loss (or who lose three or more jobs) than for those who experience their first loss (Chen, Marks, and Bersani 1994). And, finally, the trauma of being unemployed is likely to result in long-term negative consequences for well-being (Young 2012).

In a classic but still valid study, Brenner (1978) calculated the impact for a sustained 1 percent rise in unemployment in the United States from about 1940 to the early 1970s. The corresponding increases in various physical and emotional ills are shown in Table 10.3. Similarly, other researchers (Luo et al. 2011) examined suicide rates from 1928 to 2007 and found that the rates generally rose during economic recessions and fell during times of economic expansion.

The detrimental physical and emotional consequences of unemployment also are seen in other nations. In England, researchers found an association between unemployment and rates of illness (including cardiovascular disease), mortality, and suicide (Bartley, Sacker, and Clarke 2004). A Ghana study found that unemployed men were 27 percent less likely to report good health than those employed (Sulemana, Anarfo, and Doabil 2019). And a study of four nations—Australia, Germany, the United Kingdom, and the United States—concluded that unemployment has a significant negative effect on mental health in all four nations (Cygan-Rehm, Kuehnle, and Oberfichtner 2017).

## Interpersonal Relationships

A number of studies support the notion that both work-related stress and unemployment *can adversely affect interpersonal relationships.* Work in stressful conditions can lead to marital tension and conflict at home (Story and Repetti 2006; Ferguson 2011). The stress can be rooted in various factors, including the general conditions under which the work is performed and the kind of relationships the worker has with co-workers. A particularly stressful condition is shift work, which may *create both personal stress and interpersonal problems* (Grosswald 2003; Presser 2004). Researchers have found that shift work tends to increase conflict in the family, depress marital happiness and interaction, and increase various problems such as conflict over sexual and child-rearing matters and a lower quantity and quality of parent-child interaction (Demerouti, Geurts, Bakker, and Euwema 2004; Han, Miller, and Waldfogel 2010).

Underemployment is also stressful and is associated with varying degrees of both physical and emotional health (Cassidy and Wright 2008). Moreover, the strains and frustrations of stressful work conditions or of underemployment often carry over into family life, increasing tension and conflict and decreasing satisfaction.

Unemployment tends to place even more strain on an individual's relationships, including relationships within the family. During the Great Depression, when the unemployment rate went as high as one-fourth of the labor force, many workers blamed themselves for their unemployment, became disillusioned with themselves, and began to have trouble within their homes (Komarovsky 1940). Even in less serious economic recessions, workers are embarrassed by being unemployed, may begin to withdraw from social contacts, and may direct some of their hostility toward members of their families. It is, of course, not merely the embarrassment and stress of being unemployed but also the strain of trying to meet the expenses of food, clothing, housing, and health care that contributes to the conflict between spouses and between parents and children.

Not all the problems are due to unemployment or job dissatisfaction. Some situations are simply a *conflict between work and family responsibilities* (Voydanoff 2004; Forma 2009). For men, the conflict generally focuses on excessive work time—they are spending too much of their time and energy on their work. For women, the conflict is more likely to be one of scheduling problems or fatigue and irritability. In any case, the outcome is a certain amount of conflict between family members.

## Contributing Factors

The factors that contribute to unemployment are generally different from the factors involved in work dissatisfaction, alienation, and work hazards. Although we focus on the latter factors, we also examine the political economy of unemployment.

### Social Structural Factors

*The Capitalist Economy.* We noted earlier that people in a capitalist economy are motivated by profit. *In business and corporations, profit tends to be the "bottom line."* That is, the goal is profit, and managers do whatever is necessary to maximize profits. This bottom-line approach has led owners, executives, and managers to act in ways that have adverse consequences for large numbers of people. One type of action is longstanding: the subservience of workers' needs to organizational needs. Three other actions changed in nature or increased greatly after 1980: union busting, downsizing, and the use of temporary workers.

The *subservience of workers' needs to organizational needs* is illustrated by the other three actions. Workers need well-paying and meaningful jobs, but union busting, downsizing, and the use of temporary workers are ways to meet the organization's need for profits at the expense of the workers' needs. In addition, workers may be abused and exploited by tyrannical managers and supervisors who focus on efficiency and productivity rather than the workers' needs for self-esteem, encouragement, and fulfillment (Lubit 2004).

*Union busting has been going on since the unions were first formed,* but a change occurred in the 1980s (Rosenblum 1995). In 1981, the Reagan administration fired and permanently replaced more than 1,200 striking air-traffic controllers. Thereafter, an increasing number of companies dealt with strikes by hiring permanent replacements rather than by negotiating with the union.

*Downsizing and outsourcing also reflect the drive to maximize profits.* Downsizing, however, has taken on a different character—because it increases profits, it now occurs independently of whether a company is doing well or poorly and of whether the economy is booming or in recession (Simone and Kleiner 2004). Ironically, executives are rewarded for downsizing, because to the extent that profits increase as a result of the lower costs of a smaller workforce, executive bonuses go up. Similarly, outsourcing has economic benefits not only to the company but to the economy as a whole (Smith 2006). There is, therefore, little incentive on the part of either business or government to regulate the practice.

Finally, *there is increasing use of temporary and part-time workers.* Temporary employment grew rapidly during the 1980s and 1990s, accounting for about 2.5 percent of all nonfarm workers by the turn of the century (Bureau of Labor Statistics website). There are a variety of reasons why workers take temporary jobs (Jong et al. 2009). Some prefer them because of the circumstances of their lives. But for many, temporary work is a reflection of employers' desire for flexibility and lower costs rather than the worker's preferences.

A June 2019 report from the Bureau of Labor Statistics put the number of part-time workers at 26.9 million, 17.1 percent of the labor force. The majority preferred part-time work (because of such things as child care or other family responsibilities, being in school or training, and health). But a substantial minority were involuntary part-time workers, unable to find full-time work because of the economy.

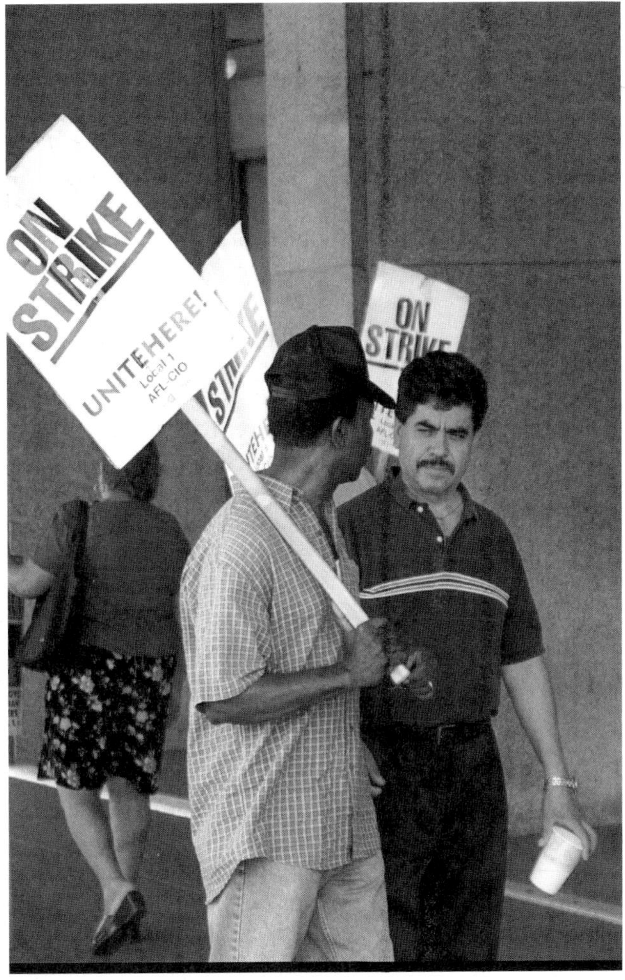


The power of labor unions has been weakened by antilabor government policies.
Andrew Resek/McGraw Hill

*The Political Economy of Work.* The traditional notion of man as the breadwinner assumed that a man's work would allow him to support his family. One of the problems of work today is that *a large number of jobs provide inadequate support and benefits to enable a family to live well.* A substantial number of Americans have to work longer hours or hold more than one job in order to provide sufficient income for their families. The Bureau of Labor Statistics noted that in 2019, 8.0 million Americans held two or more jobs, and 60 percent of them had two full-time jobs!

Many workers also struggle with wages that have not kept pace with inflation, or they have to contend with reduced employee benefits. Median household income in the United States reached a peak in 1999, then declined through 2014 until it began rising again in 2015. By 2019, it was $68,703. One reason for the lack of steady growth in household incomes is the increasing number of workers in low-wage work (Surowiecki 2013). As noted in Chapter 6, it is not possible to adequately support a family if the breadwinner works for the minimum wage. Unfortunately, it is extremely difficult to get legislation passed that raises the minimum. Ironically, when adjusted for inflation, the minimum wage was lower by 2012 than it was in the late 1960s (Shierholz 2013). And to add to the irony, worker productivity increased continuously over that period. Had the minimum wage kept pace with increases in productivity, it would now exceed $20 per hour rather than $7.25, the Federal level in early 2021.

*The Political Economy of Unemployment.* It is important to distinguish between *structural and discriminatory unemployment.* Discriminatory unemployment involves high unemployment rates for particular groups, such as women and minorities, and is discussed in the chapters that deal with those groups. Structural unemployment is the result of the *functioning of the political-economic system itself.*

Structural unemployment takes various forms. Since the Great Depression, the American economy has been regulated basically in accord with the theories of the English economist John Maynard Keynes. In Keynes's view, governments can *control the swings of the economy,* greatly moderating the inflationary and deflationary trends, programs, and taxation. There is *an inverse relationship between unemployment and inflation.* When the rate of inflation is high, the government may take steps that will result in an increase in unemployment. Some unemployment is necessary, and some fluctuations are inevitable. Yet because of the moderating impact of government intervention, fluctuations need not be as severe as they were earlier in U.S. history.

The unemployment rates shown in Table 10.1 reflect in large part the government's efforts to regulate the economy. There will always be some unemployment in a capitalist economy. The amount can be controlled and perhaps lessened by government intervention, but unemployment cannot be eliminated.

In addition to the overall rate of unemployment, the functioning of the political-economic system contributes to the high rates of unemployment in particular areas or in particular occupations at certain times. *Government spending* can create many jobs and then eliminate those jobs when the priorities change. For example, massive federal funding of the space program in the 1960s created many jobs, some of which vanished when the priorities changed in the 1970s.

*Technological changes* such as automation or the introduction of computers into a business can displace workers and lessen the need for them in the future. Old industries in the United States are in serious trouble. Numerous workers in the auto and steel industries have lost their jobs or have been indefinitely laid off. The problem may worsen as humans are replaced by robots in basic industries. Pioneered by the Japanese, robots are effective mechanisms of production in such industries as automobile manufacturing.

*The Organizational Context of Work: Unions.* The union movement has been instrumental in bringing about higher wages, fringe benefits, and safer conditions for workers (Doyle 2002). For example, in 2019, union members had median weekly earnings of $1,095, compared to $892 for non-members (Bureau of Labor Statistics 2020b). A study of the 50 states found an inverse correlation between the proportion of the working poor and the level of unionization (i.e., that fewer the unions the more working poor). There is also an inverse relationship between unionization and income inequality, and it exists both in the United States and in countries round the world (Jacobs and Myers 2014; Kerrissey 2015). Finally, research by Flavin and Shufeldt (2016) found evidence that union members have higher levels of life satisfaction than those who are not members.

Given this research, then, it is not surprising that with the dramatic decline in union membership since the 1970s, inequality between wage earners has increased considerably (Western and Rosenfeld 2011) and the subjective well-being of people has declined somewhat (Flavin, Pacek, and Radcliff 2010). Various factors have brought about the decline of unions. Some losses occurred as a result of layoffs in manufacturing. In addition, unions have faced adverse rulings by conservative federal judges and the National

Labor Relations Board (NLRB) regarding the right of unions to organize and strike. Meanwhile, management often has been supported by the legal system in efforts to keep unions out or to break existing unions. The globalization of the economy also has weakened the bargaining power of unions by allowing employers to opt for foreign locations for a part or all of the work. Finally, some unions have failed to engage in vigorous recruiting efforts.

The obstacles faced by unions are illustrated by a study of an Arizona miners' strike (Rosenblum 1995). The miners, who were largely Mexican Americans, went on strike against one of the world's largest copper producers. The strike was a reaction to the company's demand that cost-of-living adjustments and some other benefits be eliminated. The company replaced all the workers, and the replacements voted to decertify the union. The National Labor Relations Board ruled in favor of the company when the union protested.

Union membership has declined, then, not because workers have become disillusioned with their unions but because of various social factors and processes. If the unions continue to decline, there may be an increase in the kinds of work problems we have discussed.

*Contemporary Work Roles and Environments.* Job dissatisfaction and alienation reflect the *nature of work roles and work environments* in contemporary society. Workers suffer when they lack such benefits as positive relationships at the workplace, clear definitions of their work, physical comfort in the work environment, and just treatment (Gershon et al. 2009). They particularly suffer when they feel they have no control over their work lives and no security in their jobs, a situation that is exacerbated by a growing tendency to use part-time and temporary workers.

Work roles in American society result from a combination of factors, including *technological developments, efforts to maximize profits, and the bureaucratization of work.* The disposable worker is one consequence of the effort to maximize profits. At least three consequences of the technological developments bear upon the meaningfulness of work. First, technology brought with it *highly specialized tasks,* with the result that many workers focus on a narrow range of tasks and may have little or no sense of the overall project.

Second, and associated with the intense specialization, many jobs are stressful. A survey of American workers found that 5 percent reported being "extremely" stressed at work, 14 percent said they were stressed "quite a bit," and 33 percent regarded themselves as "somewhat" stressed (Yung 2004). The other 47 percent reported their stress level at work as "a little or not at all." Reasons for the stress include too much responsibility, too many demands, too much pressure, and jobs that involve *extremely repetitious, routine tasks.* Quite a few workers must *come to terms with the boredom of their work.* The tactics they use include such activities as daydreaming, playing, singing, and talking.

Barbara Garson (1975) described the *coping mechanisms* utilized by people who work in routine jobs ranging from typists, to keypunchers, to workers who stack Ping-Pong paddles all day, to tuna cleaners in a seafood plant. The deadly routine of many jobs is portrayed in the account of Cindy, a girl who worked for a time in the Ping-Pong factory.

> My job was stacking the Ping-Pong paddles into piles of fifty. Actually I didn't have to count all the way up to fifty. To make it a little easier they told me to stack them in circles of four with the first handle facing me. When there got to be thirteen handles on the second one from the front, then I'd know I had fifty. . . . As soon as I'd stack 'em, they'd unstack 'em. Maybe it wouldn't have been so bad if I could have seen all the piles I stacked at the end of

> the day. But they were taking them down as fast as I was piling them up. That was the worst part of the job (Garson 1975:1–2).

Such jobs are stressful. They may also be physically and emotionally harmful. Jobs that involve the continued use of a particular muscle can lead to *repetitive strain injury* (Breslin et al. 2013). A wide variety of jobs, from those in a chicken processing factory to those in telecommunications organizations expose workers to repetitive strain injury, which can be physically debilitating and emotionally stressful.

Third, technological developments are associated with *depersonalization* within the workplace. Workers tend to be *isolated* in certain kinds of jobs. For instance, isolation may occur when the work is computerized or automated. In such cases, the workers may have to pay closer attention to their work, have less interaction with people, and engage in fewer tasks that require teamwork.

Work roles also are affected by *bureaucratization of work.* Perhaps the majority of Americans work in bureaucratic organizations, which tend to be *authoritarian.* A defining characteristic of a bureaucracy is the hierarchy of authority. Workers in an authoritarian organization are likely to experience negative emotions and attitudes ranging from job dissatisfaction to alienation. People prefer to be *involved in decisions that affect them and their work.* Their satisfaction with their work, their motivation, and their effectiveness all can be enhanced by participation in the decision-making process (Barak and Levin 2002).

Participation gives the worker some control over his or her work. The more control that workers have, the more likely they are to be satisfied and the more likely the work is to enhance their health, while less control means less satisfaction and more physical and emotional problems are likely (Spector 2002; Gelsema et al. 2006; Brand, Warren, Carayon, and Hoonakker 2007).

Unfortunately, workers are unlikely to have the opportunity for participation and a sense of control in many bureaucratic organizations. Lacking that opportunity, they are likely to have lower levels of job satisfaction, lower morale, and lower levels of motivation.

In addition to the frustrations of working in an authoritarian organization, workers must deal with a certain amount of *built-in conflict* that bureaucracies tend to generate. In theory, such conflict is unnecessary because the chain of command is clear: All workers are experts in their own jobs, and there are rules to cover all tasks and any problems. In reality, a certain amount of conflict is invariably found in work roles. There may be *role ambiguity* (a lack of clear information about a particular work role) that results in lower job satisfaction and higher stress levels (McCleese and Eby 2006). There may be *role conflict* because different groups in the workplace have different expectations for a particular work role or because the role expectations are excessive. Role conflict, like role ambiguity, leads to lower satisfaction and higher stress levels. The important point is that these problems are not the result of the individual worker's cantankerous nature but of contradictions that are part of the work role itself. The individual falls victim to the role and suffers the consequences of lowered satisfaction and higher stress levels.

*The Political Economy of Work Hazards.* Some jobs necessarily entail more risk than others, and others entail more risk than necessary. Many work-related illnesses and injuries could be prevented or at least minimized if the health and well-being of workers took priority over profit. Historically, untold numbers of American workers have died in the name of profit and with the approval or apathy of the government.

The government has not yet engaged in the vigorous efforts needed to maintain a safe work environment. Both the federal and state governments have been lax in the

Despite the efforts of OSHA to protect the health and lives of workers, hazards still exist.
©Stockbyte/PunchStock

criminal prosecution of companies in which workers die because of inadequate safety measures. Further, the federal government tends to prosecute employers on civil rather than criminal grounds.

One government program that has been effective is the Occupational Safety and Health Administration (OSHA). OSHA (1996) was established in 1970 to protect the health and lives of workers. OSHA inspectors work with other professionals such as investigators, engineers, and physicians to establish and enforce safety standards. Overall, the workplace death rate has been cut by more than half since 1970; more than 100,000 workers could have died on the job but did not because of the improved safety and health conditions required by OSHA.

Although the results of OSHA are impressive, accidents and deaths in the workplace continue to be a problem. As long as the issue remains a civil rather than a criminal matter, work hazards probably will continue to put many workers at risk.

## Social Psychological Factors

*Attitudes.* Attitudes toward unions hurt many workers. We noted that union power may be diminishing along with declining membership. In addition, public opinion about unions and union leaders is not strongly positive. Polls by the Pew Research

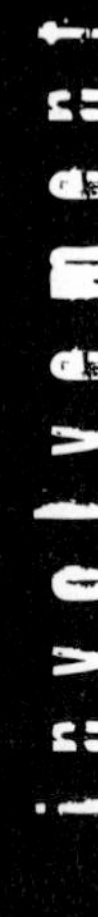

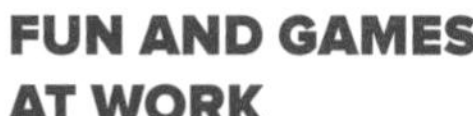

## FUN AND GAMES AT WORK

As various studies in this chapter indicate, many Americans find little pleasure in their jobs, though most expect their work to be enjoyable and fulfilling. By young adulthood, most people have worked at some job. Consider how much enjoyment and fulfillment you have received from your own work experiences. With respect to any job (or jobs) you have had, think about your feelings toward the work, the impact that the work had on your life, and the problems and satisfactions connected to the work. Imagine that someone is interviewing you about your experiences. Write out your answers to the following questions about a job you have had or now have.

What did you most like about the job?

What did you most dislike about the job?

How would you feel about working at the job for all or the major portion of your life? Why?

How were you treated by others in your work role?

Did the job make any difference in the way you feel about yourself? Why or why not?

How could the job be made more meaningful to workers?

Gather with other class members working on this project and summarize the results. What do the results say about the amount of worker dissatisfaction and alienation in America? If the only jobs available were the kinds discussed by the class, would most Americans prefer not to work? Could all the jobs be made into meaningful and fulfilling experiences?

Center show that since 1985 the proportion of Americans who have a favorable view of unions has fluctuated a little above and below the 50 percent level; in 2018 it was 55 percent (Desilver 2018). In other words, at any given point in time roughly half of Americans look favorably and half look unfavorably on the union movement.

fallacy

The negative attitudes that many Americans have about unions sometimes lead them into the *fallacy of circular reasoning,* as exemplified by the following exchange between two students in a social problems class:

"Unions hurt the economy and they hurt the workers."
"But the workers are much better off than they were in the past, before they had unions."
"They're not better off than they would be without the unions."
"How do you know? How can you say that?"
"Because unions hurt people. They keep workers from getting the best deal for themselves in the free market."

Negative thinking about unions is interesting in view of the union movement's achievements. The power of labor unions, along with government intervention, has helped eliminate many lethal work situations and has greatly improved the conditions of labor. Without the support of the public, labor unions will find themselves increasingly unable to gain further benefits for their members and for labor as a whole. Public opinion vacillates, of course, and may shift again in a more favorable direction. However, the decline in public approval of labor unions is an unwelcome sign to people who strive to improve the lot of workers.

Another attitude that enters into work problems is the sense of superiority that people might have toward certain workers. The attitudes of many Americans toward service workers, manual laborers, and clerical workers range from patronizing to contemptuous. If some workers are dissatisfied or alienated, it is in part because others *treat them with little or no respect because of their jobs.* For example, we have seen many instances of secretaries and clerks being treated with contempt by their superiors or by customers who feel they should quickly respond to demands from those who "pay your salary."

*Socialization.* One of the more important reasons Americans desire interesting work that makes full use of their skills and abilities is that they have been socialized to expect it. *The socialization process in the United States involves an emphasis on achievement,* and that achievement involves a job that will enable you to do better than your parents and to fulfill yourself (Chang et al. 2006). Work–the right kind of work–is an integral part of the American dream. That is why parents will forgo some of their own pleasure in order to send their children through college, and why professionals frequently prefer for their children to follow them in some kind of professional career.

In other words, you learn at an early age that if you are going to engage seriously in the pursuit of happiness that is your right, you must secure the kind of work that is conducive to the pursuit. As long as work is an integral part of individual fulfillment, and as long as the economy does not yield sufficient numbers of jobs that facilitate fulfillment, Americans will continue to have the quality of their lives diminished by the contradiction between socialized expectations and the realities of society.

*The Ideology and Reality of Work.* A final factor in work problems is the incongruity between the ideology about work and the reality of work. One line of thought, which dates back to the first Protestants, insists on the *value of all work.* The classic devotional writer William Law (1906:32) said, "Worldly business is to be made holy unto the Lord, by being done as a service to Him, and in conformity to His Divine will." This ideology regards work as a sacred obligation and implies that all work is equally good.

Although American ideology emphasizes the value of work and the equal value of all work, in practice not all work is given equal value. As we noted in the previous section, some kinds of work are disparaged by people who have jobs with higher prestige. Many Americans accept the ideology that work of any kind is intrinsically superior to nonwork, only to find themselves disparaged by other Americans who have "better" jobs. This ideology compounds the problems of the unemployed, who tend to define a social problem as personal and blame themselves for their plight. In addition, the work ideology may make the unemployed feel guilty about not working, even though they are the victims of a political-economic system rather than blameworthy violators of the American way.

## Solutions: Public Policy and Private Action

The problems of work can be attacked in a number of different ways. First, with regard to unemployment, the challenge is not to bring the unemployment rate down to zero; this won't happen (even economists do not mean zero unemployment when they use the term "full employment"). The challenge is to keep the rate low by maintaining a strong economy while supporting those who are unemployed.

Government programs to train, or retool, and find jobs for the unemployed are one form of support. Although such programs often benefit people, they also are usually controversial in terms of cost and effectiveness. Finding an effective job-training program is as much a political as a technical matter and, thus, requires a strong commitment from politicians.

Unemployment benefits are another form of support. Such benefits depend on action by both federal and state governments. Contrary to what some people believe, unemployment benefits are not automatically available to anyone who loses a job. The determination and distribution of the benefits are set by the individual states (Desilver 2020). In some states, relatively few of the unemployed actually get benefits.

The government could also require other kinds of benefits for workers. Time off from work is a benefit that is important to the well-being of workers (Etzion 2003). But American workers have fewer days of paid vacation than workers in many other nations. After a year on the job, blue-collar workers tend to receive an annual paid vacation of 5 days, and white-collar workers receive 10 days. Longer paid vacations come only after years on the job. In contrast, European nations give workers substantial paid vacations—35 days in Austria and Portugal (Davis 2017).

Various measures can alleviate the problem of work-family conflict. These measures can be voluntarily undertaken by firms or mandated by the government. Work-family conflict can be minimized, for example, among those people who are able to work from their homes (e.g., via computer), those parents who are able to work part-time for a few years without jeopardizing their careers, and those workers who have more control over their hours and work conditions (Work and Family Newsbrief 2003; Hill, Martinson, and Ferris 2004).

Regarding the problem of work hazards, governmental and union actions have significantly reduced the incidence of occupational injuries and illnesses. The Occupational Safety and Health Administration of the Department of Labor acts as a watchdog group to enforce safety regulations. As a result of OSHA's activity, the rate of injuries and the number of workers killed on the job have both declined dramatically. Some employers resent the OSHA regulations and complain about government intervention in their business. Yet the data on diminishing injuries and deaths support the continuing efforts of OSHA to provide workers with a safe working environment.

Various measures can help address the problems of job dissatisfaction and alienation. From this chapter's discussion about the causes of the problems, you can see that more challenging work, greater worker participation and control, and more worker autonomy are needed. In addition, the quality of the relationship between bosses and coworkers is closely related to job satisfaction. Workers who are on good terms with and feel supported by others at the workplace have higher levels of satisfaction than do other workers (Doyle 2019). Thus, programs that engage in team-building and conflict resolution skills can enhance the quality of workplace relationships.

*Job enrichment* efforts also can reduce dissatisfaction and alienation. Job enrichment involves such changes as more worker responsibility and less direct control over the worker. It also includes the upgrading of skills required for a job and enlargement of the job so that the worker is not confined to a single, highly specialized task. Some job enrichment programs have resulted in higher job satisfaction, higher levels of worker morale, fewer grievances, and less absenteeism and turnover.

Still another measure for dealing with dissatisfaction and alienation is *flextime,* which made its debut in America in 1970 after being used successfully in Europe. There are at least three different types of flextime systems, varying by the amount of choice given to the worker. In one type, the employer lets the workers choose from a range of times to start their eight-hour workdays. A second type allows employees to choose their own schedules. Once chosen and approved, the schedules must be followed for a specified length of time. In a third type, employees can vary their own schedules on a daily basis without prior approval of supervisors. All types have limits within which employees must function. Millions of Americans now work under flextime, and the results include greater satisfaction, higher morale, increased productivity, and less stress driving to work (Kelloway and Gottlieb 1998; Lucas and Heady 2002). At the same time, one researcher found that employees who request flextime, particularly when the reason is something other than childcare, were evaluated more negatively than those not making such a request (Munsch 2016). Employers must make it very clear that any request for flextime will be treated with respect and can be made with impunity.

Dissatisfaction and alienation also can be addressed through *participatory management or organizational democracy, which involves worker participation in the decision-making process.* Of course, there are many executive decisions that must be made without such participation. But employees may participate in the decision-making process in four areas: setting organizational goals, solving problems, selecting from alternative courses of action, and making changes in the organization. In more extreme forms of involvement, employees participate in decisions about hiring and firing and about their own wages and benefits.

Employees may participate in the decisions as individuals, as part of manager-employee pairs, or as members of a group of managers and employees. Such participation fulfills the needs of employees for some degree of control over their lives, for more meaningful work, and for the kind of involvement that attacks the problem of alienation. Participation programs can be costly to implement and conflict with the traditional management-worker relationship. However, they can improve productivity, quality control, and a company's market share of the product (Levin 2006).

A final measure is *employee ownership,* including the more radical form of *employee takeover of a company.* Thousands of companies now offer workers an employee stock ownership plan (ESOP). There are three types of employee ownership plans in the United States. In *direct ownership,* employees simply own shares in the company. This is the most common form of employee ownership in the United States (Blasi and Kruse 2006). In *trust ownership,* employees acquire some portion of shares over time as stock is transferred to them as a part of their benefits. In *cooperative ownership,* employees get votes in accord with the number of shares they hold; this type of ESOP gives the employees some control of the enterprise. These plans generally lead to increased job satisfaction and worker performance (Yates 2006).

In a few cases, employees have assumed ownership and full responsibility for a company or have been allowed to work without supervisory personnel. The results tend to be uniformly positive: higher productivity, lower costs, and greater worker satisfaction and morale.

*Follow-Up.* Some critics say that Americans expect too much from their work. They not only want good pay, they also want their jobs to be fulfilling. What do you think? Should people just be grateful that they have paying jobs, and find their fulfillment in after-work activities?

## Summary

The American economy, the nature of work, and the nature of the workforce all have changed over time in America. Some recent changes in the economy that are detrimental to many Americans are corporate downsizing, increased use of temporary workers, declining union strength, reduced corporate tax obligations, and decline in income for some families. The labor force and the division of labor have increased substantially. The educational level and the proportion of females in the labor force are also increasing. The work ethic remains strong, but workers now insist that their jobs be a source of fulfillment and not solely a source of income.

Work is a social problem because of unemployment and underemployment, work hazards, and dissatisfaction and alienation. Each year millions of Americans are unemployed, though the rate varies for different groups and different occupations. Many Americans are not deeply dissatisfied with or alienated from work, but many also desire a job different from the one they have. Among the hazards of work are work-induced stress and work-related injuries and illnesses.

Work is intimately related to the quality of life because it involves the worker's health. Work-induced stress, injuries and illnesses, and job dissatisfaction can all adversely affect the worker's health. Unemployment tends to be a traumatic, stressful experience that adversely affects the worker's interpersonal relationships and health.

Capitalism with its emphasis on profit is one of the factors that contributes to problems in the American economy. Subservience of workers' needs to organizational needs, union-busting, downsizing, and increased numbers of temporary jobs all reflect the drive for profit. Structural unemployment is also a product of the capitalistic system, which includes the natural swings of the economy, technological change, government spending priorities, and the growth of multinational corporations. The nature of work roles in the American technological, bureaucratic society produces much dissatisfaction, stress, and conflict. Work hazards are frequently more common than necessary because companies give priority to profit, not to worker health and safety.

Among social psychological factors that add to the problems of work are the attitudes of Americans toward unions and toward other Americans whose jobs they regard as inferior to their own. The contradiction between the ideology and reality of work is another contributing factor. The ideology glorifies work and working and places an equal value on all work. The reality is disparagement of some work and a political-economic system that guarantees a certain amount of unemployment.

## Key Terms

Capitalism
Division of Labor
Downsizing
Labor Force
Underemployment
Unemployment Rate
Work Ethic

## Study Questions

1. How have the economy, work, and the workforce been changing in America?
2. What are some consequences for workers of the globalization of the economy?
3. Discuss whether the meaning of work is changing.
4. How much and what kinds of unemployment are there in the United States?
5. How serious are the problems of work dissatisfaction and of hazards at work?
6. How do work problems affect people's health and interpersonal relationships?
7. How does the political-economic system affect the problems related to the American economy and work?
8. In what ways do contemporary work roles increase job dissatisfaction and alienation?
9. What kinds of attitudes toward work, workers, and unions contribute to the problems of work?
10. Discuss the contradiction between the ideology and the reality of work in America.
11. What can Americans do to reduce unemployment, job hazards, and job dissatisfaction?

## Internet Resources/Exercises

1. Explore some of the ideas in this chapter on the following sites:

**http://www.dol.gov** The U.S. Department of Labor site has the latest numbers from the Bureau of Labor Statistics plus reports on every aspect of work in the United States.

**http://www.bls.gov/mlr** The Monthly Labor Review site provides abstracts of all articles from 1988 to the present.

**http://aflcio.org/** News and information about various aspects of work, including safety, from the AFL-CIO.

2. The text points out that studies are inconclusive about the degree of worker satisfaction. Use a search engine to research the topic "worker satisfaction." What would you conclude about the topic on the basis of the text materials and the materials you found?

3. Use the government sites listed above to explore work and working conditions in other nations. What kinds of problems exist in other nations that are largely or totally absent in the United States? What kinds of benefits do workers have in other nations that are lacking in the United States? On the whole, which nations do you believe have the best working conditions?

## For Further Reading

Blank, Rebecca M., Sheldon H. Danziger, and Robert F. Schoeni, eds. *Working and Poor: How Economic and Policy Changes Are Affecting Low-Wage Workers.* New York: Russell Sage Foundation, 2008. Various authors discuss all aspects of the economic well-being of low-skilled workers, including their opportunities, their patterns of consumption, and how they are affected by government policies.

Bruder, Jessica. *Nomadland: Surviving America in the Twenty-First Century.* New York: W. W. Norton, 2018. A study of transient workers who move around the country to find work, providing employers with a low-cost labor pool.

Heckscher, Charles, and Paul Adler. *The Corporation as a Collaborative Community.* New York: Oxford University Press, 2006. An examination of the way the vital quality of "community" (in the form of loyalty)—both within and between businesses—has been eroded through such things as downsizing and restructuring, and a description of the new form of community that is emerging.

Janoski, Thomas, David Luke, and Christopher Oliver. *The Causes of Structural Unemployment.* Cambridge, UK: Polity Press, 2014. A discussion of the causes of unemployment in modern industrial nations, including the impact of the global economy and what can be done to address the problem.

Maynard, Douglas C., and Daniel C. Feldman, eds. *Underemployment: Psychological, Economic, and Social Challenges.* New York: Springer, 2011. An examination of the problem of underemployment from various points of view, including the issue of why underemployment is found even in healthy economies and the effects of underemployment on economic growth and human well-being.

Rubery, Jill, and Damian Grimshaw. *The Organisation of Employment: An International Perspective.* New York: Palgrave Macmillan, 2003. A readable introduction to the way employment and labor markets are organized in advanced capitalist countries. Compares such things as trends in labor market participation, vocational training systems, the regulation of the labor market, and the ways firms deal with work and employment.

Zlolniski, Christian. *Janitors, Street Vendors, and Activists: The Lives of Mexican Immigrants in Silicon Valley.* Berkeley, CA: University of California Press, 2006. An exploration of the use of Mexican immigrants for low-wage jobs in the high-tech industry, showing both how the workers are exploited and how they are affecting such things as the political process and union activity.

## References

Amadeo, K. 2016. "How outsourcing jobs affects the U.S. economy." The Balance website.

Amin, A. 2004. "Regulating economic globalization." *Transactions of the Institute of British Geographers* 29:217–33.

Ananat, E. O., and A. Gassman-Pines. 2021. "Work schedule unpredictaility." *Journal of Marriage and Family* 83:10–26.

Barak, M. E. M., and A. Levin. 2002. "Outside of the corporate mainstream and excluded from the work community: A study of diversity, job satisfaction, and well-being." *Community, Work and Family* 5:133–57.

Bartik, T. J., and S. N. Houseman. 2008. *A Future of Good Jobs? America's Challenge in the Global Economy.* Kalamazoo, MI: Upjohn Institute for Employment Research.

Bartley, M., A. Sacker, and P. Clarke. 2004. "Employment status, employment conditions, and limiting illness." *Journal of Epidemiology and Community Health* 58:501–6.

Berkshire, J. C., et al. 2011. "Bad economy has strained many nonprofit workers." *Chronicle of Philanthropy* 24 (5).

Bernhard-Oettel, C., M. Sverke, and H. De Witte. 2006. "Comparing three alternative types of employment with permanent full-time work." *Work and Stress* 19:301-18.

Blasi, J., and D. Kruse. 2006. "The political economy of employee ownership in the United States." *International Review of Sociology* 16:127-47.

Bovier, P. A., F. Arigoni, M. Schneider, and M. B. Gallacchi. 2009. "Relationships between work satisfaction, emotional exhaustion and mental health among Swiss primary care physicians." *European Journal of Public Health* 19:611-17.

Brand, J. E., J. R. Warren, P. Carayon, and P. Hoonakker. 2007. "Do job characteristics mediate the relationship between SES and health?" *Social Science Research* 36:222-53.

Brenner, M. H. 1978. "The social costs of economic distress." In *Consultation on the Social Impact of Economic Distress,* pp. 3-6. New York: American Jewish Committee, Institute of Human Relations.

Breslin, F. C., et al. 2013. "The demographic and contextual correlates of work-related repetitive strain injuries among Canadian men and women." *American Journal of Industrial medicine* 56:1180-89.

Broome, K. M., and J. B. Bennett. 2011. "Reducing heavy alcohol consumption in young restaurant workers." *Journal of Studies on Alcohol and Drugs* 72:117-24.

Bureau of Labor Statistics. 2018. "Contingent and alternative employment arrangements." BLS website.

——. 2020a. "Employer-reported workplace injuries and illnesses–2019." BLS website.

——. 2020b. "Union members summary." BLS website.

Burgard, S. A., J. E. Brand, and J. S. House. 2007. "Toward a better estimation of the effect of job loss on health." *Journal of Health and Social Behavior* 48:369-84.

Campione, W. 2008. "Employed women's well-being: The global and daily impact of work." *Journal of Family and Economic Issues* 29:346-61.

Caroli, E., and M. Godard. 2016. "Does job insecurity deteriorate health?" *Health Economics* 25:131-47.

Caskey, J. P. 1994. *Fringe Banking: Check-Cashing Outlets, Pawnshops, and the Poor.* New York: Sage.

Cassidy, T., and L. Wright. 2008. "Graduate employment status and health: A longitudinal analysis of the transition from student." *Social Psychology of Education* 11:181-91.

Chang, E., C. Chen, E. Greenberger, D. Dooley, and J. Heckhausen. 2006. "What do they want in life? The life goals of a multi-ethnic, multi-generational sample of high school seniors." *Journal of Youth & Adolescence* 35:302-13.

Chen, H., M. R. Marks, and C. A. Bersani. 1994. "Unemployment classifications and subjective well-being." *Sociological Review* 42 (February):62-78.

Cho, Y. 2018. "The effects of nonstandard work schedules on workers' health." *International Journal of Social Welfare* 27:74-87.

Cygan-Rehm, K., D. Kuehnle, and M. Oberfichtner. 2017. "Bounding the causal effect of unemployment on mental health." *Health Economics* 26:1844-61.

Dalgard, O. S., et al. 2009. "Job demands, job control, and mental health in a 110-year follow-up study." *Work & Stress* 23:284-96.

Davis, C. 2017. "World's most paid vacation days." *Huffington Post,* December 6.

Demerouti, E., S. Geurts, A. Bakker, and M. Euwema. 2004. "The impact of shiftwork on work-home conflict, job attitudes, and health." *Ergonomics* 47:987-1002.

Desilver, D. 2016. "More older Americans are working, and working more, than they used to." Pew Research Center website.

——. 2018. "Most Americans view unions favorably, though few workers belong to one." Pew Research Center website.

——. 2020. "Not all unemployed people get unemployment benefits." Pew Research Center website.

Dixon, K. A., and C. E. Van Horn. 2003. "The disposable worker: Living in a job-loss economy." *Heldrich Work Trends Survey* 6, no. 2.

Dooley, D., K. A. Ham-Rowbottom, and J. Prause. 2001. "Underemployment and depression." *Journal of Health and Social Behavior* 41:421-36.

Doyle, A. 2019. "What are the most satisfying jobs?" The Balance Careers website.

Doyle, R. 2002. "Bad things happen." *Scientific American,* June, p. 26.

Engardio, P. 2006. "Outsourcing: Job killer or innovation boost?" *Business Week Online,* November 9.

Etzion, D. 2003. "Annual vacation: Duration of relief from job stressors and burnout." *Anxiety, Stress, and Coping* 16:213-26.

Ferguson, M. 2011. "You cannot leave it at the office: Spillover and crossover of coworker incivility." *Journal of Organizational Behavior* 33:571–88.

Fitzgerald, S. R., J. A. Haythornthwaite, S. Suchday, and C. K. Ewart. 2003. "Anger in young black and white workers." *Journal of Behavioral Medicine* 26:283–96.

Flavin, P., A. C. Pacek, and B. Radcliff. 2010. "Labor unions and life satisfaction." *Social Indicators Research* 98:435–49.

Flavin, P., and G. Shufeldt. 2016. "Labor union membership and life satisfaction in the United States." *Labor Studies Journal* 41:171–84.

Forma, P. 2009. "Work, family and intentions to withdraw from the workplace." *International Journal of Social Welfare* 18:183–92.

Fragoso, Z. L., et al. 2016. "Burnout and engagement." *Workplace Health and Safety,* June 9.

Friedland, D. S., and R. H. Price. 2003. "Underemployment: Consequences for the health and well-being of workers." *American Journal of Community Psychology* 32:33–45.

Galinsky, E., et al. 2005. *Overwork in America*. New York: Families and Work Institute.

Garson, B. 1975. *All the Livelong Day: The Meaning and Demeaning of Routine Work*. New York: Penguin.

Gelsema, T. I., et al. 2006. "A longitudinal study of job stress in the nursing profession." *Journal of Nursing Management* 14:289–99.

Gershon, R. R. M., B. Barocas, A. N. Canton, X. Li, and D. Vlahov. 2009. "Mental, physical, and behavioral outcomes associated with perceived work stress in police officers." *Criminal Justice and Behavior* 36:275–89.

Griswold, D. 2010. "Global markets keep U.S. economy afloat." CATO Institute website.

Grosswald, B. 2003. "Shift work and negative work-to-family spillover." *Journal of Sociology and Social Welfare* 30:30–42.

Grunberg, L., R. Anderson-Connolly, and E. S. Greenberg. 2000. "Surviving layoffs." *Work and Occupations* 27 (February):7–31.

Han, W., D. P. Miller, and J. Waldfogel. 2010. "Parental work schedules and adolescent risky behaviors." *Developmental Psychology* 46:1245–67.

Harrison, B. 1994. Lean and Mean: *The Changing Landscape of Corporate Power in the Age of Flexibility*. New York: Basic Books.

Hatton, E. 2011. *The Temp Economy: From Kelly Girls to Permatemps in Postwar America*. Philadelphia, PA: Temple University Press.

Hauke, A., J. Flintrop, E. Brun, and R. Rugulies. 2011. "The impact of work-related psychosocial stressors on the onset of musculoskeletal disorders in specific body regions." *Work & Stress* 25:243–56.

Hill, E. J., V. Martinson, and M. Ferris. 2004. "New-concept part-time employment as a work-family adaptive strategy for women professionals with small children." *Family Relations* 53:282–92.

Hira, R. 2009. "U.S. workers in a global job market." *Issues in Science and Technology* 25:53–58.

Hochberg, A. 2009. "Overqualified and underemployed in 'survival jobs.'" National Public Radio website.

Ilg, R., and E. Theodossiou. 2012. "Job search of the unemployed by duration of unemployment." *Monthly Labor Review,* March, pp. 41–49.

Jacobs, D., and L. Myers. 2014. "Union strength, neoliberalism, and inequality." *American Sociological Review* 79:752–74.

Jiang, L., and T. M. Probst. 2016. "The moderating effect of trust in management on consequences of job insecurity." *Economics and Industrial Democracy,* July 6.

Jong, J., et al. 2009. "Motives for accepting temporary employment." *International Journal of Manpower* 30:23–52.

Junna, L., H. Moustgaard, and P. Martikainen. 2021. "Unemployment from stable, downsized and closed workplaces and alcohol-related mortality." *Addiction* 116:74–82.

Kalleberg, A. L. 2009. "Precarious work, insecure workers: Employment relations in transition." *American Sociological Review* 74:1–22.

Kelloway, E. K., and B. H. Gottlieb. 1998. "The effect of alternative work arrangements on women's well-being." *Womens Health* 4:1–18.

Kerrissey, J. 2015. "Collective labor rights and income inequality." *American Sociological Review* 80:626–53.

Komarovsky, M. 1940. *The Unemployed Man and His Family*. New York: Dryden Press.

Kulbarsh, P. 2016. "Police suicide statistics." Officer.com website.

Law, W. 1906. *A Serious Call to a Devout and Holy Life*. New York: E. P. Dutton.

Lenski, G. E. 1966. *Power and Privilege*. New York: McGraw-Hill.

Levin, H. 2006. "Worker democracy and worker productivity." *Social Justice Research* 19:109-21.

Lubit, R. 2004. "The tyranny of toxic managers." *Ivey Business Journal,* March/April.

Lucas, J. L., and R. B. Heady. 2002. "Flextime commuters and their driver stress, feelings of time urgency, and commute satisfaction." *Journal of Business and Psychology* 16:565-71.

Luo, F., et al. 2011. "Impact of business cycles on U.S. suicide rates, 1928-2007." *American Journal of Public Health* 101:1139-46.

McCleese, C. S., and L. T. Eby. 2006. "Reactions to job content plateaus." *Career Development Quarterly* 55:64-76.

Meyer, L. B. 2003. "Economic globalization and women's status in the labor market." *Sociological Quarterly* 44:351-83.

Moen, P., and Y. Yu. 2000. "Effective work/life strategies." *Social Problems* 47:291-326.

Morin, R., and R. Kochhar. 2010. "Lost income, lost friends—and loss of self-respect." Pew Research Center website.

Mossakowski, K. N. 2009. "The influence of past unemployment duration on symptoms of depression among young women and men in the United States." *American Journal of Public Health* 99:1826-32.

Munsch, C. L. 2016. "Flexible work, flexible penalties." *Social Forces* 94:1567-91.

Nixon, A. E., et al. 2011. "Can work make you sick? A meta-analysis of the relationships between job stressors and physical symptoms." *Work & Stress* 25:1-22.

Nunley, J. M., et al. 2016. "The effects of unemployment and underemployment on employment opportunities." *ILR Review,* June 22.

Occupational Safety and Health Administration. 1996. "Information about OSHA." OSHA website.

Pellegrini, L. C., and R. Rodriguez-Monguio. 2013. "Unemployment, medicaid provisions, the mental health industry, and suicide." *The Social Science Journal* 50:482-90.

Pew Research Center. 2016. "The state of American jobs." Pew Research Center website.

——. 2019. "Views of the economic system and social safety net." Pew Research Center website.

Presser, H. B. 2004. "The economy that never sleeps." *Contexts* 3:42-49.

Rauscher, K. J., C. W. Runyan, M. D. Schulman, and J. M. Bowling. 2008. "U.S. child labor violations in the retail and service industries." *American Journal of Public Health* 98:1693-99.

Reine, I., M. Novo, and A. Hammarstrom. 2004. "Does the association between ill health and unemployment differ between young people and adults?" *Public Health* 118:337-45.

Reynolds, J. 2004. "When too much is not enough: Actual and preferred work hours in the United States and Abroad." *Sociological Forum* 19:89-120.

Rosenblum, J. D. 1995. *Copper Crucible: How the Arizona Miners' Strike of 1983 Recast Labor-Management Relations in America*. Ithaca, NY: ILR Press.

Ross, J. A., et al. 2016. "Ergonomics and beyond." *Human Factors* 58:777-95.

Scharber, H. 2014. "Does 'out of work' get into the womb?" *Journal of Health and Social Behavior* 55:266-82.

Schneider, D., and K. Harknett. 2019. "Consequences of routine work-schedule instability for worker health and well-being." *American Sociological Review* 84:82-114.

Shierholz, H. 2013. "Lagging minimum wage is one reason why Americans' wages have fallen behind productivity." Economic Policy Institute website.

Siegrist, J. 1995. "Emotions and health in occupational life." *Patient Education and Counseling* 25 (July):227-36.

Simone, A., and B. H. Kleiner. 2004. "Practical guide to workplace reduction." *Management Research News* 27:125-32.

Smith, D. 2006. "Offshoring: Political myths and economic reality." *The World Economy* 29:249-56.

Spector, P. E. 2002. "Employee control and occupational stress." *Current Directions in Psychological Science* 11:133-36.

Stokes, B. 2015. "Americans agree on trade: Good for the country, but not great for jobs." Pew Research Center website.

Story, L. B., and R. Repetti. 2006. "Daily occupational stressors and marital behavior." *Journal of Family Psychology* 20:680-89.

Sulemana, I., E. B. Anarfo, and L. Doabil. 2019. "Unemployment and self-rated health in Ghana." *International Journal of Social Economics* 46:1155-70.

Surowiecki, J. 2013. "The pay is too damn low." *The New Yorker,* August 12 & 19.

Terkel, S. 1972. *Working.* New York: Avon Books.

Theodossiou, E. 2012. "U.S. labor market shows gradual improvement in 2011." *Monthly Labor Review,* March, pp. 3-23.

Thottam, J. 2004. "When execs go." *Time,* April 26, pp. 40–41.

U.S. Bureau of Economic Analysis. 2020. "U.S. international trade in goods and services." BEA website.

U.S. Census Bureau. 1975. *Historical Statistics of the United States, Colonial Times to 1970.* Washington, DC: Government Printing Office.

U.S. Department of Labor. 2000. *Futurework: Trends and Challenges for Work in the 21st Century.* Department of Labor website.

Vaisey, S. 2006. "Education and its discontents: Overqualification in America, 1972-2002." *Social Forces* 85:835–64.

Voydanoff, P. 2004. "The effects of work demands and resources on work-to-family conflict and facilitation." *Journal of Marriage and Family* 66:398–412.

Watson, B., and L. Osberg. 2018. "Job insecurity and mental health in Canada." *Applied Economics* 50:4137–52.

Weisbrot, M. 2000. "Globalism for dummies." *Harper's Magazine,* May, pp. 15–19.

Weismantle, M. 2001. "Reasons people do not work." *Current Population Reports.* Washington, DC: Government Printing Office.

Western, B., and J. Rosenfeld. 2011. "Unions, norms and the rise in U.S. wage inequality." *American Sociological Review* 76:513-37.

Work and Family Newsbrief. 2003. "Telework found to reduce conflict: Those who work from home at least two to three days a week report having lower levels of work-family conflict than those who don't." *Work and Family Newsbrief,* p. 3.

Yates, J. 2006. "Unions and employee ownership." *Industrial Relations* 45:709–33.

Young, C. 2012. "Losing a job: The nonpecuniary cost of unemployment in the United States." *Social Forces* 91:609–34.

Yung, K. 2004. "Job stresses starting to take toll." *San Diego Union-Tribune,* May 24.

CHAPTER 11

# Education

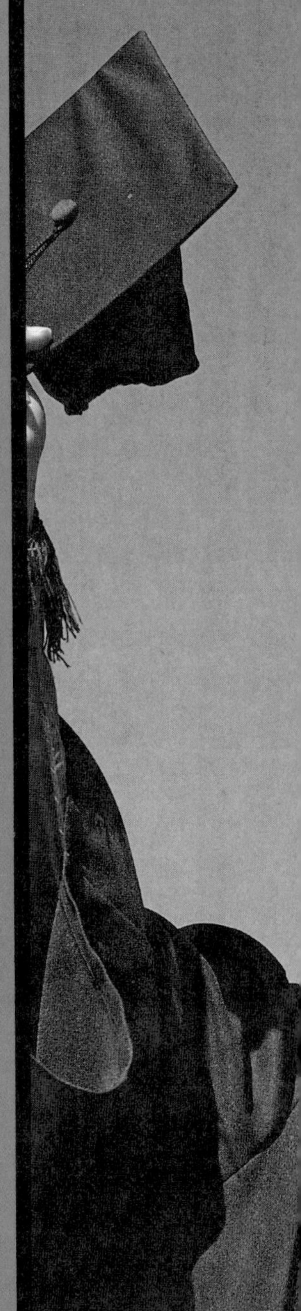

OBJECTIVES

1. Know the purposes of education.
2. Discuss the levels of educational attainment and the payoff of that attainment for Americans.
3. Explain how inequalities, the lack of expected payoff, and mediocrity make education a problem.
4. Understand how social institutions, the organization of education, and certain attitudes and values contribute to the problems of education.
5. Suggest some ways to deal with the problems of education.

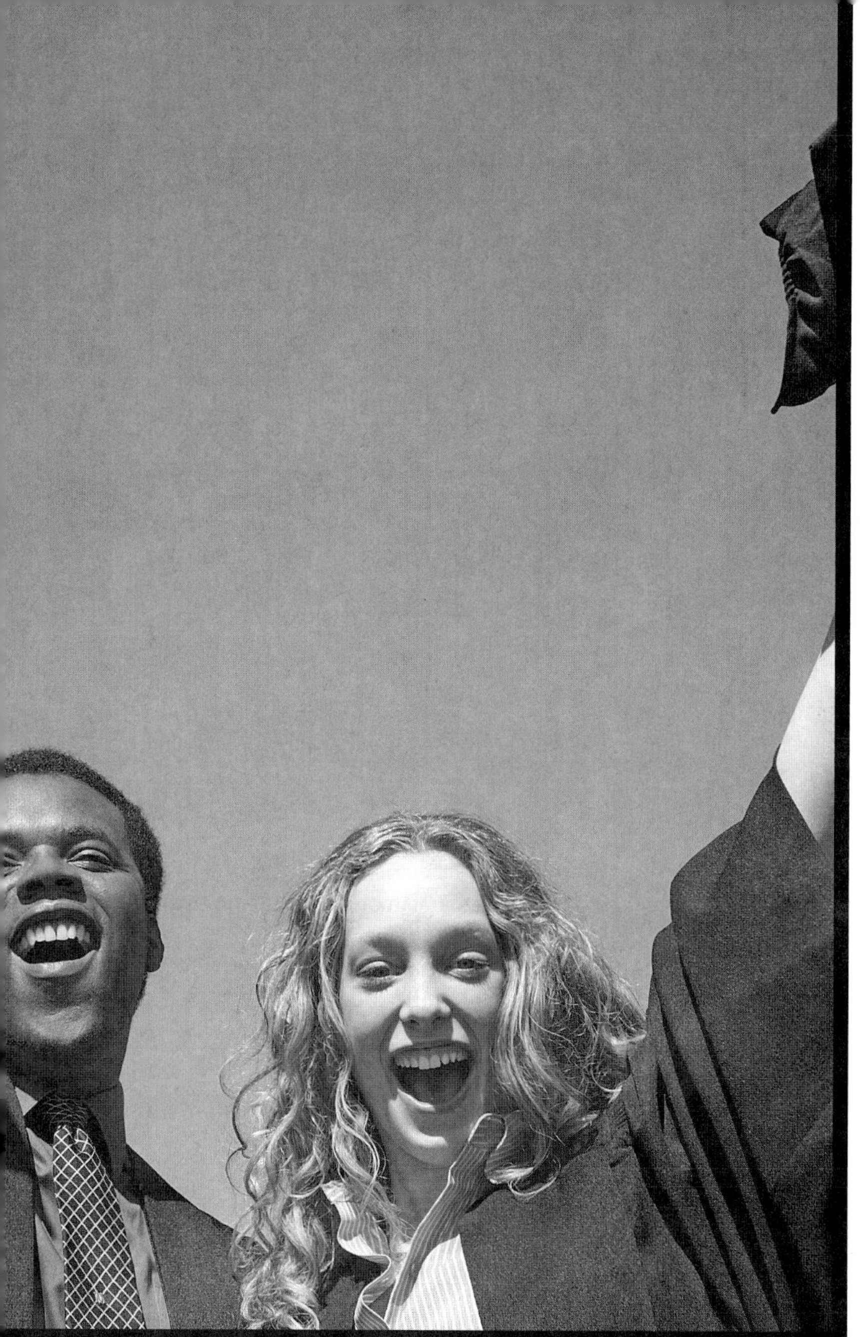

Don Hammond/Design Pics

### "I Kept My Mouth Shut"

In theory, all Americans have an equal chance to prove themselves in school. In practice, you are disadvantaged if you come from a poor or minority-group family. Marcia is an undergraduate student who comes from a middle-class family. She remembers with some regret about the time she learned how others are disadvantaged:

*I was in the first grade when I learned that we weren't all really equal at school. It was recess and I was playing on the monkey bars. One of my classmates was playing beside me. Her name was Ramona. She came from a poor family. I didn't think about it at the time, but she was very ill-kept. Neither she nor her clothes were very clean. But I liked her. I enjoyed playing with her at recess.*

*As we were playing, and Ramona was turning around on the bars, some of the other girls began to make fun of her and talk about her dirty underwear. I felt sorry for her and mad at the other girls for saying such mean things to her. I hollered to them: "She can't help it if her underwear is dirty." No sooner had I said it than the strong voice of our teacher came booming at us: "Yes, she can."*

*I could see the embarrassment on Ramona's face. She got off the monkey bars and went over and sat by herself on a bench for the rest of the recess. I'm ashamed to say that the teacher really intimidated me. I felt really bad about Ramona, but I was very careful to keep my mouth shut about it after that. I didn't want to incur the teacher's wrath, and I didn't want all the other girls to reject me.*

*I think it was about the fourth grade when I no longer saw Ramona. I don't know if she dropped out or her family moved or what. I do know that she never did well in school. But I don't think it was because she wasn't smart. Ramona just never had much of a chance.*

## Introduction

Historically, Americans have viewed education as an answer to many social ills; but a series of Gallup polls since 1974 shows a trend of declining public confidence in public schools. In 1974, 58 percent said they had a great deal or quite a lot of confidence in the nation's schools; by 2018, only 29 percent affirmed confidence in public schools while 48 percent expressed confidence in higher education.

Americans apparently have a sense that education is a problem as well as a solution to other problems. When education is in trouble, it is a very serious matter because education is the foundation of American life.

In what sense has education become a problem? In this chapter we first look at the functions of education and the high value typically placed on education. We also show how the high value is reflected in the continually "higher" amount of education attained by Americans.

In light of the functions and value of education, we look at how certain problems such as unequal opportunities bear upon the quality of life of Americans. We then examine some structural and social psychological factors that contribute to the problems and conclude with some examples of efforts to resolve the problems.

## Why Education?

What do Americans expect their educational system to achieve for them personally and for their society? In 1787 the Northwest Ordinance included a provision for the encouragement of education on the grounds that "religion, morality, and knowledge" are "necessary to good government and the happiness of mankind." The significance of this, as Parker (1975:29) pointed out, is that "a people, not yet formed into a nation, declare education to be an essential support of free government and set aside western lands for schools and education."

Thus, one function of education is to create *good and effective citizens* (Tyack 2003). There is some dispute about what it means to be a good citizen, however. Some people believe that education should produce citizens who will accept traditional values and protect the "American way of life" (which obviously means different things to different people). Education achieves this function when it transmits the **culture** from one generation to the next, that is, when it *socializes the young into the basic values, beliefs, and customs of the society.* Others believe that education should equip the citizenry to reshape their society so that the flaws and inequities are eliminated. In any case, education has been held to be essential in the process of creating effective citizens in the republic.

**culture**
the way of life of a people, including both material products (such as technology) and nonmaterial characteristics (such as values, norms, language, and beliefs)

A second function of education is to provide the individual with the *possibility for upward mobility* (Creusere, Zhao, Huie, and Troutman 2019). For a long time Americans have associated education with good jobs. Most students in colleges and universities are there to prepare for the better-paying and more prestigious jobs, not for the love of learning. Education achieves this function when it *instructs the young in knowledge and skills.*

The third function of education is personal development, including a sense of personal control (Schieman and Plickert 2008). Education *liberates people from the bonds of ignorance and prepares them to maximize their intellectual, emotional, and social development.* This function is important to educators, but few people set educational goals with personal development in mind.

Whatever their views of the primary aim of education, most Americans would probably agree that all three functions are legitimate. The schools should produce good citizens. They should help the individual to better himself or herself, and they should prepare the individual to maximize his or her own development. Because all three functions are related to the *quality of life* of the individual, if any person or group is not given the opportunity to secure an education that fulfills the functions, education becomes a social problem. Quality of life is diminished when the individual lacks the tools necessary to participate effectively in political processes, to achieve some measure of success in work or a career, or to develop his or her potential to its fullest.

## Educational Attainment and Payoff

Because of its importance to quality of life, you would expect Americans to secure an increasing amount of education over time. Most do aspire to a high level, but what about the **attainment?** Once attained, does education yield the expected payoff? Is the high value on education reflected in concrete results?

**attainment**
as distinguished from educational "achievement," the number of years of education completed by a student

### Levels of Attainment

In 1870, 57 percent of youths 5 to 17 years old were enrolled in school, and 1.2 percent were in high schools. In 2018, 93.5 percent of 5- to 6-year-olds, 97.0 percent of 7- to 9-year-olds, 98.2 percent of 10- to 13-year-olds, 98.6 percent of 14- to 15-year-olds, and 92.3 percent of 16- to 17-year-olds were enrolled in school (Digest of Educational Statistics website).

A few generations ago, completion of elementary school was considered a good *level of attainment.* Today, completion of high school is the minimal level considered appropriate. As Figure 11.1 shows, an increasing proportion of the population has been reaching that level. In fact, an increasing proportion of the population is attaining a college degree. And many students find they need or desire an advanced degree—between 1985 and 2014, enrollment in graduate programs increased more than 73 percent to 2.9 million students (Kena et al. 2016); by 2019, graduate enrollment was 3.05 million. The increasing amount of education is reflected in the data on different age groups in Table 11.1. Compare, for example, the rates for people aged 65 and older with those in the 35 to 49 age group.

Another way to look at the increasing education attainment is to note the diminishing *dropout rate.* Students begin to drop out of school after the fifth grade. Since the 1920s, the proportion dropping out, especially before completing elementary school, has decreased greatly. But there is still a substantial number who drop out—2.1 million between the ages of 16 and 24 in 2018 (Zhang 2020). The likelihood of dropping out varies among different groups. Males are more likely to drop out than are females. Students in the lower socioeconomic strata are more likely than those in higher strata to drop out. And minorities have higher rates (8 percent of Hispanics and 6.4 percent of African Americans) than do whites (4.2 percent).

One factor that has aided educational attainment is the proliferation of two-year colleges. Their enrollment increased fivefold from 1960 to 1970 and more than doubled

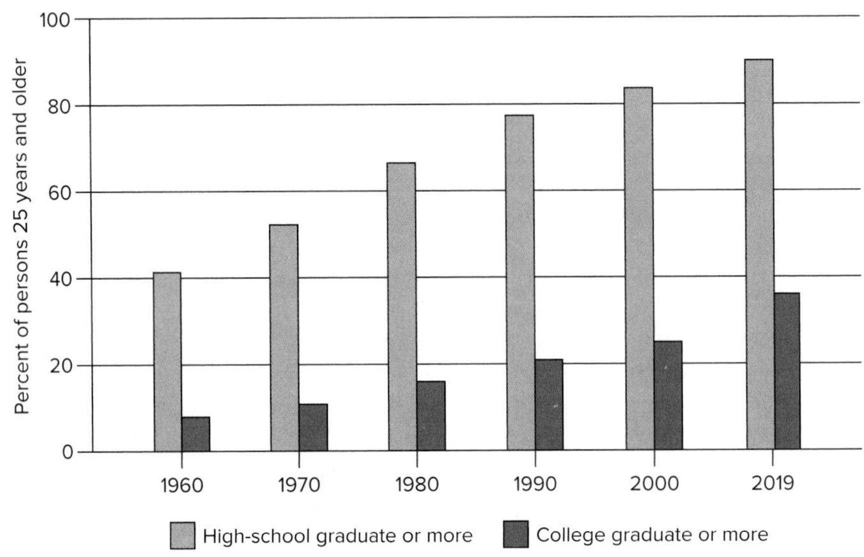


**FIGURE 11.1**
Educational Attainment of Adults (25 years and older).
Source: Digest of Educational Statistics website.

**TABLE 11.1**
Years of School Completed, by Age, Sex, Race, and Hispanic Origin, 2017 (persons 18 years old and older)

| | **Percent of Population** | | | |
|---|---|---|---|---|
| | **High School Graduate** | **Some College, but No Degree** | **Associate's Degree** | **Bachelor's or Higher Degree** |
| Total | 27.1 | 20.4 | 5.3 | 32.0 |
| Age | | | | |
| 25–34 years | 25.5 | 18.5 | 10.4 | 36.1 |
| 35–49 years | 26.9 | 15.9 | 7.5 | 35.8 |
| 50–59 years | 31.1 | 16.3 | 10.8 | 32.0 |
| 60–64 years | 30.7 | 17.4 | 10.3 | 31.5 |
| 65 years and over | 34.6 | 15.7 | 7.4 | 26.7 |
| Sex | | | | |
| Male | 30.8 | 18.9 | 8.3 | 29.3 |
| Female | 28.5 | 19.2 | 10.2 | 30.3 |
| Race/Ethnicity | | | | |
| White | 29.4 | 19.0 | 10.2 | 33.9 |
| Black | 34.3 | 22.9 | 9.3 | 20.3 |
| Asian | 18.3 | 7.8 | 6.2 | 50.3 |
| Hispanic | 30.7 | 17.2 | 6.8 | 13.6 |

SOURCE: Digest of Educational Statistics website.

from 1970 to 1980 (Figure 11.2). After 1980, enrollment continued to rise, but much more slowly. By 2018, there were 5.7 million students enrolled in two-year colleges in the nation. Community colleges offer both preparation for four-year colleges and universities and numerous terminal programs. Many students use the community college experience to decide on their educational and career goals.

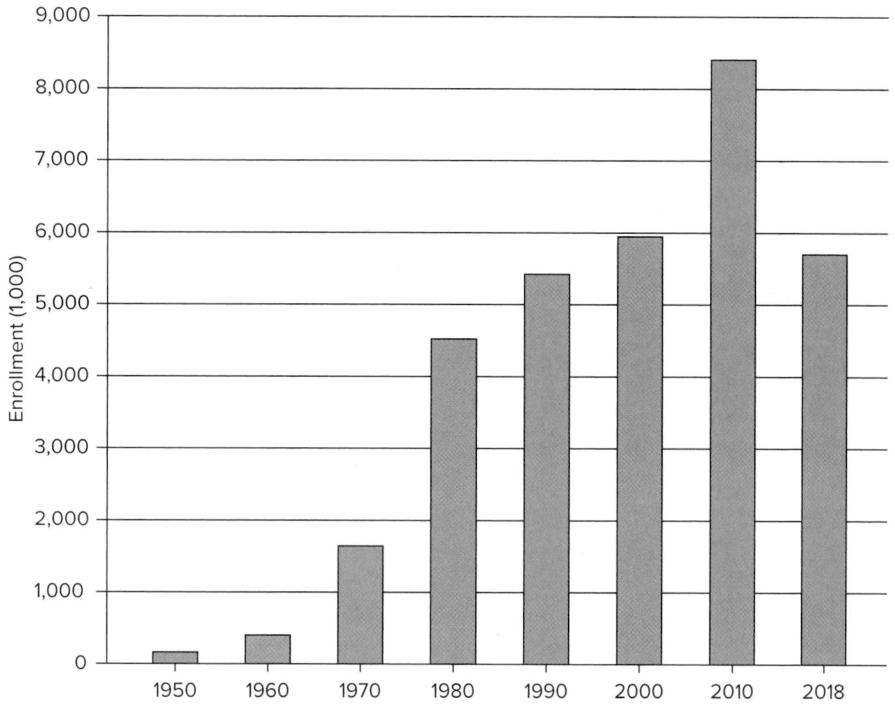


**FIGURE 11.2**
Enrollment in Community (Two-Year) Colleges, 1950–2018.

Source: Digest of Educational Statistics website.

## Attainment and Payoff

In some ways you cannot talk about the *payoff of education*. You cannot, for instance, measure the personal development of individuals and correlate that with education. However, there is a positive relationship between happiness and educational level; that is, the higher the level of education, the more likely you are to be happy. In a Gallup poll, about 90 percent of those with some college or more said they were very or fairly happy, compared to 79 percent of those with a high-school or less level of education (McCarthy 2020). Of course, happiness and life satisfaction are not measures of personal development—the fulfillment of an individual's potential. At best, you can say that the greater happiness and satisfaction reported by the better educated may reflect a tendency toward greater fulfillment of potential.

Similarly, there is only minimal evidence that education creates an effective citizenry. We know, for instance, that there is a *direct correlation between level of education and voter participation*. In fact, there are dramatic differences in voting rates between people in differing educational categories. The percentage of people with advanced degrees who vote is more than double the percentage of those who have a high-school or less education.

More educated people are also more likely to hold democratic values and to support democratic practices. Although such relationships indicate positive contributions of education to citizenship, they do not tell us whether education helps people to detect and reject demagoguery and to participate meaningfully in the defense of freedom and the shaping of a just social order. Education does increase political participation and understanding. However, the more educated people usually are the political and corporate heads who accept and maintain the institutional policies and practices that can contribute to the various social problems of the nation.

## EDUCATIONAL ATTAINMENT, BY COUNTRY

A nation cannot successfully modernize or implement a political democracy without an educated populace. People must be educated in order to function effectively in the kinds of jobs associated with an industrial economy, and they must be educated in order to participate meaningfully in a democratic political process.

An economist argued that economic growth cannot begin in a country until at least 6 percent of the population is enrolled in primary school (Peaslee 1969). As the country continues to modernize, increasing educational levels are required. Thus, nations like the United States that are the most economically and technologically developed typically have the highest average levels of educational attainment.

Political leaders are aware of the crucial importance of education and in most nations are attempting to provide expanded educational opportunities. There are still some dramatic disparities, however. Among 36 OECD (Organization for Economic Cooperation and Development) countries, from 87 to 100 percent of 5- to 7-year-old children are enrolled in school (National Center for Education Statistics 2020). But for 15- to 19-year-old youth, enrollment varied from 95 percent in Belgium to 59 percent in Columbia.

Enrollment in higher education has also expanded greatly throughout the world. In fact, enrollment rates in developing countries are now higher than the rates were in Europe a few decades ago (Schofer and Meyer 2005). Table 11.2 shows the percent of adults aged 25 to 64 who have earned a vocational or bachelor's degree in a number of countries. As with many things, the United States is neither the most nor the least educated nation in the world. Unfortunately, data are not available for most of the developing nations. But their educational opportunities are more limited than those in the developed countries. As long as such disparities exist, it is unlikely that the inequalities between nations in such factors as income, employment, and standard of living will diminish.

There is more evidence with respect to the third function of education—providing a means of upward mobility. A strong relationship exists between levels of education and income (Table 11.3). Those differences persist throughout people's careers, so that the lifetime earnings of those with high levels of education are considerably greater than those at lower educational levels (Tamborini, Kim, and Sakamoto 2015).

fallacy

Does this mean that an individual can maximize his or her income by maximizing education? In general, yes. But to assume that *anyone* can reach the highest levels of income by maximizing education is the *fallacy of non sequitur.* Your background, including your racial or ethnic identity, and the economy are among the factors that affect your chances. We discuss this situation in some detail later in this chapter, but our point here is that the high correlation between education and income does not mean that education is the open road to success. People who attain high levels of education are likely to be those whose parents had a relatively high level of education. There is mobility in the United States, but education is more useful to the privileged as a means of passing on their privileges to their children than as a means for the underdog to be upwardly mobile.

Some people have argued that education is of no use in reducing inequality in America, that schools do virtually nothing to help the poor be upwardly mobile, and that education has little effect on the future incomes of people. Rather, they feel that economic opportunities depend upon the state of the economy; one's family background; and various other noneducational factors, such as the contacts one is able to make.

It is true that education alone is not sufficient to deal with economic inequality in America, and it is true that the best way to "get ahead" in America is to start from a high socioeconomic position (obviously something over which the individual has no control). This argument overstates the case, however. The advantaged child will not

| Earned Country | Percent of Adults, 25–64 Years, Who Have Vocational Degree | Bachelor's or Higher Degree |
|---|---|---|
| Australia | 11.5 | 29.8 |
| Austria | 7.3 | 12.7 |
| Canada | 24.9 | 27.7 |
| France | 11.9 | 18.9 |
| Germany | 11.1 | 17.0 |
| Greece | 8.8 | 17.9 |
| Japan | 20.2 | 26.4 |
| Mexico | 1.2 | 16.9 |
| Norway | 2.4 | 36.2 |
| Spain | 9.7 | 22.7 |
| Switzerland | 10.8 | 25.8 |
| United Kingdom | 10.0 | 31.0 |
| United States | 10.4 | 32.6 |

**TABLE 11.2**
Educational Attainment, by Country

SOURCE: Digest of Educational Statistics website.

**TABLE 11.3**
Median Income of Households, by Educational Attainment, 2019

| Educational Attainment | Income |
|---|---|
| Less than 9th grade | $30,355 |
| 9th to 12th grade (no diploma) | $31,326 |
| High school graduate | $48,708 |
| Some college, no degree | $61,911 |
| Associate's degree | $69,573 |
| Bachelor's degree | $100,164 |
| Master's degree | $117,439 |
| Professional degree | $162,127 |
| Doctorate degree | $142,347 |

SOURCE: Digest of Educational Statistics website.

maintain his or her advantage without an education, and at least some people gain new advantages through education (Hao and Pong 2008). Most Americans recognize this, particularly those who have themselves benefitted from education. Thus, parents with a college education are likely to pass on to their children a sense of need for a similar level of attainment. As a result, students whose parents went to college are more likely to enroll in college themselves and are also likely to expect that their education will yield some kind of prestigious work (Goyette 2008).

You may conclude, then, that although many people are upwardly mobile through educational attainment, those most likely to benefit from education are already in the middle and upper strata. In terms of mobility, the payoff from education is not equally likely for all groups.

## Education and the Quality of Life

Ideally, as we have shown, education performs a number of valued functions that enhance the quality of life for Americans. Nevertheless, education is a problem because there are inequalities and the expected payoff does not always occur.

### Inequality of Opportunity and Attainment

Besides the inequality of attainment we have touched on, there is *inequality of opportunity*—a debatable and ambiguous notion, as you will see. Such inequalities contradict *the American value of education and the ideology of equal opportunities* for all. Ideally, every American ought to have equal opportunity to maximize his or her education. However, minorities and the poor do not attain the same educational levels as white males. Is this inequality of attainment a reflection of unequal opportunities or of some characteristics of the groups themselves? You have seen in previous chapters that the answer is both but that the characteristics of the groups do not include an inferior level of intelligence. Part of the reason a son of a poor white farmer does not go to college may be his own lack of motivation, but even that lack must be seen as a social phenomenon that is rooted in a complex situation in which multiple factors work together. In other words, unequal educational attainment does not mean that those groups with lower levels of attainment are incapable of extending their education. It is important to keep this aspect in mind as we explore the ways in which educational opportunities and attainment are distributed in society.

*The Meaning of Unequal Opportunities.* There is debate over the meaning of inequality of opportunity. Most Americans, including most social scientists, would affirm the *ideal of equal educational opportunity* for all. But what does that ideal mean? Does it mean that a child should have the opportunity to attend a nonsegregated school? Does it mean that all children should be schooled with equal amounts of money? Does it mean that the proportion of people of various kinds (minorities and those from different socioeconomic strata) in the differing educational levels should be the same as their proportion in the total population? Does it mean that each child should have access to the same quality and the same amount of education? Does it mean that the same amount of education should yield the same payoff in terms of income or personal development?

Or are all these matters important? If, for instance, you define equality as all children attending nonsegregated schools, there may still be considerable inequality of funding among various schools. If you define equality as equal funds per student, children could still attend segregated schools or be less likely to attend college if they are Black or poor.

Because the meaning of unequal opportunities is debated, it is unlikely that we can settle on a definition that will be acceptable to everyone. Nevertheless, it is important to select a meaning so that we can explore the extent of inequality in America. For our purposes, equality of educational opportunity means that every child has access to quality education and is not deterred from maximizing that education by social background or economic factors. Social background factors include race, ethnic origin, sex, and socioeconomic status. Economic factors include the funding of education and the cost to the student. In brief, equality means that all Americans, whatever their background, have the opportunity to attain fairly equal amounts of education. It also means that students attend schools that are equally funded and that the cost of education (college or graduate school) does not force some students to drop out before they have reached their goal. In these terms, how much inequality is there?

*Inequality of Attainment.* We have given figures in previous chapters on *differences in educational attainment.* A measure of inequality may be the proportion of various groups that has attained different levels of education. Table 11.1 shows some of the differences. Note, for example, the proportions of those having a college degree. The proportion for whites is more than double, and the proportion for Asians is triple, that of Hispanics. Overall, the table makes it clear that whites and Asians get far more education than do African Americans and Hispanics.

A word of caution is in order here. Variations exist among Hispanics in the extent to which educational attainment is low. A Pew Research Center (2013) report on the educational attainment of Hispanics found that those from a Venezuelan background were the most educated (50 percent have a bachelor's degree or more) and those from a Salvadoran background the least educated (8 percent have a bachelor's degree and 74 percent have less than a high school diploma). The reasons for these variations are unclear, but they do caution us against the assumption that ethnicity per se is the only important variable in understanding attainment levels of America's minorities.

*Funding and Costs.* The second aspect of unequal opportunities is the *funding and cost of education.* Children do not have equal educational opportunities if they attend schools with unequal resources or if they are forced to drop out at some point because they cannot pay for the cost of their education.

There are considerable inequalities of resources, both among the states and among school districts within a state. In 2016, the average expenditure per pupil ranged from $7,276 in Utah to $23,150 in New York (Digest of Educational Statistics website). The school expenditures in a state, of course, tend to reflect such things as the overall wealth of the state, the cost of living in the state, and the personal income of the residents of the state. The expenditures also reflect the ideology of the people and the state government. Although Utah spends less than any other state per pupil on education, there are many other states with a lower median household income. In any case, the amount spent on a child's education varies enormously between the states.

We are cautious about our conclusions. A particular school in a state with lower-than-average funding may offer an immeasurably better education than a ghetto school in New York, but to conclude from this example that the lower-than-average state offers a better education is the *fallacy of dramatic instance.* The point is not that every school in the better-funded state is better than every school in the more poorly funded state. Rather, overall, the schools in the better-funded state have an advantage in resources for educating students, so that the typical student is likely to experience an education backed by greater resources.

fallacy

Funding also varies considerably within states. Schools have been funded by the property tax (discussed in more detail later in this chapter). Property tax funding means that a school district populated largely by people from lower-income groups who live in cheaper homes will have a low tax base. School districts that encompass affluent areas, on the other hand, may actually have a lower rate of taxation (number of dollars of school tax per assessed value of the property) but a much higher per-pupil income. An affluent school district may have double, triple, or quadruple the funds per pupil than an adjacent poor school district has. Should the funds available for a child's schooling be considerably less because of the neighborhood in which he or she happens to be born?

Similarly, you may ask whether an individual should drop out of college because of inadequate financial resources even though he or she is quite capable of doing the work. There is not sufficient money to provide scholarships and loans for all students who would like to go to college, and the cost of attending college has risen rapidly. For a number of decades, now, the cost of a college education has been rising much faster than the overall cost of living. This increase means that millions of American families have annual incomes less than the cost of room, board, and tuition at an average private university. Obviously, many Americans are priced out of the better colleges and universities in the nation. Moreover, the disparity between those who can and those who cannot afford college is expected to grow. There are no signs yet that the spiraling costs of higher education will stop.

There are, of course, sources of aid for those from lower-income families. This does not mean that all can afford college. There is not enough aid available to offset the cost for every low-income family that wants the help. At the same time, the group hardest hit by the rising costs are those from middle-income families (Houle 2014). Their family income is too high for them to receive tuition waivers but not high enough to avoid the huge debt acquired by borrowing money to attend college.

In sum, the quality of life for many Americans is depressed because of unequal opportunities at all levels of education. Many children cannot afford to go to a better college or even to any college. Their level of attainment will be less than their abilities warrant and often less than they desire. Those same children probably attended elementary and secondary schools that spent less on them than other schools could spend. Inequality in education exists from kindergarten to the university.

### The Atmosphere: Learning or Surviving?

**atmosphere**
the general mood and social influences in a situation or place

Another kind of inequality that contradicts the American ideology of equal opportunity involves the **atmosphere** of the school. Some atmospheres are conducive to learning, some inhibit learning, and some require the student to focus on surviving, on merely getting through the institution with body and sanity intact.

*Education as Boring.* One frequently heard criticism is that education is boring (Wurdinger 2005; Kass, Vodanovich, and Khosravi 2011). For example, boredom often results when students are required to memorize large amounts of data that are not integrated with each other and not linked to important principles or ideas. Thus, history students may be required to memorize names, dates, and events without discussing their significance for understanding the processes of social life.

Boredom can afflict students at any level. The slowest students may be bored because they cannot grasp the materials. Others may be bored because they see no point to what they are doing. Gifted children may also suffer from boredom (Long 2013). Gifted elementary students typically master from a third to a half of the curriculum in five basic subjects before they even begin the school year. Boredom leads to a variety of negative consequences. Students may behave as if they lack interest or the ability to focus their attention (Webb 2000). Or they may cut classes or even drop out of school (Fallis and Opotow 2003).

*The Atmosphere of Fear.* Perhaps worse even than boredom is the *atmosphere of fear* in which some students must function. Without a safe environment, teachers find it difficult to teach and students find it difficult to learn. Unfortunately, a considerable amount of crime and violence exists in the schools.

In the previous edition of this text, we wrote that it is no longer true that students are safer at school than away from school. That is still true. In the 2017-2018 school year, according to a national survey, students aged 12 through 18 experienced 33 nonfatal victimizations per 1,000 students at school and 16 per 1,000 students away from school (Wang et al. 2020). The survey reported the following about school victimizations for the year 2017-2018:

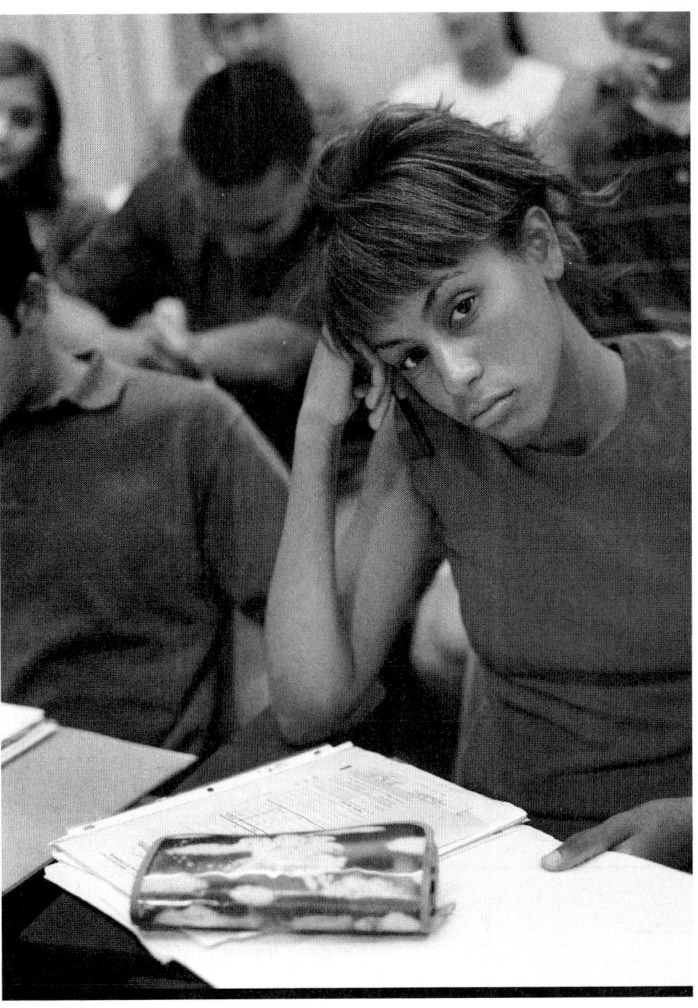

Education doesn't yield a high payoff when students are bored.
BananaStock/JupiterImages/PictureQuest

- Students aged 12 through 18 experienced 836,100 nonfatal victimizations at school.
- There were 28 school-related homicides and 13 suicides.
- A fourth of 5th-grade students attended schools where physical conflicts or bullying occurred at least monthly.
- 5 percent of 5th-grade students attended schools where theft and widespread classroom disorder occurred monthly.
- 80 percent of public schools reported that one or more incidents of violence, theft, or other crimes had taken place.
- 15 percent of public schools reported that cyberbullying had occurred among students at least weekly.

The kind of atmosphere created by such problems contributes to the difficulty of learning, to dropping out of school, to poor social adjustment, to lower academic performance, to emotional problems such as eating disorders, and to entertaining thoughts of suicide (Peguero 2011; Mundy et al. 2017; Day et al. 2021). Moreover, they are likely to have long-term negative consequences. For example, a survey of adults who had been bullied between the ages of 9 and 16 years found elevated rates of psychiatric disorders (such as phobias, anxiety, depression) among the victims (Copeland et al. 2013).

It is also important to keep in mind that all these problems are more severe in poor, inner-city schools where they create what Shanker (1994) called the "crab bucket syndrome." This syndrome refers to the fact that inner-city students who try to free themselves from the culture of gangs, drugs, and violence and do good work face enormous pressure, harassment, and even violence as others try to pull them back into the bucket. In one inner-city school, names of outstanding students were kept secret prior to an awards ceremony lest the honorees refuse to show up out of fear. One recipient had to be ordered to the stage to receive his reward; he walked up amid the sneering catcalls of others.

**ritualized deprivation**
a school atmosphere in which the motions of teaching and learning continue, while the students are more concerned about surviving than learning

*Ritualized Deprivation.* Another condition that exists in many American classrooms is described as **ritualized deprivation.** The teacher performs in a substandard fashion and may be with the children for only a short period of time. The building and facilities are substandard and contain little if anything to stimulate curiosity or motivate the intellect. The school offers a daily ritual—some of the motions of teaching and learning are present. However, the ritual occurs in such a deprived context that the student is more concerned about surviving the process than learning.

The kind of school that has an atmosphere of ritualized deprivation is most likely to be found in the urban ghetto or other dominantly low-income area. Kozol (1992) describes such a school in Chicago. It is a high school with no campus and no schoolyard, though it does have a track and playing field. Forty percent of its 1,600 students are chronic truants. Only a fourth who enter ever graduate. It has some good teachers, but others who the principal admits "don't belong in education." He is not allowed to fire them, so they continue teaching.

Kozol sat in on a 12th-grade English class. The students were learning to pronounce a randomly selected list of words that are difficult, for example, "fastidious," "auspicious," and "egregious." He asked a boy who was having difficulty pronouncing "egregious" if he knew what the word meant. The boy had no idea. The teacher never asked the students to define the words or to use them in a sentence, only to try to pronounce them.

Thus, the ritual goes on. The students in the school struggle not only with fear, threats, and drugs, but with teachers who take them through pointless exercises. There seems to be little learning, just survival.

## The Payoff: A Great Training Robbery?

One of the American expectations about education is that it will pay off in terms of upward mobility (Grubb and Lazerson 2004). Historically, the correlation between education and income has been strong, but in the early 1970s a *contradiction developed between education and the economy.* Educational attainment outstripped the capacity of the economy to absorb the graduates into jobs commensurate with their training. Even when the unemployment rate is very low, many workers cannot find employment that utilizes the skills and training they have (Livingston 1998). *The disparity between educational attainment and the skill demands of the workplace means that some workers are underemployed.*

The problem is compounded by the cost of getting the education in the first place. Most college students must resort to loans to pay for their education. Federal student loans are available for up to $57,000 for an undergraduate degree and $138,500 for graduate degrees (Zinn 2020). It is daunting, to say the least, to begin one's work life with a debt of tens of thousands of dollars or even $100,000 or more.

Some parents also take out loans to help their children pay the costs of education. There is no limit on how much they can borrow. The upshot is, in 2020, Americans owed $1.7 trillion in college debt (Carey 2020).

It might appear, then, that borrowing money to complete a college degree is not worth the risks. We disagree. Keep in mind the strong correlation between education and income (Table 11.3). Also keep in mind that those in occupations that require higher levels of education will gain more, and more rapid, increases in income than

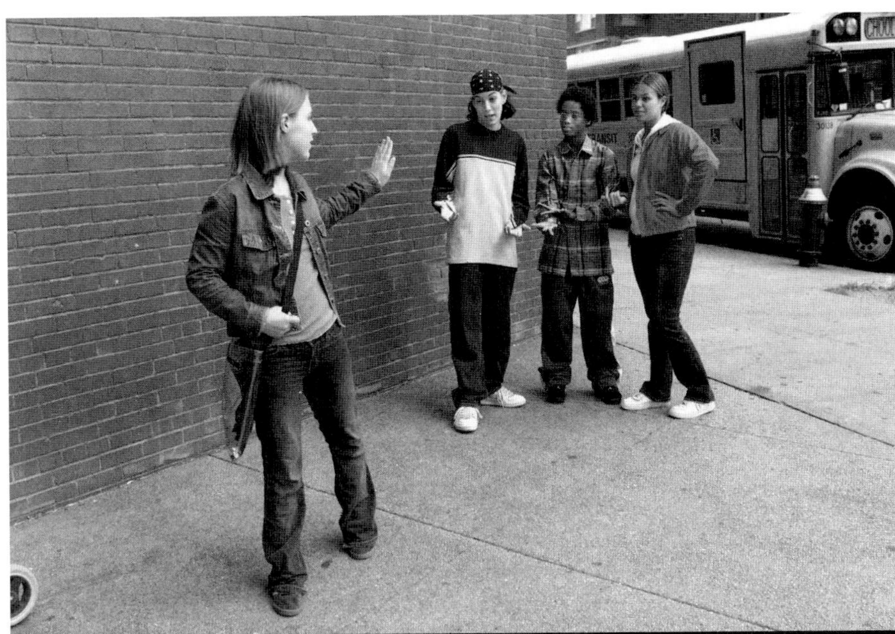

Fear of threats and violence create a difficult school environment.
Ken Karp/McGraw Hill

those in lower-level occupations. This means that over a lifetime, those with a bachelor's degree will have about double, and those with a doctorate will have about triple, the total income of those with only a high school diploma. In short, it is still true that education is associated with upward social mobility (Pfeffer and Hertel 2015).

You also should keep in mind that the diminished payoff refers strictly to employment and income. Unfortunately, Americans have focused so strongly on the economic payoff that many consider their college education useless if it does not yield a desirable, well-paying job. Only in this sense can we speak of an "oversupply" of college graduates. We could argue that all or at least the majority of Americans would profit by some college because higher education can enable the individual to think more deeply, explore more widely, and enjoy a greater range of experiences; but as long as education is valued only for its economic payoff, any failure to yield that payoff will depress the quality of life of those involved.

## American Education: A Tide of Mediocrity?

Periodically, there are severe criticisms of American education. Over the past few decades, a series of reports criticized education at every level, and all the reports suggested that the educational system is marred by mediocrity. This mediocrity means a *contradiction between the American value of and expectations about education,* on the one hand, and *the functioning of the educational system,* on the other hand.

The criticisms cover every aspect of education. For example, a report on the condition of education in 1999 looked at the quality of teaching (*Education Week* 2000). The report concluded that millions of American students have teachers who lack the minimum requirements set by the states to teach in public schools. Various loopholes and waivers are used (probably under the pressure of obtaining sufficient numbers of teachers) to put teachers into classes for which they are inadequately prepared. A follow-up study (*Education Week* 2003) described efforts to recruit and retain competent teachers, but also pointed out that the efforts were not directed toward the problem in high-poverty, high-minority, or low-achieving schools. Students in those schools were still far more likely than others to have incompetent, inexperienced, or inadequately trained teachers.

By 2020, the situation had not improved significantly. The journal gave an overall grade of "C" to the nation's schools (*Education Week* 2020). Massachusetts led the nation with a score of 91.3 out of 100 points. New Mexico had the lowest score–67.2 points. There are, then, substantial differences between the states on the quality of their educational systems.

One area of concern to critics is achievement in math and science. International data show that mathematical literacy of American students were below the average of OECD nations, ranking about halfway between the highest (China) and the lowest (Dominican Republic) (Zhang et al. 2020). In science, the United States was slightly higher than the OECD average, but still lower than 11 other nations. In part, the American scores reflect the fact that a larger proportion of American students who take the tests come from a disadvantaged social class background (Robelen 2013). But even correcting for that difference, American students are behind those of a number of nations in math and science.

A substantial number of Americans see yet another deficiency in the schools–the lack of a religious perspective. A Gallup poll reported that 61 percent of Americans support allowing daily prayer at school (Rifkin 2014). In response to the perception that the schools are spiritually deficient, there is a growing number of Christian schools. The Digest of Education Statistics website reports over 5 million students enrolled in elementary and secondary religious schools. A little over 2 million of these were in Catholic schools. What is the quality of education in these schools?

The nation, of course, has always had religiously based schools. *The parochial school tradition has been strong among Roman Catholics and Lutherans.* Some people believe that such private schools offer a better education. However, a study that compared achievement in grades four and eight between public and private schools found little difference in reading and math scores (Braun, Jenkins, and Grigg 2006). Eighth-grade students in private schools did score higher on reading. Otherwise, when taking into account characteristics of the students (such as gender and race/ethnicity), the differences in reading and math scores were insignificant.

Such scores are not, of course, the only measure of effectiveness. We need to raise the question of how religious schools, and conservative Christian schools in particular, teach the various disciplines, including the sciences. Since the schools teach pupils to think and behave in accord with particular religious doctrines, religious ideology enters into every facet of the curriculum. Such schools may teach creationism instead of (not along with) evolution and Darwinism.

In short, religious ideology is pervasive throughout the educational process, and for that reason critics charge that the Christian schools not only fail to address the issue of mediocrity, but also increase the amount of miseducation in the nation. They say the schools promote racial segregation (some began in the 1960s in the face of court-required integration), use outmoded methods of teaching (discipline is often strict), and give students distorted views of human knowledge (everything is filtered through religious doctrine).

To some extent, one's evaluation of the conservative Christian schools depends on one's values. It seems clear, however, that the schools do violate some of the basic principles of education, including free inquiry. The emphasis is not on raising questions and learning to think creatively, but on accepting answers and learning to think narrowly in accord with a particular religious doctrine.

## Contributing Factors

Why are there inequalities in educational opportunities and attainment? Why hasn't education yielded the expected payoff for some people? As you will see, part of the answer does lie in the structure and processes of the educational system. A greater part of the answer lies in nonschool factors. The problems of education are only partially a problem of the schools.

### Social Structural Factors

*Social Class, Family Background, and Educational Inequality.* In our discussion of poverty, we pointed out that *families in the lower strata* of society are different in a number of respects from those in the middle and upper strata. Certain characteristics of the lower-strata family tend to depress **cognitive development.** Consider, for example, such a simple fact as the number of books in the family home. There are likely to be far fewer in lower-strata homes, and a study of families in 42 nations discovered a strong relationship between the number of books in a home and the children's academic performance (Evans, Kelley, and Sikora 2014).

**cognitive development** growth in the ability to perform increasingly complex intellectual activities, particularly abstract relationships

Children who come from lower-strata families, then are more likely to enter school with an intellectual disadvantage that tends to depress their performance and academic achievement (Petrill, Pike, Price, and Plomin 2004; Noble, Farah, and McCandliss 2006). Their school work is further hurt by the fact that they come to school with a background that includes poor health care, parents who are minimally involved with them, few preschool opportunities, unsafe neighborhoods, and some degree of malnourishment (Alvarado 2016; Burdick-Will 2016). As a result, they may be *unprepared to learn* when they come to kindergarten. They lack the vocabulary and sentence structure skills necessary for success in school. Even if they attend equally good schools and receive equal treatment from teachers, children from such a disadvantaged background cannot have educational opportunity equal to that of others.

Thus, *the position of the family in the stratification system has a close relationship to the educational attainment of the children.* Parental educational attainment and parental influence and expectations for children strongly affect children's educational aspirations and achievement (Räty 2006; Keller and Tillman 2008; Augustine 2014). In turn, the parental behavior is related to social class; the higher the social class, the more likely parents are to have high attainment, hold high expectations, and positively influence the child to attain a high degree of education. The greater the parental income and the fewer children in the family (both of which tend to characterize the higher strata), the more willing the parents are to pay for higher education (Steelman and Powell 1991).

*Socioeconomic background affects a child at every point in his or her academic career.* Students from low-income backgrounds are less likely to graduate from high school, less likely to go to college even if they do graduate (in part because they are more likely to marry at an early age), less likely to complete college if they enroll, and less likely to go to a prestigious school regardless of their ability or aspirations (Davies and Guppy 1997; Roscigno, Tomaskovic-Devey, and Crowley 2006). Children from high-income families, in contrast, can gain admission to elite colleges and universities even though academically they do not do as well as some from low-income families who are rejected (Golden 2006). Among other things, the well-to-do gain admission through donations to the school, and because they are the children of alumni or celebrities or politicians.

**achievement**
as distinguished from educational "attainment," the level the student has reached as measured by scores on various verbal and nonverbal tests

Socioeconomic status is also one of the prime factors in unequal educational **achievement** at all levels of education, from elementary school through college (Hossler, Schmit, and Vesper 1999; Lee and Burkham 2002; Owens 2018). We are not saying that students from a lower socioeconomic background can never succeed. Some poor youths who have had strong parenting and sufficient opportunities have risen above their circumstances and carved out a better life for themselves (Furstenberg et al. 1999).

Yet the poor will always have a greater struggle. The struggle begins at the "starting gate" of kindergarten. The children enter a lower-quality school with less well-prepared and less-experienced teachers, less positive attitudes on the part of those teachers, and little in the home or neighborhood to nurture whatever motivation and aspirations they have (Lee and Burkham 2002). For such children, the school may be an alien setting. They and their teachers from the middle strata of society may be totally unprepared to deal with each other. The teachers may react to the children's range of experiences with astonishment and perplexity. The children may not even be able to distinguish the various colors when they enter school, and they may appear to have little grasp of abstract qualities such as shape and length. They may be unfamiliar with such cultural phenomena as Frosty the Snowman and *Green Eggs and Ham,* which teachers may take for granted are known to all students. Most teachers' training does not prepare them for these kinds of students.

As these children progress through school, their academic problems become more rather than less serious. Learning depends increasingly on the ability to deal with abstractions. What is a society? What is a nation? What happened in the past? Children from a deprived background may even have difficulty with such fundamental distinctions as bigger and smaller, higher and lower, round and square.

Such children could be looked upon as a challenge, but teachers may be more likely to react to them with despair or contempt. Indeed, one of the reasons that children from poor families do not achieve in school is that their *teachers may not like them.* Poor children have, if anything, a greater need for acceptance and warmth but are less likely to receive it than are middle-class children.

In addition to socioeconomic level, a number of other family background factors are important in achievement. One is the extent to which parents are involved in the process of education. The more that parents are involved in their children's education, the higher the children's level of achievement tends to be (Jimerson, Egeland, Stroufe, and Carlson 2000). "Involvement" includes such things as attending school functions, meeting with teachers, seeing that their children have adequate meals and rest so they are prepared to learn, and expecting their children to be diligent students with aspirations for high educational attainment.

For example, a study of more than 2,000 sixth-grade students in 11 middle schools in North Carolina found that the students' perceptions of their parents' expectations about school behavior was reflected in the students' math and reading scores three years later (Bowen, Hopson, Rose, and Glennie 2012). Specifically, the students were asked how upset their parents would be about such matters as a D or F on a report card, cutting classes, being late with homework, getting suspended, engaging in a fight or classroom misbehavior, and arguing with their teachers. Students who believed their parents would be very upset with such behavior tended to get higher reading and math scores than those who perceived a lesser amount of upset from parents.

involvement

## WHAT IS THE PURPOSE OF EDUCATION?

In recent decades, the proportion of majors in such disciplines as English, philosophy, history, and modern languages has dropped considerably. In many American colleges and universities, students can graduate without studying such subjects as European history, American literature, or the civilizations of ancient Greece and Rome. What do these facts say about the purpose of education? To what extent do colleges and universities help Americans fulfill the functions of education noted at the beginning of this chapter?

Interview a number of students and faculty members at your school. Ask them what they believe to be the purposes of education. Then ask them to what extent your school has goals that fulfill those purposes. Ask them to identify both their personal educational goals (in the case of faculty, their goals in teaching) and what they believe to be the true goals of the school. If your school promotes the disciplines noted in the previous paragraph, ask your respondents how they feel about the place of history, literature, and philosophy in the education of people.

What is education for, according to your respondents? Do you agree or disagree? Would you affirm or modify the three purposes of education discussed in this chapter?

Finally, *living with both biological parents* is associated with higher levels of achievement than living with a stepparent or a single parent (Cavanagh, Schiller, and Riegle-Crumb 2006; Jeynes 2006). Children who live with a single parent or a stepparent during adolescence receive less encouragement and less help with schoolwork and achieve less than children living with both birth parents (Hanson 1999; Xu 2008). Among those in single-parent households, grades are lower than for those living with both parents, and grades are lowered even more by father absence than by mother absence (Mulkey, Crain, and Harrington 1992; DeBell 2008).

*The Organization of Education.* The gap between children from the lower socioeconomic strata and those from the middle and upper strata tends to increase with the level of school. This finding suggests that the schools *may somehow contribute to educational inequality—children who are disadvantaged by their social background when they enter school become even more disadvantaged as they progress through school.*

At least two factors contribute to the disadvantage. One is the quality of teaching. Many instructors are teaching subjects for which they are not trained (*Education Week* 2000). Where there is a shortage of teachers or a need for quick action, teachers may be hired with emergency or substandard certification. Such teachers are more likely to be in schools serving the lower strata. Even if the teachers are competent, other problems may thwart the learning process. A national study of K–12 teachers reported that two out of five were disheartened and disappointed with their jobs (Yarrow 2009). More than half of them were teaching in low-income schools, and they were frustrated with the administration, classroom disorder, and an overemphasis on testing. Another national survey reported that teacher job satisfaction dropped 23 percent between 2008 and 2012 (Resmovits 2013). In 2012, only 39 percent of teachers reported being very satisfied with their jobs. Still another problem is the middle-class background of so many teachers, making it difficult for them to understand, relate to, and help children from disadvantaged backgrounds (Halvorsen, Lee, and Andrade 2009). They may believe that children from low-income families are uninterested in learning when, in fact, there is evidence that even in the face of negative teacher attitudes and low expectations for them, many if not most disadvantaged children in elementary school want teachers who care about them and help them learn (Lewis and Kim 2008).

A second factor is the *evaluation and labeling of ability.* This grouping by ability, or *tracking,* of students has been common in public schools, beginning in the first grade. It is a controversial practice. Proponents point out that tracking is necessary for dealing with the boredom and lack of adequate progress among bright students when course work proceeds too slowly in order to accommodate slower students. Tracking allows students to proceed at their own pace. "Detracking," they argue, not only hurts the brighter students but also can harm the self-confidence of low achievers when they are forced to compete with the bright students (Loveless 1999).

Opponents of tracking argue that high achievers do not benefit that much, and low achievers are stigmatized and deprived of opportunities for success (Oakes 2005; Cantu 2019). Tracking also hurts minorities, a disproportionate number of whom are placed in the low-achieving tracks. Once in a low-achievement track, it is difficult for students to escape it. Among other things, they take the kind of classes that ensure that they will remain in the same track, and their teachers tend to label them as low achievers and to expect them to perform accordingly.

Both the advocates and the critics of tracking make valid claims. Putting a student in a high track, or in an advanced or honors class, has a positive impact on that student's performance (Karlson 2015). Unfortunately, the opposite is also true—putting a student in a low track can depress educational aspirations. Consequently, the question should not be one of tracking or not tracking. Rather, the real question is how to organize schools and classrooms in light of the fact that children learn differently and at different rates. The important point to keep in mind is that inequality of achievement during the first years of school does not mean that the low achievers lack the capacity to attain high educational levels. Low achievement, as we have shown, tends to follow from a particular kind of social and family background. We also have shown, in previous chapters, the effects of labeling. If the low achiever is labeled as one with a low capacity, both the reaction of the teacher and the self-expectations of the child are negatively affected. In effect, labeling becomes a form of the *fallacy of personal attack,* blaming the students rather than the system for their lack of achievement.

fallacy

The effects of labeling on children's achievement are dramatized in an elementary school experiment that showed that teachers' expectations about the intellectual abilities of their students were reflected in the students' IQ scores (Rosenthal and Jacobson 1968). A student whom the teacher expected to do poorly tended to get lower scores, and a student whom the teacher expected to do well got higher scores. The performance of people, whether children or adults, can be significantly influenced by the expectations of others and can reflect those expectations more than any innate abilities.

Thus, labels can become *self-fulfilling prophecies,* retarding or stifling the achievement of able students. Is there any evidence that the labels are inaccurate? Can't teachers detect and encourage children who are bright but who perform poorly on achievement tests? No doubt some teachers can and do. However, children from lower socioeconomic backgrounds may have a capacity that is masked by their initial disadvantage and by their subsequent experiences and performance in the school. The evidence is scattered and, in some cases, indirect. We will furnish some evidence when we discuss the effects of desegregation in the last section of this chapter.

*The Politics of School Financing.* We have noted the large differences in the money allocated per child among various school districts. Although money per se is not the answer to all the problems of education, the funding per child makes a difference in the quality of teachers hired and the physical conditions of the school. These factors, in turn, raise attendance rates and student achievement (Condron and Roscigno 2003; Pinkerton 2003).

Both the amount of funding and the equitable distribution of the funding among districts are important. As far as the amount is concerned, some resist any increase on various grounds (such as the notion that teachers are already overpaid). It is instructive to note that between 1979 and 2013, funding for prisons and jails increased 324 percent, while funding for pre-K-12 education increased by 107 percent (Wheaton 2016). Every state in the union increased correction funding far more than education funding.

As far as distribution is concerned, one way to deal with the inequality is to *equalize the money available* to various districts. Such equalization cannot occur because public education is financed largely by the property tax. As a result, pupils in wealthier districts with more expensive homes have more money available for their education. Moreover, when states make cuts in funding for education, the poor districts may suffer a disproportionate loss. In 2011–2012, Pennsylvania cut more than a billion dollars from the state's budget for schools (Litvinov 2015). And the cuts were four times larger ($532 per student) in the 50 poorest districts than in the wealthiest districts ($113 per student).

The result of such practices is that throughout the nation children in more advantaged areas are likely to have clean, well-staffed schools with good facilities and up-to-date books and technological aids, whereas children in more disadvantaged areas are likely to attend class in dilapidated school buildings staffed by less than fully qualified teachers and supplied with outdated textbooks and few, if any, technological aids. The differences in resources are illustrated by the availability of computers. A child today whose early education is devoid of computer use lacks an important resource and has a serious deficiency in his or her education. Yet schools in poorer areas are likely to have far fewer computers available to the students than are schools in more advantaged districts. The point is that *even if the student in a lower socioeconomic area overcomes the handicaps of a disadvantaged family, he or she faces obstacles to educational attainment in the school itself.*

In principle, many Americans support the idea of equalizing the funds available to school districts—but how would that be done? Some have argued that it can be accomplished only by eliminating the property tax as the basis for funding. They point out that no child should be denied a quality education simply because his or her parents happen to live in a poorer area.

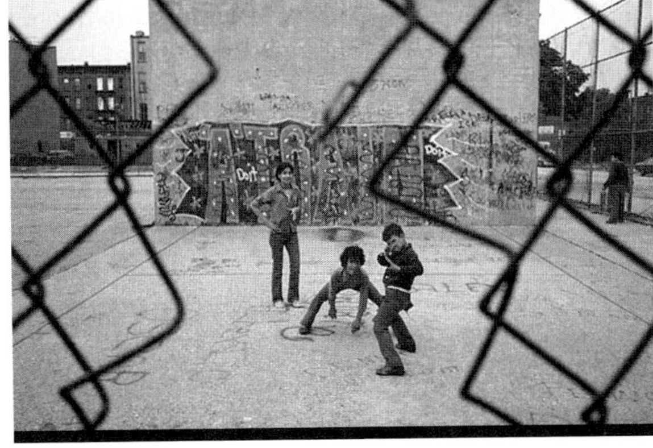

Poorer school districts cannot provide the resources enjoyed by wealthier districts.

National Archives and Records Administration (NWDNS-412-DA-13449)

Such arguments finally have begun to effect change in a number of states. In the late 1980s and early 1990s, a number of state courts ruled that existing methods of financing schools were unconstitutional. Montana, Kentucky, Michigan, and Texas were the first states to construct alternative financing systems. In Kentucky, the court decision led to a comprehensive school-reform effort that included channeling more money into poorer schools and restructuring the state education department so that its primary task is to assist local school districts rather than issue directives to them. An assessment of the situation a few years later concluded that more financial resources were available to districts but that patterns of resource allocation had not changed (Adams 1997). Clearly, the process of gaining equity in funding will be a slow and difficult one. And simply getting more equitable funding may or may not be sufficient to improve the quality of education. In 2004, Maryland began providing more resources for school districts that had larger shares of disadvantaged students (Chung 2015). The funding was more equitable, but so far it has not made a difference in student performance.

There is another aspect to the politics of financing—the extent to which political leaders give high priority to education. School districts get revenues from local, state, and federal sources. Of all revenues received by the public schools, states provide the most, and the federal government the least. When support at one of the levels declines for whatever reason, education is likely to suffer.

*The Economics of Education.* The politics of school financing interact closely with the economics of education. As with so many important areas of American life, *education is affected by the ups and downs of the economy,* and political and economic factors are intertwined as they affect the educational process. Educational decisions may be made on the basis of economic considerations. For example, a Texas survey found that 68 percent of the elementary teachers had students who were promoted to the next grade even though they had failed the class, and 61 percent of middle school and junior high teachers had students who moved on without repeating a course they had failed (Shanker 1996). In part, the practice was justified by the social stigma attached to being held back, but another part of the justification was economic: It costs a good deal to fail students and add a year or more to their schooling.

Economic factors can become even more powerful in times of recessions, when political leaders look with jaundiced eyes at the costs of education and resist any changes that involve more money. Inflation also can be troublesome. Inflation may rapidly outstrip the fiscal resources of schools and result in problems regarding salaries and the purchase of supplies.

As we pointed out in the previous section, *economic problems are also political problems.* Not everyone and not everything suffers equally in times of economic difficulty—political leaders make decisions that bear upon the resources available. The governor of a state must decide whether education, mental health, highway maintenance, or a number of other areas will receive priority consideration when budgets must be cut.

Obviously, the problems of education cannot be separated from other problems in a time of national economic difficulty. When resources are scarce, the decision to more fully fund one area—such as education—is a decision not to adequately fund another area—such as health programs. A faltering economy, therefore, inevitably means an intensification of at least some social problems.

## Social Psychological Factors

*Attitudes.* We have already noted some *attitudes that contribute to educational problems.* Parental attitudes are particularly important, because parental expectations are one of the factors in a child's educational achievement (Jacobs and Harvey 2005). Minority parents generally are very positive in their attitudes. A Pew Research Center survey reported that 86 percent of Hispanic parents and 79 percent of Black parents, compared to only 67 percent of white parents, consider a college degree to be very important (Stepler 2016). Such attitudes may help account for the increasing educational attainment of those groups.

Social class differences, on the other hand, remain problematic. Even if children from lower-class families aspire to high levels of attainment, they may not be able to realize their aspirations (Collins, Collins, and Butt 2015; Trinidad 2019). And, unfortunately, they have living examples in their network of friends and acquaintances that prove the futility of high aspirations. Only 5 percent of Americans aged 25 to 34 whose parents had less than a high-school education have a college degree (Porter 2015).

The attitudes of students toward schoolwork also affect their achievement. A national survey comparing pupils in the 5th and 11th grades found that 66 percent of 5th graders, but only 28 percent of 11th graders, strongly agreed that schoolwork is important (Calderon 2017). And when asked if they did their best in schoolwork, only 35 percent of 5th graders and 17 percent of 11th graders said they did. These attitudes are reinforced by a teen culture that disparages academic success. Large numbers of students strive to be a part of some social clique, such as the "populars" or "jocks" or "partyers," each of which tends to scorn high academic achievement.

*The attitudes of teachers also contribute to educational problems.* The attitudes of teachers are rooted in the conditions under which they must work. Low salaries, inadequate resources, and other poor working conditions may lead teachers to change professions. Others remain in teaching, but they develop jaded attitudes about their work and education generally; and sinking teacher morale usually is accompanied by lower student achievement (Black 2001).

*Values.* Many educational problems, such as segregation and school financing, are difficult to resolve because they involve a conflict of values. In essence, Americans have tried to address educational issues in the context of a *clash between the value on individualism and the value on egalitarianism* (Hochschild and Scovronick 2003). "Individualism" means that Americans expect their schools to be the means to individual advancement, and this belief translates into such attitudes as "I should be able to choose the kind of school–public or private–that my children attend without being penalized by the tax system" and "I should be able to veto any policies or practices that I deem harmful to my child's education." "Egalitarianism," on the other hand, means that Americans expect their schools to help equalize opportunities for all students, and this belief translates into such attitudes as "Poor schools should get as much money as rich schools" and "No child should be denied entrance into any school because of the child's color or social standing."

Resolving the issues that are caught up in the matrix of clashing values will never be easy. Rather, such clashing values illustrate why efforts to deal with social problems are typically accompanied by intergroup conflict.

## A Concluding Note on Inequality in Education

We have suggested that if the various factors we identified are all taken into account, then children of different racial, ethnic, and socioeconomic backgrounds should be able to show about the same levels of achievement. Earlier research by the Office of Education supports this conclusion. Figure 11.3 shows the achievement scores for sixth graders when various factors in their backgrounds are taken into account. If we look only at the scores of unequalized whites, Asian Americans, American Indians, African Americans, Mexicans, and Puerto Ricans in the United States, we see considerable differences in their achievement. The Puerto Rican students had the lowest average score and the white students the highest, about 50 percent higher.

Suppose we control for socioeconomic background. What will the differences be for children of different racial and ethnic groups but the same socioeconomic level? The answer is in the second set of points in Figure 11.3, labeled "Equalized for socioeconomic status." The spread narrows considerably, showing that a good part of the differences that were observed among the groups was really rooted in different socioeconomic backgrounds. As we continue to move to the right in the figure, each set of points takes progressively more background factors into account,

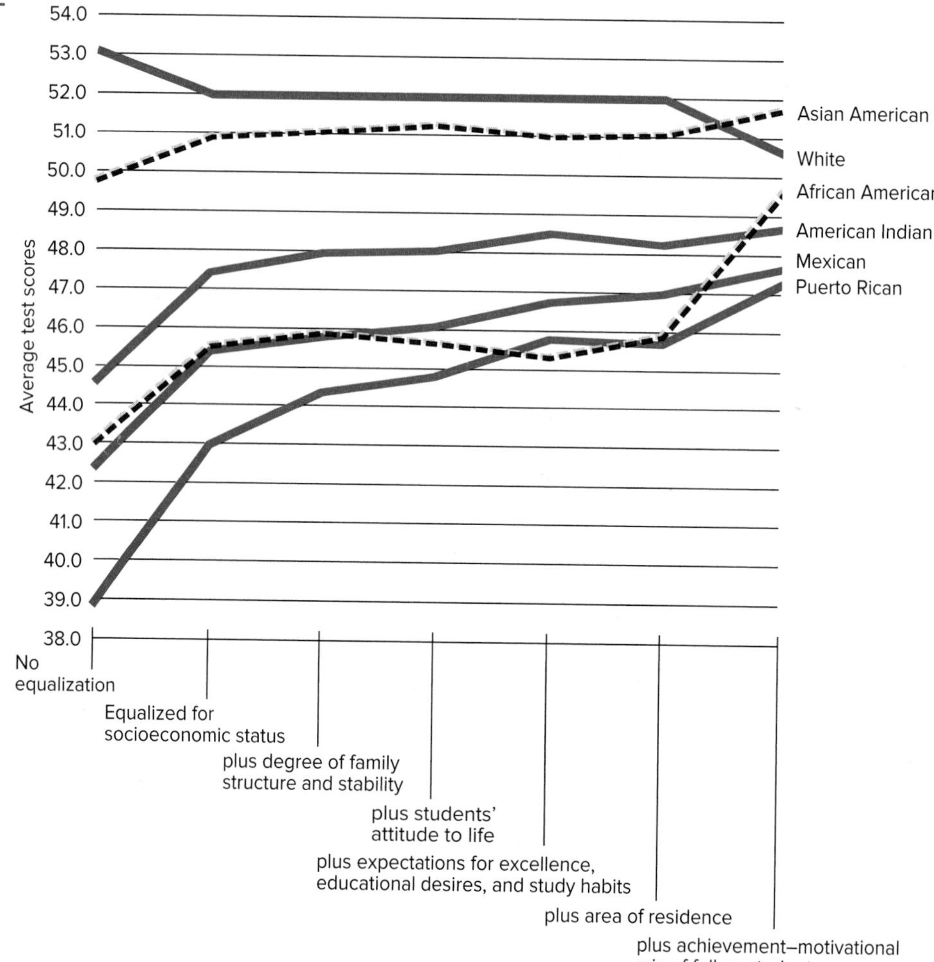


**FIGURE 11.3**
Racial and Ethnic Group Achievement Means of Sixth-Grade Pupils, Adjusted for Social Background Conditions.

Source: Adapted from Mayeske, G. W. et al., A Study of Achievement of Our Nation's Schools (Washington, DC: Government Printing Office, 1973), p. 137.

and the differences in scores diminish correspondingly. The third set of points adjusts the scores to equalize for socioeconomic status *plus* degree of family structure and stability. The next set of points adds the students' attitude to life (as described in this chapter). The fifth set of points takes in the students' expectations for excellence, educational desires, and study habits. The sixth adds to those factors the area of residence. The last set includes the achievement-motivational mix of fellow students, which means if the students were to come from the same socioeconomic background, have the same family experiences, and exhibit the same social psychological processes, the differences between the scores of the various racial and ethnic groups would be about 1 percent.

Thus, unequal educational achievement in the United States is a sociocultural matter, not a racial-genetic one (Farkas 2004; Sampson, Sharkey, and Raudenbush 2008; Cheadle 2008). As efforts have been made to help disadvantaged minorities, the gap between their scores and those of white, non-Hispanic children has narrowed. For example, comparing math scale scores on standardized tests for 9-year-olds, in 1972 whites scored on average 35 points higher than African Americans and 23 points higher than Hispanics; by 2017, the gaps were 25 and 19, respectively (Digest of Educational Statistics website). For 13-year-olds, the gaps between white-minority scores were 46 points for African Americans and 35 points for Hispanics in 1972, but down to 33 points for African Americans and 24 points for Hispanics in 2017. Such results underscore both the social nature of the problem and the importance of social action for addressing it.

## Solutions: Public Policy and Private Action

Our analysis suggests a variety of ways to attack the various problems of education. Clearly, it must be a multifaceted attack. Undoubtedly, parental involvement is one of the crucial factors in children's educational attainment. Among other parental factors, having high expectations for the children's education, creating an educationally rich environment in the home, and helping with homework will make a difference in how much children achieve academically (Wilder 2014; Otani 2020).

Another obvious need is *reform of school financing* (Martin et al. 2018). The inequities between school districts must be addressed. Whatever their background or socioeconomic status, students should have equal access to quality education.

In addition, a variety of other efforts and proposals exist that hold promise: vouchers, quality enhancement measures, efforts to reduce racial and ethnic inequality, and compensatory and other innovative programs. Some are quite controversial.

### Use of Vouchers and Tax Credits

A good deal of controversy exists over the *use of school vouchers and tax credit programs* (Medler 2002). A **voucher system** enables parents to use tax funds to send their children to private as well as public schools. Tax credit programs offer state tax credits for contributions to organizations that award scholarships to children from families with limited resources. In some states, tax credit scholarship programs send more low-income students to private schools than do voucher programs (Figlio and Hart 2011). Any program that enables children to go to private rather than public schools raises issues, including the capacity of private schools to absorb all those who want to attend them (Zehr 2011). But the most controversial issue is whether being able to choose the school that one's child attends will result in higher-quality education not only for that child but for all children.

**voucher system**
a system that allows parents to use tax money to send their children to a school, private or public, of their choice

Thus, in terms of voucher systems, proponents argue that the system will bring about higher academic achievement, increased parental involvement in children's education, better use of tax monies, and pressure on the public schools to improve the quality of education. Opponents argue that vouchers will mainly subsidize parents who can already afford to send their children to private schools, violate the separation of church and state (because most private schools are religious), and ultimately destroy the public school system. But states that have tried to implement a voucher system have encountered problems of administration and of courts that have declared it unconstitutional. Furthermore, studies of the educational outcomes in states that have set up voucher systems have not found clear, positive effects on students' academic achievement, nor improved performance by the public schools, and have reported mixed results for students overall (Anrig 2008; Usher and Kober 2011). The potential for voucher or tax credit programs to improve education substantially is not supported by the evidence we have thus far.

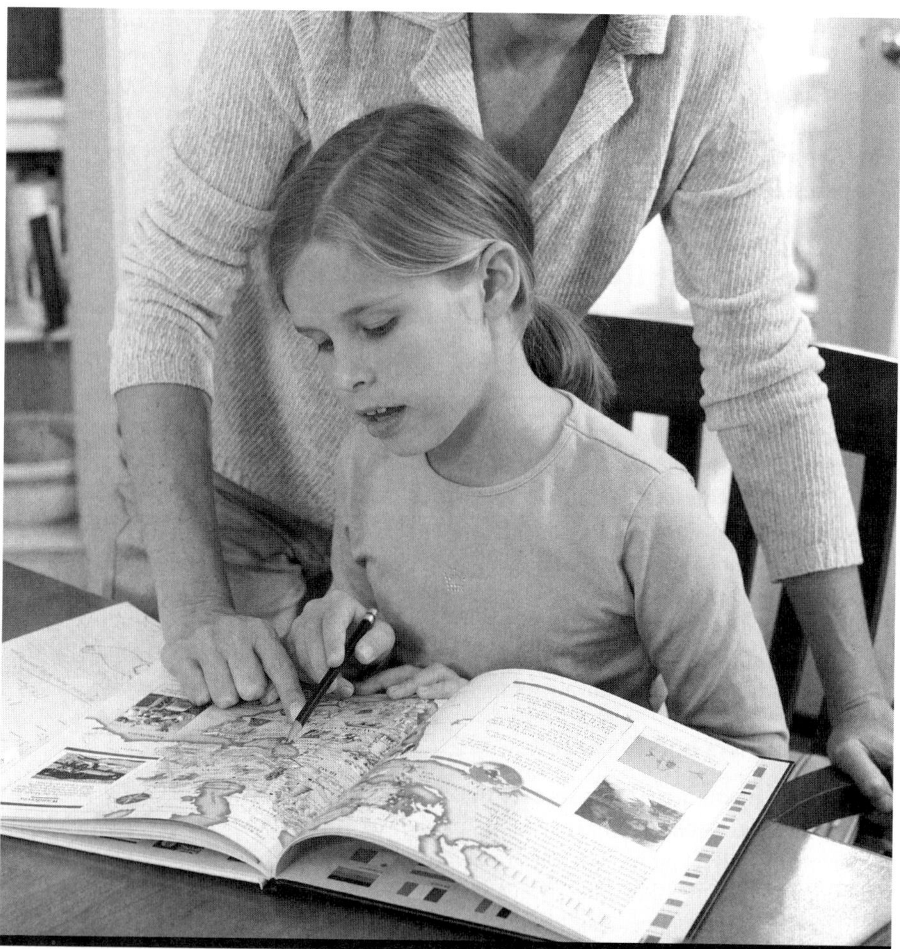

Some parents have sought to maximize their children's education by homeschooling them.

Big Cheese Photo/PunchStock

## Quality Enhancement Measures

A variety of suggestions exist for enhancing the quality of education. Lengthening the number of days in the school year could help poor children, who lose ground in the summer when they lack the intellectual demands of the classroom (Cline 2018). Establishing standards-based education, which includes testing and accountability for meeting minimum standards in subject areas, has yielded gains in student achievement in a number of states (Editorial Projects in Education Research Center 2006). Improving the school atmosphere by ensuring student safety and making schools drug- and gun-free could facilitate learning (Ingersoll and LeBoeuf 1997). Providing all children with the opportunity to attend preschool can enhance both their emotional and intellectual well-being, and can be particularly helpful to those from disadvantaged backgrounds (Scott and Delgado 2005; Arnold et al. 2006). Finally, placing all children in small classes can improve performance, because from kindergarten on those in small classes do better academically than those in large classes (Finn, Gerber, Achilles, and Boyd-Zaharias 2001; Konstantopoulos 2009).

Some analysts believe that all such efforts are only "tinkering" with the system, and that *what is needed is a complete restructuring of the schools and even the community itself*

(Emery 2006). There are varied ideas on what restructuring would involve, but most advocates agree that it requires decentralization (whether in the form of school-site management, a choice plan, or some variation on privatization).

Restructuring through decentralization gives parents and local schools greater control over the educational process. The idea is that schools will function better when they reflect the realities of the community in which they are embedded rather than conforming to some uniform set of policies and procedures. This worked well in an experiment with elementary schools in Chicago (Bryk et al. 2010). The schools were given local control with greater discretionary funding, resulting in improved student learning as reflected in reading and math scores. Decentralization also worked well for "community schools" in Oregon (Samuels 2012). As an example, one school that served low-income students utilized various nonprofit and county agencies to provide such things as homework assistance, academic enrichment, free breakfast and dinner for students, a food pantry, health screenings, dental care, and information on how to make use of various social services.

A different way to enhance quality is to start from scratch with a school—namely, establish a **charter school.** *Charter schools are nonreligious public schools that are approved by the local school district but are free of many regulations and policies that apply to other public schools.* Charter schools can be converted public schools or entirely new facilities. They are operated by educators, parents, and/or community members. In essence, the district and the school negotiate a contract or "charter" that covers a specified number of years and that spells out the school's mission, program, goals, type of student body, and method of accountability.

**charter school**
a nonreligious public school approved by the local school district but free of many regulations and policies that apply to other public schools

The first state charter-school law was passed in Minnesota in 1991 (National Study of Charter Schools 2000). By 2017, America had 7,200 charter schools with an enrollment of 3.1 million students (Zhang et al. 2020). Most of the schools are relatively small, enrolling between one and two hundred students.

Some charter schools are successful, as measured by improved scores on standardized tests, whereas others do no better or even worse than the traditional public schools (American Federation of Teachers 2002; Shah 2011; Gulosino and Liebert 2020). An analysis of 2003 test scores found that students at charter schools had lower scores in both reading and mathematics than did students in regular public schools (Robelen 2006). And a California study concluded that the state's charter schools neither closed the achievement gap for minorities nor had any positive effect on the performance of other public schools (Schutz 2007). Finally, a survey of the research on the effect of charter schools concluded that charter schools overall are producing higher gains in math achievement than are traditional schools, but reading achievement is about the same as in traditional schools (Betts and Tang 2016).

One quality-enhancement measure that seemed promising was the "No Child Left Behind Act" of 2002, which required all schools receiving federal money to meet certain standards and to educate low-income students to improve student test scores every year (Moran 2002). Students in a school in which scores did not improve for two consecutive years could receive free transportation to a school that did meet the standards. Unfortunately, the federal government failed to adequately fund the program.

In addition to inadequate funding, the program was severely criticized on various other grounds and was finally revised into the Every Student Succeeds Act (ESSA), which was passed in 2015 (Welch 2016). ESSA is too new to know how it will affect the quality of education. It tries to address the needs of all students—the gifted and the challenged, the poor and the well-to-do, and those from the various racial/ethnic groups. It requires state educational systems to be clear about what they expect students to learn, help all students meet or exceed the standards, regularly assess whether schools are teaching the standards, and make information about the schools (including assessment results) publicly available (Chenoweth 2016).

## Reducing Racial and Ethnic Inequality

Racial and ethnic inequalities in education must be reduced in order to create a society of equal opportunity. One crucial step is desegregation of schools. In the 1954 case *Brown v. Board of Education of Topeka, Kansas,* the U.S. Supreme Court ruled that segregated education imposed by governments was not legal. This ruling reversed a 19th-century decision that argued that "separate but equal" facilities may be provided by the states. The 1954 decision, which declared that separate facilities were inherently unequal and thus unconstitutional, furnished momentum for the movement to desegregate the nation's public schools.

Does desegregation help disadvantaged students? There is evidence that achievement levels of Black children are raised by attending desegregated schools (Mickelson 2001, 2015). There is also evidence that Black students who attend more segregated schools do not achieve as much academically as those who attend integrated schools (Kogachi and Graham 2020).

Unfortunately, after some small and slow gains from the 1960s to the 1980s (in 1988, a third of Black students were in schools where the majority of students were white), the desegregation process went into reverse. *Segregated housing patterns, white flight to the suburbs, resistance to busing children from their neighborhoods in order to integrate schools, and the establishment of private schools all helped subvert the desegregation efforts* (Saporito and Sohoni 2006). By 2018, 40 percent of African American students attended intensely segregated (90–100 percent) nonwhite schools (Orfield and Jarvie 2020). With the increase in segregation, the gap between white and minority test scores increased again (Berends and Penaloza 2010).

Some efforts have been made to bring white children to Black schools rather than the reverse, but those efforts were stopped by the courts. Court decisions also dismantled affirmative action programs, decreasing the enrollment of minorities in higher education. The result is a pattern of resegregation over the past two decades (Cohen 2004). On average, white students attend schools that are 78 percent white, Black students attend schools that are only 30 percent white, and Hispanic students attend schools that are only 28 percent white (Orfield and Lee 2005).

State and local governments need to devise plans to reverse the resegregation process. In the area of higher education, for example, the state of Texas initiated a plan that brought more minorities to colleges and universities (Yardley 2002). In essence, the plan guarantees slots in state universities to the top 10 percent of graduates in each high school without regard to SAT scores or grade-point averages. A student in the top 10 percent of a disadvantaged school may have a lower SAT score and/or grade-point average than a student who ranks at the 75th percentile of another high school. However, the student from the disadvantaged school will still be guaranteed a place in a public college or university.

**compensatory programs** programs designed to give intensive help to disadvantaged pupils and increase their academic skills

## Compensatory and Other Innovative Programs

**Compensatory programs** are aimed at *disadvantaged pupils.* They focus on skills such as reading and speech and attempt to offer an intensive program of help so that the disadvantaged pupil can approach the level of others in the school. Some compensatory programs are remedial. They attempt, among other benefits, to reduce the number of students per teacher, to provide the student with extra help (including after-school hours), and to use special teaching materials. The Head Start program stimulates learning of verbal and social skills among preschool disadvantaged children (Zhai, Brooks-Gunn, and Waldfogel 2011).

Another program aimed at disadvantaged children is called CIS, or Communities in Schools (Cantelon and LeBoeuf 1997). The program uses resources from the local, state, and national levels to provide at-risk youths with four items basic to the child's well-being and academic performance:

A personal one-on-one relationship with a caring adult.

A safe place to learn and grow.

A marketable skill.

An opportunity to give something back to peers and the community.

Evaluations of the CIS program find that a majority of students with high absenteeism and low grades prior to their participation have lower dropout rates and improved attendance, grades, and graduation rates (ICF International 2010).

## The Deschooling Movement

The *deschooling movement* aims at providing students with a situation in which they will maximize their learning. The movement emphasizes the necessity of a break with the existing educational structure and the creation of new schools where the children can be free to learn.

The most common manifestation of deschooling today is *homeschooling*. People decide for various reasons to teach their children at home rather than send them to the schools (Stevens 2001). Initially, most homeschooling was done by conservative Christians who felt that their children were not given sufficient moral guidance in the schools (Hawkins 1996). As a 5-year-old girl explained to the authors, she would not go to public school because "they don't teach about God there." The second wave of homeschoolers, however, includes more people who are either dissatisfied with the quality of teaching in the schools or with the potential for emotional or physical harm to their children in the schools (Cloud and Morse 2001).

According to the Digest of Educational Statistics website, there were 1.69 million children, aged 5 through 17, being homeschooled in 2016. The number is 3.3 percent of all children in that age bracket. How well are these children educated? There is not a great deal of evidence, but what we have suggests that homeschooled children do well on the whole. They score well on standardized tests of achievement, and they appear to be as socially and emotionally adjusted as children in public or private schools (Collom 2005; Ray 2013).

Undoubtedly, some children receive an inadequate education through homeschooling; but, on average, those who are homeschooled appear to be benefiting. Parents who opt for it, however, need to recognize the extent to which they are committing themselves to their children's lives. Parenting is a consuming task as it is; when homeschooling is added, parenting becomes more than a full-time job.

*Follow-Up.* In what ways were your parents involved in your elementary and high school education? Which of these ways were helpful? Were any harmful? What will you do differently to enhance your own children's education?

## Summary

Education is a problem when it fails to fulfill its expected functions: creating good and effective citizens, providing the possibility for upward mobility, and facilitating individual development. For these purposes education is highly valued by Americans. Lack of education is frequently associated with failure to achieve one's ambitions in life.

America has become an increasingly educated society. Whether this education has yielded the expected payoffs is not always clear. The greater degree of happiness reported by the highly educated may reflect a tendency toward greater fulfillment of individual potential. Education increases political participation and understanding. There is a strong relationship between education and income, but those most likely to benefit from education are already in the middle and upper strata.

Education is a problem because there are inequalities, and the expected payoff does not always occur. Educational attainment is unequally distributed among various groups. Educational funding is unequally distributed among states and school districts within states. The cost of education prices many Americans out of the better colleges and universities. The learning atmosphere of some schools (critics would say nearly all schools) is rigid and joyless and precludes individual schedules of learning; sometimes students suffer an atmosphere of fear and threat or ritualized deprivation.

A series of reports have charged that American education is in danger of being overwhelmed by mediocrity. The mediocrity affects education at every level and applies to student performance, faculty performance, administrative functioning, and academic programs. Many Americans believe that a particular kind of deficiency afflicts the schools—a non- or anti-Christian bias—and they have opted to send their children to Christian schools.

Among the social structural factors that contribute to the problems of education, social class and family background are particularly important. The organization of education also makes a difference in students' achievement and attainment. Particularly important are the distribution of funds, the assignment of teachers, the socioeconomic composition of the student body, and the evaluation and labeling of ability. The inequitable distribution of funds is a political issue that must be resolved by political action. Finally, the quality of education varies with the economy. Both recessions and inflation drain the resources available to schools.

Attitudes of parents, students, and teachers are important social psychological factors that contribute to the problems of education. The attitudes of parents and students toward school and intellectual activities, and toward the educational potential of the students are strongly related to achievement. Teacher attitudes can inhibit or facilitate student achievement.

Our analysis implies that when the various contributing factors are taken into account, children of different social backgrounds have the same capacity for achievement. The Office of Education survey supports this position. Given the same socioeconomic background, family background, attitudes, and the like, there is only about a 1 percent difference in the achievement scores of the various racial and ethnic groups.

## Key Terms

**Achievement**
**Atmosphere**
**Attainment**
**Charter School**
**Cognitive Development**
**Compensatory Programs**
**Culture**
**Ritualized Deprivation**
**Voucher System**

## Study Questions

1. What are three functions of education?
2. Discuss the levels of educational attainment in America and the varied payoffs from that attainment.
3. How much inequality of opportunity is there in America, and how does it affect attainment?
4. What kinds of school atmosphere contribute to the problems of education?
5. Is education a "great training robbery"? Why or why not?
6. Explain the meaning of "a tide of mediocrity."
7. In what ways is family background important for education?
8. What aspects of the organization of education contribute to the education problem?
9. What are the political and economic factors involved in educational problems?
10. Discuss attitudes and values involved in education problems.
11. What are ways to resolve education problems?

## Internet Resources/Exercises

1. Explore some of the ideas in this chapter on the following sites:

**http://nces.ed.gov** Site of the National Center for Education Statistics, a government effort to collect and analyze data about education in the United States and other nations.

**http://www.eric.ed.gov** Access to ERIC, the comprehensive collection of research and ideas about all facets of education.

**http://www.edweek.org** Site of *Education Week* on the Web, a weekly journal with news, evaluation, and analyses of various aspects of education.

2. Select an educational level that interests you, from preschool through graduate school, and research it on the Internet. Find five things that are fitting or useful at that level and five things that are troublesome or problematic. Comparing your two lists, how would you evaluate the educational level you have researched?

3. The text points out that American elementary and high school students do not score as high on tests of math and science as do students in many other nations. Find information on math and/or science education in Japan or one of the European nations. What are they doing that can help explain the higher scores? What recommendations would you make for American schools in order to close the gap in the scores?

## For Further Reading

Asquith, Christina. *The Emergency Teacher: The Inspirational Story of a New Teacher in an Inner-City School.* New York: Skyhorse Publishing, 2014. A touching, insightful account of an attempt to adequately teach students in one of the worst schools in Philadelphia in the face of numerous, frustrating obstacles.

Banks, James A., ed. *Diversity and Citizenship Education: Global Perspectives.* New York: Jossey-Bass, 2007. Case studies and examples of successful programs and practices from 12 nations in which there are schools that have addressed the problems of education of a diverse population for living and working together as citizens of one nation.

Graham, Patricia Albjerg. *Schooling America: How the Public Schools Meet the Nation's Changing Needs.* New York: Oxford University Press, 2006. An examination of the way in which public education, from kindergarten through college, changed in the United States over the 20th century in order to meet changing expectations; includes accounts of both failure and success in the process.

Kupchik, Aaron. *Homeroom Security: School Discipline in an Age of Fear.* New York: New York University Press, 2010. Shows how the challenge of maintaining security in the schools has led to the use of various surveillance methods and punitive measures to control behavior, which, in turn, has negative consequences for the atmosphere of the school, for student behavior, and for the way students will function in society when they become adults.

Lois, Jennifer. *Home Is Where the School Is: The Logic of Home-schooling and the Emotional Labor of Mothering.* New York: New York University Press, 2013. Analysis of the mother's role in home-schooling, and the emotional and temporal demands with which the mothers must cope.

Oakes, Jeannie and Marisa Saunders, eds. *Beyond Tracking: Multiple Pathways to College, Career, and Civic Participation.* Cambridge, MA: Harvard Education Press, 2008. An argument for the radical reform of secondary education in the United States by providing multiple pathways that recognize the diversity of the population and our responsibility to adequately address the needs of the poor and minorities.

Sexton, Robert. *Mobilizing Citizens for Better Schools.* New York: Teachers College Press, 2004. An in-depth analysis of the changes in Kentucky schools after the state's Supreme Court declared the school system unconstitutional. Includes lessons learned that can be used in other states.

Smith, Mary Lee. *Political Spectacle and the Fate of American Schools.* New York: Routledge/Falmer, 2003. Case studies that illustrate the ways in which educational policies and practices have been shaped by political considerations as much as by reasoning, research, and discussion.

## References


Adams, J. E., Jr. 1997. "Organizational context and district resource allocation." *Journal of Education Finance* 23 (Fall):234–58.

Alvarado, S. E. 2016. "Delayed disadvantage: Neighborhood context and child development." *Social Forces* 94:1847–77.

American Federation of Teachers. 2002. *Do Charter Schools Measure Up?* Washington, DC: American Federation of Teachers.

Anrig, G. 2008. "An idea whose time has gone." *Washington Monthly,* April.

Arnold, D. H., et al. 2006. "Preschool-based programs for externalizing problems." *Education and Treatment of Children* 29:311–39.

Augustine, J. M. 2014. "Maternal education and the unequal significance of family structure for children's early achievement." *Social Forces* 93:687–718.

Berends, M., and R. B. Penaloza. 2010. "Increasing racial isolation and test score gaps in mathematics." *Teachers' College Record.* TCR website.

Betts, J. R., and Y. E. Tang. 2016. "A meta-analysis of the literature on the effect of charter schools on student achievement." Society for Research on Educational Effectiveness website.

Black, S. 2001. "Morale matters." *American School Board Journal* 188:40–43.

Bowen, G. L., L. M. Hopson, R. A. Rose, and E. J. Glennie. 2012. "Students' perceived parental school behavior expectations and their academic performance." *Family Relations* 61:175–91.

Braun, H., F. Jenkins, and W. Grigg. 2006. *Comparing Private Schools and Public Schools Using Hierarchical Linear Modeling.* Washington, DC: Government Printing Office.

Bryk, A. S., et al. 2010. *Organizing Schools for Improvement: Lessons from Chicago.* Chicago, IL: University of Chicago Press.

Burdick-Will, J. 2016. "Neighborhood violent crime and academic growth in Chicago." *Social Forces.* Published on-line.

Calderon, V. J. 2017. "How to keep kids excited about school." Gallup Poll website.

Cantelon, S., and D. LeBoeuf. 1997. "Keeping young people in school: Community programs that work." *Juvenile Justice Bulletin,* June.

Cantu, G. C. 2019. "Tracking in secondary education." *Theory and Research in Education* 17:202–12.

Carey, K. 2020. "A parent trap? New data offers more dire view of college debt." *New York Times,* December 24.

Cavanagh, S. E., K. S. Schiller, and C. Riegle-Crumb. 2006. "Marital transitions, parenting, and schooling." *Sociology of Education* 79:329–54.

Cheadle, J. E. 2008. "Educational investment, family context, and children's math and reading growth from kindergarten through the third grade." *Sociology of Education* 81:1–31.

Chenoweth, K. 2016. "ESSA offers changes that can continue learning gains." *Phi Delta Kappan* 97:38–42.

Chung, H. 2015. "Education finance reform, education spending, and student performance." *Education and Urban Society* 47:412–32.

Cline, S. 2018. "Is summer breaking America's schools?" *U.S. News & World Report,* June 7.

Cloud, J., and J. Morse. 2001. "Home sweet school." *Time*, August 27, pp. 47–54.

Cohen, A. 2004. "The supreme struggle." *New York Times,* January 18.

Collins, M., G. Collins, and G. Butt. 2015. "Social mobility or social reproduction?" *Educational Review* 67:196–217.

Collom, E. 2005. "The ins and outs of homeschooling." *Education and Urban Society* 37:307–35.

Condron, D. J., and V. J. Roscigno. 2003. "Disparities within: Spending inequality and achievement in an urban school district." *Sociology of Education* 76:18–36.

Copeland, W. E., et al. 2013. "Adult psychiatric outcomes of bullying and being bullied by peers in childhood and adolescence." *JAMA Psychiatry* 70:419–26.

Creusere, M., H. Zhao, S. B. Huie, and D. R. Troutman. 2019. "Postsecondary education impact on intergenerational income mobility." *Journal of Higher Education* 90:915–39.

Davies, S., and N. Guppy. 1997. "Fields of study, college selectivity, and student inequalities in higher education." *Social Forces* 75 (June):1417–38.

Day, W., et al. 2021. "The impact of teasing and bullying victimization on disordered eating and body image disturbance among adolescents." *Trauma, Violence & Abuse.* Published online.

DeBell, M. 2008. "Children living without their fathers." *Social Indicators* 87:427–43.

Editorial Projects in Education Research Center. 2006. "State policies on standards-based education over the past decade found to have a positive relationship with gains in student achievement." Education Week website.

*Education Week*. 2000. *Quality Counts 2000: Who Should Teach?* Education Week website.

——. 2003. "To close the gap, quality counts." Education Week website.

——. 2020. *Quality Counts 2020*. Education Week website.

Emery, M. 2006. *The Future of Schools: How Communities and Staff Can Transform Their School Districts*. New York: Rowman & Littlefield.

Evans, M. D. R., J. Kelley, and J. Sikora. 2014. "Scholarly culture and academic performance in 42 nations." *Social Forces* 92:1573–1605.

Fallis, R. K., and S. Opotow. 2003. "Are students failing in school or are schools failing students?" *Journal of Social Issues* 59:103–20.

Farkas, G. 2004. "The black-white test score gap." *Contexts* 3:12–19.

Figlio, D., and C. Hart. 2011. "Does competition improve public schools?" *Education Next* 11:74–80.

Finn, J. D., S. B. Gerber, C. M. Achilles, and J. Boyd-Zaharias. 2001. "The enduring effects of small classes." *Teachers College Record* 103:145–83.

Furstenberg, F. F., Jr., T. D. Cook, J. Eccles, G. H. Elder Jr., and A. Sameroff. 1999. *Managing to Make It: Urban Families and Adolescent Success*. Chicago, IL: University of Chicago Press.

Golden, D. 2006. *The Price of Admission: How America's Ruling Class Buys Its Way into Elite Colleges—and Who Gets Left Outside the Gates*. New York: Crown.

Goyette, K. 2008. "College for some to college for all: Social background, occupational expectations, and educational expectations over time." *Social Science Research* 37:461–84.

Grubb, W. N., and M. Lazerson. 2004. *The Education Gospel: The Economic Power of Schooling*. Cambridge, MA: Harvard University Press.

Gulosino, C., and J Liebert. 2020. "Examining variation within the charter school sector." *Peabody Journal of Education* 95:300–29.

Halvorsen, A., V. E. Lee, and F. H. Andrade. 2009. "A mixed-method study of teachers' attitudes about teaching in urban and low-income schools." *Urban Education* 44:181–224.

Hanson, T. L. 1999. "Does parental conflict explain why divorce is negatively associated with child welfare?" *Social Forces* 77 (June):1283–316.

Hao, L., and S. Pong. 2008. "The role of school in the upward mobility of disadvantaged immigrants' children." *The Annals of the American Academy of Political and Social Science* 620:62–89.

Hawkins, D. 1996. "Homeschool battles." *U.S. News and World Report*, February 12, pp. 28–29.

Hochschild, J. L., and N. Scovronick. 2003. *The American Dream and the Public Schools*. New York: Oxford University Press.

Hossler, D., J. Schmit, and N. Vesper. 1999. *Going to College: How Social, Economic, and Educational Factors Influence the Decisions Students Make*. Baltimore, MD: Johns Hopkins University Press.

Houle, J. N. 2014. "Disparities in debt." *Sociology of Education* 87:53–69.

ICF International. 2010. "Communities in Schools national evaluation." ICF International website.

Ingersoll, S., and D. LeBoeuf. 1997. "Reaching out to youth out of the educational mainstream." *Juvenile Justice Bulletin* (February).

Jacobs, N., and D. Harvey. 2005. "Do parents make a difference to children's academic achievement? Differences between parents of higher and lower achieving students." *Educational Studies* 31:431–48.

Jeynes, W. H. 2006. "The impact of parental remarriage on children." *Marriage & Family Review* 40:75–102.

Jimerson, S., B. Egeland, L. A. Stroufe, and B. Carlson. 2000. "A prospective longitudinal study of high school dropouts." *Journal of School Psychology* 38:525–49.

Karlson, K. B. 2015. "Expectations on track?" *Social Forces* 94:115–41.

Kass, S. J., S. J. Vodanovich, and J. Y. Khosravi. 2011. "Applying the job characteristics model to the college education experience." *Journal of the Scholarship of Teaching and Learning* 11:56–68.

Keller, U., and K. H. Tillman. 2008. "Post-secondary educational attainment of immigrant and native youth." *Social Forces* 87:121–52.

Kena, G., et al. 2016. "The condition of education 2016." National Center for Education Statistics website.

Kogachi, K., and S. Graham. 2020. "Numerical minority status in middle school and racial/ethnic segregation in academic classes." *Child Development* 91:2083–2102.

Konstantopoulos, S. 2009. "What is the impact of class size on student learning?" *Teachers College Record*. TCR website.

Kozol, J. 1992. *Savage Inequalities: Children in America's Schools*. New York: Crown.

Lee, V. E., and D. Burkam. 2002. *Inequality at the Starting Gate: Social Background Differences in Achievement as Children Begin School*. Washington, DC: Economic Policy Institute.

Lewis, J. L., and E. Kim. 2008. "A desire to learn: African-American children's positive attitudes toward learning within school cultures of low expectations." *Teachers College Record* 110:1304–29.

Litvinov, A. 2015. "'These kids are just pawns': The rising toll of inequitable school funding." *NEA Today*, July 20.

Livingston, D. W. 1998. *The Education-Jobs Gap: Underemployment or Economic Democracy*. Boulder, CO: Westview Press.

Long, C. 2013. "Are we failing gifted students?" *NEA Today*, September 18.

Loveless, T. 1999. "Will tracking reform promote social equity?" *Educational Leadership* 56 (April):28–32.

Martin, C., et al. 2018. "A quality approach to school funding." Center for American Progress website.

McCarthy, J. 2020. "Happiness not quite as widespread as usual in the U.S." Gallup Poll website.

Medler, A. 2002. "The maturing politics of education choice." *Teachers College Record* 104:173–95.

Mickelson, R. A. 2001. "Subverting Swann: Tracking as second generation segregation in Charlotte, North Carolina." *American Educational Research Journal* 38:215–52.

——. 2015. "The cumulative disadvantages of first- and second-generation segregation for middle school achievement." *American Educational Research Journal* 52:657–92.

Moran, C. 2002. "Federally mandated school choice has few takers locally." *San Diego Union-Tribune*, September 3.

Mulkey, L. M., R. L. Crain, and A. J. C. Harringon. 1992. "One-parent households and achievement: Economic and behavioral explanations of a small effect." *Sociology of Education* 65 (January):48–65.

Mundy, L. K., et al. 2017. "Peer victimization and academic performance in primary school children." *Academic Pediatrics* 17:830–36.

National Center for Education Statistics. 2020. "The condition of education, 2020." NCES website.

National Study of Charter Schools. 2000. "The state of charter schools 2000." National Study of Charter Schools website.

Noble, K. G., M. J. Farah, and B. D. McCandliss. 2006. "Socioeconomic background modulates cognition-achievement relationships in reading." *Cognitive Development* 21:349–68.

Oakes, J. 2005. *Keeping Track: How Schools Structure Inequality*. 2nd ed. New Haven, CT: Yale University Press.

Orfield, G., and C. Lee. 2005. *Why Segregation Matters: Poverty and Educational Inequality*. Cambridge, MA: The Civil Rights Project at Harvard University.

Orfield, G., and D. Jarvie. 2020. "Black segregation matters." The Civil Rights Project at UCLA website.

Otani, M. 2020. "Parental involvement and academic achievement among elementary and middle school students." *Asia Pacific Education Review* 21:1–25.

Owens, A. 2018. "Income segregation between school districts and inequality in students' achievement." *Sociology of Education* 91:1–27.

Parker, F. 1975. "What's right with American education." In Myth and Reality, 2nd ed., ed. G. Smith and C. R. Kniker, pp. 29–36. Boston, MA: Allyn and Bacon.

Peaslee, A. L. 1969. "Education's role in development." *Economic Development and Cultural Change* 17:293–318.

Peguero, A. A. 2011. "Violence, schools, and dropping out." *Journal of Interpersonal Violence* 26:3753–72.

Petrill, S. A., A. Pike, T. Price, and R. Plomin. 2004. "Chaos in the home and socioeconomic status are associated with cognitive development in early childhood." *Intelligence* 32:445–60.

Pew Research Center. 2013. "Educational attainment by Latino origin group, 2013." Pew Research Center website.

Pfeffer, F. T., and F. R. Hertel. 2015. "How has educational expansion shaped mobility trends in the United States?" *Social Forces* 94:143–80.

Pinkerton, J. P. 2003. "A grand compromise." *Atlantic Monthly*, January/February, pp. 115–16.

Porter, E. 2015. "Education gap between rich and poor is growing wider." *New York Times*, September 22.

Räty, H. 2006. "What comes after compulsory education?" *Educational Studies* 32:1–16.

Ray, B. D. 2013. "Homeschooling associated with beneficial learning and societal outcomes but educators do not promote it." *Peabody Journal of Education* 88:324–41.

Resmovits, J. 2013. "Teacher survey shows record low job satisfaction in 2012." *Huffington Post*, February 21.

Rifkin, R. 2014. "In U.S. support for daily prayer in schools dips slightly." Gallup Poll website.

Robelen, E. 2013. "Global-achievement study casts U.S. scores in better light." *Education Week,* January 15.

Robelen, E. W. 2006. "NAEP reanalysis finds lag in charter school scores." *Education Week*. Education Week website.

Roscigno, V. J., D. Tomaskovic-Devey, and M. Crowley. 2006. "Education and the inequalities of place." *Social Forces* 84:2121–45.

Rosenthal, R., and L. Jacobson. 1968. "Self-fulfilling prophecies in the classroom: Teachers' expectations as unintended determinants of pupils' intellectual competence." In *Social Class, Race, and Psychological Development,* ed. M. Deutsch, I. Katz, and A. R. Jensen, pp. 219–53. New York: Holt, Rinehart, and Winston.

Sampson, R. J., P. Sharkey, and S. W. Raudenbush. 2008. "Durable effects of concentrated disadvantage on verbal ability among African-American children." *Proceedings of the National Academy of Sciences USA* 105:845–52.

Samuels, C. A. 2012. "Oregon community schools model shows staying power." *Education Week,* March 13. Education Week website.

Shanker, A. 1994. "The crab bucket syndrome." *New York Times,* June 19.

Schieman, S., and G. Plickert. 2008. "How knowledge is power: Education and the sense of control." *Social Forces* 87:153–83.

Schofer, E., and J. W. Meyer. 2005. "The worldwide expansion of higher education in the twentieth century." *American Sociological Review* 70:898–920.

Schutz, D. 2007. "Essay review: Pay your money and take your 'school choice.'" *Teachers College Record.* TCR website.

Scott, M. S., and C. F. Delgado. 2005. "Identifying cognitively gifted minority students in preschool." *Gifted Child Quarterly* 49:199.

Shah, N. 2011. "Academic gains vary widely for charter networks." *Education Week*. Education Week website.

Saporito, S., and D. Sohoni. 2006. "Coloring outside the lines: Racial segregation in public schools and their attendance boundaries." *Sociology of Education* 79:81–105.

Steelman, L. C., and B. Powell. 1991. "Sponsoring the next generation: Parental willingness to pay for higher education." *American Journal of Sociology* 96 (May):1505–29.

Stepler, R. 2016. "Hispanic, black parents see college degree as key for children's success." Pew Research Center website.

Stevens, M. L. 2001. *Kingdom of Children: Culture and Controversy in the Homeschooling Movement.* Princeton, NJ: Princeton University Press.

Tamborini, C. R., C. Kim, and A. Sakamoto. 2015. "Education and lifetime earnings in the United States." *Demography* 52:1383–1407.

Trinidad, J. E. 2019. "Stable, unstable, and later self-expectations' influence on educational outcomes." *Educational Research and Evaluation* 25:163–78.

Tyack, D. 2003. *Seeking Common Ground: Public Schools in a Diverse Society.* Cambridge, MA: Harvard University Press.

Usher, A., and N. Kober. 2011. "Keeping informed about school vouchers." Center on Education Policy Report.

Wang, K., et al. 2020. *Indicators of School Crime and Safety.* U.S. Department of Education.

Webb, J. T. 2000. "Mis-diagnosis and dual diagnosis of gifted children." Paper presented at the Annual Conference of the American Psychological Association.

Welch, C. E. 2016. "Every Student Succeeds Act (ESSA)." *Parenting for High Potential* 5:2–5.

Wheaton, D. 2016. "Prisons get higher funding boost than schools." *San Diego Union-Tribune*, July 31.

Wilder, S. 2014. "Effects of parental involvement on academic achievement." *Educational Review* 66:377–97.

Wurdinger, S. D. 2005. *Using Experiential Learning in the Classroom.* New York: Rowman and Littlefield.

Xu, J. 2008. "Sibship size and educational achievement." *Comparative Education* 52:413–36.

Yardley, J. 2002. "The 10 percent solution." *New York Times,* April 14.

Yarrow, A. L. 2009. "State of mind: America's teaching corps is made up of three groups with distinct attitudes about their profession." *Education Week,* October 19. Education Week website.

Zehr, M. A. 2011. "Capacity issue looms for vouchers." *Education Week,* June. Education Week website.

Zhai, F., J. Brooks-Gunn, and J. Waldfogel. 2011. "Head Start and urban children's school readiness." *Developmental Psychology* 47:134–52.

Zhang, J., et al. 2020. *The Condition of Education 2020.* U.S. Department of Education.

Zinn, D. 2020. "Student loan limits." Forbes website.

CHAPTER 12

# Family Problems

OBJECTIVES

1. Know the ways in which the American family is changing.
2. Discuss the functions of the family.
3. Identify the kinds and the extent of family problems.
4. Show how family problems affect the quality of life for family members.
5. Explain the ways in which social arrangements, including norms and roles, contribute to family problems.
6. Learn the significance of attitudes, values, and ideologies in perpetuating family problems.

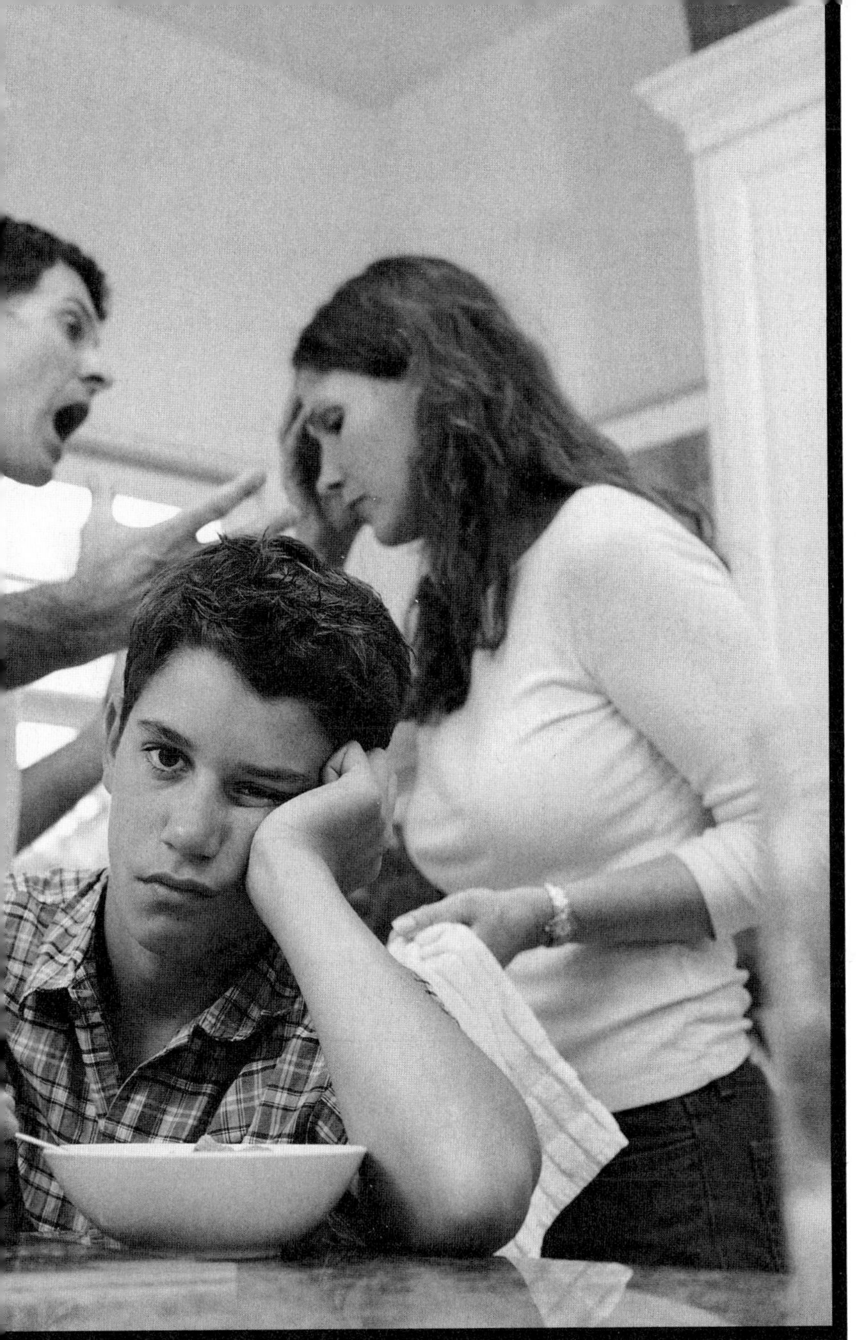
BananaStock/PunchStock

## "I Survived the Abuse"

Patricia is a self-confident, middle-aged, professional woman. Yet she could have turned out quite differently because she grew up in a home in which she suffered ongoing verbal abuse from her mother. To most people, Patricia's mother was a genteel southern lady. Patricia knew a different side of her mother:

*My mother was beautiful. She looked like a movie star. I grew up with her and my grandparents after she divorced my father when I was an infant. And I remember the verbal abuse vividly. She never shouted. She never sneered. In her pleasant, soft voice, she simply said things that were gut-wrenching to me. Like the time she took me to buy some shoes, and told the clerk in a giggly voice that he should just bring a shoe box because he probably didn't have shoes that were big enough to fit my feet. Do you know what that does to an adolescent girl?*

*When I was a teenager, my mother and I were about the same size. She would buy dresses for herself, then try them on me. I didn't say, "Let me try them on," because I never volunteered nor wanted to do it. I knew what her reaction would be. It was always the same—she would look at me in her dress, sigh, and shake her head as though it were hopeless. It was her way of letting me know how ugly I was compared to her. She also let me know this once when we were looking at a picture of us together when I was younger. She said it was too bad I was smiling and showing my big, ugly teeth.*

*One thing that saved me was my schoolwork. I was always good in school. I loved to read. I studied hard. My mother acknowledged my intelligence, but said it was a good thing I was smart because I would never be pretty. So I grew up thinking I was the world's best example of the ugly duckling. Except I expected to stay ugly. And in my mother's book, it was looks, not brains, that were a woman's most important asset. But at least I knew I was not a total loss.*

*The other thing that saved me was my husband. It took me a long time to accept his compliments as sincere. I still remember the first time he told me I was beautiful. I thought he was just trying to con me into something. Eventually, I began to see myself in a different light. And now when I look at pictures of myself as a child, my first thought is: "That's no ugly duckling. You were a lovely child. How could your mother have done that to you?"*

*A lot of my childhood pictures show a girl who is unsmiling and unhappy. That's the way I was. In some ways, I feel that I lost a good deal of my childhood. But I feel good about myself now. Most of the time, anyway. I still have occasional doubts. But I have a man in my life who keeps telling me I am beautiful. And I have a career that is going well. I only wish I had a mother whom I felt really loved me. But I guess you can't have everything.*

## Introduction

Is the family a dying institution? Some observers say yes, arguing that the family is doomed. Others go further, maintaining that the family *should* be doomed because it no longer functions in a useful way. The family, according to this argument, contributes more misery than benefit because it is ill adapted to modern social life.

Still others argue that the family is essential and ineradicable. What is needed, they argue, is help for troubled families, not radical changes or the abolition of family life. In this chapter we consider the argument that the family is doomed. Then, taking the position that it is not doomed, we look at the family as a problem. In previous chapters we asked how the family contributed to other problems. Now we examine the nature and extent of family problems. We also describe how those problems affect the quality of life. Finally, we identify the structural and social psychological factors that contribute to family problems and inquire into ways to resolve the problems.

## Is the Family Doomed?

**family**
a group united by marriage, blood, and/or adoption in order to satisfy intimacy needs and/or to bear and socialize children

**nuclear family**
husband, wife, and children, if any

A **family** is a group united by marriage, blood, and/or adoption in order to satisfy intimacy needs and/or bear and socialize children. The family, thus, is a crucial factor in both individual well-being and social life. Nevertheless, if prophecies could kill, the family would have died long ago. The popular and the professional literature continues to forecast the *death of the family,* at least the death of the **nuclear family** consisting of a married couple, and their children, if any. The evidence used to support the notion that the nuclear family is dying typically includes factors such as **divorce rates,** birthrates, runaway children, people who abandon their spouses and/or children, and **cohabitation** (in 2020, the U.S. Census Bureau reported 8.8 million cohabiting couples). The high rate of family disruption, combined with various other changes going on, makes family life appear to be in peril to some observers. At the same time, the fact that alternative forms of family life, including cohabitation, have proliferated suggests that *intimate relationships* must and will continue. Some people are merely finding alternate ways to express their intimacy needs.

**divorce rate**
typically, the number of divorces per 1,000 marriages

**cohabitation**
living together without getting married

## Alternative Forms of the Family

Many alternatives to the traditional nuclear family have been explored by Americans (Lauer and Lauer 1983). One alternative is group marriage, which has been tried in some communes. In this arrangement, all males and females have access to each other for sex and companionship. Other proposed alternatives include trial marriages with renewable contracts for specified periods of time, and "open marriages" in which each partner has the right to sexual and companionate relationships with someone other than the spouse.

Another arrangement, which has increased enormously since the 1970s, is cohabitation. As we just noted, 8.8 million unmarried couples are living together. In fact, the majority of people who marry have cohabited for an average 32 months before the marriage (Kuperberg 2019). Those who cohabit but don't marry may go on to cohabit with a new partner one or more times after their first cohabitation (Eickmeyer and Manning 2018).

Whether cohabitation leads to marriage depends, in part, upon whether one or both parties in the arrangement view themselves as being in a time of life when they are preparing to have a family or when they are taking risks to chart the course of their future (Rogers, Willoughby, and Nelson 2016). Those who view cohabitation as a preparation for marriage may be cautious because of the high divorce rate or because they have been previously married and divorced. What happens if a cohabiting woman gets pregnant? If the pregnancy was unintended, or the couple disagreed on the desirability of a child, they may end their relationship (Guzzo and Hayford 2014). In other cases, the couple may opt to marry. And still others may decide to continue to cohabit and raise the child. As a result, a substantial number of cohabiting couples have children in the home. Census Bureau data show that in 2020 2.8 million of the cohabiting couples had children under 18 in the home.

Although some couples cohabit as a test for whether to marry or not, a number of studies have found that, contrary to expectations, cohabitation does not enhance the chances for a more stable or more satisfying marriage (Heaton 2002). In fact, compared to those who married, cohabitors have higher rates of violence and abuse, lower rates of relationship happiness, higher rates of depression, less commitment to the relationship, a greater chance of breaking up even if the relationship is relatively satisfying, and lower levels of emotional and behavioral well-being of children living with them (Skinner, Bahr, Crane, and Call 2002; Brown 2004; Stanley, Whitton, and Markham 2004; Shackelford and Mouzos 2005). In addition, those who cohabit before marriage report less satisfying relationships after marriage and are more likely to have an extramarital affair (Treas and Giesen 2000).

However, more recent studies found no difference in divorce rates between those who had and those who had not cohabited before marriage (Manning and Cohen 2012; Rosenfeld and Roesler 2019). It is possible, as the researchers speculate, that as cohabitation has become widespread (about two-thirds of newlyweds cohabit prior to their first marriage), there is no longer a relationship between cohabiting and marital stability. And another study (Kuperberg 2014) concluded that a substantial part of the reason for higher rates of breakup was the young age at which a couple begins to cohabit (as we shall note below, the younger the age at marriage, the more likely there will be a divorce). We must wait on any firm conclusions until we have additional research. Moreover, even if stability is no longer an issue, there are still the questions of the quality of the relationship and of the well-being of children.

To return to the initial question: Is the family doomed? Clearly, the American family is changing in important ways. Yet, as we discuss later in this chapter, most Americans retain some traditional values about the family. Both in the United States and in Western European countries, cohabitation rates have increased dramatically, but the vast majority of people still marry at some point (Billari and Liefbroer 2016). Indeed, even those who divorce are likely to remarry. It's been estimated that about 20 percent of Americans marry two or more times during their lives (Siordia 2014). We take the position that, despite the critics and the changes, the family remains strong and crucial to the well-being of people. At the same time, it is clear that fewer people opt for the traditional form of the family in which there is a breadwinner husband, a housewife, and children. Precisely how, then, is the American family changing?

## The Changing American Family

Among the important changes in American families in recent times are *increases* in (1) age at first marriage, (2) proportion of young adults remaining single, (3) divorced adults, (4) adults living alone, (5) unmarried couples, (6) families maintained by adults with no spouse present, (7) children living with only one parent, (8) wives and mothers working, and (9) dual-career families (in which both husband and wife pursue careers, with minimal, if any, interruption of the wife's career for childbearing). At the same time, there has been a *decrease* in the number of children couples have. One effect of the various changes has been to dramatically alter the typical composition of American households over the past decades. As Figure 12.1 shows, the proportion of households with married couples has declined significantly, while the proportions of other kinds of families and of nonfamily households

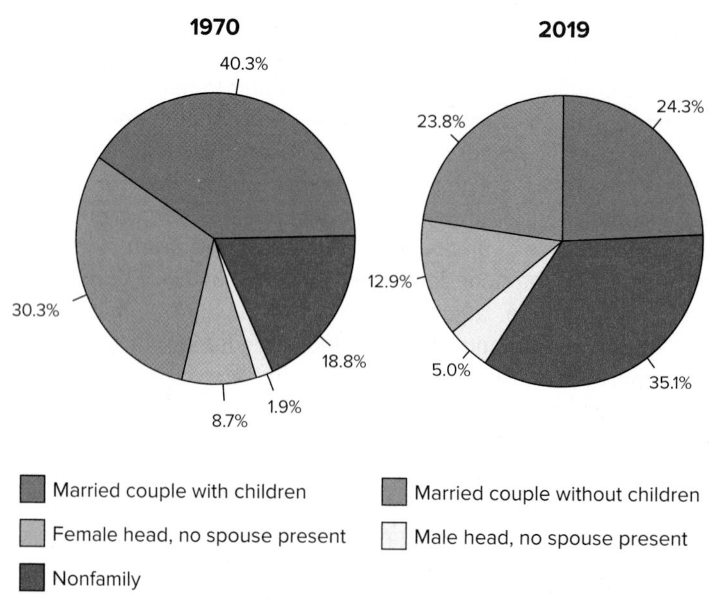


**FIGURE 12.1**
Composition of American Households, 1970 and 2019.
Source: U.S. Census Bureau website.

(such as people living alone, friends living together, and same-sex couples) have increased significantly. Consider some specific data (U.S. Census Bureau website):

- From 1970 to 2020, the proportion of people who were never married increased from 18.9 percent to 35.8 percent of adult males and from 13.7 percent to 30.0 percent of adult females.
- From 1970 to 2020, the proportion of Americans who were married dropped from 71.1 percent to 50.4 percent.
- From 1970 to 2019, the birthrate per 1,000 women decreased from 87.9 to 58.3; the average size of families is smaller than it has ever been.
- Since 1970, the proportion of all births that occur out of wedlock has more than tripled: 4 of 10 births are to unmarried women.
- The divorce rate rose dramatically after 1965; it declined from a high of 5.2 per 1,000 people in 1980 to 2.9 per 1,000 people in 2018, but is still higher than the rate of 2.5 per 1,000 people in 1965.
- Among women, 66.4 percent of those with children under age 6 and 76.8 percent of those with children between ages 6 and 17 are in the labor force.

Although such changes may be interpreted as threatening to the traditional nuclear family, you also must consider other evidence. First, many of the statistics that we just cited reflect a reversal rather than a continuation of a trend. For example, the divorce rate has tended to decrease since 1980. Second, most Americans marry at some time in their lives. Only a minority of those who are single are so by choice. Third, the bulk of Americans rate a good marriage and family life as extremely important to them (Whitehead and Popenoe 2001). Fourth, most Americans are satisfied with their own family life. A 2019 Gallup Poll reported that 76 percent of Americans are very satisfied, and another 17 percent are somewhat satisfied, with their family life (Brenan 2019).

Indeed, married people generally are happier and healthier than the nonmarried. More than 130 studies have reported that both married men and married women are happier and less stressed (as measured by such factors as alcoholism rates, suicide rates, and physical and emotional health) than are the unmarried (Lauer and Lauer 2022).

Clearly, then, Americans still value the traditional nuclear family. Just as clearly, there is an increasing tendency to prefer nontraditional roles, particularly an egalitarian arrangement (in which husband and wife both work and share responsibility for home and children).

## Functions of the Family

Whether Americans opt for a traditional or a nontraditional family arrangement, they face certain problems. The problems reflect not only the expectations and values about family life but also the *functions of the family*. Those functions, like other aspects of the family, have changed over time. At one time the family was primarily responsible for matters such as education, religious training, recreation, and providing the necessities of life. Those functions have been largely assumed by other institutions. However, the family continues to be an important factor in *regulating sexual behavior, reproduction, and rearing children.*

Another important function of the family is to provide a *primary group* for individuals. The **primary group,** consisting of the people with whom you have intimate, face-to-face interaction on a recurring basis, is of enormous importance. In a classic study, a children's home created "artificial" families after it was noted that the children

**primary group**
the people with whom one has intimate, face-to-face interaction on a recurring basis, such as parents, spouse, children, and close friends

were having developmental problems (Stanton and Schwartz 1961). Previously, all the children had been cared for by all the attendants, who carefully avoided too much involvement with any one child so as not to appear to have favorites. However, when this arrangement was abandoned and the home was divided into family groups of about four children and a "mother," the results were "astonishing."

> The need for individual attachment for the feelings which had been lying dormant came out in a rush. In the course of the one week all six families were completely and firmly established . . . the children began to develop in leaps and bounds. The most gratifying effect was that several children who had seemed hopeless as far as the training for cleanliness was concerned suddenly started to use the pot regularly and effectively (Stanton and Schwartz 1961:236).

Primary groups are important for adults as well as children. You have a personal status in primary groups. You gain an understanding of the kind of person you are and learn the kind of norms by which you are to live. Primary groups, in other words, are crucial to your well-being as a functioning human. For most Americans, the family is a primary group *par excellence.*

When problems arise in the family, they arise in the group that is important to your well-being, that provides you with important emotional support, and that is of central importance to your life satisfaction and happiness (Lauer and Lauer 2022). The family is not always a solution; it is also a problem, as we will explain later in this chapter. The point is that the family is a central aspect of your well-being; thus, when family life becomes problematic, you are threatened at the very foundation of the quality of your life.

## The Extent of Family Problems

The family becomes a problem when it does not fulfill its purposes, particularly its purpose as a primary group. The American ideal is that the family should be *structurally complete.* Children should have both a father and a mother in the home. The family should be a *supportive group,* providing emotional support for each member. "Ideal" in this context does not mean "perfect" (and therefore unrealistic). Rather, the ideal is defined as realistic and expected. When the actual situation falls short of the ideal, the *quality of life* is diminished. Expectations are thwarted, the most important primary group is disrupted, and family members experience stress.

For many people today, the expectations are thwarted more than once. In your lifetime, you might live in five, six, or more different families, each of which could fail in some way to fulfill your needs for structure and support. If your parents were divorced when you were young, and you lived with one parent for a while, then a stepparent for some years, you would have three different family experiences before adulthood. As an adult, if you cohabited, married, divorced, and remarried one or more times your family experiences would rise to six or more.

Consider next the extent of structural and supportive problems. *Structural problems* relate to the breaking up of husband and wife and/or parent and child. *Supportive problems* involve the lack of emotional support.

### Disrupted and Reconstituted Families

*Divorce rates,* one measure of structural problems, have fluctuated in the United States, but the *general trend of number of divorces per 1,000 population from 1860 to 1980 was upward.* A surge occurred after World War II and again after 1965, so that by the mid-1970s the United States had the highest divorce rate in the Western world.

| Divorces | 1960 | 1965 | 1970 | 1975 | 1980 | 1985 | 1990 | 1995 | 2000 | 2018 |
|---|---|---|---|---|---|---|---|---|---|---|
| Total (1,000) | 393 | 479 | 708 | 1,026 | 1,189 | 1,190 | 1,182 | 1,169 | 944 | 782 |
| Rate per 1,000 population | 2.2 | 2.5 | 3.5 | 4.8 | 5.2 | 5.0 | 4.7 | 4.4 | 4.1 | 2.9 |
| Rate per 1,000 married women, 15 years and over | 9.2 | 10.6 | 14.9 | 20.3 | 22.6 | 21.7 | 20.9 | 19.8 | 18.8 | n.a. |
| Percent divorced, 18 years and over: | | | | | | | | | | |
| Male | 2.0 | 2.5 | 2.5 | 3.7 | 5.2 | 7.6 | 7.2 | 8.0 | 8.8 | 8.3 |
| Female | 2.9 | 3.3 | 3.9 | 5.3 | 7.1 | 10.1 | 9.3 | 10.3 | 10.8 | 10.9 |

**TABLE 12.1**
Divorces, 1960 to 2018

SOURCE: U.S. Census Bureau website.

However, as Table 12.1 shows, the rates began to decline after 1980. The 2018 figure of 2.9 was lower than any since the late 1960s. Even so, millions of Americans continue to be affected by divorce. Children as well as adults are affected. According to the U.S. Census Bureau, in 1970, 85 percent of children lived with both parents; by 2019, as seen in Table 12.2, only 70.1 percent lived with both parents.

During the 1960s and 1970s, divorce was the major cause of single-parent families. In recent years, births to unmarried mothers are the largest factor. Single-parent families are also the result of death, separation, and abandonment. The combination of all these factors has meant a dramatic increase in the number of single-parent families since 1970. The United States now has a higher proportion of single-parent families than most other developed nations–27 percent (Charmi 2021). The proportion varies by race: 19 percent of white families, 53 percent of African American families, 13 percent of Asian families, and 29 percent of Hispanic families. We show later in this chapter some of the consequences of living in a single-parent family.

About three-fourths of people who divorce eventually remarry. If the remarriage includes children from a previous marriage of one or both partners, a **stepfamily** is formed. According to the Census Bureau, in 2018 there were 3.9 million households (11.8 percent of all households) with one or more stepchildren in them. At some point in the future, according to some demographers, the stepfamily could become the main type of American family.

**stepfamily**
a family formed by marriage that includes one or more children from a previous marriage

Strain and conflict with or about stepchildren is common in such families (Stoll, Arriaut, Fromme, and Felker-Thayer 2005). As a result, the marital relationship is stressed,

| | Percent Living with | | | |
|---|---|---|---|---|
| | Both Parents | Mother Only | Father Only | Neither Parent |
| All races | 70.1 | 21.4 | 4.5 | 4.0 |
| Non-Hispanic White | 78.2 | 14.0 | 4.5 | 3.3 |
| African American | 42.2 | 45.7 | 5.1 | 7.0 |
| Asian | 85.8 | 9.8 | 2.4 | 2.0 |
| Hispanic | 68.0 | 24.3 | 4.1 | 3.6 |

**TABLE 12.2**
Living Arrangements of Children Under 18 Years, by Race and Hispanic Origin

SOURCE: U.S. Census Bureau website.

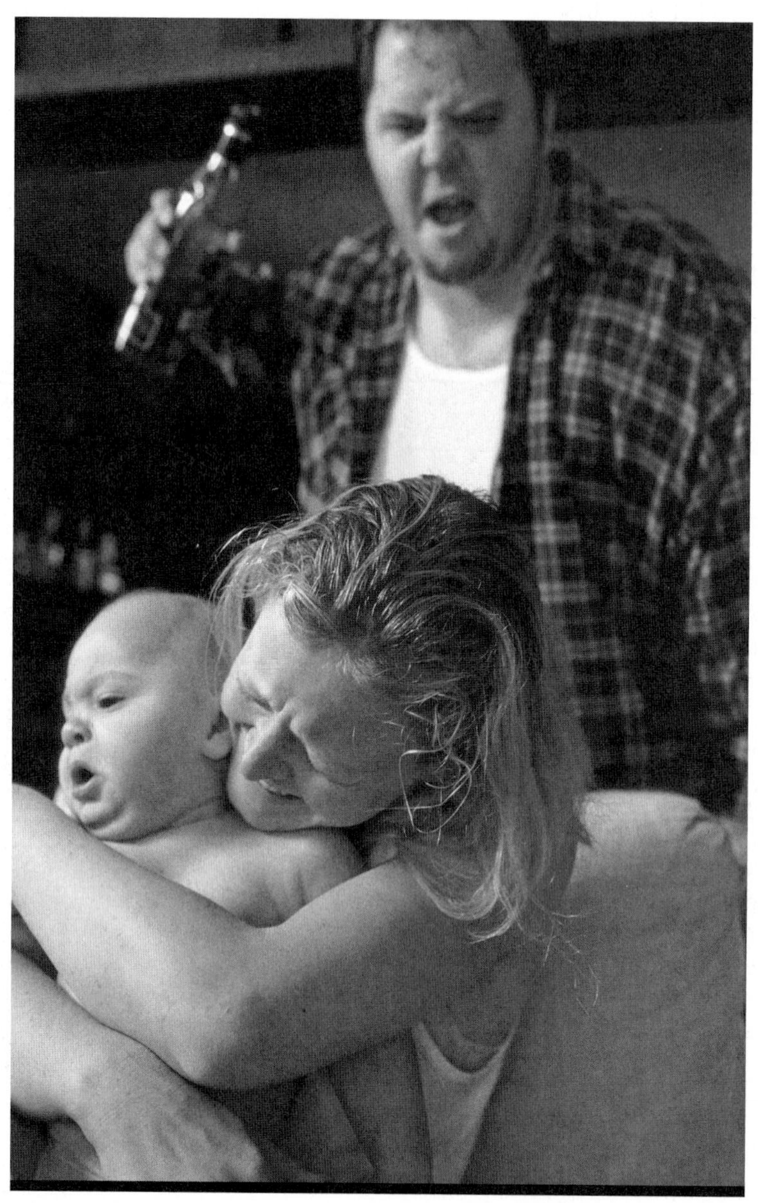

Severe violence occurs in some families.

Ingram Publishing/SuperStock

and the divorce rate among second marriages is even higher than that among first marriages. Twenty percent of first marriages, but 31 percent of second marriages, end in divorce within 5 years (AVVO Staff 2015). After 10 years, the figures are 32 percent for first marriages and 46 percent for second marriages.

## Family Violence

Information on the amount of *violence in families* shows that it is not a rare phenomenon. Violence, of course, represents an alarming example of the failure of supportiveness. It is found in every kind of family, and includes everything from name-calling and put-downs to threats, physical assaults, and forced sex (Straus et al. 2020). A substantial number of Americans are victims of abuse in the family. A survey of children in Michigan's public schools reported that 18 percent were investigated by child protective services by the time they reached third grade (Ryan et al. 2018). And more than a million women report domestic violence each year (Morgan and Truman 2020). Almost a fourth of murders are against a family member, and aggravated assaults by family members comprise about 10 percent of all aggravated assaults (Durose et al. 2005). Over their lifetime, 36.4 percent of women have been the victims of sexual violence, physical violence, or stalking (Smith et al. 2018.)

*The likelihood of being a victim of family violence varies by a number of demographic characteristics.* Nearly three-fourths of the victims are females. Whites and African Americans have higher rates of victimization than do Hispanics and those of other races. And those in the 35- to 54-year-old age group have higher rates than do other age groups.

Studies of *spouse abuse* and *child abuse* were rare until the 1960s. Since then, numerous studies, including some national surveys, have been undertaken. The first national survey of family violence occurred in 1975, and the second took place in 1985 (Gelles and Straus 1988). The researchers found that the overall rates declined during this 10-year period, perhaps because of such factors as an increase in the average age at marriage (violence is more common among younger couples), a more prosperous economy (financial stress increases violence), and less willingness to tolerate violence in the family (shelters for battered women rose from 4 to more than 1,000).

global comparison

## MARITAL QUALITY AND WELL-BEING OF CHILDREN

The family is a central element for individual well-being. In nations throughout the world, the more stable and harmonious family life, the higher the life satisfaction of family members. Four researchers surveyed 2,625 male and 4,118 female college students from 39 nations on six continents (Gohm, Oishi, Darlington, and Diener 1998). They categorized the nations by whether they have a collectivist or individualist culture. In individualist cultures (such as the United States, Germany, Australia, Japan, and Spain), people perceive their lives as depending largely on their own actions. They see society as a collection of individuals rather than as a highly integrated group. They believe that the course of their individual lives has no necessary relationship to the course of social life. Thus, they see possibilities for individual success and happiness even if the society as a whole is deteriorating.

In collectivist cultures (such as China, Brazil, India, and Tanzania), people perceive their lives as inextricably bound up with what happens in groups and in the nation as a whole. They cannot conceive of individual success that is independent of the groups to which they belong. Individual happiness, for them, is not as important as group well-being.

The researchers thought that the well-being of the college students in their survey might vary not only by the kind of family in which they grew up but also by the kind of culture in which they lived. Some of their results are shown in Figure 12.2.

Clearly, there were both cultural and state-of-marriage differences in student well-being. Generally, students in individualist cultures scored higher on a life satisfaction test than did students in collectivist cultures. But regardless of the type of culture, students from intact homes (with two natural parents or a remarriage) in which there was low interparental conflict tended to score higher than those from homes with a single parent or with high interparental conflict. The highest scores of all were those in homes headed by a married couple with low conflict.

In sum, for people everywhere, the family is important for individual well-being. If the family is functioning well, the well-being of each member is maximized. If the family is functioning poorly, all members are adversely affected.

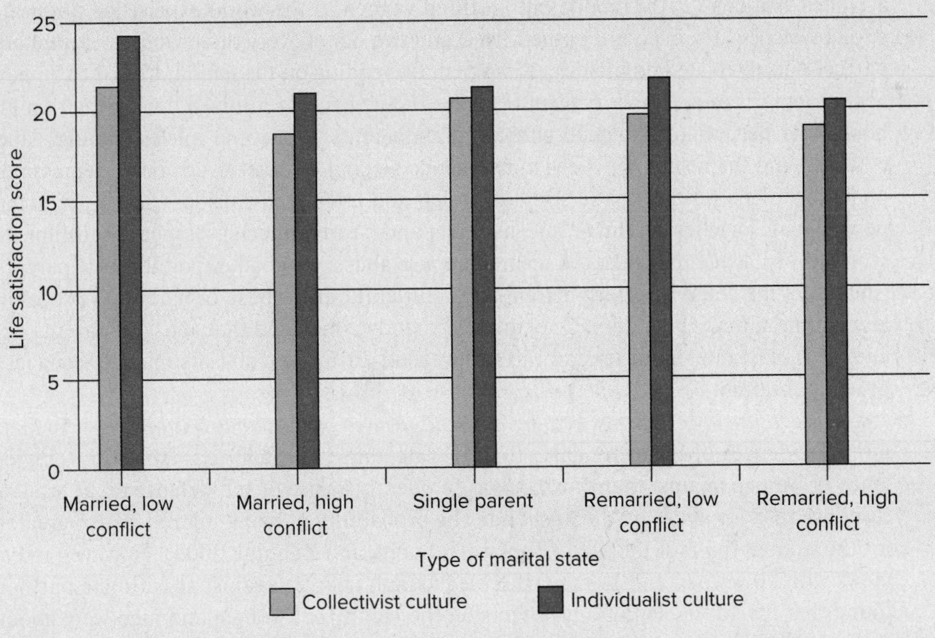


**FIGURE 12.2** Marital Status and Child Well-Being in 39 Nations.

Source: Gohm et al. 1998.

Still, there is a *high level of violence in intimate relationships generally and in families in particular.* Moreover, children who witness violence between parents are also victims, for it is a traumatizing experience to see one's parents in a violent confrontation. A national survey found that more than 1 in 9 (11 percent) children saw some kind of family violence in the year prior to the survey, including 1 in 15 (6.6 percent) who were exposed to violence between their parents (Hamby, Finkelhor, Turner, and Ormrod 2011). The researchers concluded that about a fourth of children are exposed to at least one form of family violence during their lifetime.

Of course, family violence is not an exclusively American problem. In Canada, for example, a survey of women in Quebec found that 6.1 percent had suffered physical violence and 6.8 percent had experienced sexual violence perpetrated by their male partners (Rinfret-Raynor et al. 2004). A Korean national study found that 29.5 percent of women had experienced violence from their husbands, resulting in serious mental health problems among the victims (Kim, Park, and Emery 2009). In the Middle East, wife abuse is not only pervasive but widely accepted (Boy and Kulczycki 2008); nearly 90 percent of ever-married women accept at least one reason that justifies wife beating.

Family violence is, then, a worldwide problem. A United Nations report on violence against children around the world found that "physical violence against children in the home is widespread in all regions" (Pinheiro 2006:52). For instance, 38.5 percent of students aged 11 to 18 in the Kurdistan Province of Iran reported being victimized by violence at home that caused physical injuries, and in Korea "kicking, biting, choking and beating by parents are alarmingly common, with a high risk of physical injury–and for a small proportion, disability–as a result" (Pinheiro 2006:52).

Sexual victimization in the family also occurs throughout the world. According to a United Nations (2015) report, one in three women in the world experience physical/sexual violence at some point in their lives, and two out of every three victims of intimate partner-/family-related homicides are women. Depending on the nation, from 7 to 36 percent of females and 3 to 29 percent of males report being victimized during their childhood. The perpetrators include parents, grandparents, aunts and uncles, siblings, and cousins. And the results for the victims include alcohol or other drug abuse, depression, panic disorders, posttraumatic stress disorder, and attempted suicide. Clearly, for some people in all societies "intimate" means threat and harm as much as it means fulfillment.

Family violence may take the form of spouse abuse, child abuse, or abuse of parents (including the abuse of elderly parents by adult children). Abuse of parents is probably less common than the others. One university study concluded that abuse of parents occurs in at least one out of ten families (Stevenson 2016). The abusers may be teenagers or adult children.

*Spouse abuse involves wives beating husbands as well as husbands beating wives.* In fact, more incidences of husband abuse than of wife abuse are reported. However, the violence of women against their husbands is frequently a case of self-defense or, at least, a response to prior abuse by the husband. The probability of being injured is also greater for the woman than for the man (Bookwala, Sobin, and Zdaniuk 2005). However, interviews with 90 women and 10 men who filed assault charges against an intimate partner found that the adverse emotional effects on the victimized women and men were about the same (McFarlane, Willson, Malecha, and Lemmey 2000).

Child abuse, another form of family violence, is more likely when one of the natural parents is missing. Children in a single-parent home, or those with a stepparent, are much more likely to be victims of abuse (Snyder and Sickmund 1999). Estimates of the amount of child abuse in the nation vary widely. One problem in getting reliable figures is that mandatory reporting laws were not passed in the states until the 1960s. Government data call the abuse "maltreatment" and show that there are hundreds of thousands of substantiated cases each year. The rate of maltreatment is slightly higher for girls than for boys (Forum on Child and Family Statistics 2020). By age, the highest rate occurs for children 1 year or younger. By race/ethnicity, the highest rate occurs for American Indians, followed by African Americans, whites, Hispanics, and Asian Americans (whose rate is very low).

These numbers are undoubtedly conservative. How many cases go unreported? One way to obtain more accurate information is to ask the victims themselves. For child abuse, this means asking them when they are older whether they have ever been abused. Some still will not remember or will have repressed the memory, so even the results from victimization research will underestimate the amount. A national study of adolescent health asked American youth, among other things, about their experiences of maltreatment (Hussey, Chang, and Kotch 2006). Being left home alone as a child (a possible case of neglect) was named by 41.5 percent. It was the most common kind of maltreatment. In addition, 28.4 percent reported experiencing physical assault, 11.8 percent said they had been physically neglected, and 4.5 percent reported sexual abuse. Clearly, maltreatment is more prevalent than the number of cases officially substantiated by state agencies.

Incest, which we discussed briefly in chapter 4, is likely to be an extremely traumatizing experience for a child, and the effects tend to be long-lasting with a high proportion of the victims suffering posttraumatic stress disorder (Celbis et al. 2020). A study of 17 incest survivors who became mothers found that the women had poorer relations with their own mothers and lower psychological adjustment than a comparable set of mothers who had not been sexually victimized (Fitzgerald et al. 2005). In addition, although the incest survivors appeared to be mothering as well as the others, they did not see themselves as being very effective mothers.

Girls are more likely than boys to be victims (Celbis et al. 2020), but we do not know how many victims there are in the United States. A survey of 1,672 male and female adolescents in Korea, however, reported that 3.7 percent had been victimized (Kim and Kim 2005). The families of the victims had high levels of other kinds of problems, such as mental illness, criminal behavior, and alcoholism. The victims, compared to adolescents not so victimized, had higher rates of emotional and social problems.

Besides the observable and measurable supportive problems in family violence, a considerable amount of supportive failure cannot be measured–intense conflict or alienation within families. In addition is the problem of neglect, which affects over a half million children each year. Neglectful parents abuse their children psychologically through lack of feeling and caring. They are emotionally distant from their children. They may be struggling to retain their own sanity or totally absorbed in their own pleasures. For whatever reason, they provide none of the support that parents typically give. Neglected children may never learn to trust adults. They may suffer various physical ailments because of inadequate nutrition, clothing, and sleep. They are likely to have retarded intellectual development and be insecure, withdrawn, and unable to express emotions.

## Family Problems and the Quality of Life

The effect of family problems on the *quality of life* is sometimes obvious and sometimes not. As with all social problems, the effects impact more than just those immediately involved in the problem. For example, consider the economic costs associated with divorce. Research by David Schramm and his associates (Schramm et al. 2013) assessed the economic costs of divorce in terms of various kinds of state help available to those who find themselves financially strapped after a divorce. They found that Texas spent some $3.2 billion on the consequences of divorce each year, representing about 12 percent of the total budget in 2008. In other words, even Texas families that remain intact are helping, through their taxes, to sustain those involved in family disruption. Thus, there is an economic cost of divorce for all citizens.

Moreover, other and often even more severe problems occur. Physical violence against a person by someone in his or her primary group produces emotional trauma as well as physical pain. *Alienation from those in one's primary group is emotionally traumatic.*

Less obvious is the effect of a broken home on children and their parents. Parenting is demanding and stressful even when there are two parents in the home. Not surprisingly, both single parents and their children face a broad range of stresses, including feelings of responsibility, task, and emotional overload on the part of the parent; and emotional, interpersonal, and school problems on the part of the children (Dunifon and Kowaleski-Jones 2002; Bramlett and Blumberg 2007).

Supportive problems mean, by definition, that family members endure some degree of stress. But the consequences of structural problems are less clear. Consequently, much of this section examines structural problems. You will discover that supportive problems also have some not-so-obvious consequences for the quality of life.

Most of the effects that we discuss later in this section involve a *contradiction between interaction patterns and American values.* Supportive problems mean that interaction patterns within the family contradict the value of emotional and physical health. Structural problems result in interaction patterns that contradict the value of social adjustment. Because children who grow up in broken homes lack experience with either a mother or a father, they often have various problems of adjustment and have to cope with such problems as illness, poverty, and deviant behavior more than others do.

The structural characteristics peculiar to the stepfamily, on the other hand, can lead to different types of problems (Lauer and Lauer 1999). Each member of a stepfamily may have lost an important primary relationship. Children may be angry about the loss and focus that anger on the stepparent. The noncustodial parent may interfere with the stepfamily's adjustment. The children and the stepparent also might compete for the custodial parent's attention and affection; the stepparent, after all, is entering an ongoing relationship as an "extra" member. The stepparent and children may even have difficulty because the role of stepparent is still somewhat ambiguous. Is the stepparent to be like a parent, a friend, or a teacher? Finally, the children may try to work their natural parents one against the other to gain various ends. Thus, both in single-parent and stepfamilies, interaction patterns may diminish the quality of life.

## Physical and Emotional Difficulties

Physical and mental illnesses are rooted, in part, in family arrangements. Children growing up with both biological parents receive more social, emotional, and material support than children in any other kind of family. In contrast, broken homes (structural failure) and homes in which parents frequently quarrel (supportive failure) have been linked to stress in children, often resulting in physical or emotional illness (Vandervalk et al. 2004).

*Divorce.* For adults, adjustment to divorce has *striking similarities to the bereavement process.* Contrary to a popular notion that divorce may be an avenue to freedom and therefore an exhilarating experience (at least once the legal procedure has been

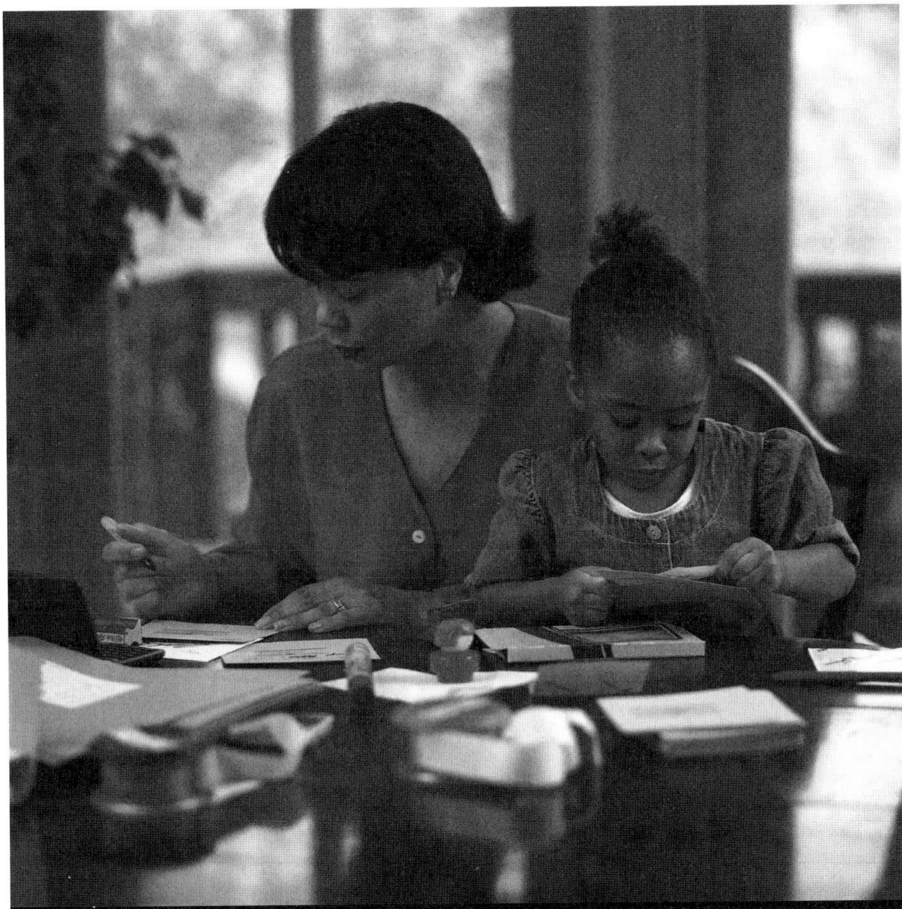

An increasing number of Americans struggle in their role of single parent.

Keith Brofsky/Photodisc/Getty Images

completed), divorced people typically face a painful process of adjustment not unlike that which occurs after a death in the family. In both death and divorce, a *primary relationship has been disrupted,* and the disruption of a primary relationship is always traumatic. The consequences include a sense of loss and bewilderment, various kinds of deprivation (including financial and emotional support), and susceptibility to emotional problems such as depression (Hilton and Kopera-Frye 2006; Hogendoorn, Leopold, and Bol 2020). The disruption, incidentally, is not only with an intimate partner but also with one's children. Thus, nonresident fathers have much higher emotional distress than either single mothers or married parents (Yuan 2016).

Particularly in the first months, divorce is more likely to bring emotional and physical disturbances than a sense of freedom. In fact, various studies report that divorced people have higher rates of suicide, accidents, death from various causes, physical and mental ailments, and alcoholism (Yip and Thorburn 2004; Lorenz, Wickrama, Conger, and Elder 2006; Stack and Scourfield 2015). Of course, these problems are not always the result of a divorce. In some cases, they existed prior to, and helped bring about, the divorce, but they also can result from the divorce (Wade and Prevalin 2004). Those who divorce are highly likely to experience at least some of these negative outcomes in the short run and, for some people, the outcomes may persist for years or decades.

Because of such outcomes, divorce is a major health problem in the nation (Chatav and Whisman 2007). It is not surprising that divorced people, compared to those not divorced, report themselves as less happy and as having more insecurity in their relationships (Schneller and Arditti 2004).

The distress of divorce involves not just the couple but also their friends and family members. The parents of those who divorce may experience problems with depression (Kalmijn and De Graaf 2012). Adult children whose parents divorce later in life report a change to a negative relationship with one or both of their parents during the initial stages of the divorce (Greenwood 2012). But young children and adolescents suffer the most. The negative consequences for young children and adolescents whose families are disrupted by divorce include the following problems:

- Children in divorced families are more likely to be anxious, depressed, and withdrawn than those in intact families, and their mental health problems tend to persist when they become adults (Kim 2011; Colen and Pereira 2019).
- Children in divorced families are more likely to have behavior problems, sleep disorders, fear of abandonment, and aggressive tendencies (Amato and Cheadle 2008; Guinart and Grau 2014).
- Adolescents from divorced homes are more likely to engage in delinquent behavior, use alcohol and illegal drugs, and pursue a life style that tends to result in various health problems (Holmes, Jones-Sanpei, and Day 2009; Thuen et al. 2015).
- Adolescents in divorced families worry about having enough money to meet both present and future needs and aspirations (Koerner, Korn, Dennison, and Witthoft 2011).
- Young women from divorced families rate themselves as less attractive and report more dissatisfaction with their bodies than do women from intact families (Billingham and Abrahams 1998).
- Children in divorced families tend to receive less maternal warmth and empathy (the conflict and pain of most divorces leave little energy for nurturance of children), which contributes to various emotional and behavior problems (Kline, Johnston, and Tschann 1991).
- Children in divorced families rate themselves lower in social competence, and, in fact, are likely to have poorer interpersonal skills (Peretti and di Vitorrio 1993; Kim 2011).
- Children and adolescents in divorced families tend to have lower levels of educational attainment and achievement and more problems in school than children from intact families (Center for Marriage and Families 2005; Sun and Li 2011; Soria and Linder 2014; Ferrer and Pan 2020).
- Children in divorced families have lower levels of emotional well-being when they become adults (Amato and Sobolewski 2001; Wauterickx, Gouwy, and Bracke 2006).
- Children in divorced families have more negative attitudes about marriage, less optimism about the possibility of a long-lasting, healthy marriage, and, in fact, have a higher probability of divorce when they become adults and marry (Wolfinger 2005; Whitton, Rhoades, Stanley, and Markman 2008).

Children also face *problems of adjustment.* They confront questions from peers, particularly when they are in elementary school, about why they have only one parent at home. They have to adjust to a change in primary relationships and possibly to restricted interaction with one of the parents (generally the father). They may have to cope with parental conflict, which often continues after the divorce, and with attempts by each parent to gain the child's loyalty and affection at the expense of the other. It is not surprising, then, that children whose parents are divorced are prone to both emotional and physical problems.

The severity of the negative consequences for children depend on a number of factors, including how well the parents handle the divorce. Some older research showed that the consequences are more severe for younger children. This may be because divorce is harder on the parents of young children (Williams and Dunne-Bryant 2006). The emotional strain of becoming a single parent (even with shared custody) and of being separated from one's child for a good deal of the time make the adjustment to divorce more difficult than it is for those without children or without children in the home.

Nevertheless, the discord that leads to divorce is probably more stressful for the child than is divorce itself. Parents who stay together "for the children's sake" may actually harm the children more than if they were to separate. A home with continual conflict or emotional coldness can be more damaging to the children than a home that is broken. Children from divorce-disrupted families have higher rates of depression and withdrawal than others, but the rates are even higher for those who live in a home with persistent conflict than for those who live in a single-parent home. A study of college students concluded that being in a conflicted home as a child significantly increased the chances of subsequent distress and emotional disorders such as depression and alcohol abuse (Turner and Kopiec 2006). Consequently, if the family is a severely dysfunctional one, the children may actually benefit by a divorce (Strohschein 2005).

Thus, the intact home may have supportive problems that are far more damaging to the child or to the spouses than a structural problem would be. In other words, structural problems of broken homes are associated with various kinds of physical and emotional problems, but the intact home is not free of such problems.

What about the stepfamily? Does remarriage mitigate the negative health effects of divorce? As noted earlier, the stepfamily has its own peculiar set of problems. In the short run, stepchildren do tend to exhibit more behavior problems, but in the long run they can function as well as children in intact families (Jensen et al. 2018).

*Abuse.* The effects of abuse tend to lead to both *short-term and long-term trauma.* Abused children may become withdrawn and isolated; feel shame, guilt, or unworthiness; and become anxious and depressed (Cole 1995; Stroebel et al. 2012). They are also likely to exhibit, to a greater degree than nonabused children, a variety of problem behaviors, such as quick anger, frequent fighting, resisting of parental authority, school problems, and violence (Kotch et al. 2008; Ryan et al. 2018). And they may suffer impaired brain functioning (Teicher 2002). Many of the negative consequences occur because of emotional abuse as well as physical abuse (Panuzio et al. 2007; Melançon and Gagné 2011).

The problems of abused children tend to persist into adulthood. Physical or sexual abuse during childhood is associated with a wide assortment of problems among adults: physical ailments, emotional problems, problems of establishing meaningful intimate relationships, substance abuse, posttraumatic stress disorder, becoming an abuser, and attempted suicide (Afifi et al. 2008; Larsen, Sandberg, Harper, and Bean 2011; Nguyen,

Karney, and Bradbury 2017; Strom et al. 2021). Emotional and physical problems also occur in children who witness violence between their parents and/or who try to intervene in the adult violence (Jarvis, Gordon, and Novaco 2005). When they grow up and marry, abused children tend to have lower marital satisfaction and a higher probability of marital disruption (Whisman 2006).

*Adults as well as children suffer physical and emotional harm from both psychological and physical abuse* (Taft et al. 2006). Abused adults have higher rates of impaired mental health, impaired physical functioning and health, and problems in social functioning (Laffaye, Kennedy, and Stein 2003; Loxton, Schofield, and Hussain 2006). A study of Hispanic women in the southeastern part of the United States asserted that so many of the women are victims of domestic violence that the abuse is a "major health problem" for them (Murdaugh, Hunt, Sowell, and Santana 2004).

Thus, the damage from abuse can be severe. The physical harm ranges from bruises and broken bones to permanent brain damage and even death. The emotional harm is more difficult to measure. Yet some indication may be seen in the high rates of both mental disorders and attempted suicide.

## Poverty

We previously noted that *female-headed families* are more likely to experience *poverty* than male-headed families. Because most single-parent families have a female head, they have a higher probability of being in poverty than do other households. Moreover, the never-married single mother is even more likely than the divorced single mother to be in poverty. Because of low welfare payments and low wages in available jobs, the single mother may be caught in a bind: Whether she works or stays home and receives welfare, she may find herself and her family living in poverty (Tucker and Lowell 2015). In recent years, the rate of poverty among families headed by a female with no husband present has been more than twice that of the general population. About half of the millions of children living in poverty are in female-headed families.

Children who grow up in poverty have challenges in many areas of their lives. Here, we look briefly at one area that is important because it will tend to perpetuate their poverty as they grow older—education. Poverty is associated with lower educational achievement, which, in turn, results in lower earnings in the labor market when the child eventually goes to work (Borjas 2011). In part, the lower educational achievement reflects the fact that children living in poverty are unprepared for school; fewer than half of poor children are ready for school at age 5 compared to 75 percent of children not living in poverty (Isaacs 2012). And once in school, 22 percent of children who lived some of the time in poverty and 32 percent of those spending more than half their childhood in poverty drop out before finishing high school, compared to 6 percent of those who have never been poor (Hernandez 2011).

## Deviant Behavior

Sexual variance, drug and alcohol abuse, and juvenile delinquency have been associated with disturbed family life (Bjarnason et al. 2003; Fagan 2003). We pointed out in earlier chapters that prostitutes and drug and alcohol abusers often have a background of disturbed relationships with their parents. There are, in fact, higher rates of a wide range of deviant behavior among children in single-parent homes (Ellis et al. 2003;

Barton 2006; Wen 2008; Magnuson and Berger 2009). Compared to those in two-parent families, children in single-parent families:

- have higher rates of antisocial behavior, aggression, anxiety, depression, and school problems.
- are less likely to complete high school.
- are more likely to get involved in early sexual activity and adolescent pregnancy.
- are more likely to use illicit drugs.
- are likely to have poorer mental and physical health.

The deviant behavior is likely to continue into adulthood. Researchers examined the records of a group of 1,575 children over a period of years. The children had all been physically or sexually abused or neglected in their early years. By the time they were in their mid- to late-20s, 49 percent had been arrested, compared to 38 percent of those in a control group of the same age, gender, race, and social class, and 18 percent had been arrested for a violent crime (National Institute of Justice 1996, 2014).

## Maladjustment

People who come from disturbed families tend to have various difficulties that we subsume under the category of **maladjustment:** antisocial behavior (such as aggression and bullying), insecurity, overconformity to one's peers, a tendency to withdraw from relationships, difficulties in relating to others, problems with one's personal identity, and various problems as adults. The maladjustment affects all areas of a child's life. Divorce, severe parental conflict, and abuse all are associated with higher rates of conduct disorder and problems with both adults and peers (Flisher et al. 1997; Bing, Nelson, and Wesolowski 2009). Such children have problems trusting others, and therefore it is difficult for them to establish effective relationships.

**maladjustment** poor adjustment to one's social environment

The problems of maladjustment continue to afflict the children as they grow into adulthood. Adults who were physically punished during childhood tend to have more physical and verbal aggression with their spouses, to be more controlling of their spouses, and to be less able to see things from the spouse's perspective (Cast, Schweingruber, and Berns 2006). And a significant number of abused children will become abusers, including the abuse of their own children.

From the point of view of the child, *abuse is a form of rejection.* It is, however, not the only way in which parents can reject and distress a child. Parental hostility is a form of supportive failure that can result in maladjustment as the child attempts to relate to others. Inconsistency–including inconsistency in discipline–in how the parent treats the child is another form of supportive failure. Inconsistency means the child lives in a capricious environment, and no one functions well with chronic uncertainty. Consequently, parents who are inconsistent in the way in which they relate to and discipline their children foster various kinds of maladjustment, including depression, hostility, and difficulties in relating to peers and adults (Carrasco et al. 2015).

The *child's sense of self-esteem,* so important in his or her social functioning, is crucially related to family experiences. Self-esteem tends to be high when a child has nurturing parents and a harmonious family environment (Brummelman and Sedikides 2020). Parents build self-esteem through such actions as affirming and supporting their children, showing their children how to constructively express their feelings, taking an interest in their children's activities, showing respect for their children's point of view, and teaching their children how to exercise self-control and handle responsibility. In contrast, supportive failure, including abuse, is related to low self-esteem, and low self-esteem tends to lead to emotional and interpersonal problems.

## Contributing Factors

The factors we examine in this section contribute to both structural and supportive problems. Some families suffer from both types of problems. The two types can be independent, but more often are interdependent. Structural problems, for instance, may either make supportive failure more likely or reflect supportive failure in the past.

### Social Structural Factors

*Social Norms.* An important factor in the divorce rate is that divorce is more "respectable" now than it was in the past. In other words, the *norms about divorce have changed.* In the past, religion and the law both said, in effect, "You should not get a divorce. You should make every effort to work it out and stay together." Today the norms about divorce reflect a loosening of the laws ("no-fault" divorce) and greater tolerance among religious groups. In contrast to the *stigma* formerly attached to divorce and to divorced people, most Americans now agree that divorce is an acceptable option if the marriage isn't working out. This new attitude is based on the norm of happiness, the notion that each individual has the right, if not the obligation, to be happy. The *fallacy of non sequitur* may be involved in the process: "I have a right to be happy; therefore, I must get a divorce." Even if you agree to the individual's right to happiness, it doesn't follow that divorce is necessary. All marriages have troubled times. Couples who have achieved long-term, satisfying marriages point out that happiness comes by working through problems, not by avoiding or leaving them (Lauer and Lauer 1986). Of course, some marriages may be hopeless, but many break up too quickly because people believe the marriage is infringing on their right to happiness.

fallacy

Age at marriage is one of the more important factors in marital instability. One study reported that 59 percent of women who married when they were younger than 18 years, compared to 36 percent of those who married when they were 20 years or more, either separated or divorced within 15 years (Bramlett and Mosher 2001).

Both structural and supportive problems are more common among the very young. In fact, adolescent marriage and parenthood has been called a case of "children raising children." Not only is the marriage more likely to break up, but problems of childrearing are likely to be serious, including a greater probability of child abuse.

Why do adolescents marry at a young age? Social norms define the appropriate time for marriage. For most Americans, that time has been soon after high school graduation or, at the latest, soon after college. In the 1950s, people lowered the ideal age for getting married. Females who were not married by the time they were 20 could develop a sense of panic that they would become old maids. Males who waited until their late 20s or after to get married might be suspected of having homosexual tendencies or an inadequate sex drive (which was an affront to their manhood). Subsequently, however, the norm about marital age has reverted to earlier notions. It is now acceptable for an individual to be and to remain single. Yet the average age for marriage is still relatively young, and the single individual may not be wholly acceptable to many businesses and corporations who still prefer their young executives to be married.

As long as these attitudes persist, structural and supportive problems due to marriage at a young age will continue.

Norms also contribute to the amount of family violence in the nation. A common norm in families is that it is proper to hit someone who is misbehaving and who does not respond to reason. Many Americans consider the use of physical punishment in the rearing of children as virtually an obligation. Recall the old saying "Spare the rod and spoil the child." It is not surprising, then, that most American parents spank their children (Walters 2019). And in some cases it is applied with a vengeance. But as a French-Canadian study showed, rather than being an effective method of discipline, harsh punishment—both physical and verbal—only increases the likelihood of aggression by the child against the parent (Pagani et al. 2009).

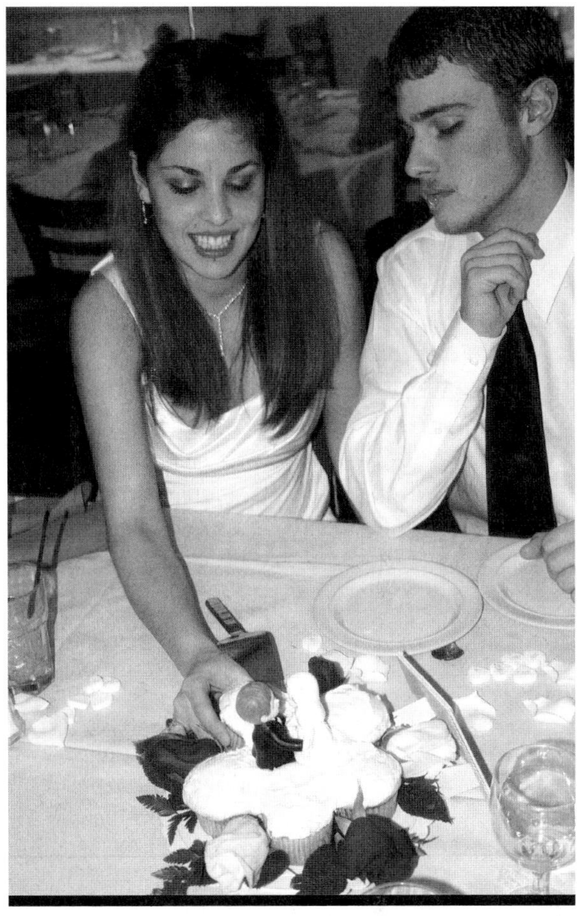

Divorce rates are higher among those who marry at a young age.
Christopher Kerrigan/McGraw Hill

*Role Problems.* A number of *role problems* contribute to both structural and supportive problems. Indeed, whatever else may be true of modern marital roles, they place an *emotional burden on people that is probably unprecedented in human history.* Modern couples often do not have the proximate interpersonal resources available to those in extended families or to those in small, preindustrial communities. Instead, they rely heavily on each other for advice, intimacy, and emotional support in times of difficulty or crisis.

Moreover, the marital role is ambiguous as well as demanding. *Role obligations* in a changing society are not as clear-cut as those in more traditional settings. Couples who disagree on role obligations of husband and wife are more prone to divorce than are those who agree. The nature of these obligations is not as important as whether the couple agrees on them and whether each feels that the other is fulfilling them. A gap between expectations and perceived behavior increases dissatisfaction.

The majority of American couples are willing to participate in activities once regarded as the domain of the opposite sex, but some may not want to give up their own traditional gender roles. A husband's expectations may still carry more weight than a wife's in determining the division of labor. Wives may be more accepting of noncompliance with expectations than husbands are. Again, however, the crucial factor is not whether the couple is traditional or nontraditional, but whether they agree on their arrangement of role obligations.

For women, *role flexibility* is important for well-being. That is, women need to be free to choose whether to work outside the home. The number who make that choice will probably continue to increase inasmuch as women who work full time outside the home have greater work satisfaction than women engaged in full-time housekeeping (Treas, van der Lippe, and Tai 2011).

The divorce rate is higher among women who work outside the home (South 2001). Financial independence allows women to escape from unhappy unions, such as those in which they perceive severe inequity in the relationship. When wives work outside the home, then, negotiation over role obligations may be required to effect a more equal sharing of both responsibilities and privileges. In particular, working wives expect an equitable sharing from their husbands of responsibility for household tasks, and they are much more likely to be happy with their marriage when they perceive such sharing exists (Frisco and Williams 2003; Khawaja and Habib 2007).

Finally, role problems can be critical in the reconstituted family. Exactly what is the relationship between stepparent and stepchild? People often bring unrealistic expectations to stepfamilies. Women who become stepmothers, for example, tend to expect themselves to:

- somehow compensate the children for the distress caused by the death or divorce.
- create a happy and close-knit family unit.
- maintain happiness and contentedness in all family members.
- demonstrate through appropriate behavior that the notion of the wicked stepmother is just a myth.
- love, and be loved by, the stepchildren almost immediately as if the stepchildren were her own natural children (Lauer and Lauer 1999).

People who impose such role obligations on themselves, or who have them imposed by others, are certain to encounter problems. Thus, stepmothers vexed by role problems have higher rates of depression and anxiety than biological mothers (Doodson and Davies 2014).

*Family Continuity.* People who are reared in problem families tend to perpetuate the problems in their own families. Those who come from families in which one or more parents died tend to have rates of disruption similar to those who come from intact families. But people who come from families in which the parents were divorced or separated have higher marital disruption rates than do those coming from intact families (Amato and DeBoer 2001). And those who grow up in families that have parental conflict or parental infidelity are more likely to engage in infidelity themselves when they are adults (Weiser et al. 2015).

Similarly, family violence tends to be continued from one generation to the next (Stith et al. 2000; Coohey 2004). Parents who abuse their children were often abused by their own parents. The battered child of today is likely to become the battering parent of tomorrow, perpetuating the problem of family violence. Marital abuse also is transmitted from one generation to another. The husband who abuses his wife is likely to be a man predisposed to violence because he learned such behavior from his parents. He may have been abused, or he simply may have witnessed violence between his parents (Carlson 1990). Unfortunately, some children learn from watching their parents that those who love you also hit you, and that this action is an appropriate means to get your own way and deal with stress. Such children are *modeling their behavior* after that of their parents, although that behavior may be considered undesirable or immoral by most others.

Even if the child does not grow up to be an abuser, *the mere fact of witnessing violence between one's parents tends to lead to problems of adjustment.* This effect occurs in infants as young as 1 to 3 years of age (McDonald et al. 2006). And the effects can persist into adulthood. Witnessing violence in the home is associated with such maladies as depression and other emotional ills, delinquency and behavior problems, and posttraumatic stress disorder (O'Keefe 1994; Crusto et al. 2010). And boys that witness violence between their parents have higher rates of dating violence (Gage 2016).

A family can perpetuate its problems into the next generation simply because it is such an important factor in the *socialization* of the child. The family is an important place for learning what it means to be a male or a female, how to function as a parent, and generally how to relate to others. Thus, there is some continuity in parent-child relationships and husband-wife relationships from generation to generation.

*Stratification and Family Problems.* Families in different social classes exhibit different problems. For one, *divorce is more common in the lower strata than in the middle and upper strata.* A government survey found that the proportion of women whose marriage broke up within 10 years was 44 percent in the low-income group, 33 percent in the middle-income group, and 23 percent in the high-income group (Bramlett and Mosher 2002). Because of the relationship between racial and ethnic background and income, variations exist in the probability of divorce among racial and ethnic groups. The same government study reported that the proportion of marriages that broke up within 10 years was 32 percent for white women, 47 percent for Black women, 20 percent for Asian women, and 34 percent for Hispanic women.

The relationship between income and divorce may seem contrary to common sense, as the well-to-do can afford the costs of divorce more easily than the poor, but financial problems put enormous strains on marital and family relationships. In fact, income is one of the best predictors of family stability. The increasing rates of structural failure as you go down the socioeconomic ladder reflect the greater potential for financial difficulties. Economic difficulties, in turn, tend to generate more discord in the home, increasing the amount of hostile, contemptuous, and angry behavior (Williams, Cheadle, and Goosby 2015; Masarik et al. 2016).

Another factor that bears on the divorce rate is jointly owned property and financial investments, both of which are more likely to be held by people in the middle- and upper-income levels. Divorce is more difficult and expensive when it involves a division of assets. Middle- and upper-income people are also more likely to have a network of friends and relations who will resist their divorce and who may support them as they try to work through their problems.

Finally, the combination of the higher rates of unmarried mothers and higher divorce rates means that fewer children in the lower socioeconomic strata live with both parents (Table 12.3). Thus, the undesirable consequences of living in a disrupted or single-parent home are more prevalent in the lower socioeconomic strata.

| Family Income | Percent with Both Parents |
|---|---|
| Under $10,000 | 29.0 |
| $10,000 to $19,999 | 36.0 |
| $20,000 to $29,999 | 49.9 |
| $30,000 to $49,999 | 62.6 |
| $50,000 to $74,999 | 73.7 |
| $75,000 to $99,999 | 83.6 |
| $100,000 and over | 91.2 |

**TABLE 12.3**
Proportion of Children Living with Both Parents, by Income

SOURCE: U.S. Census Bureau website.

Supportive failure is suggested by data on abuse and neglect. A certain amount of abuse occurs in middle- and upper-class families, but both neglect and abuse seem to be more prevalent in the lower than in the middle or upper strata (Kruttschnitt, McLeod, and Dornfeld 1994; Berger 2005).

*The Family in a Changing Structure.* Rapid change of the social structure creates its own problems, including problems for families. Certain kinds of change can affect the divorce rate. If roles are in a state of flux, the potential for conflict within the family is increased and the probability of divorce becomes greater. Rapid change may involve confusion and ambiguity about what it means to be a husband, a wife, or a parent, which leads to more stress, more conflict, and more structural and supportive problems.

Most observers agree that the current society is in a time of rapid change. Any family can put down an anchor somewhere and suddenly find that there is nothing solid to hold it in place. A family moves into a neighborhood in the hope of having a better life, only to find the neighborhood deteriorating. A family moves to a new city because the father or mother is offered a better job, only to face unemployment when an economic reversal occurs. To compound the problem, the family has no roots in the area and the family members are wholly dependent on each other for emotional support. Moreover, even if the new job opportunity works out well, the family still may be strained by the lack of a social support system. Thus, the divorce rate in the United States is positively related to urbanity, population change, and lack of church membership (Amato and Rogers 1997; Vaaler, Ellison, and Powers 2009), all of which are indicators of a lack of integration into a local community.

## Social Psychological Factors

*Attitudes.* In general, Americans' attitudes about the single-parent family have become somewhat less negative over time (Usdansky 2009). Nevertheless, the single-parent family is considered, at best, less than what is desirable and, at worst (particularly in the case of an unmarried-mother single-parent family), something that exists but should not exist or be approved. Such attitudes contribute to the problems of the single-parent family if the parent and/or children sense the disapproval or rejection of others. In essence, the disapproval or rejection means a loss of social support, and social support is essential for well-being even in the best of circumstances.

Attitudes are also a factor in problems of abuse. Men who sexually abuse their children come up with a variety of rationales that minimize or even justify the incest (Dietz 2020). In situations in which there is no intercourse, they may dismiss the seriousness of the relationship on the grounds that it "wasn't really sex." In situations in which intercourse occurs, they may define it as an adult-to-adult rather than an adult-to-child relationship or maintain that the child was a willing participant who gave permission for the incest.

Some Americans agree that violence in intimate relationships is acceptable or even necessary at times (Simon et al. 2001). Although few Americans believe that women are the *cause* of their own abuse, a fourth still believe that at least some women *want* to be abused, and most are convinced that women can end abusive relationships (Worden and Carlson 2005). Abusive husbands maintain their spouses deserve the beatings for some reason (Lancer 2017). *Blaming the victim is one of the more common characteristics of husbands who abuse their wives.* A small proportion of abused women agree that they deserved to be beaten.

How could a woman justify wife beating? Unfortunately, many victims have attitudes that lead them to remain in a violent relationship (Marano 1996; Barnett 2001). Some of these attitudes are understandable: The women may fear that they will lose their children (courts have been known to award custody to the father when a battered woman leaves the home), or be unable to protect their children, or risk their own lives. The risk to their own lives is a real one: Abusers threaten to kill their wives if they try to leave, and in fact, more abuse victims are killed when trying to leave their abusers than at any other time.

Battered women may have rationales that are difficult to counteract. Ferraro and Johnson (1983) interviewed more than 100 battered women. The women who opted to remain in their relationships justified the decision in six ways, many of which involve fallacious modes of thinking. Some of the women had a "salvation ethic"; they viewed their husbands as troubled or "sick" individuals who needed them in order to survive. Some said that the problem was beyond the control of either the women or their husbands; the violence was caused by some external factor or factors such as work pressure or loss of a job. Of course, this is the *fallacy of non sequitur*. It does not follow that a man will necessarily abuse his wife when he has problems with his work. A third explanation involved a denial of injury; some women insisted that the beatings were tolerable and even normal. Fourth, some of the women used the *fallacy of personal attack against themselves,* blaming themselves for the abuse. They said that the violence could have been averted if they had been more passive and conciliatory. A fifth reason was the women's insistence that they had no other options; some of the women believed that they were too dependent on their husbands either financially or emotionally. Finally, some of the women used the *fallacy of an appeal to authority,* claiming that a "higher loyalty"—such as a religious faith or a commitment to a stable family—motivated them. Such attitudes may be rationalizations that disguise a deeper reason for maintaining an abusive relationship, or they may be potent factors in their own right. In any case, they are used by the victims to justify and perpetuate the violence.

fallacy

fallacy

fallacy

Finally, *attitudes toward the self* are important factors in abuse. Mothers who abuse their children tend to have lower levels of self-esteem than other mothers do (Wolfner and Gelles 1993). Husbands who abuse their wives tend to be dissatisfied with their lives, believe that the man should be the head of the family but lack the resources to be the head, and assault their wives in order to establish their control over them (Felson and Messner 2000; Atkinson, Greenstein, and Lang 2005).

If negative attitudes can contribute to family conflict and disruption, positive attitudes can contribute to family health and stability. Stafford (2016) found that people who consider their marriages as sacred tend to put more effort into protecting their marriages. This enhances the spouse's marital satisfaction and the probability of maintaining a healthy and lasting union.

*Values and Homogamy.* When you marry, you undoubtedly hope that the relationship will last and be rewarding to both you and your spouse. Is marital happiness more likely to happen if you and your spouse have similar or dissimilar backgrounds? The answer to this question has been debated by social scientists. Some have argued that couples with *dissimilar backgrounds* **(heterogamy)** will be attracted to each other and will *complement* each other so that the marriage is more rewarding and successful. Others have argued that *similar backgrounds and shared rather than different values* (**homogamy**) are more likely to produce a rewarding and lasting marriage.

**heterogamy**
marriage between partners with diverse values and backgrounds

**homogamy**
marriage between partners with similar values and backgrounds

Research generally supports the view that homogamy is more conducive to a lasting marriage. Although homogamy does not mean that the couple must have similar backgrounds in every respect, it appears that the greater the similarity, the greater the likelihood of a satisfactory marriage (Mullins, Brackett, Bogle, and Pruett 2004). This

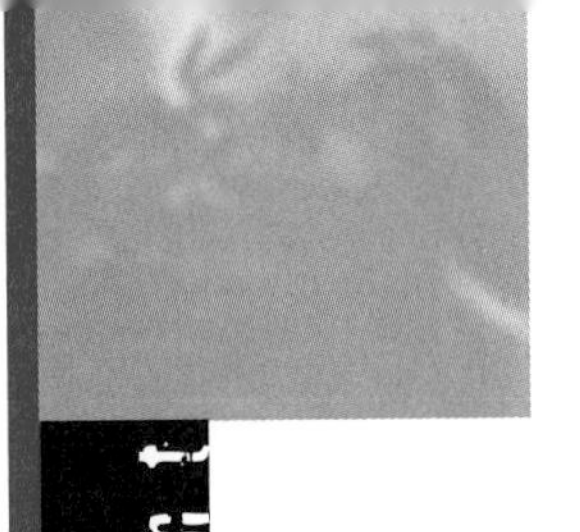

involvement

## ONE BIG HAPPY FAMILY

Some utopian communities that have arisen in the United States have considered traditional family arrangements detrimental to human well-being. The 19th-century Oneida community, for instance, was founded on the notion of "Bible communism." Private property was abolished, including the private property of a spouse or child. The entire community was a family. Every adult was expected to have sex relations with a great variety of others. Women who bore children cared for them for the first 15 months and then placed them in the children's house where they were raised communally and taught to regard all adults in the community as their parents.

Obtain literature about utopian communities of the present or past (see Lauer and Lauer 1983). For example, you might investigate Bethel, Brook Farm, Oneida, Ephrata, the Icarians, the Rappites, the Shakers, or any one of numerous contemporary communes. Consider what kinds of family arrangements they have created. Do any of these arrangements solve the kinds of problems discussed in this chapter? Why or why not? Do the utopian arrangements appear to create other kinds of problems? Would the utopian arrangement be practical for an entire society? What is your own ideal after reading about the utopians and the alternatives mentioned earlier in this chapter?

kind of relationship is more likely to result when there is similarity in family background, socioeconomic background, cultural background, personality traits, and religion. Homogamy tends to correlate with marital happiness. Perhaps the more similarity between spouses, the fewer areas of conflict. In any case, shared rather than dissimilar values are important in securing a satisfactory marriage. Structural and supportive problems are more likely to occur when the couple come from dissimilar backgrounds and hold diverse values.

*The Value of Success.* The American *value of success* can lead to supportive failure in the family. Merton (1957:136) showed how the "goal of monetary success" pervades society so that Americans "are bombarded on every side by precepts which affirm the right or, often, the duty of retaining the goal even in the face of repeated frustration." In families, schools, and the mass media, Americans are urged to pursue the goal with unrelenting diligence. Most Americans share this value of success. Even in the lower socioeconomic strata, where people often do not *expect* success, they still *wish* for it.

Monetary success often requires long hours at work and minimal contact with family. What are the consequences? A survey of employees in a Fortune 500 company found that the more time an individual spent at work, the greater was the interference with family life and the higher was the level of distress (Major, Klein, and Ehrhart 2002). In addition, family members may feel neglected by the person who is working the long hours. Clearly, then, a strong emphasis on success that leads to spending long hours at work can result in supportive failure in the family. Individuals who are attaining such success may be neglecting their families. Individuals who are severely frustrated in their attempts to attain success may react with violence in the family setting. In either case, the family members are the victims of a value that is deeply ingrained in American society.

*Ideology of the Family.* Unfulfilled or conflicting expectations about role obligations can lead to marital dissatisfaction and dissolution (Pasley, Kerpelman, and Guilbert 2001). *The American ideology of the "good" family generates a set of expectations* that may create problems if the expectations are not met. Two versions of this ideology exist, each of which can give rise to unrealistic or conflicting expectations.

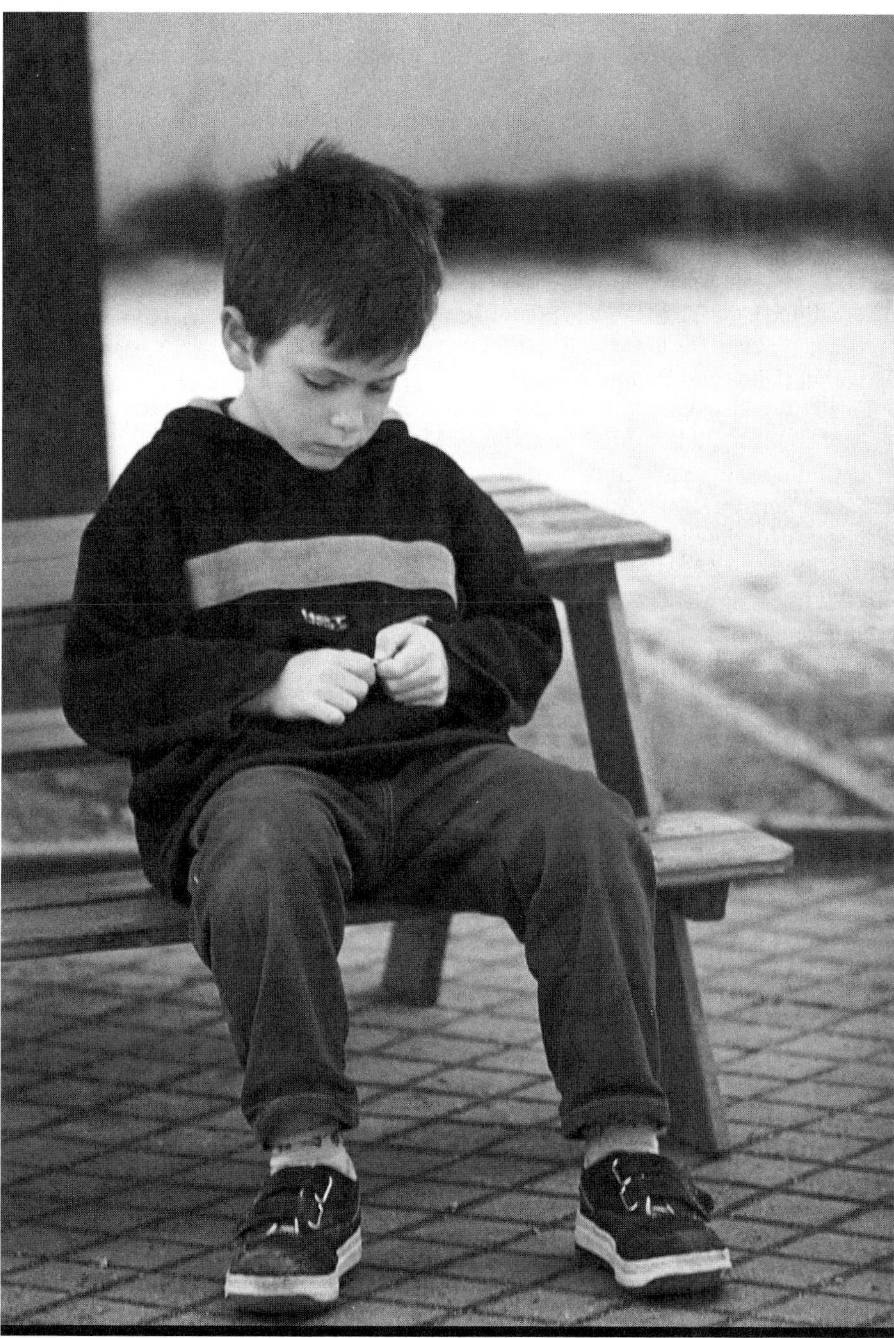

Many Americans believe that lack of time together is the family's greatest threat.

Laurence Mouton/Photoalto/PictureQuest

One version asserts that *a good family is a happy family* and that *happy families are harmonious* and free of conflict. Further, the family is a kind of miniature society in which all important human relationships and feelings can be experienced. Each person can find within the family a complete range of experiences in the context of harmony and happiness. This view of family life is unrealistic, and the result is a higher rate of emotional stress when conflict is suppressed because of the ideology.

A different version of the ideology of the good family stresses the need to express feelings and engage in creative conflict. This ideology has grown out of small-group work and says, in effect, that the good family maintains *healthy relationships* and that healthy relations can be obtained only when people give *free expression to their feelings.* People should "level" with each other and accept each other.

If the first ideology errs by condemning conflict in the family, the second one errs by encouraging too much *anger and aggression* in the home. Giving free expression to feelings may provide you with a sense of release and relief, but it does not enhance the quality of your interpersonal relationships. The free expression of anger is likely to lead to verbal and even physical aggression. In marriage, the higher and more severe the level of aggression, the lower your satisfaction and the more likely you are to experience disruption (Ulloa and Hammett 2015).

Finally, two ideologies worsen the problem of abuse within the family. One is the *ideology that the man should be the breadwinner.* Men who accept this ideology and equate breadwinning with masculinity may resort to violence if their wives earn a significant part of the family income (Atkinson et al. 2005). In such cases, the violence is an attempt to reassert male dominance in the relationship and in the family.

The other is the *ideology of nonintervention,* which asserts that outsiders should not interfere in family affairs. People who might aid a woman being beaten by a man would not interfere if that same man were beating his wife. People who might stop a woman from abusing a child would not intervene if that child were her own.

The ideology of nonintervention affects the police as well. As Ferraro (1989) found, the police may use their ideologies about battered women and family fights to evaluate specific incidents. The police officers with whom Ferraro worked believed that if battered women opted to stay in their situations, it was not the responsibility of the police to control the violent behavior. One male officer even insisted that because a man's home is his castle, he should be able to do whatever he wants there. Furthermore, the officer asserted, most wife abuse is provoked by the woman herself. Thus, in spite of a presumptive arrest policy (arrests are required when there is probable cause and the offender is present), the police frequently did not arrest the offender. Rather, they would reassure the woman and tell her to call them if anything further happened.

We should note that educational efforts are changing the ideology, so that most victims have positive and helpful experiences with the police now (Apsler, Cummins, and Carl 2003). But negative experiences still exist (Johnson 2007; Kim and Gray 2008). And such experiences can make some women hesitant about trying to get help from the police. Research with victims who came to a battered women's shelter found that two-thirds of the women had contact with the police some time during the previous six months, but most did not have as much contact as they had needed (Fleury, Sullivan, Bybee, and Davidson 1998). The women gave various reasons for not calling the police, including *fear of even greater violence* and *previous negative experiences with the police themselves.*

## Solutions: Public Policy and Private Action

As with all problems, *both therapeutic and preventive measures* can be applied to family problems. Therapeutic measures include the more traditional counseling services as well as newer efforts involving discussion and interaction in small-group settings. Public policy could require intervention, counseling, and needed protection in cases of abuse and divorce. Such measures, of course, attempt to resolve problems after they have already begun.

What kind of preventive measures could be taken? That is, what measures might minimize the number of family problems in the nation? Consider, first, what government and business can do. Much has been said about "family values" in the political arena in recent years. The question is, what are political and business leaders doing to strengthen American families?

We pointed out in the chapters on poverty and work some of the ways in which government and business can help families that are poor (some of the problems of family life are intertwined with the problem of poverty) and can address the problems created by work conditions (e.g., too much time at work and too stressful work both have negative impacts on family life). Some other nations do far better than the United States on these and other matters; some countries offer day care for workers' children and paid time off for new parents (Remery, van Doorne-Huiskes, and Schippers 2003). If businesses do not adopt such family-friendly policies on their own, they may need to do so by government mandate (Gray and Tudball 2003). Single-mother families are particularly in need of help because most have already suffered the pain of disruption and because they have the highest poverty rate of any group in the nation. The United States desperately needs policies and programs that support and help single working mothers through such benefits as child care and flexible work hours (Albelda, Himmelweit, and Humphries 2004).

The arguments against government-mandated policies include the resistance to any expansion of government into the private sector and the claim that the additional costs will harm business. The answer to the first argument is simply that if the government does not require these changes, they will not happen. With a few exceptions, business leaders are not known for voluntarily taking steps to enhance the well-being of workers when those steps involve additional costs. With regard to the second argument, a survey of 120 employers in New York found that the employers who offered flexible sick leave and child care assistance had significant reductions in turnover, offsetting some of the costs involved in the benefits (Baughman, DiNardi, and Holtz-Eakin 2003).

Numerous other courses of action also fall into the category of preventive measures. For example, states could experiment with a legalized system of trial marriage. Couples would contract to marry for a specific period of time and then have the option of renewing the contract. However, you need to be aware of the nature of experiments. They are searches—often blind gropings—for answers, and not firm guidelines. Some experiments may work, but others may not (and perhaps may even make a problem worse).

A contrary approach would be to make it harder to divorce. Some states presently allow *covenant marriages,* in which spouses sign a legal contract that they will not seek divorce except for abuse or adultery. If they want to divorce for any other reason, they agree to first undergo counseling and wait two years before finalizing the decision. A researcher tracking 600 newly wed couples, half of whom were in covenant marriages, reported that after the first two years the rate of divorce was much lower among those in the covenant marriages (Perina 2002).

Beneficial *family life education* at all stages of the life cycle, through the schools and the mass media, could change negative attitudes about single-parent families and the legitimacy of violent behavior as well as break down harmful ideologies about the "good" family. Family life education could also change some norms, and new norms can affect family life in crucial ways. For example, consider our norms about roles and the division of labor in the home. It is true that husbands today are more willing than in the past to agree with greater role freedom for their wives. Yet even women who have careers still tend to take major responsibility for home and children. Americans are egalitarian in theory but not yet in practice.

A great many false or counterproductive ideas can be attacked through educational programs. *Marriage enrichment programs* can help couples confront and work through the common issues in marriage and family life. Such programs teach couples, for example, how to create and maintain good communication patterns, handle conflict constructively, work out an equitable division of labor in the home, and manage their finances.

The problem of family violence needs to be addressed through the law, education, and practical aids like shelters for battered women. These efforts need to be buttressed by bringing about ideological changes in the culture. Religious groups can help in these efforts; a lower amount of domestic violence occurs among families who report regular attendance at religious services than among those who are not regular or who are nonattenders (Ellison, Bartkowski, and Anderson 1999; Cunradi, Caetano, and Schafer 2002).

fallacy

Ideologies of the family in which authorities and others (such as neighbors or relatives) regard domestic violence as a private matter need to be changed. If domestic violence is a private matter, then people will be hesitant to intervene and offer help to the victim, particularly when the ideology is combined with the *fallacy of personal attack*. The fallacy of personal attack is the argument that the woman has done something to deserve the violence. A former victim of abuse told us that she stayed in her marriage for many years because everyone she knew, including her priest and her own family, kept telling her that she must be doing something wrong to make her husband act so violently! Education through schools and the mass media can change people's understanding of family violence, get rid of the old ideologies, and lead to an open confrontation of the problem. Spouse and child abuse must be seen for what they are: crimes of violence and not justifiable acts within the confines of a group–the family–that is off limits to outsiders.

Finally, shelters for battered women also address the problem of violence. They provide many services, including emergency shelter, crisis counseling, support groups, child care, and assistance with housing, employment, and education. These shelters help reduce the amount of domestic violence. The very existence of shelters warns batterers that their wives have an alternative to remaining in an abusive relationship. The number of shelters increased over the past few decades; by 2020 there were over 1,500 in the nation. But the number is too small and the funding is too little to meet the demands. Even when the shelters have room, they may require women to find alternative housing within weeks; and the waiting lists for public or subsidized housing can be anywhere from seven months to years. The lack of alternatives ultimately forces many of the women to return to the men who battered them. Additional shelters would allow more women to escape abusive relationships, and the shelters also would stand as a visible reminder to men that violence against women is no longer tolerable.

*Follow-Up.* Set up a debate in your class on the topic "Divorce is too easily attained and too readily accepted in the United States today."

## Summary

Family problems are so common that some observers have argued that the family is doomed. Those who predict the end of the present type of family suggest a number of alternatives, such as group marriages, trial marriages, open marriages, or cohabitation. But most Americans continue to marry and establish homes, and to prefer that option over alternatives.

The problems of the family stem from the fact that it is one of the most important primary groups. Americans believe the family to be the cornerstone of society and that an ideal family provides stability, support, and continuity for American values. We identify two basic types of problems: structural (disruption and reconstitution of families) and supportive (lack of emotional support).

Several kinds of data suggest the extent and seriousness of family problems. Structural problems may be measured by the divorce rate, by the number of single-parent families, and by the number of reconstituted families that contain a stepparent-stepchild relationship. Supportive problems are evident in the amount of family violence, including child abuse.

All family problems diminish the quality of life. Physical and emotional difficulties may result from family conflict. Additional problems of adjusting to a broken home result from separation or divorce. And problems of adjustment to new and ambiguous roles must be confronted in the stepfamily. Poverty is more frequently associated with a female-headed than with a two-parent family, and the poverty tends to be perpetuated because the child from a single-headed family does not perform as well academically as other children do. Several kinds of deviant behavior have been associated with disturbed family life: sexual deviance, drug and alcohol abuse, and juvenile delinquency. People who come from families with problems tend to develop various kinds of maladjustment: antisocial behavior, interpersonal problems, and low self-esteem.

Norms that are permissive about divorce and that encourage young marriages are two social structural factors that contribute to family problems. Role problems contribute to marital dissatisfaction and thereby lead to both structural and supportive failure. Family problems are especially likely to occur when there is disagreement on role obligations and when expectations are in conflict and unfulfilled for one or both spouses. The stepfamily has its own peculiar set of problems, stemming from the difficulties of the stepparent-stepchild relationship. The family itself also contributes to future family problems. Because parents act as role models for their children, the children may learn patterns of behavior that will create future problems.

Family problems are generally more prevalent in the lower social strata, partly because of financial strains and partly because of different norms and roles. Rapid social change is yet another structural cause of family problems.

Among the social psychological factors, attitudes are important. A number of attitudes contribute to family problems, including negative attitudes about single-parent families and attitudes that justify abuse. Values are also a significant factor in family problems. A couple with similar values based on similar backgrounds is more likely to have a satisfactory marriage. The value of success in American culture, on the other hand, puts a strain on marriages and family life because certain occupations can consume family members who are striving for that success.

Two "good family" ideologies generate expectations and behavior that strain marriage and family relationships. One says the good family is happy and free of conflict, which can lead to a suppression of conflict and guilt. The other claims that in the good family, people can freely express their feelings, including aggression; this ideology can perpetuate debilitating conflict. Both ideologies tend to result in supportive problems. Families need a balance between excessive openness and free expression of feelings, on the one hand, and suppression and guilt, on the other hand. Finally, the ideologies that the man should be the breadwinner and that outsiders should not intervene in family affairs both worsen the problem of abuse within the family.

## Key Terms

**Cohabitation**
**Divorce Rate**
**Family**
**Heterogamy**
**Homogamy**
**Maladjustment**
**Nuclear Family**
**Primary Group**
**Stepfamily**

## Study Questions

1. What are some alternative forms of the family?
2. In what ways is the American family changing?
3. What are the important functions of the modern family?
4. What are the various kinds of problems that afflict families, and how extensive are those problems?

5. How does family disruption affect the physical and emotional well-being of people?
6. How do family problems relate to deviant behavior and maladjustment in families?
7. What norms contribute to family problems?
8. Explain the role problems that can result in both structural and supportive difficulties in families.
9. What are the relationships between the stratification system and family problems?
10. Name and explain the kinds of attitudes, values, and ideologies that contribute to family problems.
11. What are the therapeutic and preventive measures that can address family problems in the United States?

## Internet Resources/Exercises

1. Explore some of the ideas in this chapter on the following sites:

**www.nationalmarriageproject.org** Resources and reports from the National Marriage Project at the University of Virginia.

**http://www.childtrends.org** Site offering publications and links to information that helps strengthen families and increases the well-being of children.

**http://www.divorcemag.com** News, information, and links about all aspects of divorce.

2. Most of the information in this chapter involves what can go wrong in a family. Search the Internet for information about healthy family life. What are the characteristics and qualities of such families? Design a one-day "healthy family" seminar based on your findings.

3. Choose one or more nations other than the United States and find information about divorce laws and/or divorce statistics. How do your findings compare with information in this chapter on divorce in the United States? How would you explain any differences and similarities between nations?

## For Further Reading

Booth, Alan, and Ann C. Crouter, eds. *Just Living Together: Implications of Cohabitation on Families, Children, and Social Policy.* Mahwah, NJ: Lawrence Erlbaum Associates, 2002. An exploration, by a variety of experts, of individual, familial, and social causes and consequences of cohabitation.

Casper, Lynne M., and Suzanne M. Bianchi. *Continuity and Change in the American Family.* Thousand Oaks, CA: Sage, 2002. An examination of various facets of change and continuity in family life in America in the last half of the 20th century, including cohabitation, work, parenting, and single-mother families.

DePaulo, Bella. *Single Parents and Their Children.* CreateSpace Independent Publishing Platform. 2015. Although this is a self-published book, the author is an academic psychologist who brings together a number of her own and others' writings, based on research and experience, of life in the single-parent family.

Florsheim, Paul, and David Moore. *Lost and Found: Young Fathers in the Age of Unwed Parenthood.* New York: Oxford University Press, 2020. Focuses on a group of young fathers, listening to their stories, and putting the results together to understand fatherhood in our nation today.

Hertz, Rosanna. *Single by Choice: How Women Are Choosing Parenthood Without Marriage and Creating the New American Family.* New York: Oxford University Press, 2006. Based on in-depth interviews with 65 middle-class, single women who chose to be single mothers, Hertz explores different ways to become a mother and how the women balance parenthood with work.

Lauer, Robert H., and Jeanette C. Lauer. *'Til Death Do Us Part: How Couples Stay Together.* New York: Haworth Press, 1986. A study of 362 couples who have been married 15 years or more, showing how they keep their marriage intact. Compares happy, long-term marriages to those in which one or both partners are unhappy.

Wolfinger, Nicholas H. *Understanding the Divorce Cycle: The Children of Divorce in Their Own Marriages.* New York: Cambridge University Press, 2005. Explores the ways in which the divorce of one's parents affects every facet of one's intimate relationships; includes a discussion about the effects of no-fault divorce laws.

## References

Afifi, T. O., et al. 2008. "Population attributable fractions of psychiatric disorders and suicide ideation and attempts associated with adverse childhood experiences." *American Journal of Public Health* 98:946–52.

Albelda, R., S. Himmelweit, and J. Humphries. 2004. "The dilemmas of lone motherhood." *Feminist Economics* 10:1-7.

Amato, P. R., and D. D. DeBoer. 2001. "The transmission of marital instability across generations." *Journal of Marriage and Family* 63:1038-51.

Amato, P. R., and J. E. Cheadle. 2008. "Parental divorce, marital conflict and children's behavior problems." *Social Forces* 86:1139-61.

Amato, P. R., and J. M. Sobolewski. 2001. "The effects of divorce and marital discord on adult children's psychological well-being." *American Sociological Review* 66:900-21.

Amato, P. R., and S. J. Rogers. 1997. "A longitudinal study of marital problems and subsequent divorce." *Journal of Marriage and the Family* 59 (August):612-24.

Apsler, R., M. R. Cummins, and S. Carl. 2003. "Perceptions of the police by female victims of domestic partner violence." *Violence against Women* 9:1318-35.

Atkinson, M. P., T. N. Greenstein, and M. M. Lang. 2005. "For women, breadwinning can be dangerous." *Journal of Marriage and Family* 67:1137-48.

AVVO Staff. 2015. "Marriage and divorce statistics." AVVO website.

Barnett, O. W. 2001. "Why battered women do not leave." *Trauma, Violence, and Abuse* 2:3-35.

Barton, P. E. 2006. "The dropout problem." *Educational Leadership* 63:14-18.

Baughman, R., D. DiNardi, and D. Holtz-Eakin. 2003. "Productivity and wage effects of 'family-friendly' fringe benefits." *International Journal of Manpower* 24:247-59.

Berger, L. M. 2005. "Income, family characteristics, and physical violence toward children." *Child Abuse and Neglect* 29:107-33.

Billari, F. C., and A. C. Liefbroer. 2016. "Why still marry?" *The British Journal of Sociology*. Published online.

Billingham, R., and T. Abrahams. 1998. "Parental divorce, body dissatisfaction, and physical attractiveness ratings of self and others among college women." *College Student Journal* 32 (March):148-52.

Bing, N. M., W. M. Nelson, and K. L. Wesolowski. 2009. "Comparing the effects of amount of conflict on children's adjustment following parental divorce." *Journal of Divorce & Remarriage* 50:159-71.

Bjarnason, T., et al. 2003. "Alcohol culture, family structure, and adolescent alcohol use." *Journal of Studies on Alcohol* 64:200-208.

Bookwala, J., J. Sobin, and B. Zdaniuk. 2005. "Gender and aggression in marital relationships." *Sex Roles* 52:797-806.

Borjas, G. J. 2011. "Poverty and program participation among immigrant children." *Future of Children* 21:247-66.

Boy, A., and A. Kulczycki. 2008. "What we know about intimate partner violence in the Middle East and North Africa." *Violence against Women* 14:53-70.

Bramlett, M. D., and S. J. Blumberg. 2007. "Family structure and children's physical and mental health." *Health Affairs* 26:549-58.

Bramlett, M. D., and W. D. Mosher. 2001. "First marriage dissolution, divorce, and remarriage: United States." *Advance Data,* May 31. Washington, DC: Department of Health and Human Services.

Bramlett, M. D., and W. D. Mosher. 2002. *Cohabitation, Marriage, Divorce, and Remarriage in the United States.* Washington, DC: Government Printing Office.

Brenan, M. 2019. "Americans largely satisfied with 10 personal life aspects." Gallup Poll website.

Brown, S. I. 2004. "Family structure and child well-being." *Journal of Marriage and Family* 66:351-67.

Brummelman, E., and C. Sedikides. 2020. "Raising children with high self-esteem." *Child Development Perspectives* 14:83-89.

Carlson, B. E. 1990. "Adolescent observers of marital violence." *Journal of Family Violence* 5:285-99.

Carrasco, M. A., et al. 2015. "Intraparental inconsistency." *Family Relations* 64:621-34.

Cast, A. D., D. Schweingruber, and N. Berns. 2006. "Childhood physical punishment and problem solving in marriage." *Journal of Interpersonal Violence* 21:244-61.

Celbis, O., et al. 2020. "Evaluation of incest cases." *Journal of Child Sexual Abuse* 29:79-89.

Center for Marriage and Families. 2005. "Family structure and children's educational outcomes." Institute for American Values website.

Charmi, J. 2021. "320 million children in single-parent families." InterPress Service News Agency website.

Chatav, Y., and M. A. Whisman. 2007. "Marital dissolution and psychiatric disorders." *Journal of Divorce & Remarriage* 47:1-13.

Cole, C. V. 1995. "Sexual abuse of middle school students." *School Counselor* 42 (January):239-45.

Colen, F., and M. G. Pereira. 2019. "Psychological morbidity, social intimacy, physical symptomatology, and lifestyle in adult children of divorced parents." *Journal of Divorce and Remarriage* 60:183–93.

Coohey, C. 2004. "Battered mothers who physically abuse their children." *Journal of Interpersonal Violence* 19:943–52.

Crusto, C. A., et al. 2010. "Posttraumatic stress among young urban children exposed to family violence and other potentially traumatic events." *Journal of Traumatic Stress* 23:716–24.

Cunradi, C. B., R. Caetano, and J. Schafer. 2002. "Religious affiliation, denominational homogamy, and intimate partner violence among U.S. couples." *Journal for the Scientific Study of Religion* 41:139–51.

Dietz, P. 2020. "Denial and minimization among sex offenders." *Behavioral Sciences and the Law* 38:571–85.

Doodson, L. J., and A. P. C. Davies. 2014. "Different challenges, different well-being." *Journal of Divorce & Remarriage* 55:49–63.

Dunifon, R. E., and L. Kowaleski-Jones. 2002. "Who's in the house?" *Child Development* 73:1249–64.

Durose, M. R., et al. 2005. *Family Violence Statistics.* Washington, DC: Government Printing Office.

Eickmeyer, K., and W. D. Manning. 2018. "Serial cohabitation in young adulthood." *Journal of Marriage and Family* 80:826–40.

Ellis, B. J., et al. 2003. "Does father absence place daughters at special risk for early sexual activity and teenage pregnancy?" *Child Development* 74:801–21.

Ellison, C. G., J. P. Bartkowski, and K. L. Anderson. 1999. "Are there religious variations in domestic violence?" *Journal of Family Issues* 20 (January):87–113.

Fagan, A. A. 2003. "Short- and long-term effects of adolescent violent victimization experienced within the family and community." *Violence and Victims* 18:445–59.

Felson, R. B., and S. F. Messner. 2000. "The control motive in intimate partner violence." *Social Psychology Quarterly* 63:86–94.

Ferraro, K. J. 1989. "Policing woman battering." *Social Problems* 36 (February):61–74.

Ferraro, K., and J. M. Johnson. 1983. "How women experience battering: The process of victimization." *Social Problems* 30 (3):325–39.

Ferrer, A., and Pan, Y. 2020. "Divorce, remarriage and child cognitive outcomes." *Journal of Divorce & Remarriage* 61:636–62.

Fitzgerald, M. M., et al. 2005. "Perceptions of parenting versus parent-child interactions among incest survivors." *Child Abuse and Neglect* 29:661–81.

Fleury, R. E., C. M. Sullivan, D. I. Bybee, and W. S. Davidson II. 1998. "'Why don't they just call the cops?' Reasons for differential police contact among women with abusive partners." *Violence and Victims* 13 (Winter):333–46.

Flisher, A. J., et al. 1997. "Psychosocial characteristics of physically abused children and adolescents." *Journal of the American Academy of Child and Adolescent Psychiatry* 36 (1):123–31.

Forum on Child and Family Statistics. 2020. *America's Children in Brief: Key National Indicators of Well-Being, 2020.* Washington, DC: Government Printing Office.

Frisco, M. L., and K. Williams. 2003. "Perceived housework equity, marital happiness, and divorce in dual-earner households." *Journal of Family Issues* 24:51–73.

Gage, A. J. 2016. "Exposure to spousal violence in the family, attitudes and dating violence perpetration among high school students in Port-au-Prince." *Journal of Interpersonal Violence* 31:2445–74.

Gelles, R. J., and M. A. Straus. 1988. *Intimate Violence.* New York: Simon and Schuster.

Gohm, C. L., S. Oishi, J. Darlington, and E. Diener. 1998. "Culture, parental conflict, parental marital status, and the subjective well-being of young adults." *Journal of Marriage and the Family* 60 (May):319–34.

Gray, M., and J. Tudball. 2003. "Family-friendly work practices." *Journal of Industrial Relations* 45:269–91.

Greenwood, J. L. 2012. "Parent-child relationships in the context of mid- to late-life parental divorce." *Journal of Divorce & Remarriage* 53:1–17.

Guinart, M., and M. Grau. 2014. "Qualitative analysis of the short-term and long-term impact of family breakdown on children." *Journal of Divorce & Remarriage* 55:408–22.

Guzzo, K. B., and S. R. Hayford. 2014. "Fertility and the stability of co-habiting unions." *Journal of Family Issues* 35:547–76.

Hamby, S., D. Finkelhor, H. Turner, and R. Ormrod. 2011. "Children's exposure to intimate partner violence and other family violence." *Juvenile Justice Bulletin,* October.

Heaton, R. B. 2002. "Factors contributing to increasing marital instability in the United States." *Journal of Family Issues* 23:392–409.

Hernandez, D. J. 2011. "Double jeopardy: How third-grade reading skills and poverty influence high school graduation." Research report, Annie E. Casey Foundation.

Hilton, J. M., and K. Kopera-Frye. 2006. "Loss and depression in cohabiting and noncohabiting custodial single parents." *The Family Journal* 14:28–40.

Hogendoorn, B., T. Leopold, and T. Bol. 2020 "Divorce and diverging poverty rates." *Journal of Marriage and Family* 82:1089–1109.

Holmes, E. K., H. A. Jones-Sanpei, and R. D. Day. 2009. "Adolescent outcome measures in the NLSY97 family process data set." *Marriage & Family Review* 45:374–91.

Hussey, J. M., J. J. Chang, and J. B. Kotch. 2006. "Child maltreatment in the United States." *Pediatrics* 118:933–42.

Isaacs, J. B. 2012. "Starting school at a disadvantage." Research report, Center on Children and Families at Brookings.

Jarvis, K. L., E. E. Gordon, and R. W. Novaco. 2005. "Psychological distress of children and mothers in domestic violence emergency shelters." *Journal of Family Violence* 20:389–402.

Jensen, T. M., et al. 2018. "Stepfamily relationship quality and children's internalizing and externalizing problems." *Family Process* 57:477–95.

Johnson, I. M. 2007. "Victims' perceptions of police response to domestic violence incidents." *Journal of Criminal Justice* 35:498–510.

Kalmijn, M., and P. J. De Graaf. 2012. "Life course changes of children and well-being of parents." *Journal of Marriage and Family* 74:269–80.

Khawaja, M., and R. R. Habib. 2007. "Husbands' involvement in housework and women's psychosocial health." *American Journal of Public Health* 97:860–66.

Kim, H. S. 2011. "Consequences of parental divorce for child development." *American Sociological Review* 76:487–511.

Kim, H., and H. Kim. 2005. "Incestuous experience among Korean adolescents." *Public Health Nursing* 22:472–82.

Kim, J., and K. A. Gray. 2008. "Leave or stay? Battered women's decision after intimate partner violence." *Journal of Interpersonal Violence* 23:1465–82.

Kim, J., S. Park, and C. R. Emery. 2009. "The incidence and impact of family violence on mental health among South Korean women." *Journal of Family Violence* 24:193–202.

Kline, M., J. R. Johnston, and J. M. Tschann. 1991. "The long shadow of marital conflict: A model of children's post-divorce adjustment." *Journal of Marriage and the Family* 53 (February):297–309.

Koerner, S. S., M. Korn, R. P. Dennison, and S. Witthoft. 2011. "Future money-related worries among adolescents after divorce." *Journal of Adolescent Research* 26:299–317.

Kotch, J. B., et al. 2008. "Importance of early neglect for childhood aggression." *Pediatrics* 121:725–31.

Kruttschnitt, C., J. D. McLeod, and M. Dornfeld. 1994. "The economic environment of child abuse." *Social Problems* 41 (May):299–315.

Kuperberg, A. 2014. "Age at coresidence, premarital cohabitation, and marriage dissolution." *Journal of Marriage and Family* 76:352–69.

Kuperberg, A. 2019. "Premarital cohabitation and direct marriage in the United States." *Marriage & Family Review* 55:447–75.

Laffaye, C., C. Kennedy, and M. B. Stein. 2003. "Posttraumatic stress disorder and health-related quality of life in female victims of intimate partner violence." *Violence and Victims* 18:227–38.

Lancer, D. 2017. "The truth about abusers, abuse, and what to do." *Psychology Today,* June.

Larsen, C. D., J. G. Sandberg, J. M. Harper, and R. Bean. 2011. "The effects of childhood abuse on relationship quality." *Family Relations* 60:435–45.

Lauer, R. H., and J. C. Lauer. 1983. *The Spirit and the Flesh: Sex in Utopian Communities.* Netuchen, NJ: Scarecrow.

——. 1986. *'Til Death Do Us Part: How Couples Stay Together.* New York: Haworth.

——. 1999. *Becoming Family: How to Build a Stepfamily That Really Works.* Minneapolis, MN: Augsburg.

——. 2022. *Marriage and Family: The Quest for Intimacy.* 10th ed. New York: McGraw Hill.

Lorenz, F. O., K. A. Wickrama, R. D. Conger, and G. H. Elder Jr. 2006. "The short-term and decade-long effects of divorce on women's midlife health." *Journal of Health and Social Behavior* 47:111–25.

Loxton, D., M. Schofield, and R. Hussain. 2006. "Psychological health in midlife among women who have ever lived with a violent partner or spouse." *Journal of Interpersonal Violence* 21:1092–1107.

Magnuson, K., and L. M. Berger. 2009. "Family structure states and transitions." *Journal of Marriage and Family* 71:575–91.

Major, V. S., K. J. Klein, and M. G. Ehrhart. 2002. "Work time, work interference with family, and psychological distress." *Journal of Applied Psychology* 87:427-36.

Manning, W. D., and J. A. Cohen. 2012. "Premarital cohabitation and marital dissolution: An examination of recent marriages." *Journal of Marriage and Family* 74:377-87.

Marano, H. E. 1996. "Why they stay." *Psychology Today,* May-June, pp. 57-78.

Masarik, A. S., et al. 2016. "Couple resilience to economic pressure over time and across generations." *Journal of Marriage and Family* 78:326-45.

McDonald, R., et al. 2006. "Estimating the number of American children living in partner-violent families." *Journal of Family Psychology* 20:137-42.

McFarlane, J., P. Willson, A. Malecha, and D. Lemmey. 2000. "Intimate partner violence." *Journal of Interpersonal Violence* 15 (February):158-69.

Melançon, C., and M. Gagné. 2011. "Father's and mother's psychological violence and adolescent behavioral adjustment." *Journal of Interpersonal Violence* 26:991-1011.

Merton, R. K. 1957. *Social Theory and Social Structure.* New York: Free Press.

Morgan, R. E., and J. L. Truman. 2020. "Criminal victimization, 2019." Bureau of Justice Statistics website.

Mullins, L. C., K. P. Brackett, D. W. Bogle, and D. Pruett. 2004. "The impact of religious homogeneity on the rate of divorce in the United States." *Sociological Inquiry* 74:338-54.

Murdaugh, C., S. Hunt, R. Sowell, and I. Santana. 2004. "Domestic violence in Hispanics in the southeastern United States." *Journal of Family Violence* 19:107-15.

National Institute of Justice. 1996. "The cycle of violence revisited." *Research Preview,* February.

——. 2014. "From juvenile delinquency to young adult offending." NIJ report.

Nguyen, T. P., B. R. Karney, and T. N. Bradbury. 2017. "Childhood abuse and later marital outcomes." *Journal of Family Psychology* 31:82-92.

O'Keefe, M. 1994. "Linking marital violence, mother-child/ father-child aggression, and child behavior problems." *Journal of Family Violence* 9 (March):63-78.

Pagani, L., et al. 2009. "Risk factor models for adolescent verbal and physical aggression toward fathers." *Journal of Family Violence* 24:173-82.

Panuzio, J., et al. 2007. "Relationship abuse and victims' posttraumatic stress disorder symptoms." *Journal of Family Violence* 22:177-85.

Pasley, K., J. Kerpelman, and D. E. Guilbert. 2001. "Gendered conflict, identity disruption, and marital instability." *Journal of Social and Personal Relationships* 18:5-27.

Peretti, P. O., and A. di Vitorrio. 1993. "Effect of loss of father through divorce on personality of the preschool child." *Social Behavior and Personality* 21:33-38.

Perina, K. 2002. "Covenant marriage: A new marital contract." *Psychology Today,* March-April, p. 18.

Pinheiro, P. S. 2006. *World Report on Violence against Children*. Geneva, Switzerland: United Nations.

Remery, C., A. van Doorne-Huiskes, and J. Schippers. 2003. "Family-friendly policies in the Netherlands." *Personnel Review* 32:456-73.

Rinfret-Raynor, M., A. Riou, S. Cantin, C. Drouin, and M. Dube. 2004. "A survey on violence against female partners in Quebec, Canada." *Violence against Women* 10:709-28.

Rogers, A. A., B. Willoughby, and L. J. Nelson. 2016. "Young adults' perceived purposes of emerging adulthood." *The Journal of Psychology* 150:485-501.

Rosenfeld, M. J., and K. Roesler. 2019. "Cohabitation experience and cohabitation's association with marital dissolution." *Journal of Marriage and Family* 81:42-58.

Ryan, J. P., B. A. Jacob, M. Gross, B. E. Perron, A. Moore, and S. Ferguson. 2018. "Early exposure to child maltreatment and academic outcomes." *Child Maltreatment* 23:365-75.

Schneller, D. P., and J. A. Arditti. 2004. "After the breakup: Interpreting divorcer and rethinking intimacy." *Journal of Divorce & Remarriage* 42:1-37.

Schramm, D. G., et al. 2013. "Economic costs and policy implications associated with divorce." *Journal of Divorce & Remarriage* 54:1-24.

Shackelford, T. K., and J. Mouzos. 2005. "Partner killing by men in cohabiting and marital relationships." *Journal of Interpersonal Violence* 20:1310-24.

Simon, T., et al. 2001. "Attitudinal acceptance of intimate partner violence among U.S. adults." *Violence and Victims* 16:115-26.

Siordia, C. 2014. "Married once, twice, and three or more times." *Journal of Divorce & Remarriage* 55:206-15.

Skinner, K. B., S. J. Bahr, D. R. Crane, and V. R. A. Call. 2002. "Cohabitation, marriage, and remarriage." *Journal of Family Issues* 23:74–90.

Smith, S. G., et al. 2018. "The national intimate partner and sexual violence survey." Centers for Disease Control and Prevention website.

Snyder, H. N., and M. Sickmund. 1999. *Juvenile Offenders and Victims: 1999 National Report*. Washington, DC: Office of Juvenile Justice and Delinquency Prevention.

Soria, K. M., and S. Linder. 2014. "Parental divorce and first-year college students' persistence and academic achievement." *Journal of Divorce & Remarriage* 55:103–16.

South, S. J. 2001. "Time-dependent effects of wives' employment on marital dissolution." *American Sociological Review* 66:226–45.

Stack, S., and J. Scourfield. 2015. "Recency of divorce, depression, and suicide risk." *Journal of Family Issues* 36:695–715.

Stafford, L. 2016. "Marital sanctity, relationship maintenance, and marital quality." *Journal of Family Issues* 37:119–31.

Stanley, S. M., S. W. Whitton, and H. J. Markham. 2004. "Maybe I do: Interpersonal commitment and premarital or nonmarital cohabitation." *Journal of Family Issues* 25:496–519.

Stanton, A. H., and M. S. Schwartz. 1961. "The mental hospital and the patient." In *Complex Organizations*, ed. A. Etzioni, pp. 234–42. New York: Holt, Rinehart and Winston.

Stevenson, L. 2016. "Child to parent abuse." Community Care website.

Stith, S. M., et al. 2000. "The intergenerational transmission of spouse abuse." *Journal of Marriage and Family* 62:640–54.

Stoll, B. M., G. L. Arriaut, D. K. Fromme, and J. A. Felker-Thayer. 2005. "Adolescents in stepfamilies." *Journal of Divorce & Remarriage* 44:177–89.

Straus, H. E., et al. 2020. "Assessment of intimate partner violence abuse ratings by recently abused and never abused women." *BMC Women's Health* 20. Published online.

Stroebel, S. S., et al. 2012. "Father-daughter incest." *Journal of Child Sexual Abuse* 21:176–99.

Strohschein, L. 2005. "Parental divorce and child mental health trajectories." *Journal of Marriage and Family* 67:1286–1300.

Strom, I. F., et al. 2021. "Trajectories of alcohol use and alcohol intoxication in young adults exposed to childhood violence and later problematic drinking behavior." *Journal of Family Violence* 36:223–33.

Sun, Y., and Y. Li. 2011. "Effects of family structure type and stability on children's academic performance trajectories." *Journal of Marriage and Family* 73:541–56.

Taft, C. T., et al. 2006. "Examining the correlates of psychological aggression among a community sample of couples." *Journal of Family Psychology* 20:581–88.

Teicher, M. H. 2002. "Scars that won't heal: The neurobiology of child abuse." *Scientific American*, March, pp. 68–75.

Thuen, F., et al. 2015. "Growing up with one or both parents." *Journal of Divorce & Remarriage* 56:451–74.

Treas, J., and D. Giesen. 2000. "Sexual infidelity among married and cohabiting Americans." *Journal of Marriage and the Family* 62 (February):48–60.

Treas, J., T. van der Lippe, and T. C. Tai. 2011. "The happy homemaker? Married women's well-being in cross-national perspective." *Social Forces* 90:111–32.

Tucker, J., and C. Lowell. 2015. "National snapshot: Poverty among women & families." National Women's Law Center website.

Turner, H. A., and K. Kopiec. 2006. "Exposure to interparental conflict and psychological disorder among young adults." *Journal of Family Issues* 27:131–58.

Ulloa, E. C., and J. F. Hammett. 2015. "Temporal changes in intimate partner violence and relationship satisfaction." *Journal of Family Violence* 30:1093–1102.

United Nations. 2015. "The world's women." United Nations website.

Usdansky, M. L. 2009. "A weak embrace: Popular and scholarly depictions of single-parent families, 1900–1998." *Journal of Marriage and Family* 71:209–25.

Vaaler, C. E., C. G. Ellison, and D. A. Powers. 2009. "Religious influences on the risk of marital dissolution." *Journal of Marriage and Family* 71:917–34.

Vandervalk, I., E. Spruijt, M. De Goede, W. Meeus, and C. Maas. 2004. "Marital status, marital process, and parental resources in predicting adolescents' emotional adjustment." *Journal of Family Issues* 25:291–317.

Wade, T. J., and D. J. Pevalin. 2004. "Marital transitions and mental health." *Journal of Health and Social Behavior* 45:155–70.

Walters, A. S. 2019. "Why we still spank our children in the U.S." *The Brown University Child and Adolescent Behavior Letter* 35:8.

Wauterickx, N., A. Gouwy, and P. Bracke. 2006. "Parental divorce and depression." *Journal of Divorce & Remarriage* 45:43–68.

Weiser, D. A., et al. 2015. "Family background and propensity to engage in infidelity." *Journal of Family Issues*. Published online.

Wen, M. 2008. "Family structure and children's health and behavior." *Journal of Family Issues* 29:1492–1519.

Whisman, M. A. 2006. "Childhood trauma and marital outcomes in adulthood." *Personal Relationships* 13:375.

Whitehead, B. D., and D. Popenoe. 2001. *The State of Our Unions: The Social Health of Marriage in America.* National Marriage Project website.

Whitton, S. W., G. K. Rhoades, S. M. Stanley, and H. J. Markman. 2008. "Effects of parental divorce on marital commitment and confidence." *Journal of Family Psychology* 22:789–93.

Williams, D. T., J. E. Cheadle, and B. J. Goosby. 2015. "Hard times and heart break." *Journal of Family Issues* 36:924–50.

Williams, K., and A. Dunne-Bryant. 2006. "Divorce and adult psychological well-being." *Journal of Marriage and Family* 68:1178–96.

Wolfinger, N. H. 2005. *Understanding the Divorce Cycle: The Children of Divorce in Their Own Marriages.* New York: Cambridge University Press.

Wolfner, G. D., and R. J. Gelles. 1993. "A profile of violence toward children." *Child Abuse and Neglect* 17 (March):197–212.

Worden, A. P., and B. E. Carlson. 2005. "Attitudes and beliefs about domestic violence." *Journal of Interpersonal Violence* 20:1219–43.

Yip, P. S., and J. Thorburn. 2004. "Marital status and the risk of suicide." *Psychological Reports* 94:401–7.

Yuan, A. S. V. 2016. "Father-child relationships and nonresident fathers' psychological distress." *Journal of Family Issues* 37:603–21.

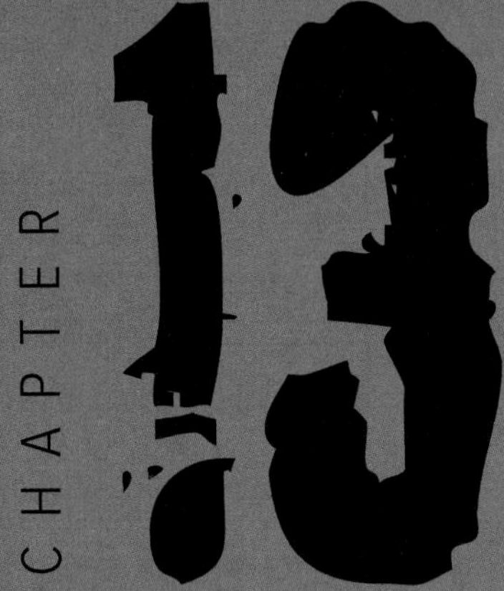

CHAPTER 13

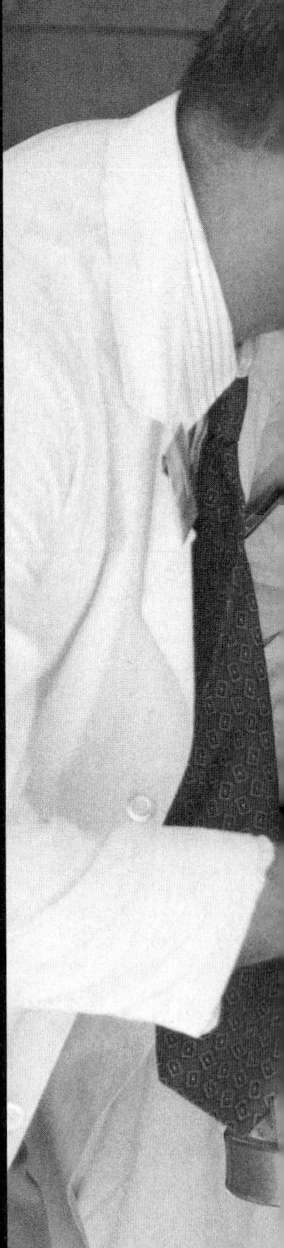

# Health Care and Illness

## Physical and Mental

OBJECTIVES

1. Understand the meaning and extent of physical and mental illness.
2. Know the kinds of undesirable consequences of illness, including suffering, disrupted interpersonal relationships, constraints on personal freedom, and economic costs.
3. Discuss the ways in which Americans receive inadequate health care, including deinstitutionalization.
4. Show how roles and social institutions affect the health care problem.
5. Describe the attitudes, values, and ideologies that contribute to the health care problem.
6. Identify some ways to address America's health care problem.

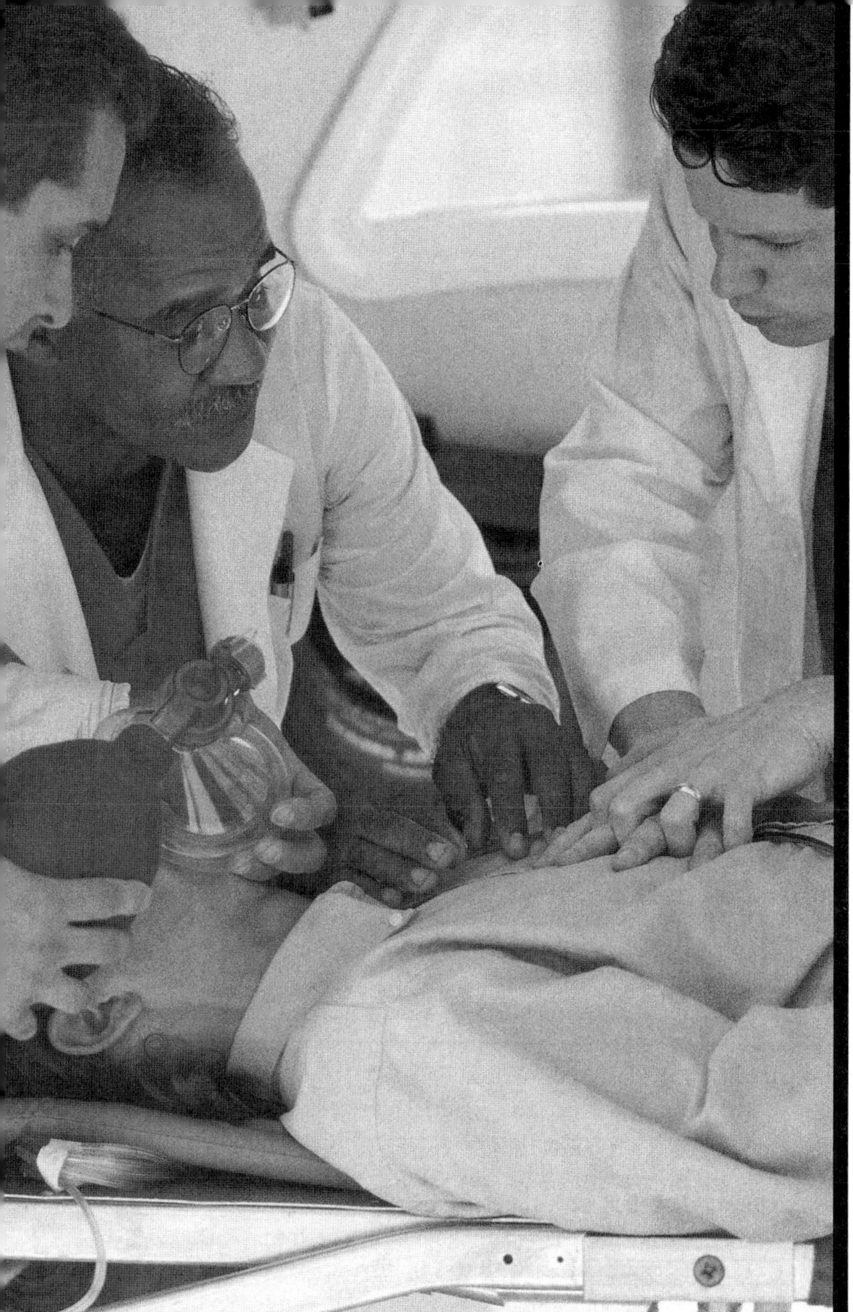
Photodisc Collection/Getty Images

### "If You Want to Live a Long Life"

Tami, in her 40s, has what she calls a "bizarre, cruel disease." She also says the disease may be helping her live a long life: "If you want to live a long life, get a chronic disease and take care of it." Tami's story illustrates both the trauma of chronic illness and the ability of some people to triumph over the trauma and live a reasonably normal life:

*I have lupus. It is intermittent and recurrent, and I know it can destroy my life, my will to live, and my ability to cope. In lupus, your body and soul are enmeshed in a web of pain and desperation. When the symptoms first appeared, people thought I was a hypochondriac. Doctors said nothing was wrong with me. They labeled me a neurotic, and I began to think of myself that way. Friends and family saw me looking well one moment and distressed the next. My internist finally turned me over to a psychiatrist. Nothing helped.*

*Then I got a new physician, and I had the shock of learning that I had a complicated, chronic illness that would alter all my plans and dreams for my life. I was both relieved and in panic. It was a relief to finally identify the problem. It was panic to know what the problem was. I suddenly had to confront the possibility of my own death. A feeling of emptiness spread throughout my body.*

*Before I got sick, I was full of life. Now I was physically, emotionally, and spiritually exhausted. At times, I could barely raise my arms to attend to personal needs. My husband remained optimistic. My daughter was angry. But as time passed, I was forced to make a decision: I had to try to take charge of my life, or waste away into nothing. I began a program of educating myself. Slowly, I got stronger. I went into remission. No one knows if it was the treatment or my changed attitudes or just a natural process.*

*I harbor no false hopes. I know I'm not cured. Sometimes, when the sun is shining I feel sad. I want to go out and bask in it. I want to forget that the sun is my enemy, that it can kill someone with lupus. But I get over the sadness. I can't make the lupus disappear by an act of my will, but I can refuse to let it destroy my spirit. I don't know what the future holds. For now, I just focus my energy on what I can control, and live moment to moment.*

## Introduction

If you were living before 1910, were sick, and randomly chose a doctor, your chances of benefiting from that doctor's ministrations were less than 50 percent. Your chances today are much better, but they vary according to such factors as whether you are physically or mentally ill, live in the city or a rural area, and are poor or well-to-do. The unequal probabilities of all Americans having good health and good health care contradict the *value of equality*. Inequality of care, then, is one reason health care is a social problem.

Another reason health care and illness are social problems is that both physical and mental illness may be induced by social factors. For instance, poverty may force an individual to live in an unhealthy physical environment. Rapid social change may generate anxiety, depression, or other mental disorders.

Adverse effects on health are serious because Americans place a *high value on good health*. Indeed, good health is one of the most important factors in happiness and life satisfaction (Michalos, Zumbo, and Hubley 2000; Van Kessel and Hughes 2018). Yet many Americans are less than fully satisfied with the health care system: In a national poll, 42 percent of Americans cited cost or access as an urgent health problem (Rifkin 2015).

**prevalence**
the number of cases of an illness that exist at any particular time

**incidence**
the number of new cases of an illness that occur during a particular period of time

**epidemiology**
the study of factors that affect the incidence, prevalence, and distribution of illnesses

In this chapter, we examine health care and illness by first drawing the distinction between physical and mental illnesses and then discussing their **prevalence** in American society. (Prevalence is the number of cases of a disease that exist at any particular time; **incidence** is the number of new cases that occur during a particular period of time.) Next, we show how the problem affects the quality of life. Then we consider the **epidemiology** of physical and mental illness–the factors that affect the incidence, prevalence, and distribution of illnesses. Finally, we discuss ways to deal with the problem.

## Nature of the Problem: Health Care and Illness

Are Americans unnecessarily concerned about their health and health care system? After all, we spend more on health care (measured either on a per capita basis or as a proportion of the gross domestic product) than any other industrial nation (Park 2008).

Nevertheless, although there have been considerable improvements in health in the nation, Americans have a higher infant-mortality rate and lower life expectancy than those in many other developed nations (Brill 2013). A survey that compared the United States with 16 other wealthy, developed nations reported that the American system was at, or near, the bottom in life expectancy and in the prevalence and mortality rates for various diseases (Woolf and Aron 2013).

As we examine the nature and extent of physical and mental illness, keep in mind that the two are not really separable (Jacobsen et al. 2002; Whooley 2006; Keyes and Simoes 2012). Physical illness can cause emotional problems. Mental illness can be manifested in physical distress (Ruo et al. 2003). Both physical and mental illness have social causes. However, the methods used to assess the extent of physical and mental illnesses are different and must be discussed separately.

## Physical Illness

Important indicators show that Americans have made significant advances in health matters. For instance, **life expectancy,** the average number of years a person can expect to live, has increased dramatically (Table 13.1). In 1900, life expectancy was less than two-thirds of the present figure. In large part, this increase in life expectancy *reflects reduced infant mortality and lower rates of infectious diseases.* It isn't that the majority of people only lived until their late 40s in the early 1900s. Rather, the large number of infant deaths combined with the high rate of infectious diseases among the middle-aged severely depressed the average length of life. Sanitation, better diet, reduced fertility, and advancing medical knowledge and technology greatly reduced both the prevalence and the seriousness of infectious diseases. Despite the progress, however, physical illness is a major problem. It is even a problem for the young. According to the National Center for Health Statistics (2019), 8.4 percent of children under 18 years of age suffered from asthma, 12 percent had a skin allergy, 6.1 percent had a food allergy, 15.2 percent had a respiratory allergy, and 4.4 percent had three or more ear infections.

**life expectancy**
the average number of years a newborn can expect to live

**TABLE 13.1**
Expectation of Life at Birth, 1900–2020

| Year | Total | Male | Female |
|---|---|---|---|
| 1900 | 47.3 | 46.3 | 48.3 |
| 1910 | 50.0 | 48.4 | 51.8 |
| 1920 | 54.1 | 53.6 | 54.6 |
| 1930 | 59.7 | 58.1 | 61.6 |
| 1940 | 62.9 | 60.8 | 65.2 |
| 1950 | 68.2 | 65.6 | 71.1 |
| 1960 | 69.7 | 66.6 | 73.1 |
| 1970 | 70.9 | 67.1 | 74.8 |
| 1980 | 73.7 | 70.0 | 77.5 |
| 1990 | 75.4 | 72.0 | 78.8 |
| 2000 | 76.8 | 74.1 | 79.3 |
| 2010 | 78.3 | 75.7 | 80.8 |
| 2020 | 80.0 | 77.9 | 82.4 |

SOURCE: *Historical Statistics of the United States, Part I* (Washington, D.C.: Government Printing Office, 1975), p. 55, and U.S. Census Bureau website.

| Cause | Percent of Deaths among | | | | |
|---|---|---|---|---|---|
| | Whites | Hispanics | Blacks | Asians | American Indians |
| Diseases of the heart | 23.3 | 20.0 | 23.3 | 21.3 | 18.1 |
| Malignant neoplasms | 21.4 | 20.6 | 20.8 | 25.1 | 17.0 |
| Cerebrovascular diseases | 5.0 | 5.5 | 5.7 | 7.5 | 3.8 |
| Chronic lower respiratory diseases | 6.4 | 2.8 | 3.3 | 2.8 | 4.9 |
| Accidents | 5.8 | 8.5 | 5.9 | 4.5 | 11.6 |
| Alzheimer's disease | 4.7 | 3.7 | 2.7 | 3.6 | 2.0 |
| Diabetes mellitus | 2.5 | 4.7 | 4.4 | 4.2 | 5.8 |
| Influenza and pneumonia | 2.0 | 2.0 | 1.7 | 3.1 | 2.0 |

SOURCE: Heron 2019.

**TABLE 13.2**
Leading Causes of Death, by Race/Ethnicity

Table 13.2 shows the diseases primarily responsible for death. Cardiovascular diseases, including high blood pressure, coronary heart disease, rheumatic heart disease, and strokes, afflict millions of Americans and have been at the top of the list since the beginning of the 20th century.

*Chronic diseases are the major cause of death in the United States.* A national survey found that 45 percent of American adults are living with one or more chronic conditions (e.g., high blood pressure and diabetes) (Fox and Duggan 2013). Chronic diseases are of long duration and may be classified along a number of dimensions (Rolland 1987). They may be *progressive* (worsening over time) or *constant.* Lung cancer is progressive, whereas stroke is constant. Their onset may be *acute* (short-term) or *gradual* (occurring over an extended period of time). Stroke is acute, whereas lung cancer is gradual. They may be *fatal* (lung cancer), *possibly fatal or life-shortening* (stroke), or *nonfatal* (kidney stones). Although heart disease and cancer are the leading causes of death, the most common chronic conditions are arthritis and sinusitis. Dementia, including Alzheimer's disease, afflicts a third or more of those people who live to age 85 (St. George-Hyslop 2000). Increasing concern has developed over health problems created by obesity, which has become increasingly prevalent since at least 1999. In 2018, 42.4 percent of American adults were obese and 9.2 percent were "severely" obese (Hales et al. 2020).

There is also concern about a *resurgence of infectious diseases.* Infectious disease mortality declined during the first eight decades of the 20th century from 797 deaths per 100,000 to 36 deaths per 100,000 (Armstrong, Conn, and Pinner 1999). However, the rates began to increase in the 1980s and 1990s. Today, infectious diseases are a serious problem throughout the world (see the Global Comparison box in this chapter). Infectious diseases cause more deaths worldwide than heart disease and cancer combined. In addition to increasing rates of such diseases as tuberculosis, at least 30 previously unknown diseases have emerged in recent decades, including Lyme disease (caused by a tick bite), pandemics (AIDS and the COVID-19 discussed next), Legionnaires' disease (caused by air-conditioning systems), toxic shock syndrome (caused by ultra-absorbent tampons), severe acute respiratory syndrome (SARS, caused by a virus), and Zika (also caused by a virus, passed on by the bite of certain mosquitoes or by sexual relations with an infected person). Among the pernicious effects of Zika is brain damage of the fetus in a pregnant woman. What these varied outbreaks mean is that new infections whose source may be obscure and for which there is no known treatment continue to appear. Infections are caused by bacteria, including bacteria that mutate, and by new strains of diseases like tuberculosis that are resistant to antibiotics and other drugs now available (Simon 2006; Barry and Cheung 2009). If we are entering a new era of infectious diseases for which we have no effective antibiotics, it is possible that by 2050 there will be as many as 10 million deaths each year from microbes that are drug resistant (Khatchadourian 2016).

*The health problems you are likely to face vary according to your gender.* In general, women have higher rates of acute diseases (such as respiratory ailments and viral infections), short-term disabilities, and nonfatal chronic diseases. Men have more injuries, more visual and hearing problems, and higher rates of life-threatening chronic diseases such as cancer and the major cardiovascular diseases.

*Health problems also vary according to racial or ethnic origin.* This may be due as much to socioeconomic differences as to racial factors per se (Haywood, Crimmins, Miles, and Yang 2000). Table 13.2 shows some interesting variations between racial and ethnic groups in the causes of death. Note, for instance, that Hispanics and Asian Americans are the only groups for which cancer causes more deaths than does heart disease. Whites are more likely than others to die from chronic lower respiratory diseases, but less likely than the others to die from diabetes. Still, for all groups except American Indians, heart disease and cancer account for close to half of all deaths.

Finally, *health problems vary by age and tend to intensify with age.* Older people are more likely than those in other age groups to define their health as only "fair" or "poor"; 26.6 percent Americans aged 75 and older do so (National Center for Health Statistics 2019). The fact that people are living longer does not mean that they all have a better quality of life.

*Pandemics.* Pandemics are infectious diseases that spread over many countries. In modern times, the most deadly pandemics were/are the Spanish Flu of 1918–1919 that infected a third of the world's population, and killed somewhere between 20 and 50 million people; HIV/AIDS, first reported in 1981, that has infected more than 65 million and killed more than 30 million people; and COVID-19, that, as of February 2021, has infected 104 million people worldwide, including 26.5 million Americans, and killed 2.3 million people, including 448,000 Americans. We will discuss AIDS and COVID-19, which are ongoing, to understand the seriousness of pandemics on people's well-being.

**AIDS**
acquired immune deficiency syndrome, a disease in which a viral infection causes the immune system to stop functioning, inevitably resulting in death

*AIDS.* **AIDS** is caused by a virus (HIV) that attacks certain white blood cells, eventually *causing the individual's immune system to stop functioning.* The individual then falls prey to one infection after another. Even normally mild diseases can prove fatal. Many AIDS patients develop rare cancers or suffer serious brain damage.

*There is no cure for AIDS.* Drugs can prolong the lives of some AIDS victims, but each infection takes its toll, and the immune system continues to collapse. In the advanced stages of HIV infection, 15 to 20 percent of patients develop a type of dementia that involves slow mental functioning (National Institute of Neurological Disorders and Stroke 2019). Eventually, the individual succumbs and dies.

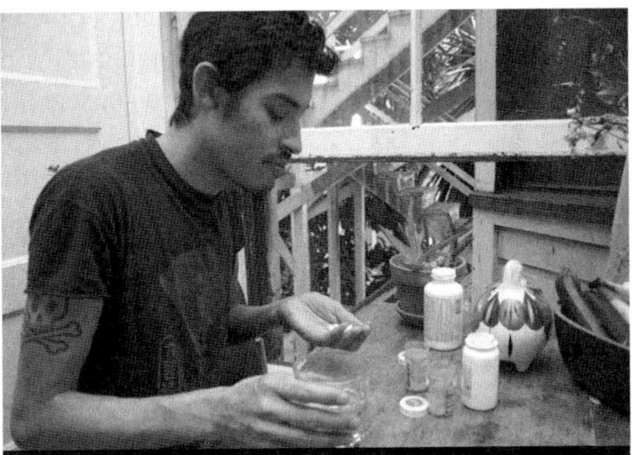

In spite of the "cocktail" of drugs available to treat AIDS patients, the disease continues to have a devasting impact on society.
Christopher Kerrigan/McGraw Hill

How does AIDS spread? The two primary ways are through sex (oral, anal, or vaginal) with someone infected with the AIDS virus and by sharing drug needles and syringes with an infected person. Some people were infected through blood transfusions before blood was tested for the virus. Infected mothers can transmit the disease to their babies before or during birth or while breast feeding. Primarily, then, the *virus is spread through blood or semen.*

## THE WORLDWIDE CHALLENGE OF INFECTIOUS DISEASES

Most research money in the United States is devoted to the study of chronic diseases, the primary cause of death for Americans. In many of the developing nations, particularly in Africa, infectious diseases are more prevalent and far more likely to be the cause of death. Worldwide, about 11 million people a year die from infectious disease (Figure 13.1). Some of these diseases are relatively rare in the United States and other Western nations. Many, not shown in the figure because they afflict fewer numbers (such as tropical diseases), are unknown in the United States. Nevertheless, the developed nations are vulnerable to these diseases because of such things as international travel and bioterrorism (Becker, Hu, and Biller-Andorno 2006).

Both new and reemerging infectious diseases afflict both the developed and the developing nations (Peleman 2004). Their spread is rapid because of such factors as pathogens that are resistant to antibiotics and disease-carrying insects that are resistant to insecticides.

The problems of dealing with these diseases are illustrated by efforts to stop malaria in Africa. For a number of years, mosquito-killing insecticide reduced the number of deaths from malaria. But the insects could not be effectively controlled in the long run, and the incidence of malaria increased again in the 1990s. As Figure 13.1 shows, malaria once again is a serious health problem, causing about a million deaths a year. Children account for a majority of the deaths.

An increasingly more deadly infection worldwide is tuberculosis (Weber 2016). Scientists estimate that a third of the world's population is infected with tubercle bacilli, and that there are 8 to 10 million new cases of tuberculosis each year. The great majority of the new cases and the deaths occur in the developing nations. Tuberculosis is difficult to treat because bacterial mutations make it resistant to any single drug, and drugs that are effective at one point in time eventually become ineffective as the bacilli become resistant.

Although the U.S. death rate from tuberculosis is now quite low, the disease presents a challenge to Americans as well as to other nations because of the new strains that are resistant to formerly effective drugs. Tuberculosis

In the United States, the number of new AIDS cases peaked in the early 1990s, then declined. More than a million Americans have been diagnosed with HIV, and tens of thousands of new cases are diagnosed each year. In 2017, there were 38,281 new cases (National Center for Health Statistics 2019). Homosexual activity is the most common way the disease is contracted. Thus, 81 percent of new infections in 2017 were men.

Some people believe that the concern over AIDS is overdrawn. Certainly, it seems an exaggeration to say that AIDS is an *epidemic.* The incidence is low compared to other diseases. Death rates are down. Moreover, there are ways to minimize the risks. Health experts advise the use of condoms as one of the best preventive measures (condoms are not foolproof, however). Others argue that the disease can be eliminated only if people change their sexual and drug-use behavior. Unfortunately, too many people ignore the preventive measures. People continue to share drug needles and to have unprotected sex (in some cases, even those who know they are HIV positive) (Semple, Patterson, and Grant 2002; Osmond, Pollack, Paul, and Catania 2007). It is likely that AIDS will continue to be a matter of concern for the foreseeable future.

*COVID-19.* In contrast to AIDS, COVID-19 infections had continued to increase by early 2021. COVID-19 is a highly infectious and dangerous respiratory disease (Lewis 2020). It spreads mainly from person to person among people in close contact (within about 6 feet). The virus spreads by respiratory droplets that are released when someone who carries the virus coughs, sneezes, breathes, sings, or talks.

is also more likely to develop in people who are infected with HIV (the virus that causes AIDS). As a result, tuberculosis could once again become a leading cause of death in the world (as it was in the early years of the 20th century). In any case, it is clear that, looking at the world as a whole, infectious diseases are still a major (and increasingly serious) health problem.

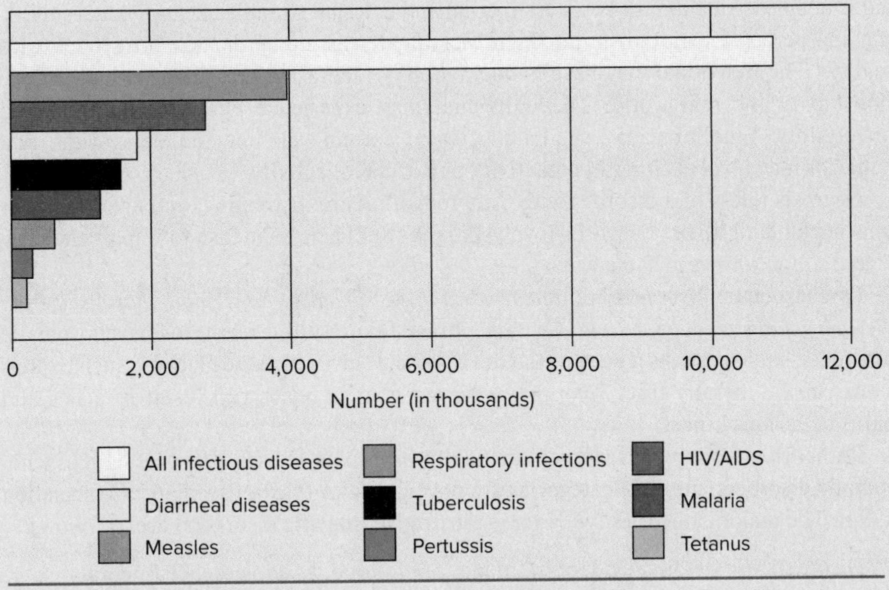


**FIGURE 13.1** Worldwide Deaths, by Selected Infectious Diseases.
Source: World Health Organization website 2007.

An important way to contain the virus is for people to wear masks when they are in public, avoid crowds, and wash hands frequently. Unfortunately, the Trump administration regularly downplayed the seriousness of the pandemic and wearing masks became a political issue—to refuse to wear one was a sign of loyalty to, and belief in, the president, while wearing one was a sign of trust in the scientists who were trying to contain the virus.

As we shall discuss later in this chapter, COVID-19 has taken a heavy toll on the economy and on Americans' emotional well-being. As of early 2021, vaccines had been developed but vaccinations were slowly administered.

And the course of the disease was still uncertain.

## Mental Illness

*Types of Mental Illness.* Some sociologists prefer the term "mental disorder" to mental illness. "Illness" suggests to them a medical model, a problem deeply rooted in an individual that may also have an organic basis. "Disorder" suggests to them a problem that is more social in its origin and resolution. We believe that both perspectives are valid in part. A particular individual's problem may be a biologically based illness, or it may be behavior that results from the actions and reactions of others (see the discussion of labeling at the end of this chapter). Or it may be a combination of both. Thus, we use the terms "mental illness" and "mental disorder" interchangeably to avoid any simplistic assumptions about the problems.

Before 1980, mental disorders were separated into three broad categories: psychoses, neuroses, and psychosomatic disorders. This breakdown is still a useful way to get a general sense of the kinds of disorders that afflict people. In a **psychosis,** the individual is unable to distinguish between internal and external stimuli. The individual's thinking and perceptions are disordered. In everyday terms, he or she has "lost touch with reality." The individual may have hallucinations or fantasize in a way that has no relationship to the real world. The individual may experience chronic perplexity and uncertainty. Emotions may vacillate between extreme elation and depression, and behavior may involve either hyperactivity or extreme inactivity.

**psychosis**
a disorder in which the individual fails to distinguish between internal and external stimuli

**Neurosis** refers to a disorder with symptoms that are distressing, and are defined as unacceptable or alien. Neuroses involve anxiety sufficiently intense to impair the individual's functioning in some way.

**neurosis**
a mental disorder involving anxiety that impairs functioning

**Psychosomatic disorders** are *impairments in physiological functioning that result from the individual's emotional state.* Certain phrases express the reality of psychosomatic disorders, such as he "is a pain in the neck" or she "gives me a headache." Such expressions can be literally true. *Your emotional reactions to others* can result in aches and pains of various kinds.

**psychosomatic disorder**
an impairment in physiological functioning that results from the individual's emotional state

Rather than a simple division of mental illness into psychoses, neuroses, and psychosomatic disorders, multiple categories are now used (American Psychiatric Association 1994). The major categories (with some illustrative, specific disorders) are as follows:

Disorders usually first evident in infancy, childhood, or adolescence (mental retardation, conduct disorders, eating disorders).

Organic mental disorders (alcohol-induced amnesia).

Substance use disorders (alcohol or drug abuse).

Schizophrenic disorders (various forms of **schizophrenia,** a psychosis that involves a thinking disorder, particularly hallucinations and fantasies).

Paranoid disorders (various forms of paranoia).

Mood disorders (depression; **bipolar disorder,** in which the individual fluctuates between emotional extremes).

**schizophrenia**
a psychosis that involves a thinking disorder, particularly hallucinations and fantasies

**bipolar disorder**
a disorder involving fluctuation between emotional extremes

Anxiety disorders (panic disorder, phobias).

Somatoform disorders (the conversion of emotional into physical problems, as in hysteria).

Dissociative disorders (multiple personality).

Psychosexual disorders (paraphilias).

Disorders of impulse control (pathological gambling, kleptomania).

Personality disorders (narcissism, an absorbing preoccupation with one's own needs, desires, and image).

*Extent of Mental Illness.* *Mental illness is a problem in all societies.* It is found among preindustrial people and in small, relatively isolated communities as well as in modernized societies. How many Americans suffer from mental disorders? There are two ways to estimate. We can examine the data on *hospitalization rates,* or we can research communities to get estimates of *"true" prevalence* ("true" because only a minority of people with mental disorders are hospitalized).

Rates of hospitalization must be interpreted cautiously because they reflect changing styles of treatment as well as changing levels of prevalence. Therapy with new drugs became common in the late 1950s. In the 1960s, **deinstitutionalization**—a movement

**deinstitutionalization**
a movement to change the setting of treatment of mental disorders from hospitals to the community through rapid discharge of patients

## involvement

### EXCEPT ME AND THEE?

There is an old saying that all the world is crazy except "me and thee, and sometimes I am not too sure of thee." As we point out in this chapter, it is probable that only a minority of the population is free of any psychiatric symptoms. To say that someone has symptoms, of course, does not mean that the individual requires psychiatric care or has problems functioning in his or her responsibilities. Nevertheless, the ideal for Americans would be the very best health—freedom from all symptoms.

How do you stack up? You can test yourself on a set of symptoms suggested by Walter Gove and Michael Geerken (1977). For the symptoms listed, write "often," "sometimes," or "never" beside each to indicate how often you have experienced them during the past few weeks.

1. I felt anxious about something or someone.
2. I was bothered by special fears.
3. I felt that people were saying things behind my back.
4. I felt it was safer not to trust anyone.
5. I couldn't take care of things because I couldn't get going.
6. I was so blue or depressed that it interfered with my daily activities.
7. I was bothered by nervousness.
8. I was in low spirits.
9. I was bothered by special thoughts.
10. I was so restless I couldn't sit for long in a chair.
11. I felt that nothing turned out the way I wanted it to.
12. I felt alone even when I was among friends.
13. I felt that personal worries were getting me down, making me physically ill.
14. I felt that nothing was worthwhile anymore.

Give yourself two points for each "often," one point for each "sometimes," and no points for each "never."

Your total score can range between 0 and 28. A score of 0 would mean that you are completely free of psychiatric symptoms. A score of 28 would mean that you have serious levels of those symptoms. If the entire class participates in this exercise, each score can be given anonymously to the instructor, who can give you the range and compute the average for the entire class. What do you think the results say about the prevalence of psychiatric symptoms in the population? Do you think students' scores would be higher or lower than those of the population at large? Why?

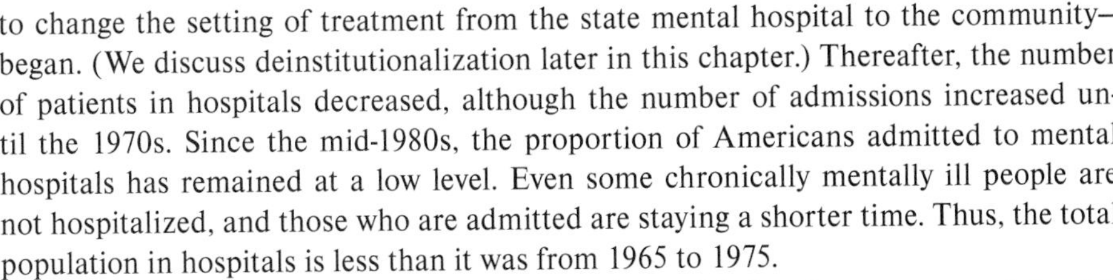

to change the setting of treatment from the state mental hospital to the community—began. (We discuss deinstitutionalization later in this chapter.) Thereafter, the number of patients in hospitals decreased, although the number of admissions increased until the 1970s. Since the mid-1980s, the proportion of Americans admitted to mental hospitals has remained at a low level. Even some chronically mentally ill people are not hospitalized, and those who are admitted are staying a shorter time. Thus, the total population in hospitals is less than it was from 1965 to 1975.

Surveys are a better way to estimate prevalence. National surveys report the following (Substance Abuse and Mental Health Services Administration 2019; Terlizzi and Zablotsky 2020):

- 19.2 percent of adults received mental health treatment in 2018.
- The prevalence of mental health treatment varies by racial/ethnic group: 13.6 percent of whites, 12.9 percent of Hispanics, and 13.6 percent of African Americans.
- In 2017, 4.5 percent of adults had a "serious" mental disorder.
- The prevalence of serious mental disorders varies by gender (3.3 percent of men and 5.7 percent of women) and age (7.5 percent of those 18–25 years, 5.7 percent of those 26–44 years, 4.0 percent of those 45–64 years, and 1.5 percent of those 65 years or older).

In 2017, 4.3 percent of American adults had serious thoughts of suicide during the preceding year.

In 2019, 18.5 percent of adults had symptoms of depression in the past two week. Women had higher rates than men; 18- to 29-year-olds had higher rates than any other age group; and Asian Americans had higher rates than other racial/ethnic groups.

*Variations exist in both the prevalence of the different disorders and in the at-risk background factors.* The prevalence doesn't remain stable over time. The rates of some disorders are going up. For example, anxiety disorders have increased among children and young adults (Twenge 2000). Rates of depression have also increased. As far as at-risk background factors are concerned, socioeconomic status and gender are both important. Rates tend to be higher among the lower social classes, and rates vary between men and women. In general, men have more problems with substance abuse and higher rates of antisocial personality disorder, whereas women have more anxiety disorders and depression. Depression affects twice as many women as men. This higher rate among women, incidentally, seems to be universal. An examination of 29 different nations found that females have more depression than males in all of them (Hopcroft and Bradley 2007).

Finally, mental disorders are so prevalent that they cost the nation more than $200 billion each year (McCarthy 2016). The cost includes such things as the care of nursing home residents, long-term patients in mental hospitals, and prisoners.

## Health Care, Illness, and the Quality of Life

One effect that illness has on the quality of life is this: People must endure considerable stress and suffering because of illness, which is a contradiction to Americans' value of good health. In addition, illness affects interpersonal relationships, involves people in inadequate health care, interferes with individual freedom, and costs the individual and the nation economically.

### Stress and Suffering

The obvious impact of illness on the quality of life is the *stress and suffering* that illness imposes on people. As an extreme example, consider Anton Boisen's (1936:3) account of his psychotic episode:

> [T]here came surging in upon me with overpowering force a terrifying idea about a coming world catastrophe. Although I had never before given serious thought to such a subject, there came flashing into my mind, as though from a source without myself, the idea that this little planet of ours, which has existed for we know not how many millions of years, was about to undergo some sort of metamorphosis. It was like a seed or an egg. In it were stored up a quantity of food materials, represented by our natural resources. But now we were like a seed in the process of germinating or an egg that had just been fertilized. We were starting to grow. Just within the short space of a hundred years we had begun to draw upon our resources to such an extent that the timber and the gas and the oil were likely soon to be exhausted. In the wake of this idea followed others. I myself was more important than I had ever dreamed of being; I was also a zero quantity. Strange and mysterious forces of evil of which before I had not had the slightest suspicion were also revealed. I was terrified beyond measure and in terror I talked. . . . I soon found myself in a psychopathic hospital. There followed three weeks of violent delirium which remain

> indelibly burned into my memory. . . . It seemed as if I were living thousands of years within that time. Then I came out of it much as one awakens out of a bad dream.

Of course, mental illness does not have to be that dramatic in order to have a negative impact on one's life. Even a relatively mild illness can be stressful to the afflicted individual and to that individual's relationships. And chilldren whose parents have mental health problems are at risk of higher levels of distress throughout their adult lives (Kamis 2020).

Physical illness also involves *stressful disruptions* in a person's life. If the person's work is disrupted, he or she may experience economic anxiety. If the illness is chronic, the individual may struggle with his or her identity (what kind of person am I?) and with alterations in lifestyle. Even the threat of serious physical illness, as illustrated by a survey of Americans during the COVID-19 pandemic, can have a negative impact on people's well-being (Barroso 2020). Rates of depression and anxiety rose during the COVID-19 pandemic, particularly among young adults (Wallis 2020). Protracted or chronic illness also affects the rest of the family (Lundwall 2002). Taking care of a chronically ill individual is demanding and stressful (Adams, Aranda, Kemp, and Takagi 2002). The marital relationship may suffer (Dashnaw 2019). Family patterns may be altered and highly constrained by the sick member, particularly if other family members must become caregivers over an extended period of time. For example, a study of the parents of children with cancer reported a significant worsening of the parents' health following the diagnosis of the cancer (Wiener et al. 2016).

Because physical and mental health are intertwined, physical health problems can generate *long-term fears* and even *serious emotional problems.* A substantial number of people experience high levels of psychological distress before or after surgery (Glosser et al. 2000). People diagnosed with serious diseases such as AIDS may develop high levels of anxiety and depression, problems with their work and social lives, and thoughts of suicide (Griffin, Rabkin, Remien, and Williams 1998).

Heart attack victims and cancer patients may have problems readjusting to normal routines. They often experience depression and anxiety even when the prognosis for the future is good, and they may have serious reservations about returning to a normal routine (Peleg-Oren and Sherer 2001). Patients with arthritis report a *significantly lower quality of life* than those without chronic disease (Anderson, Kaplan, and Ake 2004).

Serious *emotional problems* often are involved in cases of *organ transplants* (Dew et al. 2001). Severe depression and even psychosis have been reported. Men who receive organs from women may fear that their characters will be altered or that they will be feminized. Some patients develop fantasies about the transplanted organ and think of it almost in human terms as a living being within them. Some develop an image of the organ as a malevolent or hostile being; others conceive of it as life-giving. Not every patient has such serious problems, of course, but some long-term fears are probably common.

The *disabled* also endure stress and suffering because they are often *socially disvalued.* Social devaluation is particularly acute when the disability is visible. The visibly disabled individual may be treated as inferior and may be subject to serious disadvantages in job opportunities. Such experiences result in insecurity and anxiety.

The close relationship of physical and mental illness works both ways, because emotional problems can lead to physical illness. It is well-known, for example, that chronic negative emotions such as hostility, cynicism, and anxiety are risk factors for heart disease (Grewal, Gravely-Witte, Stewart, and Grace 2011; Stauber et al. 2012). To some extent, the problem can become a vicious circle for the individual, who may become entangled in the interaction between physical and mental disorders.

## Interpersonal Relationships

**stigma**
that which symbolizes disrepute or disgrace

There is a contradiction between the *sick role* and Americans' attitudes and values about desirable behavior; this contradiction can result in disrupted interpersonal relationships. Although people realize that illness is inevitable, they are reluctant to allow illnesses of others to disturb their routines. Furthermore, some illnesses, such as cancer and various kinds of mental illness, carry a social **stigma** (Angermeyer, Beck, Dietrich, and Holzinger 2004; Sandelowski, Lambe, and Barroso 2004; Wright, Wright, Perry, and Foote-Ardah 2007). The stigma means that the mentally ill person faces negative reactions (including rejection) from others (sometimes including family members) (Liegghio 2017).

The *strain on interpersonal relationships* when one of the interactants is ill is also seen in patterns of family relationships. Both physical and mental illness can lead to disruption in the family. In families with a chronically ill member, the ill member can become a focal point of family life. If the mother is ill, the husband and children may experience an emotional void in their lives. If the father is ill, there is a likelihood of economic problems and a lowered standard of living. Moreover, the father may tend to monopolize the attention of his wife, leaving the children feeling neglected. If the family develops a subculture of illness, they withdraw into themselves, isolated from outsiders.

Not all families respond to serious illness in this way, of course. Some families become more integrated, and the members experience a greater richness of family life. Others experience a temporary breakdown but recover and return to normal. Still others disintegrate in the face of the challenge, especially if the family was already weakly integrated. In every case, however, illness presents a serious challenge to the family.

One reason serious illness tends to disrupt family life is that it *precludes proper role functioning.* The physically or emotionally ill may be incapable of adequately fulfilling the role of spouse, parent, or breadwinner (Peleg-Oren and Sherer 2001). The normal functioning of family life may give way to a focus on the ill person. In extreme cases, most activities of family members reflect the ill person's needs and limitations.

As with the interplay between mental and physical illness, the relationship between interpersonal relations and illness can become a vicious circle. Poor interpersonal relationships can be a factor in the onset of a mental disorder, and mental disorders adversely affect interpersonal relationships. On the other hand, *good interpersonal relationships are associated with better health* (Berkman 2000). Those who have satisfying, close relationships have better mental and physical health, fewer problems of drug and alcohol abuse, and higher levels of satisfaction with their lives.

In sum, there is a relationship between patterns of interaction and health. Illness, whether physical or mental, tends to be associated with disturbed interpersonal relationships. The relation between interaction and illness may be a vicious circle: bad interpersonal relationships being a factor in the onset of illness, and illness being a factor in causing disturbed relationships.

## Inadequate Care

The value of good health is contradicted by the *inadequate care* that many Americans receive for both physical and mental illnesses (a national study about the latter concluded that *most* people with mental disorders are either untreated or poorly treated) (Wang et al. 2005). Inadequate care may result from a variety of factors. One important factor is the *lack of health insurance,* including 5.2 percent of all children under the age of 18 (Barnett and Vornovitsky 2016). Medicare provides seniors with some coverage, but, despite the Affordable Care Act, in 2015 10.5 percent of Americans under the age of 65 were uninsured (Figure 13.2).

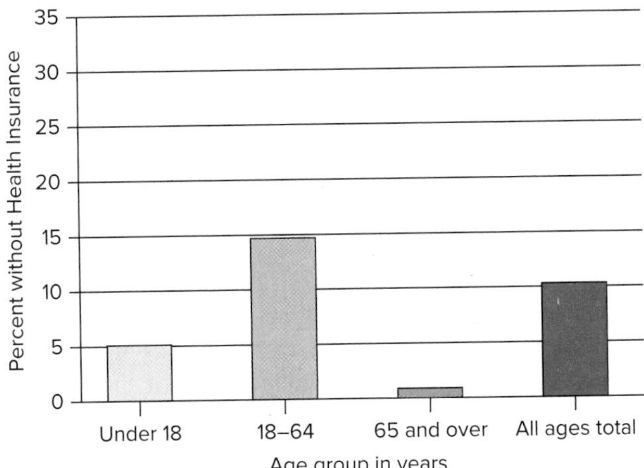


**FIGURE 13.2**
Percent of Persons without Health Insurance Coverage, 2019.
Source: Cohen et al. 2020.

The proportion who lack health insurance varies by racial/ethnic group as well as by age. In 2015, non-Hispanic whites had the lowest uninsured rate (6.7 percent) and Hispanics had the highest (16.2 percent) (Barnett and Vornovitsky 2016). The African American rate was 11.1 percent and the Asian American was 7.5 percent.

Lack of insurance can lead people to delay or avoid needed health care, or to find questionable or useless kinds of care (e.g., the use of a copper bracelet to treat arthritis). In 2018, 11.9 percent of Americans delayed or did not receive medical care because of the cost (National Center for Health Statistics 2019).

*Errors by the medical establishment are another factor in inadequate care.* Errors include **iatrogenic** problems, those caused by the physician in the course of a patient's treatment. Physicians may misdiagnose a case, prescribe the wrong medication, and even order unnecessary surgery (Pilippo et al. 1999; Shojania, Burton, McDonald, and Goldman 2003; Waldman and Smith 2012). A survey of research into medical errors concluded that 250,000 or more occur every year, making medical error the third leading cause of death in the United States (Anderson and Abrahamson 2017). In a five-year study of patient safety in 10 North Carolina hospitals, researchers found 588 incidents of patient harm among the 2,341 patients admitted (Landrigan et al. 2010). This amounts to 25 harmful incidents per 100 patients. The incidents included such things as severe bleeding during surgery, serious breathing problems due to an incorrectly performed procedure, injury and nerve damage resulting from a fall, and vaginal cuts caused by a device used to help deliver babies.

**iatrogenic**
caused by the physician in the course of his or her treatment of a patient

Women seem to be particularly prone to iatrogenic problems. One study concluded that 81.2 percent of the caesarean sections performed in four hospitals were unjustified (Gomez and Carrasquilla 1999). Another study drew the same conclusion about 70 percent of the hysterectomies performed on 497 California women (Broder, Kanouse, Mittman, and Bernstein 2000).

Hospital personnel, including medical lab technicians, also make mistakes. An analysis of critical care patients reported that medication error was the most common kind of medical error (MacFie, Baudouin, and Messer 2016). A study of medication in 36 hospitals reported that nearly one of five doses were in error–given at the wrong time, not given, given in the wrong amount, or were an unauthorized drug (Barker et al. 2002). A national study concluded that on average a hospital patient suffers at least one medication error each day, and that such errors harm 1.5 million patients and kill thousands each year in the United States (Aspden, Wolcott, Bootman, and Cronenwett 2007). And a survey of 134 Wisconsin hospitals found that 3.4 percent of the children discharged had one or more medical injuries, injuries resulting from medications, procedures, devices, implants, or grafts (Meurer et al. 2006).

Overall, medical errors probably cause more deaths than car accidents, breast cancer, suicide, homicide, or AIDS. A study by HealthGrades, an organization that rates doctors and hospitals, reported that 195,000 patients die in hospitals each year from preventable errors (Allen 2004). "Preventable errors" include such problems as overdoses, postsurgical infections, and slow medical staff responses to signs of infection or other life-threatening problems. When errors in the hospital setting are combined with errors generally in health care, medical error, as we noted earlier, is the third leading cause of death in the United States (Makary and Daniel 2016)!

The value of good health is also contradicted by the actual state of the science of medicine. Contrary to the expectations and attitudes of many Americans, *medicine is an inexact science.* Many symptoms, such as extreme fatigue or a pain in the back, are difficult to diagnose. Moreover, diagnoses are affected by who—in terms of age, sex, and race—physicians expect to have certain diseases (Lutfey et al. 2010). For example, a physician could miss the diagnosis of coronary heart disease in a middle-aged woman because such individuals are not known as high risks for the problem. Diagnosing mental disorders is even more problematic. Psychiatry is a field of *competing ideologies* rather than a science of mental therapy. There are various schools of therapy with different ideologies of health and illness and different views about diagnostic categories. A psychiatrist's diagnosis of a case will depend partly on *which school of therapy* he or she follows, but even within a particular ideology, diagnosis of mental disorders is difficult.

fallacy

A psychiatric diagnosis also may be influenced by stereotyped thinking. That is, the diagnosis may be a perfect illustration of the *fallacy of non sequitur:* "because this is a woman, her symptoms show her to be hysterical," and so forth. It isn't that the therapist consciously thinks in those terms, of course, but the diagnosis does reflect stereotypes, whether the stereotype involves gender, race, or social class (Dixon, Gordon, and Khomusi 1995; Wang, Demler, and Kessler 2002).

In addition to the influence of the gender, race, or social class of the patient, there are a number of other reasons why psychiatric diagnoses may be inaccurate (Brenner 2018). The therapist needs, but may not have, the necessary information about the patient's medical history. This requires time, and the patient may have insurance that limits the number of times he or she can see the therapist. Furthermore, any particular set of symptoms could indicate more than one mental health issue. For example, some of the symptoms of ADHD also apply to bipolar disorder, depression, and PTSD. Finally, the patient may actually have more than one condition, such that the effort to come up with a single issue is not possible.

In addition to incompetence, errors, and the fact that medicine is an art as well as a science, many Americans do not receive the quality of care they desire because of the *maldistribution of medical care.* Both economic and geographic factors enter into the maldistribution. *Maldistribution of doctors* means that people in certain areas have less access to doctors than those in other areas. There are a disproportionate number of doctors and nurses in cities and in the more well-to-do areas of the cities, leaving many rural areas and impoverished urban neighborhoods with inadequate care. For example, in 2018 the number of physicians per 10,000 population varied among the states from a low of 19.1 in Mississippi to a high of 45.0 in Massachusetts (Gooch 2019).

## Deinstitutionalization

The inadequate care of the mentally ill has been compounded by the deinstitutionalization movement that began in the mid-1950s (Lamb 1998). Partly because of newly available drugs, state and county hospitals began discharging a great many patients, including some with serious mental disorders and some who could not be effectively treated without 24-hour care. The goal was to provide a more humane, more effective, and less costly method of treating the disorders by using a community setting rather than a mental hospital. The drugs would keep the patients from harming others or themselves and enable them to function relatively well while they recovered. Their recovery would be facilitated by more normal living conditions. Further, their civil rights would be respected. In other words, the movement seemed to offer a new and enlightened approach that would transform the care of the mentally ill. Unfortunately, the reality diverged sharply from the ideal, adding to the problem of inadequate care.

One goal was met: A great many patients were released from hospitals. Patients who now go into hospitals are likely to stay only a short time compared to those who were institutionalized before 1960. As a result, the hospitals are treating more people than formerly, but they also have fewer patients in residence at any one time.

Nevertheless, deinstitutionalization has not only failed to solve many problems, it has also created new ones. In fact, many observers regard the movement as a total failure because it has basically taken the mentally ill out of the hospitals and put them on the streets or in the jails (Isaac and Armat 1990; Gilligan 2001). An estimated third of the homeless have a severe mental illness (National Coalition for the Homeless 2017). And more than 2 million deinstitutionalized mentally ill receive no treatment and hundreds of thousands are in prisons or jails (Amadeo 2016).

Studies of the homeless illustrate the way in which deinstitutionalization has failed. Homeless shelters are available, but they are hardly adequate to provide treatment for the mentally ill even if the staff had the time. Thus, large numbers of the deinstitutionalized mentally ill are lost and homeless or in jails. The problem is compounded by laws that make it difficult to involuntarily hospitalize the mentally ill. Thus, the legal basis for the deinstitutionalization movement—the rights of patients—keeps some mentally ill individuals at liberty until they act violently toward themselves or others (National Coalition for the Homeless 2017). Unfortunately, most individuals with severe mental disorders require medication, and the disorders are likely to impair their judgment and make it unlikely that they will voluntarily submit to treatment.

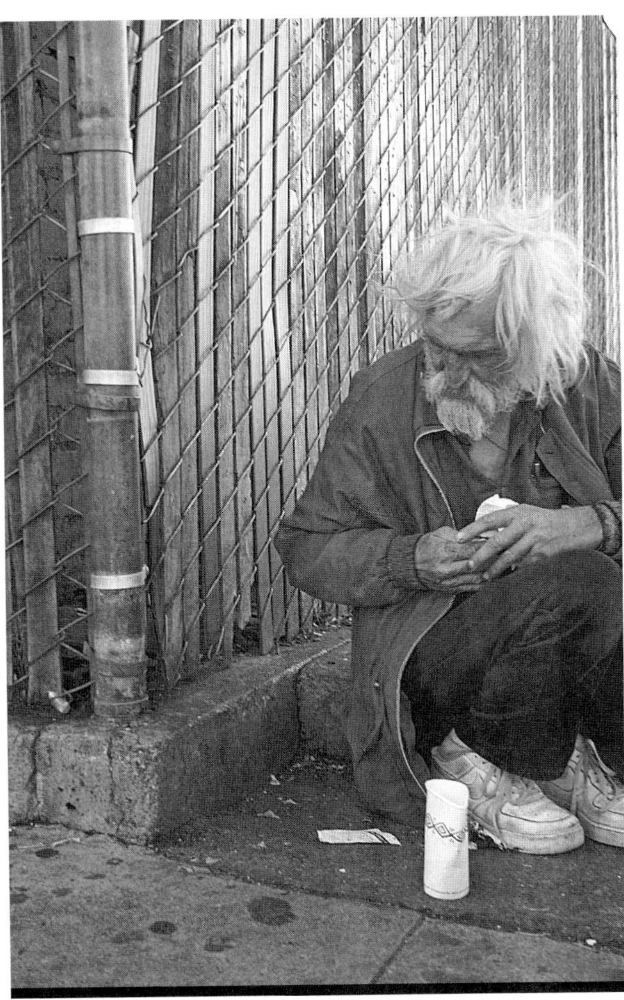

As a result of deinstitutionalization, many severely mentally ill patients have become homeless.
Christopher Kerrigan/McGraw Hill

## Individual Freedom

Americans are an individualistic people. They cherish the *freedom of the individual* and tend to react strongly to anything that threatens that freedom. However, there is sometimes a contradiction between the value of individual freedom and the value of good health. Some religious groups, for example, resist medical procedures such as blood transfusions and vaccinations on the grounds that these procedures violate their religious beliefs. If they are forced to undergo such medical treatment, their religious convictions and freedom of choice are violated. However, a counterargument is made that they may jeopardize the health or the lives of others by their refusal; thus, their freedom cannot extend to the point at which it affects the well-being of others. The same issue of individual freedom versus public well-being arises in such issues as providing a health identification number for every individual, mandatory notification of the parents of adolescents who use health care services, and the right of noncompliance with treatment of tuberculosis and other infectious diseases (Netter 2003; Adams 2004; Senanayake and Ferson 2004).

The issue of freedom is also raised by advances in biological engineering. The 1972 National Sickle Cell Anemia Control Act required people to submit to a screening blood test to determine the likelihood of their producing children with sickle cell anemia. Many people felt that this law was a clear invasion of privacy. Many more would probably consider it an invasion of privacy if the next step were taken: preventing people with certain genetic deficiencies from having children or even from marrying. Certain genetic diseases can be controlled only by forbidding certain couples to have children. Which, then, is more important: individual freedom or public health and welfare?

The history of medicine is marked by ongoing conflict between the advocates of medical advance and those who defend the freedom of the individual. Greater advances in medicine will intensify the conflict and compound the problems.

## Economic Costs

An increasing amount of the nation's *economic resources* is channeled into the effort to combat illness and promote good health. And the costs are growing rapidly. Americans spent $4,121 per capita (or a total of nearly $1.2 trillion) for health care in 2000 and $8,990 per capita (or a total of $2.96 trillion) in 2017 (National Center for Health Statistics 2019). The cost of health is not limited to expenditures, of course. There are also such factors as the loss of income and productivity when people are ill. Mental disorders alone cost the nation hundreds of billions of dollars each year in lost earnings.

The personal cost can be massive. About a fifth of Americans live in families in which health care costs more than 10 percent of family income (Banthin and Bernard 2006). And 7.3 percent are living in families in which the costs are 20 percent or more of family income. Such burdensome costs often result from long-term chronic diseases and from diseases requiring the use of *sophisticated medical technology*. Even with health insurance, an individual or a family may *find the cost of illness oppressive*. Why the dramatic increase in costs? There are various factors that help explain the increase in expenditures since 1950 (Dieleman et al. 2017): increasing population; an increasing number of the aged; increase in chronic diseases such as diabetes and heart disease; expensive new technological methods of treatment; and increase in how often people use health care services.

Thus, an increasing portion of the economic resources of individuals, families, and the nation are consumed by medical care (Toner and Stolberg 2002). The cost of that care includes the value of goods and services not produced because of illness. For example, workers with depression cost employers an estimated $44 billion per year in lost productive time (Stewart et al. 2003). Physical illness also results in lost productive time; in a national study, 13 percent of the workforce experienced a loss in productive time during a two-week period because of a common pain condition (headaches, back pain, arthritis pain, etc.) (Stewart et al. 2003). Finally, the interdependence between the economy and the nation's health was dramatically illustrated by the dire economic consequences of the COVID-19 pandemic (Casselman 2020). Unemployment soared as businesses either shut down or experienced a sharp drop in sales. Many Americans could not pay their mortgages or buy a sufficient amount of food. As of early 2021, the long-term consequences are unknown. Some observers are optimistic, while others see years of struggle ahead. But all agree that the pandemic has been disastrous for our economic well-being.

## Contributing Factors

We have pointed out that there are sociocultural factors in illness. In this section we examine some of those factors in detail. We show that sociocultural factors are involved not only in the **etiology** (causes of diseases) but also in inadequate care and the maldistribution of care.

**etiology**
the causes of a disease

### Social Structural Factors

*Roles.* Many studies have shown that *stress* leads to a variety of physical and mental health problems, including cardiovascular disease, digestive problems, heightened susceptibility to infection, problems of the skeletal-muscular system, and mental disorders (Mayer, Craske, and Naliboff 2001; House 2002). Stress can be a product of roles that are excessively demanding, contradictory, or overly restrictive. Not everyone who occupies a particular role will experience the same amount of stress, nor will everyone who occupies a particular role get sick. Nonetheless, *certain roles are considered stress-inducing* because they have been associated with a disproportionate amount of illness, particularly the female role and certain occupational roles in American society.

Women seem to have more health problems than men. Health statistics consistently show that women in the United States and other Western nations have higher rates of **morbidity,** health service usage, and certain mental disorders (Ladwig, Marten-Mittag, Formanek, and Dammann 2000; Kendler, Thornton, and Prescott 2001; National Center for Health Statistics 2019). In part, biological differences are a factor in the differential rates (Massey 2021). But the differences also reflect the fact that women generally suffer more distress (sadness, anger, anxiety, aches, etc.) than men, and this, in turn, may be rooted in the female role.

**morbidity**
the prevalence of a specified illness in a specified area

One characteristic of the female role is that *women are more emotionally involved than are men in the lives of the people around them* (Shih and Eberhart 2010). Women are more likely than men to be stressed by "network" events (events in the lives of loved ones) such as the death of a spouse, divorce, and illness of a family member. The cost of this caring is greater vulnerability to stress and illness.

The *traditional role of married women* is another reason for higher rates of illness (DeStafano and Colasanto 1990). Married women have higher rates of mental disorders than married men, but single or widowed women tend to have lower rates than their male counterparts. (Among both sexes, married people have lower rates than unmarried people [see, e.g., King and Reis 2012; Uecker 2012].)

We have noted that the majority of married women now work outside the home. Is it, then, a problem of overload? Overload (retaining the primary responsbility for child and home care while also working outside the home) can lead to physical and mental health problems (Jonsson et al. 2020). But that does not mean a married mother should not work. In fact, working enhances rather than diminishes women's health (Schnittker 2007; Glynn et al. 2009).

Women, then, *need multiple roles* in order to maximize their health (Ahrens and Ryff 2006). But they also need to have some control over what obligations their various roles entail. *Role satisfaction* is basic to well-being. Thus, women who are confined to, but dissatisfied with, the traditional role of housewife have higher rates of health problems, whereas women who are working mothers, and whose husbands assume some of the responsibilities associated with the traditional female role, have fewer health problems (Gutierrez-Lobos 2000).

We noted in Chapter 10 that certain occupational roles generate considerable physical and/or mental risks. In some cases, the occupational role may carry intrinsic risks—for example, mining occupations or high-pressure sales jobs. In other cases, the risks reflect the particular shape the role is given by the people in the workplace. For example, an engineer told us:

> I love my work. But I hate this job. My boss terrorizes everyone. If it was just the work I do, I would love going in. But I get a feeling of dread when I go through the gates every morning because I never know from one day to the next what new craziness we'll all have to endure from the boss. His demands are unreasonable, and you can't sit down and discuss things with him. He has managed to turn enjoyable work into a daily grind.

**socialization**
the process by which an individual learns to participate in a group

*The Family Context of Illness.* Among the institutional arrangements that contribute to illness are family patterns of interaction and **socialization** (the process by which an individual learns to participate in a group). We noted in the previous section that married people of both sexes have lower rates of mental illness than the unmarried. The mental health of the married couple depends on the quality of the marriage, however. When the intimate relationship between a man and a woman is defined by both as basically rewarding, the pair is more likely to enjoy positive mental and physical health (Lee and Bulanda 2005; Kaplan and Kronick 2006; Tower and Krasner 2006). Infidelity or a conflicted relationship, in contrast, is associated with major depression (Cano and O'Leary 2000).

For children, both physical and mental health are crucially related to the *quality of the relationship between the child and parents* (Feeney 2000). Children who have a good relationship with their parents and who feel themselves to be an integral part of family life are less likely to engage in various kinds of health risk behavior, including the use of alcohol, tobacco, and other drugs (Thuen et al. 2015).

Family disruption is stressful for children and typically leads to higher rates of physical and emotional problems. A study of 2-year-olds, for example, reported a higher proportion of accidents and higher rates of treatment for physical illnesses among those in single-parent and stepfamilies than those in intact homes (Dunn, Golding, Davies, and O'Connor 2000).

The adverse effects of a troubled family life may continue into adulthood. Thus, researchers found that the mental health of mothers of newborn infants had an impact on their children's romantic relationships 30 years later (Slominski, Sameroff, Rosenblum, and Kasser 2011). Mothers with mental health problems were more likely to raise children who had difficulty establishing meaningful, secure, romantic attachments.

Siblings as well as parents are important to a child's well-being. Thus, in a community study, researchers found that children who had siblings with a substance abuse problem were more likely both to use drugs themselves and to suffer from depression (Reinherz et al. 2000). They also found more depression among children whose parents were depressed.

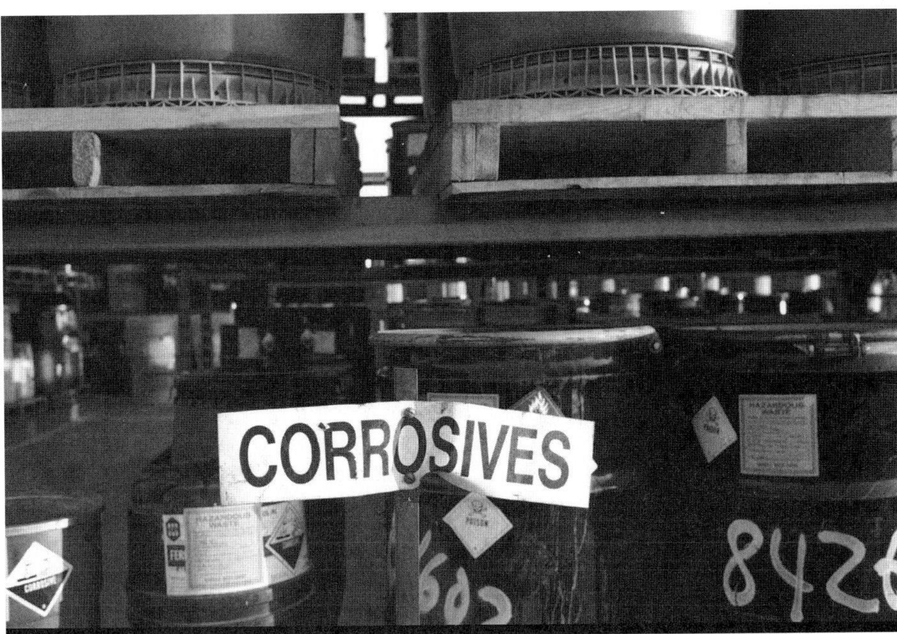


Many workers are exposed to carcinogenic materials in their workplace.

Kent Knudson/PhotoLink/Getty Images

*The Industrial Economy.* Certain aspects of the American economy, and indeed of the world economy, are involved in the onset of illness. In an increasingly industrial, technological world, people and materials move around the globe in great numbers. An infectious virus can now travel around the world in a few hours.

In the modern economy, both agricultural workers (because of the use of artificial fertilizers, herbicides, and pesticides) and other workers are exposed to materials that are **carcinogenic** (cancer-causing). Some common carcinogens in nonagricultural occupations are shown in Table 13.3. People who work in industries using carcinogenic materials are more likely to get cancer than are others.

**carcinogenic**
causing cancer

An industrial economy also exposes the citizenry to illness through *different kinds of pollution.* Lead poisoning can have disastrous effects on children: mental retardation, behavioral difficulties, perceptual problems, and emotional instability. Lead poisoning is most common among ghetto children, who ingest chips of paint from flaking walls or other substances containing lead (Richardson 2002). Use of lead in paint was discontinued for the most part by 1950, but leaded paint still exists in older buildings. Craving for such unnatural substances—a condition called **pica**—is frequently associated with impoverished living. In rural areas, pica may lead to eating dirt and clay, which is not healthful but is probably less damaging than leaded paint.

**pica**
a craving for unnatural food, such as dirt or clay

The most familiar pollutant to many Americans is automobile exhaust, which contains carbon monoxide. Carbon monoxide poisoning can lead to apathy, headaches, perceptual problems, retardation, and even psychosis. However, the precise effects of carbon monoxide poisoning are unclear. The amount of carbon monoxide released into the air from automobile exhaust varies considerably from one area to another. We discuss chemical pollutants further in Chapter 15.

Noise is another kind of pollution linked to the industrial economy that can have deleterious effects. The noise level endured by some workers can create mental stress, as can road traffic noise and the noise associated with living near an airport (Stansfeld and Matheson 2003). Children appear to be particularly vulnerable

| Agent | Organ Affected | Occupation |
|---|---|---|
| Wood | Nasal cavity and sinuses | Woodworkers |
| Leather | Nasal cavity and sinuses; urinary bladder | Leather and shoe workers |
| Iron oxide | Lung; larynx | Iron ore miners; metal grinders and polishers; silver finishers; iron foundry workers |
| Nickel | Nasal sinuses; lung | Nickel smelters, mixers, and roasters; electrolysis workers |
| Arsenic | Skin; lung; liver | Miners; smelters; insecticide makers and sprayers; tanners; chemical workers; oil refiners; vintners |
| Chromium | Nasal cavity and sinuses; lung; larynx | Chromium producers, processors, and users; acetylene and aniline workers; bleachers; glass, pottery, and linoleum workers; battery makers |
| Asbestos | Lung (pleural and peritoneal mesothelioma) | Miners; millers; textile and shipyard workers |
| Petroleum, petroleum coke, wax, creosote, shale, and mineral oils | Nasal cavity; larynx; lung; skin; scrotum | Workers in contact with lubricating oils, cooling oils, paraffin or wax fuel oils or coke; rubber fillers; retort workers; textile weavers; diesel jet testers |
| Mustard gas | Larynx; lung; trachea; bronchi | Mustard gas workers |
| Vinyl chloride | Liver; brain | Plastic workers |
| Bis-chloromethyl ether, chloromethyl methyl ether | Lung | Chemical workers |
| Isopropyl oil | Nasal cavity | Isopropyl oil producers |
| Coal soot, coal tar, other products of coal combustion | Lung; larynx; skin; scrotum; urinary bladder | Gashouse workers, stokers, and producers; asphalt, coal tar, and pitch workers; coke oven workers; miners; still cleaners |
| Benzene | Bone marrow | Explosives, benzene, or rubber cement workers; distillers; dye users; painters; shoemakers |
| Auramine, benzidine, alpha-naphthylamine, magenta, 4-aminodiphenyl, 4-nitrodiphenyl | Urinary bladder | Dyestuffs manufacturers and users; rubber workers (pressmen, filtermen, laborers); textile dyers; paint manufacturers |

**TABLE 13.3**
Common Occupational Carcinogens

SOURCE: American Public Health Association; *Health and Work in America* (Washington, DC: Government Printing Office, 1975).

to noise pollution. Environmental noise can impair reading comprehension, long-term memory, and motivation and may also be associated with elevated blood pressure (Haines, Brentnall, Stansfeld, and Klineberg 2003; Stansfeld and Matheson 2003). A study of German children concluded that high exposure to traffic noise, especially at nighttime, stimulates bodily processes that increase the problem of bronchitis (Ising et al. 2004).

As we noted in Chapter 10, *fluctuations in the state of the economy* also have been identified as having adverse effects on people's health. Unemployment is associated with health problems and increased mortality rates in all societies (Brenner 2005; Maitoza 2019). In fact, a study of 42 nations showed that unemployment lowers well-being even in those countries with high levels of social security (Ouweneel 2002).

*The Politics of Illness.* Usually people do not think of illness as a political issue, but *government policy* is a crucial factor in health care. For example, after President Obama signed the Affordable Care Act in 2010, there was an immediate political response from opponents that was designed to sabotage the legislation (Lanford and Quadagno 2016). Lawsuits were filed in 26 states that challenged some of the key provisions. Among those provisions was the expansion of Medicaid in order to insure those in the lower-income brackets. But the Supreme Court ruled that provision unconstitutional, and many states opted not to expand. In addition, a succession of bills to repeal the act were introduced in Congress. Criticism has been so strong and so vocal that a substantial number of Americans disapprove of the law. While the law significantly reduced the proportion of those without any health insurance, the future of health insurance is uncertain because of the ongoing political wrangling.

*Political factors also enter into the struggle against various health problems and diseases.* American infant mortality rates, for example, are higher than the rates of many other nations, and the rate for African Americans is more than double that for whites (National Center for Health Statistics 2019). Yet the African Americans most at risk—those in impoverished areas—are least likely to have the political influence necessary to secure federal funds for infant health programs.

Another example is provided by a physician, Jane Hightower (2008). She was concerned about the health problems of some of her patients, and eventually traced the source to the mercury-laden fish they had eaten. Although the toxic nature of mercury is well-known, industry and government had colluded to obscure the danger of eating the fish, working to protect the profits of those who caught and sold the fish rather than the health of those who were consuming it. Thus, scientific findings may be ignored or downplayed or rejected by politicians and businesspeople (and by scientists whose work is funded by corporations—recall the notorious few scientists whose work was funded by tobacco companies and who persisted in downplaying the hazards of smoking in the face of overwhelming evidence to the contrary).

Funding for research into causes and cures of diseases reflects political as well as scientific and humanitarian considerations. Of course, political decisions may reflect ideological considerations as well as economic ones, as well illustrated by the controversy over stem cell research during the Bush administration (Rosenberg 2002). Stem cells are obtained from human embryos, which are destroyed in the process. The medical value of embryonic stem cells lies in the fact that they can become any type of cell in a child or adult, which means that they have the potential to cure a variety of diseases that result from particular cells in the body being disabled or destroyed (diabetes, Parkinson's disease, cirrhosis of the liver, etc.).

But the embryos are destroyed in the process, and many of those who believe that human life begins at conception consider the destruction of an embryo an act of murder. Based on this reasoning, the government limited federal funding of research to existing stem cell lines, which most researchers considered inadequate and of poor quality. This decision was reversed in the Obama administration, which once again allowed the creation of new stem cell lines.

From a strictly scientific point of view, the years when no new stem cell lines could be created were a setback to important medical research. From an ideologically informed view, depending on your beliefs, they were either years of high moral ground or of the subservience of medical considerations to political ones. In any case, it is clear that political decisions are at least as important as scientific ones in research that bears upon the health of Americans.

Finally, there is the issue of governmental regulations that can reduce exposure to a number of known health threats. Fagin and Lavelle (1999) ask why no regulations exist on such actions as the use of certain toxic weed killers that have been linked with cancer and birth defects in farming communities, the use by dry cleaners of a chemical that pollutes homes, and "dry clean only" labels in clothing that can now be cleaned by cheaper and safer water-based alternatives. Of course, the answer to these and the other examples they cite is that political considerations outweigh public health needs.

*The Stratification of Illness.* When we speak of the stratification of illness, we are referring to the *different patterns of illness* and *variations in health care among the socioeconomic strata.* People in the lower strata tend to have more, and more serious, health problems than those in the middle and upper strata. With regard to physical health problems, for example, those in the lower strata have higher rates of chronic illnesses such as asthma, hypertension, diabetes, and heart disease; suffer more days of restricted activity due to illness; are less likely to use health care services (including fewer visits to physicians and dentists); are less likely to use preventive health measures such as vaccinations; are more likely to report daily pain as a result of financial worries; and have higher risks of death from all causes in each age category (Stringhini et al. 2010; Johnson and Schoeni 2011; Ferraro, Schafer, and Wilkinson 2016; National Center for Health Statistics 2019).

Ironically, then, poor and uneducated Americans have the fewest resources to meet medical expenses and the greatest likelihood of discovering that they have a serious, chronic, disabling, or even fatal illness. The pattern of physical illness in American society—more problems and less help as people descend the socioeconomic ladder—is likely to continue because of both the lack of information and resources among the poor and the concentration of medical services outside the areas where they live.

The pattern for mental illness is similar. In general, the rates of psychiatric disorders are higher in the lower strata (Wheaton and Clarke 2003; Strohschein 2005; Wickrama, Conger, Lorenz, and Jung 2008; McLaughlin et al. 2012).

The higher rates of illness in the lower strata reflect in part their lower likelihood of having health insurance and regular health care. They also reflect, however, the greater number and intensity of stressors in their lives: more role problems, more family disorganization, more financial stress, a greater number of stressful life events, and a more unhealthy lifestyle (such as smoking, abuse of drugs and alcohol, and poor eating habits) (Grzywacz, Almeida, Neupert, and Ettner 2004; Clouston et al. 2015; Mirowsky and Ross 2015; Lippert 2016).

*Social Change and Health.* As a society changes, the nature of health problems also changes. For example, new technologies (such as vaccines, new drugs, better tests, new kinds of surgery) clearly affect our health status. Many of them contribute to better health. But some can have adverse effects as well. The Internet, for instance, can enhance people's ability to understand health issues. It can also cloud understanding by offering conflicting or erroneous information. Also the compulsive use of the Internet by teenagers leads to problems of mental health (Ciarrochi et al. 2016). Adults who are compulsive users can also develop mental health issues such as depression (Dokoupil 2012).

It is not only change per se that can be problematic. The *rate of change* also affects our well-being. One effort to measure the effects of rate is the Social Readjustment Rating Scale. A respondent indicates which of the 43 events composing the scale have occurred to him or her within the last year. The events include role changes (such as death of spouse, divorce or marriage, beginning or stopping work) and changes in institutional participation (school, church activities, financial status). Each event is rated in terms of how much adjustment it requires. Scores range from 100 for the most stressful event (death of a spouse) to 11 for the least stressful (a minor violation of the law). The total score reflects the number and kinds of events that have occurred in an individual's life during the previous year.

Considerable research since the early 1970s supports the thesis. For example, a high rate of change in life events can result in depression or neurotic disorders (Medhi and Das 2015), in alcohol abuse (Saha et al. 2017), and in a lessening of the body's ability to ward off disease (Zautra, Okun, Robinson, and Lee 1989), and various other physical and emotional disorders (Turner and Lloyd 1999; McQuaid et al. 2000; Tiet et al. 2001; Malik and Malik 2016).

Note, however, that although a rapid rate of change does increase stress, the stress may be moderated if the people perceive the changes as desirable. It is *undesirable life events,* rather than change per se, that are likely to cause illness. People may function in a context of rapid change with minimal effects on their physical and mental health as long as they desire the changes that are occurring (and, perhaps, as long as they have areas of stability in the midst of the change).

## Social Psychological Factors

*Attitudes and Values.* Certain attitudes and values of individuals who are ill, of the public, and of medical personnel affect rates of illness and the nature of health care. Negative attitudes toward one's work can increase the risk of illness. An individual's work is a focal point of his or her existence as well as one of the most time-consuming areas of life. If it is defined in negative terms, the risk of illness is increased (Spector 2002).

A particular personality type, identified by a cluster of attitudes and values, has an increased probability of coronary heart disease (Eaker et al. 2004). Men who are ambitious, highly competitive, and self-driving and who impose frequent deadlines on themselves have a higher incidence of coronary heart disease than do men with opposite characteristics (Rosenman 1990). All these characteristics are admired in American society; they are long-standing American values. Unfortunately, when accepted and followed diligently, they are also the precursors of illness.

The sick person's attitudes about his or her illness and prospects for recovery are another important factor. Some people are skeptical about the ability of medical care to deal with their health problems (Borders et al. 2004). Such skepticism is stronger among young, white males in the lower socioeconomic strata. In contrast, other people believe that their prospects for recovery from illness are very good. They rely confidently on medical help and, in some cases, also believe that God is at work to bring about healing. Positive attitudes, especially ones that are grounded in spirituality, are associated with shorter and fewer illnesses, improved immune functioning, better mental health, and longer life (Oxman, Freeman, and Manheimer 1995; Braam et al. 2004; Kliewer 2004).

The attitudes of other people may be as important as the ill person's own attitudes. We have noted the stigma associated with certain kinds of physical and mental illness, a stigma that creates adverse reactions in individuals who are ill. For example, people with Parkinson's disease tend to feel ashamed and want to withdraw from public situations because, among other difficulties, they are unable to control their saliva and have difficulty speaking (Angulo et al. 2019). They are aware of the embarrassment and unease created in people with whom they interact.

fallacy

Mental illness tends to be even more of a stigma, so much so that many Americans who would benefit from therapy either refuse to seek help or drop out before the therapy is complete (Corrigan 2004). The stigma of mental illness is fueled by a number of myths (Socall and Holtgraves 1992; Wahl 2003). The myths are a form of the *fallacy of personal attack,* because they stigmatize current and past mental patients. The following are some of the common myths:

A person who has been mentally ill can never be normal.

Persons with mental illness are unpredictable.

Mentally ill persons are dangerous.

Anyone who has had shock treatment must be in a really bad way.

When you learn that a person has been mentally ill, you have learned the most important thing about his or her personality.

A former mental patient will make a second-rate employee.

These statements are myths. Note, however, that although the vast majority of people with serious mental illness are no more dangerous than those in the general population, there is a subgroup of the mentally ill that does pose a risk of acting violently (Swanson et al. 2002; Knezevic et al. 2017). People with a history of violent behavior, those who do not take their medication, and those with a problem of substance abuse are more likely than other people to engage in violent behavior. Yet for the great majority of the mentally ill, all the statements just listed, including the statement that they are dangerous, are myths.

The myths illustrate the way in which people who are troubled or different tend to be labeled. Thomas Scheff (1966) made the most thorough use of labeling theory to analyze mental illness. According to Scheff, the mentally ill are *rule breakers,* though the rules they break are different from the rules criminals break. The mentally ill break rules that govern normal social interaction, rules that define "common decency" and indicate an acceptance of social reality as defined by the group. Everyone occasionally breaks such rules with impunity. You may, for example, overreact to an insult, refuse to talk to someone who has angered you, or talk too loudly or too softly. The person who consistently breaks the rules of conventional interaction runs the risk of being labeled mentally ill.

Yet not everyone who breaks the rules is labeled mentally ill. In fact, most rule breaking is "denied and is of transitory significance" (Scheff 1966:51). A certain amount of rule breaking always goes unnoticed or unpunished. The response of other people varies in accord with the kinds of rules that are broken. Loud speech, for example, is less likely to be negatively sanctioned than the refusal to speak at all.

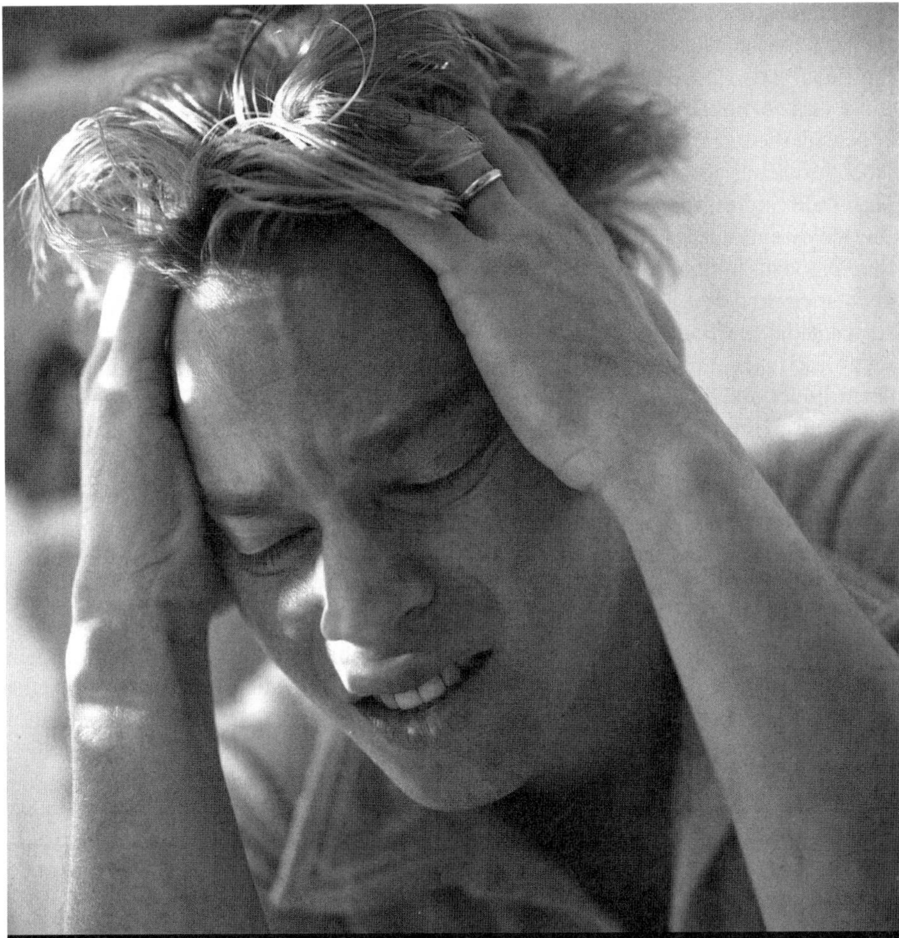

Many people who need treatment avoid it because of the stigma associated with mental illness.
Scott T. Baxter/Getty Images

How do people know when to label someone as mentally ill when there are various kinds of behavior that break rules? Scheff points out that *stereotyped imagery of mental illness* is learned early in life and that these stereotypes are reinforced in normal interaction. People avoid behavior that is a stereotype of mental illness and thereby reinforce the image of that behavior as a symptom of mental illness. Furthermore, they evaluate others according to the stereotype.

If an individual behaves in accord with the stereotype, he or she may be labeled mentally ill and rewarded for playing out the stereotyped role. Moreover, the individual may be punished for any attempt to abandon the role and adopt more conventional behavior. This objection occurs because people desire a *predictable social order;* that is, they expect to know how a mentally ill person behaves even if they do not define that behavior as desirable. Just as criminals who avow they are beginning new, law-abiding lives are likely to be treated with some suspicion (their behavior is no longer predictable), the mentally ill who seem to be recovering may be told that they are not as well as they think. In other words, once an individual is labeled as ill, the responses of other people tend to perpetuate the behavior involved.

Scheff denied that his is a complete explanation of mental illness. His aim was not to supplant psychiatric approaches but to supplement them and to stimulate new thinking about mental illness.

Evidence shows that labels do have a significant impact (Markham 2003). Even when the label may enhance sympathetic understanding and help among those with whom the individual has relatively close ties, it is likely to lead to rejection and discrimination by those with whom the individual has more casual ties (Perry 2011). In addition to having to cope with the social stigma, those who are labeled may accept the labels as legitimate and label themselves accordingly. This has further negative consequences. Moses (2009) studied 54 adolescents who were receiving integrated mental health services. Only a minority of the adolescents engaged in self-labeling using psychiatric terms; the majority talked about their problems in nonpathological terms or indicated that they were uncertain or confused about their problems. Those who self-labeled, compared to the others, scored higher on self-stigma and depression. Thus, labeling is a powerful social factor, and even if it does not directly lead to mental illness, it clearly seems to have negative outcomes (Rosenfield 1997).

Attitudes and values also affect medical care of physical illness. The *distribution of physicians* in the United States does not reflect medical need. Physicians, of course, are attracted to places that have desirable resources, abundant professional opportunities, and an active medical community. They also cluster in areas where they are likely to maximize their income. This pattern has been characteristic for some time, and it implicitly means that many Americans are receiving inadequate medical care. Apparently, physicians' attitudes toward working with the less affluent and the value physicians place on income outweigh their commitment to good medical care for all.

The attitudes and values of physicians have inhibited development of governmental programs that would reduce the maldistribution of medical care. Although most physicians now accept and even support Medicare, the American Medical Association (AMA) vigorously opposed the program when it was first proposed. Earlier, organized medicine had opposed Blue Cross plans for many of the same reasons. In both cases the financial benefits to physicians have been enormous. The programs also have provided more Americans with better medical care. Yet this result has often been in spite of, rather than because of, the attitudes and values of physicians.

## Solutions: Public Policy and Private Action

As in the case of drug and alcohol abuse, more money and effort have been expended on the treatment of ill health than on its prevention. In order to change this focus, there needs to be an expansion or improvement of existing programs and the development of new, innovative programs. An example of an existing program that can be expanded is the neighborhood health center, which addresses the maldistribution of care by bringing medical services to previously neglected groups. Poor people, minority groups, and residents of rural areas have benefited from these federally funded centers (Wright et al. 2000). However, the centers have faced difficulties in maintaining a stable professional staff and receiving adequate funding from the federal government.

### Health Care Reform

As we noted earlier in this chapter, in 2010 Congress enacted the Affordable Care Act (popularly called "Obamacare") to address some of the serious deficiencies in the American health care system. One of those deficiencies involved the tens of millions of Americans without any health insurance. The ACA significantly reduced the number of uninsured Americans. Still, by 2019 one out of seven adults remained uninsured (Cha and

Cohen 2020). This lack of health insurance has detrimental effects on both the uninsured individual and on society. As far as the individual is concerned, the need for insurance is dramatized by the fact that when uninsured people reach the age of 65, their health improves significantly because of Medicare (McWilliams, Meara, Zaslavsky, and Ayanian 2007). But the need is also dramatized by the fact that the uninsured are more likely than those with insurance to die before they reach the age of 65 (Wilper et al. 2009).

With regard to social effects, the uninsured are treated by hospitals in their emergency rooms. The costs of such care are borne by the hospitals; this means that those costs are passed on to insurance companies, who then pass them on to those they insure in the form of higher premiums. In other words, to have a segment of the population uninsured raises the costs of health care for the insured.

The Affordable Care Act reduced the number of those without insurance by, among other things, allowing more of the poor to secure coverage (Sommers 2016). But the lack of insurance is still a deficiency in the system. And there are other deficiencies. One is the lack of adequate care throughout the nation (recall, for example, the wide variation in number of physicians and dentists among the states). Another is the rapidly rising costs to the nation (the United States spends a larger proportion of its gross domestic product on health care than any of the major industrialized nations) and to individuals (in the form of increasingly higher insurance premiums and higher out-of-pocket expenses for care not covered by insurance). The societal cost of health care can be, and has been, exacerbated by overuse of the system. For example, an investigation of a Texas city found that in one year Medicare spent $15,000 per enrollee, nearly twice the national average and $3,000 more per year than the average person in the city earned (Gawande 2009). The problem was overuse—far more doctor visits, tests, and medical procedures than in a nearby city in the same state. Clearly, any system can be misused or abused. Regulation and oversight are necessary.

While the challenges are vexing, the need is pressing. In fact, since the administration of Franklin D. Roosevelt, most presidents have argued for some kind of national health insurance program (Pear 2009). Until very recently, however, all efforts at reform failed because of the power of various interest groups. Now those interest groups, including employers, business groups, and insurers, appear ready for change. Still to be hammered out is what kind of change is acceptable. Some want the federal government to offer a plan that would compete with private insurers, but others find this idea abhorrent. Some would prefer the coverage to be dealt with at the state level, but others argue that the states cannot or will not accept such responsibility. Some want whatever system is implemented to be regulated by the free market, but others argue that the system will require close federal regulation. Virtually everyone agrees on one point—health care reform is desperately needed and the federal government will have a crucial role in the reform.

## Innovations in the Delivery of Health Care

There is a need for ongoing innovations that effectively deliver health care. For example, an innovation that has emerged in the face of escalating costs is the *managed-care plan, which includes health maintenance organizations (HMOs), point-of-service (POS) plans, and preferred provider organizations (PPOs).* The original idea of the HMO was to offer people a comprehensive, prepaid health care plan. The individual pays an annual fee and receives total medical care, including necessary hospitalization and/or surgery. There are different kinds of HMOs, but one of the important distinctions for the quality of care is that of the not-for-profit versus the investor-owned HMO. A national survey found that patients in the not-for-profit HMOs were more likely to be very satisfied with their care than were patients in the investor-owned groups (Tu and Reschovsky 2002).

There are problems with care by an HMO. One is that administrators who are not physicians or therapists are making decisions about the kind and the length of treatment that will be allowed. Their decisions may be based on keeping costs at a minimum rather than on doing what the physician or therapist considers best for the patient.

Another problem is *capitation,* which means that the doctor receives a fixed monthly amount for each patient (Kuttner 1998). Any additional costs incurred in the treatment of patients must be absorbed by the physician or group of physicians involved. Therapists face the same dilemma in treating mental disorders.

Dissatisfaction with HMOs has led to a growth in the use of the point-of-service (POS) and preferred provider organization (PPO) plans. The *point-of-service* plan allows a patient to go to a health care provider outside the HMO, but the patient must bear the additional cost. The *preferred provider organization* is composed of a network of physicians and hospitals that offer care at discounted rates. A particular PPO may contract with HMOs to treat their patients. The difference is that the physicians remain in their own offices and have patients other than those who come from the HMO.

## Innovations in Treatment

Innovations in treatment are also needed. There are, of course, continuing technological innovations that facilitate diagnosis and treatment of various physical illnesses, but there is a need for innovations that consider the close relationships between physical and mental health and between mind and body. The mind plays a key role in health, a fact that needs further exploration and exploitation (Jacobs 2001).

Innovations in the treatment of mental disorders also have been developed in an effort to achieve quicker, more effective results. One approach is the *community support system* (Roskes, Feldman, Arrington, and Leisher 1999). In essence, a variety of services, supports, and opportunities are set up within communities to enable mental patients to function. Among other benefits, the support system can include therapy, health and dental care, a crisis-response service, housing, income maintenance, family and community support, and protection and advocacy services. Community support systems can be more effective than hospitalization in dealing with mental illness (Chinman, Weingarten, Stayner, and Davidson 2001).

Another program offers support to the patient's family when the family is the primary caretaker of the chronically ill person (Bull and McShane 2002). Family care, which is an alternative to hospitalization, generates various kinds of stress. Groups of families entrusted with the care of a chronically ill member meet for support, skill training, and information. With the aid of a mental health professional, the families are able to form a support group that enables each of them to cope with the difficult task.

## Prevention

It is usually much less costly and always more beneficial to people to *prevent illnesses* than to treat them once they have emerged. Preventive medical care includes such things as the neighborhood or community health centers that provide checkups for early detection or prevention of physical illness. Similarly, "preventive psychiatry" has emerged as an effort at early detection of mental disorders. Any realistic effort at prevention has to address the sources of stress in society. Stress-inducing roles must be changed. Help must be provided for troubled families. Economic deprivation must be eliminated. Government policy and its agencies must be responsive to health needs rather than to business interests. And people need to be educated about, and encouraged to pursue, those kinds of activities that foster better health, including such things as recreation, finding a social support system, and being a part of groups and organizations like churches that provide a network of friends (Koenig and Vaillant 2009).

One program of prevention that gained momentum in the 1980s is aimed at minimizing or eliminating smoking. Spurred by reports from the surgeon general and anti-smoking groups, the federal government has banned or restricted smoking in all federal facilities. Many states have done the same, or have gone even further. California, for example, forbids smoking in all public buildings, including restaurants. Such measures, along with increased education and higher taxes on cigarettes, have resulted in a substantial decline in the number of Americans who smoke.

Finally, *a crucial aspect of prevention is lifestyle.* In fact, the three leading causes of death in America are all related to lifestyle. In 2000, the leading causes of death were tobacco (18.1 percent of all deaths), poor diet and physical inactivity (16.6 percent of all deaths), and alcohol consumption (3.5 percent of all deaths) (Mokdad, Marks, Stroup, and Gerberding 2004). Or to put the matter in positive terms, national data show that people with four kinds of low-risk behavior (never smoked, a healthy diet, adequate physical activity, and moderate alcohol consumption) lived an average 11.1 years longer than those with none of the low-risk behaviors (Ford, Zhao, Tsai, and Li 2011). Nevertheless, in spite of considerable information about the value of a healthy lifestyle, *the lifestyle of Americans has tended to become less rather than more healthy.* Only 23.2 percent of adults engage in both aerobic activity and muscle strengthening exercises (Hales et al. 2020). Nearly half of adults do neither. In addition, there is a high rate of obesity in the nation: 18.5 percent of children and adolescents, and 41.2 percent of adult women and 38.1 percent of adult men (National Center for Health Statistics 2019). The high rate of obesity is a significant factor in the nation's relatively poor world ranking in longevity (Preston and Stokes 2011). Obesity makes people more vulnerable to disability and various diseases, including arthritis, diabetes, and cancer (Ferraro and Kelley-Moore 2003; Calle, Rodriguez, Walker-Thurmond, and Thun 2003; Leveille, Wee, and Iezzoni 2005). And obesity is a causal factor in at least 2.8 million premature deaths each year (Johnson 2005; Holland 2020).

The point is, you have a good deal of control over your own health, and you choose to ignore that control at your own peril. A healthy lifestyle is essential for both physical and mental health.

*Follow-Up.* In what ways do you try to manage your lifestyle in an attempt to prevent illness? What more could you do?

## Summary

Good health is a primary value of Americans. Some advances have been made, as indicated by the increasing life expectancy. The main problem of physical health today is chronic diseases rather than the infectious diseases that plagued society in earlier times. Millions of Americans are limited in their activities because of chronic conditions. There is general agreement about the classification of mental disorders, which are found in all societies.

Illness affects the quality of life in many ways. The illness itself and the inadequate care that many Americans receive cause stress and suffering. Interpersonal relationships are adversely affected. Individual freedom is threatened by certain medical advances. Often, heavy economic costs are involved for the nation and for individuals. Both physical and mental illnesses cause fears and anxiety. There is, in fact, a close relationship between physical and mental illness; each can be a factor in bringing about the other, so the individual can be caught in a vicious circle.

Structural factors contribute to the problem. Certain stress-inducing roles have been associated with illness, especially the female role and certain occupational roles. Patterns of interaction and socialization in the family can promote or inhibit good physical and mental health. The industrial economy exposes people to carcinogenic materials and to various pollutants. Fluctuations in the economy generate stress. Political decisions reflect economic interests rather than health needs.

Health care problems are more serious for individuals in the lower than the higher socioeconomic strata. People in the lower strata suffer higher rates of mental and physical illness and receive less adequate care for both. Also, different kinds of illness characterize the various socioeconomic strata.

One other important structural factor is change, and the rate of change, of the structure itself. There is evidence that rapid change may result in illness. A crucial factor in the effects of a changing structure is whether the people define the changes as desirable.

Among social psychological factors, attitudes and values are related to illness. The ill person's attitudes about the illness and his or her prospects for recovery are important. Negative attitudes toward work and certain attitudes rooted in traditional American values increase the probability of illness. Once a person is ill, negative attitudes of other people can inhibit recovery—a problem stressed by labeling theory. The attitudes and values of physicians have contributed to the maldistribution of care and have delayed federal programs designed to correct that maldistribution. These attitudes and values are supported by the ideology of free enterprise, which stresses governmental noninterference in medical care.

## Key Terms

AIDS
Bipolar Disorder
Carcinogenic
Deinstitution-alization
Epidemiology
Etiology
Iatrogenic
Incidence
Life Expectancy
Morbidity
Neurosis
Pica
Prevalence
Psychosis
Psychosomatic Disorder
Schizophrenia
Socialization
Stigma

## Study Questions

1. What are the various kinds of physical and mental illness, and how prevalent are they?
2. What kinds of suffering are associated with illness?
3. How does problematic health affect interpersonal relationships?
4. In what sense can it be said that Americans have inadequate health care? How has deinstitutionalization contributed to this problem?
5. How does illness affect individual freedom?
6. What are the economic costs of health and illness?
7. How do gender and occupational roles contribute to health and illness?
8. In what ways is the health problem affected by the family, the economy, and the polity?
9. What kinds of attitudes and values on the part of those who are ill, the public, and health personnel affect rates of illness and the nature of health care?
10. What innovations could help ameliorate the health problem?

## Internet Resources/Exercises

1. Explore some of the ideas in this chapter on the following sites:

**http://www.cdc.gov/nchs** The National Center for Health Statistics site has the most comprehensive collection of health data available.

**http://www.mentalhealth.org** The site of the U.S. Substance Abuse and Mental Health Services Administration, with full coverage of news and data about mental health.

**http://medlineplus.gov** The National Library of Medicine site, which has information about all health topics.

2. Many nations have national health coverage. Search the Internet for programs in at least two industrialized nations. Compare information about coverage and health conditions in those nations with the United States. What facts could you use to support or to reject a national health program in this country?

3. There is an ongoing struggle in the United States between consumer advocate groups, big business, and politicians over government regulations or potential regulations that bear upon health. Research a recent controversial issue. What were the arguments pro and con for federal regulation? What measures were taken by various groups to get acceptance for their position? Did the outcome, in your judgment, benefit or harm public well-being? Report your findings to the class.

## For Further Reading

Bendelow, Gillian. *Health, Emotion and the Body.* Cambridge, UK: Polity, 2009. An examination of the relationship between physical and mental illness, focusing on stress as the key factor in understanding the interaction between body and mind, and emphasizing the fact that illness is a social and emotional phenomenon.

Blanc, Paul D. *How Everyday Products Make People Sick.* Berkeley, CA: University of California Press, 2007. A discussion of the kinds of everyday products, such as glue, bleach, a rayon scarf, or the wood in a patio deck, that can be hazardous to your health, including the difficulty of getting controls or alerting the public to the dangers.

Budrys, Grace. *Unequal Health: How Inequality Contributes to Health and Illness.* Lanham, MD: Rowman and Littlefield, 2003. Illustrates the various ways in which differing kinds of inequality, separately and in combination with each other, significantly affect health and illness throughout an individual's lifetime.

Emanuel, Ezekiel J. *Which Country has the World's Best Health Care?* New York: Public Affairs, 2020. Analysis of healthcare systems in 11 countries in an effort to discover how well they perform and what factors go into making them succeed.

Himmelstein, David, Steffie Woolhandler, and Ida Hellender. *Bleeding the Patient: The Consequences of Corporate Health Care.* Monroe, ME: Common Courage Press, 2001. A critique of profit-driven health care, showing the varied ways in which patients are victimized by the system.

Kreider, Katherine. *The Big Fix: How the Pharmaceutical Industry Rips Off American Consumers.* New York: Public Affairs, 2003. A detailed study of the prescription drug industry, including the methods used to market the drugs and the reasons that prices are so high.

Whitaker, Robert. *Mad in America: Bad Science, Bad Medicine, and the Enduring Mistreatment of the Mentally Ill.* Cambridge, MA: Perseus Publishing, 2002. A history of how psychiatrists have treated schizophrenics, underscoring the fact that treatment is a trial-and-error process that changes from generation to generation.

## References

Adams, B., M. P. Aranda, B. Kemp, and K. Takagi. 2002. "Ethnic and gender differences in distress among Anglo American, African American, Japanese American, and Mexican American spousal caregivers of persons with dementia." *Journal of Clinical Geropsychology* 8:279–301.

Adams, K. E. 2004. "Mandatory parental notification: The importance of confidential health care for adolescents." *Journal of the American Medical Women's Association* 59:87–90.

Ahrens, C. J., and C. D. Ryff. 2006. "Multiple roles and well-being." *Sex Roles* 55:801–15.

Allen, S. 2004. "Report puts hospital deaths from preventable errors at 195,000." *San Diego Union-Tribune,* July 27.

Amadeo, K. 2016. "Deinstitutionalization: How does it affect you today?" The Balance website.

American Psychiatric Association. 1994. *Diagnostic and Statistical Manual of Mental Disorders,* 4th ed. Washington, DC: American Psychiatric Association.

Anderson, J. P., R. M. Kaplan, and C. F. Ake. 2004. "Arthritis impact on U.S. life quality." *Social Indicators Research* 69:67-91.

Anderson, J., and K. Abrahamson. 2017. "Your health care may kill you." *Studies in Health Technology and Informatics* 234:13-17.

Angermeyer, M. C., M. Beck, S. Dietrich, and A. Holzinger. 2004. "The stigma of mental illness." *International Journal of Social Psychiatry* 50:153-62.

Angulo, J., et al. 2019. "Shame in Parkinsons disease." *Journal of Parkinson's Disease* 9:489-99.

Armstrong, G. L., L. A. Conn, and R. W. Pinner. 1999. "Trends in infectious disease mortality in the United States during the 20th century." *Journal of the American Medical Association* 281 (January 6): 61-66.

Aspden, P., J. Wolcott, J. L. Bootman, and L. R. Cronenwett, eds. 2007. *Preventing Medication Errors.* Washington, DC: National Academies Press

Banthin, J. S., and D. M. Bernard. 2006. "Changes in financial burdens for health care." *Journal of the American Medical Association* 296:2712-19.

Barker, K. N., E. A. Flynn, G. A. Pepper, D. W. Bates, and R. L. Mikeal. 2002. "Medication errors observed in 36 health care facilities." *Archives of Internal Medicine* 162:1897-903.

Barnett, J. C., and M. S. Vornovitsky. 2016. "Health insurance coverage in the United States: 2015." U.S. Census Bureau website.

Barroso, A. 2020. "About half of Americans say their lives will remain changed in major ways when the pandemic is over." Pew Research Center website.

Barry, C. E., and M. S. Cheung. 2009. "New tactics against tuberculosis." *Scientific American,* March, pp. 62-69.

Becker, K., Y. Hu, and N. Biller-Andorno. 2006. "Infectious diseases—a global challenge." *International Journal of Medical Microbiology* 296:179-85.

Berkman, L. F. 2000. "From social integration to health." *Social Science and Medicine* 51:843-58.

Boisen, A. T. 1936. *The Exploration of the Inner World.* New York: Harper and Bros.

Borders, T. F., et al. 2004. "Older persons' evaluations of health care." *Health Services Research* 39:35-52.

Braam, A. W., et al. 2004. "Religious involvement and 6-year course of depressive symptoms in older Dutch citizens." *Journal of Aging and Health* 16:467-89.

Brenner, G. H. 2018. "6 reasons for common psychiatric diagnostic mistakes." *Psychology Today,* May.

Brenner, M. H. 2005. "Commentary: Economic growth is the basis of mortality rate decline in the 20th century—experience of the United States 1901-2000." *International Journal of Epidemiology* 34:1214-21.

Brill, S. 2013. "Bitter pill." *Time,* March 4.

Broder, M. S., D. E. Kanouse, B. S. Mittman, and S. J. Bernstein. 2000. "The appropriateness of recommendations for hysterectomy." *Obstetrics and Gynecology* 95 (February):199-205.

Bull, M. J., and R. E. McShane. 2002. "Needs and supports for family caregivers of chronically ill elders." *Home Health Care Management and Practice* 14:92-98.

Calle, E. E., C. Rodriquez, K. Walker-Thurmond, and M. J. Thun. 2003. "Overweight, obesity, and mortality from cancer in a prospectively studied cohort of U.S. adults." *New England Journal of Medicine* 348:1625-38.

Cano, A., and K. D. O'Leary. 2000. "Infidelity and separations precipitate major depressive episodes and symptoms of nonspecific depression and anxiety." *Journal of Consulting and Clinical Psychology* 68:774-81.

Casselman, B. 2020. "U.S. economy stumbles as the Coronavirus spreads widely." *New York Times,* December 3.

Cha, A. E., and R. A. Cohen. 2020. "Reasons for being uninsured among adults aged 18-64 in the United States, 2019." National Center for Health Statistics website.

Chinman, M. J., R. Weingarten, D. Stayner, and L. Davidson. 2001. "Chronicity reconsidered: Improving person-environment fit through a consumer-run service." *Community Mental Health Journal* 37:215-29.

Ciarrochi, J., et al. 2016. "The development of compulsive internet use and mental health." *Developmental Psychology* 52:272-83.

Clouston, S. A. P., et al. 2015. "Educational inequalities in health behaviors." *Journal of Health and Social Behavior* 56:323-40.

Cohen, R., et al. 2020. "Health insurance coverage." National Center for Health Statistics website.

Corrigan, P. 2004. "How stigma interferes with mental health care." *American Psychologist* 59:614-25.

Dashnaw, D. 2019. "Chronic illness and marriage problems." Couples Therapy Inc. website.

DeStafano, L., and D. Colasanto. 1990. "Unlike 1975, today most Americans think men have it better." *Gallup Poll Monthly,* February, 293.

Dew, M. A., et al. 2001. "Prevalence and risk of depression and anxiety-related disorders during the first three years after heart transplantation." *Psychosomatics* 42:300–13.

Dieleman, J. L., et al. 2017. "Factors associated with increases in US health care spending." *Journal of the American Medical Association* 318:1668–78.

Dixon, J., C. Gordon, and T. Khomusi. 1995. "Sexual symmetry in psychiatric diagnosis." *Social Problems* 42 (August):429–49.

Dokoupil, T. 2012. "Is the onslaught making us crazy?" Newsweek, July 16.

Dunn, J., J. Golding, L. Davies, and T. G. O'Connor. 2000. "Distribution of accidents, injuries, and illnesses by family type." *Pediatrics* 106:68–72.

Eaker, E. D., L. M. Sullivan, M. Kelly-Hayes, R. B. D'Agostino, and E. J. Benjamin. 2004. "Anger and hostility predict the development of atrial fibrillation in men in the Framingham Offspring Study." *Circulation* 109:1267–71.

Fagin, D., and M. Lavelle. 1999. *Toxic Deception: How the Chemical Industry Manipulates Science, Bends the Law, and Endangers Your Health.* Monroe, ME: Common Courage Press.

Feeney, J. A. 2000. "Implications of attachment style for patterns of health and illness." *Child: Care, Health, and Development* 26:277–88.

Ferraro, K. F., and J. A. Kelley-Moore. 2003. "Cumulative disadvantage and health: Long-term consequences of obesity?" *American Sociological Review* 68:707–29.

Ferraro, K. F., M. H. Schafer, and L. R. Wilkinson. 2016. "Childhood disadvantage and health problems in middle and later life." *American Sociological Review* 81:107–33.

Ford, E. S., G. Zhao, J. Tsai, and C. Li. 2011. "Low-risk lifestyle behaviors and all-cause mortality." *American Journal of Public Health* 101:1922–29.

Fox, S., and M. Duggan. 2013. "The diagnosis difference." Pew Research Center website

Gawande, A. 2009. "The cost conundrum." *The New Yorker,* June 1, pp. 36–44.

Gilligan, J. 2001. "The last mental hospital." *Psychiatric Quarterly* 72:45–61.

Glosser, G., et al. 2000. "Psychiatric aspects of temporal lobe epilepsy before and after anterior temporal lobectomy." *Journal of Neurological and Neurosurgical Psychiatry* 68 (1):53–8.

Glynn, K., et al. 2009. "The association between role overload and women's mental health." *Journal of Womens' Health* 18:217–23.

Gomez, O. L., and G. Carrasquilla. 1999. "Factors associated with unjustified Caesarean section in four hospitals in Cali, Colombia." *International Journal of Quality Health Care* 11 (October):385–89.

Gooch, K. 2019. "50 states ranked by most active physicians per 100,000." Becker's Hospital Review website.

Gove, W. R., and M P. Geerken. 1977. "The effect of children and employment on the mental health of married men and women." *Social Forces* 56:66–76.

Grewal, K., S. Gravely-Witte, D. E. Stewart, and S. L. Grace. 2011. "A simultaneous test of the relationship between identified psychosocial risk factors and recurrent events in coronary artery disease patients." *Anxiety Stress and Coping* 24:463–75.

Griffin, K. W., J. G. Rabkin, R. H. Remien, and J. B. W. Williams. 1998. "Disease severity, physical limitations, and depression in HIV-infected men." *Journal of Psychosomatic Research* 44 (February):219–27

Grzywacz, J. G., D. M. Almeida, S. D. Neupert, and S. L. Ettner. 2004. "Socioeconomic status and health: A micro-level analysis of exposure and vulnerability to daily stressors." *Journal of Health and Social Behavior* 45:1–16.

Gutierrez-Lobos, K. 2000. "The gender gap in depression reconsidered." *Social Psychiatry and Psychiatric Epidemiology* 35:202–10.

Haines, M. M., S. L. Brentnall, S. A. Stansfeld, and E. Klineberg. 2003. "Qualitative responses of children to environmental noise." *Noise Health* 5:19–30.

Hales, C. M., et al. 2020. "Prevalence of obesity and severe obesity among adults." National Center for Health Statistics website.

Haywood, M. D., E. M. Crimmins, T. P. Miles, and Y. Yang. 2000. "The significance of socioeconomic status in explaining the racial gap in chronic health conditions." *American Sociological Review* 65:910–30.

Heron, M. 2019. "Deaths: Leading causes for 2017." National Center for Health Statistics website.

Hightower, J. M. 2008. *Diagnosis Mercury: Money, Politics and Poison*. Washington, DC: Island Press.

Holland, K. 2020. "Obesity facts." Healthline website.

Hopcroft, R. L., and D. B. Bradley. 2007. "The sex difference in depression across 29 countries." *Social Forces* 85:1483–1507.

House, J. S. 2002. "Understanding social factors and inequalities in health." *Journal of Health and Social Behavior* 43:125–42.

Isaac, R. J., and V. C. Armat. 1990. *Madness in the Streets: How Psychiatry and the Law Abandoned the Mentally Ill*. New York: Free Press.

Ising, H., H. Lange-Asschenfeldt, H. J. Moriske, J. Born, and M. Eilts. 2004. "Low frequency noise and stress." *Noise Health* 6:21–28.

Jacobs, L. A. 2001. "What makes a terrorist?" *State Government News* 44:10–14.

Jacobsen, P. B., et al. 2002. "Predictors of posttraumatic stress disorder symptomatology following bone marrow transplantation for cancer." *Journal of Consulting and Clinical Psychology* 70:235–40.

Johnson, C. K. 2005. "Obesity goes from no. 2 killer to no. 7." *San Diego Union-Tribune,* April 20.

Johnson, R. C., and R. F. Schoeni. 2011. "Early-life origins of adult disease." *American Journal of Public Health* 202:2317–24.

Jonsson, K. R., et al. 2020. "Determinants and impact of role-related time use allocation on self-reported health among married men and women." *BMC Public Health* 20:1204.

Kamis, C. 2020. "The long-term impact of parental mental health on children's distress trajectories in adulthood." *Society and Mental Health*. Online article.

Kaplan, R. M., and R. G. Kronick. 2006. "Marital status and longevity in the United States population." *Journal of Epidemiology and Community Health* 60:760–65.

Kendler, K. S., L. M. Thornton, and C. A. Prescott. 2001. "Gender differences in the rates of exposure to stressful life events and sensitivity to their depressogenic effects." *American Journal of Psychiatry* 158:587–93.

Keyes, C. L. M., and E. J. Simoes. 2012. "To flourish or not: Positive mental health and all-cause mortality." *American Journal of Public Health* 102:2164–72.

Khatchadourian, R. 2016. "The unseen." *The New Yorker,* June 20

King, K. B., and H. T. Reis. 2012. "Marriage and long-term survival after coronary artery bypass grafting." *Health Psychology* 31:55–62.

Kliewer, S. 2004. "Allowing spirituality into the healing process." *Journal of Family Practice* 53:616–24.

Knezevic, V. 2017. "Prevalence and correlates of aggression and hostility in hospitalized schizophrenic patients." *Journal of Interpersonal Violence* 32:151–63.

Koenig, L. B., and G. E. Vaillant. 2009. "A prospective study of church attendance and health over the lifespan." *Health Psychology* 28:117–24.

Kuttner, R. 1998. "Must good HMOs go bad?" *New England Journal of Medicine* 338 (May 21):16–22.

Ladwig, K. H., B. Marten-Mittag, B. Formanek, and G. Dammann. 2000. "Gender differences of symptom reporting and medical health care utilization in the German population." *European Journal of Epidemiology* 16:511–18.

Lamb, H. R. 1998. "Deinstitutionalization at the beginning of the new millennium." *Harvard Review of Psychiatry* 6 (May–June):1–10.

Landrigan, C. P., et al. 2010. "Temporal trends in rates of patient harm resulting from medical care." *New England Journal of Medicine* 363:2124–34

Lanford, D., and J. Quadagno. 2016. "Implementing Obamacare." *Sociological Perspectives* 59:619–39.

Lee, G. R., and J. R. Bulanda. 2005. "Change and consistency in the relation of marital status to personal happiness." *Marriage and Family Review* 38:69–84.

Leveille, S. G., C. C. Wee, and L. I. Iezzoni. 2005. "Trends in obesity and arthritis among baby boomers and their predecessors, 1971–2002." *American Journal of Public Health* 95:1607–13.

Lewis, T. 2020. "Covid-19 misinformation that won't go away." *Scientific American,* November.

Liegghio, M. 2017. "'Not a good person': Family stigma of mental illness from the perspectives of young siblings." *Child & Family Social Work* 22:1237–45.

Lippert, A. M. 2016. "Stuck in unhealthy places." *Journal of Health and Social Behavior* 57:1–21.

Lundwall, R. A. 2002. "Parents' perceptions of the impact of their chronic illness or disability on their functioning as parents and on their relationships with their children." *The Family Journal* 10:300–7.

Lutfey, K. E., et al. 2010. "Physician cognitive processing as a source of diagnostic and treatment disparities in coronary heart disease." *Journal of Health and Social Behavior* 51:16–29.

MacFie, C. C., S. V. Baudouin, and P. B. Messer. 2016. "An integrative review of drug errors in critical care." *Journal of the Intensive Care Society* 17:63–72.

Maitoza, R. 2019. "Family challenges created by unemployment." *Journal of Family Social Work* 22:187–205.

Makary, M. A., and M. Daniel. 2016. "Medical error—the third leading cause of death in the U.S." *BMJ* 353:21–39.

Malik, N., and S. Malik. 2016. "Relationship of life events and psychiatric symptoms among adolescents." *Pakistan Journal of Medical Research* 55:44.

Markham, D. 2003. "Attitudes towards patients with a diagnosis of 'borderline personality disorder.'" *Journal of Mental Health* 12:595–612.

Massey, S. C., et al. 2021. "Sex differences in health and disease." *Cancer Letters* 498:78–87.

Mayer, E. A., M. Craske, and B. D. Naliboff. 2001. "Depression, anxiety, and the gastrointestinal system." *Journal of Clinical Psychiatry* 61:28–36.

McCarthy, J. 2016. "One in eight U.S. adults say they smoke marijuana." Pew Research Center website.

McLaughlin, K. A., et al. 2012. "Socioeconomic status and adolescent mental disorders." *American Journal of Public Health* 102:1742–50.

McQuaid, J. R., et al. 2000. "Correlates of life stress in an alcohol treatment sample." *Addictive Behaviors* 25 (January- February):131–37.

McWilliams, J. M., E. Meara, A. M. Zaslavsky, and J. Z. Ayanian. 2007. "Health of previously uninsured adults after acquiring Medicare coverage." *Journal of the American Medical Association* 298:2886–94.

Medhi, D., and P. D. Das. 2015. "Clinical study on role of life events in genesis of neurotic disorders and depression." *Open Journal of Psychiatry and Allied Sciences* 67:138–42.

Meurer, J. R., H. Yang, C. E. Guse, M. C. Scanlon, and P. M. Layde. 2006. "Medical injuries among hospitalized children." *Quality and Safety in Health Care* 15:202–7.

Michalos, A. C., B. D. Zumbo, and A. Hubley. 2000. "Health and the quality of life." *Social Indicators Research* 51:245–86.

Mirowsky, J., and C. E. Ross. 2015. "Education, health, and the default American lifestyle." *Journal of Health and Social Behavior* 56:297–306.

Mokdad, A. H., J. S. Marks, D. F. Stroup, and J. L. Gerberding. 2004. "Actual causes of death in the United States, 2000." *Journal of the American Medical Association* 291:1238–45.

Moses, T. 2009. "Self-labeling and its effects among adolescents diagnosed with mental disorders." *Social Science & Medicine* 68:570–78.

National Center for Health Statistics. 2019. *Health, United States, 2018.* Hyattsville, MD: National Center for Health Statistics.

National Coalition for the Homeless. 2017. "Mental illness and homelessness." NCH website.

National Institute of Neurological Disorders and Stroke. 2019. "Neurological complications of AIDS fact sheet." NINDS website.

Netter, W. J. 2003. "Curing the unique health identifier." *Jurimetrics* 43:165–86.

Osmond, D. H., L. M. Pollack, J. P. Paul, and J. A. Catania. 2007. "Changes in prevalence of HIV infection and sexual risk behavior in men who have sex with men in San Francisco." *American Journal of Public Health* 97:1677–83.

Ouweneel, P. 2002. "Social security and well-being of the unemployed in 42 nations." *Journal of Happiness Studies* 3:167–92.

Oxman, T. E., D. H. Freeman Jr., and E. D. Manheimer. 1995. "Lack of social participation or religious strength and comfort as risk factors for death after cardiac surgery in the elderly." *Psychosomatic Medicine* 57 (January-February):5–15.

Park, A. 2008. "America's health checkup." *Time,* December 1, pp. 41–51.

Pear, R. 2009. "Health care reform." *New York Times,* May 28.

Peleg-Oren, N., and M. Sherer. 2001. "Cancer patients and their spouses." *Journal of Health Psychology* 6:329–38.

Peleman, R. A. 2004. "New and re-emerging infectious diseases." *Current Opinion in Anaesthesiology* 17:265–70.

Perry, B. 2011. "The labeling paradox." *Journal of Health and Social Behavior* 52:460–77.

Pilippo, S., L. Mustaniemi, H. Lenko, R. Aine, and J. Maenpaa. 1999. "Surgery for ovarian masses during childhood and adolescence." *Journal of Pediatric and Adolescent Gynecology* 12 (November):223–27.

Preston, S. H., and A. Stokes. 2011. "Contribution of obesity to international differences in life expectancy." *American Journal of Public Health* 101:2137–43.

Reinherz, H. A., R. M. Giaconia, A. M. Hauf, M. S. Wasserman, and A. D. Paradis. 2000. "General and specific childhood risk factors for depression and drug disorders by early adulthood." *Journal of the American Academy of Child Adolescent Psychiatry* 39 (February):223-31.

Richardson, J. W. 2002. "Poor, powerless and poisoned." *Journal of Children and Poverty* 8:141-57.

Rifkin, R. 2015. "In U.S., healthcare insecurity at record low." Gallup Poll website.

Rolland, J. S. 1987. "Chronic illness and the life cycle: A conceptual framework." *Family Process* 26 (2):203-21.

Rosenberg, D. 2002. "Stem cells: Slow progress." *Newsweek,* August 12.

Rosenfield, S. 1997. "Labeling mental illness: The effects of received services and perceived stigma on life satisfaction." *American Sociological Review* 62 (August):660-72.

Rosenman, R. H. 1990. "Type A behavior pattern: A personal overview." *Journal of Social Behavior and Personality* 5 (1):1-24.

Roskes, E., R. Feldman, S. Arrington, and M. Leisher. 1999. "A model program for the treatment of mentally ill offenders in the community." *Community Mental Health Journal* 35:461-72.

Ruo, B., et al. 2003. "Depressive symptoms and health-related quality of life." *Journal of the American Medical Association* 290:215-21.

Saha, A., et al. 2017. "Stressful life events and severity of alcohol consumption in male psychiatric inpatients." *Industrial Psychiatry Journal* 26:13-18.

Sandelowski, M., C. Lambe, and J. Barroso. 2004. "Stigma in HIV-positive women." *Journal of Nursing Scholarship* 36:122-28.

Scheff, T. 1966. *Being Mentally Ill.* Chicago, IL: Aldine.

Schnittker, J. 2007. "Working more and feeling better: Women's health, employment, and family life, 1974-2004." *American Sociological Review* 72:221-38.

Semple, S. J., T. L. Patterson, and I. Grant. 2002. "Gender differences in the sexual risk practices of HIV1 heterosexual men and women." *AIDS and Behavior* 6:45-54.

Senanayake, S. N., and M. J. Ferson. 2004. "Detention for tuberculosis: Public health and the law." *Medical Journal of Australia* 180:573-76.

Shih, J. H., and N. K. Eberhart. 2010. "Gender differences in the associations between interpersonal behaviors and stress generation." *Journal of Social and Clinical Psychology* 29:243-55.

Shojania, K. G., E. C. Burton, K. M. McDonald, and L. Goldman. 2003. "Changes in rates of autopsy-detected diagnostic errors over time." *Journal of the American Medical Association* 289:2849-56.

Simon, H. B. 2006. "Old bugs learn some new tricks." *Newsweek,* December 11.

Slominski, L., A. Sameroff, K. Rosenblum, and T. Kasser. 2011. "Longitudinal pathways between maternal mental health in infancy and offspring romantic relationships in adulthood." *Social Development* 20:762-82.

Socall, D. W., and T. Holtgraves. 1992. "Attitudes toward the mentally ill: The effects of label and beliefs." *Sociological Quarterly* (3):435-45.

Sommers, B. D., et al. 2016. "Changes in utilization and health among low income adults after Medicaid expansion or expanded private insurance." *JAMA Internal Medicine.* Published online.

Spector, P. E. 2002. "Employee control and occupational stress." *Current Directions in Psychological Science* 11:133-36.

St. George-Hyslop, P. H. 2000. "Piecing together Alzheimer's." *Scientific American,* December, pp. 76-83.

Stansfeld, S. A., and M. P. Matheson. 2003. "Noise pollution: Non-auditory effects on health." *British Medical Bulletin* 68:243-57.

Stauber, S., et al. 2012. "A comparison of psychosocial risk factors between 3 groups of cardiovascular disease patients referred for outpatient cardiac rehabilitation." *Journal of Cardiopulmonary Rehabilitation and Prevention.* PubMed website.

Stewart, W. F., J. A. Ricci, E. Chee, D. Morganstein, and R. Lupton. 2003. "Lost productive time and cost due to common pain conditions in the U.S. workforce." *Journal of the American Medical Association* 290:2443-54.

Stringhini, S., et al. 2010. "Association of socioeconomic position with health behaviors and mortality." *Journal of the American Medical Association* 303:1159-66.

Strohschein, L. 2005. "Household income histories and child mental health trajectories." *Journal of Health and Social Behavior* 46:359-75.

Substance Abuse and Mental Health Services Administration. 2019. "Behavioral Health Barometer: United States, 2017." SAMHSA website.

Swanson, J. W., et al. 2002. "The social-environmental context of violent behavior in persons treated for severe mental illness." *American Journal of Public Health* 92:1523–31.

Terlizzi, E. P., and B. Zablotsky. 2020. "Mental health treatment among adults." National Center for Health Statistics website.

Thuen, F., et al. 2015. "Growing up with one or both parents." *Journal of Divorce & Remarriage* 56:451–74.

Tiet, Q., et al. 2001. "Relationship between specific adverse life events and psychiatric disorders." *Journal of Abnormal Child Psychology* 29:153–64.

Toner, R., and S. G. Stolberg. 2002. "Decade after health care crisis, soaring costs bring new strains." *New York Times,* August 11.

Tower, R. B., and M. Krasner. 2006. "Marital closeness, autonomy, mastery, and depressive symptoms in a U.S. Internet sample." *Personal Relationships* 13:429

Tu, H. T., and J. D. Reschovsky. 2002. "Assessment of medical care by enrollees in for-profit and nonprofit health maintenance organizations." *New England Journal of Medicine* 346:1288–93.

Turner, R. J., and D. A. Lloyd. 1999. "The stress process and the social distribution of depression." *Journal of Health and Social Behavior* 40 (December):374–404.

Twenge, J. M. 2000. "The age of anxiety? Birth cohort change in anxiety and neuroticism, 1952–1993." *Journal of Personality and Social Psychology* 79:1007–21.

Uecker, J. E. 2012. "Marriage and mental health among young adults." *Journal of Health and Social Behavior* 53:67–83.

Van Kessel, P., and A. Hughes. 2018. "Americans who find meaning in these four areas have higher life satisfaction." Pew Research Center website.

Wahl, O. F. 2003. "News media portrayal of mental illness." *American Behavioral Scientist* 46:1594–1600.

Waldman, J. D., and H. L. Smith. 2012. "Strategic planning to reduce medical errors." *Journal of Medical Practice Management* 27:230–36.

Wallis, C. 2020. "The mental toll of COVID-19." *Scientific American,* December.

Wang, P. S., et al. 2005. "Twelve-month use of mental health services in the United States." *Archives of General Psychiatry* 62:629–40.

Wang, P. S., O. Demler, and R. C. Kessler. 2002. "Adequacy of treatment for serious mental illness in the United States." *American Journal of Public Health* 92:92–98.

Weber, L. 2016. "An entirely curable disease is a top 10 killer around the world." *Huffington Post,* October 13.

Wheaton, B., and P. Clarke. 2003. "Space meets time: Integrating temporal and contextual influences on mental health in early adulthood." *American Sociological Review* 68:680–706.

Whooley, M. A. 2006. "Depression and cardiovascular disease." *Journal of the American Medical Association* 295:2874–81.

Wickrama, K. A. S., R. D. Conger, F. O. Lorenz, and T. Jung. 2008. "Family antecedents and consequences of trajectories of depressive symptoms from adolescence to young adulthood." *Journal of Health and Social Behavior* 49:468–83.

Wiener, L., et al. 2016. Impact of care-giving for a child with cancer on parental health behaviors, relationship quality, and spiritual faith." *Journal of Pediatric Oncology Nursing* 33:378–98.

Wilper, A. P., et al. 2009. "Health insurance and mortality in US adults." *American Journal of Public Health* 99:2289–95.

Woolf, S. H., and L. Y. Aron. 2013. "The US health disadvantage relative to other high-income countries." *Journal of the American Medical Association* 309:771–72.

World Health Organization. 2007. "Climate and health." WHO website.

Wright, E. R., D. E. Wright, B. L. Perry, and C. E. Foote-Ardah. 2007. "Stigma and the sexual isolation of people with serious mental illness." *Social Problems* 54:78–98.

Wright, P. J., R. H. Fortinsky, K. E. Covinsky, P. A. Anderson, and C. S. Landefeld. 2000. "Delivery of preventive services to older black patients using neighborhood health centers." *Journal of the American Geriatric Society* 48 (February):124–30.

Zautra, A. J., M. A. Okun, S. E. Robinson, and D. Lee. 1989. "Life stress and lymphocyte alterations among patients with rheumatoid arthritis." *Health Psychology* 8 (1):1–14.

PART

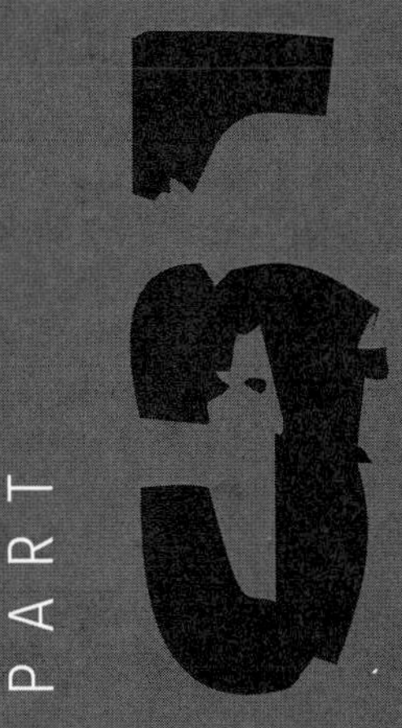

# Global Social Problems



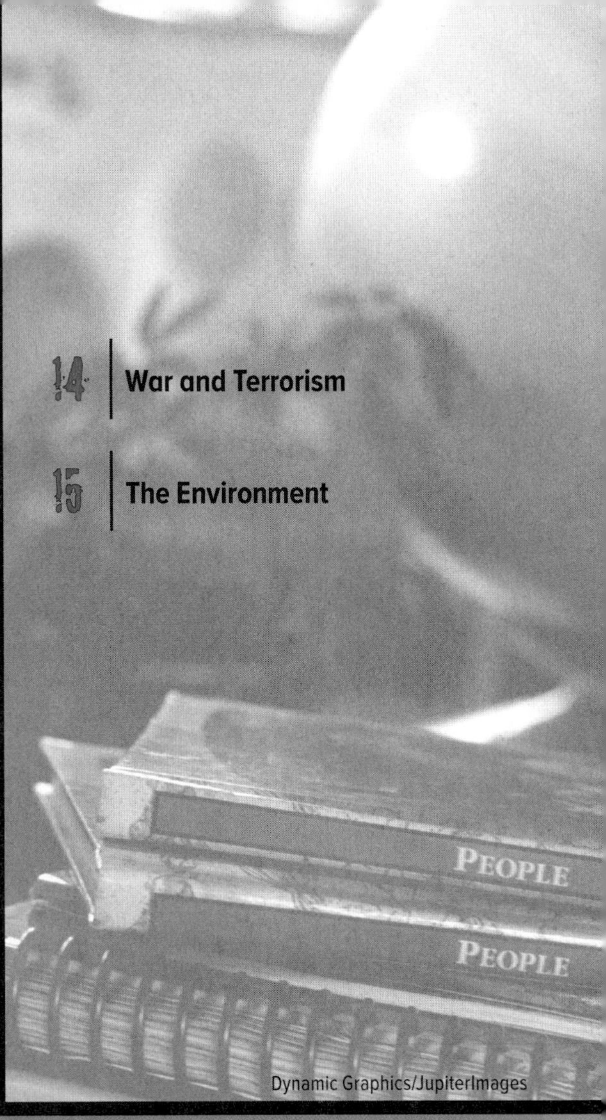


Dynamic Graphics/JupiterImages

Is there hope for civilization? Ever since the invention of gunpowder, pessimists have been predicting that humans will destroy themselves with their own technology. Their pessimism doesn't seem all that far-fetched, particularly because war, terrorism, and environmental problems all pose serious threats to the quality of human life, if not to the very existence of the human race.

In this final part, we examine these problems. We cannot discuss them meaningfully without seeing them in their global context. The threat they pose goes beyond any particular nation and inevitably includes all nations. We examine war and terrorism first. Then we explore the vexing environmental problems that are not only threatening but also involve painful dilemmas.

CHAPTER

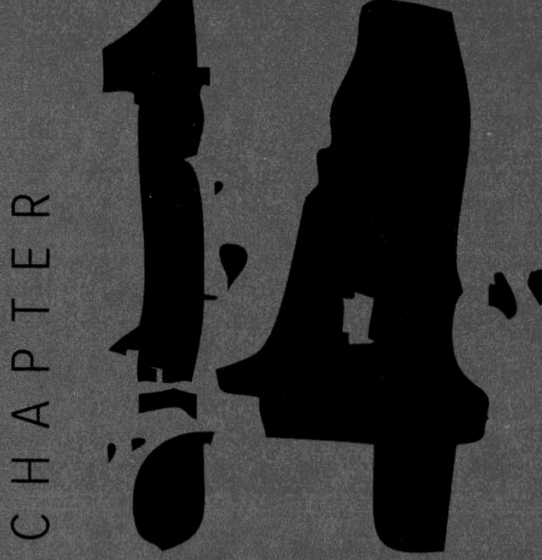

# War and Terrorism

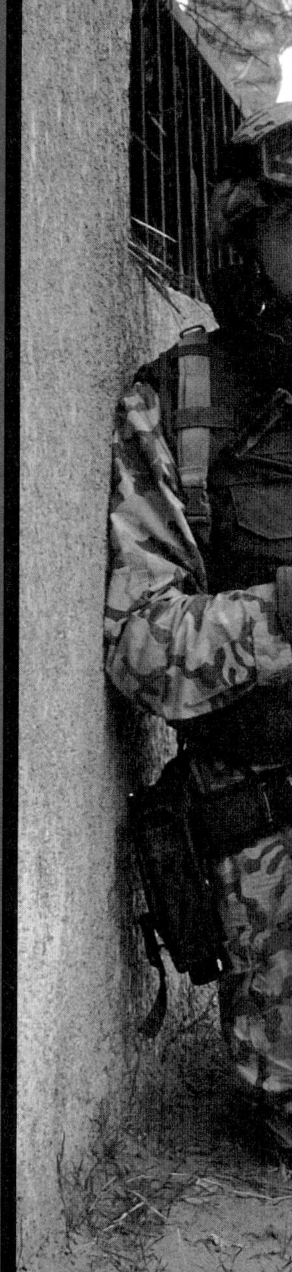

## OBJECTIVES

1. Distinguish between war, civil war, and terrorism, and know the extent of each.
2. Discuss the varied ways in which war and terrorism detract from the quality of life.
3. Identify the political and economic factors that contribute to the problems of war and terrorism.
4. Explain the kinds of attitudes and ideologies that legitimate war and terrorism.
5. Suggest steps that can be taken to address the problems of war and terrorism.

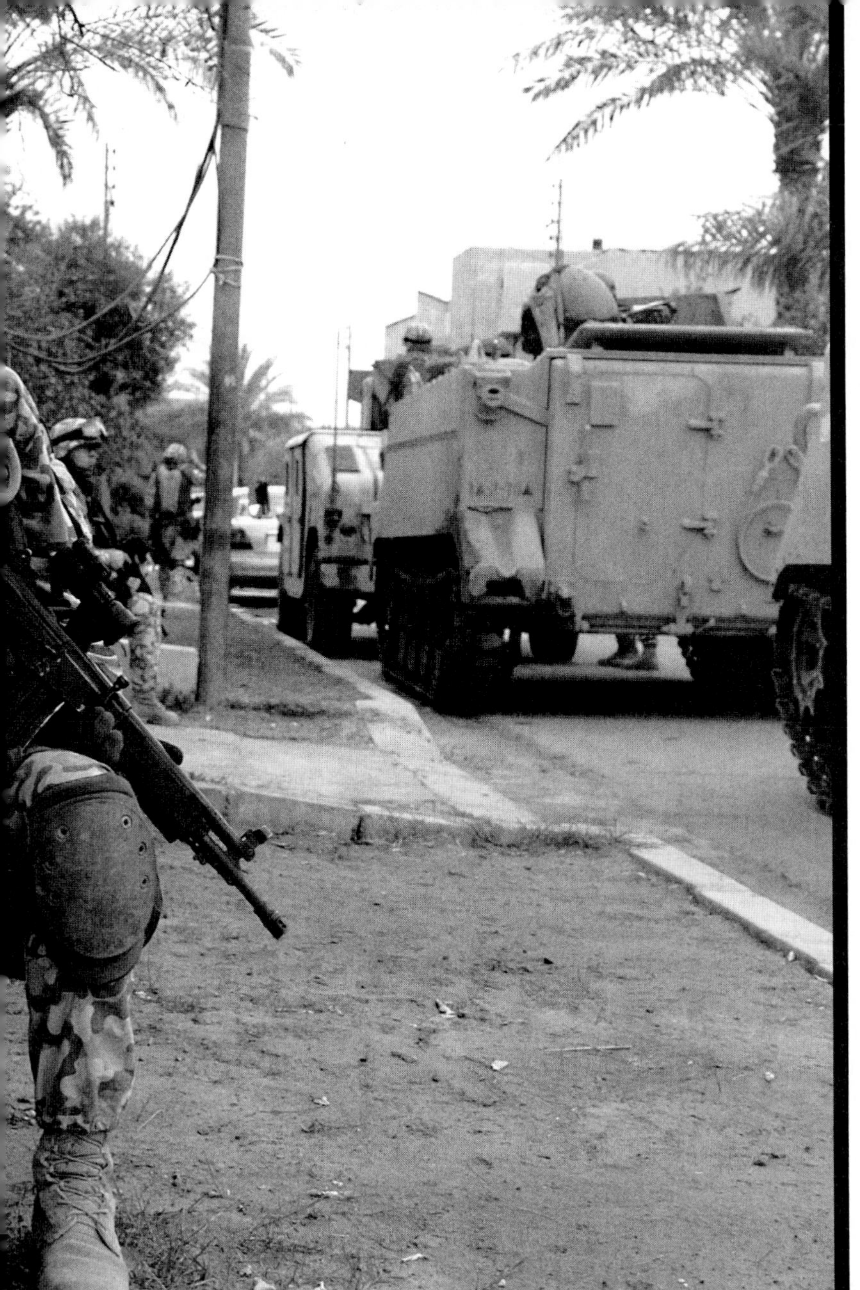
Department of Defense photo by Sgt. David Foley, U.S. Army

## "I Didn't Want to See It"

Steve is 22. He is a veteran of the 1991 war against Iraq. In many ways, Steve is fortunate. He was not wounded, and he has not suffered from post-traumatic stress syndrome. He returned home to a wife and baby girl with minimal problems of adjustment. But in another way, Steve also suffers from the war. His suffering is the memory of things he wished he had never seen:

*When we chased the elite Iraqi forces back into their own country and literally overwhelmed them, we all felt a sense of pride and exultation. It was the sweet taste of victory. A victory that cost us very little in terms of lives. I wish I had come home immediately after that. But we were stationed for a time within the borders of Iraq, guarding against any return of their forces. That's when I saw the real costs of the war. I didn't want to see it. But I couldn't avoid it.*

*Every day we would face Iraqi children begging for food. We saw hundreds of refugees camped out in the desert, living in burned-out cars and trucks. When I came through one of the refugee camps, I nearly got ill.*

*But it was the children that really got to me. I have my own little girl. I couldn't help but think about her when I saw those Iraqi kids. Some of them would look at our guns and start crying. And then there were the mothers holding crying babies who needed food or medicine. And there was nothing at all we could do.*

*One day an Iraqi professor came up to us. She spoke English, and she went on and on about how miserable their lives were. They had no food, she said, and nothing but dirty water to drink. They had no drugs, no hospitals, and no way to treat people who were wounded or sick.*

*I tell you, the combat was frightening at times. But it was far easier than dealing with those hurting people. I don't think I'll ever be able to forget the children begging for food. I'm home. I'm safe. I guess the war is still going on for some of them.*

## Introduction

On September 11, 2001, four American passenger jets were hijacked by terrorists. Two of the planes crashed into the Twin Towers of the World Trade Center and a third slammed into the Pentagon. A fourth plane, headed for the White House, went down in Pennsylvania after passengers tried to stop the hijackers. With more than 3,000 deaths from this terrorist attack, "war" took on a new meaning for Americans.

The next month, the United States launched an attack on Afghanistan, where the perpetrators of the September 11 attack were believed to be in hiding. And in March 2003, the United States and Great Britain invaded Iraq, calling it Operation Iraqi Freedom and justifying the action on the grounds that the Iraqi government had ties with the terrorists and also had weapons of mass destruction that were threatening our two nations. Over the next few years, opposition to the war grew dramatically. By 2007, when asked about the nation's most pressing problems, more Americans named the war in Iraq than any other issue. By 2016, the United States was still involved in conflicts with the radical Islamic group, ISIS, but was not officially at war with another nation. By 2020, a Gallup poll found the economy to be the most important problem for the nation. But "terrorism and national security" came in second: 44 percent of those surveyed said they were "extremely" important issues, and another 39 percent said they were "very" important (Brenan 2020). So war and terrorism have been, and continue to be, considered a more important problem than many other issues facing the nation.

In this chapter, we begin by looking at the nature and extent of the problem. We show the ways that war and terrorism detract from the quality of life. We identify the sociocultural factors that contribute to the problem. Finally, we discuss some proposals for minimizing or eliminating war and terrorism.

## War, Civil War, and Terrorism

When you hear the word "war," your first thought may be of armies from two opposing nations clashing with each other. However, this definition doesn't best describe present-day wars, which are more likely to be civil wars or wars of terrorism.

### The New Face of War

Modern warfare is no longer confined to opposing armies facing each other on the battlefield. Nor is it merely a matter of nuclear powers confronting each other with the threat of mass destruction. Rather, the small armaments that have flooded the world can be used by dissidents to destroy a nation's infrastructure. And:

> Civilians are targets as much as combatants, often more so. . . . Children fight alongside adults. The front line may be someone's bedroom. Hospitals and libraries are fair game. Even humanitarian aid workers become pawns (Musser and Nemecek 2000:47).

Not only have the struggles spread from the battlefield to the bedroom, but increasingly they have involved civil wars and terrorism. *Civil war* is rebellion by dissident groups within a nation. If the groups are small, they may simply engage in acts of domestic terrorism (discussed in Chapter 4). **International terrorism** is politically motivated violence against citizens of political entities different from those of the perpetrators in order to coerce and intimidate others into accepting the perpetrators' goals. Terrorism is not new, but the September 11, 2001, attacks made Americans painfully aware both of its destructive potential and of their vulnerability to it.

**international terrorism**
politically motivated violence against citizens of political entities different from those of the perpetrators in order to coerce and intimidate others into accepting the perpetrators' goals

The "new face" of war also includes some controversial methods of waging war. One is the use of drones to target and kill individuals deemed a threat (Kaag and Kreps 2014; Horowitz 2016). Those who oppose the drones argue, among other things, that killing someone outside a war zone is an assassination and therefore it is illegal. They also note that drones are known to have killed the wrong targets, including innocent bystanders. Those who support drones argue that they provide us with a safer way to confront and destroy our enemies.

Another controversial method is the use of such techniques as waterboarding to torture captured enemy combatants in order to gain information (Del Rosso 2014). Proponents insist that any such method is legitimate in the defense of freedom. Opponents stress the point that such a method is inconsistent with a humane, democratic society, and only gets the victim to say anything that will stop the torture, whether or not the information is accurate.

## The Extent of the Problem

*Wars and Civil Wars.* When the United States is not involved in war, Americans tend to think that the era is one of relative peace. Yet at any point in time the world experiences a large number of armed conflicts, including both wars and minor armed conflicts. A **war** is defined as a major armed conflict between nations or between organized groups within a nation in which 1,000 or more people are killed (Renner 1997). Minor armed conflicts may involve the same kind of weaponry and fighting, but they result in fewer deaths. The total number of armed conflicts has fluctuated over time, but between 2006 and 2015 there has always been at least 30 each year; in 2019, there were 32 active conflicts (Stockholm International Peace Research Institute 2020).

**war**
a major armed conflict between nations or between organized groups within a nation in which a thousand or more people are killed

Most wars in recent decades involve the developing nations of the world, but the United States and other developed nations can be drawn into the conflicts under certain circumstances. One such circumstance occurred in late 1990, when Iraq invaded and took over Kuwait. When Iraq refused to respond to U.N. demands to withdraw, a multinational force began a massive air bombardment in January 1991, thus starting the Gulf War.

Although the war was brief, the damage was massive and it should serve as a reminder that war is always possible. In fact, current events threaten future wars. Pakistan and India continue to struggle over Kashmir. Palestinians and Israelis continue to kill each other. Islamic terrorists in various parts of the world are calling on all Muslims to engage in a holy war against Israel and the United States. And the list goes on. The point is that *you live in a world that is never free of war or the threat of war.*

The bloodiest wars in recent times have been civil wars and wars involving just two nations (Renner 1999). More than 1.5 million died in the civil war in the Sudan (97 percent of them civilians), more than 1 million died in the Mozambican civil war from 1981 to 1994, nearly 4 million died in the war that broke out in the Democratic Republic of the Congo in 1998, and about 1.5 million died in the Soviet intervention in Afghanistan between 1978 and 1992. The incidence of civil wars has increased since the end of World War II (Fearon and Laitin 2002). Rebellion against dictators occurred in the "Arab spring" of 2011. It began in December 2010 when a Tunisian street vendor committed suicide after local officials confiscated his vegetable cart. Thousands of Tunisians went into the streets to demand the end of the 23-year dictatorship of the nation. Their action prompted similar protests in Egypt, Libya, and other Arab nations, leading to the downfall of a number of dictatorial governments. Tens of thousands died as the protests turned into civil wars. Overall, millions have died in civil wars over the last 60 years.

We should note that "civil war" does not mean that only one nation is involved. In the civil war that ravaged Syria beginning in 2012, Russia and Iran gave support to the existing regime, while the United States and others supported the rebels. In the modern era, few, if any, civil wars are ignored by the rest of the world. In some cases, that results in a nation simultaneously having to deal with both civil war and war with one or more other nations. Consider, for example, the war between Yemen and Saudi Arabia (Gambrell 2021). Yemen was once two nations. The war began as a civil war in 2014, when Houthis (a Shiite muslim group) in the north seized the capital and then tried to take control of the entire nation. Saudi Arabia and a few other countries entered the war against the Houthis the next year. The United States backed the Saudis. Iran supported the Houthis. By early 2021, 130,000 have died from the war, and tens of thousands of children have died from starvation or disease.

*Terrorism.* For most Americans prior to September 11, 2001, terrorism was something that was a problem elsewhere. Little was made in our news media about terrorism other than the acts of various leftist movements, the Irish Republican Army, and the attacks on U.S. embassies in Kenya and Tanzania in 1998 that killed 301 people. Since the end of the Cold War, attacks by leftist groups have declined, while those by Islamist groups have increased dramatically (Robison, Crenshaw, and Jenkins 2006). The September 11 attack was the worst terrorist attack ever in terms of the number killed.

Nevertheless, Americans have suffered far fewer attacks and far fewer casualties than the rest of the world. Globally, the number of terrorism deaths has ranged from 7,827 in 2010 to 44,490 in 2014. In 2017, an estimated 26,445 died from terrorism (Ritchie et al. 2019).

Of course, the main purpose of terrorism is not merely to kill people. It is to use the killings and the destruction to dramatize a condition that the terrorists find unacceptable (Northern Ireland remaining under British control, Israel's domination of Palestinians, American troops in Muslim countries, etc.), and to warn people that none of them is safe as long as the condition persists. Thus, terrorist attacks in recent years have included a school in Russia in which 323 people, half of them children, were killed; suicide bombings in Egyptian resorts; the bombing of four commuter trains during morning rush hour in Madrid, Spain; the bombing of the Australian embassy in Jakarta, Indonesia; subway bombings in London, England; and more than 400 small bombs exploding in cities and towns in Bangladesh.

It is unlikely that terrorist attacks will decline significantly in the near future. An important reason is that there is no single group or cause involved. Even though the radical Islamist group responsible for the 9/11 attack, al-Qaida, has been greatly weakened by the killing of Osama bin Laden and other key leaders and the disruption of base operations in Afghanistan, the group is still regarded as a significant terrorist threat because of other radical groups with whom it cooperates and shares resources. In addition, a number of smaller, loosely organized terrorist groups have emerged in various parts of the world. Thus, at this point terrorism appears to be something with which we will have to deal for an unforeseeable number of years.

Although bombings have been the most common form of terrorism, there is concern that other, possibly even more destructive, forms will emerge, including biological terrorism (Kuhr and Hauer 2001). A vast number of biological, chemical, and radioactive materials are capable of causing mass illness and death, and terrorists are capable of securing many if not most of these materials.

## War, Terrorism, and the Quality of Life

Like the impact of violence at the interpersonal and intergroup levels, it is not possible to fully capture in writing the impact of war and terrorism. To give you a sense of what people are doing to each other through such violence, consider a few reported experiences. You will see that war and terrorism destroy and dehumanize.

### Human Destruction and Injury

*Human destruction* reaches a peak in war. The 20th century was the bloodiest in human history. More than 100 million deaths occurred, compared to 19.4 million in the 19th century and 3.7 million from the 1st to the 15th centuries (Renner 1999:10). The figures for American casualties in various wars are shown in Table 14.1. From the Civil War (including Union troops only) to the present, nearly 1 million American military personnel have died as a result of wars. And nearly 1.5 million more have been wounded.

Increasingly, civilians are the main victims of war through a combination of direct injuries, starvation, and disease. Civilians accounted for half of all war-related deaths in the 1950s, three-fourths of deaths in the 1980s, and nearly 90 percent of deaths in 1990 (Renner 1993:9). Estimates of the number of civilians who died in the war against Iraq range from 100,000 to 600,000 or more. In addition, more than a million Iraqi citizens fled their homes and their country to escape the violence.

Similarly, an analysis of death in the Congo's civil war reported that for every combat death there were 62 nonviolent deaths, 34 of them children (Lacey 2005). These deaths are caused by such things as malnutrition and various diseases resulting from the chaos and deprivation.

Civilians are also the main victims in terrorist attacks. The great majority of Americans killed by terrorists have been civilians. The thousands of Palestinians

**TABLE 14.1**
War Casualties of American Military Personnel (in thousands)

| War | Battle Deaths | Nonbattle Deaths | Wounded |
|---|---|---|---|
| Civil War* | 140 | 224 | 282 |
| World War I | 53 | 63 | 204 |
| World War II | 292 | 114 | 671 |
| Korean War | 34 | 3 | 103 |
| Vietnam War | 47 | 11 | 153 |
| Persian Gulf War | ** | ** | 1 |
| War on Iraq | 4.4 | 0.9 | 32.0 |
| War on Afghanistan | 2.2 | 0.4 | 20.0 |

*Union troops only
**Fewer than 500
SOURCES: U.S. Census Bureau website; U.S. Department of Defense website.

and Israeli casualties in the ongoing terrorist attack-retaliation cycle in Israel and the occupied territories also have been mainly civilians.

In addition, *children are increasingly the likely victims of war and terrorism.* Children are victims in a number of ways. First, they are often among those killed. Second, they suffer severe and sometimes permanent injuries, are left without parents and/or homes, or fall prey to hunger and disease. Third, children are recruited for, or forced into, being combatants in wars and terrorist activities. Hundreds of thousands of children, some as young as 7 years old, have fought in armed conflicts or participated in terrorist attacks around the world. Palestinian children, for example, are taught the virtue of self-sacrifice, are encouraged to throw stones at Israeli soldiers and to become suicide bombers, and are assured that if they die they will receive the reward of martyrs (Burdman 2003). Finally, children may be victimized when women who participate in war have babies with birth defects. Women who served in Vietnam, for example, were far more likely to have children with birth defects than were other women (Brooks 1999).

A United Nations report summarized the situation with regard to children and war and terrorist activities as follows (United Nations General Assembly 2006:4):

> Today, in over 30 situations of concern around the globe, children are being brutalized and callously used to advance the agendas of adults. It has been estimated that over 2 million children have been killed in situations of armed conflict; another 6 million have been rendered permanently disabled; and, more than 250,000 children continue to be exploited as child soldiers. Increasingly, children and women are the casualties of war, with the fatalities of civilians disproportionately higher than ever before in the history of warfare.

The report also notes that thousands of girls are raped and sexually exploited, and both boys and girls are being seized and taken away from their homes and communities in large numbers. Such suffering and death of children are among the most agonizing effects of war (see "I Didn't Want to See It" at the beginning of this chapter).

Various factors account for the human destruction in war. The obvious factor, of course, is the use of weaponry, including bombs. Even when bombs are aimed at military targets, a certain number will hit civilians. For instance, the 1991 war against

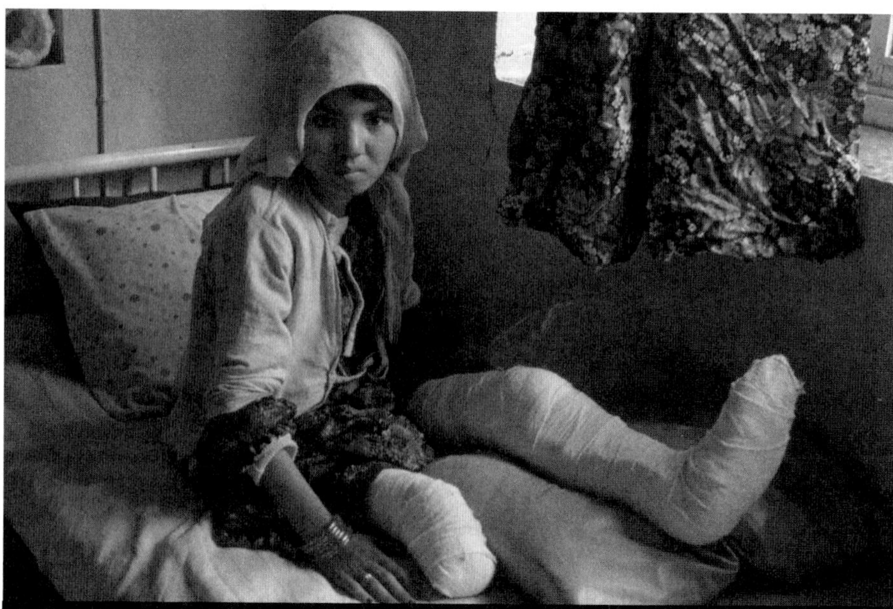

Each year, land mines kill or maim more than 25,000 people, many of them children like this young Afghan girl.

Peter Turnley/Corbis/Getty Images

Iraq, with its "smart" bombs and missiles that hit military targets with pinpoint accuracy, was heralded as an example of the wonders of modern military technology. However, many hospitals also were hit, including the only hospital in the nation that performed kidney transplants and advanced heart surgery (Burleigh 1991). In addition, the destruction of power plants prevented some hospitals from operating even basic equipment like incubators and refrigerators.

Land mines are also responsible for many civilian deaths and injuries. There are more than 100 million land mines in more than 70 countries; an estimated 10 million mines are in Afghanistan alone (Rieder and Choonara 2012). The mines remain lethal for decades (Henig 2012), and more are being planted every year. Land mines kill or maim at least one person every hour (Williams 2004). One in every 236 people in Cambodia is an amputee because of land mines. A study of victims of land mines admitted to an emergency surgical center in Cambodia from 2003 to 2006 found that a little over a fourth were children (Bendinelli 2009). Compared to the adults, the children were more likely to require a blood transfusion; suffer blindness; be maimed in their upper limbs; and die from their injuries. As with war generally, women and children are at greater risk from land mines than are soldiers.

Land mines cause suffering and destruction indirectly as well. An investigation of the Nuba people in the Sudan found serious problems resulting from the mere existence of the mines (Sultan 2009). Knowing that the mines had been planted, the Nubas avoided the area. That meant they no longer had the same access to water or to farmland. Greater numbers concentrated in more inaccessible areas, resulting in economic hardship, loss of local markets, insufficient food, and outbreaks of disease among both animals and humans.

Despite the dire consequences, and despite the fact that 134 countries have signed a mine ban treaty and 18 countries have destroyed their stockpiles, 47 other countries (including the United States, China, and Russia) have not signed the treaty and have stockpiled as many as 200 million mines.

The more recent version of land mines is the *improvised explosive device,* or IED (Bryce 2006). IEDs are homemade bombs designed to kill or incapacitate the opposition. They can be hidden and camouflaged so effectively that they are extremely difficult to detect. They are usually triggered by the victims, but can also be triggered remotely. They have emerged as major weapons in the war in Iraq. About 3 percent of American combat deaths in World War II were due to mines or booby traps. The figure for the Vietnam War was 9 percent. But in Iraq, IEDs accounted for fully 65 percent of U.S. combat deaths and about half of all nonfatal injuries.

Another reason for the destructiveness of war is that, throughout human history, conquering armies have considered the vanquished to be undeserving of humane treatment. Girls and women experience a higher probability of being raped. Rape occurs in all wars, including civil wars. A survey of households in Sierra Leone reported that 94 percent contained at least one person who had suffered abuse in the previous 10 years of the nation's civil war, and one of eight of the households contained someone who had been victimized by some kind of war-related sexual violence (Physicians for Human Rights 2002). Such rape in wartime, like rape generally, is most often a hostile act. Farr (2009) calls it "extreme war rape." The point is that the rapists intend to inflict emotional and physical injury on their victims. Farr examined war rape in 27 countries engaged in armed conflicts and concluded that extreme war rape was found in all of them.

Finally, war is destructive because, in their quest for military power or military victory, governments may act in ways that harm their own people. In 1993 the Department of Energy acknowledged that the United States had conducted about 800 radiation tests on humans between 1945 and 1970—and some of these people were unaware of the risks (Wheeler 1994). Part of the justification for the research, which was often supported financially by the Department of Defense or the Atomic Energy Commission, was the presumed threat of nuclear war and, thereby, the need to know the effects of radiation on the human body as well as ways to counter those effects.

Wars always have been destructive, but they are more destructive now than they were in the past. Clearly, one reason for the increasing number of people killed, as well as the increasing proportion of civilians among those killed, is the *changed nature of war,* which now involves the total population of nations rather than military personnel only.

Another reason for the increased destructiveness of war is the *increasingly sophisticated nature of military technology* compared to past weaponry. It is now possible to kill people in numbers that are staggering. In World War I, fewer than 3 people per 100,000 were killed by bombs in England and Germany. In World War II, nearly 300 people per 100,000 were killed by bombs (Hart 1957:44). World War II also saw the introduction of atomic weapons. Two Japanese cities, Hiroshima and Nagasaki, were each decimated by a single bomb. About 140,000 people in Hiroshima and 70,000 in Nagasaki died immediately or within a few weeks, and another 130,000 died within five years after the attack (Committee for the Compilation of Materials on Damage Caused by the Atomic Bombs in Hiroshima and Nagasaki 1981). It is sobering to realize that whereas the Hiroshima bomber delivered 25,800 tons of TNT-equivalent explosives, a bomber today can deliver *literally hundreds of times more destructive power.* It's estimated that one nuclear bomb now could result in 6.42 million deaths and 3.06 million injuries (Buck 2018). To repeat, that's just *one* bomb!

In addition to the destruction of bombs and bullets, there is the horror of biological and chemical warfare. During the Iran-Iraq war from 1980 to 1988, the Iraqis used mustard gas, breaking a 63-year-old international agreement that forbids the use of any chemical weapons (Willems 2002). The gas initially causes sneezing and coughing and sometimes nausea and vomiting. Within hours, the victim suffers tightness in the chest and shortness of breath as a result of respiratory inflammation. Painful blisters appear on the body, causing patches of skin to fall off. Some victims recover, but some die and others suffer bone marrow or gastrointestinal problems for years.

The destructiveness of war goes beyond that inflicted by weaponry. As studies of Palestinian and Lebanese children have shown, children who witness military violence may become more aggressive and antisocial in their behavior (Qouta, Punamäki, Miller, and El-Sarraj 2007; Tarabah et al. 2015). An investigation of American soldiers who were parents found that when the soldiers were combat deployed the rate of maltreatment of their children by their spouses rose significantly (Gibbs, Martin, Kupper, and Johnson 2007). And the rates of violence within a society tend to go up in the aftermath of war. Some of the violence involves homicides by veterans (Purdy 2008). But, for reasons unknown, the violence extends to nonveterans as well, particularly when the war is defined as illegitimate by the citizenry (Bebber 1994; Bunte, Connell, and Powell 2019). Thus, when the United States launched military operations during the 1980s, rates of murder, rape, and aggravated assault rose dramatically. However, *the increase in the rate of criminal violence occurred only in the years immediately after the four military operations.*

Another consequence of war is the increased rates of physical problems among veterans. About 1 out of every 10 living veterans was seriously injured while serving in the military (Morin 2011). Most of the injuries happened during combat. Compared to veterans who were not seriously injured, the seriously injured are more than twice as likely to report difficulty readjusting to civilian life and nearly twice as likely to say their current health is only poor to fair. Veterans of the Gulf War developed a number of persistent physical symptoms: chronic fatigue, skin rashes, muscle and joint pain, shortness of breath, headaches, and diarrhea (Clark 1994; Gray et al. 2002). And Gulf War veterans who may have been exposed to nerve agents in Iraq have elevated rates of death from brain cancer (Bullman, Mahan, Kang, and Page 2005).

Finally, the destruction of human life and well-being is affected by the threat of war as well as by war itself. *The production and storage of weapons of war are hazardous even if the weapons are never used.* Radioactive wastes from the production of nuclear weapons contaminate water and soil, posing hazards to human health (Baverstock 2005; Shrader-Frechette 2005). Arms plants in the United States have been known to routinely release large amounts of radioactive particles into the air. Some government nuclear-production facilities disposed of radioactive waste as though it were harmless; the result was the contamination of some water supplies. Even apart from carelessness, however, no nation has yet solved the problem of safely disposing of the wastes. The result is an increased risk of cancer, leukemia, and genetic damage.

## Psychological and Interpersonal Disruption and Dehumanization

*Psychological and interpersonal disruption and dehumanization* occur during and after war and terrorist attacks—both of which are disruptive for military and civilian personnel. No one escapes the trauma.

*The Trauma for Civilians.* Civilian trauma of the severest kind followed the atomic bombings of the Japanese cities of Hiroshima and Nagasaki during World War II. Hiroshima was a city accustomed to crises, having experienced periodic disastrous floods. Nevertheless, the social order of the city collapsed after the atomic bomb was dropped. The city was rebuilt mainly through the work of migrants from the hinterland rather than through the efforts of the surviving residents. The survivors

> suffered from extreme shock and fatigue that lingered for a year. . . . Demoralization was so extreme that industrial alcohol was sold as a substitute for saki; many citizens died or went blind from drinking it (Dentler and Cutright 1965:420).

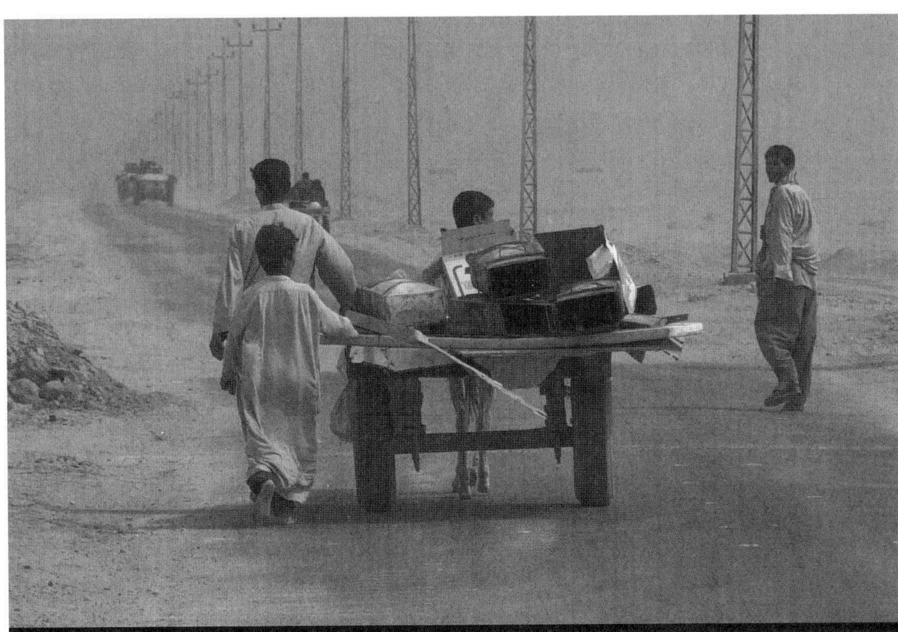

Civilians are the emotional and physical victims of war in massive numbers.

U.S. Navy photo by Photographer's Mate 1st Class Arlo K. Abrahamson

Drugs were used to escape reality. Children who survived developed a fear of becoming attached to others and of having their own children when they became adults. Crimes of violence and thefts of precious water and other scarce goods were common. Four months after the bomb had been dropped, the number of reported crimes for one month was as high as all reported crime throughout the entire war. Years later, the survivors were still not capable of leading normal, happy lives. Most of them carried a *deep sense of guilt,* including the guilt of surviving when so many had died.

Hiroshima became a city of chaos, pain, crime, anxiety, and deep-rooted fear. So many people continued to feel sick a month after the bomb fell that a rumor spread that the bomb had left a poison that would give off deadly fumes for seven years (Hersey 1946:94). Such rumors, of course, intensified the already pervasive anxiety and fear of the people and contributed to an atmosphere that drained people of the necessary psychological strength to function normally and proceed with the work of rebuilding.

The suffering need not be on the scale of Hiroshima for people to experience the emotional trauma of war. Civilians in war zones suffer emotional problems in large numbers (Cardozo, Vergara, Agani, and Golway 2000), and the problems may continue even after they are out of the war zone. Increased depression and posttraumatic stress disorder were found in a study of 124 Cambodian refugees living in Utah (Blair 2000). A team of researchers interviewed nearly a thousand Cambodians living in a refugee camp on the Thailand-Cambodia border. Many of them had witnessed the murder of a family member, had been raped, or had been physically assaulted during the civil war in their country. More than 80 percent felt depressed (with 55 percent meeting the criteria for clinical depression) and 15 percent had symptoms of posttraumatic stress syndrome (Mollica et al. 1994). Similarly, a survey of Guatemalan refugees living in Mexico 20 years after a long civil conflict in Guatemala found that the refugees had high rates of mental problems, including anxiety, depression, and posttraumatic stress disorder (Sabin et al. 2003). Widespread mental health problems not only exist among civilians who endured the war in Bosnia, but worsened among some of them as they aged (Carballo et al. 2004). Among Iranian Kurds, being exposed to chemical weapons during the Iran-Iraq war of the 1980s resulted in long-term high rates of major anxiety, severe depression, and posttraumatic stress syndrome (Hashemian et al. 2006). Finally, a national survey in Iraq found that 17 percent of the adult population suffered some kind of mental disorder, particularly depression, phobias, posttraumatic stress syndrome, and anxiety (Rubin 2009). And nearly 70 percent of those with one of the disorders said they had thoughts about suicide.

Civilians can suffer even if they are not directly exposed to conflict, because great numbers of civilians flee an oncoming battle and become refugees in another area or another country. In 2016, when the Syrian civil war raged, about 6 in 10 Syrians were displaced from their homes (Connor 2016). Worldwide, an estimated 70.8 million people were displaced from their homes as of 2019 (Stockholm international Peace Research Institute 2020). Whatever trauma a war inflicts on the civilian population, the effects are even stronger for those displaced (Shemyakina and Plagnol 2013).

*Children as well as adults are traumatized by war.* Consider, for example, what it must have been like to have been a Jewish child in a Nazi concentration camp during World War II.

Or consider what life is like for Lebanese children who have grown up in a land wracked by war and civil war. Those children who experienced the death of a family member or the forced displacement of their family, or who saw their home destroyed or someone killed, were about 1.7 times more likely than other children to be nervous or depressed and to exhibit aggressive behavior (Chimienti, Nasr, and Khalifeh 1989). Continued shelling and killing were also responsible for depression among Lebanese mothers, and their depression, in turn, was associated with the illness of their children (Bryce, Walker, Ghorayeb, and Kanj 1989). Among young people injured by shelling in 1996, half suffered some kind of impairment and 29 percent who had been enrolled in school did not continue their education (Mehio Sibai, Shaar Sameer, and el Yassir 2000).

Many children and young people in the Middle East have never experienced an extended time of peace. It is little wonder, then, that children in the Gaza Strip who have been exposed to war conflict have a high rate of emotional and behavioral problems (Thabet and Vostanis 2000). Studies of children in other war situations yield similar results (Brajs-Zganec 2005; Hoge et al. 2007).

*The Trauma for Combatants.* During the latter days of World War II, the American Air Force launched a massive air attack on German positions near Saint Lo, France. The famous war correspondent Ernie Pyle was there to record his reaction as the planes began to come:

> [T]hey came in a constant procession and I thought it would never end. . . . I've never known a storm, or a machine, or any resolve of man that had about it the aura of such a ghastly relentlessness. . . . It seems incredible to me that any German could have come out of the bombardment with his sanity. When it was over I was grateful, in a chastened way that I had never before experienced, for just being alive (Commager 1945:441, 444).

In part, because of the horror of battle, there is *a high rate of posttraumatic stress disorder, major depression, and drug abuse among veterans* (Dohrenwend et al. 2006; Eisen et al. 2012; Shen, Arkes, and Williams 2012). They may reexperience the war trauma in dreams, have recurring images and thoughts related to the trauma, feel a lack of involvement in life, experience guilt about having survived in situations in which others died, and struggle with sleep disturbances. The rates are higher, and the symptoms are more severe, among veterans who experienced combat and those who were prisoners of war (Neria et al. 2000; Wallis 2004; Solomon, Dekel, and Zerach 2008).

It is possible that the rate of traumatization among combatants is increasing. Hayman and Scaturo (1993) reported higher rates of posttraumatic stress disorder among Vietnam veterans than those reported by studies of veterans of other wars. A study of Gulf War veterans also noted rates of disability compensation two to three times higher than those of World War II, the Korean conflict, or the Vietnam War (Haley, Maddrey, and Gershenfeld 2002). There is as yet no explanation for these increasing rates.

The psychological problems vary in their severity but affect a substantial number of veterans. Among the returning troops who fought in Afghanistan or Iraq, 21.8 percent had posttraumatic stress disorder, and 17.4 percent struggled with depression (Seal et al. 2009). The rate of those with a mental health problem varied considerably depending on the number of times deployed: 12 percent after the first deployment, 19 percent after the second, and 27 percent after the third or fourth (Thompson 2008). Those who experienced combat also were at increased risk for heavy weekly drinking, binge drinking, alcohol-related health problems, and suicide (Jacobson et al. 2008; Doran et al. 2018). In addition to all these risks, women veterans who bear children also have an elevated risk of postpartum depression (Combellick 2020).

In addition to the personal distress, veterans experience a variety of interpersonal problems, including decreased satisfaction with romantic, marital, and family relationships; increased sexual dissatisfaction; higher rates of extramarital affairs; higher rates of intimate partner violence; higher rates of divorce; a diminished capacity to work once they return to civilian life; and higher rates of homelessness and suicide (MacLean 2010; Solomon, Shimrit, Zerach, and Horesh 2011; London, Allen, and Wilmoth 2013; Hoyt, Wray and Rielage 2014; Peterson et al. 2015; Department of Defense 2016; Karney and Trail 2016). Younger soldiers may be more likely than older ones to develop serious problems. A study of 57 veterans of the Vietnam War found that those who were adolescents (17 to 19 years old) at the time of their tour of duty were more likely than older soldiers to have problems of adjustment (Harmless 1990). The younger soldiers experienced later on a greater number of conflicted relationships and work problems. Finally, parents who are exposed to war tend to exhibit less warmth and more harshness toward their children which, in turn, is a factor in the emotional distress of the children as they age (Eltanamly 2021).

As we noted in Chapter 13, there is an integral relationship between physical and emotional health. Continued emotional problems will adversely affect physical health. Thus, an examination of 605 male combat veterans of World War II and the Korean War found that posttraumatic stress symptoms were associated with increased onset of various physical problems, including arterial, gastrointestinal, skin, and musculoskeletal disorders (Schnurr, Spiro, and Paris 2000).

Combatant trauma stems from more than battle conditions, however. Military personnel may be traumatized and dehumanized by their own acts. Consider, for example, some of the acts that took place during World War II, such as mass extermination of and "medical" experiments on Jews. Some of the worst acts of the war were committed in the infamous *concentration camps,* especially Dachau (Gellhorn 1959:235–42). For example, Nazi Germans wanted to know how long their pilots could survive without oxygen. At Dachau they put prisoners into a car and pumped out the oxygen. Some prisoners survived for as long as 15 minutes. Nazi Germans also wanted to see how long pilots could survive in cold water if they were shot down over the English Channel or some other body of water. Thus, prisoners were placed in vats of ice water that reached to their necks. Some subjects survived for two and a half hours. Both experiments resulted in painful deaths for all the subjects.

Inhuman punishments were meted out to prisoners at Dachau who violated such rules as standing at attention with their hats off when an SS trooper passed within six feet. Prisoners were lashed with a bullwhip, hung by bound hands from a hook, or placed in a box that prevented them from sitting, kneeling, or lying down.

Perhaps the most disquieting aspect of all was the crematorium. A reporter who was in Dachau after it had been captured by the Allies wrote her reaction on seeing piles of dead bodies:

> They were everywhere. There were piles of them inside the oven room, but the SS had not had time to burn them . . . the bodies were dumped like garbage, rotting in the sun, yellow and nothing but bones, bones grown huge because there was no flesh to cover them, hideous, terrible, agonizing bones, and the unendurable smell of death. . . . Nothing about war was ever as insanely wicked as these starved and outraged, naked, nameless dead (Gellhorn 1959:240).

Dehumanizing acts are not confined to any one people. Americans learned during the Vietnam War that they too are capable of atrocities. That war was particularly vicious for soldiers because there were no "lines" in the usual sense of the word. The enemy was everywhere and could not be distinguished from allies. Americans and some Vietnamese were fighting other Vietnamese. As we heard a Vietnam veteran put it: "After a while you get so sick of the trouble that you start killing everyone. It gets so you don't feel so bad about shooting at a six-year-old kid because the kids are throwing grenades at you." The South Koreans who fought with the Americans and South Vietnamese reportedly wiped out entire villages, including men, women, and children, when they suspected that enemy forces were present. In Iraq, American guards at Abu Ghraib prison subjected Iraqi prisoners to abuse and humiliation of a kind that enraged people throughout the Arab world and led President Bush to express a "deep disgust" and a promise to bring to justice the guards who were responsible (Roston and McAllister 2004).

Soldiers who perform such acts may have *serious psychological problems* once they reflect on what they have done. They have treated other human beings as objects, dehumanizing them, and they are appalled at their own actions. Even soldiers who do not participate in such actions may be traumatized. Just being in combat seems to bring some individuals to the point of irrationality, if not insanity. Since the time of the ancient Greeks, soldiers have succumbed to madness as a result of the horrors of combat (Gabriel 1987). Anything from fatigue to hysterical paralysis to psychosis may afflict them.

*Terrorism and Trauma.* *Terrorist acts* also generate emotional trauma (Pfefferbaum et al. 2001, 2002; Verger et al. 2004). Once attacks occur, the fear of future attacks erodes social trust, creating a kind of social unease (Godefroidt 2020). Even if there were no fear of future attacks, however, the attacks themselves are destructive to people's well-being. A number of studies of Americans after the September 11, 2001, attacks reported an increase in emotional distress, including depression (Stein et al. 2004; Knudsen, Roman, Johnson, and Ducharme 2005). Telephone interviews with 1,008 Manhattan residents between one and two months after the attacks found that 7.5 percent reported symptoms consistent with posttraumatic stress syndrome and 9.7 percent reported symptoms of depression (Galea et al. 2002). Some of these symptoms existed prior to the attacks, but the researchers were able to determine that the rate of posttraumatic stress syndrome tripled in the weeks following the attacks. Researchers have found persistent posttraumatic stress disorder and other emotional problems a decade later among those with high exposure to the terrorist attacks (Neria, DioGrande, and Adams 2011).

Other research showed an increase in smoking and in alcohol and marijuana use after the attacks (Vlahov et al. 2004), and a survey of adolescents reported a sharply increased sense of vulnerability to dying than was found among adolescents prior to the attacks (Halpern-Felsher and Millstein 2002). These negative consequences can persist for years afterward (Richman, Cloninger, and Rospenda 2008).

Studies of other nations also find various kinds of trauma resulting from exposure to terrorist acts. A survey of Jewish and Palestinian citizens in Israel found that those exposed to terrorist acts had higher rates of depression and of posttraumatic stress disorder (Hobfoll, Canetti-Nisim, and Johnson 2006). And a study of Israeli adolescents found that being exposed to terrorism significantly increased the level of violent behavior by the youth (Even-Chen and Itzhaky 2007).

## Environmental Destruction

**environmental destruction** alterations in the environment that make it less habitable or useful for people or other living things

As you will see in the next chapter, a precarious balance exists between natural resources and the growing demand for energy. *Conservation of natural resources throughout the world is essential, but there is a contradiction between this need and the willingness of people to engage in war,* because war always involves a certain amount of **environmental destruction.** The environment has been called "an invisible casualty of war" (Hynes 2011), and the increasing destructive power of weaponry has made war an ever-greater disaster for the land.

Before the war, Vietnam was the "rice bowl of Asia," but the land was so decimated by bombing that the nation had to import rice after the war. The military also sprayed millions of gallons of herbicides on fields and forests in an effort to flush out guerrillas. We do not yet know the long-term effects on the environment, but the short-term effects included serious disruption of agriculture.

The Gulf War also turned into an environmental disaster when the Iraqis dumped hundreds of millions of gallons of crude oil into the Persian Gulf and set fire to hundreds of wellheads in Kuwait. At one point, Kuwaiti officials estimated that the fires were burning 6 million gallons of oil a day, about 9 percent of the total world consumption of petroleum (Renner 1991:28). The smoke caused daytime April temperatures to drop as much as 27 degrees below normal and created severe smog as far as 1,000 miles away. Black rain (soot washed out of the air) coated people, animals, buildings, and crops with a black, oily film (Renner 1991:28).

The longer the warfare lasts, the more severe the environmental consequences. In 2001, the United States and other nations launched an attack on Afghanistan to unseat the ruling Taliban because they had harbored terrorists. The Taliban were defeated and a new government was installed within a matter of months, but the nation had already endured 23 years of wars and the warfare of opposing factions. The resulting environmental destruction has been severe (Garcia 2002). Irrigation canals were destroyed, dense forests were decimated, and a number of species of birds and mammals are close to extinction. Without the trees, the ground has eroded. Dust often hangs in the air, blocking sunlight and causing respiratory problems and other diseases.

Although much of the environmental destruction is the result of intensive bombing, the evidence suggests that such bombing contributes little to winning a war. A study of the strategic bombing of Germany during World War II concluded that at least 300,000 Germans were killed (including adults and children) and 780,000 injured; 155,546 British and American airmen also died in the assaults. Nevertheless, "the slaughter made little contribution to victory" (Wilensky 1967:25), and although the United States dropped more bombs in Vietnam than all the Allied forces dropped in World War II, the United States did not win in Vietnam.

As with other effects, it is not only wartime itself that results in environmental destruction; the years of preparation and the years following a war also have deadly consequences for the environment. Thus, it may take decades to repair the damage in nations such as Vietnam and Afghanistan. A 2002 report noted that more than half a century after the naval battles of World War II, the oil, chemicals, and unexploded ammunition on sunken ships in the Pacific still pose a serious peril to people and fisheries (Wolters Kluwer Editorial Staff 2002). Land also continues to be contaminated by materials from World War II, including land on which armaments were made. Each new war adds to the peril.

You will see in Chapter 15 that one of the serious environmental problems is that of toxic waste dumps. One of the worst polluters is the U.S. government's various weapons laboratories and assembly plants (Morain 1990). Experts estimate that it will require decades and hundreds of billions of dollars to clean up toxic wastes at federal facilities throughout the nation. At other sites, including military bases, a range of toxic wastes such as pesticides, asbestos, old fuel, chemicals, and even radioactive materials threaten the environment and pose hazards to human health and life. In fact, the hazards may be far greater than those created by bombings.

## The Economic Costs

War is *one of the greatest devourers of economic resources.* For the first two decades of the 21st century, the United States appropriated an estimated $6.4 trillion (Crawford 2019). And the War on Terror added $2.4 trillion to the total (Amadeo 2020).

Consider also the cost of stockpiling weaponry and preparing for possible wars. The lengthy arms race between the United States and the Soviet Union that lasted until 1996 cost Americans a staggering $5.5 trillion (Newman 1998). A look at military spending throughout the world (see "Global Comparison") makes it clear that an enormous amount of the world's resources is being channeled into paying for past wars and preparing for future wars.

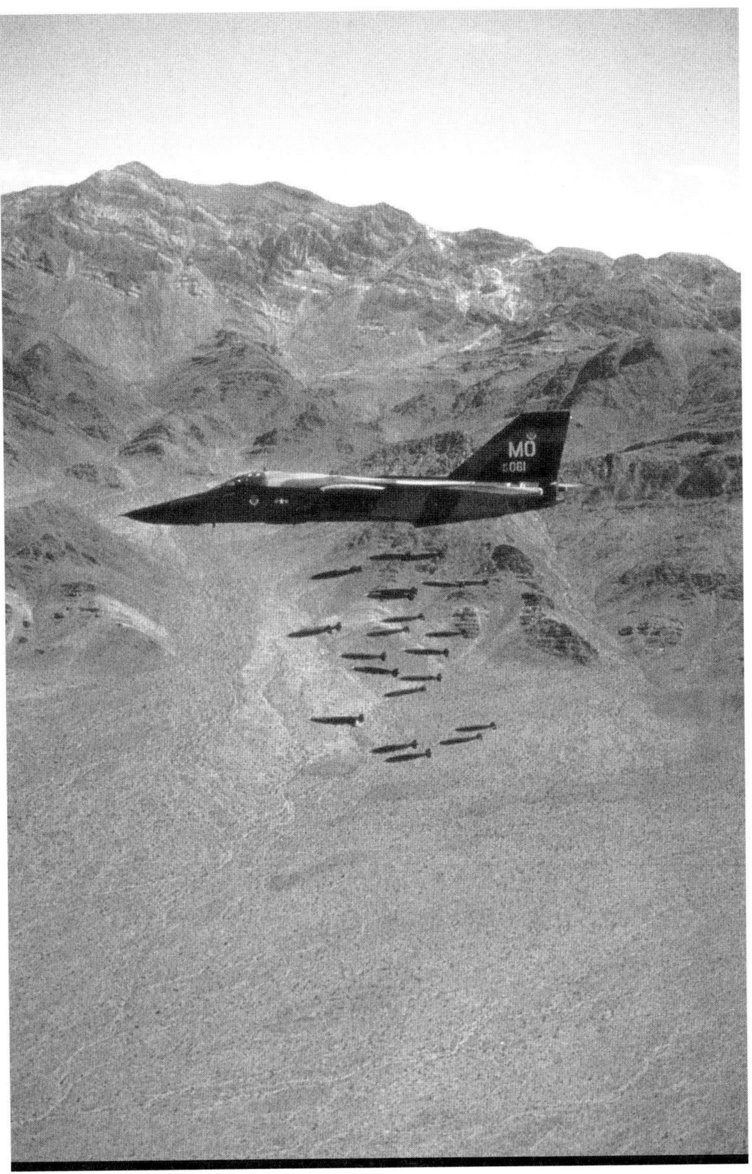


Some people argue that military spending increases the number of jobs. Others point out that the same expenditure of funds in other sectors would create far more jobs.

Purestock/SuperStock

One reason for the *high cost of preparedness* is the technological advances made in weaponry, which cost considerably more than weapons of the past (Wood 2004). Still, it is sobering to realize that the world's per capita military spending is larger than the per capita gross domestic national product of some of the poorest nations of the world. Some nations allocate more to their military than they do to health and/or education. It's all part of a frantic effort by most of the nations of the world to gain **military parity** if not military superiority.

**military parity** equality or equivalence in military strength

The economic costs are more than the money spent, of course. Indirect economic costs include the money spent to combat the emotional and physical problems resulting from war and preparations for war. Indirect costs also result from so much money being funneled into the military. It is estimated that every $1 billion spent on defense creates

8,555 jobs and adds $565 million to the economy (Amadeo 2020). But it's also estimated that if the $1 billion were given to the citizenry as a tax cut, it would raise demand for goods sufficiently to create 10,779 jobs.

What if the United States invested the billions spent on military preparedness in electronics, education, health, and other sectors that benefit human beings? What if those nations in which substantial numbers of adults are illiterate and chronically hungry invested their resources in health, education, and industrial development? What could be accomplished?

Consider first what needs to be accomplished. Each year:

- Hundreds of thousands of children become partially or totally blind because of vitamin A deficiency.
- Millions of children die of diseases that could have been prevented by relatively inexpensive immunization.
- Millions of children die before they reach the age of 5.
- Millions of children are deprived of a primary education.
- Hundreds of millions of women are illiterate.
- Hundreds of millions of people are chronically malnourished.
- More than a billion people lack access to safe drinking water.

If only a relatively small part of the billions of dollars expended every year on the military were diverted to social programs, many of these needs could be addressed. Weighing the cost of modern military equipment and personnel against nonmilitary needs can dramatize this trade-off (Military Education 2016). For example, the cost of one submarine is the same as the sum of the total annual income of 46,516 average households; plus the cost of four years of college education for 109,597 students; plus the cost of health insurance for 152,591 families; plus the cost of 10,370 new homes!

Ironically, we live in a world in which there are more soldiers than physicians per capita, a world in which military technology makes the distance between western Europe and Russia a matter of minutes while poor women in Africa must walk for hours each day just to get the family's water supply. A military mentality results in an enormous waste of resources that could be channeled into the enhancement of the quality of life of people throughout the world.

*Terrorism also has economic costs, and it has become particularly costly since September 11, 2001.* The most dramatic economic loss was the World Trade Center—about $40 billion (Friedman 2002). But the costs of terrorism involve far more than the facilities damaged or destroyed. Since September 11, 2001, governments and businesses have invested huge sums of money to increase security (Moritsugu 2001). Businesses also must bear the costs of such things as reduced revenues (because of decreased activity of consumers who may fear leaving their homes), higher insurance rates, and impeded international trade because of tighter security at borders. A survey that looked at the cost of terrorism estimated that for Standard and Poor's 500 companies alone, the direct and indirect costs are $107 billion a year for the United States (Byrnes 2006).

There is also the additional cost to the government. The Department of Homeland Security spends tens of billions of dollars each year. The money is used for a wide variety of purposes, including better screening of baggage and people at airports, more vaccines and bioterrorism antidotes, tighter border security, new bomb-detection machines, and more FBI agents. Clearly, the threat of terrorist activity has made the world as a whole, including the United States, a much different economic environment.

## War, Terrorism, and Civil Liberties

*The right of free speech* is a longstanding American value. However, there *is a contradiction between this value and the perceived need for consensus and security during a war and in the face of terrorism.* In fact, governments tend to frame the issue in such terms: We must choose between freedom and security because we cannot have a full measure of both (Donohue 2008). Davenport (1995) examined events in 57 nations over a 34-year period and found that "increasing the resources given to the army enhanced the likelihood that censorship and political restrictions would be applied by governments." These restrictions occurred in nations with democratic as well as autocratic governments.

In the United States, both citizens and government officials have participated in the suppression of civil liberties during wartime. During World War I there was mob violence against dissenters and numerous prosecutions of people who spoke out against American involvement. In the later years of the Vietnam War, there were cases of mass protests against the war, mob violence against war protestors, massive arrests of demonstrators, and resultant court cases in which the issue of civil liberties was fought.

Violations of civil liberties were less severe for most Americans during World War II, but some German Americans were imprisoned in the early days of the war, and Japanese Americans were almost totally deprived of their civil rights. In 1942, more than 100,000 Japanese Americans were relocated from their homes into detention camps in isolated areas. They had committed no crimes. There was no evidence that they supported Japan rather than America in the war, but they were defined as potential sources of subversion. Longstanding prejudice against the Japanese Americans and jealousy of their landholdings, especially on the West Coast, played into this decision. The relocations caused serious economic and psychological problems for many of the victims. The wholesale deprivation of civil liberties was upheld as legal by the U.S. Supreme Court, which ruled that the government did not have to respect traditional rights during a national emergency.

Unfortunately, if a war is considered legitimate or if terrorism is considered an imminent danger by the majority of people, they may passively or even gladly accept restrictions on their civil liberties (Davis 2007). Furthermore, their institutions, including religion and the mass media, may actively help build consensus. During the Gulf War, the mass media facilitated consensus by not informing the public of Middle Eastern history, by "the jingoistic behavior of American reporters and anchorpersons," and by biased reporting (Stires 1991). For example, just before the bombing began in January 1991, polls showed that the American public was evenly divided between using military and economic sanctions against Iraq to try to force it out of Kuwait, but a content analysis of network news programs between August 8, 1990, and January 3, 1991, reported that of 2,855 minutes of coverage of the Gulf crisis, only a little over 1 percent noted grassroots dissents from presidential policies, only 1 of 878 news sources was a peace organization, and more professional football players than peace activists were asked about their attitudes toward the war (Stires 1991:141–42).

*Terrorism poses as severe a threat to civil liberties as does war* (Lacayo 2003; Hunter 2016). Government actions following the September 11, 2001, attacks alarmed civil libertarians (Liptak, Lewis, and Weiser 2002). More than 1,200 people suspected of violating immigration laws or of being material witnesses to terrorism were detained for weeks or months without being charged. The attorney general altered federal rules to allow the monitoring of communications between inmates and their lawyers if the government believed there was a reasonable suspicion of terrorist information. The government considered trying suspected terrorists by military tribunals rather than in the courts.

## MILITARISM: "A WORLD GONE INSANE"

We were discussing the problem of war in a social problems class, focusing on the militarism of American society. A student objected: "Let's not make this an American problem. It's a *world* problem. Even the poorest nations are spending their resources on the military. We live in a world gone insane with arms."

He was right. Militarism is not a problem of any single nation but of the entire world. From the poorest to the richest of nations, military expenditures are consuming resources that could be used to enhance the quality of life of the citizenry.

In 2019 military expenditures of the nations of the world totaled an estimated $1.92 trillion (Stockholm International Peace Research Institute 2020). The United States was by far the biggest spender—38.2 percent of the world total. By contrast, China, which ranked second in terms of total military spending, accounted for 13.6 percent of the total. After China, the top military spenders were Russia, Saudi Arabia, France, and the United Kingdom.

Those who defend the amount the United States spends on the military point out that the expenditures are necessary and that as the richest country in the world we can afford them. Whether they are necessary is a matter of considerable debate. Whether we, or other nations, can afford them must be examined in light of both the total amount (imagine what those enormous sums could do for such things as health care, education, and the infrastructure) and of the proportion of the nation's gross domestic product consumed by military spending.

When we look at the proportion of the gross domestic product represented by military spending (see Figure 14.1), the United States is not at the top of the list. There are eight nations that spend a larger proportion (Central Intelligence Agency 2016). And the nation that spent the highest proportion in recent years is also one of the poorer nations—South Sudan's military spending was 10.3 percent of its gross domestic product.

Of course, whether a nation can "afford" its military expenditures is a matter of values. But one measure of well-being in a nation is the infant mortality rate (number of deaths of children under five years of age per 1,000 live births in a given year). Higher rates typically reflect poverty and inadequate health care. For 2018, the infant mortality rate in the United States was 7 per 1,000 live births. Compare that with the rates in some nations that are considerably poorer than the United States but that spend a higher proportion of their GDP on the military: Jordan, 16; Algeria, 23; Iraq, 27; South Sudan, 99 (World

Within weeks of the attack, Congress passed what the attorney general called the "Patriot Act," which gave officials nearly unprecedented peacetime authority to "nullify the constitutional rights of individual citizens" (Van Deerlin 2003). And the administration created the Department of Homeland Security, which is responsible for preventing terrorist attacks and reducing the nation's vulnerability to terrorism. The department must gather information on citizens to fulfill its mandate. Invasive surveillance measures by government agents increased immediately after September 11 (Gould 2002). They continued under the Patriot Act and the department. And the fears of civil libertarians seemed to be justified because the Patriot Act was used by prosecutors to deal with people charged with common crimes (Caruso 2003). The Patriot Act expired in 2015, and was replaced by the USA Freedom Act, which modified some of the Patriot Act's provisions and allowed many of the questionable practices to continue.

In 2005, news broke that President Bush had authorized domestic spying by the National Security Agency without court approval (Condon 2005). The president defended the need for such spying (including such things as eavesdropping on telephone calls and

Health Organization 2018). Improvements in infant mortality rates and other health matters, in educational opportunities, and in other economic benefits cannot be implemented when military spending consumes so much of a nation's resources, a situation that one of our students called "a world gone insane with arms."

Not to be overlooked in this is the fact that the United States is also one of the world's leading suppliers of arms. As Table 14.2 shows, the total amount of arms sales to other nations has fluctuated since 1995, but more often than not has remained in excess of $1 trillion.

| Year | Total Amount (millions of dollars) |
|---|---|
| 1995 | $12,100 |
| 1996 | 11,710 |
| 1997 | 15,663 |
| 1998 | 13,179 |
| 1999 | 16,888 |
| 2000 | 10,436 |
| 2001 | 12,001 |
| 2002 | 10,240 |
| 2003 | 9,315 |
| 2004 | 10,681 |
| 2005 | 10,985 |
| 2010 | 8,098 |
| 2020 | 17,000 |

**TABLE 14.2**
U.S. Military Sales Deliveries to Other Countries

SOURCES: U.S. Census Bureau website; Stockholm International Peace Research Institute website.

e-mail between the United States and other nations) and called the leaking of the program a "shameful act." Had the news not leaked out, the spying would have probably continued. But after resisting the critics for some time the president relented and declared in early 2007 that the government would disband the warrantless surveillance program and that future spying would be overseen by the secret court that governs clandestine spying in the nation.

Not everyone is concerned about the violations of civil liberties that have occurred since 2001. In fact, some observers argue that Americans face a trade-off. As one jurist put it, "it stands to reason that our civil liberties will be curtailed. They *should* be curtailed to the extent that the benefits in greater security outweigh the costs in reduced liberty" (Posner 2001:46). And, in fact, many Americans agree. The greater the perceived threat of terrorism, the more people are willing to give up civil liberties in order to gain more security (Davis and Silver 2004).

For civil libertarians, this argument is the *fallacy of non sequitur.* To say that Americans need increased security does not mean that the government must necessarily curb

fallacy

traditional civil liberties. As the American Civil Liberties Union (2002) argued, without civil rights and privacy protections, "What's to stop the Department [of Homeland Security] from abusing the very citizens it is responsible for protecting?"

Undoubtedly the debate will continue. The extent to which civil liberties are curtailed by the effort to deal with terrorism remains to be seen.

## Contributing Factors

War and terrorism are complex phenomena. Some thinkers have tried to make them, like violence, a simple outgrowth of a *human need for aggression.* Yet, like aggression and violence, they are linked with *cultural values and patterns.* Some societies, for example, have no notions of organized warfare. The Hopi Indians traditionally had no place for offensive warfare and did not idealize the warrior as did other tribes. Furthermore, the Hopi conceived of the universe as a harmonious whole, with gods, nature, people, animals, and plants all working together for their common well-being.

Why do people support wars? In particular, why do they support wars in view of the consequences we have described? Why do people support terrorism? What makes a terrorist willing to commit suicide in order to hurt or kill civilians? In the following sections, we examine various factors that help answer these vexing questions.

### Social Structural Factors

*The Economics of War and Terrorism.* The idea that wars have an *economic cause* is an ancient one. The Greek philosophers Plato and Aristotle both argued that economic factors are fundamental in the outbreak of war. Plato believed that the quest for unlimited wealth brings on not only war but a number of other human problems. Aristotle saw economic competition as the root of wars. In particular, poverty is the "parent" of both revolution and crime. The same economic inequality that leads to revolution within a nation results in wars between nations.

**Marxist**
pertaining to the system of thought developed by Karl Marx and Friedrich Engels, particularly emphasizing materialism, class struggle, and the progress of humanity toward communism

Marxists also argue that war has an economic basis. The **Marxist** view is that war is a *mechanism for maintaining inequalities* in a struggle for control of raw materials and markets. The inequalities are necessary because capitalism requires an ever-expanding market to endure. Warfare is one way to ensure that a nation will have control over adequate resources and an expanding market. Consequently, war is an inevitable outcome of capitalism.

Although the Marxist explanation of war is debatable, economic factors are probably always at work in war and in preparations for war, including civil wars (Cunningham and Lemke 2014; Goodman 2020). High military budgets mean considerable profits to a number of industries, offering them literally hundreds of billions of dollars in military prime contracts. With such funds at stake, it is not surprising that there are intense lobbying efforts in Congress to maintain and even increase military expenditures. One way that members of Congress can pump money into their districts or states is to maintain a military presence (in the form of a base) or secure military contracts for local industries. The military presence may no longer be needed and the military contracts may be wasteful, but the economic benefits to the district or state outweigh such considerations.

Economic factors are also at work in civil wars and terrorism. Some nations experience sharp economic inequality between racial, ethnic, or religious groups. *These racial, ethnic, or religious divisions may form the basis for civil war or terrorist activities* (Bonneuil and Auriat 2000; Reynal-Querol 2002).

A prime example is the Palestinian suicide bombers in Israel (Ratnesar 2002). Between 2000 and 2002, more than 70 bomb attacks or suicide bombings killed or injured hundreds of civilians. Although even some top leaders of the Palestinians have condemned the bombings, the majority of Palestinians defend the killing of Israeli citizens on the grounds that Palestinians are killed by Israeli troops.

Why do the majority of Palestinians defend what many people in the world community denounce as terrorism? They do so because these terrorist activities have developed in a context of what a United Nations human rights official has called daily experiences of discrimination, inequality, and powerlessness. Palestinians have lost land, work opportunities, freedom of movement, and access to water. The ongoing cycle of violence and retaliation between Palestinians and Israelis has greatly increased Palestinian poverty. After 2006, a political and economic boycott of the elected Palestinian administration increased unemployment, poverty, and conflict and also made access to health care more restrictive (Rahim et al. 2009). By 2014, according to a World Bank (2014) report, unemployment in the Palestinian territories was 26.3 percent, and about a fourth of the population was living in poverty. The cycle of violence and the cycle of increasing inequality have fed on each other.

*The Politics of War: Militarism.* From a political point of view, there are advantages to both militarism and war. The presence of a foreign threat, whether real or fabricated by politicians, can create cohesion within a society, including support for both domestic and foreign policies that might otherwise be resisted. One important source of unity in American foreign policy has been the support of both Republicans and Democrats for anticommunist policies.

In the international arena, a strong military gives a nation higher status and more power. The nuclear arsenal of the United States, for example, is a "big stick" that can be used to facilitate the nation's diplomatic efforts and economic trade relations with its allies as well as its enemies. Some observers see this as necessary and proper in order to spread democracy in the world. Others see American foreign policy over the last century or so (including the 2003 war on Iraq) as an expression of imperialism. Chalmers Johnson (2004) argued that the nation has been on a steady path to imperialism, building an empire not through colonies but by establishing military bases throughout the world–there are around 800 U.S. bases outside the nation's borders. Imperialism is manifest in such things as the justification of interference in the affairs of other nations (including the overthrow of governments that are said to be hostile to our interests) and of preemptive war (Walt 2005).

Militarism is seen not only in foreign policy, but also in the resources allocated to defense. Some defend the defense budget on the basis that it has consumed an increasingly smaller proportion of the total federal budget. Yet the U.S. military budget is vastly higher than that of any other nation. In fact, it is close to half of all military spending in the world. As a proportion of the gross domestic product, however, the U.S. budget is not the highest but is still about 60 percent higher than that of the world average (Figure 14.1). Moreover, through arms sales the United States, along with Britain, France, Russia, and China, is contributing to the high level of weaponry throughout the world. Two-thirds of arms sales are to developing nations, which desperately need their resources for social, educational, and health programs (Grimmett 2006).

Why is an arms buildup, or the maintenance of high levels of arms, in other nations of concern? When the communist governments in Eastern Europe fell during the 1990s and the United States and Russia engaged in an arms limitation agreement in 1990, a

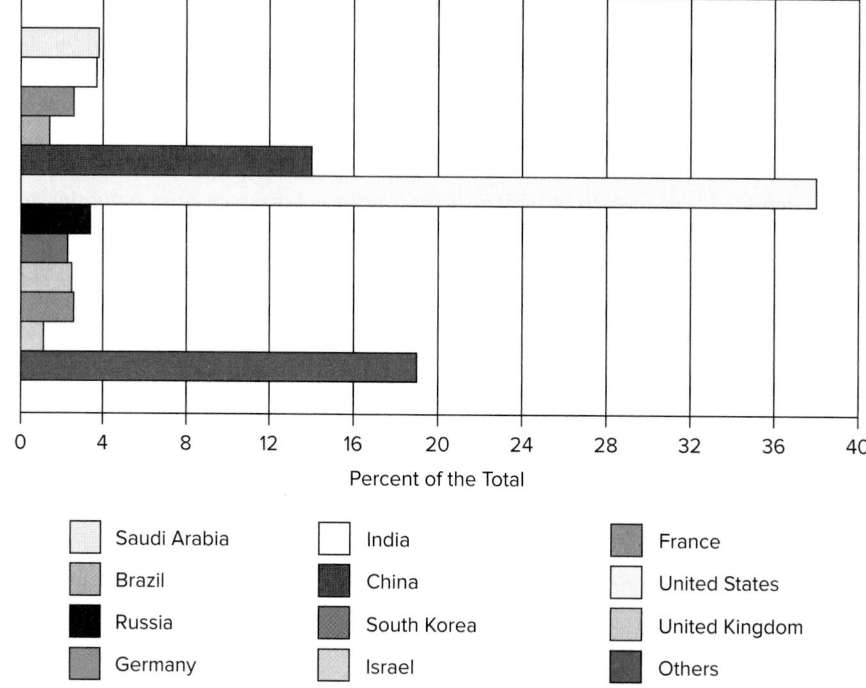


**FIGURE 14.1**
Share of Military Expenditures, 2019, by Country.
Source: Stockholm International Peace Research Institute website.

new era of peace appeared to be at hand. Wars and civil conflicts continued in various parts of the world, but there seemed little likelihood of a world war breaking out. Since 2001, however, peace once again appears to be precarious. The U.S. wars against Afghanistan and Iraq have angered many Muslims throughout the world. Anti-American sentiment worldwide is at a high level (Fuller 2011). And it is particularly high in predominantly Muslim nations (Stokes 2014).

In addition, a number of nations continue to build up their weaponry. Iran and North Korea, neither of which is friendly to the United States or the West in general, are working hard to build new biological, chemical, and nuclear weapons along with long-range missiles. In short, militarism is flourishing throughout the world.

*The Politics of Terrorism: Autonomy.* Throughout the world are groups who both desire and lack political autonomy—the right of people to govern their own affairs. Generally, when people press for autonomy, they believe that their interests are not adequately represented (or are even ignored) by the current government. Indeed, the United States became a nation under such circumstances.

The lack of political autonomy is a major factor in terrorism. For example, much bloodshed occurred in the struggle by East Timor to gain independence from Indonesia and the attempt by Yugoslavia to suppress the political autonomy of Kosovo. East Timor was finally granted the right to govern itself, and the Yugoslav Republic broke apart when U.N. forces took military action to stop the political oppression of minorities.

The early years of the 21st century are rife with examples of the struggle for political autonomy, including:

- Terrorist acts arising from the dispute between India and Pakistan over Kashmir, and the desire of Kashmir to be independent.
- The Chechnyan revolt against Russia.

- Terrorist acts by Palestinians who want to be free of Israeli control.
- Terrorist acts by the Irish who want Northern Ireland to be free of English control.
- Basque separatists' terrorist acts against Spain.
- Terrorist acts by Islamic extremists who want the Muslim world to be free of all influence and control by the West.

A careful analysis of every suicide terrorist attack in the world from 1980 through the early 2000s concludes that suicide bombers are not primarily the result of Islamic fundamentalism (Pape 2005). The great bulk of suicide bombings take place in the context of campaigns that strive to get rid of foreign military forces from territory that the terrorists regard as their own. Moreover, contrary to assumptions, suicide bombers are not impoverished, uneducated religious fanatics, but more often are educated, middle-class political activists.

In support of these conclusions, Pape notes such things as the fact that prior to Israel's invasion of Lebanon in 1982 there was no Hezbollah suicide campaign against Israel. Nor were there any suicide attacks in Iraq until after the American invasion in 2003. Other observers agree that suicide bombers are driven primarily by the conviction that only through such desperate tactics as killing themselves in order to kill and instill fear into the enemy can their people achieve the political ends that are needed for their well-being (Brym 2007).

Sometimes governments get involved in helping terrorists—providing such things as sanctuary, personnel, weapons, and economic aid—with whose cause they sympathize. According to the U.S. Department of State (2019), Iran, North Korea, Syria, and Cuba are *state sponsors of terrorism*. This means that these countries have repeatedly provided support for acts of international terrorism through such means as training, arms, and giving shelter for individual terrorists and terrorist groups. But there is also a cluster of independent, cell-based units that do not rely on particular states for their support (Benjamin and Simon 2005). Instead, terrorist groups use various methods to gain financial support for their activities, including "charities" and illegal enterprises such as drugs, extortion, and kidnapping (Perl 2006).

## Social Psychological Factors

*Attitudes.* Militarism and war are legitimated by a number of attitudes. The concept of a "just war" has a long history in the West. A just war is one that meets a number of tests, such as whether it has a just cause and whether all peaceful alternatives have been exhausted. If the war is just, the people are expected to support it fully. Shortly before the 1991 war against Iraq, some religious leaders questioned whether the notion of a just war is still valid in the face of the awful destructiveness of modern weapons (Day 1991). Indeed, Stires (1991) called the subsequent war against Iraq a "sanctioned massacre" because of the way in which the U.S. military technology overwhelmed the Iraqi forces. In spite of disparities in the military technology of nations and the incredible destructiveness of modern weapons, most people accept the notion that at least some wars are just.

The attitude that the United States has a mission to be "number one" in the world helps the country justify militarism. National pride is involved in attaining a place of military superiority. Gibson (1994) has argued that this need for being a "winner" facilitated U.S. involvement in Grenada, Panama, and the Persian Gulf. These military actions reflected the American dream of "redeeming Vietnam and recovering from all

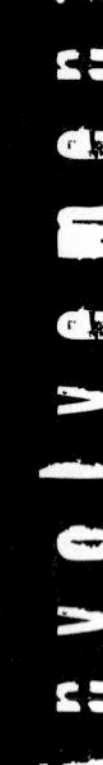

## "WHAT A GREAT WAR THAT WAS"

A friend of ours served as a navigator in the Air Force during World War II. "Those," he says "were some of the best days of my life." He recalls his days in the military as a time of adventure. He does not desire war, but neither does he think of it in terms of the detrimental consequences discussed in this chapter.

Interview a number of armed forces veterans. If possible, find veterans who served in different wars, and include some who did have combat experience as well as some who did not. How do they describe the experience of war? Do they mention any of the consequences discussed in this chapter? Would they be willing to serve in another war or to have their children serve? Note any differences based on service in different wars or on combat versus noncombat experience. If everyone felt as your respondents did, would the probability of future wars be greater or less?

the other disappointments and traumas of the late 1960s and 1970s" (Gibson 1994:269). After the Gulf War in particular, Americans purchased a spate of military-type items: commemorative handguns, rifles, knives, and T-shirts and uniforms. Many of those who made the purchases were celebrating the restoration of the nation as the supreme military power of the world.

*International misperception* is a set of attitudes that legitimate both militarism and war. In a classic analysis, White (1966) identified six forms of misperceptions that recur in cases of international wars:

1. The *diabolical-enemy image* imputes flagrant evil to the enemy, who is conceived to be thoroughly criminal in behavior. In 2002, when President Bush urged new action against Iraq, he said that the Iraqi regime not only raped women to intimidate them but also tortured dissenters and their children and that President Saddam Hussein was a "dangerous and brutal man" who sought to acquire the destructive technologies that matched his hatred (Kozaryn 2002). Ironically, portraying the enemy as diabolically cruel can justify using the same behavior against the enemy (Dutton, Boyanowsky, and Bond 2005). Thus, Americans tortured captured terrorists with little, if any, question being raised about the moral or legal legitimacy of the practice (Shane and Mazzetti 2009).
2. The *virile self-image* implies preoccupation with one's strength and courage and the need to avoid humiliation by determined fighting.
3. The *moral self-image* affirms the nation's goodness; Americans are the people of God and the enemy is of the devil. This attitude is the *fallacy of personal attack* and ignores the fact that among the enemy are many innocent, decent people who also are victims of the struggle between the nations.

fallacy

4. *Selective inattention* means that only the worst aspects of the enemy are noticed; at the same time Americans attend to the best aspects of themselves, reinforcing the idea of the war as a conflict between black and white, good and evil.
5. *Absence of empathy* means the inability to understand how the situation looks from the other's viewpoint. An American might wonder, for example, how any German could fight on behalf of Hitler, or how any South Vietnamese could not welcome the American effort to save Vietnam from communism. People on both sides of

a war fail to understand how the war could be justified by those on the other side. In the 1991 war against Iraq, Americans denied their contribution to the problem (later reports indicated that the United States had assured the Iraqis it would not interfere if they invaded Kuwait, and it had built up the Iraqi forces during the 1980s) and placed the blame totally on Iraq's shoulders.

6. *Military overconfidence* refers to the conviction that our side can win. In the case of the 1991 war against Iraq, the Iraqi leaders boasted (and no doubt believed to some extent) that the enemy would be soundly and humiliatingly defeated. Similarly, top American political leaders predicted that the 2003 war against Iraq would be swift, would result in a decisive victory for the United States, and would establish democracy in that nation.

These attitudes can be found on both sides of a conflict and are encouraged by the opposing leaders. For decades, American leaders portrayed the Soviet Union as an evil empire that threatened the nation's fundamental (and righteous) values. On the other hand, *Pravda,* the Soviet Communist Party's daily newspaper, discussed attempts at arms control with the United States in terms of dealing with "militaristic ambitions," "hotheads in the Pentagon," and "insane anti-logic" (Lichter, Lichter, Amundson, and Fowler 1987:12).

Misperceptions were also at work in the 2003 war against Iraq (Kull, Ramsay, and Lewis 2003). Many Americans accepted the notion that Iraq was involved in the September 11, 2001, terrorist attacks, that Iraq had developed and was prepared to use weapons of mass destruction, and that a good part, if not most, of world opinion favored the American position. The news media, particularly Fox News, helped shape these misperceptions. People who watched Fox network were three times more likely to hold those misperceptions than were people who watched other networks. Misperceptions were also fostered among the Iraqi people. They were told that the United States was the "Satan" of the world and that American forces would be soundly defeated if they invaded Iraqi soil.

In any confrontation between nations, the perceptions on both sides are remarkably similar, and people will support war to the extent that they accept such attitudes. Because both sides have the same attitudes, the attitudes obviously cannot be realistic. Nevertheless, they have typically been defined as valid and have served to legitimate international violence.

We noted earlier in this chapter that the majority of Palestinians support the suicide bombers and other acts of terror against Israel. Even though most Muslim leaders (both religious and political) condemn terrorism, the people take the attitude that the terrorists are only acting in defense of the Palestinian people and are doing nothing worse than what is being done to them.

Other terrorists also justify their actions on the grounds that they are really defending rights and seeking the well-being of the oppressed. They may also believe that change is nonexistent or too slow and that attention needs to be called to their cause (Jacobs 2001).

*War, Terrorism, and Ideology.* *Ideologies* support militarism and war. In particular, Bacevich (2010) has identified an ideology about national security to which every president since 1945 has subscribed. The ideology consists of four assertions. First, the world needs to avoid chaos through order. Second, only the United States has the necessary power and resources to create and maintain global order. Third, only the United States is capable of identifying the principles (which, of course, are American principles) that are valid for a proper global order. Fourth, most of the world understands and accepts this role for the United States. Such an ideology, Bacevich argues, is why the United States repeatedly has gotten, and will continue to get, involved in wars.

This ideology was a part of the rationale for initiating the war against Iraq in 1991. It was necessary, Americans were told, for the United States to take steps to protect the world against dictators like Saddam Hussein. Of course, the ideology is used selectively. In other situations in which dictators and totalitarian governments have initiated action against another country or against a segment of their own country, the United States has responded only with moral support or arms. In Iraq, however, the ideology was used to justify a massive assault.

The Islamic extremists who resort to terrorism use a fundamentalist interpretation of the Koran to help motivate their followers (Del Castillo 2001; Hassan 2001). They represent what one researcher called "political Islam" rather than "personal religiosity" (Haddad 2003). For them, religion and politics are intertwined and inseparable. Their ideology includes a rejection of Western culture, a belief in Islamic law as a basis for the state, and the assertion that believers who are martyred in the cause of pursuing those aims are ensured entrance to eternal paradise. Many of the extremists received their education in fundamentalist religious schools, where they learned only a particular interpretation of the Koran and little that was modern except for the use of armaments. Women and girls as well as men and boys are recruited to be suicide bombers. A study of suicide bombers in the Boko Haram movement in Africa found that more than half the bombers were women or girls, some as young as the age of 7 (Markovic 2019).

## Solutions: Public Policy and Private Action

Inequalities of wealth and power among nations and between groups within nations, political and ideological conflicts, and economic factors all contribute to the likelihood of war and terrorism. An important step toward solving the problem would be to negotiate treaties that reduced the weaponry and armaments in the world. Current stockpiles, which are more than sufficient to eradicate life on the earth, need to be cut back. Military spending must be reduced. The sale of weapons of mass destruction is not an acceptable way to boost the supplier nation's economy. The massive number of weapons in the world also aids the cause of terrorists, who are able to secure sufficient arms to carry out their attacks.

Nations that thwart the effort to reduce arms or that abet terrorism can be subjected to economic sanctions through the United Nations. Such sanctions should be used judiciously. They eventually worked against Libya, which seems to have withdrawn from the ranks of those countries that sponsor terrorism (Collins 2004). Sanctions did not work to overthrow the Iraqi regime of Saddam Hussein, however. The main outcome of the sanctions was "enormous human suffering, including massive increases of child mortality and widespread epidemics" (Gordon 2002:44).

One problem with fighting terrorism is the sophisticated and strong financial infrastructure of some groups (Basile 2004). Terrorists have the economic resources they need to train their people, purchase arms, and pay the expenses needed to carry out their missions. International cooperation will be necessary to break up the financial base of terrorism because it is rooted in both legitimate and illegitimate businesses and charities and it transfers money around the world through poorly regulated banking networks.

Although the United States has tried to take the lead in committing the world's nations to a concerted fight against terrorism, cooperation will be difficult because of unilateral actions the country has taken in the name of its own interests (Cameron 2002). The 1989 Convention on the Rights of the Child was ratified by every nation except Somalia and the United States. The Comprehensive Test Ban Treaty of 1996 to halt nuclear testing and the development of new nuclear weapons was ratified by all the NATO nations and Russia but rejected by the United States. The United States rejected the Ottawa Treaty to Ban Landmines, while 142 other countries approved it. In 2002, the Bush administration gave notice that the United States was pulling out of the 1972 Anti-Ballistic Missile Treaty, which limited the testing and deployment of antimissile weapons. A day later, Russia announced that it was no longer bound by the 1993 START II agreement, which outlawed multiple-warhead missiles and other weapons in the strategic arsenals of the two nations. The Trump administration further hurt the chances for arms reduction by criticizing and withdrawing from a number of treaties without offering anything to replace them (Larison 2020).

In essence, U.S. foreign policy in recent decades reflects more a determination to protect what political leaders define as the nation's self-interest (defined, in part at least, in terms of the international misperceptions described earlier) than a desire to be a leader in the construction of world peace. It is questionable how long the nation can continue to press for cooperation in fighting terrorism while asserting its right to take unilateral action on other issues whenever it pleases.

The United States also needs to stop the ongoing sale of arms to nations throughout the world. Armaments may simply be a symptom of deep conflicts between people, but curbing the availability of arms is still crucial for three reasons. First, arms proliferation tends to gain a momentum of its own; no nation is satisfied with just being equal to others but wants an advantage over its enemies or potential enemies.

Second, if arms are readily available, nations will more likely rely on them than on diplomacy and negotiations to settle their disputes (recall that in Chapter 4 we noted that the availability of a weapon makes it more likely that it will be used). Third, when arms are readily available, the ensuing hostilities are likely to be far more devastating

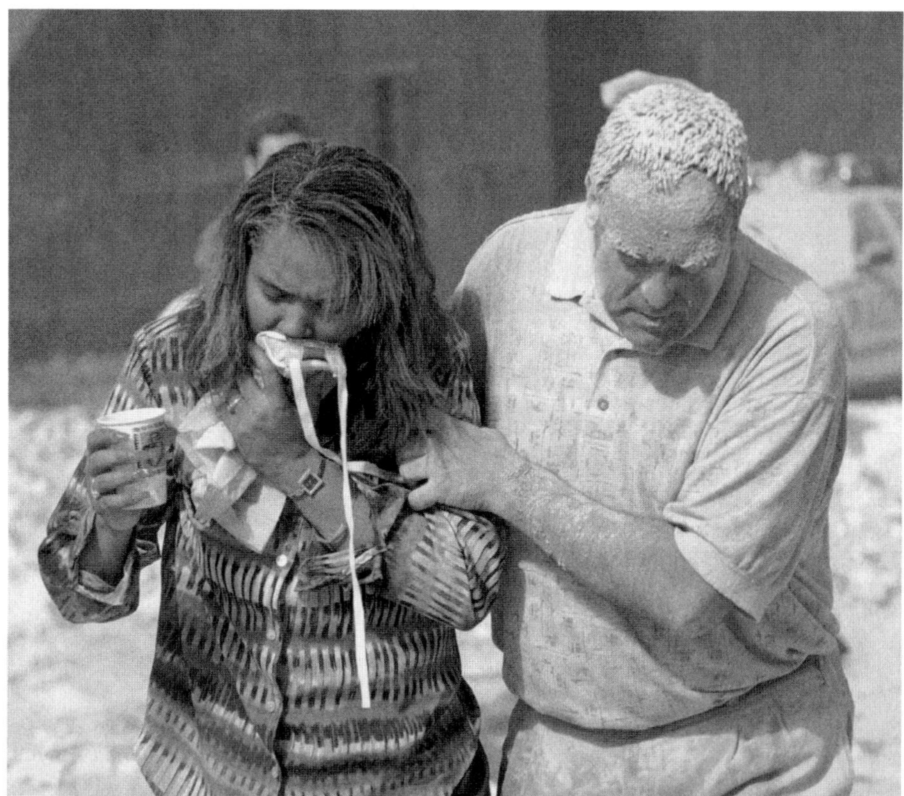

Innocent bystanders are the main victims of terrorist attacks.

Library of Congress Prints and Photographs Division [LC-DIG-ppmsca-01813]

than they would be otherwise. For instance, the United States and the Soviet Union both shipped large amounts of arms to Somalia during the Cold War, each trying to lure the country into its sphere of influence. After the Cold War ended, a civil war broke out in Somalia in 1991, decimating the country and turning it into a nightmare of heavily armed, competing factions.

Of course, it is risky for any nation to demilitarize unless its potential adversary does the same, but there is some evidence to suggest that the risk is minimal. In the process called *Graduated Reciprocation in Tension-Reduction* (GRIT), one nation initiates an action that visibly reduces the way it threatens the other nation without at the same time endangering its own security. The action is an invitation to the other side to reciprocate (Elms 1972). Will such reciprocation occur? Following the 1962 Cuban missile crisis, President John F. Kennedy announced that the United States would stop atmospheric nuclear tests and would resume them only if another country's action compelled it to do so. The next day the Soviet Union agreed to a Western-backed proposal in the United Nations to send observers to Yemen (a proposal the Soviets had been blocking). America reciprocated by agreeing to restore the Hungarian delegation to full status in the United Nations. A few days later Khrushchev announced that Russia would stop producing strategic bombers. Shortly thereafter the "hot line" between the White House and the Kremlin was installed. This series of concessions was the result of each side taking a step that led the other to reciprocate.

Subsequently, Soviet President Gorbachev initiated a number of efforts to reduce tensions and to engage in arms reductions. The United States responded to each effort positively. Neither nation used concessions by the other as an opportunity to attack or even to gain an advantage by further buildup.

In contrast, the reverse process occurred in the Israeli-Palestinian conflict. Each side believed it had the right to—indeed, that it *must*—retaliate against the other after each attack. Clearly, such a process has no end (Brym and Araj 2006). There can be a graduated reciprocation in tension building as well as in tension reduction.

In addition to a halt to unilateral action and the breaking of international agreements, and to actively working to reduce arms and demilitarize the world, there is a need in the United States for changed attitudes and ideologies. More contact between peoples—cultural, educational, and political contact—could alter some of the misperceptions that abound in the world. Education should include an international perspective, so that Americans become increasingly aware of the smallness of the world and of the similarities among human beings everywhere. Instead of viewing other countries as adversaries or as problems, Americans should view them as partners working together on common problems. If the United States strives to be a world leader, let it be a leader in peace and in promoting the well-being of people rather than a leader who uses strength for pursuing self-interest.

The effort to avoid war and terrorism and to reduce the costs of preparing for war entails a great deal of work and frustration, but the alternatives to making the effort are grim. A noted man of peace, Martin Luther King Jr., put it this way:

> In a day when sputniks dash through outer space and guided ballistic missiles are carving highways of death through the stratosphere, nobody can win a war. The choice today is no longer between violence and nonviolence. It is either nonviolence or nonexistence (quoted in Weinberg and Weinberg 1963:74).

*Follow-Up.* What kind of measures would you like to see become a matter of public policy to maximize your own protection from terrorist attacks?

## Summary

Americans are greatly concerned about war and terrorism. Warfare is no longer just a matter of opposing armies on the battlefield, but increasingly involves civil wars and terrorist activities.

War diminishes the quality of life of people and destroys the lives of many. From the Civil War to the present, nearly a million American military personnel have died as a result of wars. And nearly 1.5 million more have been wounded. During the 20th century, the bloodiest of all centuries, wars killed more than a hundred million people. War and terrorism cause psychological disruption and dehumanization of everyone involved. As illustrated by posttraumatic stress disorder, the effects last after the war or terrorist act is over. Much environmental destruction is involved. The economic costs of war, of preparation for possible wars, and of terrorism are staggering. The costs of fighting war and stopping terrorism inevitably mean that certain social needs will be neglected. War and terrorism always pose a threat to civil liberties, as illustrated by sanctions against dissenters and the detention of Japanese Americans in isolated camps during World War II and measures taken by the U.S. government after the September 11, 2001, attacks.

Social structural and social psychological factors help bring about war and terrorist activities and motivate people to support them. Economic factors are involved in wars and terrorism. Military spending is highly profitable to some industries, and people who profit from such spending tend to exercise considerable power in the government. Severe economic inequality between racial, ethnic, or religious groups within nations can give rise to civil war or terrorism.

Militarism is a political factor that can lead to war. The military influence in America is strong. The military, the government, and the corporations have some shared interests. This military-industrial-governmental linkage tends to maintain high levels of defense spending. Arms races tend to be self-perpetuating because each side views developments of the other with alarm and responds with its own efforts, which then become the stimuli to the other side to make further advances.

The desire for autonomy is a political factor in terrorism. People everywhere want the right to govern themselves and may assert that right through civil war or terrorist activities when they believe their interests are not represented in the government.

A number of attitudes justify war and terrorism, including the notion of a just war, the idea that Americans have a mission to be number one in the world, the set of attitudes called "international misperception" held by people on both sides of a potential conflict, and the belief that terrorist acts are a necessary form of self-defense. Finally, the ideology that Americans must protect national security by taking responsibility for creating and maintaining a global order that is consistent with American ideals supports militarism and war, and Islamic extremists use a religion-based ideology to justify terrorist acts.

## Key Terms

Environmental Destruction
International Terrorism
Marxist
Military Parity
War

## Study Questions

1. How extensive is the problem of war and terrorism?
2. How has the amount of human destruction and injury during war changed over time?
3. What is meant by "psychological and interpersonal disruption and dehumanization" as a consequence of war and terrorism?
4. What effects does the problem have on the environment?
5. What are the economic costs?
6. How do war and terrorism affect civil liberties?
7. How do economic factors enter into war and terrorism?
8. What kinds of political factors contribute to the problem?
9. What attitudes and ideologies legitimate wars and terrorism?
10. What steps could be taken to diminish the possibility of war and terrorist acts?

## Internet Resources/Exercises

1. Explore some of the ideas in this chapter on the following sites:

**https://library.bu.edu/security/thinktanks** The International Terrorism and Security Research site has news, essays, and links to other sites that deal with terrorism throughout the world.

**http://www.fbi.gov** The FBI site features the latest news and information about terrorist activities.

**http://www.iwpr.net** The Institute for War and Peace Reporting site has news about conflicts throughout the world.

2. Go to the site of the Institute for War and Peace Reporting. Summarize the various wars and armed conflicts currently reported there. Where are the trouble spots in the world? What are the more common kinds of conflicts–wars between nations or civil wars? What materials in the text could you use to help understand the reasons for the conflicts?

3. Search the Internet for a particular aspect of terrorism, such as the history of terrorism, terrorism in the United States, the war on terrorism, or terrorist groups. Make a report to the class showing how your findings fit in with, or modify, the text materials.



## For Further Reading

Cole, David, and James X. Dempsey. *Terrorism and the Constitution: Sacrificing Civil Liberties in the Name of National Security.* 2nd ed. Washington, DC: First Amendment Foundation, 2002. Two constitutional scholars show how civil liberties are threatened by the government's response to real or perceived threats, from the communists of the 1950s to the Islamic terrorists of the 21st century.

Grynberg, Michal, ed. *Words to Outlive Us: Eyewitness Accounts from the Warsaw Ghetto.* New York: Henry Holt, 2002. Detailed accounts from individual diaries, journals, and other writings show life in the Jewish community from the first bombardments of the capital to the razing of the Jewish ghetto. The struggles, deprivations, and suffering are graphically portrayed in these previously unpublished accounts.

Harwayne, Shelley. *Messages to Ground Zero: Children Respond to September 11, 2001.* Portsmouth, NH: Heinemann, 2002. A compilation of poems, drawings, and essays that illustrate children's reactions to the terrorist attacks, ranging from admiration for the heroic rescuers to personal feelings of anxiety and grief.

Honigsberg, Peter Jan. *Our Nation Unhinged: The Human Consequences of the War on Terror.* Berkeley, CA: University of California Press, 2009. A professor of law analyzes the ways in which executive power was abused, the Constitution was subverted, and civil liberties were eroded as the government responded to the September 11, 2001, attacks by terrorists.

Howard, Russell, and Reid Sawyer, eds. *Terrorism and Counterterrorism: Understanding the New Security Environment.* Guilford, CT: McGraw-Hill/Dushkin, 2002. A collection of articles by terrorism experts analyzing terrorism from many perspectives, including suggestions on how to deal with the current terrorist groups.

Margulies, Joseph. *Guantanamo and the Abuse of Presidential Power.* New York: Simon & Schuster, 2006. A close examination of a major point of contention over civil liberties–the American prison at Guantanamo Bay, Cuba, including abuses at the prison and the efforts of the president to defend the situation by extending the bounds of presidential authority.

Tirman, John. *The Deaths of Others: The Fate of Civilians in America's Wars.* New York: Oxford University Press, 2011. Beginning with the seldom-recognized fact that the millions of foreign civilians who have died in America's wars receive little notice, Tirman explores the extent of those deaths in various wars, the ways in which our tactics brought about such destruction, and the reason for minimal concern on the part of the American people for such a massive amount of killing.

## References

Amadeo, K. 2020. "War on terror facts, cost, and timeline." The Balance website.

American Civil Liberties Union. 2002. "ACLU says Homeland Security Bill step backward." Press release. American Civil Liberties Union website.

Bacevich, A. J. 2010. *Washington Rules: America's Path to Permanent War.* New York: Henry Holt.

Basile, M. 2004. "Going to the source: Why Al Qaeda's financial network is likely to withstand the current war on terrorist financing." *Studies in Conflict and Terrorism* 27:169–85.

Baverstock, K. 2005. "Science, politics and ethics in the low dose debate." *Medicine, Conflict and Survival* 21:88–100.

Bebber, C. C. 1994. "Increases in U.S. violent crime during the 1980s following four American military actions." *Journal of Interpersonal Violence* 9 (March):109–16.

Bendinelli, C. 2009. "Effects of landmines and unexploded ordnance on the pediatric population and comparison with adults in rural Cambodia." *World Journal of Surgery* 33 (May):1070–74.

Benjamin, D., and S. Simon. 2005. *The Next Attack: The Failure of the War on Terror and a Strategy for Getting It Right*. New York: Times Books.

Blair, R. G. 2000. "Risk factors associated with PTSD and major depression among Cambodian refugees in Utah." *Health and Social Work* 25 (February):23–30.

Bonneuil, N., and N. Auriat. 2000. "Fifty years of ethnic conflict and cohesion: 1945–94." *Journal of Peace Research* 37:563–81.

Brajs-Zganec, A. 2005. "The long-term effects of war experiences on children's depression in the Republic of Croatia." *Child Abuse & Neglect* 29:31–43.

Brenan, M. 2020. "Economy tops voters' list of key election issues." Gallup Poll website.

Brooks, C. 1999. "Study prompts VA to help ill kids of female Vietnam vets." *San Diego Union-Tribune,* September 4.

Bryce, J. W., N. Walker, F. Ghorayeb, and M. Kanj. 1989. "Life experiences, response styles, and mental health among mothers and children in Beirut, Lebanon." *Social Science and Medicine* 28 (7):685–95.

Bryce, R. 2006. "Man versus mine." *Atlantic Monthly* (January/February):44–46.

Brym, R. J. 2007. "Six lessons of suicide bombers." *Contexts* 6:40–45.

Brym, R. J., and B. Araj. 2006. "Suicide bombing as strategy and interaction." *Social Forces* 84:1969–86.

Buck, K. 2018. "Interactive map reveals how many people would die if a nuclear bomb landed on your house." Metro News website.

Bullman, T. A., C. M. Mahan, H. K. Kang, and W. F. Page. 2005. "Mortality in U.S. Army Gulf War veterans exposed to 1991 Khamisiyah chemical munitions destruction." *American Journal of Public Health* 95:1382–88.

Bunte, J. B., N. M. Connell, and Z. A. Powell. 2019. "War abroad and homicide at home." *Social Forces* 97:1839–63.

Burdman, D. 2003. "Education, indoctrination, and incitement: Palestinian children on their way to martyrdom." *Terrorism and Political Violence* 15:96–123.

Burleigh, N. 1991. "Watching children starve to death." *Time,* June 10, pp. 56–58.

Byrnes, N. 2006. "The high cost of fear." *Business Week,* November 6, p. 16.

Cameron, F. 2002. "Utilitarian multilateralism." *Politics* 22:68–75.

Carballo, M., et al. 2004. "Mental health and coping in a war situation." *Journal of Biosocial Science* 36:463–77.

Cardozo, B. L., A. Vergara, F. Agani, and C. A. Golway. 2000. "Mental health, social functioning, and attitudes of Kosovar Albanians following the war in Kosovo." *Journal of the American Medical Association* 284:569–77.

Caruso, D. B. 2003. "Patriot Act reach now extends beyond terrorism." *San Diego Union-Tribune,* September 15.

Central Intelligence Agency. 2016. *The World Factbook*. CIA website.

Chimienti, G., J. A. Nasr, and I. Khalifeh. 1989. "Children's reactions to war-related stress." *Social Psychiatry and Psychiatric Epidemiology* 24 (6):282–87.

Clark, C. 1994. "VA secretary vows to find cause of Gulf War syndrome." *San Diego Union-Tribune,* March 30.

Collins, S. D. 2004. "Dissuading state support of terrorism." *Studies in Conflict and Terrorism* 27:1–18.

Combellick, J. L., et al. 2020. "Postpartum depression in a cohort of post-9/11 women veterans" *Military Behavioral Health* 8:345–52.

Commager, H. S., ed. 1945. *The Pocket History of the Second World War.* New York: Pocket Books.

Committee for the Compilation of Materials on Damage Caused by the Atomic Bombs in Hiroshima and Nagasaki. 1981. *The Physical, Medical, and Social Effects of the Atomic Bombings,* trans. Eisei Ishikawa and David L. Swain. New York: Basic Books.

Condon, G. E. 2005. "Bush says spying is needed to guard U.S." *San Diego Union-Tribune,* December 20.

Connor, P. 2016. "About six-in-ten Syrians are now displaced from their homes." Pew Research Center website.

Crawford, N. C. 2019. "United States budgetary costs and obligations of post-9/11 wars through FY2020." Watson Institute website.

Cunningham, D. E., and D. Lemke. 2014. "Beyond civil war: A quantitative examination of causes of violence within countries." *Civil Wars* 16:328–45.

Davenport, C. 1995. "Assessing the military's influence on political repression." *Journal of Political and Military Sociology* 23 (Summer):119–44.

Davis, D. W. 2007. *Negative Liberty: Public Opinion and the Terrorist Attacks on America.* New York: Russell Sage Foundation.

Davis, D. W., and B. D. Silver. 2004. "Civil liberties vs. security: Public opinion in the context of the terrorist attacks on America." *American Journal of Political Science* 48:28–46.

Day, A. 1991. "Morality, war: Do they mix?" *Los Angeles Times,* January 15.

Del Castillo, D. 2001. "Pakistan's Islamic colleges provide the Taliban's spiritual fire." *Chronicle of Higher Education* 48:A19–21.

Del Rosso, J. 2014. "The toxicity of torture." *Social Forces* 93:383–404.

Dentler, R. A., and P. Cutright. 1965. "Social effects of nuclear war." In *The New Sociology,* ed. I. L. Horowitz, pp. 409–26. New York: Oxford University Press.

Department of Defense. 2016. "DOD releases 2014 annual report on suicide." DOD website.

Dohrenwend, B. P., et al. 2006. "The psychological risks of Vietnam for U.S. veterans." *Science* 313:979–82.

Donohue, L. K. 2008. *The Cost of Counterterrorism: Power, Politics, and Liberty.* Cambridge, UK: Cambridge University Press.

Doran, N. et al. 2018. "Predictors of suicide risk in Iraq and Afghanistan Veterans." *Military Behavioral Health* 6:215–25.

Dutton, D. G., E. O. Boyanowsky, and M. H. Bond. 2005. "Extreme mass homicide: From military massacre to genocide." *Aggression and Violent Behavior* 10:437–73.

Eisen, S. V., et al. 2012. "Mental and physical health status and alcohol and drug use following return from deployment to Iraq or Afghanistan." *American Journal of Public Health* 102:566–73.

Elms, A. C. 1972. *Social Psychology and Social Relevance.* Boston, MA: Little, Brown.

Eltanamly, H., et al. 2021. "Parenting in times of war." *Trauma, Violence & Abuse* 22:147–60.

Even-Chen, M. S., and H. Itzhaky. 2007. "Exposure to terrorism and violent behavior among adolescents in Israel." *Journal of Community Psychology* 35:43–55.

Farr, K. 2009. "Extreme war rape in today's civil-war-torn states." *Gender Issues* 26:1–41.

Fearon, J., and D. Laitin. 2002. "A world at war." *Harper's Magazine,* March, p. 84.

Friedman, S. 2002. "9/11 boosts focus on interruption risks." *National Underwriter Property and Casualty—Risk and Benefits Management* 106:17.

Fuller, G. E. 2011. "US can blame itself for anger in the Middle East and start making peace." *Christian Science Monitor,* February 4.

Gabriel, R. A. 1987. *No More Heroes: Madness and Psychiatry in War.* New York: Farrar, Straus, and Giroux.

Galea, S., et al. 2002. "Psychological sequelae of the September 11 terrorist attacks in New York City." *New England Journal of Medicine* 346:982–87.

Gambrell, J. 2021. "Biden says he's ending US support for Saudi Arabia's war in Yemen." *The Baltimore Sun,* February 05.

Garcia, M. 2002. "War-stripped, barren Afghan environment will take years to recover." *Knight Ridder/Tribune News Service,* February 11. Knight Ridder/Tribune website.

Gellhorn, M. 1959. *The Face of War.* New York: Simon and Schuster.

Gibbs, D. A., S. L. Martin, L. L. Kupper, and R. E. Johnson. 2007. "Child maltreatment in enlisted soldiers' families during combat-related deployments." *Journal of the American Medical Association* 298:528–35.

Gibson, J. W. 1994. *Warrior Dreams: Violence and Manhood in Post-Vietnam America.* New York: Hill and Wang.

Godefroidt, L. 2020. "How fear drives us apart." *Terrorism and Political Violence* 32:1482–1505.

Goodman, P. 2020. "The 8 main reasons for war." Owlcation website.

Gordon, J. 2002. "Cool war: Economic sanctions as a weapon of mass destruction." *Harper's Magazine,* November, pp. 43–49.

Gould, J. B. 2002. "Playing with fire: The civil liberties implications of September 11th." *PAR* 62:74–79.

Gray, G. C., et al. 2002. "Self-reported symptoms and medical conditions among 11,868 Gulf War–era veterans." *American Journal of Epidemiology* 155:1033–44.

Grimmett, R. F. 2006. "Conventional arms transfers to developing nations, 1998–2005." *CRS Report for Congress,* October 23.

Haddad, S. 2003. "Islam and attitudes toward U.S. policy in the Middle East." *Studies in Conflict and Terrorism* 26:135–54.

Haley, R. W., A. M. Maddrey, and H. K. Gershenfeld. 2002. "Severely reduced functional status in veterans fitting a case definition of Gulf War syndrome." *American Journal of Public Health* 92:46–47.

Halpern-Felsher, B. L., and S. G. Millstein. 2002. "The effects of terrorism on teens' perceptions of dying." *Journal of Adolescent Health* 30:308–11.

Harmless, A. 1990. "Developmental impact of combat exposure: Comparison of adolescent and adult Vietnam veterans." *Smith College Studies in Social Work* 60 (March):185–95.

Hart, H. 1957. "Acceleration in social change." In *Technology and Social Change,* ed. F. R. Allen et al., pp. 27–55. New York: Appleton-Century-Crofts.

Hashemian, F., et al. 2006. "Anxiety, depression, and posttraumatic stress in Iranian survivors of chemical warfare." *Journal of the American Medical Association* 296:560–66.

Hassan, N. 2001. "An arsenal of believers: Talking to the 'human bombs.'" *The New Yorker,* November 19, pp. 36–42.

Hayman, P. M., and D. J. Scaturo. 1993. "Psychological debriefing of returning military personnel: A protocol for post-combat intervention." *Journal of Social Behavior and Personality* 8 (5):117–30.

Henig, D. 2012. "Iron in the soil: Living with military waste in Bosnia-Herzegovina." *Anthropology Today* 28:21–23.

Hersey, J. 1946. *Hiroshima.* New York: Alfred A. Knopf.

Hobfoll, S. E., D. Canetti-Nisim, and R. J. Johnson. 2006. "Exposure to terrorism, stress-related mental health symptoms, and defensive coping among Jews and Arabs in Israel." *Journal of Consulting and Clinical Psychology* 74:207–18.

Hoge, C. W., A. Terhakopian, C. A. Castro, S. C. Messer, and C. C. Engel. 2007. "Association of posttraumatic stress disorder with somatic symptoms, health care visits, and absenteeism among Iraq war veterans." *American Journal of Psychiatry* 164:150–53.

Horowitz, M. C. 2016. "Public opinion and the politics of the killer robots debate." Research & Politics website.

Hoyt, T., A. M. Wray, and J. K. Rielage. 2014. "Preliminary investigation of the roles of military background and posttraumatic stress symptoms in frequency and recidivism of intimate partner violence perpetration among court-referred men." *Journal of Interpersonal Violence* 29:1094–1110.

Hunter, L. Y. 2016. "Terrorism, civil liber- ties, and political rights." *Studies in Conflict and Terrorism* 39:164–93.

Hynes, H. P. 2011. "The invisible casualty of war." *Peace Review* 23:387–95.

Jacobs, L. A. 2001. "What makes a terrorist?" *State Government News* 44:10–14.

Jacobson, I. G., et al. 2008. "Alcohol use and alcohol-related problems before and after military combat deployment." *Journal of the American Medical Association* 300:663–75.

Johnson, C. 2004. *The Sorrows of Empire: Militarism, Secrecy, and the End of the Republic.* New York: Metropolitan Books.

Karney, B. R., and T. E. Trail. 2016. "Associations between prior deployments and marital satisfaction among army couples." *Journal of Marriage and Family.* Published online.

Knudsen, H. K., P. M. Roman, J. A. Johnson, and L. J. Ducharme. 2005. "A changed America? The effects of September 11th on depressive symptoms and alcohol consumption." *Journal of Health and Social Behavior* 46:260–73.

Kozaryn, L. D. 2002. "Bush says Saddam Hussein 'must be stopped.'" U.S. Department of Defense website.

Kaag, J., and S. Kreps. 2014. *Drone Warfare.* New York: Polity Press.

Kuhr, S., and J. M. Hauer. 2001. "The threat of biological terrorism in the new millennium." *American Behavioral Scientist* 44:1032–41.

Kull, S., C. Ramsay, and E. Lewis. 2003. "Misperceptions, the media, and the Iraq war." *Political Science Quarterly* 118:569–98.

Lacayo, R. 2003. "The war comes back home." *Time,* May 12, pp. 30–34.

Lacey, M. 2005. "Beyond the bullets and blades." *New York Times,* March 20.

Larison, D. 2020. "Trump's arms control farce." *The American Conservative,* October.

Lichter, S. R., L. S. Lichter, D. R. Amundson, and J. M. Fowler. 1987. "The truth about Pravda: How the Soviets see the United States." *Public Opinion* (March–April):12–13.

Liptak, A., N. A. Lewis, and B. Weiser. 2002. "After Sept. 11, a legal battle on the limits of civil liberty." *New York Times,* August 4.

London, A. S., E. Allen, and J. M. Wilmoth. 2013. "Veteran status, extramarital sex, and divorce." *Journal of Family Issues* 34:1452–73.

MacLean, A. 2010. "The things they carry: Combat, disability, and unemployment among U.S. men." *American Sociological Review* 75:563–85.

Markovic, V. 2019. "Suicide squad: Boko Haram's use of the female suicide bomber." *Women & Criminal Justice* 29:283–302.

Mehio Sibai, A., N. Shaar Sameer, and S. el Yassir. 2000. "Impairments, disabilities and needs assessment among non-fatal war injuries in South Lebanon, Grapes of Wrath, 1996." *Journal of Epidemiology and Community Health* 54 (January):35–39.

Military Education. 2016. "The true cost of military equipment spending." Military Education website.

Mollica, R. F., et al. 1994. "The effect of trauma and confinement on functional health and mental health status of Cambodians living in Thailand-Cambodia border camps." *Journal of the American Medical Association* 270:581–86.

Morain, D. 1990. "Complex, costly cleanups may snarl base closings." *Los Angeles Times,* June 19.

Morin, R. 2011. "For many injured veterans, a lifetime of consequences." Pew Research Center website.

Moritsugu, K. 2001. "U.S. economy struggles to bear brunt of terrorism's costs." Knight Ridder/Tribune News Service. Knight Ridder/Tribune website.

Musser, G., and S. Nemecek. 2000. "A new kind of war." *Scientific American,* June, p. 47.

Neria, Y., et al. 2000. "Posttraumatic residues of captivity." *Journal of Clinical Psychiatry* 61 (January):39–46.

Neria, Y., L. DioGrande, and B. G. Adams. 2011. "Posttraumatic stress disorder following the September 11, 2001, terrorist attacks." *American Psychologist* 66:429–46.

Newman, R. J. 1998. "A U.S. victory, at a cost of $5.5 trillion." *U.S. News and World Report,* July 13.

Pape, R. 2005. *Dying to Win: The Strategic Logic of Suicide Terrorism.* New York: Random House.

Perl, R. F. 2006. "International terrorism: Threat, policy, and response." *CRS Report for Congress,* August 16.

Peterson, R., et al. 2015. "Identifying homelessness among veterans using VA administrative data." *PLoS One,* July 14. PLoS One website.

Pfefferbaum, B., et al. 2001. "Traumatic grief in a convenience sample of victims seeking support services after a terrorist incident." *Annals of Clinical Psychiatry* 13:19–24.

——. 2002. "Exposure and peritraumatic response as predictors of posttraumatic stress in children following the 1995 Oklahoma City bombing." *Journal of Urban Health* 79:354–63.

Physicians for Human Rights. 2002. "War-related sexual violence in Sierra Leone." Physicians for Human Rights website.

Posner, R. A. 2001. "Security versus civil liberties." *Atlantic Monthly,* December, pp. 46–47.

Purdy, M. 2008. "Personal tragedies illuminate the consequences of war." *Nieman Reports* 62:68–69.

Qouta, S., R. Punamäki, T. Miller, and E. El-Sarraj. 2007. "Does war beget child aggression?" *Aggressive Behavior* 34:231–44.

Rahim, H. F. A., et al. 2009. "Maternal and child health in the occupied Palestinian territory." *The Lancet* 373:967–77.

Ratnesar, R. 2002. "Revenge: Arafat—and why the rage keeps burning." *Time,* April 8.

Renner, M. 1991. "Military victory, ecological defeat." *World Watch* (July–August):27–34.

——. 1993. *Critical Juncture: The Future of Peacekeeping.* Washington, DC: Worldwatch Institute.

——. 1997. *Small Arms, Big Impact.* Washington, DC: Worldwatch Institute.

——. 1999. "Ending violent conflict." In *State of the World 1999,* ed. L. R. Brown et al., pp. 151–68. New York: W. W. Norton.

Reynal-Querol, M. 2002. "Ethnicity, political systems, and civil wars." *Journal of Conflict Resolution* 46:29–54.

Richman, J. A., L. Cloninger, and K. M. Rospenda. 2008. "Macrolevel stressors, terrorism, and mental health outcomes." *American Journal of Public Health* 98:323–29.

Rieder, M., and I. Choonara. 2012. "Armed conflict and child health." *Archives of Disease in Childhood* 97:59–62.

Ritchie, H., et al. 2019. "Terrorism." OurWorldData website.

Robison, K. K., E. M. Crenshaw, and J. C. Jenkins. 2006. "Ideologies of violence: The social origins of Islamist and leftist transnational terrorism." *Social Forces* 84:20 09–26.

Roston, E., and J. F. O. McAllister. 2004. "Humiliation in an Iraqi jail." *Time,* May 10, p. 20.

Rubin, A. J. 2009. "Iraqi surveys start to unveil the mental scars of war, especially among women." *New York Times,* March 8.

Sabin, M., R. L. Cardozo, L. Nackerud, R. Kaiser, and L. Varese. 2003. "Factors associated with poor mental health among Guatemalan refugees living in Mexico 20 years after civil conflict." *Journal of the American Medical Association* 290:635.

Schnurr, P. P., A. Spiro III, and A. H. Paris. 2000. "Physician-diagnosed medical disorders in relation to PTSD symptoms in older male military veterans." *Health Psychology* 19 (January):91–97.

Seal, K. H., et al. 2009. "Trends and risk factors for mental health diagnoses among Iraq and Afghanistan veterans using Department of Veterans Affairs health care, 2002–2008." *American Journal of Public Health* 99:1651–58.

Shane, S., and M. Mazzetti. 2009. "In adopting harsh tactics, no look at past use." *New York Times,* April 22.

Shemyakina, O. N., and A. C. Plagnol. 2013. "Subjective well-being and armed conflict." *Social Indicators Research* 113:1129–52.

Shen, Y., J. Arkes, and T. V. Williams. 2012. "Effects of Iraq/Afghanistan deployments on major depression and substance use disorder." *American Journal of Public Health* 102:S80–S87.

Shrader-Frechette, K. 2005. "Radiobiology and gray science: Flaws in landmark new radiation protections." *Science and Engineering Ethics* 11:167–69.

Solomon, Z., D. Shimrit, G. Zerach, and D. Horesh. 2011. "Marital adjustment, parental functioning, and emotional sharing in war veterans." *Journal of Family Issues* 32:127–47.

Solomon, Z., R. Dekel, and G. Zerach. 2008. "The relationships between posttraumatic stress symptom clusters and marital intimacy among war veterans." *Journal of Family Psychology* 22:659–66.

Stein, B. D., et al. 2004. "A national longitudinal study of the psychological consequences of the September 11, 2001, terrorist attacks." *Psychiatry* 67:105–17.

Stires, L. K. 1991. "The Gulf 'war' as a sanctioned massacre." *Contemporary Social Psychology* 15 (December):139–43.

Stockholm International Peace Research Institute. 2020. *SIPRI Yearbook, 2020.* Stockholm International Peace Research Institute website.

Stokes, B. 2014. "Which countries don't like America and which do." Pew Research Center website.

Sultan, D. H. 2009. "Landmines and recovery in Sudan's Nuba Mountains." *Africa Today* 55:45–61.

Tarabah, A., et al. 2015. "Exposure to violence and children's desensitization attitudes in Lebanon." *Journal of Interpersonal Violence.* Published online.

Thabet, A. A., and P. Vostanis. 2000. "Posttraumatic stress disorder reactions in children of war." *Child Abuse and Neglect* 24 (February):291–98.

Thompson, M. 2008. "America's medicated army." *Time,* June 16, pp. 38–42.

U.S. Department of State. 2019. "Country reports on terrorism." U.S. Department of State website.

United Nations General Assembly. 2006. "Report of the special representative of the Secretary-General for children and armed conflict." United Nations website.

Van Deerlin, L. 2003. "Abandoning the bill of rights." *San Diego Union-Tribune,* June 11.

Verger, P., et al. 2004. "The psychological impact of terrorism." *American Journal of Psychiatry* 161:1384–89.

Vlahov, D., S. Galea, J. Ahern, H. Resnick, and D. Kilpatrick. 2004. "Sustained increased consumption of cigarettes, alcohol, and marijuana among Manhattan residents after September 11, 2001." *American Journal of Public Health* 94:253–54.

Wallis, C. 2004. "Hidden scars of battle." *Time,* July 12, p. 35.

Walt, S. M. 2005. *Taming American Power: The Global Response to U.S. Primacy.* New York: W. W. Norton.

Weinberg, A., and L. Weinberg, eds. 1963. *Instead of Violence.* New York: Grossman.

Wheeler, D. L. 1994. "An ominous legacy of the atomic age." *Chronicle of Higher Education,* January 12.

White, R. K. 1966. "Misperception and the Vietnam war." *Journal of Social Issues* 22 (July):1–19.

Wilensky, H. L. 1967. *Organizational Intelligence.* New York: Basic Books.

Willems, J. L. 2002. "7 Mustard gas: Signs, symptoms and treatment." *Journal of Toxicology: Clinical Toxicology* 40:250–51.

Williams, J. 2004. "Facts that should change the world." *New Statesman,* May 10, p. 21.

Wolters Kluwer Editorial Staff. 2002. *Oil Spill Intelligence Report,* April 11. Wolters Kluwer website.

Wood, D. 2004. "Defense spending a threat to world economic stability." *San Diego Union-Tribune,* January 19.

World Bank. 2014. "Economic monitoring report to the ad hoc liaison committee." World Bank website.

World Health Organization. 2018. "Health statistics." WHO website.

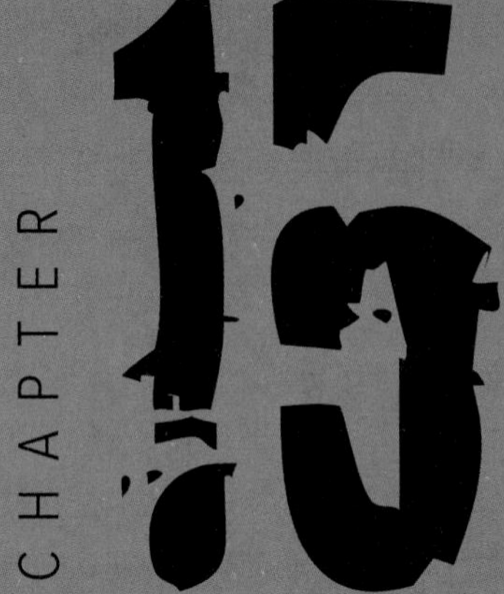


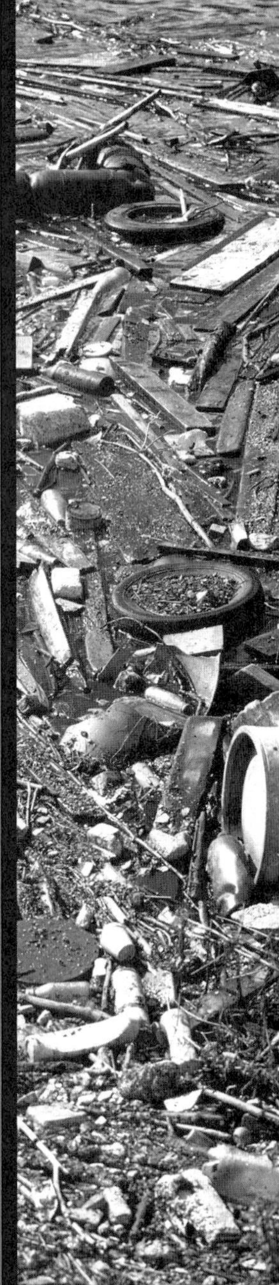

# The Environment

OBJECTIVES

1 Understand the nature of the ecosystem.

2 Identify the types and extent of environmental problems.

3 Discuss the ways in which environmental problems threaten the desired quality of life.

4 Explain the social structural and social psychological factors that underlie environmental problems.

5 Suggest some ways to deal with the problems of environmental pollution and environmental depletion.

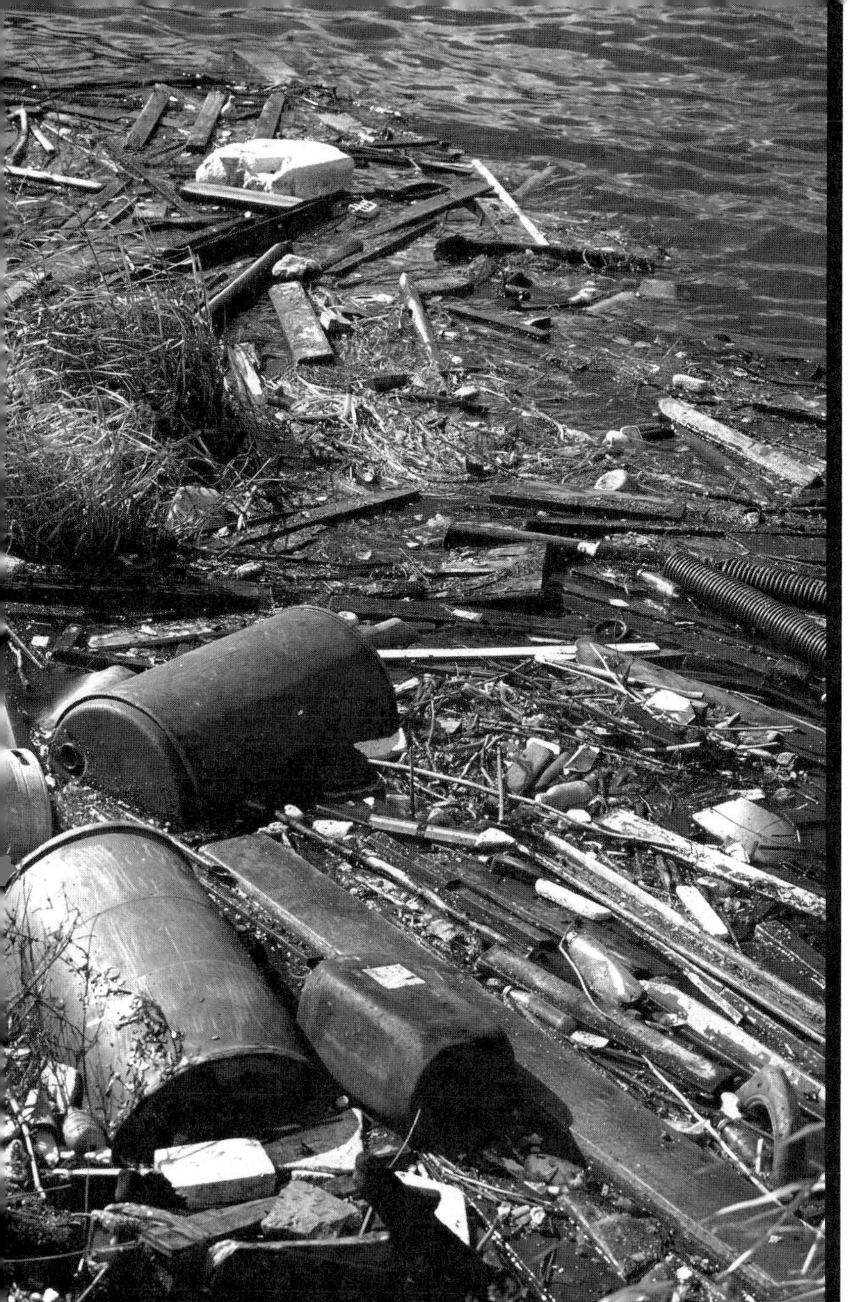

Steve Allen/Brand X Picture/Alamy Stock Photo

## "We're Not Safe Here Anymore"

Karl is a civilian employee on an air force base in a western state. Karl lives in a home that was occupied by his great-grandparents—built long before the air force base. Yet Karl isn't sure whether his children or his grandchildren will live in this place.

*I can't imagine living anywhere else. But I can't imagine my children or grandchildren living here. I don't even want them to. We're not safe here anymore. The hazardous wastes from the base have contaminated our water supply. We can't grow our gardens anymore. We can't drink the water. We don't even feel safe taking a bath in it.*

*And it's not just the water. When you know that stuff is all around you, you feel like you're living in poison. Of course, I try not to think about it most of the time. But you can't keep it out of your mind altogether. And whenever I do think about it, I can feel myself getting nervous. Or sometimes I just get depressed.*

*I love this place. It's my home. But sometimes I hate it. At least, I hate what's happened to it. I don't know yet what we're going to do. But I do know that even if my wife and I don't leave, our kids will. And that will be the end of generations of my family on this land.*

## Introduction

In 2004, the Nobel Peace Prize was awarded to an environmentalist activist, Wangari Maathai of Kenya. She founded and led a movement to plant millions of trees to replenish the dwindling forests that provide Africans with cooking fuel. To many observers, declaring an environmentalist the winner of the Peace Prize seemed strange. But Christopher Flavin, president of Worldwatch Institute, declared it a most fitting award, because "the insecurity the world struggles with today is inextricably linked to the ecological and social problems" that Maathai strives to address (Flavin 2005:xix). In other words, although Americans tend not to consider them as serious as other matters we have addressed in this book, the problems we deal with in this chapter are crucial to the security and general well-being of people everywhere.

We look first at the ecosystem to set the stage for an understanding of environmental problems. Then we examine various kinds of environmental problems and how extensive they are. We show how these problems affect the quality of life and what structural and social psychological factors contribute to them. Finally, we consider several proposed as well as actual efforts to resolve these problems.

## The Ecosystem

**ecosystem**
a set of living things, their environment, and the interrelationships among and between them

The **ecosystem** refers to the interrelationships between all living things and the environment. The emphasis is on the interdependence of all things: people, land, animals, vegetation, atmosphere, and social processes. Commoner (1971:16–17) called the ecosystem of the earth a "machine" and described some of the crucial interrelationships:

> Without the photosynthetic activity of green plants, there would be no oxygen for our engines, smelters, and furnaces, let alone support for human and animal life. Without the action of the plants, animals, and microorganisms that live in them, we could have no pure water in our lakes and rivers. Without the biological processes that have gone on in the soil for thousands of years, we would have neither food crops, oil, nor coal. This machine is our biological capital, the basic apparatus on which our total productivity depends. If we destroy it, our most advanced technology will become useless and any economic and political system that depends on it will founder. The environmental crisis is a signal of this approaching catastrophe.

Nature is not "out there" to be conquered for human benefit. Rather, people, nature, and the earth form a delicately balanced system. What is done at one place can have serious consequences for the system at that place or in other places. For example, companies that drill for natural gas in Texas and Oklahoma use fracking—pumping massive amounts of water and other materials into the ground to crack rock and release the gas (Kuchment 2016). An increase in the amount of drilling has resulted in a dramatic jump in the number of earthquakes in the region. Between 2008 and 2015, Texas had a sixfold and Oklahoma had a 160-fold increase in the number of earthquakes, some of which have resulted in injuries and damage to buildings and highways.

The interrelationships between human activity and the environment are also illustrated by the problems of acid rain and the threat to the ozone layer. The problem of acid rain was originally caused by sulfur dioxide emissions from coal-burning plants and factories and by nitrogen oxides from automobile exhaust and some industries. These chemicals, as they rise, mix with water vapor to form sulfuric and nitric acids that then fall to the earth as rain or snow. Acid rain threatens lakes and forests, kills fish and birds, reduces crop yields, contributes to health problems, and damages buildings and monuments (see the U.S. Environmental Protection Agency website; see also Bright 2000; Leslie 2003; Youth 2003). Moreover, the damage may occur hundreds or thousands of miles away from where the sulfur dioxide emissions occurred.

In recent decades, tougher air pollution regulations have significantly reduced sulfur dioxide emissions. Some damaged lakes and forests are beginning to recover. However, acid rain continues to be a problem, but more in the form of nitric acid rather than sulfuric acid (Tennesen 2010). The nitric acid is produced not only by coal-burning plants and automobiles but also by farming (bacteria work on fertilizer to create nitric acid).

The threat to the ozone layer is another example of current environmental problems. Ozone is a rare form of oxygen that is poisonous to human beings at ground level but is necessary in the upper atmosphere to absorb the deadly ultraviolet radiation of the sun. There is a natural balance of ozone distribution from ground level to the stratosphere. However, human activity disturbs that natural balance. High-voltage electrical equipment, including electrostatic air cleaners used to reduce other kinds of air pollution, create ground level ozone, and higher than normal concentrations at ground level pose health problems to the eyes, throat, and lungs.

The ozone in the upper atmosphere is reduced as a result of a number of human activities, including the use of nitrogen fertilizers, supersonic airplanes, fluorocarbons from aerosol spray cans (now banned in most nations), and nuclear explosions in the atmosphere. The effects of a depleted ozone layer are far reaching, involving changes in the earth's climate, destruction of some plant and animal life, reduced crop yields, increased incidence of skin cancer, possible genetic damage to plants and humans, and an impact on the food chain of the oceans (McGinn 1999; Singh and Agrawal 2008).

Environmental problems dramatize the interdependence in the ecosystem. A poet once wrote that one cannot stir a flower without troubling a star. It is imperative that individuals make every effort to evaluate all the implications of human action for their delicately balanced ecosystem.

## Types of Environmental Problems

Environmental problems can be divided into two types: **environmental pollution** and **environmental depletion.** "Pollution" refers to degradation of air, land, water, climate (global warming), aesthetic environment (eye pollution), and sound environment (noise pollution). "Depletion" refers to the diminishing supply of natural resources, illustrated well by the challenge of meeting the ever-increasing demand for energy.

**environmental pollution**
harmful alterations in the environment, including air, land, and water

**environmental depletion**
increasing scarcity of natural resources, including those used for generating energy

**pollutant**
anything that causes environmental pollution

### Environmental Pollution

Pollution is any alteration of the environment that is harmful to the ecosystem and/or to human well-being. **Pollutants,** those things that cause the pollution, are by-products of human activity (e.g., industrial production, war, farming, and the use of hazardous materials). In this chapter, we discuss numerous kinds of pollution and pollutants. It is important to keep in mind that in an ecosystem the overall impact of pollutants is greater than the impact of particular pollutants in particular places.

Pollution can occur in two ways: through catastrophes and through the slower, more insidious poisoning that occurs as a result of various processes and activities. The catastrophes dramatize the problem. In 1984, vapors from a deadly chemical used to manufacture pesticides escaped through a faulty valve into the air in Bhopal, India.

Within a few hours, more than 2,500 people were dead, and thousands were critically ill. It was one of the worst industrial disasters in history. The accident underscored the horrendous consequences of exposure to toxic substances. Yet even more important than the catastrophes are the countless ways in which industries are exposing millions of people to high levels of toxic materials. Many of the victims in Bhopal died quickly. Others died more slowly or suffered long-term health problems as the result of regular exposure to toxic materials in the air, water, and land. Twenty years later, in 2004, survivors and their supporters demonstrated because people were still suffering, and 24 years later, in 2008, hundreds of tons of toxic waste still lay within a warehouse on the grounds of the old factory (Sengupta 2008). And three decades later, residents continued to exhibit both physical and mental health problems arising from the disaster (Howard 2014; Murthy 2014).

*Air Pollution.* Millions of tons of pollutants are released into the air every year in the United States and are visible in the smog that darkens urban areas. Much other pollution is not visible to the naked eye because it results from the discharge of gases and tiny particulate matter into the air. In some areas, atmospheric conditions tend to concentrate pollutants in the air. Even when winds blow the pollutants away from the populated area in which they are generated, damage still occurs.

Major air pollutants include suspended particulates (dust, pollen, ash, soot, chemicals, etc.), sulfur dioxide (from industrial processes), carbon monoxide (from motor vehicle exhaust, forest fires, decomposition of organic matter, etc.), and nitrogen dioxide (from motor vehicle exhaust, atmospheric reactions, etc.). The burning of fossil fuels—oil, natural gas, and coal—is the primary source of air pollution (Flavin and Dunn 1999).

While many people think of air pollution in terms of outside air, *a major problem throughout the world is indoor air pollution* (World Health Organization 2005). In developing countries, the indoor smoke resulting from burning solid fuels pollutes indoor air and is responsible for much illness and early death. In the United States and other developed nations, there are numerous sources of indoor pollution, including the polluted outdoor air but also including numerous everyday products found in all buildings, from offices to homes (Figure 15.1). For example, formaldehyde, which emits toxic vapors that can lead to respiratory ailments and cancer, is used in a great many products, including bed sheets, permanent press shirts, fingernail hardeners and polishes, latex paints, plywood and particle-board cabinets, and plastic-laminated kitchen counters (Environmental Protection Agency 2021a). We don't know how many homes are polluted by excessive levels of formaldehyde, but a survey of homes in Japan reported that a fourth of them had concentration levels above the value set by the Ministry of Health, Labor, and Welfare as acceptable (Osawa and Hayashi 2009).

*Water Pollution.* There are eight different kinds of water pollution (Sampat 2000). First is organic sewage, which requires dissolved oxygen in order to be transformed into carbon dioxide, water, phosphates, nitrates, and certain plant nutrients. Less oxygen is needed if the sewage is treated, but the amount of treatment varies and in some places there is no treatment at all.

**eutrophication**
overfertilization of water due to excess nutrients, leading to algae growth and oxygen depletion

**Eutrophication,** a second kind of water pollution, is overfertilization of water from excess nutrients, leading to algae growth and oxygen depletion. Eutrophication threatens aquatic life. It has already killed great numbers of fish in the United States and in other nations.

A third type of water pollution results from infectious agents. Many water-borne bacteria that cause disease have been eliminated in the United States, but there is still danger from infectious viruses such as hepatitis. Organic chemicals such as insecticides,

| OUTDOOR SOURCES | BUILDING EQUIPMENT | COMPONENTS/ FURNISHINGS | OTHER POTENTIAL INDOOR SOURCES |
|---|---|---|---|
| **Polluted Outdoor Air**<br>• Pollen, dust, mold spores<br>• Industrial emissions<br>• Vehicle and nonroad engine emissions (cars, buses, trucks, lawn and garden equipment)<br>**Nearby Sources**<br>• Loading docks<br>• Odors from dumpsters<br>• Unsanitary debris or building exhausts near outdoor air intakes<br>**Underground Sources**<br>• Radon<br>• Pesticides<br>• Leakage from underground storage tanks | **HVAC Equipment**<br>• Mold growth in drip pans, ductwork, coils, and humidifiers<br>• Improper venting of combustion products<br>• Dust or debris in ductwork<br>**Other Equipment**<br>• Emissions from office equipment (volatile organic compounds [VOCs], ozone)<br>• Emissions from shop, lab, and cleaning equipment | **Components**<br>• Mold growth on or in soiled or water-damaged materials<br>• Dry drain traps that allow the passage of sewer gas<br>• Materials containing VOCs, inorganic compounds, or damaged asbestos<br>• Materials that produce particles (dust)<br>**Furnishings**<br>• Emissions from new furnishings and floorings<br>• Mold growth on or in soiled or water-damaged furnishings | • Science laboratory supplies<br>• Vocational art supplies<br>• Copy/print areas<br>• Food prep areas<br>• Smoking lounges<br>• Cleaning materials<br>• Emissions from trash<br>• Pesticides<br>• Odors and VOCs from paint, caulk, adhesives<br>• Occupants with communicable diseases<br>• Dry-erase markers and similar pens<br>• Insects and other pests<br>• Personal care products<br>• Stored gasoline and lawn and garden equipment |

**FIGURE 15.1** Typical Sources of Indoor Air Pollutants.
Source: U.S. Environmental Protection Agency website.

pesticides, and detergents cause a fourth kind of water pollution. These chemicals may also be highly toxic to aquatic life.

Inorganic and miscellaneous chemicals constitute a fifth category of water pollutants. These chemicals can alter the life of a body of water, kill fish, and create unpleasant tastes when the water is used as a drinking supply. Sixth, sediments from land erosion may cause pollution. These sediments can diminish the water's capacity to assimilate oxygen-demanding wastes and block the sunlight needed by aquatic plants.

Radioactive substances, a seventh kind of pollutant, are likely to become more serious if nuclear power plants to generate electricity become more common. The eighth kind of water pollution is waste heat from power plants and industry. Overheated water holds less oxygen, and fish and other aquatic life are generally very sensitive to temperature changes.

Not only are lakes and rivers being polluted, but the oceans are as well. Oil spills and the dumping of waste into the oceans have made many beaches unsafe for swimming.

Millions of barrels of oil are poured into the ocean each year from the cleaning of the bilges of tankers. In addition, thousands of oil-polluting incidents occur every year from such problems as tanker accidents. Incidents in and around U.S. waters result in various amounts of spillage. According to the Environmental Protection Agency, there are almost 14,000 oil spills each year in the United States alone.

**pesticide**
a chemical used to kill insects defined as pests

**herbicide**
a chemical used to kill plant life, particularly weeds

*Land Pollution.* **Pesticides, herbicides,** chemical wastes, radioactive fallout, acid rain, and garbage all infect the soil. Some chemicals used in pesticides, herbicides, and a number of manufactured products are hazardous to human health and are highly stable, remaining in the soil for decades (McGinn 2000).

The pesticide DDT, for example, was banned in the United States after it was found to interfere with the formation of normal eggshells in certain birds, adding to the potential extinction of some species. It is incredibly stable, having been detected in Antarctic penguins, in the blood and fat of most Americans, and in carrots and spinach sold in supermarkets more than a decade after being banned.

Nor is the threat posed only by the "active" ingredients in pesticides. The so-called inert ingredients can constitute up to 99 percent of the contents, and many of those ingredients are biochemically active. For example, an unlisted ingredient in Dibrom, a mosquito pesticide, is naphthalene, which may cause cancer and developmental problems in children (Epstein 2003).

The problem of pesticides is compounded by the fact that the pests tend to develop a resistance to them; thus, increasing quantities are required over time. And if the natural enemies of a particular pest disappear, a pest control program may require monstrous increases in dosage of the pesticide.

*Climate Change.* Air pollution from carbon dioxide, methane, nitrous oxide, and a number of other gases is a primary factor in the so-called greenhouse effect (McKeown and Gardner 2009). The gases trap solar energy in the atmosphere, which, in turn, leads to global warming. Few if any scientists deny that global warming is occurring (although there is still a small amount of disagreement about the extent to which human activity is a factor in the warming). A report from the National Aeronautics and Space Administration (2020) dramatizes changes that are occurring. Atmospheric carbon dioxide is at the highest level ever and is increasing. Records of the earth's average surface temperature have been kept increasing since 1951; 2016 and 2020 are tied for the warmest years on record. The global sea level has risen about 8 inches in the last century. And ice sheets and glaciers are shrinking. Greenland lost an average of 279 billions tons of ice each year between 1993 and 2019.

As the warming continues, the impact on human life will be severe (McKeown and Gardner 2009). Scientists warn that there will be:

- Increased flooding and intensity of storms on coastal areas;
- An increase in extremes, with more of both droughts and flooding;
- Reduced fresh water supplies and food production;
- Damage to ecosystems, including extinctions; and
- Increases in malnutrition, disease, and mortality.

Although, as we noted, there is some disagreement about the extent to which human activity contributes to the warming, the great majority of scientists argue convincingly that humankind has seriously affected the climate (Collins et al. 2007). For example, some of the greenhouse gases have no natural source; they are the products of processes initiated by humans. And even those that have a natural source are increased greatly by human activity. Thus, most of the increase in carbon dioxide (which had remained at roughly the same level for 100,000 years prior to the industrial revolution) is due to the burning of coal, oil, and natural gas. In short, although some politicians and skeptical observers demur, the scientific community is virtually one voice in proclaiming both the severity of, and the central role of human activity in, the problem.

*Noise Pollution.* Prolonged exposure to noise of sufficient intensity can not only damage hearing but can also disturb sleep, create irritability, diminish the ability to concentrate on work, disrupt activity and communication, and cause accidents (National Academy of Engineering 2010). Many things—from traffic to industrial processes to vacuum cleaners—contribute to noise pollution. You may find the noise level in a particular situation as anything from annoying to painful. For most people, the noise environment is worsening. Indeed, hundreds of millions of people throughout the world are exposed to unacceptable noise levels at work and at home (Skanberg and Ohrstrom 2002).

*Aesthetic Damage.* An aesthetically pleasing environment is one component of a high quality of life (Sirgy, Efraty, Siegel, and Lee 2001). An attractive environment can affect mood and influence health-promoting behavior like exercise (Craig, Brownson, Cragg, and Dunn 2002). It is no minor point, then, that pollution involves *deterioration of the beauty of the environment* as well as actual physical damage.

Air pollution, for instance, leads to the deterioration of buildings, statues, and paintings. It can inhibit visibility, obscure scenic views, and produce noxious odors. This kind of aesthetic damage—whether from air and water pollution or from litter—is the effect on the environment that most people first recognize. Whatever the source, aesthetic damage signals that the environment is less pleasing, that the beauty of the natural world has been scarred by human activity.

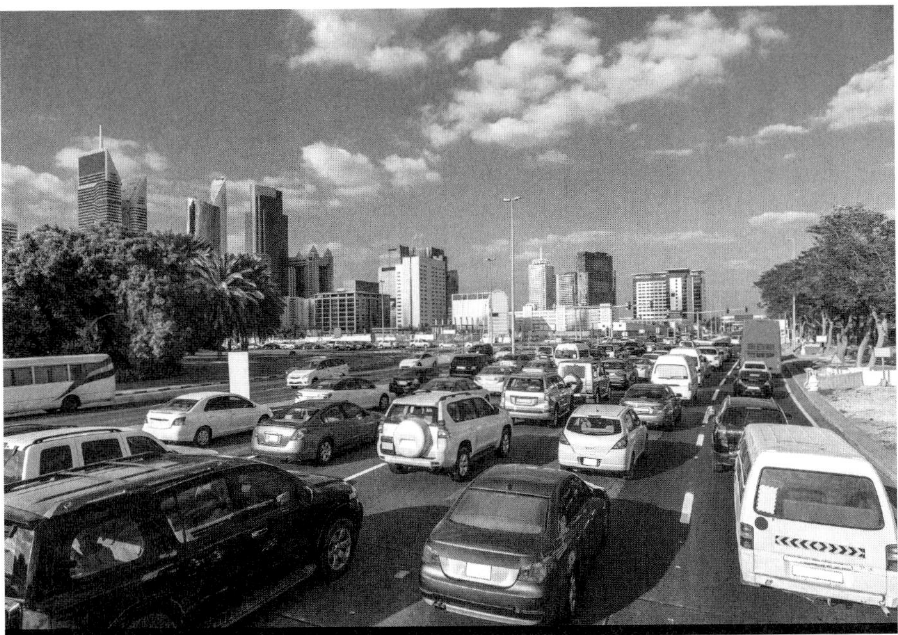

Energy consumption per capita is higher in the United States than it is in any other country in the world.

S-F/Shutterstock

**TABLE 15.1**
Energy Production and Consumption, 1950–2020

| Year | Total Production (quad. Btu) | Total Consumption (quad. Btu) | Consumption/ Production Ratio |
|---|---|---|---|
| 1950 | 35.5 | 34.6 | 0.97 |
| 1960 | 42.8 | 45.1 | 1.05 |
| 1970 | 63.5 | 67.9 | 1.07 |
| 1975 | 61.4 | 72.0 | 1.17 |
| 1980 | 67.2 | 78.4 | 1.17 |
| 1985 | 67.7 | 76.7 | 1.13 |
| 1990 | 70.7 | 84.6 | 1.20 |
| 1995 | 71.2 | 91.5 | 1.29 |
| 2000 | 71.3 | 100.0 | 1.40 |
| 2005 | 69.9 | 100.3 | 1.44 |
| 2010 | 75.0 | 98.0 | 1.31 |
| 2020 | 104.0 | 99.6 | 0.96 |

SOURCE: U.S. Energy Information Administration website.

## Environmental Depletion

*The Dwindling Natural Resources.* Air, water, and land can be restored, but the problem of dwindling resources is another matter. If the air is cleaned, it may become just as useful as before it was polluted. But once a mine has been exhausted, an oil well pumped dry, or a patch of soil ruined for farming, you have lost a resource that cannot be reclaimed easily or quickly, if at all.

For a long time Americans tended to think that the nation had virtually unlimited natural resources. In 1973, a group of oil-producing nations temporarily suspended the sale of oil to other nations, and Americans confronted the fact that no nation in the modern world can be self-sufficient by virtue of its own natural resources. The United States does not have sufficient oil in its own reserves to meet its needs. Nor does it have sufficient supplies of various other natural resources. In 2019, the United States imported 100 percent of 17 minerals used in various manufacturing processes and products (U.S. Geological Survey 2020). And the nation imported varying amounts of dozens of other minerals, ranging from 21 percent of iron and steel slag to 96 percent of bismuth.

*Energy Production and Consumption.* An integral part of the pollution problem and the dwindling of resources is the production and consumption of energy. As Table 15.1 shows, energy consumption has risen rapidly in the United States. Although the United States does not have the highest per capita usage of energy, our usage accounts for 17 percent of the world's energy consumption.

# How Big Are These Environmental Problems?

How serious are the environmental problems of this country? Using the same two categories of environmental pollution and environmental depletion, consider what the data reveal.

## Environmental Pollution

The federal Environmental Protection Agency (EPA) has established standards for six "criteria" air pollutants: sulfur dioxide, particulate matter, carbon monoxide, ozone, lead, and nitrogen dioxide. Many states and cities have adopted the Pollutant Standards Index (PSI), which indicates when any of the six criteria pollutants are at a level considered to be adverse to human health. These six criteria pollutants are not the only sources of the problem but are the ones used by the federal government to evaluate air quality.

In general, enforcement of *air pollution standards* has been reducing the amount of the pollutants released into the air (Environmental Protection Agency 2021b). From 1970 through 2019, the combined emissions of the six common pollutants declined by 77 percent even though the gross domestic product and energy consumption have increased significantly. Also, from 2000 through 2019, the number of unhealthy air days in major cities declined by 77 percent.

Such progress is hopeful but it should not obscure the fact that serious problems remain. In many places–particularly the developing nations–it is a more serious problem than in the United States. It is estimated that more than a billion people are exposed to outdoor air pollution each year, mainly in urban areas where about half the world's population now lives (United Nations Environment Programme 2016). This urban air pollution is responsible for a million premature deaths each year.

As noted earlier, *indoor air pollution* is also a serious problem. According to the World Health Organization (2016), between 3 and 4 million deaths each year are caused by indoor air pollution. And about one out of every eight deaths worldwide is linked with either indoor or outdoor air pollution.

In the United States and other developed nations, indoor air pollution can cause the "*sick building syndrome.*" In a sick building, the workers suffer from acute physical and/or psychological discomfort that is eased when they leave the building (Thorne et al. 2001). The sick building syndrome includes a variety of symptoms: mucous membrane irritation, eye irritation, headaches, nausea, feelings of lethargy, fatigue, the inability to concentrate, breathing difficulties, and fainting (Abdul-Wahab 2011). The syndrome is due to such factors as inadequately maintained air conditioning and heating systems; pests (e.g., cockroaches and dust mites); moisture and mold in ceiling tiles, carpet, insulation, and furnishings; improper ventilation; and toxic vapors from copy-machine liquids, paint, flooring, and cleaning agents (Mendell et al. 2006).

In severe cases, the air quality inside the building may be far worse than the urban air outside the building. It is not known how many buildings are sick, but a number of surveys indicate that from 40 percent to 55 percent of office occupants will experience one or more sick building symptoms each week (Hood 2005).

Nor are people's homes necessarily safe. We have noted that formaldehyde is toxic and that a wide range of materials and products used in homes contain formaldehyde. In the 1970s, about half a million homes were insulated with urea formaldehyde. In addition, there are other toxic chemicals in virtually all homes, making them one of the more hazardous places to be. Some of the chemicals in the home may not be toxic in themselves but can combine with common kinds of air pollution to cause health problems (Hughes 2004).

Another problem in homes and other buildings is the *presence of radon gas, which can cause lung cancer after long periods of exposure* (Pawel and Puskin 2004; Centers for Disease Control and Prevention 2021). The Environmental Protection Agency claims that millions of homes and buildings contain high levels of the gas (EPA website). The gas is odorless and colorless and can be detected only by appropriate testing. Radon is produced by the decay of uranium in rocks and soil.

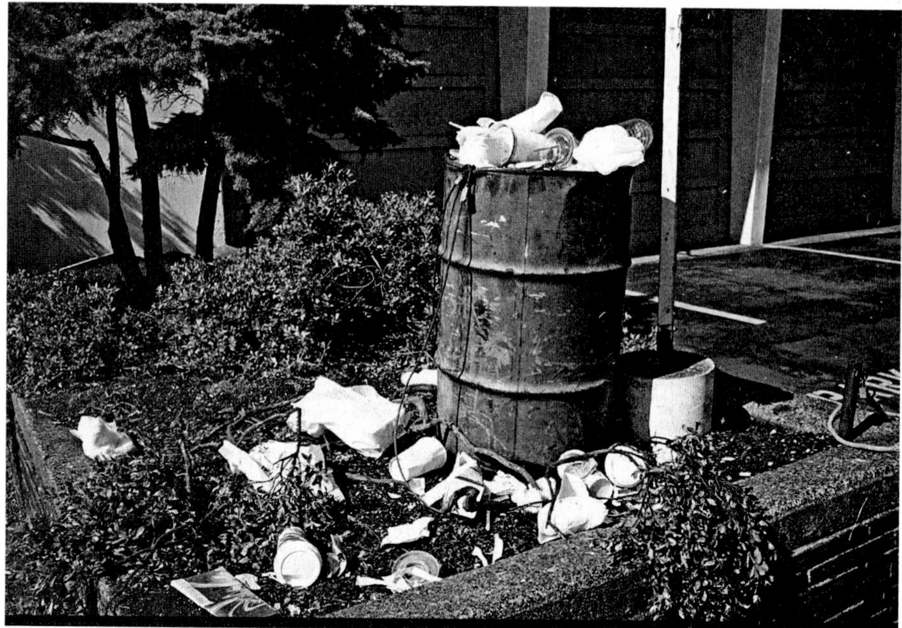

Per capita, Americans discard almost twice as much garbage as do people in Western Europe or Japan.

S. Meltzer/PhotoLink/Getty Images

Electromagnetic radiation is another possible form of air pollution. We say "possible" because the issue is controversial. Various studies have come out with contradictory results. For example, diverse researchers have found that the use of cell phones slows cognitive function, or speeds up cognitive functioning, or has no effect on cognitive functioning (Rich 2010). Research funded by the telecommunications industry is much more likely than independent research to find no harm in cell phone use.

The problem is compounded by the fact that we don't know what levels, if any, are unsafe for humans. Some early researchers reported possible increases in cancer and Alzheimer's disease, but a more recent survey of various studies concluded that there is no consistent evidence that low-level radio-frequencies (the kind that most people would be exposed to) have adverse health effects (Elwood and Wood 2019). At most, there may be a very weak connection between exposure and illness, but the issue is still unresolved (Brodsky et al. 2003; Moulder, Foster, Erdreich, and McNamee 2005; Kheifets, Afifi, and Shimkhada 2006; Genuis 2008). On the other hand, there is increasing evidence that the radiation can adversely affect brain functioning, including learning and memory (Narayanan et al. 2019).

Some advances have also been made in *water pollution control.* The volume of pollutants discharged into the nation's waterways has decreased, and thousands of acres of lakes and thousands of miles of rivers and streams have been restored and made safe for swimming and fishing. The problem remains serious, however. Many of America's rivers and streams are polluted by high levels of phosphorus and nitrogen. Water pollution also includes the oil spills noted earlier. And serious pollution occurs from various toxic materials dumped into the oceans and waterways and from nitrogen and phosphorus from agricultural runoff. The greenhouse gases that fuel the warming are also a threat to the ecosystem of the oceans (Lieberman 2004). Oceans contain increasing concentrations of carbon dioxide, which can hamper the efforts of many marine animals to form shells.

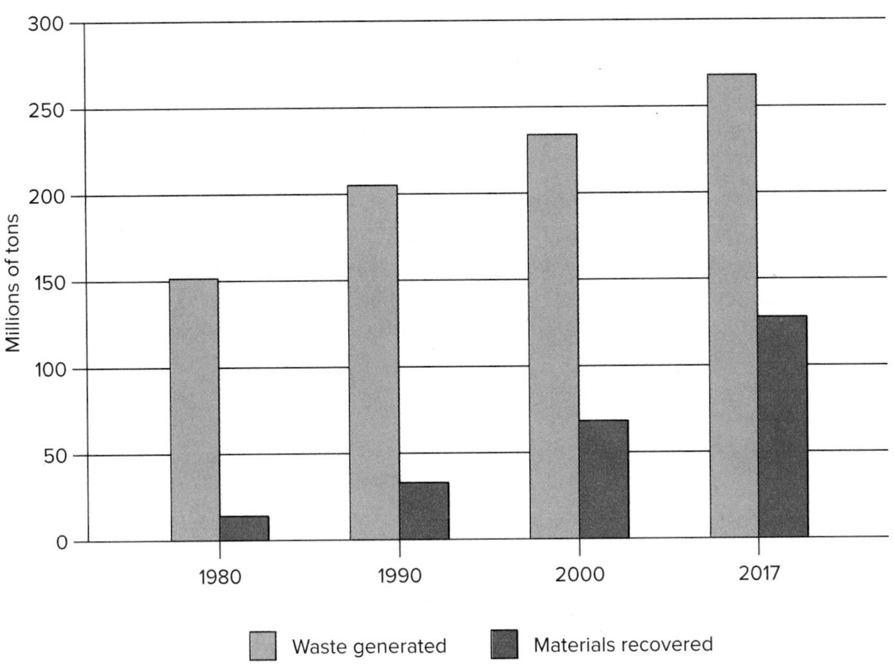


**FIGURE 15.2**
Municipal Solid Waste Generation and Recovery.
Source: EPA website.

Pollution by hazardous wastes has also declined, but the problem is still severe. Literally billions of pounds of toxic chemicals are released into the environment each year. This form of pollution intersects with the problems of racial or ethnic origin and poverty because chemical plants and toxic wastes tend to be in areas where the poor and minorities live (Pine, Marx, and Lakshmanan 2002; Pais, Crowder, and Downey 2014).

Finally, there is the staggering amount of trash and garbage discarded each year. Americans discard hundreds of millions of tons of trash and garbage every year, and the amount is increasing. As Figure 15.2 shows, the amount of waste that is recovered (recycled) is also growing. But the sheer amount of the waste that is not recycled is staggering. Consider, for example, plastics (Geyer, Jambeck, and Law 2017). An estimated 8,300 metric tons of plastics had been produced by 2015, resulting in 6,300 metric tons of waste. Only about 9 percent was recycled. The rest was either incinerated (12 percent) or thrown into landfills (79 percent).

Trash illustrates the dilemmas of environmental problems. To help clean the air, incinerators, which once burned a good part of the trash, were phased out and "sanitary" landfills became the main method of disposal. Because a good part of the trash is paper, much that is thrown away is supposedly biodegradable. That is, it will eventually break down, decompose, and become a part of the earth.

Unfortunately, biodegradation doesn't happen in landfills. Archaeologists have discovered that so-called biodegradable trash and garbage are preserved rather than destroyed in landfills, probably because the materials are tightly packed and covered, with little exposure to light or moisture (Grossman and Shulman 1990; Schwartz 2020). Most of the trash remains essentially unchanged in weight, volume, and form for decades.

## WORLD ENERGY PRODUCTION AND CONSUMPTION

Energy production and consumption are an integral part of the problems of pollution and dwindling resources. They also play an integral part in the quality of people's lives. For example, try to imagine a world without electricity and the internal combustion engine. It would still be a livable world, but as Flavin and Dunn (1999:23) put it:

> *Homo sapiens* has relied for most of its existence on a virtually limitless flow of renewable energy resources—muscles, plants, sun, wind, and water—to meet its basic needs for shelter, heat, cooking, lighting, and movement. The relatively recent transition to coal that began in Europe in the seventeenth century marked a major shift to dependence on a finite stock of fossilized fuels.

This shift affected every aspect of life—health care, education, leisure activities, and so on. People throughout the world desire the standard of living produced by the shift. As developing nations strive to achieve the standard of living now enjoyed by the developed nations, questions of practicality arise. Does the earth have enough resources for all nations to achieve such a standard? Energy use per capita varies enormously around the world (Table 15.2). Note the difference between a developing nation such as India and the developed nations such as the United States. The United States consumes over four times the amount of energy that is consumed on the entire continent of Africa!

Even among the developed nations there is a considerable difference in the amount of energy consumed per capita. Some of these differences reflect varying climates (e.g., heating and air conditioning are needed far more in some nations than in others). Yet the figures raise the question of how much energy per capita is needed for a decent standard of living. Is life in the United States, where energy consumed per capita is significantly higher than that of the United Kingdom, Austria, Germany, and Japan, far superior to that of other developed nations? Or is there a good deal of unnecessary energy use in the United States? Could Americans cut down on their energy use without seriously or even moderately diminishing the quality of their lives?

It is difficult to estimate the seriousness of all kinds of pollution, partly because measurement techniques have not been developed and partly because the potential hazards involved have been recognized only recently. Some forms of pollution, such as noise pollution and aesthetic damage, are undesirable or annoying rather than hazardous. How can their seriousness be assessed? In spite of such problems, it is clear that pollution in general is one of the serious problems confronting the nation, and it is a problem for which there are no easy answers.

### Environmental Depletion

Many experts believe that the astounding pace at which people are consuming natural resources threatens the resource capacity of the earth (Assadourian 2010). We mentioned earlier that Americans now import a major proportion of many important minerals and will import even more in the future as they continue to devour their own resources at a high rate.

The problem of depletion, of course, is international (Moyer 2010). For example, a major concern for the well-being of the earth is deforestation. Between 2000 and 2005, Africa lost 3.2 percent of its forested area, and South America lost 2.5 percent (Gardner 2006). Over the course of human history, nearly half of the earth's forests have been depleted, most of which has occurred since 1970. Tropical forests may contain as many as half of the world's plant and animal species, including many plants used for medicine. In addition, they are a major impediment to the buildup of carbon dioxide and, thereby, to global warming. About 1.3 million hectares of tropical forest are cut down each year to provide fuel and land for development and agriculture

| Country | Total (Quadrillion Btu) | Per Capita (Million Btu) |
|---|---|---|
| World total | 575.4 | 79.3 |
| United States | 97.8 | 304.3 |
| Brazil | 15.1 | 73.9 |
| Canada | 14.6 | 416.0 |
| China | 129.2 | 94.5 |
| India | 28.0 | 22.4 |
| Japan | 20.6 | 162.3 |
| Mexico/Chile | 9.1 | 65.4 |
| Australia/New Zealand | 7.0 | 257.5 |
| Russia | 31.7 | 222.6 |

**TABLE 15.2**
Energy Consumption of Selected Nations

SOURCE: U.S. Energy Information Administration website.

(Flavin and Engelman 2009). And that adds 6.5 billion tons of carbon dioxide to the earth's atmosphere each year.

Increasing energy use is another major concern. Energy use per capita is increasing in most of the nations of the world (Enerdata 2020). And as Table 15.2 shows, with the exception of China, the United States uses more energy than any nation in the world and more energy per capita than the great majority of nations. With about 4.4 percent of the world's population, the U.S. proportion of the world's consumption of energy is 17 percent!

The amount of energy Americans consume driving their vehicles is staggering, and the number of miles traveled continues to increase in spite of rising gas prices and efforts to encourage car pools. In 1970, Americans drove their cars, vans, pickups, SUVs, and motor homes 1.11 trillion miles. By 2019, the number rose to 3.26 trillion miles (U.S. Department of Transportation 2020).

How can Americans keep up with their voracious appetite for energy? Some experts believe that nuclear sources are the only hope, but reliance on nuclear power plants poses serious problems. Total reliance on nuclear power is not even feasible because of the number of plants that would have to be built and the problem of storing radioactive wastes. In addition, there is the ever-present possibility of accidents and disasters. This possibility became a reality in April 1986 when two large explosions occurred at the Chernobyl plant in the Soviet Union, "a blast heard round the world" (Flavin 1987). Within days, much of Europe reported the highest levels of radioactive fallout ever. Within two weeks, elevated levels of radioactivity were detected throughout the Northern Hemisphere. For weeks afterward, fresh vegetables in many areas of Europe were contaminated. Cows that grazed on contaminated grass soon produced milk with unhealthy levels of radioactivity. For a number of months, as many as 100 million people had to alter their diets.

The Soviet Union, of course, suffered the worst consequences. Thirty-one people were killed and 1,000 were injured immediately. Another 135,000 were evacuated from their homes. Of the 25,000 workers under the age of 35 who participated in the cleanup, 5,000 to 7,000 died (Chernousenko 1991). As many as 4 million people in the region are at high risk for cancer and other illnesses. The incidence of these illnesses began to increase within a few years after the accident (Parks 1991). Ten years after the disaster, researchers found a variety of psychosomatic symptoms and high levels of fear and stress (Specter 1996). More than two decades later, researchers linked the disaster to high rates of mental health problems, thyroid cancer (including in the Czech Republic, which had received only a moderate amount of radioactive fallout), and leukemia among the emergency workers who responded to the disaster (Murbeth, Rousarova, Scherb, and Lengfelder 2004; Bromet 2012; Ivanov et al. 2012; Tronko et al. 2012).

The Chernobyl disaster, along with subsequent accidents and near-disasters, has intensified concerns about the utility of nuclear power for generating energy. As a result, several nations—including the United States, Great Britain, and Germany—have cut back on the number of reactors in operation.

## Environmental Problems and the Quality of Life

Environmental problems confront Americans with *a number of inherent contradictions:* the value of growth and progress versus the value of freedom to choose the size of one's family; the desire for abundant energy versus the value of a clean environment; the preference for reasonably low energy prices versus the value of independence in the world arena. It is impossible to have all these options, so Americans must engage in *trade-offs* between such choices as cost and abundance, national independence and abundance, and abundance and quality of the environment.

### The Environmental Threat to Life and Health

The *environmental threat to both physical and emotional well-being* occurs from all the environmental problems named thus far.

*The Physical Threat.* The physical threat is summarized by the U.S. Public Health Service (1995:80):

> Among the numerous diseases and dysfunctions that have a known or suspected environmental component are cancer, reproductive disorders such as infertility and low birthweight, neurological and immune system impairments, and respiratory conditions such as asthma. Exposure to environmental hazards can be through air, food, or water and covers a broad range of factors such as pesticides, toxic chemicals, and radiation.

We are surrounded by hazards of all kinds, and those hazards may be even more threatening than we have realized. A "moderate" level of pollution by ambient fine particulate matter is considered generally safe by the Environmental Protection Agency. But a study of 10 years of data on Boston, Massachusetts, found that residents had a 34 percent higher chance of having a stroke within hours of experiencing a "moderate" level of the pollution (Wellenius et al. 2012). Globally, the pollution from power plants, automobiles, and other sources is a factor in about one out of every five deaths—8.7 million (Milman 2021).

Among the illnesses that severe air pollution can cause or contribute to:

Permanent lung damage in children (Gauderman et al. 2007)

Genetic abnormalities in children (Fagin 2008)

Fetal deaths (Siddika et al. 2016)

Infant mortality, including sudden infant death syndrome (Dales et al. 2004; World Health Organization 2016)

Respiratory illness and death from respiratory infections (Spix et al. 1998; Samet et al. 2000)

Cardiovascular disease (Samet et al. 2000; Miller et al. 2007)

Premature deaths (Revkin 2001; World Health Organization 2016)

Asthma attacks (Sarafino, Paterson, and Murphy 1998; Schwartz 2004)

Lung cancer (Moore 1999; Parent et al. 2007)

There is also a possible link between air pollution and autism (Roberts et al. 2013) and between air pollution and tuberculosis (Lai et al. 2016). These adverse consequences may be caused by either outdoor or indoor air pollution. We pointed out earlier in this chapter that many products and materials in the home give off toxic vapors. A similar situation exists in workplaces. Workers in particular kinds of jobs may be exposed to, or may work with, one of the chemicals known to be a factor in respiratory problems, cancer, and other illnesses.

For example, a study of 125 pregnant women who were exposed to organic solvents in their jobs found an increased risk of major fetal malformations; they were thus more likely than nonexposed women to give birth to babies with major defects (Khattak et al. 1999). The researchers also found an increased risk of miscarriage among the exposed women. Other research found that the use of cleaning products can exacerbate the problem of asthma (Vizcaya et al. 2015).

Some of the chemicals to which workers are exposed are known to be neurotoxic, causing damage to the nervous system, with resulting behavioral and emotional disorders. The problem of neurotoxins came to public attention in the 1970s when workers at a fabrics plant suffered various degrees of nerve damage. The workers had been exposed to a solvent used as an ink thinner and machine cleaner. As a result, they experienced weakness in their hands and feet (so much so that some could barely turn a key or use a screwdriver), loss of weight, and problems with walking (Anderson 1982).

Exposure to toxic materials can also lead to sterility. Male sperm counts have been declining for many decades (Swan 2006; Levine 2017). The decline may reflect the fact that industries use a number of chemicals that can result in infertility. In Costa Rica, 1,500 banana plantation workers developed permanent sterilization from exposure to a toxic pesticide (Thrupp 1991; Mostafalou and Abdollahi 2017). In the United States, children born to women who live within a quarter mile of a toxic waste dump have higher rates of birth and heart defects (Roosevelt 2004).

The depleted ozone layer raises the risk of skin cancer, whereas high ozone levels at ground level are harmful to both humans and plant life. In fact, high ozone levels are associated with breathing difficulties, asthma attacks, lung damage, and increases in the number of cardiovascular and respiratory deaths (Gryparis et al. 2004; Environmental Protection Agency 2015). In rural areas, high ozone levels reduce crop yields (Monastersky 1999).

Acid rain is a threat to forests and lakes. Eutrophication in waterways can kill massive numbers of fish, which means less food available for a world in which millions of people are starving. Ironically, some of the eutrophication problems arise from efforts to produce an adequate food supply. More than half the phosphorus that overfertilizes water comes from municipal wastes, but a substantial minority is due to urban and rural runoff. As farmers continue to apply fertilizer in increasing quantities to improve the yield of needed agricultural products, they also increase the likelihood of eutrophication of waterways and the consequent destruction of needed fish.

Routinely used pesticides and herbicides produce yet another hazard (Alarcon et al. 2005). The consequences of exposure to pesticides and herbicides include increased risk for stillbirth, birth defects, children's asthma, injury to the nervous system and reproductive organs, lung damage, problems with the immune and endocrine systems, renal disease, and cancer (Mansour 2004; Salam, Li, Langholz, and Gilliland 2004; Lebov et al. 2016).

A number of adverse consequences of global warming have already surfaced (Epstein 2000). Disease-causing bacteria, viruses, and fungi are spreading more widely; malaria and other mosquito-associated diseases have begun to appear in areas of the world where they were once absent. The problem will only intensify as the warming continues.

Finally, noise pollution is at best a nuisance and at worst a hazard to personal well-being. Excessive noise levels can result in nervousness, amnesia, conversation problems, hearing damage, high blood pressure, increased risk of cardiovascular disorders, sleep disturbance, lower work productivity, and problems in relating to others (Haines et al. 2003; Gan et al. 2016; Moteallemi, Bina, and Mortezaie 2018).

*The Emotional Threat.* The emotional threat is illustrated by the fact that people who work around hazardous materials may suffer from increased anxiety and depression (Roberts 1993). They experience stress over potential health problems–from uncertainty about the seriousness of the exposure and from a sense of powerlessness over the situation (what can an individual do to change the situation?) (Hallman and Wandersman 1992; Matthies, Hoger, and Guski 2000).

In Chapter 9, we discussed the Flint, Michigan water crisis, which exposed people to dangerous levels of lead and outbreaks of Legionnaire's disease. The crisis also took an emotional toll on the citizenry (Kruger et al. 2017). Among other things, those who were aware of the dangers posed by their drinking water were more likely to develop posttraumatic stress disorder.

Another study of psychological consequences involved a survey of Alabama residents who lived near the Gulf of Mexico where the massive BP oil spill occurred in 2010 (Gill, Picou, and Ritchie 2012). Five months after the disaster, researchers found high levels of stress generated by such things as concern over family health, economic loss, exposure to the oil, and future financial security.

Noise also detracts from emotional well-being. The New York City Department of Health and Mental Hygienes (2021) claimed that more than 30 million Americans have hearing loss from exposure to loud noise, and in New York City nearly one in six adults say they have ringing in their ears or hearing loss. A study of 2,844 children who lived near major airports in three different countries found a correlation between exposure to aircraft noise and hyperactivity and between traffic noise and conduct problems (Stansfeld et al. 2009).

## Threat to the Ecological Balance

Many of the examples given in this chapter show that human actions can result in a whole chain of consequences for the environment. One consequence can be an upsetting of the ecological balance. Alterations occur in the ecosystem that can have adverse effects on the quality of life.

One way that the ecological system has been altered is through the *disappearance of a number of species of animals and plants* as a result of human activity. Hundreds of animals and plants have become extinct. Hundreds more are endangered (in danger of becoming extinct) or threatened (likely to become endangered). The list of endangered or threatened species includes 95 mammals, 99 birds, 528 other kinds of animal life, and 943 plants (U.S. Fish and Wildlife Service 2021). A declining number of species means less diversity, represents a vast biological loss, and poses a direct threat to the quality of human life. As Tuxill (1999:7–8) wrote:

> In addition to providing the genetic underpinnings of our food supply, plant diversity keeps us healthy—one in every four drugs prescribed in the United States is based on a chemical compound originally discovered in plants. Plants also furnish oils, latexes, gums, fibers, timbers, dyes, essences, and other products that we use to clean, clothe, shelter, and refresh ourselves and that have many industrial uses as well. Health assemblages of native plants renew and enrich soils, regulate our freshwater supplies, prevent soil erosion, and provide the habitat needed by animals and other creatures.

Finally, a diminishing diversity increases the likelihood of pest infestations and outbreaks of disease.

Clearly, *people depend on biological diversity for the quality of their lives* (MacDonald and Nierenberg 2003). Still, caution needs to be exercised about the loss of species. Ecosystems are dynamic, not static. Some species would disappear regardless of human activity. On the other hand, humans need to be careful not to fall into the *fallacy of circular reasoning* by arguing that only those species disappear for which there is no use or importance. Therefore, the argument would run, those species that have become extinct are not needed anyway; humans are doing just fine without them. This line of reasoning ignores the fact that some species became extinct because of human activity rather than the natural workings of nature. People need to be concerned that the ecological balance is not upset, that they do not start a chain of consequences that will be detrimental to human life.

fallacy

Perhaps more important than the balance among the species is the possibility that humans will somehow intrude into the major processes of the ecosystem and cause irreversible damage that could threaten life—for the continuation of life demands certain processes, including reproduction, **photosynthesis,** and the recycling of minerals. The reproduction of some species has been affected by certain pollutants. For instance, the use of DDT caused the eggshells of some birds to become thinner and to crack before the young hatched, thus threatening the birds' reproductive capacity. DDT also has affected the reproductive capacity of some fish. Other pesticides and herbicides also may impair reproduction.

**photosynthesis**
a natural process essential to life, resulting in the production of oxygen and organic materials

Photosynthesis may be adversely affected by air pollution, by pesticides and herbicides, and above all, by the spread of the human population, which destroys the habitat of other species. Air pollution inhibits the plant life in which photosynthesis occurs, whereas human activity such as **urbanization** destroys plants by destroying their habitat. It is also possible that the pesticides and herbicides accumulating in the oceans will disrupt the process there as well. Photosynthesis is essential in the production of oxygen; it helps maintain the carbon dioxide balance in the atmosphere and is of fundamental importance in producing the organic material needed for supporting life. It is difficult to imagine that

**urbanization**
the increasing concentration of people living in cities

photosynthesis would halt completely. If it did, it would be a catastrophe. But whether or not the process could totally stop, it is clearly adversely affected by certain human activities.

## The Economic Costs

It is difficult to place a price tag on environmental problems. To fully assess the cost, we would have to include an enormous number of items: damage to livestock, trees, and crops; the death of wildlife; the expense of pollution-control measures; the cost of medical care for those whose health is adversely affected; the lost work time due to ill health; the expense of maintaining and refurbishing buildings and other structures that deteriorate because of pollution; and the cost of restoring the quality of the air and of waterways. The public is barely aware of the *innumerable ways in which economic resources are consumed by ecological problems.*

Consider the factors involved in analyzing and estimating these economic costs. First, the pollutants are emitted at a particular time and place. Second, they affect the environmental quality. (For example, the amount of sulfur dioxide in the air at a particular time and place may increase and may cause an increase in the number of people with respiratory problems.) Finally, a dollar cost must be assigned to the damages.

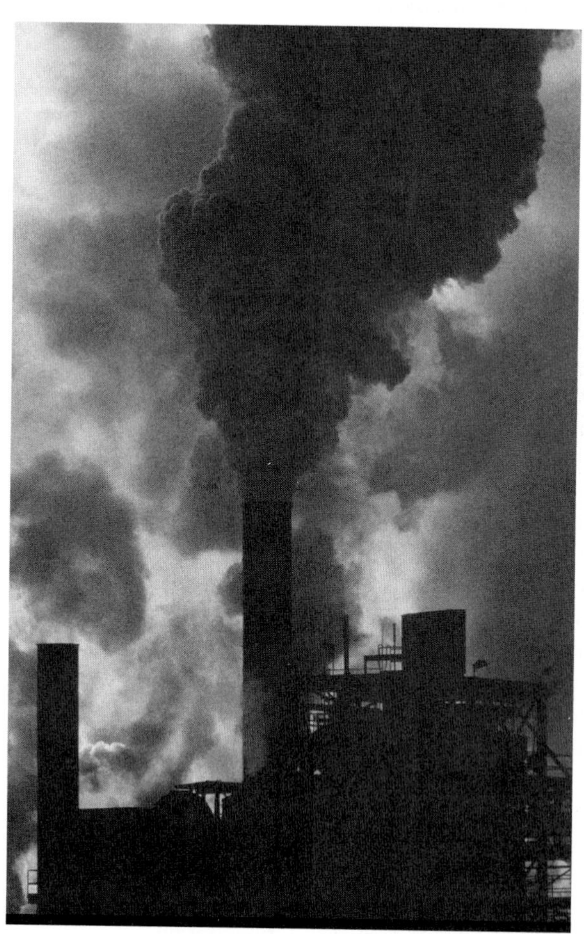

Pollution results in damage to health, property, and vegetation.

Doug Menuez/Getty Images

Every factor in this process is marked by uncertainty. We are not yet aware of all the amounts and kinds of pollutants being emitted. Nor do we yet know how all the pollutants act and interact in the environment. Thus, identifying actual damages is problematic. It is relatively easy to assign a dollar value to some damages, but extremely difficult for others. We can estimate the cost of painting a building marred by air pollution or the cost of replacing damaged crops, but what is the dollar value of a human life; a clear sky; a place for recreation; or a species that contributes to the diversity, complexity, and stability of the ecosystem?

Keeping these difficulties in mind, we can still estimate some of the economic costs of pollution. The costs, in terms of damage to property, materials, health, and vegetation, run into many billions of dollars each year for air pollution alone. One researcher (Robinson 2019) estimates that damages from air pollution cost our nation about 5 percent of the yearly gross domestic product. But because of ongoing reductions in the pollution the damages declined 20 percent from 2008 to 2014.

## Threat to World Peace

The contradictions between the demand for energy, the desire for a clean environment, the desire for reasonably low prices for energy, the struggle for natural resources, and the value on political independence are manifested on the international level in the form of a *threat to world peace.* A number of armed conflicts in the world can be traced to the struggle for control of various natural resources (Renner 2002).

In addition, the developing nations of the world are demanding to share in the affluence enjoyed by the West and Japan. Inequality among nations has become a matter of international concern. On May 1, 1974, the General Assembly of the United Nations adopted the "Declaration on the Establishment of a New International Order," which asserted a determination to work for a new and more equitable international economic order. If the widening gap between the developed and the developing nations is not eliminated, many observers fear that the result will be a world war between the relatively few rich nations and the far more numerous poor nations.

Questions arise about whether the earth's resources are sufficient and whether the environmental damage can be adequately contained if the developing nations are to achieve the same standard of living as the developed nations. On the one hand, if the gap between the rich and the poor nations is not narrowed, peace is threatened by those nations or groups of nations that would resort to violence to achieve a higher economic status (Renner 1999). On the other hand, if rich nations help poor nations achieve a higher standard of living, depleted resources and a damaged environment may drastically lower the quality of life for the entire world. It appears that the contradictions inherent in these ecological problems will continue to plague us in the future.

## Contributing Factors

Before looking at the sociocultural factors that contribute to environmental problems, you should note that some of the problems are caused by *ignorance and accidents.* Ignorance is involved because people often do not know and generally cannot anticipate the environmental consequences of their behavior. DDT, for instance, seemed beneficial because it controlled many pests, including the carriers of malaria. What was not known at the time was that DDT would impair the reproductive capacity of some fish and birds and would remain in the food chain with such persistence.

Accidents also contribute to environmental problems. It is not possible, for example, to avoid all oil spills. Weather conditions cannot be controlled. Human error cannot be totally eliminated. Thus, it was human error that led to a nuclear reaction in a uranium-reprocessing facility in Tokaimura, Japan, in 1999. The reaction lasted nearly 20 hours and had the potential for creating a Chernobyl-type disaster. And it was weather conditions—a tsunami created by an earthquake—that killed around 20,000 people in Japan in 2011 and damaged a nuclear plant that released huge amounts of radiation. It will be years before we know the full impact of this disaster.

In addition to ignorance and accidents, however, a number of sociocultural factors contribute to environmental problems. As with other social problems, both social structural and social psychological factors are involved.

### Social Structural Factors

Population Growth. *A growing population poses a threat to the environment* (Gardner, Assadourian, and Sarin 2004). Population growth accelerates the consumption of the earth's natural resources to the point that oil, natural gas, and certain minerals may eventually be exhausted. The population could even reach a number at which it would be impossible to produce enough food. The point is, any given area on the earth has a *limited carrying capacity,* that is, a limit to the number of people who can live there without causing a collapse of the biological system. If the biological system collapses, the inhabitants must either be supported by outside resources, move from the area, or face massive deaths.

Fortunately, the rate of population growth has slowed. It has slowed so much that the population of some European nations has declined and other nations may experience a decline in the future (Carr 2009). Nevertheless, the total population of the world and of most countries (even those with declining birthrates) continues to increase. The increase reflects the fact that the number of women of childbearing age has been growing and life expectancy has been rising (Engelman 2009).

As a result, the world's population is more than double what it was in 1950. The populations of the poorer nations are among those with the highest growth rates. Given their growing populations, what are the prospects for raising the standard of living in the poorer nations and for maintaining a high standard for those in the developed nations? Most scientists doubt that the earth can sustain the number of people now living at the same standard enjoyed by the average American. In fact, Assadourian (2010) estimated the earth can sustain only about 1.4 billion people at the U.S. standard.

The problems of population growth are compounded by the fact that the effects of increased population are more than additive. We noted earlier in this chapter that people generally, and Americans in particular, are consuming increased amounts of energy and other resources *per capita.* In other words, the impact per person on the environment is far greater today than it was in past years.

A second reason that a growing population has more than an additive impact on the environment is the *threshold effect.* Vegetation in an area may be able to survive a certain size of population and the air pollution created by that population. But further increase in the population might create just enough additional pollution to kill the vegetation. It becomes "the straw that breaks the camel's back."

The threshold effect can occur in all kinds of pollution with detrimental effects on all kinds of needed processes such as crop yields, fish populations, and human health (Brown and Postel 1987; Jones et al. 2020). For example, in 1982, about 8 percent of the trees in West Germany were damaged from pollution. The figure jumped to 34 percent one year later, and then to 50 percent by 1984. Something had tipped the balance and caused a sudden surge in deterioration. Several Canadian scientists showed the effects of acid rain by deliberately acidifying a small lake. Over an eight-year period, they gradually increased the concentration of acids in the lake and found a particular point at which a dramatic change occurred in the ability of the various species of fish to reproduce and survive. The effects of population may be additive to a point, and beyond that point *the increasing quantitative changes become a qualitative change.*

*The Industrial Economy.* Both pollution and depletion of the environment are rooted in the industrial economy. This finding is dramatically illustrated by the fact that the United States, with about 4.4 percent of the world's population, accounts for 16 percent of the world's carbon dioxide emissions (EPA website). Various industrial processes, from the generation of electricity to the production of goods, are responsible for a considerable part of the air pollution problem.

Water pollution is also a by-product of industrial processes. This problem includes thermal pollution, which occurs when water is taken from a waterway in large quantities and used for cooling. In the cooling process, the water absorbs heat. When this heated water is dumped back into the river or lake, it can raise the temperature to a point that is dangerous for aquatic life.

A major cause of air pollution in the United States is the *extensive use of the automobile.* The automobile also bears heavy responsibility for the rapid depletion of the world's oil reserves. America is involved in a love affair with the automobile. According to the EPA, automobiles and trucks produce 75 percent of carbon monoxide pollution in our nation and 27 percent of greenhouse gas emissions. Thirty percent of the world's autos are in the United States, accounting for half of the world's emissions from cars. And the number of cars continues to increase.

The burgeoning number and use of automobiles creates increasing pollution. Despite the fact that emissions per automobile have been greatly reduced over the past few decades, overall air quality has worsened in many cities because of the increased number of cars. Yet to drastically reduce the use of the automobile not only would be contrary to the American value of freedom and mobility, it also would cause serious economic problems. The automobile, a prime factor in environmental pollution and depletion, is an integral part of our affluent economy. Significant numbers of workers depend on the manufacture, distribution, service, and use of motor vehicles. An attack on the automobile is clearly an attack on the economy. Thus, a way must be found to deal with the environmental problem without ignoring the economic consequences.

As the automobile illustrates, the industrial economy operates at a pace that outstrips the ability to counteract the environmental problems it creates. Consider the chemical industry. Cancer is largely an environmental problem often *caused by carcinogenic chemicals* (Napoli 1998; McGinn 2002). There are approximately 2 million known chemical compounds, and thousands more are discovered each year. Some of these new compounds will be carcinogenic, but there are insufficient facilities to properly test them all.

These chemical compounds are one example of useful new products. Unfortunately, useful products can have undesirable environmental side effects. Because industrial technology can produce enormous quantities of any single product and an enormous range of products, and because the economy is set up to maximize growth, the whole situation is self-sustaining. Continual expansion is the goal. That goal is facilitated by (1) massive advertising; (2) the proliferation of products, many competing for the same market; (3) the planned obsolescence of products; and (4) lobbying at various levels of government to ensure that governmental decisions will be favorable to business and

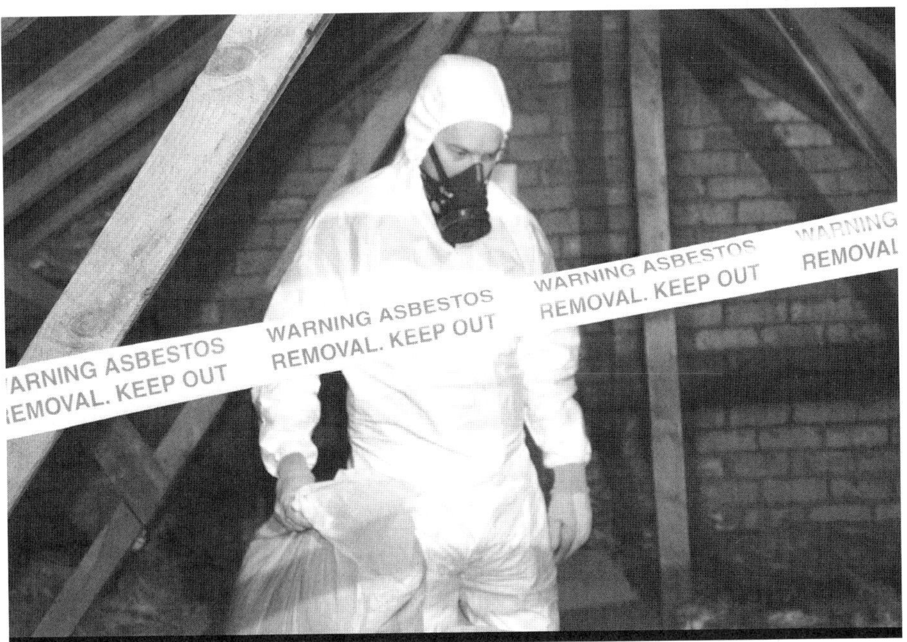


Many industrial workers are directly exposed to a variety of hazards to their health.

Alistair Forrester Shankie/E+/Getty Images

industry. "Planned obsolescence" refers to the fact that many products are specifically designed to last only a limited time. In fact, some are designed and advertised as throw-away products: clothing, pots and pans, and safety razors are to be used once or twice and then discarded. The consequences of planned obsolescence are the production of more trash that must be disposed of, the use of more resources, and the creation of more pollutants from industries that make such products.

Business and industry not only lobby for industrial growth, they also vigorously oppose pollution-control proposals and, in some cases, have managed to defeat those proposals either by lobbying or by influencing public opinion. Thus, the industrial economy intersects with the polity in environmental problems.

*The Politics of the Environment.* Environmental problems have generally not been high-priority items with politicians. This lack of attention is unfortunate, because one way to get something done about environmental problems is to create positions that have specific responsibility for those problems. For environmental problems, this solution means governmental positions. Although Americans dislike the creation of new governmental positions, without them little may be done. There is little incentive for private industry to take the lead in addressing ecological problems.

Pollution is a national problem that requires federal action. In the past, the federal government either ignored the problem or delegated responsibility to the states. This attitude changed with the creation of the Environmental Protection Agency. Today, most politicians express interest and concern for environmental issues. Unfortunately, the rhetoric is not always matched by effective action.

The political nature of environmental problems is well illustrated by what has happened in the sale of timber in the national forests. As we have already noted, deforestation is a serious problem. Among other things, trees help reduce air pollution. According to one estimate, the reduction resulted in 850 fewer deaths and 670,000 fewer cases of acute respiratory symptoms over a year's time (U.S. Forest Service 2016). The federal government, however, has a history of selling forested land at a price below the value of the timber on the land. At least until the end of the 20th century, timber sales by the government not only led to a reduction in the amount of forested land but also cost the government far more than it received from the sales. A report by the U.S. Forest Service (2016) indicates that the problem persists. The report noted that sales of forested land are made to those who are not concerned about conservation, so that "the survival of these forests and their associated ecosystem services is in question" (U.S. Forest Service 2016, p. 37).

Another example of politics affecting environmental problems involves the destruction wrought by Hurricane Katrina (Mayer 2005). The state of Mississippi wanted casinos built on the wetlands of the Gulf coast. They wanted the revenue from the casinos, but didn't want them built on dry land because of objections from local conservative moralists. The Environmental Protection Agency argued against the casinos because the wetlands are the home of aquatic life, are an important mechanism for drainage, and act as a buffer against storm damage. A U.S. senator from Mississippi was influential in having an EPA employee who was holding up the casino permits transferred. The permits were granted, the casinos were built, and the damage both to the casinos and the coast was far more severe than it would otherwise have been. In this case, politics triumphed over environmental needs. But the victory turned bitter with Katrina.

A third example of adverse environmental effects from political decisions is the Flint, Michigan, drinking water crisis that came to national attention in 2014. A political decision was made to switch the city's water supply from Lake Huron to the Flint

## NATURE BATS LAST

"Of all the problems I've studied," said one student, "the environmental problem is the most frustrating and frightening to me. It seems that no matter what you do, you're trapped. I see what it means to say that nature bats last." In spite of the seriousness of the problems and the dilemmas (such as a new technology that addresses one problem only to create another), this chapter shows that people have made some progress in dealing with environmental problems. Where does your community stand? Make a survey of the environmental problems. Check your newspaper, your library, and local officials to get information about pollution levels. Tour your area and observe the number and, if possible, kinds of pollutants that are daily being released into the atmosphere, the waterways, and the land. Use the materials in this chapter and the data you get from your survey to write an article or a letter to the editor of your local newspaper and/or your school newspaper. Even though nature always bats last, is it possible that both human beings and nature can be winners in the long run?

involvement

River. The aim was to save money during a time of fiscal struggle. However, officials failed to apply corrosion inhibitors to the water. Soon a resident had the water tested, and it was found to have high levels of lead. The proportion of children with elevated lead levels in their blood doubled in two years from 2013 to 2015 (Hanna-Attisha et al. 2016). The city switched back to water from Lake Huron in late 2015.

Thus, the stance of the government on environmental issues is crucial. Consider, finally, the problem of toxic chemicals. Whatever your background, your body is undoubtedly contaminated with toxic chemicals (Curtis and Wilding 2007). You can't avoid them because they're found in many common household products such as shower curtains, shampoo, furniture, cosmetics, and computers. This is not to say that you are in imminent danger; your body can absorb certain levels of toxic substances without harming you. The problem is we don't know precisely what those levels are, and we don't know how many of the chemicals to which we are routinely exposed are toxic.

Some scientists believe that the increasing rates of infertility among women are due, at least in part, to toxic chemicals (Schapiro 2007). We don't know all of the long-range health consequences of exposure, but future generations may provide us with information—tests of the umbilical cords of 10 newborns in 2006 found traces of carcinogenic and gene-mutating chemicals. It may be that our ever-more-sophisticated technology is exposing us to ever-more kinds and levels of toxic chemicals.

Concern about the matter led Congress to pass the Toxic Substances Control Act in 1976, which gave the government the authority to regulate chemicals that might harm people and/or the environment. However, the chemical industry influenced the legislation so that all chemicals on the market before 1979 were not subject to federal testing. In addition, the procedures set up by the law are favorable to industry. As a result, the government has assessed the risks on less than 200 of the tens of thousands of chemicals on the market today (Schapiro 2007). For many people, this means that the government is failing in its responsibility to adequately protect the citizenry.

### Social Psychological Factors

*Attitudes and the Environment.* Many people see the Earth as a resource to be mined rather than as a trust to be cared for. The measure of success is the amount of goods that can be consumed. People are admonished that they could be just as happy with less and warned that they are engaged in a process of self-destruction as they abuse the Earth for their own excessive gratification, but these warnings largely seem to fall on deaf ears. Environmentalism is honored more in theory than in practice. The prevailing attitude is "I must get all that I can out of this life," rather than "I must cherish and sustain the Earth that gives us life."

*Existing attitudes lend mixed support for environmental action.* On the one hand, fewer than half of Americans identify themselves as environmentalists (Jones 2016). On the other hand, two-thirds of Americans believe the government should do more to address the problem of climate change (Tyson and Kennedy 2020).

Given these mixed attitudes, it is not surprising that there is little public pressure for the federal government to be more aggressive in compelling business and industry to be environmentally responsible. Such attitudes will not spur politicians to take actions necessary to deal effectively with environmental problems.

fallacy

In addition, many people believe that stricter environmental regulations will force business closings and bring about a loss of jobs, a belief unsupported by evidence. There may be an occasional closing or the loss of certain jobs, but to generalize from a few cases is to commit the *fallacy of dramatic instance.* In the nation as a whole, there is no conflict between jobs and the environment (Obach 2002). On the contrary, efforts to protect the environment create new jobs. Moreover, some of the most serious environmental problems are due to industries that add relatively little to the nation's economy (Freudenburg 2009). A significant amount of toxic emissions are emitted by the chemical and primary metal industries; these account for less than 5 percent of the nation's gross domestic product and less than 1.5 percent of American jobs.

Racist attitudes contribute to a problem noted earlier: the greater exposure of minorities to hazardous materials both at work and in their homes. *Environmental racism means that African Americans, Hispanics, and other minorities are more likely to be exposed to toxic waste sites and to higher levels of air pollution* (Grineski, Bolin, and Boone 2007; Sicotte and Swanson 2007). It also means that minorities are more likely to work near toxic waste sites. In addition to racial and ethnic minorities, the poor of all races are also more likely to suffer detrimental consequences from environmental problems. The well-to-do, who have more political power than others, have the NIMBY (not-in-my-backyard) attitude that leads them to take action to minimize environmental hazards in their own places of work and housing. Thus, attitudes contribute to the greater exposure of both racial and ethnic minorities and the poor to environmental problems.

*Values and the Environment.* The value of growth, "the more the better," has been a theme of American life. Sorokin (1942:255) called this aspect of American culture "quantitative colossalism." It leads to continual expansion of the perception of the "good life," which means ever-increasing goods and services and a concomitant ever-intensifying of environmental problems.

The American value of individualism also contributes to political inaction and thus to the environmental problems. As Hardin (1971) put it in a memorable phrase, our individualism involves us in the "*tragedy of the commons.*" In the Middle Ages the "commons" was the pastureland of a village. It was owned by no one person because it was available for use by all the people of the village. The "commons" today are the world's resources, and the "tragedy" is that it is advantageous for individuals to exploit those resources but disadvantageous to all when too many individuals pursue their own advantage. Yet, with our value on individualism (rather than on group well-being), we are, said Hardin (1971:247), "locked into a system of 'fouling our own nest,'" by behaving "only as independent, rational, free-enterprisers." The value of individualism also makes Americans reluctant to yield power to government. For many Americans, political inaction is the soul of good government, but in the realm of ecology, political inaction is the harbinger of disaster.

## Solutions: Public Policy and Private Action

At the outset, we need to acknowledge that environmental problems pose numerous dilemmas. There are no easy answers. Some of the "solutions" create new problems. For instance, with the surge in population growth in the 19th century, farmers began looking for ways to increase food production. One way was through the development of nitrogen-based fertilizers, which led to enormously increased food production. But those same fertilizers were, and continue to be, responsible for "poisoning ecosystems, destroying fisheries, and sickening and killing children throughout the world" (Fisher and Fisher 2001). Thus, the needed additional food is had at the expense of air and water quality.

Still, there are many ways to alleviate the problems, including many actions that individuals can take and are taking (DeSilver 2015). For example, the amount of energy expended on home heating has declined since 1993. The proportion of light bulbs in the home that are incandescent (and therefore use more energy) has declined dramatically, from about 65 percent in 2013 to 25 percent in 2015. The amount of water used by the average household has declined since 1980. And the percentage of paper, cardboard, yard trimmings, metals, and plastics that is recycled has risen substantially.

Such actions, along with changes in business and industry, have contributed substantially to progress in addressing environmental issues in recent decades. The emission of greenhouse gases into the atmosphere and the release of toxic chemicals into the environment have both declined. Blood lead levels in children have declined. Many lakes and waterways that were unsafe for fishing or swimming are once again usable. And the amount of materials recycled has increased greatly.

Action can also be taken to address the problem of dwindling natural resources. One way is to reduce consumption. Thus, a number of European nations reduced their oil consumption between 1980 and 2008 (Mouawad 2008). The reductions ranged from 13 percent in Italy to 33 percent in Denmark. During the same period, however, oil consumption in the United States rose 21 percent.

The reduction in various kinds of pollution, increased recycling, and reduced oil consumption by the European nations all demonstrate that environmental problems can be attacked by human action. Such action must be taken by individuals, by business and industry, and by the various levels of government.

### What Can Individuals Do?

In addition to the actions of individuals mentioned above, knowledgeable people need to educate others about the seriousness of environmental pollution and depletion in order to change attitudes, values, and behavior. When people understand what they can do and the benefits of their efforts, they are more likely to engage in the appropriate behavior (Scott 1999; O'Connor, Bord, Yarnal, and Wiefek 2002).

Such education helps individuals recognize how much each one can do to alleviate the environmental problems. For example, you could stop using throwaway items such as cameras and razors. You could refuse to buy cheese that is sliced and individually wrapped in plastic. Or parents could use cloth instead of disposable diapers. There are literally hundreds of ways in which an individual could help alleviate environmental problems (Neff 2018). Many of them may seem minor but when a large number of people engage in them, they add up to substantial savings. When millions of people use automobiles that get more miles to the gallon than older models, when millions participate in recycling efforts, when millions use energy-saving appliances and methods that cut back on electricity, the savings are enormous. People could easily save a million or more barrels of crude oil every day without detracting from their standard of living.

Individuals can also work with others to find innovative ways to help the environment. An activist in San Francisco invented the "Carrotmob" (Caplan 2009). In essence, the idea is to reward businesses for green activity rather than punishing (by boycotting, for example) those that harm the environment. The first Carrotmob event took place after the activist got bids from 23 convenience stores and chose the one that promised to spend the highest proportion of profits on more energy-efficient lighting. Hundreds of shoppers were then secured to visit the store on a particular day, and the agreed-upon percentage of their purchases was used to make the store's lighting more energy efficient. Subsequently, people in other cities, including some in other nations, adopted the Carrotmob principle of reverse boycott.

## What Can Business and Industry Do?

Business and industry must cooperate with governmental efforts to clean up the environment, but they must also strive to balance growth with ecological considerations and search for *alternative, clean sources of energy* upon which to base the economy. A number of alternatives are already being studied. Some people advocate nuclear power, but a total conversion to nuclear power is not feasible. Furthermore, nuclear power confronts people with the very difficult questions of how to dispose of radioactive waste and how to ensure against leaks and accidents that can release radioactivity into the atmosphere. Other possible alternatives include solar energy (the light and heat from the sun), geothermal energy (the water and hot rock beneath the earth's surface), the use of wind-driven generators, bioheat (heat derived from burning such things as wood or pellets), designing new buildings to be more energy efficient, and using seawater or lake water for cooling (Sawin and Moomaw 2009). These alternatives are not necessarily practical in every area. Rather, the advantages and disadvantages of each of these alternatives must be explored carefully but quickly, for the supply of fossil fuels is being rapidly depleted while the demand for energy is increasing throughout the world.

## What Can the Government Do?

Government action at every level is crucial in dealing with environmental problems. The federal government could mandate higher gas mileage for all new cars. The government could effect savings in resources and simultaneously help the pollution problem by supporting the development of mass transit. Mass transit can carry 70 times the number of people as a highway, generate only 1 percent of the hydrocarbons, and cost one-tenth as much to build per mile as does a highway (Hagerman 1990). The government could follow through with a congressional mandate in the early 1990s to set standards for the distribution transformers that convert the high-voltage current transmitted over grids into lower-voltage current for home and business use (Kolbert 2006). More efficient transformers are available, and installing them in place of the less efficient ones now in use could save the nation about 12 billion kilowatt hours of electricity usage a year—enough to power all the households in Iowa for one year.

The federal government could also diminish or eliminate pollution caused by its own operations and by those supported by federal funds. It could provide direct funding and tax incentives for research into pollution control and alternative energy sources. It could impose tax penalties on businesses and corporations that damage the environment, a measure that has proven to reduce problems in the United States and other nations (Roodman 1999). It could support international treaties that set goals for cutting the emission of greenhouse gases. It could reduce the production of greenhouse gases like methane, which is the second largest contributor to global warming, by requiring the use of technology that captures the gas at landfills and waste management facilities and during the mining of fossil fuels (Hansen 2004; Jorgenson 2006).

Any action the federal government takes in behalf of the environment is likely to have effects beyond what any policy or program is designed to do. A study of the effects of a national environmental policy on nations in the European Union found that the citizens who live in nations that adopt strong pro-environment policies are more likely than others to drive less in order to help the environment (Borek and Bohon 2008). Moreover, the reduced driving occurs even when the policies are not directly related to the use of the automobile.

State and local governments also can play a significant role in addressing environmental problems by establishing recycling laws and policies. Recycling is now available in many if not most communities, but there are still those communities that do not provide a recycling service. Such a service is advantageous to the community itself as well as to the national and global effort to deal with environmental problems, for recycling means a lessening of the waste disposal problem. In addition, recycling reduces the demand for newly produced energy and materials, thereby saving our natural resources. And for some goods, such as paper, using recycled material saves energy in the manufacturing process.

Trimming waste disposal needs gets into an area that has almost reached crisis proportions in some cities. The volume of discarded material is surpassing the capacity to manage it. In addition, electronic waste has become the main contributor to high levels of lead in landfills (Saphores, Nixon, Ogunseitan, and Shapiro 2006). Recycling, which can address such problems to a considerable extent, may need to be mandatory. Will people cooperate? Unfortunately, some people will not. But most will, particularly when measures such as curbside pickup of materials are instituted (Domina and Koch 2002).

*Follow-Up.* Make a list of the actions you have personally taken to alleviate environmental problems. Which of these, or other actions, would you make a matter of law and which would you make purely voluntary?

## Summary

Environmental problems arise out of the need to maintain a balanced ecosystem—a balance between people and their natural environment. Human activity can disrupt this ecosystem to the point of destruction.

Environmental problems may be broadly classified as environmental pollution and environmental depletion. Pollution includes air pollution, water pollution, land pollution, global warming, noise pollution, and aesthetic damage. Depletion refers to dwindling natural resources, including energy.

It is difficult to measure the extent of these environmental problems. Some progress has been made but the problems remain serious.

Environmental problems involve inherent contradictions among a number of American values. We do not fully understand how these contradictions are being manifested in social life, but we know that they diminish the quality of life in a number of ways. Pollutants threaten the health and life of humans, animals, and plants. The ecological balance is threatened by the potential destruction of certain processes that are necessary to sustain life on earth. The economic costs of both pollution damage and pollution control are enormous, and the contradictions between the demand for energy, the need for a clean environment, and the aspirations of the developing world pose a threat to world peace.

Rapid population growth is one of the important threats to the environment. The effects of population growth are more than additive, as evidenced by diminishing returns and the threshold effect. In addition to population growth, the industrial economy is at the root of environmental problems. The products, by-products, and continuing growth in the industrial economy create serious environmental problems. The problems are intensified by the tendency of the government to ignore them or to set up ineffective programs and policies. Federal action is imperative if Americans are to seriously attack the problems of the environment.

Among social psychological factors, attitudes that view the earth simply as a resource to be exploited and that give minimal importance to environmental problems inhibit action. Racist attitudes intensify the problem for minorities by exposing them to more hazards at work and home. The American values of growth and individualism have supported the economic and political arrangements that contribute to the problems.

## Key Terms

Ecosystem
Environmental Depletion
Environmental Pollution
Eutrophication
Herbicide
Pesticide
Photosynthesis
Pollutant
Urbanization

## Study Questions

1. What is the ecosystem? Why is it important to us?
2. Name and explain the three types of environmental problems people face.
3. How extensive are the environmental problems?
4. In what ways do environmental problems pose a threat to life, health, and the ecological balance?
5. Discuss the economic costs of environmental problems.
6. How do environmental problems threaten world peace?
7. What are some of the undesirable effects of population growth?
8. How does the economy and polity affect environmental problems?
9. What kinds of social psychological factors contribute to environmental problems?
10. What might be done to deal with the problems of environmental pollution and environmental depletion?

## Internet Resources/Exercises

1. Explore some of the ideas in this chapter on the following sites:

**http://www.epa.gov** The U.S. Environmental Protection Agency has materials on all the environmental problems we have discussed.

**http://www.envirolink.org** The Envirolink Network offers links to thousands of resources on every environmental issue.

**http://ewg.org** Site of the Environmental Working Group, whose research is designed to improve health and protect the environment.

2. Most scientists agree that global warming is a severe and urgent problem. Some people still disagree. Search the Internet for arguments both for and against global warming as a serious problem. Summarize the points and the supporting data made by both sides. Identify any fallacies of thinking you find in the arguments.

3. Political action is imperative if environmental problems are to be effectively attacked. Use a search engine to explore the relationship between government or politics and environmental problems. Find information on government at all levels. Make a list of the 10 most helpful and 10 most harmful actions (or lack of action) taken by governments in recent years. Use the information to write a letter to your local paper urging governmental action on some environmental problem about which you are concerned.

## For Further Reading

Dasgupta, Partha. *Human Well-Being and the Natural Environment.* New York: Oxford University Press, 2001. An economist argues that human well-being depends on the natural environment, including places of beauty, as well as on material goods and knowledge.

Kolbert, Elizabeth. *The Sixth Extinction: An Unnatural History.* New York: Henry Holt & Company, 2014. A review of past mass extinctions in the earth's history, and a description of processes at work today that make a new extinction possible.

Lerner, Steve. *Sacrifice Zones: The Front Lines of Toxic Chemical Exposure in the United States.* Cambridge, MA: MIT Press, 2010. An account of a number of American communities that have, in effect, been "sacrificed" for the economic benefit of businesses that establish plants that release toxic chemicals into the environment. The plants provide needed jobs, but the health consequences for the nearby residents are devastating.

Mauch, Christof. *Shades of Green: Environmental Activism Around the Globe.* New York: Rowman & Littlefield, 2006. Shows how political, economic, religious, and scientific factors come to bear on environmental activism, including ways that such factors can suppress, dilute, or enhance environmental action in diverse social and cultural settings.

Rischard, Jean-Francois. *High Noon: 20 Global Problems, 20 Years to Solve Them.* New York: Basic Books, 2003. Examines the environmental problems that threaten the planet—global warming, biodiversity losses, depletion of fisheries, deforestation, water deficits, and maritime pollution—as well as the issues related to those problems and ways in which nations must work together to resolve the problems.

Rogers, Elizabeth, and Thomas M. Kostigen. *The Green Book: The Everyday Guide to Saving the Planet One Simple Step at a Time.* New York: Three Rivers Press, 2007. Details the numerous small ways in which each individual can contribute to a greener earth (e.g., use one less napkin a day or reduce your shower time by just one minute), and shows the dramatic impact on the environment if massive numbers of individuals practice them.

Withgott, Jay H., and Scott R. Brennan. *Environment: The Science Behind the Stories.* 5th ed. New York: Addison-Wesley, 2014. Case studies are used to illustrate and discuss every kind of environmental problem in a way that is scientifically sound yet accessible to those not scientifically trained.

## References

Abdul-Wahab, S. A., ed. 2011. *Sick Building Syndrome.* New York: Springer.

Alarcon, W. A., et al. 2005. "Acute illnesses associated with pesticide exposure at schools." *Journal of the American Medical Association* 294:455–65.

Anderson, A. 1982. "Neurotoxic follies." *Psychology Today* (July):30–42.

Assadourian, E. 2010. "The rise and fall of consumer cultures." In *State of the World 2010,* ed. L. Starke and L. Mastny, pp. 3–20. New York: W. W. Norton.

Borek, E., and S. A. Bohon. 2008. "Policy climates and reductions in automobile use." *Social Science Quarterly* 89:1293–1311.

Bright, C. 2000. "Anticipating environmental surprise." In *State of the World 2000,* ed. L. R. Brown et al., pp. 22–38. New York: W. W. Norton.

Brodsky, L. M., R. W. Habash, W. Leiss, D. Krewski, and M. Rapacholi. 2003. "Health risks of electromagnetic fields." *Critical Review of Biomedical Engineering* 31:333–54.

Bromet, E. J., 2012. "Mental health consequences of the Chernobyl disaster." *Journal of Radiological Protection* 32:71-5.

Brown, L. R., and S. Postel. 1987. "Thresholds of change." In *State of the World 1987,* ed. L. R. Brown, pp. 3-19. New York: W. W. Norton.

Caplan, J. 2009. "Boycotts are so 20th century." *Time,* June 8, p. 54.

Carr, D. 2009. "Worries over a population implosion." *Contexts* 8:58-59.

Centers for Disease Control and Prevention. 2021. "Protect yourself and your family from radon." CDC website.

Chernousenko, V. M. 1991. *Chernobyl: Insight from the Inside*. New York: Springer-Verlag.

Collins, W., et al. 2007. "The physical science behind climate change." *Scientific American,* August, pp. 64-73.

Commoner, B. 1971. *The Closing Circle*. New York: Alfred A. Knopf.

Craig, C. L., R. C. Brownson, S. E. Cragg, and A. L. Dunn. 2002. "Exploring the effect of the environment on physical activity." *American Journal of Preventive Medicine* 23:36-43.

Curtis, K., and B. C. Wilding. 2007. *Is It in Us?* New York: Body Burden Work Group and Commonweal Biomonitoring Resource Center.

Dales, R., et al. 2004. "Air pollution and sudden infant death syndrome." *Pediatrics* 113:628-31.

DeSilver, D. 2015. "How Americans are—and aren't—making ecofriendly lifestyle changes." Pew Research Center website.

Domina, T., and K. Koch. 2002. "Convenience and frequency of recycling." *Environment and Behavior* 34:216-38.

Elwood, M., and A. W. Wood. 2019. "Health effects of radiofrequency electromagnetic energy." *New Zealand Medical Journal* 132:64-72.

Enerdata. 2020. "Global energy statistical yearbook." Enerdata website.

Engelman, R. 2009. "Fertility falls, population rises, future uncertain." In *Vital Signs, 2009,* ed. L. Starke, pp. 83-85. Washington, DC: Worldwatch Institute.

Environmental Protection Agency. 2015. "Air quality guide for ozone." EPA website.

——. 2021a. "Facts about formaldehyde." EPA website.

——. 2021b. "Our nation's air." EPA website.

Epstein, D. J. 2003. "Secret ingredients." *Scientific American,* August, pp. 22-23.

Epstein, P. R. 2000. "Is global warming harmful to health?" *Scientific American,* August, pp. 50-57.

Fagin, D. 2008. "China's children of smoke." *Scientific American,* August, pp. 72-79.

Fisher, D. E., and M. J. Fisher. 2001. "N: The nitrogen bomb." *Discover,* April, pp. 50-57.

Flavin, C. 1987. "Reassessing nuclear power." In *State of the World 1987,* ed. L. R. Brown, pp. 57-80. New York: W. W. Norton.

——. 2005. "Preface." In *State of the World 2005,* ed. L. Starke, pp. xix-xxi. New York: W. W. Norton.

Flavin, C., and R. Engelman. 2009. "The perfect storm." In *State of the World 2009: Into a Warming World,* ed. L. Starke, pp. 5-12. New York: W. W. Norton.

Flavin, C., and S. Dunn. 1999. "Reinventing the energy system." In *State of the World 1999,* ed. L. R. Brown et al., pp. 22-40. New York: W. W. Norton.

Freudenburg, W. 2009. "Polluters' shell game." *Worldwatch* 22:17-21.

Gan, W. Q., et al. 2016. "Exposure to loud noise, bilateral high-frequency hearing loss and coronary heart disease." *Occupational and Environmental Medicine* 73:34-41.

Gardner, G. 2006. "Deforestation continues." In *Vital Signs: 2006-2007,* ed. L. Starke, pp. 102-103. New York: W. W. Norton.

Gardner, G., E. Assadourian, and R. Sarin. 2004. "The state of consumption today." In *State of the World 2004,* ed. L. Starke, pp. 3-23. New York: W. W. Norton.

Gauderman, W. J., et al. 2007. "Effect of exposure to traffic on lung development from 10 to 18 years of age." *The Lancet* 369:571-77.

Genuis, S. J. 2008. "Fielding a current idea: Exploring the public health impact of electromagnetic radiation." *Public Health* 122:113-24.

Geyer, R., J. R. Jambeck, and K. L. Law. 2017. "Production, use, and fate of all plastics ever made." *Science Advances*. Online article.

Gill, D. A., J. S. Picou, and L. A. Ritchie. 2012. "The Exxon Valdez and BP oil spills: A comparison of initial social and psychological impacts." *American Behavioral Scientist* 56:3-23.

Grineski, S., B. Bolin, and C. Boone. 2007. "Criteria air pollution and marginalized populations." *Social Science Quarterly* 88:535-54.

Grossman, D., and S. Shulman. 1990. "Down in the dumps." *Discover* (April):36-41.

Gryparis, A., et al. 2004. "Acute effects of ozone on mortality from the 'Air Pollution and Health: A

European Approach' project." *American Journal of Respiratory and Critical Care Medicine*. [e-published ahead of print date]. AJRCCM website.

Hagerman, E. 1990. "California's drive to mass transit." *World Watch* (September-October):7-8.

Haines, M. M., S. L. Brentnall, S. A. Stansfeld, and E. Klineberg. 2003. "Qualitative responses of children to environmental noise." *Noise Health* 5:19-30.

Hallman, W. K., and A. Wandersman. 1992. "Attribution of responsibility and individual and collective coping with environmental threats." *Journal of Social Issues* 48 (4):101-18.

Hanna-Attisha, M., et al. 2016. "Elevated blood lead levels in children associated with the Flint drinking water crisis." *American Journal of Public Health* 106:283-90.

Hansen, J. 2004. "Defusing the global warming time bomb." *Scientific American,* March, pp. 68-77.

Hardin, G. 1971. "The tragedy of the commons." In *Man and the Environment,* ed. W. Jackson, pp. 243-54. Dubuque, IA: Wm. C. Brown.

Hood, E. 2005. "Investigating indoor air." *Environmental Health Perspectives* 113:158.

Howard, S. 2014. "Bhopal's legacy." *BMJ,* December 11.

Hughes, A. 2004. "Researchers study 'sick' buildings." *Civil Engineering,* May 4, p. 33.

Ivanov, V. K., et al. 2012. "Leukemia incidence in the Russian cohort of Chernobyl emergency workers." *Radiation and Environmental Biophysics* 51:143-49.

Jones, J. M. 2016. "Americans' identification as 'environmentalists' down to 42%." Gallup Poll website.

Jones, L., et al. 2020. "Climate driven threshold effects in the natural environment." Climate Change Committee online report.

Jorgenson, A. K. 2006. "Global warming and the neglected greenhouse gas." *Social Forces* 84:1779-98.

Khattak, S., et al. 1999. "Pregnancy outcome following gestational exposure to organic solvents." *Journal of the American Medical Association* 281 (March 24-31):1106-9.

Kheifets, L., A. A. Afifi, and R. Shimkhada. 2006. "Public health impact of extremely low-frequency electromagnetic fields." *Environmental Health Perspectives* 114:1532-37.

Kolbert, E. 2006. "Untransformed." *The New Yorker,* September 25, pp. 64-65.

Kruger, D. J., et al. 2017. "Toxic trauma." *Journal of Community Psychology* 45:957-62.

Kuchment, A. 2016. "Drilling for earthquakes." *Scientific American,* July.

Lai, T., et al. 2016. "Ambient air pollution and risk of tuberculosis." *Occupational and Environmental Medicine* 73:56-61.

Lebov, J. F., et al. 2016. "Pesticide use and risk of end-stage renal disease among licensed pesticide applicators in the Agricultural Health Study." *Occupational and Environmental Medicine* 73:3-12.

Leslie, M. 2003. "Acid rain collection." *Science* 301:899.

Levine, H., et al. 2017. "Temporal trends in sperm count." *Human Reproduction Update* 23:646-59.

Lieberman, B. 2004. "Rising $CO_2$ levels threaten oceans, scientists say." *San Diego Union-Tribune,* July 16.

MacDonald, M., and D. Nierenberg. 2003. "Linking population, women, and biodiversity." In *State of the World 2003,* ed. L. Starke, pp. 38-61. New York: W. W. Norton.

Mansour, S. A. 2004. "Pesticide exposure—Egyptian scene." *Toxicology* 198:91-115.

Matthies, E., R. Hoger, and R. Guski. 2000. "Living on polluted soil." *Environment and Behavior* 32:270-86.

Mayer, J. 2005. "High stakes." *The New Yorker,* September 19, pp. 37-38.

McGinn, A. P. 1999. "Charting a new course for oceans." In *State of the World 1999,* ed. L. R. Brown et al., pp. 78-95. New York: W. W. Norton.

——. 2000. *Why Poison Ourselves?* Washington, DC: Worldwatch Institute.

——. 2002. "Reducing our toxic burden." In *State of the World 2002,* ed. L. Starke, pp. 75-100. New York: W. W. Norton.

McKeown, A., and G. Gardner. 2009. *Climate Change Reference Guide.* Washington, DC: Worldwatch Institute.

Mendell, M. J., et al. 2006. "Indicators of moisture and ventilation system contamination in U.S. office buildings as risk factors for respiratory and mucous membrane symptoms." *Journal of Occupational & Environmental Hygiene* 3:225-33.

Miller, K. A., et al. 2007. "Long-term exposure to air pollution and incidence of cardiovascular events in women." *New England Journal of Medicine* 356:447-58.

Milman, O. 2021. "'Invisible killer.'" *The Guardian,* February 9.

Monastersky, R. 1999. "China's air pollution chokes crop growth." *Science News,* March 27, Science News website.

Moore, P. 1999. "New evidence links air pollution with lung cancer." *Lancet* 353 (February 27):729.

Mostafalou, S., and M. Abdollahi. 2017. "Pesticides: An update of human exposure and toxicity." *Archives of toxicology* 91:549–99.

Moteallemi, A., B. Bina, and S. Mortezaie. 2018 "Effects of noise pollution on Samen district residents in Mashhad city." *Environmental Health Engineering and Management* 5 23–27.

Mouawad, J. 2008. "The big thirst." *New York Times,* April 20.

Moulder, J. E., K. R. Foster, L. S. Erdreich, and J. P. McNamee. 2005. "Mobile phones, mobile phone base stations and cancer." *International Journal of Radiation Biology* 81:189–203.

Moyer, M. 2010. "How much is left?" *Scientific American,* September, pp. 74–82.

Murbeth, S., M. Rousarova, H. Scherb, and E. Lengfelder. 2004. "Thyroid cancer has increased in the adult populations of countries moderately affected by Chernobyl fallout." *Medical Science Monitor* 10:300–6.

Murthy, R. S. 2014. "Mental health of survivors of 1984 Bhopal disaster." *India Psychiatry Journal* 23:86–93.

Napoli, M. 1998. "Hormone-disrupting chemicals." *HealthFacts,* November, p. 1.

Narayanan, S. N., et al. 2019. "Radiofrequency electromagnetic radiation-induced behavioral changes and their possible basis." *Environmental Science and Pollution Research International* 26 (30):30693–710.

National Academy of Engineering. 2010. *Committee on Technology for a Quieter America.* NAE website.

National Aeronautics and Space Administration. 2020. "Climate change: How do we know?" NASA website.

Neff, M. 2018. *Simple Acts to Save Our Planet.* New York: Adams Media.

New York City Department of Health and Mental Hygiene. 2021. "Noise." NYC Health website.

O'Connor, R. E., R. J. Bord, B. Yarnal, and N. Wiefek. 2002. "Who wants to reduce greenhouse gas emissions?" *Social Science Quarterly* 83:1–17.

Obach, B. K. 2002. "Labor-environmental relations." *Social Science Quarterly* 83:82–100.

Osawa, H., and M. Hayashi. 2009. "Status of the indoor air chemical pollution in Japanese houses based on the nationwide field survey from 2000 to 2005." *Building and Environment* 44:1330–36.

Pais, J., K. Crowder, and L. Downey. 2014. "Unequal trajectories: Racial and class differences in residential exposure to industrial hazard." *Social Forces* 92:1189–215.

Parent, M., M. Rousseau, P. Boffetta, A. Cohen, and J. Siemiatycki. 2007. "Exposure to diesel and gasoline engine emissions and the risk of lung cancer." *American Journal of Epidemiology* 165:53–62.

Parks, M. 1991. "Cherynobyl." *Los Angeles Times,* April 23.

Pawel, D. J., and J. S. Puskin. 2004. "The U.S. Environmental Protection Agency's assessment of risks from indoor radon." *Health Physics* 87:68–74.

Pine, J. C., B. D. Marx, and A. Lakshmanan. 2002. "An examination of accidental-release scenarios from chemical-processing sites: The relation of race to distance." *Social Science Quarterly* 83:317–31.

Renner M. 1999. "Ending violent conflict." In *State of the World 1999,* ed. L. R. Brown et al., pp. 151–68. New York: W. W. Norton.

——. 2002. "Breaking the link between resources and repression." In *State of the World 2002,* ed. L. Starke, pp. 149–73. New York: W. W. Norton.

Revkin, A. C. 2001. "EPA ties tiniest soot particles to early deaths." *New York Times,* April 21.

Rich, N. 2010. "For whom the cell tolls." *Harper's Magazine,* May, pp. 44–53.

Roberts, A. I., et al. 2013. "Perinatal air pollution exposures and autism spectrum disorder in the Children of Nurses' Health Study II participants." *Environmental Health Perspectives* 121:746–54.

Roberts, J. T. 1993. "Psychosocial effects of workplace hazardous exposures: Theoretical synthesis and preliminary findings." *Social Problems* 40 (February):74–89.

Robinson, E. 2019. "How much does air pollution cost the U.S.?" Stanford Earth website.

Roodman, D. M. 1999. "Building a sustainable society." In *State of the World 1999,* ed. L. R. Brown et al., pp. 169–88. New York: W. W. Norton.

Roosevelt, M. 2004. "The tragedy of Tar Creek." *Time,* April 26, pp. 42–47.

Salam, M. T., Y. F. Li, B. Langholz, and F. D. Gilliland. 2004. "Early-life environmental risk factors for asthma." *Environmental Health Perspectives* 112:760–65.

Samet, J. M., et al. 2000. "Fine particulate air pollution and mortality in 20 U.S. cities, 1987–1994." *New England Journal of Medicine* 343:1742–49.

Sampat, P. 2000. *Deep Trouble: The Hidden Threat of Groundwater Pollution.* Washington, DC: Worldwatch Institute.

Saphores, J. M., H. Nixon, O. A. Ogunseitan, and A. A. Shapiro. 2006. "Household willingness to recycle electronic waste." *Environment and Behavior* 38:183-208.

Sarafino, E. P., M. E. Paterson, and E. L. Murphy. 1998. "Age and impacts of triggers in childhood asthma." *Journal of Asthma* 35 (2):213-17.

Sawin, J. L., and W. R. Moomaw. 2009. "An enduring energy future." In *State of the World,* ed. L. Starke, pp. 130-50. New York: W. W. Norton.

Schapiro, M. 2007. "Toxic inaction." *Harper's Magazine,* October, pp. 78-83.

Schwartz, J. 2004. "Air pollution and children's health." *Pediatrics* 113:1037-43.

——. 2020. "Why biodegradable isn't what you think." *New York Times,* October 1.

Scott, D. 1999. "Equal opportunity, unequal results." *Environment and Behavior* 31 (March):267-90.

Sengupta, S. 2008. "Decades later, toxic sludge torments Bhopal." *New York Times,* July 7.

Siddika, N., et al. 2016. "Prenatal ambient air pollution exposure and the risk of stillbirth." *Occupational and Environmental Medicine* 73:573-81.

Singh A., and M. Agrawal. 2008. "Acid rain and its ecological consequences." *Journal of Environmental Biology* 29:15-24.

Sicotte, D., and S. Swanson. 2007. "Whose risk in Philadelphia? Proximity to unequally hazardous industrial facilities." *Social Science Quarterly* 88:515-34.

Sirgy, M. J., D. Efraty, P. Siegel, and D. J. Lee. 2001. "A new measure of quality of work life (QWL) based on need satisfaction and spillover theories." *Social Indicators Research* 55:241-302.

Skanberg, A., and E. Ohrstrom. 2002. "Adverse health effects in relation to urban residential soundscapes." *Journal of Sound and Vibration* 250:151-55.

Sorokin, P. A. 1942. *The Crisis of Our Age*. New York: E. P. Dutton.

Specter, M. 1996. "10 years later, through fear, Chernobyl still kills in Belarus." *New York Times,* March 31.

Spix, C., et al. 1998. "Short-term effects of air pollution on hospital admissions of respiratory diseases in Europe." *Archives of Environmental Health* 53 (January-February):54-64.

Stansfeld, S. A., et al. 2009. "Aircraft and road traffic noise exposure and children's mental health." *Journal of Environmental Psychology* 29:203-207.

Swan, S. H. 2006. "Does our environment affect our fertility?" *Seminars in Reproductive Medicine* 24:142-46.

Tennesen, M. 2010. "Sour Showers." *Scientific American,* September, p. 23.

Thorne, P. S., et al. 2001. "Indoor environmental quality in six commercial office buildings in the Midwest United States." *Applied Occupational and Environmental Hygiene* 16:1065-77.

Thrupp, L. A. 1991. "Sterilization of workers from pesticide exposure: The causes and consequences of DBCP-induced damage in Costa Rica and beyond." *International Journal of Health Services* 21 (4):731-57.

Tronko, M., et al. 2012. "Thyroid cancer in Ukraine after the Chernobyl accident." *Journal of Radiological Protection* 32:65-70.

Tuxill, J. 1999. *Nature's Cornucopia*. Washington, DC: Worldwatch Institute.

Tyson, A., and B. Kennedy. 2020. "Two-thirds of Americans think government should do more on climate." Pew Research Center website.

U.S. Department of Transportation. 2020. "Highway statistics 2019." DOT website.

U.S. Fish and Wildlife Service. 2021. "Endangered species." U.S. Fish and Wildlife Service website.

U.S. Forest Service. 2016. "Forest service research and development performance and accountability report." USFS website.

U.S. Geological Survey. 2020. "Mineral commodity summaries 2019." USGS website.

U.S. Public Health Service. 1995. *Healthy People 2000*. Washington, DC: Government Printing Office.

United Nations Environment Programme. 2016. "Urban air pollution." UNEP website.

Vizcaya, D., et al. 2015. "Cleaning products and short-term respiratory effects among female cleaners with asthma." *Occupational and Environmental Medicine* 72:757-63.

Wellenius, G. A., et al. 2012. "Ambient air pollution and the risk of acute ischemic stroke." *Archives of Internal Medicine* 172:229-34.

World Health Organization. 2005. "Indoor air pollution and health." WHO website.

——. 2016. "Ambient air pollution: A global assessment of exposure and burden of disease." WHO website.

Youth, H. 2003. "Watching birds disappear." In *State of the World 2003,* ed. L. Starke, pp. 14-37. New York: W. W. Norton.

# glossary

**abuse** improper use of drugs or alcohol to the degree that the consequences are defined as detrimental to the user or society

**achievement** as distinguished from educational "attainment," the level the student has reached as measured by scores on various verbal and nonverbal tests

**addiction** repeated use of a drug or alcohol to the point of periodic or chronic intoxication that is detrimental to the user or society

**adjudication** making a judgment; settling a judicial matter

**aggression** forceful, offensive, or hostile behavior toward another person or society

**AIDS** acquired immune deficiency syndrome, a disease in which a viral infection causes the immune system to stop functioning, inevitably resulting in death

**alienation** a sense of estrangement from one's social environment, typically measured by one's feelings of powerlessness, normlessness, isolation, meaninglessness, and self-estrangement

**anarchism** the philosophy that advocates the abolition of government in order to secure true freedom for people

**atmosphere** the general mood and social influences in a situation or place

**attainment** as distinguished from educational "achievement," the number of years of education completed by a student

**attitude** a predisposition about something in one's environment

**autonomy** the ability or opportunity to govern oneself

**binge drinking** having five or more drinks on the same occasion

**biological characteristic** an inherited, rather than learned, characteristic

**bipolar disorder** fluctuation between emotional extremes

**bisexual** having sexual relations with either sex or both together

**bureaucracy** an organization in which there are specific areas of authority and responsibility, a hierarchy of authority, management based on written documents, worker expertise, management based on rules, and full-time workers

**capitalism** an economic system in which there is private, rather than state, ownership of wealth and control of the production and distribution of goods; people are motivated by profit and compete with each other for maximum shares of profit

**carcinogenic** causing cancer

**catharsis** discharge of socially unacceptable emotions in a socially acceptable way

**charter school** a nonreligious public school approved by the local school district but free of many regulations and policies that apply to other public schools

**cognitive development** growth in the ability to perform increasingly complex intellectual activities, particularly abstract relationships

**cohabitation** living together without getting married

**compensatory programs** programs designed to give intensive help to disadvantaged pupils and increase their academic skills

**conflict theory** a theory that focuses on contradictory interests, inequalities between social groups, and the resulting conflict and change

**consumer price index** a measure of the average change in prices of all types of consumer goods and services purchased by urban wage earners and clerical workers

**contradiction** opposing phenomena within the same social system

**corporate welfare** governmental benefits given to corporations that are unavailable to other groups or to individuals

**critical thinking** the analysis and evaluation of information

**culture** the way of life of a people, including both material products (such as technology) and nonmaterial characteristics (such as values, norms, language, and beliefs)

**cunnilingus** oral stimulation of the female genitalia

**cybersex** sexual activity conducted via the Internet

**dehumanization** the process by which an individual is deprived of the qualities or traits of a human being

**deinstitutionalization** a movement to change the setting of treatment of mental disorders from hospitals to the community through rapid discharge of patients

**dependent variable** the variable in an experiment that is influenced by an independent variable

**detoxification** supervised withdrawal from dependence on a drug

**differential association theory** the theory that illegal behavior is due to a preponderance of definitions favorable to such behavior

**discrimination** arbitrary, unfavorable treatment of the members of some social group

**disfranchise** to deprive of the right to vote

**division of labor** the separation of work into specialized tasks

**divorce rate** typically, the number of divorces per 1,000 marriages

**domestic terrorism** the use, or threatened use, of violence by people operating entirely within the United States to intimidate or coerce the government and/or citizens in order to reach certain social or political aims

**downsizing** reduction of the labor force in a company or corporation

**ecosystem** a set of living things, their environment, and the interrelationships among and between them

**environmental depletion** increasing scarcity of natural resources, including those used for generating energy

**environmental destruction** alterations in the environment that make it less habitable or useful for people or other living things

**environmental pollution** harmful alterations in the environment, including air, land, and water

**epidemiology** the study of factors that affect the incidence, prevalence, and distribution of illnesses

**erotica** sexually arousing materials that are not degrading or demeaning to adults or children

**ethnic group** people who have a shared historical and cultural background that leads them to identify with each other

**etiology** the causes of a disease

**eutrophication** overfertilization of water due to excess nutrients, leading to algae growth and oxygen depletion

**exploitation** use or manipulation of people for one's own advantage or profit

**fallacy of appeal to prejudice** argument by appealing to popular prejudices or passions

**fallacy of authority** argument by an illegitimate appeal to authority

**fallacy of circular reasoning** use of conclusions to support the assumptions that were necessary to make the conclusions

**fallacy of composition** the assertion that what is true of the part is necessarily true of the whole

**fallacy of dramatic instance** overgeneralizing

**fallacy of misplaced concreteness** making something abstract into something concrete

**fallacy of non sequitur** something that does not follow logically from what has preceded it

**fallacy of personal attack** argument by attacking the opponent personally rather than dealing with the issue

**fallacy of retrospective determinism** the argument that things could not have worked out any other way than they did

**family** a group united by marriage, blood, and/or adoption in order to satisfy intimacy needs and/or to bear and socialize children

**fellatio** oral stimulation of the male genitalia

**forcible rape** the carnal knowledge of a female forcibly and against her will

**frequency distribution** the organization of data to show the number of times each item occurs

**gender** the meaning of being male or female in a particular society

**gender role** the attitudes and behavior that are expected of men and women in a society

**ghetto** an area in which a certain group is segregated from the rest of society; often used today to refer to the impoverished area of the inner city

**gridlock** the inability of the government to legislate significant new policies

**herbicide** a chemical used to kill plant life, particularly weeds

**heterogamy** marriage between partners with diverse values and backgrounds

**heterosexual** having sexual preference for persons of the opposite sex

**homogamy** marriage between partners with similar values and backgrounds

**homophobia** irrational fear of homosexuals

**homosexual** having sexual preference for persons of the same sex; someone who privately or overtly considers himself or herself a homosexual

**iatrogenic** caused by the physician in the course of his or her treatment of a patient

**ideology** a set of ideas that explain or justify some aspect of social reality

**incest** exploitative sexual contact between relatives in which the victim is under the age of 18

**incidence** the number of new cases of an illness that occur during a particular period of time

**independent variable** the variable in an experiment that is manipulated to see how it affects changes in the dependent variable

**innate** existing in a person from birth

**institution** a collective pattern of dealing with a basic social function; typical institutions identified by sociologists are the government, economy, education, family and marriage, religion, and the media

**institutional racism** policies and practices of social institutions that tend to perpetuate racial discrimination

**interaction** reciprocally influenced behavior on the part of two or more people

**interest group** a group that attempts to influence public opinion and political decisions in accord with the particular interests of its members

**international terrorism** politically motivated violence against citizens of political entities different from those of the perpetrators in order to coerce and intimidate others into accepting the perpetrators' goals

**labor force** all civilians who are employed or unemployed but able and desiring to work

**lesbian** a female homosexual

**life chances** the probability of gaining certain advantages defined as desirable, such as long life and health

**life expectancy** the average number of years a newborn can expect to live

**lobbyist** an individual who tries to influence legislation in accord with the preferences of an interest group

**maladjustment** poor adjustment to one's social environment

**malnutrition** inadequate food, in amount or type

**Marxist** pertaining to the system of thought developed by Karl Marx and Friedrich Engels, particularly emphasizing materialism, class struggle, and the progress of humanity toward communism

**mean** the average

**median** the score below which are half of the scores and above which are the other half

**military parity** equality or equivalence in military strength

**morbidity** the prevalence of a specified illness in a specified area

**morphological** pertaining to form and structure

**neurosis** a mental disorder involving anxiety that impairs functioning

**norm** shared expectations about behavior

**nuclear family** parents, and children, if any

**obscenity** materials that are offensive by generally accepted standards of decency

**organized crime** an ongoing organization of people who provide illegal services and goods and who maintain their activities by the aid of political corruption

**paraphilia** the need for a socially unacceptable stimulus in order to be sexually aroused and satisfied

**participant observation** a method of research in which one directly participates and observes the social reality being studied

**patronage** giving government jobs to people who are members of the winning party

**pedophile** an adult who depends on children for sexual stimulation

**personal problem** a problem that can be explained in terms of the qualities of the individual

**pesticide** a chemical used to kill insects defined as pests

**photosynthesis** a natural process essential to life, resulting in the production of oxygen and organic materials

**pica** a craving for unnatural substances, such as dirt or clay

**pimp** one who earns all or part of his or her living by acting as a manager or procurer for a prostitute

**placebo** any substance having no physiological effect that is given to a subject who believes it to be a drug that does have an effect

**pluralism** the more or less equal distribution of power among interest groups

**political alienation** a feeling of political disillusionment, powerlessness, and estrangement

**political party** an organized group that attempts to control the government through the electoral process

**pollutant** anything that causes environmental pollution

**pornography** literature, art, or films that are sexually arousing

**posttraumatic stress disorder** an anxiety disorder associated with serious traumatic events, involving such symptoms as nightmares, recurring thoughts about the trauma, a lack of involvement with life, and guilt

**poverty** a state in which income is insufficient to provide the basic necessities of food, shelter, clothing, and medical care

**poverty level** the minimum income level that Americans should have to live on, based on the Department of Agriculture's calculations of the cost of a basic diet called "the economy food plan"

**power elite model** a model of politics in which power is concentrated in political, economic, and military leaders

**predatory crimes** acts that have victims who suffer loss of property or some kind of physical harm

**prejudice** a rigid, emotional attitude that legitimates discriminatory behavior toward people in a group

**prevalence** the number of cases of an illness that exist at any particular time

**primary group** the people with whom one has intimate, face-to-face interaction on a recurring basis, such as parents, spouse, children, and close friends

**promiscuity** undiscriminating, casual sexual relationships with many people

**prostitution** having sexual relations for remuneration, usually to provide part or all of one's livelihood

**psychosis** a disorder in which the individual fails to distinguish between internal and external stimuli

**psychosomatic disorder** an impairment in physiological functioning that results from the individual's emotional state

**psychotherapeutic drugs** prescription drugs, including pain relievers, tranquilizers, stimulants, and sedatives, that are used for intoxication effects rather than medical purposes

**race** a group of people distinguished from other groups by their origin in a particular part of the world

**racism** the belief that some racial groups are inherently inferior to others

**recidivism** repeated criminal activity and incarceration

**regulatory agency** an organization established by the government to enforce statutes that apply to a particular activity

**rehabilitation** resocializing a criminal and returning him or her to full participation in society

**reification** defining what is abstract as something concrete

**relative deprivation** a sense of deprivation based on some standard used by the individual who feels deprived

**retributiveness** paying people back for their socially unacceptable behavior

**ritualized deprivation** a school atmosphere in which the motions of teaching and learning continue, while the students are more concerned about surviving than learning

**role** the behavior associated with a particular position in the social structure

**role conflict** a person's perception that two or more of his or her roles are contradictory, or that the same role has contradictory expectations, or that the expectations of the role are unacceptable or excessive

**sadomasochism** the practice of deriving sexual pleasure from the infliction of pain

**sanctions** mechanisms of social control for enforcing a society's standards

**schizophrenia** a psychosis that involves a thinking disorder, particularly hallucinations and fantasies

**self-fulfilling prophecy** a belief that has consequences (and may become true) simply because it is believed

**sex** an individual's identity as male or female

**sexism** prejudice or discrimination against someone because of his or her sex

**sexting** sending erotic or nude photos or videos of oneself to a particular person or to a number of others via a cell phone or the Internet

**sexual harassment** unwelcome sexual advances, requests for sexual favors, and other sexual behavior that either results in punishment when the victim resists or creates a hostile environment or both

**socialization** the process by which an individual learns to participate in a group

**social problem** a condition or pattern of behavior that contradicts some other condition or pattern of behavior; is defined as incompatible with the desired quality of life; is caused, facilitated, or prolonged by social factors; involves intergroup conflict; and requires social action for resolution

**socioeconomic status** position in the social system based on economic resources, power, education, prestige, and lifestyle

**sodomy** intercourse defined as "unnatural"; particularly used to refer to anal intercourse

**statutory rape** sexual intercourse with a female who is below the legal age for consenting

**stealth racism** hidden or subtle acts of prejudice and discrimination that may be apparent only to the victim

**stepfamily** a family formed by marriage that includes one or more children from a previous marriage

**stereotype** an image of members of a group that standardizes them and exaggerates certain qualities

**stigma** that which symbolizes disrepute or disgrace

**stratification system** arrangement of society into groups that are unequal with regard to such valued resources as wealth, power, and prestige

**structural functionalism** a sociological theory that focuses on social systems and how their interdependent parts maintain order

**subsidy** a government grant to a private person or company to assist an enterprise deemed advantageous to the public

**survey** a method of research in which a sample of people are interviewed or given questionnaires in order to get data on some phenomenon

**symbolic interactionism** a sociological theory that focuses on the interaction between individuals, the individual's perception of situations, and the ways in which social life is constructed through interaction

**test of significance** a statistical method for determining the probability that research findings occurred by chance

**total institution** a place in which the totality of the individual's existence is controlled by external forces

**transgender** having a gender identity different from one's anatomy

**trauma** physical or emotional injury

**underemployment** working full time for poverty wages, working part time when full-time work is desired, or working at a job below the worker's skill level

**unemployment rate** the proportion of the labor force that is not working but is available for work and has made specific efforts to find work

**urbanization** the increasing concentration of people living in cities

**values** things preferred because they are defined as having worth

**variable** any trait or characteristic that varies in value or magnitude

**violence** the use of force to kill, injure, or abuse others

**voucher system** a system that allows parents to use tax money to send their children to a school, private or public, of their choice

**war** a major armed conflict between nations or between organized groups within a nation in which a thousand or more people are killed

**white-collar crime** crimes committed by respectable citizens in the course of their work

**work ethic** the notion that your sense of worth and the satisfaction of your needs are intricately related to the kind of work you do

## D

### H

# subject index

*Page numbers in italics refer to figures or tables. Page numbers in bold refer to running glossary terms.*